P9-CDM-722

# READY, SET, GO!

WITH DONATELLE,
HEALTH: THE BASICS, 12E

The MasteringHealth Edition

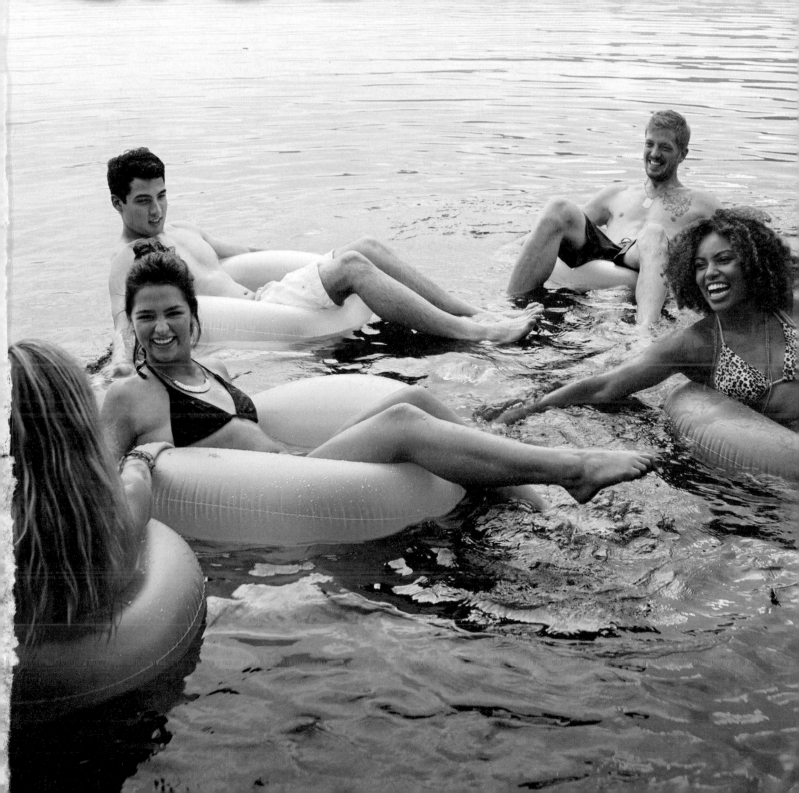

# GET YOUR STUDENTS READY!

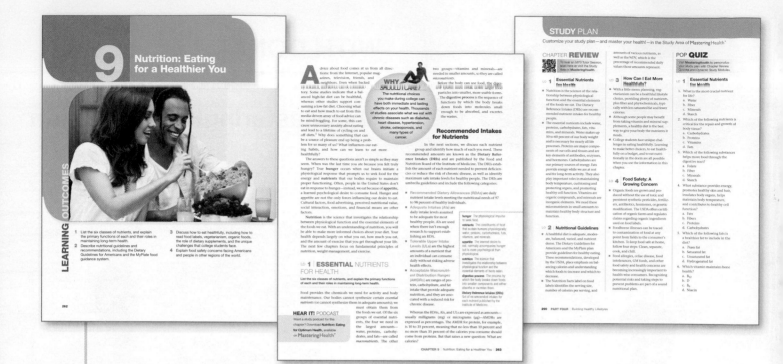

## NEW! Study Plan Tied to Learning Outcomes

Numbered learning outcomes now introduce every chapter and mini-chapter, giving students a roadmap for their reading. Each chapter concludes with a Study Plan, which summarizes key points of the chapter and provides review questions and critical thinking questions to check understanding, all tied to the chapter's learning outcomes and assignable in MasteringHealth.

## NEW! *ABC News* Lecture Launchers

New videos from *ABC News* bring personal health to life and spark discussion with up-to-date hot topics such as stress among millennials, hate crimes, and rates of heroin use. Assignable multiple-choice questions available in MasteringHealth provide wrong-answer feedback to redirect students to the correct answer.

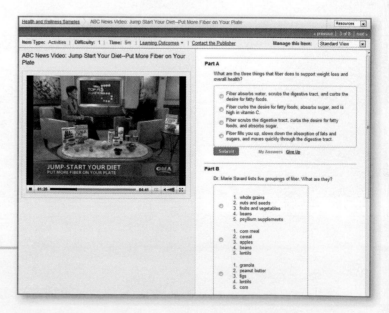

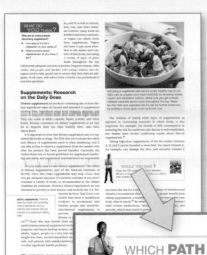

## NEW! Interactive Behavior Change Activities— Which Path Would You Take?

By scanning QR codes with their mobile devices, students gain access to an exploration of various health choices through an engaging, interactive, low-stakes, and anonymous experience. These activities show students the possible consequences of various choices they make today on their future health through a choose-your-own-adventure style interface.

WHICH **PATH** WOULD YOU TAKE **?**

Scan the QR code to see how different dietary choices YOU make today can affect your overall health tomorrow.

## UPDATED!

**A new mini-chapter, Focus On: Sexuality,** has been pulled from the previously titled Healthy Relationships and Understanding Sexuality chapter, making it easier to assign the sexuality material in connection with the Reproductive Choices chapter (contraception). Additional information on social connections is now included in the Relationships chapter.

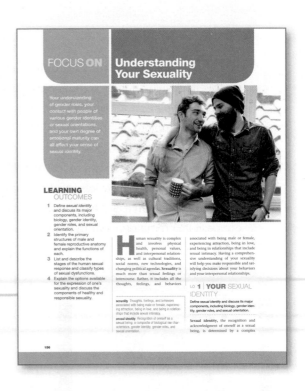

## UPDATED!

## Current Health Topics Straight from the Headlines

Current health issues are covered throughout the new edition, speaking to students' questions and concerns. New and updated material covers such areas as

- the heritability of well-being
- suicide risk factors
- the psychological and physiological effects of meditation
- technostress
- the relationship between media violence and actual violence
- social network use
- the abuse of heroin, khat, and salvia

- the characteristics of successful weight losers
- orthorexia nervosa
- CrossFit and high-intensity interval training (HIIT)
- the global burden of disease
- safe oral sex
- the human impact on the existence or extinction of other species

## UPDATED!

**Focus On: Financial Health mini-chapter** has been streamlined to focus more on the connection between wealth and health.

# GET YOUR **STUDENTS GOING**
# WITH MasteringHealth™

Mastering is the most effective and widely used online homework, tutorial, and assessment system for the sciences and now includes content specifically for health courses. Mastering delivers self-paced tutorials that focus on your course objectives, provides individualized coaching, and responds to each student's progress.

## **BEFORE** CLASS  Dynamic Study Modules and eText 2.0 Provide Students with a Preview of What's to Come

NEW! **Dynamic Study Modules** help students study effectively on their own by continuously assessing their activity and performance in real time. Students complete a set of questions with a unique answer format that also asks them to indicate their confidence level. Questions repeat until the student can answer them all correctly and confidently. Once completed, Dynamic Study Modules explain the concept using materials from the text.

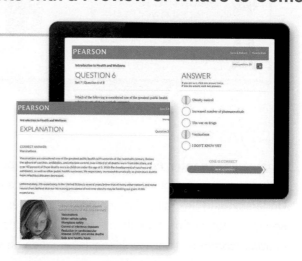

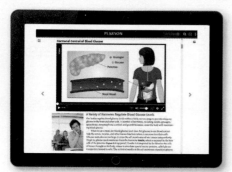

NEW! **Interactive eText 2.0,** complete with embedded media, is mobile friendly and ADA accessible.

- Now available on smartphones and tablets
- Seamlessly integrated videos and other rich media
- Accessible (screen-reader ready)
- Configurable reading settings, including resizable type and night reading mode
- Instructor and student note-taking, highlighting, bookmarking, and search

## **DURING** CLASS  Engage Students with Learning Catalytics™

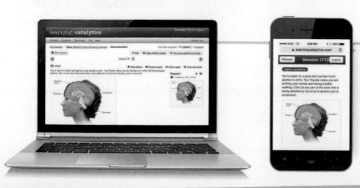

**Learning Catalytics**, a "bring your own device" student engagement, assessment, and classroom intelligence system, allows students to use their smartphones, tablets, or laptops to respond to questions in class.

# AFTER CLASS

## Easy-to-Assign, Customizable, and Automatically Graded Assignments

The breadth and depth of content available to you to assign in MasteringHealth is unparalleled, allowing you to quickly and easily assign homework to reinforce key concepts.

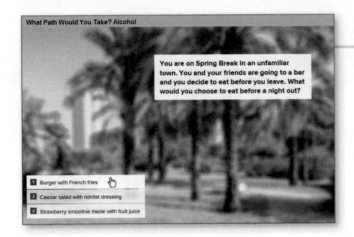

NEW! **Interactive Behavior Change Activities—Which Path Would You Take?—** allow students to explore various health choices through an engaging, interactive, low-stakes, and anonymous experience.

In activities covering topics such as alcohol, smoking, nutrition, and fitness, students receive specific feedback on the choices they make today and the possible consequences on their future health.

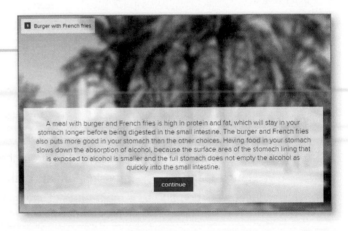

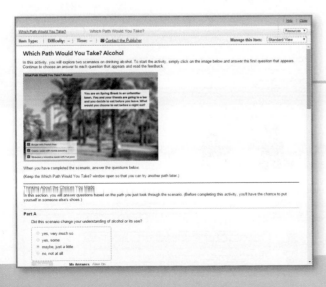

These activities are linked out to Mastering from the book and made assignable in Mastering with follow-up questions.

# AFTER CLASS

## Other Automatically Graded Health and Fitness Activities Include . . .

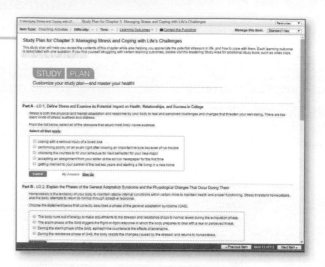

NEW! **Study Plans** tie all end-of-chapter material (including chapter review, pop quiz, and Think About It! questions) to specific numbered learning outcomes and Mastering assets. Assignable Study Plan items contain at least one multiple-choice question per learning outcome and wrong-answer feedback.

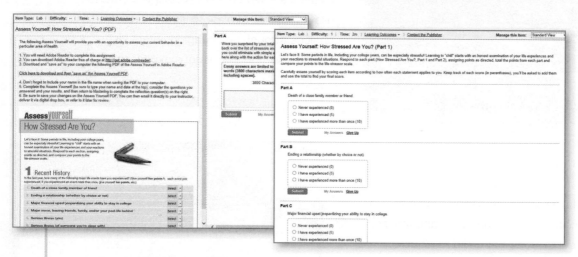

UPDATED! **Self-Assessments** from the text are available within MasteringHealth in easy-to-assign formats both in PDF format with a self-reflection section and as a multi-part activity that speaks to your gradebook.

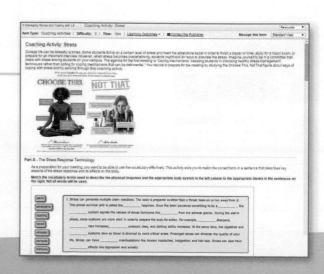

**Coaching Activities** guide students through key health and fitness concepts with interactive mini-lessons that provide hints and feedback.

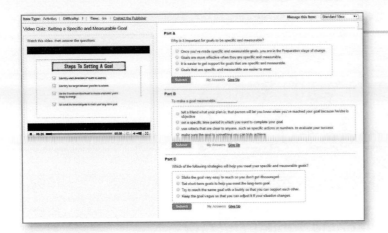

**Behavior Change Videos** are concise whiteboard-style videos that help students with the steps of behavior change, covering topics such as setting SMART goals, identifying and overcoming barriers to change, planning realistic timelines, and more. Additional videos review key fitness concepts such as determining target heart rate range for exercise. All videos include assessment activities and are assignable in MasteringHealth.

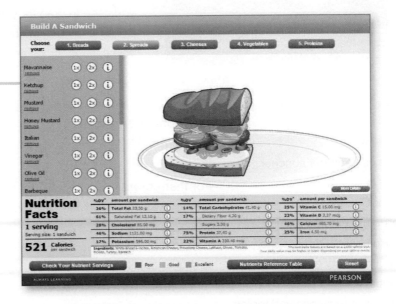

**NutriTools Coaching Activities** in the nutrition chapter allow students to combine and experiment with different food options and learn firsthand how to build healthier meals.

**Learning Outcomes**

All of the MasteringHealth assignable content is tagged to book content and to Bloom's Taxonomy. You also have the ability to add your own outcomes, helping you track student performance against your learning outcomes. You can view class performance against the specified learning outcomes and share those results quickly and easily by exporting to a spreadsheet.

# EVERYTHING YOU NEED TO TEACH **IN ONE PLACE**

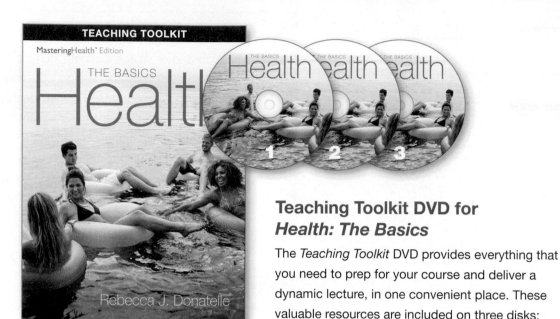

## Teaching Toolkit DVD for *Health: The Basics*

The *Teaching Toolkit* DVD provides everything that you need to prep for your course and deliver a dynamic lecture, in one convenient place. These valuable resources are included on three disks:

### DISK 1
**Robust Media Assets for Each Chapter**

- *ABC News* Lecture Launcher videos
- Behavior Change videos
- PowerPoint Lecture Outlines
- PowerPoint clicker questions and Jeopardy-style quiz show questions
- Files for all illustrations and tables and selected photos from the text

### DISK 2
**Comprehensive Test Bank**

- Test Bank in Microsoft Word, PDF, and RTF formats
- Computerized Test Bank, which includes all the questions from the printed test bank in a format that allows you to easily and intuitively build exams and quizzes

### DISK 3
**Additional Innovative Supplements for Instructors and Students**

**For Instructors**
- *Instructor Resource and Support Manual* in Microsoft Word and PDF formats
- Step-by-step MasteringHealth tutorials
- Video introduction to Learning Catalytics™
- *Great Ideas in Teaching Health & Wellness*
- *Teaching with Student Learning Outcomes*
- *Teaching with Web 2.0*

**For Students**
- Take Charge Self-Assessment Worksheets
- *Behavior Change Log Book and Wellness Journal*
- *Live Right! Beating Stress in College and Beyond*
- *Eat Right! Healthy Eating in College and Beyond*
- *Food Composition Table*

**User's Quick Guide for** *Health: The Basics*

This easy-to-use printed supplement accompanies the Teaching Toolkit and offers easy instructions for both experienced and new faculty members to get started with the rich Toolkit content and MasteringHealth.

MasteringHealth™ Edition

# HEALTH
## THE BASICS

REBECCA J. **DONATELLE**

Oregon State University

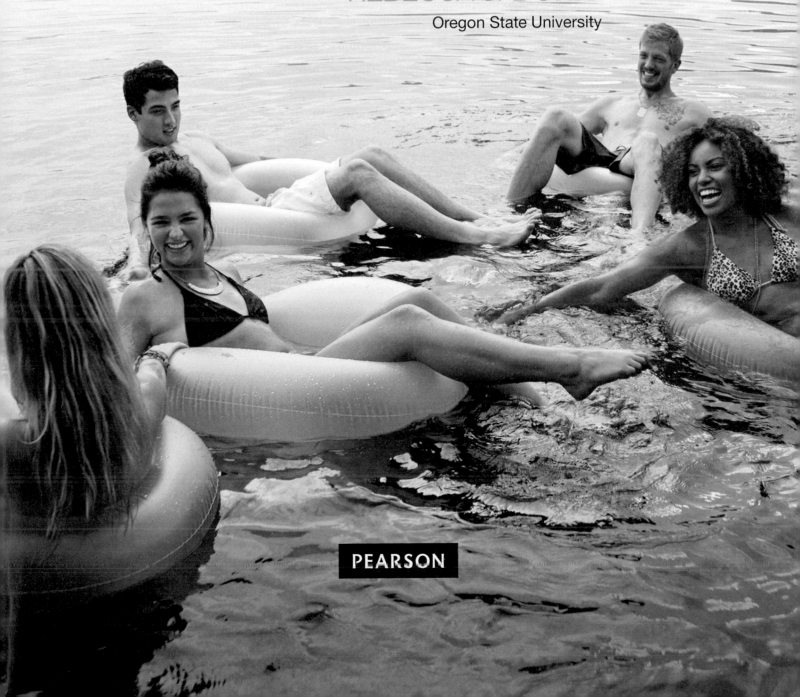

**PEARSON**

Senior Acquisitions Editor: Michelle Cadden
Project Manager: Lauren Beebe
Program Manager: Susan Malloy
Development Editors: Kari Hopperstead, Nic Albert
Editorial Assistant: Heidi Arndt
Director of Development: Barbara Yien
Development Manager: Cathy Murphy
Program Management Team Lead: Mike Early
Project Management Team Lead: Nancy Tabor
Production Management: Jeanine Furino, Cenveo®
    Publisher Services
Copyeditor: Jane Loftus
Compositor: Cenveo® Publisher Services

Art Coordinator: Eric Zeiter, Lachina
Design Manager: Marilyn Perry
Interior Designer: Jerilyn Bockorick, Cenveo®
    Publisher Services
Cover Designer: Yvo Riezebos, Tandem Creative, Inc.
Illustration: Lachina
Rights & Permissions Project Manager: William Opaluch
Rights & Permissions Management: Rachel Youdelman
Photo Researcher: Amanda Larkin, QBS Learning
Senior Procurement Specialist: Stacey J. Weinberger
Executive Product Marketing Manager: Neena Bali
Senior Field Marketing Manager: Mary Salzman

Cover Photo Credit: Dreampictures/Image Source/Corbis

**Library of Congress Cataloging-in-Publication Data**

Donatelle, Rebecca J., 1950-
 Health : the basics / Rebecca J. Donatelle. -- 12e [edition].
    pages cm
 Includes bibliographical references and index.
 ISBN 978-0-13-418326-8 (alk. paper) -- ISBN 0-13-418326-6 (alk. paper)
 1. Health--Textbooks. I. Title.
 RA776.D663 2017
 613--dc23
                    2015029437

ISBN 10: 0-13-418326-6; ISBN 13: 978-0-13-418326-8 (Student edition)
ISBN 10: 0-13-428694-4; ISBN 13: 978-0-13-428694-5 (Instructor's Review Copy)

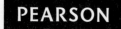

# BRIEF CONTENTS

# CONTENTS

## PART THREE | Avoiding Risks from Harmful Habits

PART FOUR | **Building Healthy Lifestyles**

PART FIVE | **Preventing and Fighting Disease**

## 12 Reducing Your Risk of Cardiovascular Disease and Cancer   354

## FOCUS ON Minimizing Your Risk for Diabetes   386

# FEATURE BOXES

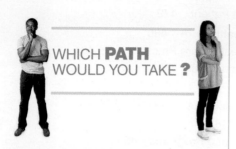
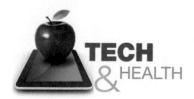
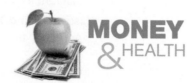
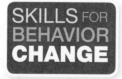

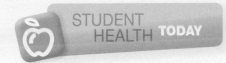
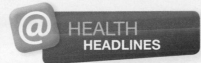

STUDENT HEALTH TODAY

HEALTH HEADLINES

HEALTH IN A DIVERSE WORLD

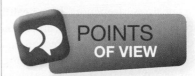

POINTS OF VIEW

Today, threats to our health and the health of our planet dominate the media and affect our daily lives on a regular basis. Looming water shortages, poor air quality, food safety concerns, violence and the threat of terrorism, chronic and infectious diseases, and other concerns have us wondering about our ability to survive and thrive. We are advised to watch what we eat, lose weight, exercise more, reduce our stress, sleep more, have healthier relationships, be vigilant against a host of threats, and do our part to protect ourselves, our communities, our resources, and our planet. The issues often seem so huge, so far-reaching and overwhelming, that you may wonder if there is anything you can do to make a difference—to ensure a life that is healthy and long and a planet that is preserved for future generations. You are not alone! Getting healthy and staying healthy is a challenge for many, but the good news is that you *can* do things to improve your health and the health of others. Regardless of your age, sex, race, the environment you live in, or the challenges you face, you can be an agent for healthy change for you, your loved ones, and the greater community. It can start now, and it can start with you!

After years of teaching and working with students of all ages and stages of life and careers, I am encouraged by the fact that so many young adults are working hard to change their own health futures and the health of their families and communities. The problem is that with so much "talk" about health on so many platforms, sifting through the "junk information" and making the right choices based on *good science* and *good sense*, can be difficult.

My goal in writing *Health: The Basics,* the MasteringHealth™ Edition, is to build upon the strengths of past editions; to utilize the most current, scientifically valid research, to examine some of the important issues and controversies about health today, and motivate students to become "actively engaged in health" at all levels. As part of the process, we have worked hard to provide students with essential tools and technologically sound resources to empower them to take a careful and realistic look at their health risks, to examine their behaviors and the factors that contribute to those behaviors, and take the steps necessary to prioritize *health* in their lives. Although prioritizing individual and community health is a priority of this text, it is important to recognize that our health is increasingly connected to the health of the global community and our planet. As such, my aim is to challenge students to think globally as they consider health risks and seek creative solutions, both large and small, to address complex health problems. There is no *one-size-fits-all recipe* for health. You can do it your way—whether that means starting slow with "baby steps" designed to change deeply engrained behaviors or gearing up for major changes that all happen at once. Remember, we didn't develop our behaviors overnight. Being patient but persistent with ourselves is often part of the process.

This book is designed to help students quickly grasp the information, focusing on key objectives that have relevance to their own lives, both now and in the future. We provide the most current, comprehensive, concise, and scientifically valid information about each health topic, put a wealth of technological tools and resources at students' fingertips to assist in decision making, encourage students to think about the issues, and help students answer these questions: What is the issue and why should I care? What are my options for action? When and how do I get started?

With each new edition of *Health: The Basics,* I am gratified by the overwhelming success that this book has enjoyed. I am excited about making this edition the best yet—more timely, more relevant, and more interesting for students. Let's face it: Our world faces unprecedented challenges to individual and community health. Understanding these challenges and having a personal plan to preserve, protect, and promote health will help ensure our *healthful* future!

## NEW TO THIS EDITION

*Health: The Basics,* the MasteringHealth Edition, maintains many features that the text has become known for, while incorporating several major revisions, exciting new features, and a more explicit connection between the text and multimedia resources in MasteringHealth. **MasteringHealth** is an online homework, tutorial, and assessment product designed to improve and assess results by helping students quickly master concepts. Students benefit from self-paced tutorials that feature immediate wrong-answer feedback and hints that emulate the office-hour experience to help keep students on track. With a wide range of interactive, engaging, and assignable activities, students are encouraged to actively learn and retain tough course concepts and apply them to real-world changes.

The multimedia created for the MasteringHealth Edition is more innovative and interactive than ever, and a tighter text and MasteringHealth integration provides students the opportunity to master course content using a variety of resources on and off the page, reflecting the manner in which students study today.

The most noteworthy changes to the text and multimedia as a whole include the following.

- **NEW! Interactive Behavior Change Activities— Which Path Would You Take?** Allow students to explore various health choices through an engaging, interactive, low-stakes, and anonymous experience. These choose-your-own-adventure-style activities show students the possible consequences of various choices they make today on their future health; these activities are accessible via the QR code from the book and made assignable in MasteringHealth™ with follow-up questions.
- **NEW! ABC News Videos** bring health to life and spark discussion with up-to-date hot topics from 2012 to 2015. MasteringHealth activities tied to the videos include multiple-choice questions that provide wrong answer feedback to redirect students to the correct answer.
- **NEW! Study Plans** tie all end-of-chapter material (including Chapter Review, Pop Quiz, and Think About It questions) to specific, numbered Learning Outcomes. Assignable Study Plan items in MasteringHealth contain at least one multiple-choice question per Learning Outcome and include wrong-answer feedback.
- **NEW! eText 2.0** complete with embedded *ABC News* videos and Health Video Tutors; eText 2.0 is mobile friendly and ADA accessible.

  - Now available on smartphones and tablets.
  - Seamlessly integrated videos.
  - Accessible (screen-reader ready).
  - Configurable reading settings, including resizable type and night reading mode.
  - Instructor and student note taking, highlighting, bookmarking, and search.

- **NEW! Focus On: Sexuality mini-chapter** has been pulled from the previously titled Healthy Relationships and Understanding Sexuality chapter, and includes expanded coverage of topics such as sexual identity, sexual response and dysfunctions, and variant sexual behavior. This new Focus On makes it easier to assign the sexuality material in connection with the Reproductive Choices chapter (contraception).
- **UPDATED! Chapter 5, Connecting and Communicating in the Modern World** (formerly titled Healthy Relationships and Understanding Sexuality), now includes more information on social connections and how we interact and relate to others, including new research on social network use, addiction and social media meanness.
- **UPDATED! Focus On: Financial Health mini-chapter** has been streamlined to focus more on the connection between money and health and includes updated coverage of college students' financial issues and how these can affect both success in college and future health.

# Chapter-by-Chapter Revisions

The MasteringHealth Edition has been thoroughly updated to provide students with the most current information and references for further exploration and includes a tighter integration between the text and multimedia resources in MasteringHealth. Learning outcomes are now explicitly tied to chapter sections and the end-of-chapter Study Plan to create a clear learning path for students. Portions of chapters have been reorganized to improve the flow of topics, and figures, tables, feature boxes, and photos have all been added, improved on, and updated. Throughout the text, all data, statistics, and references have been updated to the most recent possible. The following is a chapter-by-chapter listing of some of the most noteworthy changes, updates, and additions.

## Chapter 1: Accessing Your Health

- New and updated coverage of relapse and recovery
- Updated research on health disparities
- New info on the Affordable Care Act

## Focus On: Improving Your Financial Health

- Updated material on the link between health and wealth
- Updated coverage of financial struggles in college
- New chapter summaries and Pop Quiz

## Chapter 2: Promoting and Preserving Your Psychological Health

- Updated coverage of emotional intelligence
- New research on heritability of well-being
- Updated material on risk factors for mental illness, as well as cost and stigma
- Updated research on mood disorders
- New research on suicide and risks in the United States and abroad

## Focus On: Cultivating Your Spiritual Health

- New research on the psychological and physiological effects of meditation
- Updated research on the spiritual tendencies of undergraduates
- New coverage of the relationship between spirituality and stress reduction
- New chapter summaries and Pop Quiz

## Chapter 3: Managing Stress and Coping with Life's Challenges

- Updated research on stress in America
- Updated material on massage therapy
- New material on technostress
- New app suggestions for help relaxing

## Focus On: Improving Your Sleep

- Updated research on students and sleep
- New Student Health Today box on caffeine, sleep, and your health
- New Skills for Behavior Change on ditching blue-light devices
- New chapter summaries and Pop Quiz

## Chapter 4: Preventing Violence and Injury

- Updated research on rates of violent crime in the United States and globally
- Updated research on violence and relationship violence on U.S. college campuses
- New info on the relationship between media violence and actual violence
- Updated research on the relationship between substance abuse and violence
- Updated Skills for Behavior Change with tips for men and women on reducing dating violence

## Chapter 5: Connecting and Communicating in the Modern World

- Updated coverage of social support
- Updated discussions of social networks and social capital
- New material on relational connectedness and collective connectedness
- New research surrounding social network use, real-world connection, and addiction
- New Skills for Behavior Change on social media meanness

## Focus On: Understanding Your Sexuality

- New Focus On, "Understanding Your Sexuality," with coverage of:
  - Sexual identity and its components
  - Male and female anatomy
  - Sexual response cycles and dysfunctions
  - Varieties of sexual expression
  - Makeup of healthy and responsible sexuality
- New chapter summaries and Pop Quiz

## Chapter 6: Considering Your Reproductive Choices

- Updated statistics on contraception use and unintended pregnancy
- Coverage of new diaphragms
- Updated information on IUDs available
- Updated information on ECP availability
- Updated information on maternal health and pregnancy
- New Money & Health box on health care reform and contraceptives
- New Student Health Today box on men's involvement in birth control

## Chapter 7: Recognizing and Avoiding Addiction and Drug Abuse

- Updated research regarding the prevalence of gambling addiction in the United States
- New coverage of khat
- New information on heroin use spreading to suburban areas
- New coverage of salvia
- Updated research regarding the prevalence of drug use in college students
- Updated information on the legalization of marijuana and its surrounding debate

## Chapter 8: Drinking Alcohol Responsibly and Ending Tobacco Use

- Updated research on drinking rates
- Updated research on the dangers of alcohol use during pregnancy
- New coverage of alcohol use disorder
- New coverage of tobacco use disorder
- Updated information on e-cigarettes

## Chapter 9: Nutrition: Eating for a Healthier You

- New Health Headlines on coconut oil
- Updated information on the *Dietary Guidelines for Americans*
- Updated data on the prevalence of vegetarianism
- Updated information on food-borne pathogens

## Chapter 10: Reaching and Maintaining a Healthy Weight

- Updated statistics on overweight and obesity in the United States and globally
- New Student Health Today box on characteristics of successful weight losers
- Updated coverage and reviews of major diets and their effectiveness
- Updated coverage of prescription weight-loss drugs

## Focus On: Enhancing Your Body Image

- New Student Health Today box on "thinspiration"
- Updated statistics regarding prevalence of eating disorders in the United States
- New discussion of orthorexia nervosa
- New chapter summaries and Pop Quiz

## Chapter 11: Improving Your Personal Fitness

- Updated statistics regarding Americans meeting guidelines for aerobic exercise
- Updated research regarding physical activity and cognitive functions
- Updated research regarding physical activity and extended life span
- New coverage of Crossfit and other HIIT exercise plans

## Chapter 12: Reducing Your Risk of Cardiovascular Disease and Cancer

- New and updated coverage of the global burden of disease
- Updated statistics regarding prevalence of cancer and heart disease
- Updated coverage of disease disparity and chronic disease across communities
- New guidelines for the management and treatment of high blood pressure
- Updated research on nonmodifiable risk factors for heart disease
- Updated discussion of the role of inflammation and infectious diseases in CVD and cancer risks

- Updated information about risks of prediabetes and strategies for prevention
- Updated research on the importance of prevention for CVD, cancer, and diabetes

## Focus On: Minimizing Your Risk for Diabetes

- Updated statistics regarding the prevalence of diabetes
- Updated statistics on the economic burden of diabetes
- New chapter summaries and Pop Quiz

## Chapter 13: Protecting against Infectious Diseases and Sexually Transmitted Infections

- Updated research on environmental conditions and the spread of disease
- Updated discussion of antibiotics and superbugs
- Updated coverage of MRSA
- Updated coverage of meningitis and college students, and its prevention
- Updated research on the prevalence of STIs
- Updated discussion of vaccination and opting out
- New Student Health Today box on making oral sex safe

## Focus On: Reducing Risks for Chronic Diseases and Conditions

- Updated statistics regarding rates of bronchitis across populations
- Updated statistics regarding the prevalence of asthma and emphysema
- Updated information regarding the prevalence of migraines
- Updated discussion of IBS, IBD, Crohn's disease, and other conditions
- New chapter summaries and Pop Quiz

## Chapter 14: Preparing for Aging, Death, and Dying

- Updated statistics on health care costs for older Americans
- Updated information regarding living arrangements of older Americans
- Updated coverage of the legality and controversy surrounding physician-assisted suicide

## Chapter 15: Promoting Environmental Health

- Updated statistics on population growth and projections for the future
- Updated discussion of ecological footprints
- New coverage of the impact of human actions on the existence or extinction of other species
- Discussion of carbon tax and cap and trade policies to curb pollution
- Updated information on water use and access
- New tables on indoor air and water pollutants and their health and ecosystem effects

## Chapter 16: Making Smart Health Care Choices

- Updated coverage of the ACA, with a special emphasis on young adults/college students
- New coverage of the diverse options for health care, including independent practice associations, HMOs, and others
- New and expanded coverage of Medicare Part A, B, and D, as well as Advantage plans and Medigap plans
- Updated stats on costs of healthcare, strategies for reducing health care and future issues

## Focus On: Understanding Complementary and Integrative Health

- Updated coverage of alternative/integrative health approaches, rates of use, and considerations when making decisions about complementary and integrative health
- Updated coverage of complementary medical systems and specific methods of care
- Updated discussion of "natural" supplements
- New chapter summaries and Pop Quiz

# TEXT FEATURES AND LEARNING AIDS

*Health: The Basics* includes the following special features, all of which have been revised and improved upon for this edition:

- **Chapter Learning Outcomes** summarize the main competencies students will gain from each chapter and alert students to the key concepts and are now explicitly tied to chapter sections. Focus On mini-chapters now also include learning outcomes.
- **Study Plans** tie all end-of-chapter material (including Chapter Review, Pop Quiz, and Think About It questions) to specific numbered Learning Outcomes and Mastering-Health™ assets.
- **What Do You Think?** critical-thinking questions appear throughout the text, encouraging students to pause and reflect on material they have read.
- **Why Should I Care?** features present information on the effects poor health habits have on students in the here and now.
- **Assess Yourself** boxes help students evaluate their health behaviors. The **Your Plan for Change** section within each box provides students with targeted suggestions for ways to implement change.
- **Skills for Behavior Change** boxes focus on practical strategies that students can use to improve health or reduce their risks from negative health behaviors.
- **Tech & Health** boxes cover the new technology innovations that can help students stay healthy.
- **Money & Health** boxes cover health topics from the financial perspective.

- **Points of View** boxes present viewpoints on a controversial health issue and ask students *Where Do You Stand?* questions, encouraging them to critically evaluate the information and consider their own opinions.
- **Health Headlines** boxes highlight new discoveries and research, as well as interesting trends in the health field.
- **Student Health Today** boxes focus attention on specific health and wellness issues that relate to today's college students.
- **Health in a Diverse World** boxes expand discussion of health topics to diverse groups within the United States and around the world.
- A **running glossary** in the margins defines terms where students first encounter them, emphasizing and supporting understanding of material.
- A **Behavior Change Contract** for students to fill out is included at the back of the book.

# SUPPLEMENTARY MATERIALS

## Instructor Supplements

- **MasteringHealth** (www.masteringhealthandnutrition .com or www.pearsonmastering.com). MasteringHealth coaches students through the toughest health topics. A variety of **Coaching Activities** guide students through key health concepts with interactive mini-lessons, complete with hints and wrong-answer feedback. **Reading Quizzes** (20 questions per chapter) ensure students have completed the assigned reading before class. *ABC News* **videos** stimulate classroom discussions and include multiple-choice questions with feedback for students. Assignable **Behavior Change Video Quiz** and **Which Path Would You Take?** activities ensure students complete and reflect on behavior change and health choices. **NutriTools** in the nutrition chapter allow students to combine and experiment with different food options and learn firsthand how to build healthier meals. **MP3 Tutor Sessions** relate to chapter content and come with multiple-choice questions that provide wrong-answer feedback. **Learning Catalytics** provides open-ended questions students can answer in real time. **Dynamic Study Modules** enable students to study effectively in an adaptive format. Instructors can also assign these for completion as a graded assignment prior to class.
- **Teaching Toolkit DVD.** The Teaching Toolkit DVD includes everything instructors need to prepare for their course and deliver a dynamic lecture in one convenient place. Resources include *ABC News* videos, Health Video Tutor videos, clicker questions, Quiz Show questions, PowerPoint lecture outlines, all figures and tables from the text, PDF and and Microsoft Word files of the *Instructor Resource and Support Manual,* PDF, RTF, and Microsoft Word files of the Test Bank, the Computerized Test Bank, the User's Quick Guide, *Teaching with Student Learning Outcomes, Teaching with Web 2.0, Great Ideas! Active Ways to Teach Health and Wellness, Behavior Change Log Book and Wellness Journal, Eat Right!, Live Right!,* and *Take Charge of Your Health* worksheets.

- **ABC News Videos** and **Health Video Tutors.** New *ABC News* videos, each 3 to 8 minutes long, and 27 Health Video Tutors accessible via QR codes in the text help instructors stimulate critical discussion in the classroom. Videos are embedded within PowerPoint lectures on the Teaching Toolkit DVD and through MasteringHealth.
- *Instructor Resource and Support Manual.* This teaching tool provides chapter summaries, outlines, integrated *ABC News* video discussion questions, tips and strategies for managing large classrooms, ideas for in-class activities, and suggestions for integrating Mastering-Health and MyDietAnalysis into your course.
- **Test Bank.** The Test Bank incorporates Bloom's Taxonomy, or the higher order of learning, to help instructors create exams that encourage students to think analytically and critically. Test Bank questions are tagged to global and book-specific student learning outcomes.

## Student Supplements

- **The Study Area of MasteringHealth™** is organized by learning areas. *Read It* houses the Pearson eText 2.0 as well as the Chapter Objectives and up-to-date health news. *See It* includes *ABC News* videos and the Behavior Change videos. *Hear It* contains MP3 Tutor Session files and audio-based case studies. *Do It* contains the choose-your-own-adventure-style Interactive Behavior Change Activities—Which Path Would You Take?, interactive NutriTools activities, critical-thinking Points of View questions, and Web links. *Review It* contains Practice Quizzes for each chapter, Flashcards, and Glossary. *Live It* will help jump-start students' behavior change projects with interactive Assess Yourself Worksheets and resources to plan change.
- **eText 2.0** comes complete with embedded *ABC News* videos and Health Video Tutors. eText 2.0 is mobile friendly and ADA accessible, available on smartphones and tablets, and includes instructor and student note taking, highlighting, bookmarking, and search functions.
- *Behavior Change Log Book and Wellness Journal.* This assessment tool helps students track daily exercise and nutritional intake and suggests topics for journal-based activities.
- *Eat Right! Healthy Eating in College and Beyond.* This booklet provides students with practical nutrition guidelines, shopper's guides, and recipes.
- *Live Right! Beating Stress in College and Beyond.* This booklet gives students tips for coping with stress during college and for the rest of their lives.
- **Digital 5-Step Pedometer.** This pedometer measures steps, distance (miles), activity time, and calories, and provides a time clock.
- **MyDietAnalysis** (www.mydietanalysis.com). Powered by ESHA Research, Inc., MyDietAnalysis features a database of nearly 20,000 foods and multiple reports. It allows students to track their diet and activity using up to three profiles and to generate and submit reports electronically.

# ACKNOWLEDGMENTS

It is hard for me to believe that *Health: The Basics* is in its 12th edition! Who would have envisioned the evolution of these health texts even a decade ago? With the nearly limitless resources of the Internet, social networking sites, instantaneous access to national databases for statistics, and a myriad of interesting videos and late-breaking news reports, there is a media blitz of information to communicate with students. Each step along the way in planning, developing, and translating that information to students and instructors requires a tremendous amount of work from many dedicated people, and I cannot help but think how fortunate I have been to work with the gifted publishing professionals at Pearson. Through time constraints, decision making, and computer meltdowns, this group handled every issue, every obstacle with patience, professionalism, and painstaking attention to detail.

Susan Malloy, program manager, used her years of experience organizing and developing major health-related textbooks to direct the planning, implementing, and producing of this text. Her guidance was invaluable in making sure that the book continues to be a market-leading text. In particular, Susan's past experience in the successes of *Access to Health* and *Health: the Basics* over the years and her above-and-beyond the call of duty efforts have been greatly appreciated.

Kari Hopperstead, development editor, has worked on several editions of these books as well. Her attention to detail, fabulous work ethic, and knowledge of the health marketplace (and my books!) were invaluable in creating the structure and plan as well as providing creative direction during the pre-editorial phase.

In addition to Kari, Nic Albert did a fantastic job of providing guidance and editorial assistance in reining in an often "overzealous" author in streamlining page length and fine-tuning the many aspects of each chapter so that I didn't end up with a 1,000-page manuscript! He clearly has a solid grasp of what is important and did an excellent job of putting the pieces together in a concise and easy-to-understand manuscript.

Lastly, I would like to provide a special thank you to Lauren Beebe who has worked tirelessly and efficiently on both *Access to Health*, 14e, and *Health: The Basics*, 12e! Not only is Lauren a creative, highly skilled, and well-organized project manager; she has the temperament and professionalism to help move a project through time constraints, deadlines, and challenges, and to make sure that all of the great work from so many people comes to fruition in a top-notch product. Her skills in navigating production pitfalls, keeping the author and contributors on task, and meeting production deadlines were truly exemplary.

Further praise and thanks go to the highly skilled and hard-working, creative, and charismatic Senior Acquisitions Editor Michelle Cadden, who has helped to catapult this book into a competitive twenty-first century. From searching out and procuring cutting-edge technology to meet the demands of an increasingly savvy student to having her finger on the pulse of what instructors and students need in their classrooms today, Michelle's fresh approach and enthusiasm for the work were much appreciated, and Pearson is fortunate to have a new acquisitions editor with her experience and competence at the helm! Michelle has consistently been a key figure in moving the college/university health text to the next level.

Although these individuals were key contributors to the finished work, there were many other people who worked on this revision of *Health: The Basics*. At every level, I was extremely impressed by the work of key individuals. Thanks also to Jeanine Furino and the hard-working staff at Cenveo Publisher Services who put everything together to make a polished finished product. The talented artists at Lachina deserve many thanks for making our innovative art program a reality. Aimee Pavy, Senior Content Producer, put together our most innovative and comprehensive media package yet. Additional thanks go to the rest of the team at Pearson, especially Editorial Assistant Heidi Arndt, Development Manager Cathy Murphy, and Director of Development Barbara Yien.

The editorial and production teams are critical to a book's success, but I would be remiss if I didn't thank another key group who ultimately helps determine a book's success: the textbook representative and sales group and their hard-working, top-notch marketing leader, Executive Product Marketing Manager Neena Bali. From directing an outstanding marketing campaign to the everyday tasks of being responsive to instructor needs, Neena does a superb job of making sure that *Health: The Basics* gets into instructors' hands and that adopters receive the service they deserve. In keeping with my overall experiences with Pearson, the marketing and sales staffs are among the best of the best. I am very lucky to have them working with me on this project, and I want to extend a special thanks to all of them!

## CONTRIBUTORS
### TO THE 12TH EDITION

Many colleagues, students, and staff members have provided the feedback, reviews, extra time, assistance, and encouragement that have helped me meet the rigorous demands of publishing this book over the years. Whether acting as reviewers, generating new ideas, providing expert commentary, or revising chapters, each of these professionals has added his or her skills to our collective endeavor.

I would like to thank specific contributors to chapters in this edition. In order to make a book like this happen on a relatively short timeline, the talents of many specialists in the field must be combined. Whether contributing creative skills in writing, envisioning areas that will be critical to the current and future health needs of students, using their experiences to make topics come alive for students, or utilizing their professional expertise to ensure scientifically valid information, each of these individuals was carefully selected to help make this text the best that it can be. I couldn't do it without their help! As always, I would like to give particular thanks to Dr. Patricia Ketcham (Oregon State University), who has helped with the *Health: The Basics* series since its earliest beginnings. As associate director of health promotion in Student Health Services on campus, with specialties in health promotion and health behavior and substance abuse, Dr. Ketcham provides a unique perspective on the key challenges facing today's students. She contributed to revisions of Chapter 7, Recognizing and Avoiding Addiction and Drug Abuse; Chapter 8, Drinking Alcohol Responsibly and Ending Tobacco Use; Focus On: Enhancing Your Body Image; Chapter 14, Preparing for Aging, Death, and Dying; and Chapter 16, Making Smart Health Care Choices. Dr. Susan Dobie, associate professor in the School of Health, Physical Education, and Leisure Services at University of Northern Iowa, used her background in health promotion and health behavior and in teaching a diverse range of students to provide a fresh approach to revisions of Chapter 5, Connecting and Communicating in the Modern World; Focus On: Understanding Your Sexuality; and Chapter 6, Considering Your Reproductive Choices. Dr. Erica Jackson, associate professor in the Department of Public & Allied Health Sciences at Delaware State University, applied her wealth of fitness knowledge to update and enhance Chapter 11, Improving Your Personal Fitness. Deborah Landforce, instructor at Lane Community College, utilized her extensive background in counseling, relationships, and spirituality to provide a fresh and engaging update to Focus On: Cultivating Your Spiritual Health. With her outstanding background in nutrition science and applied dietary behavior, Dr. Kathy Munoz, professor in the Department of Kinesiology and Recreation Administration at Humbolt State University, provided an extensive revision and updating of Chapter 9, Nutrition: Eating for a Healthier You. Laura Bonazzoli, who has been a key part of developing and refining many aspects of this book over the last editions, used her considerable knowledge and skills in providing major revisions of Chapter 1, Accessing Your Health; Focus On: Improving Your Financial Health; and Focus On: Understanding Complementary and Alternative Medicine.

## REVIEWERS FOR THE 12TH EDITION

With each new edition of *Health: The Basics*, we have built on the combined expertise of many colleagues throughout the country who are dedicated to the education and behavioral changes of students. We thank the many reviewers who have made such valuable contributions to the past 11 editions of *Health: The Basics*. For the 12th edition, reviewers who have helped us continue this tradition of excellence include the following:

Tia Bennett, Northeastern State University
Daniel Czech, Georgia Southern University
Andy Harcrow, University of Alabama
Sylvette La Touche-Howard, University of Maryland
Theodore Murray, Monroe Community College
Adam Parker, Angelo State University
Carole Sloan, Henry Ford College
Glenda Warren, University of the Cumberlands
Brian Witkov, Salem State University
Sharon Woodard, Wake Forest University

## REVIEWERS FOR MASTERINGHEALTH™

We continue to thank the following members of the Faculty Advisory Board, who offered us valuable insights that helped develop MasteringHealth for the previous edition: Steve Hartman (Citrus College), William Huber (County College of Morris), Kris Jankovitz (Cal Poly), Stasi Kasaianchuk (Oregon State University), Lynn Long (University of North Carolina Wilmington), Ayanna Lyles (California University of Pennsylvania), Steven Namanny (Utah Valley University), Karla Rues (Ozarks Technical Community College), Debra Smith (Ohio University), Sheila Stepp (SUNY Orange), and Mary Winfrey-Kovell (Ball State University). For the 12th edition the following people contributed content:

Laura Bonazzoli
Lorin Hawley
Melanie Healy
John Murdzek
Dena Pistor
Karla Rues
Bruce Turchetta

Many thanks to all!
Rebecca J. Donatelle, PhD

# 1 Accessing Your Health

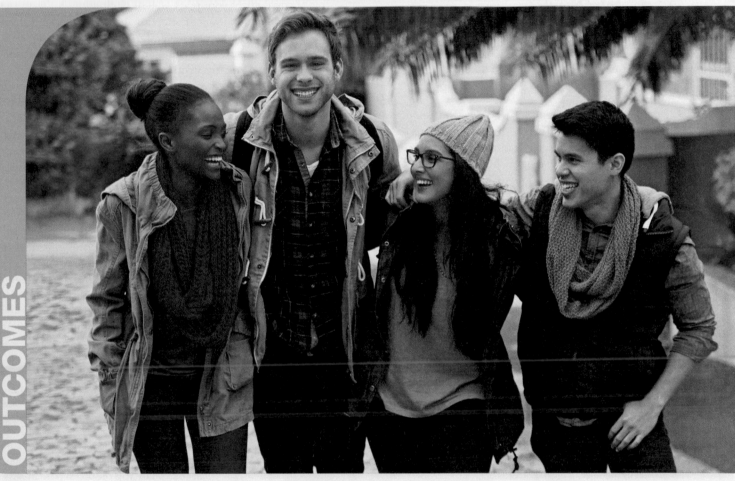

**1** Describe the immediate and long-term rewards of healthy behaviors and the effects that your health choices may have on others.

**2** Compare and contrast the medical model of health and the public health model, and discuss the six dimensions of health.

**3** Identify modifiable and nonmodifiable personal and social factors that influence your health; discuss the importance of a global perspective on health; and explain how gender, racial, economic, and cultural factors influence health disparities.

**4** Compare and contrast the health belief model, the social cognitive model, and the transtheoretical model of behavior change, and explain how you might use them in making a specific behavior change.

**5** Identify your own current risk behaviors, the factors that influence those behaviors, and the strategies you can use to change them.

**G**ot health? That may sound like a simple question, but it isn't. Health is a process, not something we just "get." People who are healthy in their fifties, sixties, and beyond aren't just lucky or the beneficiaries of hardy genes. In most cases, those who are healthy and thriving in later years set the stage for good health by making it a priority in their early years. Whether the coming decades are filled with good health, productive careers, special relationships, and fulfillment of life goals is influenced by the health choices you make—beginning right now.

## LO 1 | WHY HEALTH, WHY NOW?

Describe the immediate and long-term rewards of healthy behaviors and the effects that your health choices may have on others.

Every day, the media reminds us of health challenges facing the world, the nation—maybe even your campus or community. You might want to ignore these issues, but you can't. In the twenty-first century, your health is connected to the health of people with whom you directly interact, as well as to people you've never met, and to the well-being of your local environment, as well as the entire planet. Let's take a look at how.

## Choose Health Now for Immediate Benefits

Almost everyone knows that overeating leads to weight gain, or that drinking and driving increases the risk of motor vehicle accidents. But other choices you make every day may influence your well-being in ways you're not aware of. For instance, did you know that the amount of sleep you get each night could affect your body weight, your ability to ward off colds, your mood, your interactions with others, and your driving? What's more, inadequate sleep is one of the most commonly reported impediments to academic success (**FIGURE 1.1**). Similarly, drinking alcohol reduces your immediate health and your academic performance. It also sharply increases your risk of unintentional injuries—not only motor vehicle accidents, but also falls, drownings, and burn injuries. This is especially significant because for people between the ages of 15 and 44, unintentional injury—whether related to alcohol use or any other factor—is the leading cause of death (**TABLE 1.1**).

It isn't an exaggeration to say that healthy choices have immediate benefits. When you're well nourished, fit, rested, and free from the influence of nicotine, alcohol, and other drugs, you're more likely to avoid illness, succeed in school, maintain supportive relationships, participate in meaningful work and community activities, and enjoy your leisure time.

## Choose Health Now for Long-Term Rewards

Successful aging starts now. The choices you make today are like seeds: Planting good seeds means you're more likely to enjoy the fruits of a longer and healthier life. In contrast, poor choices increase the likelihood of a shorter life, as well as persistent illness, addiction, and other limitations on quality and quantity of life.

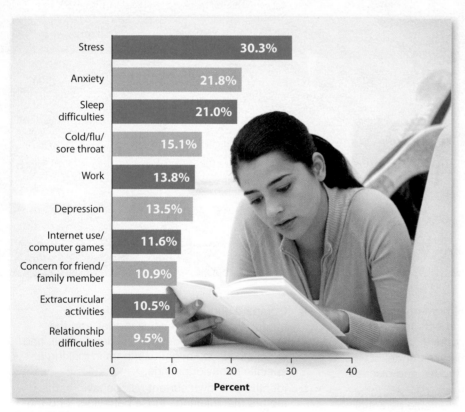

**FIGURE 1.1** Top Ten Reported Impediments to Academic Performance—Past 12 Months In a recent survey by the National College Health Association, students indicated that stress, anxiety, poor sleep, and recurrent minor illnesses, among other things, had prevented them from performing at their academic best.

**Source:** Data are from American College Health Association, *American College Health Association—National College Health Assessment II (ACHA-NCHA II) Reference Group Data Report, Spring 2014* (Hanover, MD: ACHA, 2014).

**HEAR IT!** PODCASTS

Want a study podcast for this chapter? Download **Promoting Health Behavior Change** on MasteringHealth™

## TABLE 1.1 | Leading Causes of Death in the United States, 2012, Overall and by Age Group (15 and older)

| All Ages | Number of Deaths |
|---|---|
| Diseases of the heart | 599,711 |
| Malignant neoplasms (cancer) | 582,623 |
| Chronic lower respiratory diseases | 143,489 |
| Cerebrovascular diseases (stroke) | 128,546 |
| Accidents (unintentional injuries) | 127,792 |
| **Aged 15–24** | |
| Accidents (unintentional injuries) | 11,908 |
| Suicide | 4,872 |
| Assault (homicide) | 4,614 |
| Malignant neoplasms (cancer) | 1,574 |
| Diseases of the heart | 956 |
| **Aged 25–44** | |
| Accidents (unintentional injuries) | 30,885 |
| Malignant neoplasms (cancer) | 15,011 |
| Diseases of the heart | 13,720 |
| Suicide | 12,974 |
| Assault (homicide) | 7,047 |
| **Aged 45–64** | |
| Malignant neoplasms (cancer) | 161,158 |
| Diseases of the heart | 106,493 |
| Accidents (unintentional injuries) | 36,216 |
| Chronic liver disease and cirrhosis | 20,107 |
| Chronic lower respiratory diseases | 19,745 |
| **Aged 65+** | |
| Diseases of the heart | 477,840 |
| Malignant neoplasms (cancer) | 403,497 |
| Chronic lower respiratory diseases | 122,375 |
| Cerebrovascular diseases | 109,127 |
| Alzheimer's disease | 82,690 |

**Source:** Data from M. Heron, "Deaths: Leading Causes for 2012, Table 9," *National Vital Statistics Reports* 63, no. 9 (2014), www.cdc.gov/nchs/data/nvsr/nvsr63/nvsr63_09.pdf

**Life Expectancy** According to current **mortality** rates—the proportion of deaths within a population—the average **life expectancy** at birth in the United States is projected to be 78.8 years for a child born in 2013.[1] In other words, we can expect that Americans born today will live to an average age of over 78 years, more than 30 years longer than the 47-year life expectancy for people born in the early 1900s. But

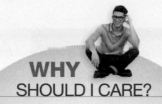

life expectancy a century ago was largely determined by our susceptibility to infectious disease. In 1900, over 30 percent of all deaths occurred among children younger than 5 years old, and the leading cause of death was infection.[2] Even among adults, infectious diseases such as tuberculosis and pneumonia were the leading causes of death, and widespread epidemics of infectious diseases such as influenza crossed national boundaries, killing millions.

With the development of vaccines and antibiotics, life expectancy increased dramatically as premature deaths from infectious diseases decreased. As a result, **chronic diseases** such as heart disease, cerebrovascular disease (which leads to strokes), cancer, and chronic lower respiratory diseases became leading causes of death. Advances in diagnostic technologies, heart and brain surgery, radiation and other cancer treatments, as well as new medications, have continued the trend of increasing life expectancy into the twenty-first century.

**mortality** The proportion of deaths to population.
**life expectancy** Expected number of years of life remaining at a given age, such as at birth.
**chronic disease** A disease that typically begins slowly, progresses, and persists, with a variety of signs and symptoms that can be treated but not cured by medication.

# 68 & 70

ARE THE **HEALTHY** LIFE EXPECTANCY AGES OF MEN AND WOMEN, RESPECTIVELY, IN THE UNITED STATES IN 2012, WHILE THE AVERAGE TOTAL LIFE EXPECTANCY AGES ARE 76 AND 81.

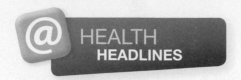
# AMERICA
*Shorter Lives, Poorer Health*

In 2013, the Institute of Medicine (IOM), part of the National Academy of Sciences, published a report comparing health and longevity in the United States to that of 16 "peer" countries—high-income democracies including Canada, Australia, Japan, and 13 countries in Western Europe. Its sobering finding was that, for decades, Americans have been dying at earlier ages than people in peer countries, and experiencing poorer health at all life stages, from birth through older adulthood.

An intriguing aspect of the findings is that Americans' reduced longevity reverses after age 75; that is, an American who lives to age 75 can actually expect to live longer than a 75-year-old from a peer country. This advantage is thought to be due to lower cancer death rates as well as better management of blood pressure and blood lipids, two factors in heart disease. Our reduced longevity overall, therefore, must be due to factors affecting us earlier in life. For example, the United States has a higher infant mortality rate than that of the peer countries. We also have a higher rate of accidental injury deaths, homicides, and drug-related deaths, all of which are more common in young or middle adulthood. Americans also have higher rates of HIV/AIDS, obesity, and diabetes, conditions that reduce the likelihood that people will ever reach age 75.

The IOM study identifies four general factors for our high rates of life-threatening diseases and injuries:

- **Our troubled health care system.** Americans are more likely to be uninsured and, whether insured or not, to find their care unaffordable or inaccessible.
- **Our unequal society.** The United States has a high level of poverty and income inequality, as well as low levels of social mobility and educational performance. Moreover, social assistance programs reach a lower percentage of Americans in need.
- **Our car culture.** Whereas many communities in peer countries are pedestrian and bike friendly, communities throughout the United States tend to be designed around motor vehicles, promoting obesity and reducing fitness.
- **Our poor behaviors.** Although our rates of smoking are lower, we're more likely to abuse drugs. We have more traffic accidents involving alcohol, have lower rates of seatbelt use, and are more likely to use firearms. We also consume the most calories per person.

If citizens of 16 peer countries can enjoy better health and longer lives, Americans can as well. Get involved by supporting increased access to health care and social services, and pedestrian-friendly community redevelopment. As you learn about health-promoting behaviors in this text, be sure to put them into practice.

**Source**: Institute of Medicine, "U.S. Health in International Perspective: Shorter Lives, Poorer Health," January 2013, www.iom.edu/~/media/Files/Report%20Files/2013/US-Health-International-Perspective/USHealth_Intl_PerspectiveRB.pdf.

---

**healthy life expectancy** Expected number of years of full health remaining at a given age, such as at birth.

**health-related quality of life (HRQoL)** Assessment of impact of health status—including elements of physical, mental, emotional, and social function—on overall quality of life.

**well-being** An assessment of the positive aspects of a person's life, such as positive emotions and life satisfaction.

Unfortunately, life expectancy in the United States is several years below that of many other nations. Why is this so? Researchers cite many complex factors, including reduced access to health care, poor health behaviors, social inequality, and poverty, all of which play roles in our high rates of obesity, certain chronic diseases, and fatal injuries.[3] For more, see **Health Headlines**.

*Healthy* Life Expectancy Healthful choices increase your **healthy life expectancy**—the number of years of full health you enjoy without disability, chronic pain, or significant illness. One aspect of healthy life expectancy is **health-related quality of life (HRQoL)**, a concept that focuses on the impact of health on physical, mental, emotional, and social function. Closely related to this is **well-being,** which assesses the positive aspects of a person's life, such as positive emotions and life satisfaction.[4]

## Your Health Is Linked to Your Community

Our personal health choices affect the lives of others because they contribute to national health and the global burden of

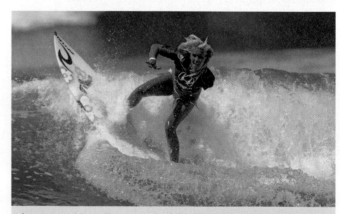

A person with an illness or disability doesn't necessarily have a low quality of life. Hawaiian surfer Bethany Hamilton lost her arm in a shark attack while surfing at age 13, but that hasn't prevented her from achieving her goals as a professional surfer.

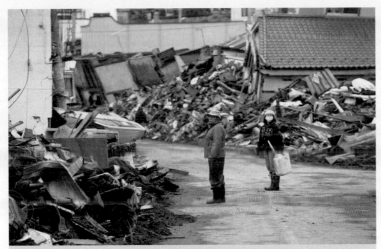

Conditions and events in one location can have far-reaching impacts. A 2011 earthquake and tsunami caused devastation in Japan and damaged the Fukushima Daiichi nuclear power plant, releasing radiation and spreading fear of widespread nuclear fallout.

Compare and contrast the medical model of health and the public health model, and discuss the six dimensions of health.

For some, the word **health** simply means the antithesis of sickness. To others, it means fitness, wellness, or well-being. As our collective understanding of illness has improved, so has our ability to understand the many nuances of health.

## Models of Health

Over the centuries, different ideals—or models—of human health have dominated. Our current model of health has broadened from a focus on the physical body to an understanding of health as a reflection not only of ourselves, but also of our communities.

**Medical Model** Prior to the twentieth century, perceptions of health were dominated by the **medical model**, in which health status focused primarily on the individual and his or her tissues and organs. The surest way to improve health was to cure the individual's disease, either with medication to treat the disease-causing agent or through surgery to remove or repair the diseased tissues. Thus, government resources focused on initiatives that led to treatment, rather than prevention, of disease.

**Public Health Model** Not until the early decades of the 1900s did researchers begin to recognize that entire populations of poor people, particularly those living in certain locations, were victims of environmental factors over which they had little control: polluted water and air, a low-quality diet, poor housing, and unsafe work settings. As a result, researchers began to focus on an **ecological** or **public health model**, which views diseases and other negative health events as a result of an individual's interaction with his or her social and physical environment.

Recognition of the public health model enabled health officials to move to control contaminants in water, for example, by building adequate sewers, and to control burning and other forms of air pollution. In the early 1900s, colleges began offering courses in health and hygiene. Over time, public health officials began to recognize and address many other forces affecting human health, including hazardous work conditions; pollution; negative influences in the home and social environment; abuse of drugs and alcohol; stress; unsafe behavior; diet; sedentary lifestyle; and cost, quality, and access to health care.

disease. For example, we've said that overeating and inadequate physical activity contribute to obesity. But obesity isn't a problem only for the individual. Along with its associated health problems, obesity burdens the U.S. health care system and the U.S. economy overall. According to the United States Centers for Disease Control and Prevention (CDC), the medical costs of obesity in the United States are nearly $150 billion each year.[5] Obesity also costs the public *indirectly* through reduced tax revenues because of income lost from absenteeism and premature death, increased disability payments because of an inability to remain in the workforce, and increased health insurance rates as claims rise for treatment of obesity and associated diseases.

Smoking, excessive alcohol consumption, and illegal drug use also place an economic burden on our communities and society. Moreover, these behaviors have social and emotional consequences, such as for people who lose their loved ones in their prime. The burden on caregivers who personally sacrifice to take care of those disabled by diseases is another part of this problem.

At the root of the concern that individual health choices cost society is an ethical question: To what extent should the public be held accountable for an individual's unhealthy choices? Should we require individuals to somehow pay for their poor choices? In some cases, we already do. We tax cigarettes and alcohol, and many states' tax exemptions for food items exclude candy and sweetened soft drinks. On the other side of the debate are those who argue that smoking, drinking, and overeating are behaviors that require treatment, not punishment. Are seemingly personal choices that influence health always entirely within our control? Before we can answer this question, we need to understand what health actually is.

**health** The ever-changing process of achieving individual potential in the physical, social, emotional, mental, spiritual, and environmental dimensions.

**medical model** A view of health in which health status focuses primarily on the individual and a biological or diseased organ perspective.

**ecological or public health model** A view of health in which diseases and other negative health events are seen as a result of an individual's interaction with his or her social and physical environment.

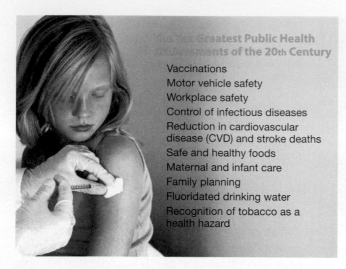

**The Ten Greatest Public Health Achievements of the 20th Century**

Vaccinations

Motor vehicle safety

Workplace safety

Control of infectious diseases

Reduction in cardiovascular disease (CVD) and stroke deaths

Safe and healthy foods

Maternal and infant care

Family planning

Fluoridated drinking water

Recognition of tobacco as a health hazard

**FIGURE 1.2** The Ten Greatest Public Health Achievements of the Twentieth Century

**Source:** Adapted from Centers for Disease Control and Prevention, "Ten Great Public Health Achievements—United States, 1900–1999," *Morbidity and Mortality Weekly Report* 48, no. 12 (April 1999): 241–43.

By the 1940s progressive thinkers began calling for policies, programs, and services to improve individual health and that of the population as a whole—shifting focus from treatment of individual illness to **disease prevention**. For example, childhood vaccination programs reduced the incidence and severity of infectious disease; safety features such as seatbelts and airbags in motor vehicles and helmet laws for cyclists reduced traffic injuries and fatalities; laws governing occupational safety reduced injuries and deaths among American workers. In 1947 at an international conference focusing on global health issues, the World Health Organization (WHO) proposed a new definition of health: "Health is the state of complete physical, mental, and social well-being, not just the absence of disease or infirmity."[6] This new definition prompted a global movement to expand our concept of health.

**disease prevention** Actions or behaviors designed to keep people from getting sick.

**health promotion** The combined educational, organizational, procedural, environmental, social, and financial supports that help individuals and groups reduce negative health behaviors and promote positive change.

**risk behaviors** Actions that increase susceptibility to negative health outcomes.

**wellness** The achievement of the highest level of health possible in each of several dimensions.

The public health model also began to emphasize **health promotion**—policies and programs that promote behaviors known to support good health. Health-promotion programs identify people engaging in **risk behaviors** (those that increase susceptibility to negative health outcomes) and create environments conducive to positive behavior change. While an emphasis on individual knowledge, attitudes, and skills are key, successful change is most likely to occur when public

policies and services, technological advances, and community support help motivate and sustain positive health behaviors. These multifaceted approaches have worked to improve our overall health status greatly in the past 100 years. **FIGURE 1.2** lists the ten greatest public health achievements of the twentieth century.

# Wellness and the Dimensions of Health

In 1968, biologist, environmentalist, and philosopher René Dubos proposed an even broader definition of health. In his Pulitzer Prize–winning book, *So Human an Animal,* Dubos defined health as "a quality of life, involving social, emotional, mental, spiritual, and biological fitness on the part of the individual, which results from adaptations to the environment."[7] This concept of adaptability, or the ability to cope successfully with life's ups and downs, became key to our overall understanding of health.

Later, the concept of **wellness** enlarged Dubos's definition of health by recognizing levels—or gradations—of health (**FIGURE 1.3**). To achieve *high-level wellness,* a person must move progressively higher on a continuum of positive health indicators. Those who fail to achieve these levels may slip into illness, premature disability, or death.

Today, the words *health* and *wellness* are often used interchangeably to describe the dynamic, ever-changing process of trying to achieve one's potential in each of six interrelated dimensions (**FIGURE 1.4**):

■ **Physical health.** This dimension includes features like the shape and size of your body, how responsive and acute your senses are, how susceptible you are to disease and disorders, as well as general body functioning, overall physical fitness, and your body's ability to heal. More recent definitions of physical health encompass a person's ability to perform *activities of daily living (ADLs),* or those activities that are essential to function normally in society—including things like getting up out of a chair, bending over to tie your shoes, or writing a check.

■ **Social health.** The ability to have a broad social network and maintain satisfying interpersonal relationships with friends, family members, and partners is a key part of overall wellness. Successfully interacting and communicating with others, adapting to various social situations, and being able to give and receive love are all part of social health.

■ **Intellectual health.** The ability to think clearly, reason objectively, analyze critically, and use brainpower

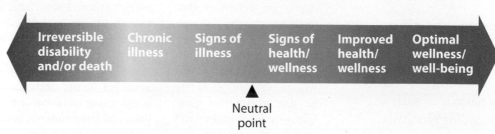

| Irreversible disability and/or death | Chronic illness | Signs of illness | Signs of health/ wellness | Improved health/ wellness | Optimal wellness/ well-being |

▲
Neutral
point

**FIGURE 1.3** The Wellness Continuum

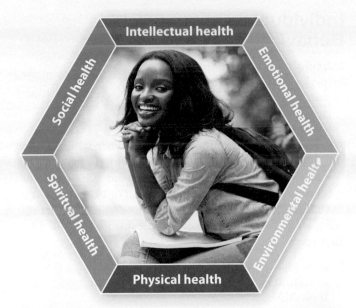

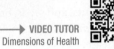

**FIGURE 1.4**
**The Dimensions of Health**
When all dimensions are balanced and well developed, they support your active, thriving lifestyle.

▶ **VIDEO TUTOR**
Dimensions of Health

effectively to meet life's challenges are all part of this dimension. This includes learning from successes and mistakes and making sound, responsible decisions. It also includes a healthy curiosity about life and an interest in learning new things.

■ **Emotional health.** This is the feeling component—being able to express emotions when appropriate, and to control them when not. Self-esteem, self-confidence, trust, love, and many other emotional reactions and responses are all part of emotional health.

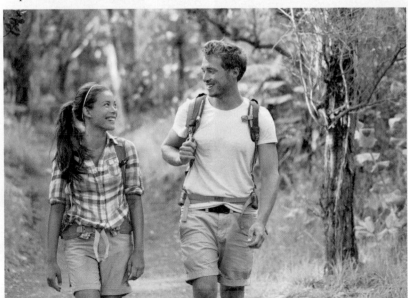

Today, health and wellness mean taking a positive, proactive attitude toward life and living it to the fullest.

■ **Spiritual health.** This dimension involves having a sense of meaning and purpose in your life. This may include believing in a supreme being or following a particular religion's rules and customs. It also may involve the ability to understand and express one's purpose in life; to feel a part of a greater spectrum of existence; to experience peace, contentment, and wonder over life's experiences; and to care about and respect all living things.

■ **Environmental health.** This dimension entails understanding how the health of the environments in which you live, work, and play can affect you; protecting yourself from hazards in your own environment; and working to preserve, protect, and improve environmental conditions for everyone.

Achieving wellness means attaining the optimal level of well-being for your unique limitations and strengths. For example, a physically disabled person may function at his or her optimal level of performance; enjoy satisfying interpersonal relationships; work to maintain emotional, spiritual, and intellectual health; and have a strong interest in environmental concerns. In contrast, those who spend hours lifting weights but pay little attention to their social or emotional health may look healthy but may lack balance in all dimensions of health. The perspective we need is *holistic,* emphasizing the balanced integration of mind, body, and spirit.

**determinants of health** The range of personal, social, economic, and environmental factors that influence health status.

## LO 3 | WHAT INFLUENCES YOUR HEALTH?

Identify modifiable and nonmodifiable personal and social factors that influence your health; discuss the importance of a global perspective on health; and explain how gender, racial, economic, and cultural factors influence health disparities.

If you're lucky, aspects of your world conspire to promote your health: Everyone in your family is slender and fit; there are fresh vegetables on sale at the neighborhood farmer's market; and a new bike trail opens along the river (and you have a bike!). If you're not so lucky, aspects of your world discourage health: Everyone in your family is overweight; your peers urge you to keep up with their drinking; there are only cigarettes, alcohol, and junk food for sale at the corner market; and you wouldn't dare walk or ride alongside the river for fear of being mugged. In short, seemingly personal choices aren't always totally within an individual's control.

Public health experts refer to the factors that influence health as **determinants of health,** a term the U.S. Surgeon General defines as "the range of personal, social, economic, and

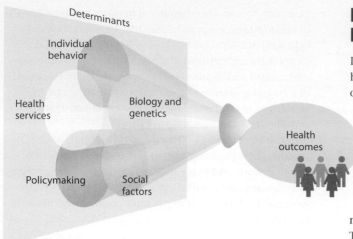

Determinants

Individual behavior

Health services

Biology and genetics

Policymaking

Social factors

Health outcomes

**FIGURE 1.5** *Healthy People 2020* **Determinants of Health** The determinants of health often overlap with one another. Collectively, they impact health of individuals and communities.

**Source:** Adapted from *Healthy People 2020* Framework, U.S. Department of Health and Human Services, Office of Disease Prevention and Health Promotion.

**health disparities** Differences in the incidence, prevalence, mortality, and burden of diseases and other health conditions among specific population groups.

environmental factors that influence health status."[8] The Surgeon General's health promotion plan, called *Healthy People,* has been published every 10 years since 1990 with the goal of improving the quality and years of life for all Americans. The overarching goals set out by the newest version, *Healthy People 2020,* are:

- Attain high-quality, longer lives free of preventable diseases.
- Achieve health equity, eliminate disparities, and improve health of all groups.
- Create social and physical environments that promote good health for all.
- Promote quality of life, healthy development, and healthy behaviors across all life stages.

*Healthy People 2020* classifies health determinants into five categories: individual behavior, biology and genetics, social factors, health services, and policymaking (**FIGURE 1.5**). *Healthy People 2020* also includes strong language about reducing **health disparities** that exist between populations based on racial or ethnic background, sex and gender, income and education, health insurance status, geographic location, sexual orientation, and disability.[9] See the **Health in a Diverse World** box for examples of groups that often experience health disparities.

# Individual Behavior

Individual behaviors can help you attain, maintain, or regain good health, or they can undermine your health and promote disease. Health experts refer to behaviors within your power to change as *modifiable determinants*. Modifiable determinants significantly influence your risk for chronic disease—responsible for 7 out of 10 deaths in the United States.[10] Incredibly, just four modifiable determinants are responsible for most chronic disease (**FIGURE 1.6**). They are:[11]

- **Lack of physical activity.** Low levels of physical activity contribute to over 200,000 deaths in the United States annually.[12]
- **Poor nutrition.** Diets low in whole foods like fruits, vegetables, nuts, and seeds, but high in sodium, processed meats, and *trans* fats are associated with the greatest burden of disease.[13]
- **Excessive alcohol consumption.** Alcohol causes 88,000 deaths in adults annually through cardiovascular disease, liver disease, cancer, and other diseases, as well as motor vehicle accidents and violence.[14]
- **Tobacco use.** Tobacco smoking and the cancer, high blood pressure, and respiratory disease it causes are responsible for about 1 in 5 deaths in American adults.[15]

One 2015 study found that smoking, low levels of physical activity, high alcohol intake, and obesity explained between

**SEE IT!** VIDEOS

What is behind an increase in measles outbreaks? Watch **Measles on the Rise** in the Study Area of MasteringHealth™

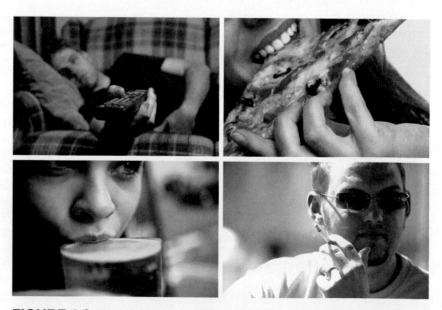

**FIGURE 1.6** **Four Leading Causes of Chronic Disease in the United States** Lack of physical activity, poor nutrition, excessive alcohol consumption, and tobacco use—all modifiable health determinants—are the four most significant factors leading to chronic disease among Americans today.

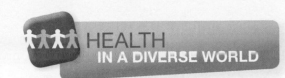

# HEALTH
## IN A DIVERSE WORLD

# THE CHALLENGE OF HEALTH DISPARITIES

The following factors can affect an individual's ability to attain optimal health:

- **Race and ethnicity.** Research indicates dramatic health disparities among people of certain racial and ethnic backgrounds. For example, African Americans have the highest rates of heart disease, colorectal cancer, and infant mortality of any ethnic group. For racial or ethnic minority groups, socioeconomic differences, stigma based on "minority status," poor access to health care, lower-quality health insurance, cultural barriers and beliefs, discrimination, and limited education and employment opportunities can all affect health status.

- **Sex and gender.** At all ages and stages of life, men and women experience major differences in rates of disease and disability. For instance, 20.5 percent of men smoke versus 15.8 percent of women, but women who smoke have higher rates of lung disease. Also, osteoporosis occurs in four times as many women as men, and men have a higher prevalence of heart disease than women until age 75. Men also have much higher rates of drug-induced deaths, as well as deaths from suicide and homicide. These factors all contribute to males having a lower life expectancy overall, as well as a lower healthy life expectancy than females.

Remote Area Medical (RAM) clinics attempt to address the problem of health disparities caused by location, poverty, and lack of insurance. At RAM clinics, rural families wait in line for hours to receive free health care from hundreds of professional doctors, nurses, dentists, and other health workers.

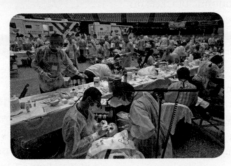

- **Economics and education.** Income and education provide resources that protect against health problems throughout life. Persistent poverty may make it difficult to buy healthy food, medications, quality housing, and access to safe, affordable exercise options. People who are uninsured or underinsured may face unaffordable payments or copayments, high deductibles, or limited care in their area. Moreover, people with low levels of education experience increased rates of illness, premature death, and risk-taking behaviors such as smoking and binge drinking.

- **Geographic location.** Whether you live in an urban or rural area and have access to public transportation or your own vehicle can have a huge impact on

what you eat, the amount of physical activity you get, and your ability to visit the doctor or dentist. Moreover, healthy life expectancy is lowest throughout the Southeastern United States, with the exception of Florida.

- **Sexual orientation.** Gay, lesbian, bisexual, or transgender individuals may lack social support, may be denied health benefits due to unrecognized marital status, and may experience unusually high stress levels and stigmatization by other groups.

- **Disability.** Disproportionate numbers of disabled individuals lack access to health care services, social support, and community resources that would enhance their quality of life.

**Source:** Data from Centers for Disease Control and Prevention, "Current Cigarette Smoking among Adults: United States, 2005–2012," *Morbidity and Mortality Weekly Report* 63, no. 2 (2014): 29–34, Available at www.cdc.gov/mmwr/preview/ mmwrhtml/mm6302a2.htm?s_cid=mm6302a2_w; L.Mosca, E. Barrett-Connor, and N. Kass Wenger, "Sex/Gender Differences in Cardiovascular Disease Prevention," *Circulation* 124 (2011): 2145–154, doi: 10.1161/CIRCULATIONAHA.110.968792; National Institute on Aging, "Osteoporosis: The Bone Thief," August 22, 2014, www.nia.nih.gov /health/publication/osteoporosis; Centers for Disease Control and Prevention, "CDC Health Disparities and Inequalities Report—United States, 2013," *Morbidity and Mortality Weekly Report* 62, Supplement 3 (November 22, 2013): 1–187, Available at www.cdc.gov/mmwr/preview/ ind2013_su.html#HealthDisparities2013; Centers for Disease Control and Prevention, "State-Specific Healthy Life Expectancy at Age 65 Years—United States, 2007–2009," *Morbidity and Mortality Weekly Report* 62, no. 28 (July 19, 2013): 561–66.

24% and 50% of the increased death rate in low-income U.S. populations.[16] Other modifiable determinants include stress levels, exposure to toxic chemicals in home and work environments, use of over-the-counter medications and illegal drugs; sexual behaviors and use of contraceptives; sleep habits; and hand washing and other simple infection-control measures.

## Biology and Genetics

Biological and genetic determinants are things you can't typically change or modify. Health experts frequently refer to these factors as *nonmodifiable determinants*. Genetically inherited traits include genetic disorders such as sickle cell disease,

hemophilia, and cystic fibrosis, as well as inherited predispositions to conditions such as allergies and asthma, cardiovascular disease, diabetes, and certain cancers. Nonmodifiable determinants also refer to certain innate characteristics, such as your age, race, ethnicity, metabolic rate, and body structure. Your sex is another key biological determinant: As compared to men, women have an increased risk for low bone density and autoimmune diseases (in which the body attacks its own cells), whereas men have an increased risk for heart disease compared to women. Your own history of illness and injury also classifies as biology, for instance, if you had a serious knee injury in high school, it may cause pain with walking and exercise, which in turn may predispose you to weight gain.

## Social Factors

Social factors include both the social and physical conditions in the environment where people are born or live. Disparities in income and education, exposure to crime and violence, the availability of healthful foods, the state of buildings and roads, the quality of air, soil, and water, and even climate are all examples.

**Economic Factors** Even in affluent nations such as the United States, people in lower socioeconomic brackets on average have substantially shorter life expectancies and more illnesses than do people who are wealthy.[17] Economic disadvantages exert their effects on human health within nearly all domains of life, including:

- Lacking access to quality education from early childhood through adulthood
- Living in poor housing with potential exposure to asbestos, lead, dust mites, rodents and other pests, inadequate sanitation, unsafe drinking water, and high levels of crime
- Being unable to pay for nourishing food, warm clothes, heat, and other basic needs
- Having insecure employment or being stuck in a low-paying job with few benefits
- Having few assets to fall back on in case of illness or injury

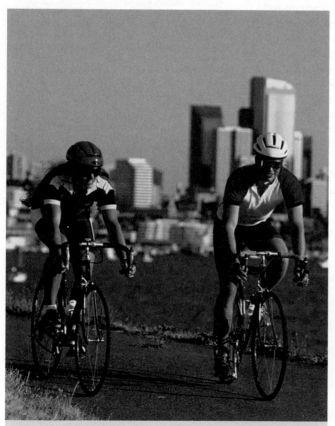

The built environment of your community can promote positive health behaviors. Wide bike paths, good signage and lighting, and major thoroughfares closed to automobile traffic encourage residents to safely incorporate healthy physical activity into their daily lives.

# ABOUT 38 MILLION

AMERICANS DO NOT HAVE HEALTH **INSURANCE**.

Economic disparities also influence access to quality health care. More than twice as many poor Americans report difficulties accessing health care compared to high-income Americans.[18]

**The Built Environment** As the name implies, the *built environment* includes anything created or modified by human beings, including buildings, roads, recreation areas, transportation systems, electric transmission lines, and communications cables.

Researchers in public health have increasingly been promoting changes to the built environment that can improve the health of community members.[19] These include increased construction of parks, sidewalks, "open streets" free of motor traffic, bike paths, and fitness centers as well as public transit systems to which commuters typically walk or bike.[20] In addition, some communities have established incentive programs to encourage the purchase of fresh produce at farmers markets in underserved communities.[21]

**Pollutants and Infectious Agents** Physical conditions also include the quality of the air we breathe, our land, our water, and our foods. When individuals and communities are exposed to toxins, radiation, irritants, and infectious agents via their environment, they can suffer significant harm.

With the rise of global travel and commerce, the health status of people in one region can affect the health of people around the world—a clear reminder of the need for a proactive international response for disease prevention and climate change.

## Access to Quality Health Services

The health of individuals and communities is also determined by access to quality health care, including not only services for physical and mental health, but also accurate and relevant health information and products such as eyeglasses, medical supplies, and medications. Although the numbers of uninsured Americans fell by 9.5 million people in 2014, the first year of enrollment under the 2010 Affordable Care Act (ACA), about 15% of American adults age 19 to 64 are estimated to

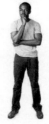

WHICH **PATH** WOULD YOU TAKE **?**

Scan the QR code to see how different choices YOU make today can affect your overall health tomorrow.

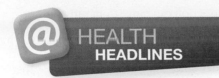
# NATIONAL HEALTH CARE REFORM

In 2010, the United States passed the Patient Protection and Affordable Care Act (ACA). While the ACA is not intended to achieve universal coverage, one of its main goals is to increase access to health insurance among uninsured Americans, primarily by expanding Medicaid eligibility. This expansion is largely funded by federal dollars, and as of December 2014, 27 states and the District of Columbia had accepted the funds and begun implementation. The law also provides tax credits to help small businesses pay to cover their employees.

One of the most contentious aspects of the ACA is the so-called individual mandate: All Americans are required to carry health insurance or face an annual (and progressively increasing) fine. The individual mandate is necessary to push young, healthy Americans into the insurance pool, thereby diluting the cost of overall care. Incidentally, coverage under your college's student health plan typically qualifies under the health care law.

Opponents have argued that compelling individuals to purchase an expensive product such as health insurance is an overreach by the federal government; however, in June 2012, the U.S. Supreme Court ruled that Congress could enact the ACA under its authority to raise and collect taxes.

Significant reforms of the ACA include a provision allowing young adults to stay on their parents' health insurance plan up to age 26 if they do not have access to coverage through an employer. In addition, all plans are required to cover certain preventive services with no co-payment or deductible.

The ACA also reforms certain insurance industry practices deemed unfair or counter to the public good, including:

- Insurers are no longer allowed to deny coverage to people with preexisting conditions.
- Insurers are not allowed to cancel coverage because the insured made an honest mistake on his or her application.
- Insurers have to publicly justify rate hikes of 10 percent or more and must spend at least 80 percent of premiums on health care as opposed to administration, marketing, etc.
- New health insurance plans cannot impose annual or lifetime coverage limits.

Regardless of whether you have the opportunity to get a student health plan through your college or university, you might qualify for care on the ACA marketplace at a lower cost. To find out if this applies to you, visit the ACA's information page for college students at https://www.healthcare.gov/young-adults/college-students/.

**Sources:** Institute of Medicine, "U.S. Health in International Perspective: Shorter Lives, Poorer Health," January 2013, www.iom.edu/~/media/Files/Report%20Files/2013/US-Health-International-Perspective/USHealth_Intl_PerspectiveRB.pdf; Kaiser Family Foundation, "Status of State Action on the Medicaid Expansion Decision, 2014," December 17, 2014, http://kff.org/health-reform/state-indicator/state-activity-around-expanding-medicaid-under-the-affordable-care-act/; U.S. Centers for Medicare & Medicaid Services, "Health Coverage Options for College Students," www.healthcare.gov/young-adults/college-students/.

remain uninsured.[22] Moreover, 30% of Americans who purchased plans in the ACA marketplace reported that they still lacked confidence that, if they became ill, they would be able to afford the care they needed.[23] Both individuals without health insurance and those with a high-deductible plan say they delay care. A survey conducted in the fall of 2014 found that 40% of Americans with a high-deductible plan had delayed needed care because of the deductible.[24] If care is delayed, a disease may not be treated until it is advanced, reducing the chance of recovery and leading to higher rates of hospitalization, longer stays, and more costly health care.

## Policymaking

Public policies and interventions can have a powerful and positive effect on the health of individuals and communities. Examples include policies banning smoking in public places, policies that require you be vaccinated before enrolling in classes, and laws that ban cell phone use while driving. Health policies serve a key role in protecting public health and motivating individuals and communities to change.

Access to health services is also affected by policymaking—including health insurance legislation. As just noted, implementation of the 2010 ACA, has begun to increase Americans' access to quality care. The ACA is discussed in the **Health Headlines** box.

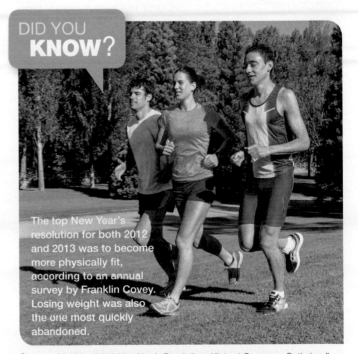

DID YOU **KNOW**?

The top New Year's resolution for both 2012 and 2013 was to become more physically fit, according to an annual survey by Franklin Covey. Losing weight was also the one most quickly abandoned.

**Source:** PR Web, "2013 New Year's Resolutions Hints at Consumer Optimism," www.prweb.com/releases/2012/10/prweb10043254.htm.

Compare and contrast the health belief model, the social cognitive model, and the transtheoretical model of behavior change, and explain how you might use them in making a specific behavior change.

While many factors influence your health status, you have the most control over your individual behaviors. Over the years, social scientists and public health researchers have developed a variety of models to illustrate how individual behavior change occurs. We explore three of those here.

## Health Belief Model

We often assume that when rational people realize their behaviors put them at risk, they will change to reduce that risk. However, it doesn't always work that way. Consider the number of health professionals who smoke, consume junk food, and act in other unhealthy ways. They surely know better, but their "knowing" is disconnected from their "doing." One classic model of behavior change suggests our beliefs may help explain why this occurs.

A **belief** is an appraisal of the relationship between some object, action, or idea (e.g., smoking) and some attribute of that object, action, or idea (e.g., "Smoking is expensive, dirty, and causes cancer" or "Smoking is relaxing and I'm too young to get cancer"). Thousands of studies over the past 50 years have provided evidence that beliefs subtly influence behavior. In the 1950s, psychologists at the U.S. Public Health Service developed the **health belief model (HBM),** which describes the ways in which beliefs affect behavior change.[25] The HBM holds that several factors must support a belief before change is likely:

**belief** Appraisal of the relationship between some object, action, or idea and some attribute of that object, action, or idea.

**health belief model (HBM)** Model for explaining how beliefs may influence behaviors.

**social cognitive model (SCM)** Model of behavior change emphasizing the role of social factors and thought processes (cognition) in behavior change.

**transtheoretical model** Model of behavior change that identifies six distinct stages people go through in altering behavior patterns; also called the *stages of change model.*

- Perceived seriousness of the health problem. The more serious the perceived effects are, the more likely action will be taken.
- Perceived susceptibility to the health problem. People who perceive themselves at high risk are more likely to take preventive action.
- Perceived benefits. People are more likely to take action if they believe that this action will benefit them.
- Perceived barriers. Even if a recommended action is perceived to be effective, the individual may believe it is too expensive, difficult, inconvenient, or time-consuming. These perceived barriers must be overcome or acknowledged as less important than the benefits.
- Cues to action. A person who is reminded or alerted about a potential health problem is more likely to take

action. These cues to action can range from early symptoms of a disorder to an e-mail from a health care provider.

People follow the HBM many times every day. Take, for example, smokers. Older smokers are likely to know other smokers who have developed serious heart or lung problems. They are thus more likely to perceive tobacco as a threat to their health than are teenagers who have just begun smoking. The greater the perceived threat of health problems caused by smoking, the greater the chance a person will quit.

However, many chronic smokers know the risks yet continue to smoke. Why? According to Rosenstock, some people do not believe they are susceptible to a severe problem—they act as though they are immune to it—and are unlikely to change their behavior. They also may feel that the immediate pleasure outweighs the long-range cost.

## Social Cognitive Model

Developed from the work of several researchers over decades, the **social cognitive model (SCM)** is most closely associated with the work of psychologist Albert Bandura.[26] Fundamentally, the model proposes that three factors interact in a reciprocal fashion to promote and motivate change: the *social environment* in which we live, *our thoughts or cognition* (including our values, beliefs, and expectations), and *our behaviors.* We change our behavior in part by observing models in our environments—from childhood to the present moment—reflecting on our observations and regulating ourselves accordingly. For instance, if we observe a family member successfully quitting smoking, we are more apt to believe we can do it, too. In addition, when we succeed in changing ourselves, we change our thoughts about ourselves, potentially promoting further behavior change: After we've successfully quit smoking, we may feel empowered to increase our level of physical activity. Moreover, as we change ourselves, we become a model for others to observe.

The SCM is often used to design health promotion programs. For example, one public health program engaged overweight and obese men in a program of goal-setting, reward setting, journaling, and social support to improve their eating and activity patterns.[27] Another recent study designed according to the SCM increased condom use in participants who viewed a video of someone modeling self-efficacy and consideration of partner expectations.[28]

## Transtheoretical (Stages of Change) Model

Why do so many New Year's resolutions fail before Valentine's Day? According to Drs. James Prochaska and Carlos DiClemente, it's because most of us aren't really prepared to take action. Their research indicates that behavior changes usually do not succeed when starting with the change itself. Instead, we must go through a series of stages to adequately prepare ourselves for that eventual change.[29] According to Prochaska and DiClemente's **transtheoretical model** of behavior change (also called the *stages of change model*), our chances of keeping those New Year's resolutions will be greatly enhanced if we have proper reinforcement and help during each of the following stages:

1. **Precontemplation.** People in the precontemplation stage have no current intention of changing. They may have tried to change a behavior before and given up, or they may be in denial and unaware of any problem.
2. **Contemplation.** In this phase, people recognize that they have a problem and begin to contemplate the need to change. Despite this acknowledgment, people can languish in this stage for years, realizing that they have a problem but lacking the time or energy to make the change.
3. **Preparation.** Most people at this point are close to taking action. They've thought about what they might do and may even have a plan.
4. **Action.** In this stage, people begin to follow their action plans. Those with a plan of action are more ready for action than are those who have given it little thought.
5. **Maintenance.** During the maintenance stage, a person continues the actions begun in the action stage and works toward making these changes a permanent part of his or her life. In this stage, it is important to be aware of the potential for relapses and to develop strategies for dealing with such challenges.
6. **Termination.** By this point, the behavior is so ingrained that constant vigilance may be unnecessary. The new behavior has become an essential part of daily living.

We don't necessarily go through these stages sequentially. They may overlap, or we may shuttle back and forth from one to another—say, contemplation to preparation, then back to contemplation—for a while before we become truly committed to making the change (**FIGURE 1.7**). Still, it's useful to recognize "where we are" with a change, so that we can consider the appropriate strategies to move us forward.

## LO 5 | HOW CAN YOU IMPROVE YOUR HEALTH BEHAVIORS?

Identify your own current risk behaviors, the factors that influence those behaviors, and the strategies you can use to change them.

Clearly, change is not always easy. To successfully change a behavior, you need to see change not as a singular *event* but as a *process* by which you substitute positive patterns for new ones—a process that requires preparation, has several stages, and takes time to occur. The following four-step plan integrates ideas from each of the above behavior change models into a simple guide to moving forward.

## Step One: Increase Your Awareness

Before you make a change, it helps to learn what researchers know about behaviors that contribute to and detract from your health. Each chapter in this book provides a foundation of information focused on these factors. Check out the Table of Contents at the front of the book to locate chapters with the information you're looking for.

This is also a good time to take stock of the health determinants in your life: What aspects of your biology and behavior support your health, and which are obstacles to overcome? What elements of your social and physical environment could you tap into to help you change, and which might hold you back? Making a list of all of the health determinants that affect you—both positively and negatively—should greatly increase your understanding of what you might want to change and what to do to make that change happen.

## Step Two: Contemplate Change

With increased awareness of the behaviors that contribute to wellness and the specific health determinants affecting you, you may be contemplating change. In this stage, the following strategies may be helpful.

### Examine Your Current Health Habits and Patterns
Do you routinely stop at fast-food restaurants for breakfast? Smoke when you're feeling stressed? Party too much on the weekends? Get to bed way past 2 A.M.? When considering a behavior you might want to change, ask yourself the following:

- How long has this behavior existed, and how frequently do I do it?
- How serious are long- and short-term consequences of the habit or pattern?
- What are some of my reasons for continuing this problematic behavior?

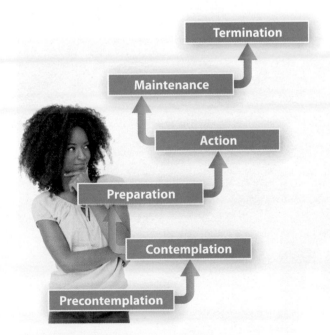

**FIGURE 1.7 Transtheoretical Model** People don't move through the transtheoretical model stages in sequence. We may make progress in more than one stage at one time, or we may shuttle back and forth from one to another—say, contemplation to preparation, then back to contemplation—before we succeed in making a change.

- What kinds of situations trigger the behavior?
- Are other people involved in this behavior? If so, how?

Health behaviors involve elements of personal choice, but they are also influenced by other determinants. Some are *predisposing factors*—thoughts, physical symptoms, family history, media messages, and other factors that make it more or less likely to change a behavior. For instance, if you've been contemplating quitting smoking, and then find out that a beloved grandparent who smokes has been diagnosed with emphysema, you're more likely to register for a smoking cessation program.

In contrast, *enabling factors* are resources, relationships, and other factors that either support or undermine your efforts to change. For example, support from a friend who quit smoking might enable your change attempt, whereas sharing an apartment with someone who smokes would enable you to continue smoking.

Finally, various *reinforcing factors* can encourage you to maintain or abandon your healthful behaviors. Encouragement and praise from others, as well as rewards you give yourself for accomplishing goals can reinforce positive behaviors. In contrast, something like gaining weight after you've quit smoking could act as a negative reinforcer, tempting you to start smoking again.

**motivation** A social, cognitive, and emotional force that directs human behavior.

### Identify a Target Behavior
To clarify your thinking around the various behaviors you might target for change, ask yourself these questions:

- **What do I want?** Is your ultimate goal to lose weight? To exercise more? To reduce stress? To have a lasting relationship? You need a clear picture of your target outcome.
- **Which change is the greatest priority at this time?** Rather than saying, "I need to eat less *and* start exercising," identify one specific behavior that contributes significantly to your greatest problem, and tackle that first.
- **Why is this important to me?** Think through why you want to change. Are you doing it because of your health? To improve your academic performance? To look better? To win someone else's approval? It's best to target a behavior because it's right for you rather than because you think it will help you win others' approval.

Successful targeting involves filling in the details. Identifying the specific behavior you would like to change—rather than the general problem—will help you set clear goals.

### Learn More about the Target Behavior
Once you've clarified what behavior you'd like to change, you're ready to learn more about that behavior. Again, the information in this textbook will help. In addition, this is a great time to learn how to find accurate and reliable health information on the Internet (see the **Tech & Health** box).

As you conduct your research, don't limit your focus to the behavior and its effects. Learn all you can about aspects of your world that might pose obstacles to your success. For instance, let's say you decide you want to meditate for 15 minutes a day. Besides learning what meditation is, how it's practiced, and what benefits you might expect from it, also identify potential obstacles. Do you live in a super-noisy dorm? Are you afraid your friends might think meditating is weird? In short, learn everything you can—positive and negative—about your target behavior now, and you'll be better prepared for change.

### Assess Your Motivation and Your Readiness to Change
Wanting to change is an essential prerequisite of the change process, but to achieve change, you need more than desire. You need real **motivation**, which isn't just a feeling, but a social and cognitive force that directs your behavior. To understand what goes into motivation, let's return for a moment to two models of change discussed earlier: the health belief model (HBM) and the social cognitive model (SCM).

Remember that, according to the HBM, your beliefs affect your ability to change. For example, when reaching for another cigarette, smokers sometimes tell themselves, "I'll stop

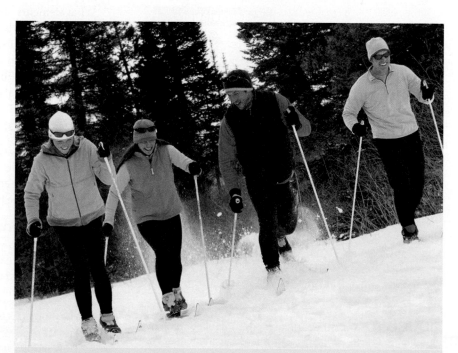

Your friends can help you stay motivated by modeling healthy behaviors, offering support, joining you in your change efforts, and providing reinforcement.

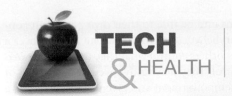

# TECH & HEALTH | SURFING FOR THE LATEST IN HEALTH

The Internet can be a wonderful resource for quickly finding answers to your questions, but it can also be a source of much *misinformation*. To ensure that the sites you visit are reliable and trustworthy, follow these tips.

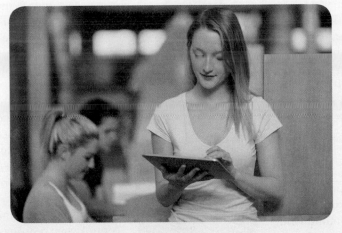

**Find reliable health information at your fingertips!**

- Look for websites sponsored by an official government agency, a university or college, or a hospital/medical center. Government sites are easily identified by their *.gov* extensions, college and university sites typically have *.edu* extensions, and many hospitals have a *.org* extension. Major philanthropic foundations, such as the Robert Wood Johnson Foundation, the Kellogg Foundation, and others, often provide information about selected health topics. In addition, national nonprofit organizations, such as the American Heart Association and the American Cancer Society, are often good, authoritative sources of information. Foundations and nonprofits usually have URLs ending with a *.org* extension. Lastly, if you're asked for personal information, look for the prefix https, indicating an encrypted (and more secure) connection.

- Search for well-established, professionally peer-reviewed journals such as the *New England Journal of Medicine* (**http://content.nejm.org**) or the *Journal of the American Medical Association (JAMA,* **http://jama.ama-assn.org**). Although some of these sites require a fee for access, you can often locate concise abstracts and information that can help you conduct a search. Your college may make these journals available to students for no cost.

- Consult the Centers for Disease Control and Prevention (**www.cdc.gov**) for consumer news, updates, and alerts.

- For a global perspective on health issues, visit the World Health Organization (**www.who.int/en**).

- There are many government- and education-based sites that are independently sponsored and reliable. Some of these include:
  1. Aetna Intelihealth: **www.intelihealth.com**
  2. FamilyDoctor.org: **familydoctor.org**
  3. MedlinePlus: **www.nlm.nih.gov/medlineplus**
  4. Go Ask Alice!: **www.goaskalice.columbia.edu**

- WebMD Health: **webmd.com**

- The nonprofit health care accrediting organization Utilization Accreditation Review Commission (URAC; **www.urac.org**) has devised more than 50 criteria that health sites must satisfy to display its seal. Look for the "URAC Accredited Health Web Site" seal on websites you visit.

- Finally, gather information from two or more reliable sources to see whether facts and figures are consistent. Avoid websites that try to sell you something, whether products like dietary supplements or services such as medical testing. When in doubt, check with your own health care provider, health education professor, or state health division website.

---

tomorrow," or "They'll have a cure for lung cancer before I get it." These beliefs allow them to continue what they're doing. As you contemplate change, consider whether your beliefs are likely to motivate you to achieve lasting change. Ask yourself the following:

- Do you believe that your current pattern could lead to a serious problem? The more severe the consequences are, the more motivated you'll be to change the behavior. For example, smoking can cause cancer, emphysema, and other deadly diseases. The fear of developing those diseases can help you stop smoking. But what if cancer and emphysema were just words to you? In that case, you could study

up on these disorders and the tissue destruction, pain, loss of function, and emotional suffering they cause. Doing so might increase your motivation: In Canada, a law requires graphic images of gangrenous limbs, diseased organs, and chests sawed open for autopsy to cover at least half of cigarette packages. Researchers estimate that this graphic labeling has reduced smoking rates in Canada by 2.9 to 4.7 percent, cutting the total number of smokers by at least one-eighth.[30]

- Do you believe that you are personally likely to experience the consequences of your behavior? For example, losing a loved one to lung cancer could motivate you to work harder to stop smoking. If you can't convince yourself that your behavior will affect you, try employing the social cognitive model to help change your beliefs and gain some motivation. For instance, you could interview people struggling with the consequences of the behavior you want to change. Ask them what their life is like, and if, when they were engaging in the behavior, they believed that it would harm them. Your health care provider may be able to put you in touch with patients who would be happy to support your behavior change plan in this way. And don't ignore the motivating potential of positive role models.

Even though motivation is powerful, to achieve change, it has to be combined with common sense, commitment, and a realistic understanding of how best to move from point A to point B. *Readiness* is the state of being that precedes behavior change. People who are ready to change possess the knowledge, skills, and external and internal resources that make change possible.

**Develop Self-Efficacy** One of the most important factors influencing health status is **self-efficacy**, an individual's belief that he or she is capable of achieving certain goals or of performing at a level that may influence events in life. In general, people who exhibit high self-efficacy approach challenges with a positive attitude and are confident that they can succeed. In turn, they may be more motivated to change and more likely to succeed. Prior success can lead to expectations of success in the future.

Conversely, someone with low self-efficacy or with self-doubts may give up easily or never even try to change a behavior. These people tend to shy away from difficult challenges. They may have failed before, and when the going gets tough, they are more likely to give up or revert to old patterns of behavior. A number of methods for developing self-efficacy follow.

To reach your behavior change goals, you need to take things one step at a time.

state their opinions and be true to their own beliefs. In contrast, people who believe that they have no control over a situation or that others control what they do have an *external* locus of control. They may easily succumb to feelings of anxiety and disempowerment and give up. For example, a recent review study found that, compared to people with an internal locus of control, people with an external locus of control are likely to suffer more significant symptoms of psychiatric illness following a natural disaster, military service, or other traumatic experience.[31]

Having an internal or external locus of control can vary according to circumstance. For instance, someone who learns that diabetes runs in his family may resign himself to facing the disease one day instead of actively working to minimize his risk. On this front, he would be demonstrating an external locus of control. However, the same individual might exhibit an internal locus of control when resisting a friend's pressure to smoke.

## Step Three: Prepare for Change

You've contemplated change for long enough! Now it's time to set a realistic goal, anticipate barriers, reach out to others, and commit. Here's how.

**Set SMART Goals** Unsuccessful goals are vague and open-ended: for instance, "Get into shape by exercising more." In contrast, SMART goals are:

- **S**pecific. "Attend a Tuesday/Thursday aerobics class at the YMCA."
- **M**easurable. "Reduce my alcohol intake on Saturday nights from three drinks to two."
- **A**ction oriented. "Volunteer at the animal shelter on Friday afternoons."
- **R**ealistic. "Increase my daily walk from 15 to 20 minutes."
- **T**ime-oriented. "Stay in my strength-training class for the full 10-week session, then reassess."

Knowing that your SMART goal is attainable—that you can achieve it within the current circumstances of your life—increases your motivation. This, in turn, leads to a better chance of success and to a greater sense of self-efficacy—which can motivate you to succeed even more.

**Use Shaping** **Shaping** is a process that involves taking a series of small steps toward a goal. Suppose you want to start jogging 3 miles every other day, but right now you get tired and winded after half a mile. Shaping would dictate a process of slow, progressive steps, like walking 1 hour every other day at a slow, relaxed pace for the first week; walking for an hour every other day, but at a faster pace that covers more distance the second

**self-efficacy** Belief in one's ability to perform a task successfully.

**locus of control** The location, *external* (outside oneself) or *internal* (within oneself), that an individual perceives as the source and underlying cause of events in his or her life.

**shaping** Using a series of small steps to gradually achieve a particular goal.

**Cultivate an Internal Locus of Control** The conviction that you have the ability to change is a powerful motivator. People who have a strong *internal* **locus of control** believe that they have power over their own actions. They are more driven by their own thoughts and are more likely to

Do you have an internal or an external locus of control?

- Can you think of some friends whom you would describe as more internally or externally controlled?
- How do people with these different views deal with similar situations?

week; and speeding up to a slow run the third week

Regardless of the change you plan, remember that your current habits didn't develop overnight, and they won't change overnight, either. Start slowly to avoid hurting yourself or causing undue stress. Keep the steps of your program small and achievable, and master one step before moving on to the next. Be flexible and willing to change the original plan if it proves to be ineffective.

## Anticipate Barriers to Change

Recognizing possible stumbling blocks in advance will help you prepare fully for change. In addition to negative social determinants, aspects of the built environment, or lack of adequate health care, a few general barriers to change include:

- **Overambitious goals.** Even with the strongest motivation, overambitious goals can undermine self-efficacy and derail change. Habits are best changed one small step at a time.
- **Self-defeating beliefs and attitudes.** Believing you're too young, fit, or lucky to worry about the consequences of your behavior can keep you from making a solid commitment to change. Likewise, thinking you are helpless to change your habits can also undermine efforts.
- **Lack of support and guidance.** If you want to cut down on your drinking, socialize with peers who drink moderately, if at all. Remember that positive role models and social support are key aspects of the social cognitive model of behavior change.

- Emotions that sabotage your efforts and sap your will. Sometimes the best laid plans go awry because you're having a bad day or fighting with someone. Emotional reactions to life's challenges are normal, but don't let the occasional lapse sabotage your efforts to change. If you're experiencing severe psychological distress, seek counseling to help you address those issues before trying to change other aspects of your health.

## Enlist Others as Change Agents

The social cognitive model recognizes the importance of our social contacts in successful change. Most of us are highly influenced by the approval or disapproval (real or imagined) of close friends, family members, and other social and cultural groups. In addition, **modeling**—learning by observing and imitating role models—can give you practical strategies, inspiration, and confidence for making your own changes. Observing a friend who is a good conversationalist, for example, can help you improve your communication skills. Change agents commonly include:

- **Family members.** From the time of your birth, your parents and other family members have influenced your food choices, activity patterns, political beliefs, and many other actions and values. Positive family units provide care and protection, are dedicated to the healthful development of all family members, and work together to solve problems. When the loving family unit does not exist or when it does not provide for basic human needs, many young people have great difficulties.
- **Friends.** As you leave childhood behind, your friends increasingly influence your behaviors. If your friends offer encouragement, or even express interest in joining with you in the behavior change, you are more likely to remain motivated. Thus, friends who share your personal values can greatly support your behavior change.
- **Professionals.** Consider enlisting support from professionals such as your health or PE instructor, coach, health care provider, or other adviser. As appropriate, consider the counseling services offered on campus, as well as community services such as smoking cessation programs, support groups, and your local YMCA.

## Sign a Contract

It's time to get it in writing! A formal *behavior change contract* serves many powerful purposes. It functions as a promise to yourself, as a public declaration of intent, as an organized plan that lays out start and end dates and daily actions, as a listing of barriers you may encounter, as a place to brainstorm strategies to overcome barriers, as a list of sources of support, and as a reminder of the benefits of sticking with the program. Writing a behavior change contract will help you clarify your goals and make a commitment to change. Fill out the Behavior Change Contract at the back

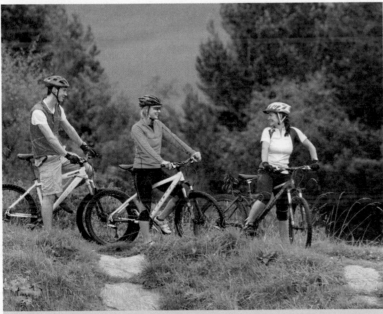

Seek out the support and encouragement of friends who have similar goals and interests to strengthen your commitment to positive health behaviors.

**modeling** Learning and adopting specific behaviors by observing others perform them.

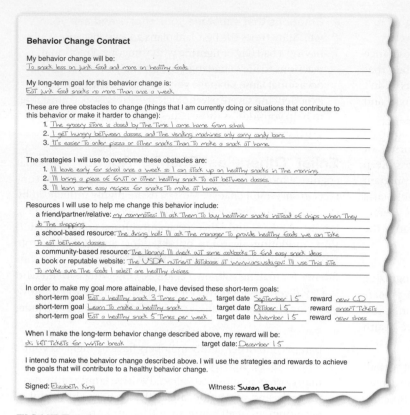

**Behavior Change Contract**

My behavior change will be:
To snack less on junk food and more on healthy foods.

My long-term goal for this behavior change is:
Eat junk food snacks no more than once a week

These are three obstacles to change (things that I am currently doing or situations that contribute to this behavior or make it harder to change):
1. The grocery store is closed by the time I come home from school
2. I get hungry between classes, and the vending machines only carry candy bars.
3. It's easier to order pizza or other snacks than to make a snack at home.

The strategies I will use to overcome these obstacles are:
1. I'll leave early for school once a week so I can stock up on healthy snacks in the morning.
2. I'll bring a piece of fruit or other healthy snack to eat between classes.
3. I'll learn some easy recipes for snacks to make at home.

Resources I will use to help me change this behavior include:
a friend/partner/relative: my roommates. I'll ask them to buy healthier snacks instead of chips when they do the shopping.
a school-based resource: The dining hall. I'll ask the manager to provide healthy foods we can take to eat between classes.
a community-based resource: The library. I'll check out some cookbooks to find easy snack ideas
a book or reputable website: The USDA nutrient database at www.ars.usda.gov. I'll use this site to make sure the foods I select are healthy choices.

In order to make my goal more attainable, I have devised these short-term goals:
short-term goal Eat a healthy snack 3 times per week    target date September 15    reward new CD
short-term goal Learn to make a healthy snack    target date October 15    reward concert tickets
short-term goal Eat a healthy snack 5 times per week    target date November 15    reward new shoes

When I make the long-term behavior change described above, my reward will be:
ski lift tickets for winter break    target date: December 15

I intend to make the behavior change described above. I will use the strategies and rewards to achieve the goals that will contribute to a healthy behavior change.

Signed: Elizabeth King    Witness: Susan Bauer

**FIGURE 1.8** Example of a Completed Behavior Change Contract
A blank version is included in the back of the book and in MasteringHealth for you to fill out.

of this book to help you set a goal, anticipate obstacles, and create strategies to overcome those obstacles. **FIGURE 1.8** shows an example of a completed contract.

# Step Four: Take Action to Change

It's time to put your plan into action! Active behavior change strategies include visualization, countering, controlling the situation, changing your self-talk, rewarding yourself, and journaling. The options don't stop here, but these are a good place to start.

**imagined rehearsal** Practicing, through mental imagery, to become better able to perform an event in actuality.

**countering** Substituting a desired behavior for an undesirable one.

**situational inducement** Attempt to influence a behavior through situations and occasions that are structured to exert control over that behavior.

**self-talk** The customary manner of thinking and talking to yourself, which can affect your self-image.

**positive reinforcement** Presenting something positive following a behavior that is being reinforced.

## Visualize New Behavior

Mental practice can transform unhealthy behaviors into healthy ones. Athletes and others often use a technique known as **imagined rehearsal** to reach their goals. Careful mental and verbal rehearsal of how you intend to act will help you anticipate problems and greatly improve the likelihood of success.

## Learn to "Counter"

**Countering** means substituting a desired behavior for an undesirable one. If you want to stop eating junk food, for example, compile a list of substitute foods and places to get them and have this ready before your mouth starts to water at the smell of a burger and fries.

**Control the Situation** Any behavior has both antecedents and consequences. *Antecedents* are the aspects of the situation that come beforehand; these cue or stimulate a person to act in certain ways. *Consequences*—the results of behavior—affect whether a person will repeat that action. Both antecedents and consequences can be physical events, thoughts, emotions, or the actions of other people. Once you recognize the antecedents of a given behavior, you can employ **situational inducement** to modify those that are working against you—you can seek settings, people, and circumstances that support your efforts to change, as well as avoid those likely to derail you. Similarly, identifying substitute antecedents that support more positive results gives you a strategy for controlling the situation.

**Change Your Self-Talk** There is a close connection between what people say to themselves, known as **self-talk,** and how they feel. According to psychologist Albert Ellis, most emotional problems and related behaviors stem from irrational statements that people make to themselves when events in their lives are different from what they would like them to be.[32]

For example, suppose that after doing poorly on a test you say to yourself, "I can't believe I flunked that easy exam. I'm so stupid." Now change this irrational, negative self-talk into rational, positive statements about what is really going on: "I really didn't study enough for that exam. I'm certainly not stupid; I just need to prepare better for the next test." Changing negative self-talk can help you recover from disappointment and take positive steps to correct the situation.

Another technique for changing self-talk is to practice blocking and stopping. For example, suppose you are preoccupied with thoughts of your ex-partner, who has recently left you. Whenever thoughts of him/her enter your head, consciously STOP them; focus on the actions you're taking right now to move forward. The **Skills for Behavior Change** box on the next page offers more strategies for changing self-talk.

**Reward Yourself** Recall from our discussion of reinforcing factors that rewarding yourself is one way to promote positive behavior change. This is called **positive reinforcement.** Types of positive reinforcement can be classified as follows:

- *Consumable reinforcers* are edible items, such as your favorite fruit or snack mix.

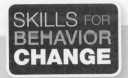
## CHALLENGE THE THOUGHTS THAT SABOTAGE CHANGE

Are any of the following thought patterns and beliefs holding you back? Try these strategies to combat self-sabotage:

▶ **"I don't have enough time!"** Chart your hourly activities for 1 day. What are your highest priorities and what can you eliminate? Plan to make time for a healthy change next week.

▶ **"I'm too stressed!"** Assess your major stressors right now. List those you can control and those you can change or avoid. Then identify two things you enjoy that can help you reduce stress now.

▶ **"I'm worried about what others may think."** Ask yourself how much others influence your decisions about drinking, sex, eating habits, and the like. What is most important to you? What actions can you take to act in line with these values?

▶ **"I don't think I can do it."** Just because you haven't done something before doesn't mean you can't do it now. To develop some confidence, take baby steps and break tasks into small segments of time.

▶ **"I can't break this habit!"** Habits are difficult to break, but not impossible. What triggers your behavior? List ways you can avoid these triggers. Ask for support from friends and family.

---

- *Activity reinforcers* are opportunities to do something enjoyable, such as going on a hike or taking a trip.
- *Manipulative reinforcers* are incentives such as getting a lower rent in exchange for mowing the lawn or the promise of a better grade for doing an extra-credit project.
- *Possessional reinforcers* are tangible rewards, such as a new electronic gadget or sports car.
- *Social reinforcers* are signs of appreciation, approval, or love, such as loving looks, affectionate hugs, and praise.

The difficulty with employing positive reinforcement often lies in determining which incentive will be most effective for you. Your reinforcers may initially come from others (*extrinsic* rewards), but as you see positive changes in yourself, you will begin to reward and reinforce yourself (*intrinsic* rewards). Keep in mind that reinforcers should immediately follow a behavior, but beware of overkill. If

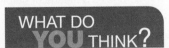

**WHAT DO YOU THINK?**

What type of reinforcers would most likely get you to change a behavior?

- Why would it motivate you?
- Can you think of options to reinforce behavior changes?

---

you reward yourself with a movie every time you go jogging, this reinforcer will soon lose its power. It would be better to give yourself this reward after, say, a full week of adherence to your jogging program.

**Journal** Writing personal experiences, interpretations, and results in a journal, notebook, or blog is an important skill for behavior change. You can log your daily activities, monitor your progress, record how you feel about it, and note ideas for improvement.

**Deal with Relapse** Relapse is often defined as a return of symptoms in a person thought to have been successfully treated for a serious disease. But relapse can also be defined as a return to a previous pattern of negative behavior (drinking, binge eating, failure to take necessary medication, etc.) after a period of time successfully avoiding that behavior. For example, an estimated 40 to 60 percent of people recovering from a substance abuse disorder suffer a relapse.[33] It doesn't mean that your program of change is a failure: Behavior change is a process, and setbacks are part of learning to change.

> **relapse** Returning to a pattern of negative behavior after a period of time successfully avoiding that behavior.

A few simple strategies can help you can get back on track after a relapse. First, figure out what went wrong. Every relapse begins with a slip—a one-time mistake.[34] What triggered that slip, and how can you modify your personal choices or the aspects of your environment that contributed to it? Second, use countering: If you've been overeating ever since your relationship ended, consciously choose behaviors that comfort you without undermining your intention to lose weight. Third, a relapse might be telling you that you need some assistance with making this change; consider joining a support group, taking a class, getting some counseling, or otherwise accessing professional help.

## Let's Get Started!

After you acquire the skills to support successful behavior change, you're ready to apply those skills to your target behavior. Create a behavior change contract incorporating the goals and skills we've discussed, and place it where you will see it every day and where you can refer to it as you work through the chapters in this text. Consider it a visual reminder that change doesn't "just happen." Reviewing your contract can help you stay alert to potential problems, be aware of your alternatives, maintain a firm sense of your values, and stick to your goals under pressure.

# ASSESS | YOURSELF

## How Healthy Are You?

Although we all recognize the importance of being healthy, sorting out which behaviors are most likely to cause problems or pose great risk can be a challenge. *Before* you decide where to start, it is important to evaluate your current health status.

Completing the following assessment will give you a clearer picture of health areas in which you excel—as well as those that could use some work. Answer each question, then total your score for each section and fill it in on the Personal Checklist at the end of the assessment. Think about the behaviors that influenced your score in each category. Would you like to change any of them? Choose the area that you'd like to improve, and then complete the Behavior

Change Contract at the back of your book. Use the contract to think through and implement a behavior change over the course of this class.

Each of the categories in this questionnaire is an important aspect of the total dimensions of health, but this is not a substitute for the advice of a qualified health care provider. Consider scheduling a thorough physical examination by a licensed physician or setting up an appointment with a mental health counselor at your school if you need help making a behavior change.

For each of the following, indicate how often you think the statements describe you.

## 1 Physical Health

| | Never | Rarely | Some of the Time | Usually or Always |
|---|---|---|---|---|
| 1. I am happy with my body size and weight. | 1 | 2 | 3 | 4 |
| 2. I engage in vigorous exercises such as brisk walking, jogging, swimming, or running for at least 30 minutes per day, three to four times per week. | 1 | 2 | 3 | 4 |
| 3. I get at least 7 to 8 hours of sleep each night. | 1 | 2 | 3 | 4 |
| 4. My immune system is strong, and my body heals itself quickly when I get sick or injured. | 1 | 2 | 3 | 4 |
| 5. I listen to my body; when there is something wrong, I try to make adjustments to heal it or seek professional advice. | 1 | 2 | 3 | 4 |

Total score for this section: _____

## 2 Social Health

| | Never | Rarely | Some of the Time | Usually or Always |
|---|---|---|---|---|
| 1. I am open, honest, and get along well with others. | 1 | 2 | 3 | 4 |
| 2. I participate in a wide variety of social activities and enjoy being with people who are different from me. | 1 | 2 | 3 | 4 |
| 3. I try to be a "better person" and decrease behaviors that have caused problems in my interactions with others. | 1 | 2 | 3 | 4 |

| | Never | Rarely | Some of the Time | Usually or Always |
|---|---|---|---|---|
| 4. I am open and accessible to a loving and responsible relationship. | 1 | 2 | 3 | 4 |
| 5. I try to see the good in my friends and do whatever I can to support them and help them feel good about themselves. | 1 | 2 | 3 | 4 |

Total score for this section: _____

## 3 Emotional Health

| | Never | Rarely | Some of the Time | Usually or Always |
|---|---|---|---|---|
| 1. I find it easy to laugh, cry, and show emotions such as love, fear, and anger, and try to express these in positive, constructive ways. | 1 | 2 | 3 | 4 |
| 2. I avoid using alcohol or other drugs as a means of helping me forget my problems. | 1 | 2 | 3 | 4 |
| 3. I recognize when I am stressed and take steps to relax through exercise, quiet time, or other calming activities. | 1 | 2 | 3 | 4 |
| 4. I try not to be too critical or judgmental of others and try to understand differences or quirks that I note in others. | 1 | 2 | 3 | 4 |
| 5. I am flexible and adapt or adjust to change in a positive way. | 1 | 2 | 3 | 4 |

Total score for this section: _____

## 4 Environmental Health

| | Never | Rarely | Some of the Time | Usually or Always |
|---|---|---|---|---|
| 1. I buy recycled paper and purchase biodegradable detergents and cleaning agents, or make my own cleaning products, whenever possible. | 1 | 2 | 3 | 4 |
| 2. I recycle paper, plastic, and metals; purchase refillable containers when possible; and try to minimize the amount of paper and plastics that I use. | 1 | 2 | 3 | 4 |
| 3. I try to wear my clothes for longer periods between washing to reduce water consumption and the amount of detergents in our water sources. | 1 | 2 | 3 | 4 |
| 4. I vote for pro-environment candidates in elections. | 1 | 2 | 3 | 4 |
| 5. I minimize the amount of time that I run the faucet when I brush my teeth, shave, or shower. | 1 | 2 | 3 | 4 |

Total score for this section: _____

## 5 Spiritual Health

| | Never | Rarely | Some of the Time | Usually or Always |
|---|---|---|---|---|
| 1. I take time alone to think about what's important in life—who I am, what I value, where I fit in, and where I'm going. | 1 | 2 | 3 | 4 |
| 2. I have faith in a greater power, be it a supreme being, nature, or the connectedness of all living things. | 1 | 2 | 3 | 4 |
| 3. I engage in acts of caring and goodwill without expecting something in return. | 1 | 2 | 3 | 4 |
| 4. I sympathize and empathize with those who are suffering and try to help them through difficult times. | 1 | 2 | 3 | 4 |
| 5. I go for the gusto and experience life to the fullest. | 1 | 2 | 3 | 4 |

Total score for this section: _____

## 6 Intellectual Health

| | Never | Rarely | Some of the Time | Usually or Always |
|---|---|---|---|---|
| 1. I carefully consider my options and possible consequences as I make choices in life. | 1 | 2 | 3 | 4 |
| 2. I learn from my mistakes and try to act differently the next time. | 1 | 2 | 3 | 4 |
| 3. I have at least one hobby, learning activity, or personal growth activity that I make time for each week, something that improves me as a person. | 1 | 2 | 3 | 4 |
| 4. I manage my time well rather than let time manage me. | 1 | 2 | 0 | 4 |
| 5. My friends and family trust my judgment. | 1 | 2 | 3 | 4 |

Total score for this section: _____

Although each of these six aspects of health is important, there are some factors that don't readily fit in one category. As college students, you face some unique risks that others may not have. For this reason, we have added a section to this self-assessment that focuses on personal health promotion and disease prevention. Answer these questions and add your results to the Personal Checklist in the following section.

## 7 Personal Health Promotion/ Disease Prevention

| | Never | Rarely | Some of the Time | Usually or Always |
|---|---|---|---|---|
| 1. If I were to be sexually active, I would use protection such as latex condoms, dental dams, and other means of reducing my risk of sexually transmitted infections. | 1 | 2 | 3 | 4 |
| 2. I can have a good time at parties or during happy hours without binge drinking. | 1 | 2 | 3 | 4 |
| 3. I eat when I am hungry and stop eating when I am full. I do not try to lose weight by starving or forcing myself to vomit. | 1 | 2 | 3 | 4 |
| 4. If I were to get a tattoo or piercing, I would go to a reputable person who follows strict standards of sterilization and precautions against blood-borne disease transmission. | 1 | 2 | 3 | 4 |
| 5. I do not engage in extreme sports that risk bodily injury. | 1 | 2 | 3 | 4 |

Total score for this section: _____

## Personal Checklist

Now, total your scores for each section and compare them to what would be considered optimal scores. Are you surprised by your scores in any areas? Which areas do you need to work on?

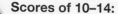

| | Ideal Score | Your Score |
|---|---|---|
| Physical health | 20 | _____ |
| Social health | 20 | _____ |
| Emotional health | 20 | _____ |
| Environmental health | 20 | _____ |
| Spiritual health | 20 | _____ |
| Intellectual health | 20 | _____ |
| Personal health promotion/ disease prevention | 20 | _____ |

### Scores of 10–14:

Your health risks are showing! Find information about the risks you are facing and why it is important to change these behaviors. Perhaps you need help in deciding how to make the changes you desire. Assistance is available from this book, your professor, and student health services at your school.

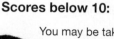

### Scores of 15–20:

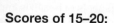

Outstanding! Your answers show that you are aware of the importance of these behaviors in your overall health. More importantly, you are putting your knowledge to work by practicing good health habits that reduce your overall risks. Although you received a very high score, still consider areas in which your scores could be improved.

### Scores below 10:

You may be taking unnecessary risks with your health. Perhaps you are not aware of the risks and what to do about them. Identify each risk area and make a mental note as you read the associated chapter in the book. Whenever possible, seek additional health resources, either on your campus or through your local community, and make a serious commitment to behavior change. If any area is causing you to be less than functional in your class work or personal life, seek professional help. Remember that these scores are only indicators, not diagnostic tools.

## YOUR PLAN FOR **CHANGE**

The **ASSESS YOURSELF** activity gave you the chance to gauge your total health status. Now that you have considered these results, you can take steps toward changing certain behaviors that may be detrimental to your health.

### TODAY, YOU CAN:

☐ Evaluate your behavior and identify patterns and specific things you are doing.

☐ Select one pattern of behavior that you want to change.

☐ Fill out the Behavior Change Contract at the back of your book. Be sure to include your long- and short-term goals for change, the rewards you'll give yourself for reaching these goals, the potential obstacles along the way, and the strategies for overcoming these obstacles. For each goal, list the small steps and specific actions that you will take.

### WITHIN THE NEXT TWO WEEKS, YOU CAN:

☐ Start a journal and begin charting your progress toward your behavior change goal.

☐ Tell a friend or family member about your behavior change goal, and ask him or her to support you along the way.

☐ Reward yourself for reaching your short-term goals, and reevaluate them as needed.

### BY THE END OF THE SEMESTER, YOU CAN:

☐ Review your journal entries and consider how successful you have been in following your plan. What helped you be successful? What made change more difficult? What will you do differently next week?

☐ Revise your plan as needed: Are the goals attainable? Are the rewards satisfying? Do you have enough support and motivation?

# STUDY PLAN

Customize your study plan—and master your health!—in the Study Area of MasteringHealth™

## CHAPTER REVIEW

To hear an MP3 Tutor Session, scan here or visit the Study Area in **MasteringHealth**.

### LO 1 | Why Health, Why Now?

- Choosing good health has immediate benefits, such as reducing the risk of injury and illnesses and improving academic performance; long-term rewards, such as disease prevention, longevity, and improved quality of life; and societal benefits, such as reducing the public costs of disability and disease.

- The average life expectancy at birth in the United States is 78.8 years. This has increased greatly over the past century; however, unhealthy behaviors continue to contribute to chronic diseases such as heart disease and stroke, among the leading causes of death for Americans.

### LO 2 | What Is Health?

- The definition of *health* has changed over time. The medical model focused on physical aspects of health and treatment of disease, whereas the current ecological or public health model focuses on social, environmental, economic, and other factors contributing to health, disease prevention, and health promotion.

- Health can be seen as existing on a continuum and encompassing the dynamic process of fulfilling one's potential in the physical, social, intellectual, emotional, spiritual, and environmental dimensions of life. Wellness means achieving the highest level of health possible in each of the health dimensions.

### LO 3 | What Influences Your Health?

- Health is influenced by factors called *determinants*. The Surgeon General's health promotion plan, *Healthy People,* classifies determinants as individual behavior, biology and genetics, social factors, policymaking, and health services. Disparities in health among different groups contribute to increased risks.

### LO 4 | How Does Behavior Change Occur?

- Models of behavior change include the health belief model, the social cognitive model, and the transtheoretical (stages of change) model. A person can increase the chance of successfully changing a health-related behavior by viewing change as a process containing several steps and components.

### LO 5 | How Can You Improve Your Health Behaviors?

- When contemplating a behavior change, it is helpful to examine current habits; learn about a target behavior; and assess motivation and readiness to change. Developing self-efficacy and an internal locus of control are essential for maintaining motivation. When preparing to change, it is helpful to set SMART goals that employ shaping; anticipate barriers to change; enlist the help and support of others; and sign a behavior change contract. When taking action to change, it is helpful to visualize the new behavior; practice countering; control the situation; change self-talk; reward oneself; and keep a log, blog, or journal.

## POP QUIZ

Visit **MasteringHealth** to personalize your study plan with Chapter Review Quizzes and Dynamic Study Modules.

### LO 1 | Why Health, Why Now?

1. What term is used to describe the expected number of years of full health remaining at a given age, such as at birth?
   a. Healthy life span
   b. Healthy life expectancy
   c. Health-related quality of life
   d. Wellness

2. What statistic is used to describe the number of deaths from heart disease this year?
   a. Morbidity
   b. Mortality
   c. Incidence
   d. Prevalence

### LO 2 | What Is Health?

3. Everyday tasks, such as walking up the stairs or tying your shoes, are known as
   a. wellness behaviors.
   b. healthy life expectancy.
   c. cues to action.
   d. activities of daily living.

4. Janice describes herself as confident and trusting, and she displays both high self-esteem and high self-efficacy. The dimension of health this relates to is the
   a. physical dimension.
   b. emotional dimension.
   c. spiritual dimension.
   d. intellectual dimension.

### LO 3 | What Influences Your Health?

5. *Healthy People 2020* is a(n)
   a. blueprint for health actions designed to improve health in the United States.
   b. projection for life expectancy rates in the United States in the year 2020.
   c. international plan for achieving health priorities for the environment by the year 2020.
   d. set of specific goals that states must achieve in order to receive federal funding for health care.

### LO 4 | How Does Behavior Change Occur?

6. The social cognitive model of behavior change suggests that
   a. understanding the seriousness of and our susceptibility to a health problem motivates change.

b. contemplation is an essential step to adequately prepare ourselves for change.

c. behavior change usually does not succeed if it begins with action.

d. the environment in which we live—from childhood to the present—influences change.

### LO 5 | How Can You Improve Your Health Behaviors?

7. Suppose you want to lose 20 pounds. To reach your goal, you take small steps. You start by joining a support group and counting calories. After 2 weeks, you begin an exercise program and gradually build up to your desired fitness level. What behavior change strategy are you using?
   a. Shaping
   b. Visualization
   c. Modeling
   d. Reinforcement

8. After Kirk and Tammy pay their bills, they reward themselves by watching TV together. The type of positive reinforcement that motivates them to pay their bills is a(n)
   a. activity reinforcer.
   b. consumable reinforcer.
   c. manipulative reinforcer.
   d. possessional reinforcer.

9. The aspects of a situation that cue or stimulate a person to act in certain ways are called
   a. antecedents.
   b. setting events.
   c. consequences.
   d. active inducements.

10. What strategy for change is advised for an individual in the preparation stage?
   a. Following an action plan
   b. Contemplating a need to change
   c. Setting realistic goals
   d. Practicing blocking and stopping

*Answers to the Pop Quiz questions can be found on page A-1. If you answered a question incorrectly, review the section identified by the Learning Outcome. For even more study tools, visit MasteringHealth.*

## THINK ABOUT IT!

### LO 1 | Why Health, Why Now?

1. How healthy is the U.S. population today? What factors influence today's disparities in health?

### LO 2 | What Is Health?

2. How are the words *health* and *wellness* similar? What, if any, are important distinctions between these terms? What is health promotion? Disease prevention?

### LO 3 | What Influences Your Health?

3. What are some of the health disparities existing in the United States today? Why do you think these differences exist? What policies do you think would most effectively address or eliminate health disparities?

### LO 4 | How Does Behavior Change Occur?

4. What is the health belief model? How may this model be working when a young woman decides to smoke her first cigarette? Her last cigarette?

### LO 5 | How Can You Improve Your Health Behaviors?

5. Using our four-step plan for behavior change, discuss how you might act as a change agent to help a friend stop smoking. Why is it important that your friend be ready to change before trying to change?

The ability to budget and manage personal finance plays a key role in psychological and physical health—in college and beyond.

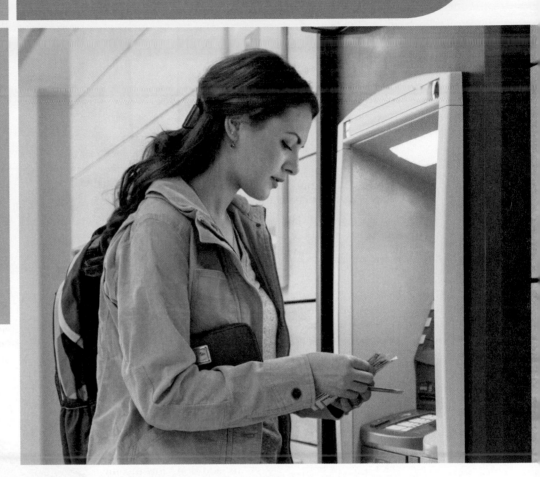

## LEARNING OUTCOMES

**1** List and explain factors that influence the relationship between health and wealth.

**2** Describe common financial struggles college students face as well as strategies families employ to make college more affordable.

**3** Explain how to successfully manage finances through budgeting, understanding debt and credit, and avoiding identity theft.

They say money can't buy happiness or love—but can it buy health? We do know that individuals of a greater **socioeconomic status (SES)** tend to live healthier and longer lives than those living in poverty.[1] The relationship between poverty and health can be demonstrated worldwide, whether it's based on individual income, the wealth of the community, or the overall gross national product of the country.[2] People living in wealthy, developed countries have much longer life expectancies than do those in poor countries (**FIGURE 1**). There also tends to be an inverse relationship between SES and overweight (body mass index); that is, the lower someone's income, the greater his/her odds for being overweight or obese. Carrying extra weight is a major risk factor for developing heart disease, stroke, and diabetes, so the relationship between body mass and overall health is important.

A higher income doesn't guarantee better health. For example, the United States has the highest household wealth and highest disposable income per capita in the world, yet lags behind many other nations in life expectancy. An assortment of other factors, from social connectedness to work-life balance,

**socioeconomic status (SES)** An individual or family's social and economic position in relation to others with regards to education, income, and occupation.

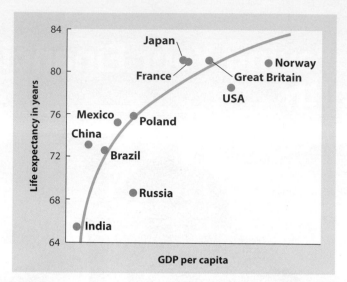

**FIGURE 1** Life Expectancy at Birth and GDP per Capita, 2011 (or nearest year)

**Source:** Based on Figure 1.1.2, "Health at a Glance 2013: OECD Indicators," The Organisation for Economic Co-operation and Development (OECD), November 2013, Available at www.oecd-ilibrary.org

→ VIDEO TUTOR
Financial Health

contribute to a population's health.[3] Still, while money may not exactly buy good health, it makes attaining it much easier. This chapter will address some of the factors that influence health and wealth and what you can do now to increase your financial health.

## LO 1 | THE LINK BETWEEN HEALTH AND WEALTH

List and explain factors that influence the relationship between health and wealth.

The relationship between health and wealth is based on a complex interplay of many interconnected factors, including what the U.S. Surgeon General defines as *determinants of health*: individual behavior, the physical environment, and access to health services. For example, research has associated higher rates of smoking, a behavior linked to a wide range of negative health effects, with lower socioeconomic status.[4] Many factors contribute

to higher smoking rates in poorer populations, including lower social support for quitting, increased likelihood of failing to complete smoking-cessation programs and drug therapies, and a weaker sense of self-efficacy.[5] We also know that tobacco ads frequently target low-income neighborhoods. In addition, low-income individuals may lack education about the risks of smoking, may turn to smoking to reduce stress, or may have become addicted at an early age after witnessing family members smoking.

Let's take a closer look at additional risks low-income individuals face and factors that influence the link between health and socioeconomic status.

## Money and Stress

We've all experienced some degree of financial anxiety or stress. Have you ever been embarrassed to admit to your friends that you can't afford a concert ticket, when everyone else is going to the show? Or have you been jealous of your roommate's new smartphone when you're stuck with an older model? While these feelings may quickly pass, on the whole we have a tendency to compare ourselves to others. Because we value money as an indicator of status and success, those with long-term financial insecurity may experience increased feelings of inferiority, low self-esteem, and self-doubt. These feelings are in part due to **relative deprivation**—the inability of lower-income groups to sustain the same lifestyle as higher-income groups in the same community.

For low-income individuals, experiencing constant feelings of inferiority, anxiety, and insecurity in a money-driven society can progress to chronic stress. In addition, not having enough money for basic needs can cause acute stress. Financial stress is associated with a plethora of negative health outcomes, such as mental health issues, cardiovascular disease, immune system issues, and infectious diseases.[6]

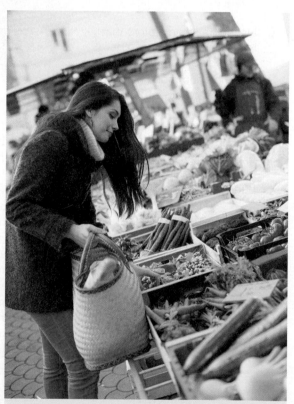

Living in an area with more farmers' markets than liquor stores provides ample access to healthy foods.

**relative deprivation** The inability of lower-income groups to sustain the same lifestyle as higher-income groups in the same community, often resulting in feelings of anxiety and inferiority.

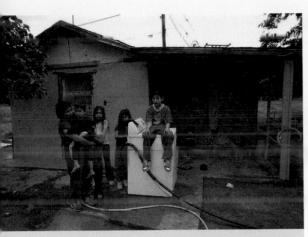

Experiencing poverty in childhood makes people susceptible to a variety of health problems, including asthma, obesity, and mental health issues.

## Money and Access to Resources

People of lower SES often live in areas where they lack access to social services and support, such as nearby medical facilities, educational opportunities, safe housing, or clean water. Researchers have found higher obesity rates in areas with a greater density of fast-food restaurants and lower obesity rates in areas with better access to healthy foods in supermarkets.[7] Areas where people lack access to affordable, nutritious foods that make up a full and healthy diet (including fruits, vegetables, and whole grains) are known as *food deserts*.[8] The difference between living in a fast food–dense neighborhood lacking supermarkets and a place that promotes good health—a safe, walkable neighborhood with a weekend farmer's market, for instance—usually comes down to money.

Researchers also link some lower-income counties in the United States with lower government spending on social services, safety, affordable housing, and education.[9] While living in a high-income area with ample access to resources won't automatically guarantee good health, it does reduce certain risk factors.

## Poverty, Early Care, and Education

Disadvantages early in life can have a lasting impact on health. For example, pregnant women of low SES may face problems with nutrition inadequacy, stress, smoking, and drug or alcohol abuse—all of which can contribute to an unhealthy fetus. Getting preconception and prenatal care includes regular medical checkups as well as stopping unhealthy habits—both of which have a major impact on the growth and development of a healthy child. (You'll learn more about preconception care and prenatal care in Chapter 6.) Low-income pregnant women may lack access to preconception and prenatal care.

Experiencing poverty in childhood is associated with increased rates of asthma, obesity, mental health issues, and other disorders.[10] Education can teach parents and children healthy habits, but quality education may be lacking in groups of lower SES as they face barriers of access and resources. Parents of low SES may also be dealing with other problems such as job insecurity, health issues, substance abuse, and high stress. Children in these homes may lack a parental model of good health-related habits.

## LO 2 | FINANCIAL STRUGGLES IN COLLEGE

Describe common financial struggles college students face as well as strategies families employ to make college more affordable.

Many first feel the burden of financial struggles in college. Students may experience increased financial pressure today at a time when money sources are dwindling. A recession followed by a period of sluggish economic growth reduced many family incomes and savings, meaning less help from parents. Increased demands on state and local governments have led to cuts to colleges and universities and resultant increases in tuition and other fees. The average cost of tuition and fees at public 4-year colleges and universities was less than $2,000 in 1990. It is now over $9,000. In just 5 years, between 2009–2010 and 2014–2015, the cost increased by a staggering 17 percent.[11] Other costs, such as course materials, housing, food, and travel expenses, can all add up.

It's not surprising that a recent survey of 15,000 college students found that 60 percent worried often or very often about meeting regular expenses, and over half also worried frequently about paying for school.[12] Over one third of undergraduate students queried in a different survey said that finances have been "traumatic or very difficult to handle" in the past year.[13] The financial burden students face can have a debilitating effect on their mental health and likelihood of graduating.

## Making College More Affordable

In a recent survey of incoming college first-year students, almost half indicated that financial aid was a major determining factor in the college they chose to attend.[14] About 25 percent of students who were admitted to their top choice school decided not to attend because they were not offered aid. Another recent study found that, on average, about 22 percent of college costs are paid for with borrowed funds.[15]

In 2013, President Obama announced plans aimed at making college more affordable. Some notable reforms included a new rating system tying financial aid to college performance; holding students receiving financial aid responsible for receiving a degree; and matching student loan repayment plans to income.[16] While some specific reforms proposed have prompted some backlash, what's clear is that financial aid is becoming increasingly important.

Families are also taking steps to make college more affordable. These steps include having students reduce spending, increase their workload, or take on

---

### WHAT DO YOU THINK?

Do you think the federal government should provide financial aid to colleges based on how well they serve low- and middle-income students?

- Should such funding be reduced if colleges don't perform well?
- What constitutes a valuable education?

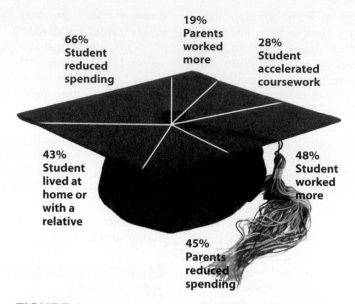

**66% Student reduced spending**

**19% Parents worked more**

**28% Student accelerated coursework**

**43% Student lived at home or with a relative**

**48% Student worked more**

**45% Parents reduced spending**

**FIGURE 2** How Families Cut Costs to Make College More Affordable

**Source:** Data are from Sallie Mae, "A Snapshot of How America Pays for College 2014," 2014, www1.salliemae.com

another roommate (**FIGURE 2**).[17] While these solutions can help, there are some drawbacks. For example, having a job in college looks good on a resume. But the difficulty of balancing work and school can cause students to spend less time on coursework or drop out altogether. In the United States, only 54 percent of first-time college students complete their degree within 6 to 8 years. Even more bleak, only 34 percent of non-first-time students finish their degree.[18] One common reason students drop out is growing debt.

## LO 3 | ACTIONS TO IMPROVE YOUR FINANCIAL HEALTH

Explain how to successfully manage finances through budgeting, understanding debt and credit, and avoiding identity theft.

- - - - - - - - - - - - - - - - - - - - - - - - -

Financial health is not about having a fancy car, the newest smartphone, or a five-bedroom house. It involves being smart about what you spend and save for the future. Life after graduation may seem far off now, but at some point you'll want sufficient savings to support a family, help your parents financially, or pay for advanced education programs

to get yourself higher up the career ladder. Being even a little bit savvy about budgeting and other financial matters will serve you well throughout life.

College is also a great step toward enhancing your socioeconomic status. According to a recent study, median income for those holding a bachelor's degree is nearly $50,000, compared to $30,000 for those with only a

high-school diploma.[19] By making smart financial choices, you can receive a degree, successfully manage debt, and learn to save money.

## Prioritizing Health Insurance

Purchasing health insurance may be low on your financial priority list. What's the point in spending your precious dollars on health care you don't need? While college-age students generally suffer low rates of chronic diseases, individuals aged 15–24 are at significant risk of accidents.[20] If you were to have an accident, being covered by a health insurance plan could be the difference between quick recovery and financial ruin. Say you were to break a leg—the costs for medical treatment without health insurance may be up to $7,500.[21] If you don't have the savings, charging $7,500 to a credit card can equal substantial debt that lingers long after your leg heals. Planning for potentially devastating outcomes from an unexpected injury or illness is one key to financial health.

## Making a Budget

Learning skills to effectively manage your money will help you become financially

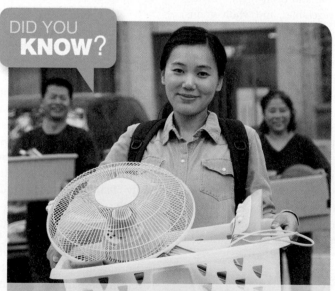

**DID YOU KNOW?**

Ninety-eight percent of American families agree that college is a valuable investment; more than 80% are willing to stretch themselves financially to obtain higher education.

**Source:** Sallie Mae, "A Snapshot of How America Pays for College 2014," 2014, www1.salliemae.com

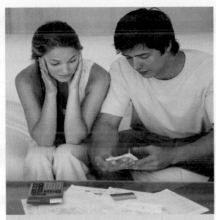

Many college students worry about finances. Smart spending, such as investing in health insurance, can buffer against unexpectedly large costs and the debt that goes along with them.

secure. Creating a **budget** during tough economic times may strike you as downright depressing. But how often do you worry vaguely about money? If you feel a little guilty or tense every time you open your wallet, then creating a budget may actually be a stress reducer by showing you how much you can afford to spend. Here are a few tips for getting started.

## Set Goals

Budgeting should be goal oriented. For students, goal number one is to avoid debt as much as possible. If you have more resources, your goal may be to graduate with no debt at all, or to save for occasional indulgences like a vacation. At other points in life, you may budget to save for buying a car, supporting a family, or retiring. Whenever your life circumstances change, draw up a new budget to match current income level, expenses, and priorities.

## Track Expenses

Start your budget by tallying what you owe for things you buy and services you use. Rent, mortgages, utilities, car loan payments, insurance premiums, and (in some cases) phone plans are examples of *fixed expenses*, meaning their cost does

## SEE IT! VIDEOS

Need tips on living cheaply? Watch

**This Frugal Family Has Mastered Living Cheaply** in the Study Area of **MasteringHealth**™

not change much in the short term. Add in tuition, books, supplies, and other fees for school. Student loan payments may be deferred, depending on the type of loan, if you are in school at least half time. But other debts such as credit card balances can't be deferred and need to be listed as monthly expenses.

Next, figure out how much you spend on food, clothing, entertainment, and personal products or services. Most of these items are **discretionary spending**, things you like, but don't necessarily need. Of course, food is essential, but be careful how you classify it. Unless you eat only at a school dining hall that has a fixed fee, chances are you are spending much more on restaurants and store-bought food than you strictly need to.

## Track Income

Income is the money you have to spend. It generally includes wages from work or interest payments from investments. It may also include financial aid payments, allowances or stipends, and other gifts. Some students will also be withdrawing money from college savings accounts to pay for living expenses and tuition.

When you earn more than you spend, you have a **budget surplus**. If expenses are greater than income, you have a **budget deficit**. As mentioned before, the goal with budgeting should be to create a surplus and build savings. College is a unique time when many people run budget deficits while earning a degree, trusting that future wage gains from their education make the debt feasible. Sometimes this leads people to feel that, because they are already going into debt, they might as well borrow as much as they can to make life easier or more fun in the short term. Avoid this thought process. Every dollar of debt you take on matters. With compound interest and loan terms, just a "few extra" thousand dollars more at the end of school can take many extra years to pay off.

## Making the Budget Numbers Add Up

Both income and expenses may be concentrated at the beginning of each academic term when scholarship and loan money arrive and tuition is due.

**budget** An estimate of spending and income over a set period of time.
**discretionary spending** Goods and services that are not life essentials.
**budget surplus** Money left over for savings after expenses have been paid.
**budget deficit** Spending more money than your income.

students receiving lump sum payments may overspend early on and find themselves unexpectedly broke before finals. Accurate budgets can smooth out spending and help you avoid that problem.

Let's say you create a budget that shows there should be $100 surplus at the end of each month, but that theoretical surplus never appears. The problem could be that you're failing to track all of your discretionary spending. Forgetting to include the purchase of a daily cup of coffee, an occasional film, and other minor expenditures can quickly add up to that missing $100 per month of savings.

To track spending accurately, watch your expenses for several weeks to a month at a time. Write everything down and keep receipts. Use the **Assess Yourself** budget worksheet at the end of the chapter and on **MasteringHealth** or try a personal finance app or computer program that tracks spending and income.

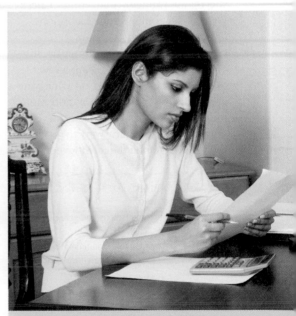

A budget helps you put limits on spending and save for your goals. No matter the income level, a budget is important.

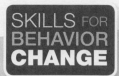

## CREATIVE WAYS TO CUT SPENDING

Little changes in behavior can add up to big savings. Consider some of the following:

▶ **Cut back on the cappuccinos.** A large espresso drink from a coffee shop can cost $4 or $5. Making coffee at home or switching your order to less costly drip varieties saves money.

▶ **Add 2 more weeks between haircuts.** If you normally book hair appointments every 4 weeks, extend that to 6. You'll end up paying for three to four fewer haircuts per year than if you scheduled monthly.

▶ **Drive less.** Carpooling saves on gas and bridge tolls. If you live in an area where car sharing or good public transportation exists, getting rid of your car entirely could save thousands of dollars. You can avoid insurance, gas, maintenance, parking fees, and car payments.

▶ **Cook more.** Cooking meals from scratch is often cheaper (and healthier) than eating out. If you live on campus and cannot cook, consider the lower-cost dining plan options available.

▶ **Use your phone on Wi-Fi.** If you don't have an unlimited data plan for your smart phone, then texting and downloading on a cellular network gets expensive fast. Avoid charges by using the phone on Wi-Fi networks whenever possible.

▶ **Carry cash instead of credit cards.** Withdraw a set amount of cash each week for daily expenses and reserve the credit cards for less frequent, big-ticket buying.

Many universities also offer free spreadsheets for student budgeting. Check your own school's website for options.

Budget cutting is hard. Nobody enjoys passing on doing things because of money woes. To be happier while reducing spending, focus on what you gain: self-discipline, control, and more money in your future. Also remind yourself that there are many ways to socialize and be entertained that are inexpensive.

Make lower-cost options part of your regular routine and reserve higher-cost things for rare treats. Once the period of adjustment is over, you will likely find that your "new financial normal" feels just fine. The **Skills for Behavior Change** box gives some examples of little things you can do to help trim spending.

## Understanding Debt and Credit Basics

It would be nearly impossible for governments, businesses, and individuals to function in the modern world without credit and debt. These tools allow huge projects such as highway systems and airports to be built all at once and then paid for gradually. Families can buy homes and cars or fund college educations, too. Used wisely, credit and debt are incredibly helpful. But overuse of credit and debt are also major contributors to recessions, job losses, and other turmoil.

**Debt** is the condition of owing money for something that was purchased. **Credit** is the ability to purchase things in advance of paying for them: Put another way, credit is a loan. The original amount borrowed is referred to as the loan **principal**. Loans also include **interest** charges. Interest is sometimes described as "rent" for using someone else's money. *Fixed interest rate loans* have payments that will not fluctuate for the life of the loan. *Variable interest rate loans* have interest rates that fluctuate over time.

## Types of Student Aid

The first experience many young adults have with loans comes when reviewing student aid packages. Financial aid options may come from the university itself, the government, or through private banks or firms. Government aid is often awarded according to financial need, whereas other aid may be awarded based on achievements in sports or academics.

Some people think "aid" and "loans" are exactly the same, but student loans, of course, are one type of aid that requires repayment. A **grant** is another aid type—money you don't repay. Most scholarships are grants. You also may have heard of Pell grants, which are issued by the federal government to some undergraduate students. **Federal work study** is another type of aid in which part-time jobs are arranged either on or off campus to help pay for education.

If you take out student loans, it is crucial to understand the details regarding repayment, deferrals (situations where you can put off repaying), interest rates, and loan length. In past decades, someone who got into financial trouble could declare bankruptcy, which nullified all current debts. But bankruptcy laws have since changed to exclude education loans, meaning debt

**debt** Money owed for goods and services that have been purchased.

**credit** The ability to buy goods and services in advance of paying for them.

**principal** Either the original loan amount or the amount left outstanding on a loan, excluding interest.

**interest** A fee paid by the borrower of a loan.

**grant** Financial student aid that does not need to be repaid.

**federal work study** A type of financial aid in which part-time jobs for students are arranged to help them pay for school.

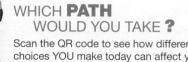

WHICH **PATH** WOULD YOU TAKE **?**

Scan the QR code to see how different choices YOU make today can affect your financial health tomorrow.

## TABLE 1 | Differences between Federal and Private Student Loans

| Loan Issue | Federal Student Loans | Private Student Loans |
|---|---|---|
| Repayment timeline | You don't start repaying federal student loans until you graduate, leave school, or enroll less than half-time. | Many private student loans require payments while you are still in school. |
| Interest rate | Fixed interest rates won't change and are often lower than private loans—much lower than credit card interest rates. | May have variable interest rates, some greater than 18%. Variable rates may substantially increase the total amount you repay. |
| Subsidies | Undergraduates with financial need may qualify for *subsidized loans* in which the government pays the interest if you are in school at least half-time. | Private student loans are not subsidized. No one pays the interest on your loan but you. |
| Credit checks | You don't need to get a credit check or have a credit history for most federal student loans. | May require a credit record, and the loan cost depends on credit score and other factors. |
| Interest tax deduction | Interest may be tax deductible. | Interest may not be tax deductible. |
| Deferrals | If you have trouble repaying your loan, you may be able to temporarily postpone or lower payments. | Private student loans may not offer *forbearance* or *deferment* options. |
| Repayment plans | There are several repayment plans, including an option to tie your monthly payment to your income. | Some, but not all, private loans offer repayment plans. |
| Loan forgiveness | You may be eligible to have some portion of your loans forgiven (removed) if you work in public service. | It is unlikely that your lender will offer a loan forgiveness program. |

**Source:** Table adapted from "What Types of Aid Can I Get?," Federal Student Aid, an Office of the U.S. Department of Education, http://studentaid.ed.gov. Accessed May 2014.

you incur in college will stick with you for a very long time.[22]

The two main categories of student loans are private and federal. Private student loans are issued by banks, credit unions, state agencies, or schools. Federal student loans are funded by the federal government. If you have a choice, pick a federal loan. They are almost always more consumer friendly than private loans when it comes to interest rates, deferral options, penalties, tax breaks, and fees. **TABLE 1** compares both types of loans.

## Credit Cards

There are just over 400 million open credit card accounts in the United States today, which averages to more than one card for every man, woman, and child.[23] Credit cards are *unsecured loans,* meaning the only thing guaranteeing their repayment is your promise. This differs from *secured loans* such as home mortgages, where the loan giver is allowed to seize an asset (for home mortgages, the house itself) if payments are not made on time.

Getting your first credit card is an important, but also potentially dangerous rite of passage. On the positive side, there are some things such as renting a car or booking a hotel that are almost impossible to do without a credit card. Likewise, many high-end cards provide purchase protection programs, so if your new phone falls into the bathtub, your card may actually compensate for the loss. On the other hand, the danger of credit cards is that they can make shopping too easy. Once spending is out of control, extra fees and compounding interest can make debt balloon fast. More than 7 percent of credit

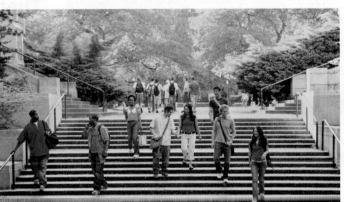

Usually, government-sponsored loans are a better deal in the long haul than private loans. Be sure you do research before you take on any loans for school.

# $15,611

IS THE AVERAGE AMOUNT OF U.S. CREDIT CARD **DEBT**.

card accounts are currently more than 90 days delinquent.[24]

## Interest and Fees

Because credit cards are loans, the banks and firms that issue them make money by charging interest on what you owe (your *account balance*) as well as other fees. Common fee types include *cash advance fees,* charged when you withdraw money from a credit card at an ATM; *annual fees,* charged once every 12 months; and *late fees,* charged when you pay your monthly bill late.

Credit card interest is calculated in a variety of ways. Some cards have variable rates, others have fixed rates. (Fixed rates can change; lenders just need to inform you in writing before they alter anything.) Add in a dizzying array of fees, and you get widespread confusion about which card is a good deal. Find the card with the fewest fees and lowest interest rate possible.

A good starting point for comparison shopping is the **annual percentage rate (APR)**, which is the officially quoted interest rate you pay over a year-long period. The Truth in Lending Act requires that all credit cards clearly state the APR. Card APRs vary greatly: One person may have a card featuring a 10 percent rate while others charge 22 or 23 percent. Think about it: A person with a 10 percent APR is charged less than *half* the interest than is someone with the higher APR.

What counts as your official "first credit card" is one created in your name only, with no cosigner who is guaranteeing that charges will be covered. The first card you have independently likely has a small **credit limit**. This is good. It allows you to build credit history without getting far into debt. Start with a single account. Most people get into trouble when they run up balances on multiple cards.

Although your first credit card may have a low credit limit, it will almost certainly have a high APR. Since you don't have any credit history yet, it is hard for companies to judge how much of a risk it is to loan to you. To compensate for this, credit cards charge you high interest.

Many credit cards do not charge interest if you pay the balance off in full each month. The period of time between the end of the credit card's billing cycle and the date payment is due is known as the *grace period*. For example, if you purchased a bus ticket in mid-December, but paid your bill in full before the due date of

---

**annual percentage rate (APR)** The yearly cost of a credit card account, including interest and certain fees, expressed as a percentage.

**credit limit** The maximum amount a person can charge on a credit card account.

**identity theft** Stealing personal information and using it without permission.

---

## WHY SHOULD I CARE?

Responsible credit card use is necessary to build a credit history with a good credit score—an evaluation of how likely a person is to default on his or her debt. Credit scores are based on factors such as length of credit history, how much current debt you have, total credit available, and how often you've recently applied for credit. Having a good credit score will aid you in renting apartments, obtaining car loans, and being approved for home mortgages. You're entitled by law to receive one free credit report each year. Take advantage of this service to make sure everything on your report is accurate, so there won't be any surprises next time you try to get approved for an apartment or loan. For information on how to check your credit report, visit the Federal Trade Commission's web page at www.consumer.ftc.gov/articles /0155-free-credit-reports.

---

January 7, you would pay no interest—even though the credit card company had lent you the funds for 3 weeks. Knowing what day of the month your payment is due can allow you to avoid most interest charges and other fees.

### Know Your Consumer Credit Rights

If your credit card application is rejected, you have the right to know why. Being rejected should be investigated, since it may indicate identity theft or a credit report mistake. After rejection, you can always apply for a credit card somewhere else. A "no" at one company doesn't automatically mean, "no" elsewhere.

For many years, credit card companies were criticized for unfair practices related to young adults. Firms paid universities for easy access to students on campus. Students received mugs, tee shirts, and other items in exchange for filling out brief applications. People of limited financial means could rapidly get multiple cards. Interest rates and fees were high, and penalties for missed payments extreme. In 2009, the Credit Card Accountability Responsibility and Disclosure (CARD) Act was enacted. It

---

included rules to prevent predatory practices aimed at young consumers, including the following:[25]

- Credit card issuers who set up on or near campus can't give students gifts in exchange for applying for cards.
  - Colleges must publicly disclose marketing contracts with credit card companies.
  - Those under age 21 must provide proof of ability to repay charges by themselves in card applications. Otherwise, the card must be cosigned by someone over age 21 who has financial means to cover potential debts.
  - If a card is cosigned, then credit limits cannot be raised without written permission of the cosigner.

The CARD Act also banned retroactive rate increases, limited fees, removed certain limits on store gift cards (like expiration dates), and required "plain language" disclosure of fees and rates.

The Consumer Financial Protection Bureau (CFPB) is a new government agency whose goal is to educate, conduct research, and enforce federal laws that protect consumers. The CFPB (www.consumerfinance.gov) is the place to look for recent developments in credit card rules and other financial information.

## Protecting against Fraud and Identity Theft

**Identity theft** occurs when someone steals personal information (name, address, social security number, credit card, or bank account numbers) and uses it without permission. Identity crimes have always existed, but they really exploded when credit cards, computers, and online banking became widespread. In 2013, identity theft cost Americans about $18 billion and impacted 13.1 million people.[26] Technology makes people particularly vulnerable to identity theft. Non-credit card fraud tripled in 2013,

# 44%

## OF IDENTITY **FRAUD** INVOLVES INTERNET TRANSACTIONS.

including compromised internet accounts (i.e., eBay, Amazon) and e-mail accounts associated with commerce sites such as PayPal.[27]

## Credit Card Theft

If you see unfamiliar charges on your statement, call the fraud number on the back of your card immediately. You will not be held responsible for charges if they happen after you report the card theft. After the first few days, you may be liable for up to $50 in charges.

## Bank (Debit) Card Theft

As with credit cards, if you report theft of ATM or debit cards before any charges have occurred, you won't be liable for any charges. Reporting a theft within 2 business days will only cost you $50. But reporting bank card fraud 2 to 60 days after a crime leaves you liable for up to $500 of losses, and if you discover the problem after 60 days, you will be unable

to recover *any* lost money.[28] Watch those bank cards and balances carefully!

## Protecting Personal Information and Avoiding Scams

Sometimes accounts are compromised through data breaches at credit card and banking facilities. The companies in question should notify you of the problem and, if necessary, close the compromised accounts and transfer your balances to new accounts.

While you don't have control over identity breaches, there are other types of fraud you can help prevent. Here are some tips:

- **Steer clear of phishers.** Phishing is an e-mail scam where someone impersonates a bank, credit card company, or other entity in an attempt to trick you into divulging account numbers or passwords. Most financial institutions will not contact you via e-mail asking for personal information. Never supply personal information without verifying the request is genuine. Look up contact information independently to verify the requester.

- **Update your smartphone operating system and computer software regularly.** When security

vulnerabilities are discovered, programmers "bug patch" them quickly to resolve threats. But you remain open to attack if you don't update to newer versions.

- **Remove key information from social media accounts.** Sharing birth dates and other life details commonly used for passwords, such as names of pets and hometowns, on social media sites makes you vulnerable to fraud. Passwords should not contain words a stranger can easily look up.

## Get a Smart Card

Traditional credit and debit cards have magnetic strip technology that is fairly easy to steal from. New smart cards contain microchips that make it harder to hijack account information. Merchants and banks in the United States have been slow to adopt smart cards, but increased fraud means they are likely to become more widely available soon.

## Password Lock Your Smartphone and PC

If you don't put a password on the home screen of your PC or other devices, they become a goldmine of names, numbers, and other information for identity thieves when stolen.

## Shred Anything with Your Credit Card Number on It

Don't throw away old card statements or communications unless the account numbers have been rendered unreadable.

## Cleaning Up Identity Theft Messes

Once you discover identity theft, place a fraud alert on your credit reports and ask for report copies to review for problems. Close any accounts that were misused or set up fraudulently. Fill out dispute forms so related debts won't be held against you. Visit the Federal Trade Commission website at www.ftc.gov to learn more about complaint forms and how to correct credit reports. You should also file a police report to document the crime.

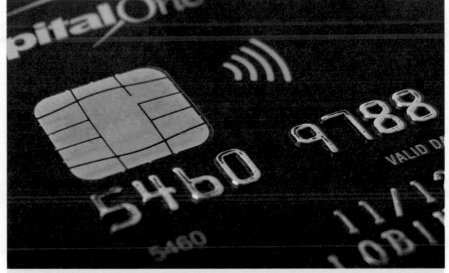

Smart debit or credit cards contain a microchip and are much more secure from fraud than are cards that only have a magnetic strip.

Use this budgeting worksheet as a starting point for tallying your income, expenses, and net income (total income minus total expenses).

| | Monthly Budget | Monthly Actual | Annual Budget |
|---|---|---|---|
| **INCOME** | | | |
| Wages from jobs | | | |
| Stipends (from parents or others) | | | |
| Student loan aid | | | |
| Scholarship awards | | | |
| Gifts | | | |
| Other/miscellaneous | | | |
| **TOTAL INCOME** | | | |
| **EXPENSES** | | | |
| Tuition | | | |
| Textbooks | | | |
| Supplies | | | |
| School fees | | | |
| Computer, tablet, Wi-Fi, etc. | | | |
| Rent or mortgage | | | |
| Utilities: gas, electric, water | | | |
| Insurance: car, health, residence | | | |
| Car: parking, gas, loan payments, maintenance, registration | | | |
| Public transportation | | | |
| Airfare (if flying to/from school regularly in the year) | | | |
| Cell phone | | | |

| | Monthly Budget | Monthly Actual | Annual Budget |
|---|---|---|---|
| **EXPENSES** *continued* | | | |
| Internet/other | | | |
| Dining plan or groceries | | | |
| Eating out | | | |
| Entertainment | | | |
| Clothing | | | |
| Personal products and services | | | |
| Miscellaneous | | | |
| **TOTAL EXPENSES** | | | |
| **NET INCOME** | | | |

## YOUR PLAN FOR **CHANGE**

The **ASSESS YOURSELF** activity allowed you to begin tracking spending, income, and saving. If you face a budget deficit, then consider some of the following steps to fix it:

**TODAY,** YOU CAN:

☐ Calculate a dollar amount you need to reduce spending to eliminate your budget shortfall.

☐ Reduce purchases of new clothing, switch to less expensive brands for food or personal products, and go to the movies and restaurants less often.

☐ Unless something is broken, postpone purchases of phones, cars, or computers.

**WITHIN THE NEXT TWO WEEKS,** YOU CAN:

☐ Research lower-cost options for Internet service providers, and consider downgrading or eliminating cable TV service.

☐ If utility bills are high, be more mindful of your water, electricity, or gas usage.

☐ Weigh costs and benefits of getting a part-time job or increasing current work hours.

☐ Look up your phone plan details. See if it is possible to switch to a lower-cost option without incurring penalties or fees.

**BY END OF THE SEMESTER,** YOU CAN:

☐ Ditch car loans. Sell the vehicle, pay off the loan, and buy a car you can afford outright.

☐ Reduce housing expenses. If you rent a residence near family, consider moving home. If that's not possible, find a cheaper apartment or roommates to reduce costs.

## CHAPTER REVIEW

 To hear an MP3 Tutor Session, scan here or visit the Study Area in **MasteringHealth**.

### LO 1 | The Link between Health and Wealth

- Wealthier populations tend to enjoy better health than lower-income populations, in part because the stress associated with poverty increases the risk for poor health. Poorer communities also have reduced access to nutritious foods and quality health care.

### LO 2 | Financial Struggles in College

- The cost of higher education has increased dramatically over the past decade. Students are borrowing, working part-time, and finding ways to decrease their expenses to make college more affordable.

### LO 3 | Actions to Improve Your Financial Health

- You can improve your financial health by prioritizing health insurance and creating a budget. Track your income and expenses—especially your discretionary expenditures—closely to avoid shortfalls.
- Strictly limit credit card purchases and pay off your balance monthly to avoid high interest charges.
- You can reduce your risk for identity theft by monitoring your personal information. If you suspect fraudulent activity on one of your accounts, contact the financial institution immediately to limit losses or liability for unauthorized charges.

## POP QUIZ

Visit **MasteringHealth** to personalize your study plan with Chapter Review Quizzes and Dynamic Study Modules.

### LO 1 | The Link between Health and Wealth

1. Which of the following statements helps to explain the association between low socioeconomic status (SES) and poor health in the United States?
   a. The lower a county's income, the greater the prevalence of underweight, which contributes to poor health.
   b. Greater government spending on social services in low SES counties fosters dependency.
   c. For low-SES individuals, experiencing constant feelings of inferiority, anxiety, and insecurity can progress to chronic stress, which is a risk factor for poor health.
   d. All of the above statements are true.

### LO 2 | Financial Struggles in College

2. A majority of college students
   a. worry about meeting regular expenses and about paying for school.
   b. admitted to their top-choice college decide not to attend because they are not offered aid.
   c. who are enrolled in college for the first time fail to earn their degree within 6 to 8 years.
   d. report that they make college more affordable by living at home or with a relative.

### LO 3 | Actions to Improve Your Financial Health

3. The interest rate you pay over a year-long period is your
   a. credit limit.
   b. annual percentage rate.
   c. annual fee.
   d. grace period.

*Answers to the Pop Quiz questions can be found on page A-1. If you answered a question incorrectly, review the section identified by the Learning Outcome. For even more study tools, visit MasteringHealth.*

# 2

# Promoting and Preserving Your Psychological Health

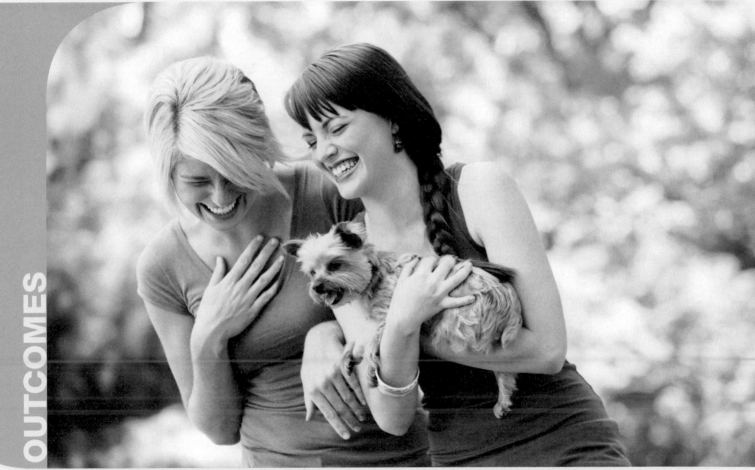

1 Define each of the four components of psychological health, and identify the basic traits shared by psychologically healthy people.

2 Discuss the roles of self-efficacy and self-esteem, emotional intelligence, personality, and happiness in psychological well-being.

3 Describe and differentiate psychological disorders, including mood disorders, anxiety disorders, obsessive-compulsive disorder, post-traumatic stress disorder, personality disorders, and schizophrenia, and explain their causes and treatments.

4 Discuss risk factors and possible warning signs of suicide, as well as actions that can be taken to help a person contemplating suicide.

5 Explain the different types of treatment options and professional services available to those experiencing mental health problems.

ost students describe their college years as among the best of their lives, but they may also find the pressure of grades, finances, and relationships, along with the struggle to find themselves, to be extraordinarily difficult. Psychological distress caused by relationship issues, family concerns, academic competition, and adjusting to college life is common. Experts believe that the anxiety-inducing campus environment is a major contributor to poor health decisions such as high levels of alcohol consumption and overeating. These, in turn, can affect academic success and overall health.

## LO 1 | **WHAT** IS PSYCHOLOGICAL HEALTH?

Define each of the four components of psychological health, and identify the basic traits shared by psychologically healthy people.

Psychological health is the sum of how we think, feel, relate, and exist in our day-to-day lives. Our thoughts, perceptions, emotions, motivations, interpersonal relationships, and behaviors are a product of our experiences and the skills we have developed to meet life's challenges. **Psychological health** includes mental, emotional, social, and spiritual dimensions (**FIGURE 2.1**).

**psychological health** The mental, emotional, social, and spiritual dimensions of health.

Most experts identify several basic elements psychologically healthy people regularly display:

- **They feel good about themselves.** They are not typically overwhelmed by fear, love, anger, jealousy, guilt, or worry. They know who they are, have a realistic sense of their capabilities, and respect themselves.
- **They feel comfortable with other people, respect others, and have compassion for others.** They enjoy satisfying and lasting personal relationships and do not take advantage of others or allow others to take advantage of them. They accept that there are others whose needs are greater than their own and take responsibility for fellow human beings. They can give love, consider others' interests, take time to help others, and respect personal differences.
- **They are "self-compassionate."** Kind and understanding of their own imperfections and weaknesses, they acknowledge their "humanness." They are mindful of the problems in life and work to be the best that they can be, given their limitations and things they can't control. They are not self-absorbed, narcissistic, or overly critical of themselves.[1]
- **They control tension and anxiety.** They recognize the underlying causes and symptoms of stress and anxiety in their lives and consciously avoid irrational thoughts, hostility, excessive excuse making, and blaming others for their problems.
- **They meet the demands of life.** They try to solve problems as they arise, accept responsibility, "cut themselves some slack" when they make mistakes, and plan ahead. They cope positively when faced with adversity or stress.

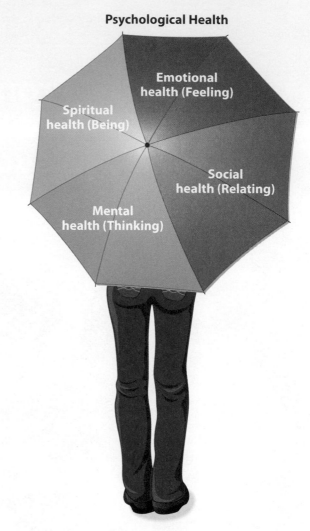

**Psychological Health**

Emotional health (Feeling)

Spiritual health (Being)

Social health (Relating)

Mental health (Thinking)

**FIGURE 2.1** Psychological Health Psychological health is a complex interaction of the mental, emotional, social, and spiritual dimensions of health. Possessing strength and resiliency in these dimensions can maintain your overall well-being and help you weather the storms of life.

They pick themselves up, bounce back, and move on, setting realistic goals, thinking for themselves, and making independent decisions. Acknowledging that change is inevitable, they welcome new experiences.

- **They curb hate and guilt.** They acknowledge and combat tendencies to respond with judgmental criticism, anger, thoughtlessness, selfishness, vengefulness, or feelings of inadequacy. They do not try to knock others aside or stand on others shoulders to get ahead, but rather reach out to help others.
- **They maintain a positive outlook.** They approach each day with a presumption that things will go well. They look to the future with enthusiasm rather than dread. Having fun and making time for themselves are

**HEAR IT!** PODCASTS

Want a study podcast for this chapter? Download **Psychological Health: Being Mentally, Emotionally, and Spiritually Well,** available on **MasteringHealth™**

| | | | |
|---|---|---|---|
| No zest for life; pessimistic/cynical most of the time; spiritually down | Shows poorer coping than most, often overwhelmed by circumstances | Works to improve in all areas, recognizes strengths and weaknesses | Possesses zest for life; spiritually healthy and intellectually thriving |
| Laughs, but usually at others, has little fun | Has regular relationship problems, finds that others often disappoint | Healthy relationships with family and friends, capable of giving and receiving love and affection | High energy, resilient, enjoys challenges, focused |
| Has serious bouts of depression, "down" and tired much of time; has suicidal thoughts | Tends to be cynical/critical of others; tends to have negative/critical friends | Has strong social support, may need to work on improving social skills but usually no major problems | Realistic sense of self and others, sound coping skills, open-minded |
| A "challenge" to be around, socially isolated | Lacks focus much of the time, hard to keep intellectual acuity sharp | Has occasional emotional "dips", but overall good mental/emotional adaptors | Adapts to change easily, sensitive to others and environment |
| Experiences many illnesses, headaches, aches/pains, gets colds/infections easily | Quick to anger, sense of humor and fun evident less often | | Has strong social support and healthy relationships with family and friends |

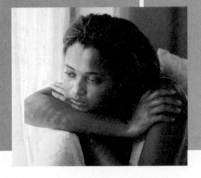
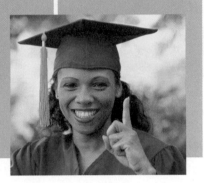

**FIGURE 2.2** Characteristics of Psychologically Healthy and Unhealthy People
Where do you fall on this continuum?

integral parts of their lives. Most of the time, they are the "glass half full" individuals.

- **They value diversity.** They do not feel threatened by those of a different gender, religion, sexual orientation, race, ethnicity, age, or political party. They are nonjudgmental and do not force their beliefs and values on others.
- **They appreciate and respect the world around them.** They take time to enjoy their surroundings, are conscious of their place in the universe, and act responsibly to preserve their environment.

In sum, psychologically healthy people possess emotional, mental, social, and spiritual **resiliency** and don't live in a world where "it's all about me." Resilient individuals have the ability to overcome challenges from major tragedies to minor disappointments and typical life obstacles we often face. They usually respond to challenges and frustrations in appropriate ways, despite occasional slips (see **FIGURE 2.2**). When they do slip, they recognize it, are kind to themselves rather than engaging in endless self-recrimination, and take action to rectify the situation.

Psychologists have long argued that before we can achieve any of the above characteristics of psychological health, we must meet certain basic human needs. In the 1960s, human theorist Abraham Maslow developed a *hierarchy of needs* to describe this idea (**FIGURE 2.3**): At the bottom of his hierarchy are basic *survival needs,* such as food, sleep, and water; at the next level are *security needs,* such as shelter and safety; at the third level—*social needs*—is a sense of belonging and affection; at the fourth level are *esteem needs,* self-respect and respect for others; and at the top are needs for *self-actualization* and self-transcendence.

According to Maslow, a person's needs must be met at each of these levels before he or she can be truly healthy. Failure to meet needs at a lower level will interfere with a person's ability to address higher-level needs. For example, someone who is homeless or worried about threats from violence will be unable to focus on fulfilling social, esteem, or actualization needs.[2]

> **resiliency** The ability to adapt to change and stressful events in healthy and flexible ways.
>
> **mental health** The thinking part of psychological health; includes your values, attitudes, and beliefs.

## Mental Health

The term **mental health** is used to describe the "thinking" or "rational" dimension of our health. A mentally healthy person perceives life in realistic ways, can adapt to change, can develop rational strategies to solve problems, and can carry out personal and professional responsibilities. In addition, a mentally

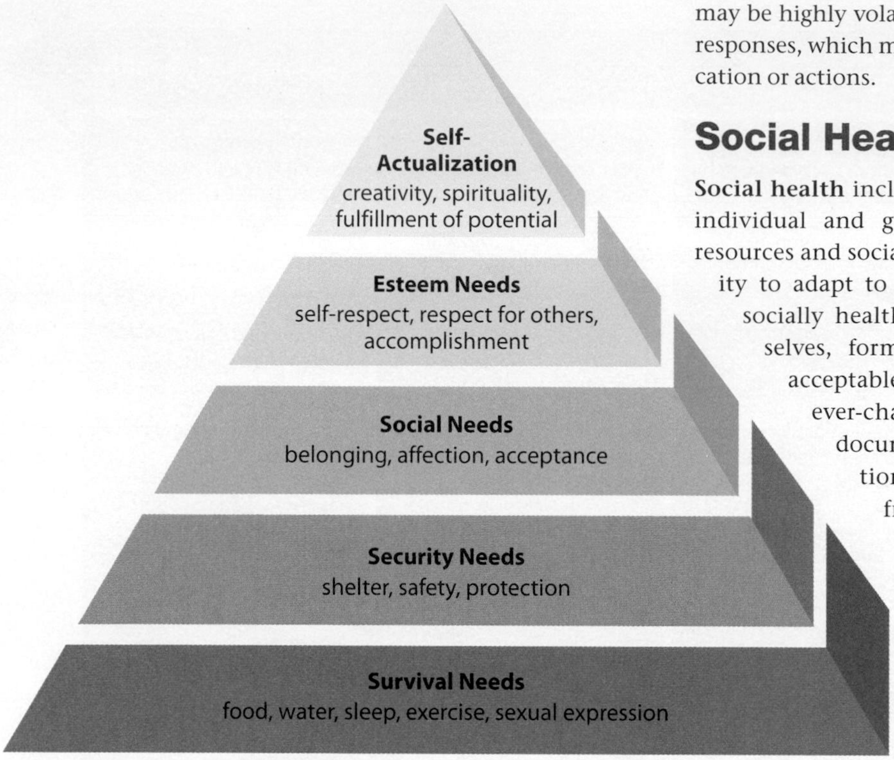
Self-Actualization
creativity, spirituality, fulfillment of potential
Esteem Needs
self-respect, respect for others, accomplishment
Social Needs
belonging, affection, acceptance
Security Needs
shelter, safety, protection
Survival Needs
food, water, sleep, exercise, sexual expression

**FIGURE 2.3** **Maslow's Hierarchy of Needs** To be psychologically healthy, basic needs must be met. Without these, life challenges can be difficult.

**Source:** From A. H. Maslow, *Motivation and Personality*, 3rd ed., eds. R. D. Frager and J. Fadiman (Upper Saddle River, NJ: Pearson Education, Inc., 1987). Reprinted by permission.

**VIDEO TUTOR** Maslow's Hierarchy of Needs

healthy person has the intellectual ability to learn and use information effectively and strive for continued growth. This is often referred to as *intellectual health,* a subset of mental health.[3]

## Emotional Health

The term **emotional health** refers to the feeling, or subjective, side of psychological health. **Emotions** are intensified feelings or complex patterns of feelings that we experience on a regular basis, including love, hate, frustration, anxiety, and joy, among others. Typically, emotions are described as the interplay of four components: physiological arousal, feelings, cognitive (thought) processes, and behavioral reactions. As rational beings, we are responsible for evaluating our individual emotional responses, their causes, and the appropriateness of our actions.

Emotionally healthy people usually respond appropriately to upsetting events. Rather than reacting in an extreme fashion or behaving inconsistently or offensively, they express their feelings, communicate with others, and show emotions in appropriate ways. In contrast, emotionally unhealthy people are much more likely to let their feelings overpower them. They may be highly volatile and prone to unpredictable emotional responses, which may be followed by inappropriate communication or actions.

**emotional health** The feeling part of psychological health; includes your emotional reactions to life.

**emotions** Intensified feelings or complex patterns of feelings.

**social health** Aspect of psychological health that includes interactions with others, ability to use social supports, and ability to adapt to various situations.

## Social Health

**Social health** includes your interactions with others on an individual and group basis, your ability to use social resources and social support in times of need, and your ability to adapt to a variety of social situations. Typically, socially healthy individuals can listen, express themselves, form healthy attachments, act in socially acceptable and responsible ways, and adapt to an ever-changing society. Numerous studies have documented the importance of positive relationships and support from family members, friends, coworkers, community groups, and significant others to overall well-being. In addition, social support has been shown to moderate the effects of stress, reduce risks of depression, and improve overall longevity.[4]

Families have a significant influence on psychological development. Healthy families model and help develop the cognitive and social skills necessary to solve problems, express emotions in socially acceptable ways, manage stress, and develop a sense of self-worth and purpose. In adulthood,

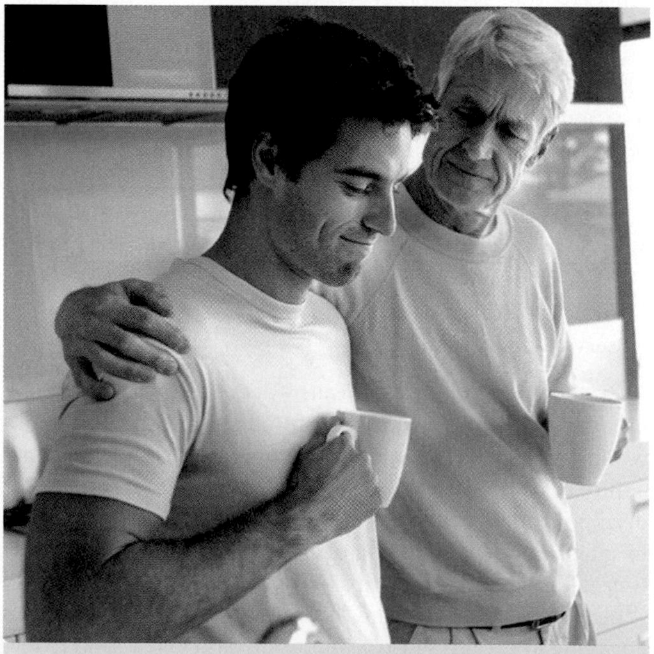

Your family members play an important role in your psychological health. As you were growing up, they modeled behaviors and skills that helped you develop cognitively and socially. Their love and support can give you a sense of self-worth and encourage you to treat others with compassion and care.

family support is one of the best predictors of health and happiness.[5] Children brought up in **dysfunctional families**—in which there is violence, distrust, anger, dietary deprivation, drug abuse, significant parental discord, or abuse—may run an increased risk of psychological problems.

The concept of **social support** is more complex than many people realize. In general, it refers to the people and services with whom we interact and share social connections (see Chapter 5 for more information on the importance of social networks and social bonds). These ties can provide *tangible support,* such as babysitting services or money to help pay the bills, or *intangible support,* such as encouraging you to share your concerns. Research shows that college students with adequate social support have improved overall well-being, including higher GPAs, higher perceived ability in math and science courses, less stress and depression, less peer pressure for binge drinking, lower rates of suicide, and higher overall life satisfaction.[6]

The communities we live in can provide social support, as can religious institutions, schools, clinics, and local businesses that work to provide support for those in need. Likewise, you are a part of a campus community with a multitude of services designed to provide support and care for your psychological health by creating a safe environment to explore and develop your mental, emotional, social, and spiritual dimensions.

## Spiritual Health

It is possible to be mentally, emotionally, and socially healthy and still not achieve optimal psychological well-being. For many people, the difficult-to-describe element that gives life purpose is the *spiritual dimension.*

The term *spirituality* is broader in meaning than religion and is defined as an individual's sense of purpose and meaning in life; it involves a sense of peace and connection to others.[7] Spirituality may be practiced in many ways, including through religion; however, religion does not have to be part of a spiritual person's life. **Spiritual health** refers to the sense of belonging to something greater than the purely physical or personal dimensions of existence. For some, this unifying force is nature; for others, it is a feeling of connection to other people; for still others, it is a god or other higher power. (**Focus On: Cultivating Your Spiritual Health** explores the role spirituality plays in your overall psychological health.)

## WHY SHOULD I CARE?

Emotional health can affect social and intellectual health. People who feel hostile, are overly negative and critical, withdrawn, or moody may become socially isolated. Because they are not much fun to be around, people may avoid them at the very time they are most in need of emotional support. For students, a more immediate concern is the impact of emotional upset on academic performance. Have you ever tried to study for an exam after a fight with a friend or family member? Emotional turmoil can seriously affect your ability to think, reason, and act rationally.

Discuss the roles self-efficacy and self-esteem, emotional intelligence, personality, and happiness in psychological well-being.

As we have seen, psychological health involves four dimensions. Attaining self-fulfillment is a lifelong, conscious process that involves enhancing each of these components. The keys to enhancing psychological health lie in developing self-efficacy and self-esteem, understanding and controlling emotions, cultivating healthy personality traits and emotional intelligence, and pursuing happiness.

## Self-Efficacy and Self-Esteem

During our formative years, successes and failures in school, athletics, friendships, intimate relationships, jobs, and every other aspect of life subtly shape our beliefs about our personal worth and abilities. These beliefs in turn become internal influences on our psychological health.

**Self-efficacy** describes a person's belief about whether he or she can successfully engage in and execute a specific behavior. **Self-esteem** refers to one's realistic sense of self-respect or self-worth. People with high levels of self-efficacy and self-esteem tend to express a positive outlook on life.

Self-esteem is internal, but it is influenced by the relationships we have with our parents and family growing up; with friends as we grow older; with our significant others as we form intimate relationships; and with our teachers, coworkers, and others throughout our lives. One of the best ways to promote self-esteem is through a support system of people who share your values, provide constructive feedback, and are caring and nurturing. The **Health Headlines** box on page 42 discusses the possible downside of having too much self-esteem.

## Learned Helplessness versus Learned Optimism
Psychologist Martin Seligman proposed that people who continually experience

**dysfunctional families** Families in which there is violence; physical, emotional, or sexual abuse; significant parental discord; or other negative family interactions.

**social support** Network of people and services with whom you share ties and from whom you get support.

**spiritual health** Aspect of psychological health that relates to having a sense of meaning and purpose to one's life, as well as a feeling of connection with others and with nature.

**self-efficacy** Describes a person's belief about whether he or she can successfully engage in and execute a specific behavior.

**self-esteem** Refers to one's realistic sense of self-respect or self-worth.

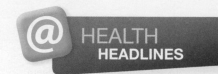
# OVERDOSING ON SELF-ESTEEM?

Fostering self-esteem in children has been seen as key to keeping them away from drugs and violence and to ensuring well-adjusted lives. However, there is a fine line between healthy self-esteem and vanity or narcissism, leading some to have an exaggerated self-image, a need for constant compliments, and a sense of feeling entitled to special treatment. A friend who posts selfies all day on Facebook or Snapchat so everyone knows what he's doing/eating/wearing may have crossed that line! Are all those posts on the edge of being narcissistic? How much is *too* much focus on self?

Dr. Jean Twenge, author of *Generation Me: Why Today's Young Americans are More Confident, Assertive, Entitled and More Miserable Than Ever*, discusses a study of over 16,000 college students who took the Narcissistic Personality Inventory between 1982 and 2006. Average scores for college students progressively increased over time—with the most recent students showing a 30 percent increase in narcissism over their peers from the early 1980s. The self-esteem generation's need for positive feedback is strong. Although the sample size was small, a University of Michigan study showed students reported liking and wanting moments that boost their self-esteem more than having sex, eating a favorite food, drinking, or nearly all other pleasurable events!

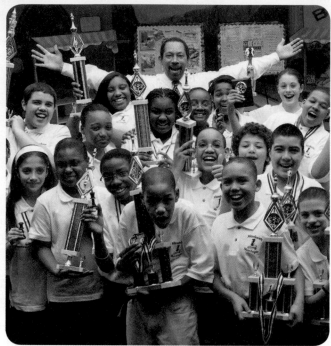

**Is too much self-esteem a bad thing?**

Call it the "gifted and talented effect" if you will, but it appears to have serious downsides. First, preliminary research indicates people who have been protected from failure and always told how special they are (perhaps by well-meaning parents and teachers) and who have extremely high levels of self-esteem might be more prone to anger, aggression, and other negative behaviors when others don't meet their gratification needs. Second, learning to lose may teach us valuable lessons. Carol Dweck, a psychology professor at Stanford University, found that after a steady diet of praise, kids collapsed at the first experience of difficulty. Failure can teach us to keep trying—and that just showing up is not enough to excel in college or the subsequent work world; in real life, there are no participation ribbons.

Psychologists continue to support the idea that self-esteem is important for positive growth and development. More research is needed to examine potential risks of too much self-esteem and the best ways to deal with it once it occurs.

**Sources:** Aspen Educational Group, "Narcissistic and Entitled to Everything—Does Gen Y Have Too Much Self-Esteem?," Accessed February 11, 2012, www.aspeneducation.com/article-entitlement.html; J. M. Twenge et al., "Egos Inflating Over Time: A Cross Temporal Meta-Analysis of the Narcissistic Personality Inventory," *Journal of Personality* 76, no. 4 (2008): 875–902; J. M. Twenge, *Generation Me: Why Today's Young Americans are More Confident, Assertive, Entitled and More Miserable Than Ever* (New York: Simon & Schuster, 2014); B. J. Bushman, S. J. Moeller, and J. Crocker, "Sweets, Sex, or Self-Esteem? Comparing the Value of Self-Esteem Boosts with Other Pleasant Rewards," *Journal of Personality* (2011), doi: 10.1111/j.1467-6494.2011.00712; M. Wei, K. Yu-Hsin Liao, T. Ku, and P. Shaffer, "Attachment, Self Compassion, Empathy, and Subjective Well-Being among College Students and Community Adults," *Journal of Personality* 79, no. 1 (2011): 191–221; A. Merryman, "Losing Is Good for You," *New York Times* (September 24, 2013), www.nytimes.com/2013/09/25/opinion/losing-is-good-for-you.html?_r=0

**learned helplessness** Pattern of responding to situations by giving up because of repeated failure in the past.

**learned optimism** Teaching oneself to think positively.

failure may develop a pattern of response known as **learned helplessness** in which they give up and fail to take action to help themselves.8 Seligman ascribes this response in part to society's tendency toward *victimology*—blaming one's problems on other people and circumstances. Although viewing ourselves as victims may make us feel better temporarily, it does not address the underlying causes of a problem. Ultimately, it can erode self-efficacy by making us feel that we cannot improve a situation.

Today, many self-help programs use elements of Seligman's principle of **learned optimism.** The idea is that we can teach ourselves to be optimistic. By changing our self-talk, examining our reactions, and blocking negative thoughts, we can "unlearn" habitual negative thought processes. Some programs practice positive affirmations with clients, teaching them the habit of acknowledging positive things about themselves.

# Emotional Intelligence

Intelligence has long been regarded as key to a successful career and healthy social life. It helps us understand the complex interaction of forces in our lives and respond in rational, reasonable ways. In the 1990's, two leading psychologists, Peter Salavey and John Mayer championed a more comprehensive view of intelligence, known as **emotional intelligence (EI)**.[9] Essentially, EI is our ability to identify, use, understand, and manage our own emotions as well as those of others. Reacting to and channeling those emotions in positive and constructive ways has been shown to improve well-being.[10] Your *emotional intelligence quotient (EQ)* is an indicator of social and interpersonal skills—your ability to successfully maneuver in sometimes emotionally charged settings. Emotional intelligence typically consists of the following:

- **Self-Awareness.** The ability to recognize your own emotions, moods, and reactions, as well as have an awareness of how others perceive or react to you.
- **Self-Regulation/Self-Management.** The ability to control your emotional impulses, think before responding, and express yourself appropriately.
- **Internal Motivation.** A drive for learning about things, being able to take initiative and follow through, as well as being trustworthy, stable, and consistent.
- **Empathy.** An awareness of what others might be going through, rather than being so engrossed in self that you are oblivious to others. Not being judgmental and rigid in thinking and reacting appropriately to others little "mental moments" is part of this element.
- **Social Skills.** Involves identifying social cues, learning to listen and respond appropriately, and knowing how to work with others for the common good and to avoid conflicts with others.

Proponents of EI suggest that developing or increasing your emotional intelligence can help you build stronger relationships, succeed at work, and achieve your goals.[11]

## Personality

Your personality is the unique mix of characteristics that distinguishes you from others. Heredity, environment, culture, and experience influence how each person develops. Personality determines how we react to the challenges of life, interpret our feelings, and resolve conflicts. A leading personality theory called the *five-factor model* distills personality into five traits, often called the "Big Five":[12]

- **Agreeableness.** People who score high are trusting, likable, and demonstrate friendly compliance and love, while low scorers are critical and suspicious.
- **Openness.** People who score high demonstrate curiosity, independence, and imagination, while low scorers are more conventional and down-to-earth.
- **Neuroticism.** People who score high in neuroticism are anxious and insecure, while those who score low show the ability to maintain emotional control.
- **Conscientiousness.** People who score high are dependable and demonstrate self-control, discipline, and a need to achieve, while low scorers are disorganized and impulsive.
- **Extroversion.** People who score high adapt well to social situations, demonstrate assertiveness, and draw enjoyment from the company of others, while low scorers are more reserved and passive.

Scores in each category are compared to those of others who have completed the tests. Scoring high on agreeableness, openness, conscientiousness, and extroversion, while scoring low on neuroticism, is often related to psychological well-being.

Most recent schools of psychological theory indicate that we have the power to understand our behavior and change it, thus molding our own personalities, even as an adult.[13] Although inhospitable social environments make it more difficult, there are opportunities for making changes and improving our long-term psychological well-being.

## Happiness and the Mind-Body Connection

Can negative emotions make us physically ill? Can positive emotions help us stay well? At the core of the mind-body connection is **psychoneuroimmunology (PNI),** the study of the interactions of behavioral, neural, and endocrine functions and the functioning of the body's immune system.

One area of study that appears to be particularly promising in enhancing both psychological and

> **emotional intelligence (EI)**
> A person's ability to identify, understand, use, and manage emotional states in positive and constructive ways.
>
> **psychoneuroimmunology (PNI)**
> The study of the interactions of behavioral, neural, and endocrine functions and the functioning of the body's immune system.

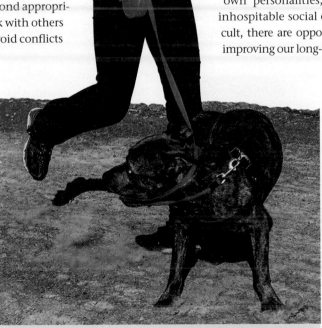

Spending time in the fresh air with your best friend is a simple thing you can do to improve psychological health.

**subjective well-being** An uplifting feeling of inner peace.

**mental illnesses** Disorders that disrupt thinking, feeling, moods, and behaviors and that impair daily functioning.

physical health is *happiness*—a collective term for several positive states in which individuals actively embrace the world around them.[14] Happiness appears to reduce the risk or limit the severity of cardiovascular disease, pulmonary disease, diabetes, hypertension, colds, and other infections, and even slow down the aging process.[15] Laughter can promote increases in heart and respiration rates and can reduce levels of stress hormones in much the same way light exercise can. For this reason, laughter has been promoted as a possible risk reducer for people with hypertension and other forms of cardiovascular disease.[16] Not all happiness is created equal though. New research indicates that happiness derived from doing kind deeds or working toward your life's purpose improves health more than happiness found in pleasure-seeking activities like watching TV.[17]

**Subjective well-being** is an overall "feel-good" state defined by three central components: *satisfaction with present life, relative presence of positive emotions,* and *relative absence of negative emotions.*[18] You do not have to be happy all the time to achieve overall subjective well-being. Everyone experiences disappointments, unhappiness, and times when life seems unfair. However, people with a high level of subjective well-being often demonstrate more *resiliency* in dealing with challenges. They can bounce back, stronger and wiser, having learned from their lessons.

Scientists suggest that people may be biologically predisposed to happiness and well-being. Numerous studies have examined the role of environment and genetics and concluded that each contributes to overall happiness and well-being. Since circumstances interact with genetic predisposition, it may be possible to influence happiness and well-being development.[19] Other psychologists, most notably Martin Seligman, suggest that we can develop well-being by practicing positive psychological actions. Seligman describes five elements of

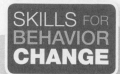

## SKILLS FOR BEHAVIOR CHANGE

### USING PERMA TO ENHANCE YOUR HAPPINESS

Implement the following strategies to enhance well-being and employ a more positive outlook:

**"P"—Positive Emotions**
▶ Consider what brings you the most happiness and engage in that behavior often.
▶ Be open to new experiences, be curious, and be kind.

**"E"—Engagement**
▶ Adopt mindfulness and appreciation for being in the present moment.
▶ Consider what activities completely absorb you and invest more time in those activities.

**"R"—Relationships**
▶ Open yourself to building new relationships and deepen existing ones.
▶ Offer others social support and accept support that is offered to you.

**"M"—Meaning**
▶ Consider, what is your legacy?
▶ Invest time in activities that bring you peace: pray, meditate, or care for others.

**"A"—Achievement**
▶ Set realistic goals and pursue them.
▶ If achievement equals skills plus effort; put forth the effort to build strong skills.

**Source:** Adapted from E. Terantin-O'Brien, IDEA Health and Fitness Association, "Applying the PERMA Model," June 2013, Available at: www.ideafit.com/fitness-library/applying-the-perma-model; M.Seligman, *Flourish: A Visionary New Understanding of Happiness and Well-Being* (New York: Free Press, 2011).

well-being (represented by the acronym PERMA) that help humans *flourish*.[20] The **Skills for Behavior Change** provides some suggestions for ways to incorporate these five principles into your own life.

## LO 3 | WHEN PSYCHOLOGICAL HEALTH DETERIORATES

Describe and differentiate psychological disorders, including mood disorders, anxiety disorders, obsessive-compulsive disorder, post-traumatic stress disorder, personality disorders, and schizophrenia, and explain their causes and treatments.

**Mental illnesses** are disorders that disrupt thinking, feeling, moods, and behaviors and cause varying degrees of impaired functioning in daily living. They are believed to be caused by a variety of biochemical, genetic, and environmental

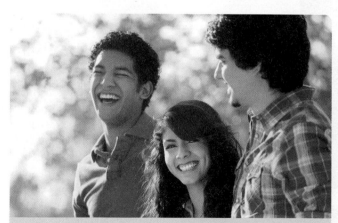

Research suggests that laughter can increase blood flow, boost the immune response, lower blood sugar levels, and facilitate better sleep. Additionally, sharing laughter and fun with others can strengthen social ties and bring joy to your everyday life.

# 22.5

PERCENT OF AMERICANS OVER THE AGE OF 18 HAVE ONE OR MORE DIAGNOSABLE **MENTAL DISORDERS**.

factors.[21] Among the most common risk factors are a genetic or familial predisposition and excessive, unresolved stress, particularly due to trauma or war or devastating natural or human-caused disaster. Changes in biochemistry due to illness, drug use, or other imbalances may trigger unusual mental disturbances. Car accidents or occupational injuries that cause physical brain trauma are among common threats to brain health. In addition, a mother's exposure to viruses or toxic chemicals while pregnant may play a part, as can having a history of child abuse or neglect.[22] Mental illnesses can range from mild to severe and can exact a heavy toll on quality of life, both for people with the illnesses and for those who interact with them.

Mental disorders are common in the United States and worldwide. The basis for diagnosing mental disorders in the United States is the *Diagnostic and Statistical Manual of Mental Disorders,* Fifth Edition (*DSM-5*). An estimated 22.5 percent of Americans aged 18 and older—just over 1 in 5 adults—suffer from one or more mental disorders in a given year.[23] About 5 percent, or 1 in 20, suffer from a serious mental illness requiring close monitoring, residential care in many instances, and medication.[24] Mental disorders are the leading cause of disability in the United States, costing more than $440 billion in direct medical care and indirect costs, such as lost productivity.[25] People with serious mental illness are often affected in the prime of life and die, on average, up to 23 years sooner than other Americans.[26] Increasing numbers of the most seriously ill find employment difficult due to mental illness stigma, receive disability payments for decades, or need caregiver support, resulting in lifelong financial support. With a lack of public prevention, early treatment, and support options, increasing numbers of the mentally ill end up on the streets of our cities or in prisons.

## Mental Health Threats to College Students

Mental health problems among college students are growing in both number and severity.[27] In the most recent National College Health Assessment survey, approximately 1 in 3 undergraduates reported "feeling so depressed it was difficult to function" at least once in the past year, and over 8 percent of students reported "seriously considering attempting suicide" in the past year.[28] More than 1 in 4 college students experience a mental health issue each year; *anxiety* is most common (41.6 percent), with *depression* (35 percent) and *relationship problems* (35.8 percent) following not far behind.[29] Although these data may appear alarming, it is important to note that increases in help-seeking behavior and wider availability of campus services, in addition to actual increases in overall prevalence of disorders, may contribute to these trends. Still, significant numbers of troubled students never seek help due to worries about stigma. It is estimated that 60 percent of adults and almost half of youth aged 8–15 with mental illnesses received no mental health services in the last year.[30] **FIGURE 2.4** shows the mental health concerns reported by American college students.

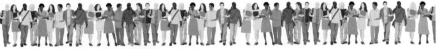

**Felt overwhelmed by all they needed to do: 86.4%**

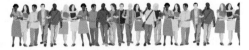

**Felt things were hopeless: 46.4%**

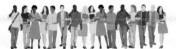

**Felt so depressed that it was difficult to function: 32.6%**

**Seriously considered suicide: 8.1%**

**Intentionally injured themselves: 6.4%**

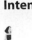

 = 2%

**Attempted suicide: 1.3%**

**FIGURE 2.4**   Mental Health Concerns of American College Students, Past 12 Months

**Source:** Data from American College Health Association, *American College Health Association, National College Health Assessment II (ACHA-NCHA II): Reference Group Data Report, Spring 2014* (Hanover, MD: American College Health Association, 2014).

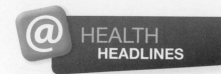

# WHEN ADULTS HAVE ADHD

Attention-deficit/hyperactivity disorder (ADHD) is often associated with school-aged children, and over 6.4 percent of children have it; however, it isn't just a childhood disease. For many people, symptoms persist into adulthood. About 4 percent of the adult population, or slightly over 12 million adults, are living with ADHD.

People with ADHD are distracted much of the time. Even when they try to concentrate, they find it hard to pay attention. Organizing things, listening to instructions, and remembering details are especially difficult.

## Effects of Adult ADHD

Left untreated, ADHD can disrupt everything from careers to relationships to financial stability. Key areas of disruption might include the following:

- **Health.** Impulsivity and trouble with organization can lead to health problems, such as compulsive eating, alcohol and drug abuse, or forgetting to take medication for a chronic condition.
- **Work and finances.** Difficulty concentrating, completing tasks, listening, and relating to others can lead to trouble at work and school. Managing finances may also be a concern because a person with ADHD may

struggle to pay bills on time, lose paperwork, miss deadlines, or spend impulsively, resulting in debt.

- **Relationships.** If you have ADHD, you might wonder why loved ones constantly nag you to tidy up, get organized, and take care of business. If your romantic partner has ADHD, you might be hurt that your loved one doesn't seem to listen to you, blurts out hurtful things, and leaves you with the bulk of organizing and planning.

## Get Educated about ADHD

If you suspect you or someone close to you has ADHD, learn as much as you can about adult ADHD and treatment options. The organization Children and Adults with attention-deficit/hyperactivity disorder (CHADD) is a good source of information and support (www.chadd.org). Adult ADHD can be a challenge to diagnose; there is no simple test for it, and it often occurs concurrently with other conditions, such as depression or anxiety. To ensure that you have the best treatment, secure a diagnosis and treatment plan from a qualified professional with experience in ADHD. ADHD can be treated, and getting the needed help can improve health, relationships, finances, and grades.

Disorder and chaos can be headaches for us all, but ADHD sufferers may find them insurmountable obstacles.

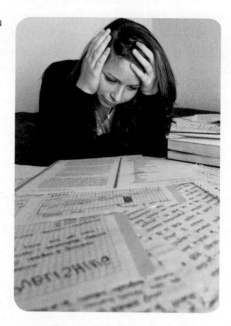

**Sources:** Centers for Disease Control and Prevention, "Attention-Deficit Hyperactivity Disorder," Updated February 2015; www.cdc.gov/ncbddd /adhd/facts.html; Healthline, "ADHD by the Numbers: Facts, Statistics, and You," September 2014, www.healthline.com/health/adhd/facts-statistics -infographic#1; Helpguide.org, "Adult ADD/ADHD: Signs, Symptoms, Effects, and Treatment," December 2014, www.helpguide.org/articles/add-adhd /adult-adhd-attention-deficit-disorder.

---

**chronic mood disorder** Experience of persistent emotional states, such as sadness, despair, hopelessness, or euphoria.

**major depression** Severe depressive disorder with physical effects such as sleep disturbance and exhaustion, and mental effects such as the inability to concentrate; also called *clinical depression*.

Although there are many types of mental illnesses, we will focus on those disorders most common among young adults, particularly college students: mood disorders, obsessive-compulsive disorder (OCD), post-traumatic stress disorder (PTSD), personality disorders, and schizophrenia. See the **Health Headlines** box for information on attention-deficit/hyperactivity disorder. (For coverage of addiction, which is classified as a mental disorder, see **Chapter 7: Recognizing and Avoiding Addiction and Drug Abuse** beginning on page 203.)

## Mood Disorders

**Chronic mood disorders** affect how you feel, such as persistent sadness or feelings of euphoria. Key examples include major depression, persistent depressive disorder, bipolar

disorder, and seasonal affective disorder. In any given year, approximately 7.4 percent of Americans aged 18 or older suffer from a mood disorder.[31]

**Major Depression** We've all had days when life's challenges push us over the proverbial edge, but short periods of feeling down are not the same as major depression. **Major depression** or *clinical depression* is the most common mood disorder, affecting approximately 6.3 percent of the U.S. population in a given year.[32]

Major depression is characterized by a combination of symptoms that interfere with work, study, sleep, appetite, relationships, and enjoyment of life. Symptoms can last for weeks, months, or years and vary in intensity.[33] Sadness and despair are the main symptoms of depression.[34] Other common signs include:

- Preoccupation with failures/inadequacies; concern over what others are thinking
- Difficulty concentrating, indecisiveness, memory lapses

- Loss of sex drive or interest in being close to others
- Fatigue, oversleeping, insomnia, and loss of energy
- Feeling anxious, worthless, or hopeless
- Withdrawal or isolation
- Significant weight loss or gain due to appetite changes
- Recurring thoughts that life isn't worth living; thoughts of death or suicide

Mental health problems, particularly depression, have gained increased recognition as obstacles to healthy adjustment and success in college. Students who have weak communication skills, who find that college isn't what they expected, or who lack motivation, often have difficulties. Stressors such as anxiety over relationships, pressure to get good grades and win social acceptance, abuse of alcohol and other drugs, poor diet, and lack of sleep can overwhelm even the most resilient students. Being far from home without the security of family and friends can exacerbate problems. International students are particularly vulnerable. In a recent survey by the American College Health Association, 12 percent of college students reported having been diagnosed with or treated for depression in the past 12 months.[35]

Depression in men is often masked by alcohol or drug abuse or by the socially acceptable habit of working excessively long hours. Typically, depressed men present less as hopeless and helpless and more as irritable, angry, and discouraged—often personifying a "tough guy" image.[36] Men are less likely to admit they are depressed, and doctors are less likely to suspect it, based on what men report during doctor's visits. Although depression is associated with an increased risk of coronary heart disease in both men and women, it is associated with a higher risk of death in women, particularly women under the age of 55.[37]

In fact, women are more than twice as likely as men to experience depression.[38] A combination of biological, genetic, psychosocial, and environmental factors are all possibly at play. Social and cultural roles that limit choice can lead to role overload as women try to juggle family, career, child-rearing and parent care, as well as managing home and hearth.[39] Newer research indicates that women may also ruminate more over negative life events and have a harder time letting things go than do men. Dwelling on negative events may lead to depression.[40]

## Persistent Depressive Disorder
**Persistent depressive disorder (PDD)**, formerly called *dysthymic disorder* or *dysthymia*, is a less severe form of chronic mild depression. Individuals with PDD may appear to function well, but may lack energy or fatigue easily; may be short-tempered, overly pessimistic, and ornery; or may not feel quite up to par, without

## WHY SHOULD I CARE?

Increases in mental health problems on campuses throughout the country have raised concerns among campus leaders and counseling centers. Mental health problems can affect every aspect of your life, including relationships, academics, career potential, and overall well-being. Stigma over mental illnesses keep many from reaching out for help. Knowing the signs and symptoms of someone who is struggling (including you) and where to go for help is key to avoiding serious problems.

any significant, overt symptoms. Genetics and a history of abuse, neglect, or trauma, as well as high stress levels are among suspected causes. People with PDD may cycle into major depression over time. For a diagnosis, symptoms must persist for at least 2 years in adults (1 year in children). This disorder affects approximately 2.5 percent of the adult population in the United States in a given year.[41] Treatment often includes selected antidepressants and highly structured psychotherapy.

## Seasonal Affective Disorder
*Seasonal depression*, typically referred to as **seasonal affective disorder (SAD)**, strikes during the fall and winter months and is associated with reduced exposure to sunlight. People with SAD suffer from extreme fatigue, irritability, apathy, carbohydrate craving and weight gain, increased sleep time, and general sadness. Several factors are implicated in SAD development, including disruption in the body's natural circadian rhythms and changes in levels of the hormone melatonin and the brain chemical serotonin.[42] Over 500,000 people in the United States suffer from SAD. Nearly three fourths of those with SAD are women in early adulthood, particularly those living at high latitudes with long winter nights.[43]

The most beneficial treatment for SAD is light therapy, which exposes patients to lamps that simulate sunlight. Other treatments include diet change (such as eating more complex carbohydrates), increased exercise, stress-management techniques, sleep restriction (limiting the number of hours slept in a 24-hour period), psychotherapy, and prescription medications.

## Bipolar Disorder
People with **bipolar disorder** (formerly called *manic depression*) often have severe mood swings, ranging from extreme highs (mania) to extreme lows (depression). Sometimes these swings are dramatic and rapid; other times they are slow and gradual. When manic, people may be overactive, talkative, and filled with energy; when depressed, they may experience some or all of the symptoms of major depression. Bipolar disorder affects approximately 2.6 percent of the adult population and 11.2 percent of 13- to 18-year-olds in the United States.[44]

Although the cause of bipolar disorder is unknown, a family history is the most likely risk,

**persistent depressive disorder** (formerly *dysthymic disorder*) Type of depression that is milder and harder to recognize than major depression; chronic; and often characterized by fatigue, pessimism, or a short temper.

**seasonal affective disorder (SAD)** Type of depression that occurs in the winter months, when sunlight levels are low.

**bipolar disorder** Form of mood disorder characterized by alternating mania and depression; also called *manic depression*.

particularly among primary relatives (parents or siblings). Environmental factors such as drug abuse, high stress, and trauma also appear to be triggers. A range of medications is used to treat bipolar disorder, depending on symptoms. Individual and family therapy are often combined with medications.[45]

## What Causes Mood Disorders?
Because mood disorders are believed to be caused by the interaction of environmental, psychological, biological, and genetic factors, an exact cause for each type is difficult to pinpoint.[46] The most promising theory of causation involves *neurotransmitters,* chemicals in the brain that cause an imbalance and lead to depression, for example; however, this theory is far from proven. Bipolar disorder is believed to have a heredity component, yet a gene for it has not been isolated. New imaging techniques show distinctly different brain activity between those with depression or bipolar disorder compared to individuals with no mood disorders.[47] Whether these differences are the result of genetic, environmental, or other brain issues remains in question.

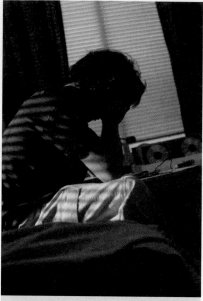

There is more to depression than simply feeling blue. When a person is clinically depressed, he or she finds it difficult to function, sometimes struggling just to get out of bed in the morning or to follow a conversation.

# Anxiety Disorders

**Anxiety disorders** are characterized by persistent feelings of threat and worry and include generalized anxiety disorder, panic disorders, and phobic disorders. The largest mental health problem in the United States, anxiety disorders affect more than 40 million people in any given year. Anxiety disorders are most prevalent among 13- to 17-year-olds, with a median age of onset of 6 years.[48] Over 14 percent of U.S. undergraduates report being diagnosed with or treated for anxiety in the past year.[49]

**anxiety disorders** Mental illness characterized by persistent feelings of threat and worry in coping with everyday problems.

**generalized anxiety disorder (GAD)** A constant sense of worry that may cause restlessness, difficulty in concentrating, tension, and other symptoms.

**panic attack** Severe anxiety reaction in which a particular situation, often for unknown reasons, causes terror.

**phobia** Deep and persistent fear of a specific object, activity, or situation that results in a compelling desire to avoid the source of the fear.

**social anxiety disorder** Phobia characterized by fear and avoidance of social situations; also called *social phobia.*

## Generalized Anxiety Disorder
One common form of anxiety disorder, **generalized anxiety disorder (GAD)**, is severe enough to interfere significantly with daily life. To be diagnosed with GAD, one must exhibit at least three of the following symptoms for more days than not during a 6-month period: restlessness or feeling keyed up or on edge, being easily fatigued, difficulty concentrating or mind going blank, irritability, muscle tension, and/or sleep disturbances.[50]

## Panic Disorder
Panic disorder is characterized by the occurrence of **panic attacks,** an acute feeling of anxiety causing an intense physical reaction. Approximately 6.7 percent of college students report being diagnosed or treated for panic attacks in the last year.[51] Panic attacks and disorders are increasing in incidence, particularly among young women.

Although highly treatable, panic attacks may become debilitating and destructive, particularly if they happen often or cause a person to avoid going out in public or interacting with others. Panic attacks typically begin abruptly, peak within 10 minutes, last about 30 minutes, and leave the person tired and drained.[52] Symptoms include increased respiration, chills, hot flashes, shortness of breath, stomach cramps, chest pain, difficulty swallowing, and a sense of doom or impending death.

## Phobic Disorders
Phobias, or phobic disorders, involve a persistent and irrational fear of a specific object, activity, or situation, often out of proportion to the circumstances. Between 5 and 12 percent of American adults suffer from specific phobias, such as fear of spiders, snakes, or riding in elevators.[53])

Another 7.4 percent of American adults suffer from **social anxiety disorder,** also called *social phobia.*[54] Social anxiety disorder is characterized by a persistent fear and avoidance of

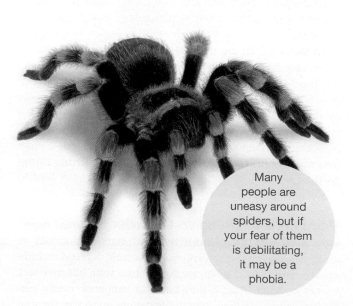

Many people are uneasy around spiders, but if your fear of them is debilitating, it may be a phobia.

social situations. Essentially, a person with social anxiety disorder dreads these situations for fear of being humiliated, embarrassed, or even looked at. These disorders vary in scope. Some individuals experience difficulties only in specific situations, such as getting up in front of the class to give a presentation. In extreme cases, a person avoids all contact with others.

### What Causes Anxiety Disorders?

Because anxiety disorders vary in complexity and degree, it is not yet clear why one person develops them and another doesn't. The following factors are often cited as possible causes:[55]

- **Biology.** Some scientists trace the origin of anxiety to the brain and its functioning. Using sophisticated positron-emission tomography (PET) scans, scientists can analyze areas of the brain that react during anxiety-producing events. Families appear to display similar brain and physiological reactivity, so we may inherit tendencies toward anxiety disorders.
- **Environment.** Anxiety can be a learned response. Experiencing a repeated pattern of reaction to certain situations can program the brain to respond in a certain way. For example, if one of your siblings had a huge fear of spiders and screamed whenever one crawled into sight during your childhood, you might develop similar anxieties.
- **Social and cultural roles.** Because men and women are taught to assume different roles, women may find it more acceptable to scream, tremble, or otherwise express extreme anxiety. Men, in contrast, may have learned to repress anxious feelings rather than act on them.

In general, anxiety disorders are highly treatable. While treatment should be tailored to the specific nature and severity of an individual's anxiety, it typically includes antianxiety medications in combination with psychotherapy. Length of treatment varies based on history and the presence of other mental disorders.

## Obsessive-Compulsive Disorder

People who feel compelled to perform rituals over and over again; who are fearful of dirt or contamination; who have an unnatural concern about order, symmetry, and exactness; or who have persistent intrusive thoughts may be suffering from **obsessive-compulsive disorder (OCD)**. Approximately 1 percent of Americans aged 18 and over have OCD.[56]

Not to be confused with being a perfectionist, a people with OCD often know their behaviors are irrational, yet are powerless to stop them. According to the *DSM-5,* OCD diagnosis requires obsessions to consume more than 1 hour per day and interfere with normal social or life activities. Although the exact cause is unknown, genetics, biological abnormalities, learned behaviors, and environmental factors have all been

considered. Obsessive-compulsive disorder usually begins in childhood or the teen years; most people are diagnosed before age 20.[57]

Although highly treatable, only one third of individuals with OCD receive treatment. Treatments vary by disorder type, severity, and other factors. The most effective treatments tend to be a combination of psychotherapy and medications designed to treat symptoms, such as antidepressants or antianxiety medication.[58]

## Post-Traumatic Stress Disorder

People who have experienced or witnessed a traumatic event may develop **post-traumatic stress disorder (PTSD)**. While only about 4 percent of Americans suffer from PTSD each year, about 8 percent will experience PTSD in their lifetimes, with women experiencing rates twice as high as men.[59] Fourteen percent of U.S. combat veterans who fought in Iraq and Afghanistan have experienced PTSD.[60] However, the "worst stressful experiences" reported most frequently by those with PTSD are not war-related, but rather the unexpected death, serious illness, or injury of someone close, and sexual assault. PTSD in women appears related to a history of abuse, rape, or assault. Natural disasters, serious accidents, violent assault, and terrorism are all causes of PTSD in both men and women.[61] PTSD is not rooted in weakness or an inability to cope; traumatic events

> **obsessive-compulsive disorder (OCD)** Form of anxiety disorder characterized by recurrent, unwanted thoughts and repetitive behaviors.
>
> **post-traumatic stress disorder (PTSD)** Collection of symptoms that may occur as a delayed response to a traumatic event or series of events.

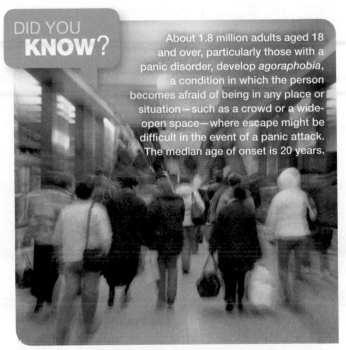

**DID YOU KNOW?**

About 1.8 million adults aged 18 and over, particularly those with a panic disorder, develop *agoraphobia*, a condition in which the person becomes afraid of being in any place or situation—such as a crowd or a wide-open space—where escape might be difficult in the event of a panic attack. The median age of onset is 20 years.

**Sources:** NIMH. "The Numbers Count: Mental Disorders in America-Social Phobias-Agoraphobia. October 1, 2013, www.lb7.uscourts.gov/documents/12-cv-1072url2.pdf

can actually cause chemical changes in the brain, leading to PTSD.[62]

Symptoms of PTSD include:

- Dissociation, or perceived detachment of the mind from the emotional state or even the body
- Intrusive recollections of the traumatic event, such as flashbacks, nightmares, and recurrent thoughts or images
- Acute anxiety or nervousness, in which the person is hyperaroused, may cry easily, or experiences mood swings
- Insomnia and difficulty concentrating
- Intense physiological reactions, such as shaking or nausea, when something reminds the person of the traumatic event

PTSD may be diagnosed if a person experiences symptoms for at least 1 month following a traumatic event. However, in some cases, symptoms don't appear until months or even years later.

Treatment for PTSD may involve psychotherapy, as well as medications to help with depression, anxiety, and sleep. Group and talk therapy is also often recommended, depending on the nature and severity of PTSD.

## Personality Disorders

**Personality disorders** are psychiatric disorders characterized by distinctive sets of traits, behaviors, and patterns that are rigid, different from cultural or social expectations, and lead to difficulties in perceiving and relating to situations and other people. Often individuals with personality disorders feel their behavior is normal and that others are to be blamed for problems in their world.[63] It is estimated that at least 10 percent of adults in the United States have some form of personality disorder.[64] People who live, work, or are in relationships with individuals suffering from personality disorders often find interactions with them to be challenging and destructive.

One common type of personality disorder is *paranoid personality disorder,* involving pervasive, unfounded suspicion and mistrust of other people, irrational jealousy, and secretiveness. Persons with this illness have delusions of being persecuted by everyone, from family members and loved ones to the government.

*Narcissistic personality disorders* involve an exaggerated sense of self-importance and self-absorption. Typically, persons with narcissistic personalities are overly needy and demanding, believing they are "entitled" to nothing but the best. Many worry about an increase in this disorder among younger generations of Americans today.[65]

Persons with *antisocial personality disorders* display a long-term pattern of manipulation and taking advantage of others, often in a criminal manner. Symptoms include disregard for the safety of others and lack of remorse, arrogance, and anger.

*Borderline personality disorder (BPD)* is characterized by severe emotional instability, mood swings, impulsiveness, and poor self-image[66] High suicide rates, unpredictable mood swings, and erratic and risky behaviors, including gambling, unsafe sex, illicit drug use, daredevil driving, and self-mutilation, are typical.[67] (For more about self-mutilation, see **Student Health Today**). Although causation is not clear, genetics and environment appear to converge to increase risks. About 2 million Americans have BPD, with the highest rates in adults aged 18–35.[68]

For treating personality disorders, individual and group psychotherapy, skill development, family education, support from peers, and medications can lead to a good long-term prognosis.[69]

## Schizophrenia

**Schizophrenia** is a severe psychological disorder that affects about 1 percent of the U.S. population.[70] Schizophrenia is characterized by alterations of the senses; the inability to sort and process incoming stimuli and make appropriate responses; an altered sense of self; and radical changes in emotions, movements, and behaviors. Typical symptoms of schizophrenia include fluctuating courses of delusional behavior, hallucinations, incoherent and rambling speech, inability to think logically, erratic movement, odd gesturing, and difficulty with activities of daily living.[71] Symptoms usually appear in men during the late teen years and twenties, while women generally present symptoms in their late twenties and early thirties.[72] Often regarded as odd or dangerous, schizophrenic individuals can have difficulties in social interactions and may withdraw.

For decades, scientists believed that schizophrenia was a form of madness provoked by the environment in which a child lived. In the mid-1980s, magnetic resonance imaging (MRI) and PET scans began allowing scientists to study brain function more closely; based on that knowledge, schizophrenia was found to be a biological disease of the brain. The brain damage occurs early in life, possibly as early as the second trimester of fetal development. Fetal exposure to toxic substances, infections, and medications have been studied as a possible risk, and hereditary links are being explored.

Even though theories that blame abnormal family life or childhood trauma for schizophrenia have been discarded in favor of biological theories, a stigma remains attached to the disease. Families of people with schizophrenia frequently experience anger and guilt. They often need information, family counseling, and advice on how to meet the schizophrenic person's needs for shelter, medical care, vocational training, and social interaction.

At present, schizophrenia is treatable but not curable. Treatments usually include some combination of hospitalization, medication, and psychotherapy. With proper medication, public understanding, support of loved ones, and access to therapy, many schizophrenics lead normal lives.

**personality disorder** Mental disorder characterized by inflexible patterns of thought and beliefs that lead to socially distressing behavior.

**schizophrenia** Mental illness with biological origins characterized by irrational behavior, severe alterations of the senses, and often an inability to function in society.

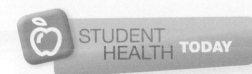

## STUDENT HEALTH TODAY — CUTTING THROUGH THE PAIN

Self-injury, also termed self-mutilation, self-harm, or nonsuicidal self-injury (NSSI), is the act of deliberately harming one's body in an attempt to cope with overwhelming negative emotions. Self-injury is an attempt at coping; it is not an attempt at suicide.

The most common method of self-harm is cutting (with razors, glass, knives, or other sharp objects). Other methods include burning, bruising, excessive nail biting, breaking bones, pulling out hair, and embedding sharp objects under the skin.

NSSI appears to be on the increase, with 17.2 percent of adolescents, 13.4 percent of young adults, and 5.5 percent of adults engaging in this behavior according to a recent study. Reports on prevalence of NSSI in college students vary, ranging from 7 percent to 15 percent. Many people who harm themselves suffer from other mental health conditions and have experienced sexual, physical, or emotional abuse as children or adults. Self-harm is also commonly associated with mental illnesses such as borderline personality disorder, depression, anxiety disorders, substance abuse disorders, post-traumatic stress disorder, and eating disorders.

Signs of self-injury include multiple scars, current cuts and abrasions, and implausible explanations for wounds and ongoing injuries. A self-injurer may attempt to conceal scars and injuries by wearing long sleeves and pants. Other symptoms can include difficulty handling anger, social withdrawal, sensitivity to rejection, or body alienation. If you or someone you know is engaging in self-injury, seek professional help. Treatment involves psychotherapy, group counseling/support, and in some cases, medication. Treatment success is often a challenge as the self-injurer must stop the behavior and learn to recognize and manage the feelings that triggered it.

If you are a recovering self-injurer, some of the following steps may be part of your treatment:

1. Start by being aware of feelings and situations that trigger your urge to hurt yourself.
2. Identify a plan of what you can do instead when you feel the urge, including alternative behaviors.

For more information, visit these resources: S.A.F.E. Alternatives, **www.selfinjury.com,** and Help Guide, **www.helpguide.org /mental/self_injury.htm**

**Sources:** American College Health Association, *ACHA–NCHA II: Reference Group Data Report, Spring 2014* (Hanover, MD: American College Health Association, 2014); M. J. Sornberger et al., "Nonsuicidal Self-Injury and Gender: Patterns of Prevalence, Methods, and Locations among Adolescents," *Suicide and Life-Threatening Behavior* 42, no. 3 (2012): 266–78; J. Whitlock et al., "Nonsuicidal Self-Injury in a College Population: General Trends and Sex Differences," *Journal of American College Health* 59, no. 8 (2011): 691–98; M. Smith and J. Segal, HelpGuide.org, "Cutting and Self-Harm," updated February 2014, www.helpguide .org/mental/self_injury.htm; S. Swannell, et al. "Prevalence of nonsuicidal self-injury in nonclinical samples: Systematic review, meta-analysis and meta-regression." *Suicide Life Threat Behavior* 44, no. 3 (2014): 272–303. doi: 10.1111/Sltb. 12070

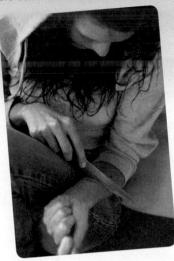

In self-injury, cutting and scratching behaviors are more common in females, while burning and hitting behaviors are more common in males.

---

## LO 4 | SUICIDE: GIVING UP ON LIFE

Discuss risk factors and possible warning signs of suicide, as well as actions that can be taken to help a person contemplating suicide.

*"Every 40 seconds a person dies of suicide somewhere in the world . . . another 20 or so more attempt suicide."* These grim statistics and others from the World Health Association's 2014 report highlight the growing international toll of suicide.[73] Each year, over 805,000 deaths are reported internationally. The young, aged 15–29, are particularly vulnerable, with suicide being the second leading cause of death in this group internationally.[74] In some of the richest countries, more than 300 percent as many men die of suicide as women. However, in low- and middle-income countries, the male-to-female suicide ratio is only 1.5 men to every woman. Globally, suicides make up 50 percent of all violent deaths for men and over 71 percent for women. The highest rates of suicide are among individuals aged 70 years and older.[75]

In the United States, older American suicide rates are comparable to overall international rates. Suicide is the third leading cause of death for 15- to 19-year-olds and the second leading cause of death for 19- to 24-year-olds.[76] The pressures, disappointments, challenges, and changes of the college years may contribute to the emotional turmoil that can lead a young person to contemplate suicide. However, young adults who do not attend college are also at risk; in fact, suicide rates for young adults are higher in the general population than among college students.[77]

### Overall Suicide Risks

Risk factors include a family history of suicide, previous suicide attempts, excessive drug and alcohol use, prolonged depression, financial difficulties, serious illness in oneself or a loved one, and loss of a loved one through death or rejection.[78] Recent research indicates that LGBT people are significantly more likely to have thought about or attempted suicide than their heterosexual counterparts, with transgender individuals having the highest rates.[79] Those raised in home and school environments where homophobic teasing is not condoned had significantly lower rates of suicide attempts, whereas those from low-income homes with less than high school education and with the presence of substance abuse had significantly more suicide attempts.[80]

Whether more likely to attempt suicide or more often successful, nearly four times as many men die by suicide as women.[81] Firearms, suffocation, and poison are the most common methods. Males are almost twice as likely as females to commit suicide with firearms, whereas younger females (age 10 to 24 years) are more likely to commit suicide by suffocation and older females (25 years and older) are more likely to commit suicide by poisoning.[82]

## Warning Signs of Suicide

People who commit suicide usually indicate their intentions, although others do not always recognize their warnings.[83] Anyone who expresses a desire to kill himself or herself or who has made an attempt is at risk. Common signs a person may be contemplating suicide include:[84]

- Recent loss and a seeming inability to let go of grief
- History of depression
- Change in personality, such as sadness, withdrawal, irritability, anxiety, tiredness, indecisiveness, apathy
- Change in behavior, such as inability to concentrate, loss of interest in classes or work, unexplained demonstration of happiness following a period of depression, or risk-taking behavior
- Change in sexual interest
- Change in sleep patterns and/or eating habits
- A direct statement (including statements posted on social media) about committing suicide, such as "I might as well end it all"
- An indirect statement (including statements posted on social media), such as "You won't have to worry about me anymore"
- Final preparations such as writing a will, giving away prized possessions, or writing revealing letters or social media posts
- Preoccupation with themes of death
- Marked changes in personal appearance

## Preventing Suicide

Most people who attempt suicide really want to live but see death as the only way out of an intolerable situation. Crisis counselors and suicide hotlines may help temporarily, but the best way to prevent suicide is to get rid of conditions and substances that may precipitate attempts, including alcohol, drugs, loneliness, isolation, and access to guns.

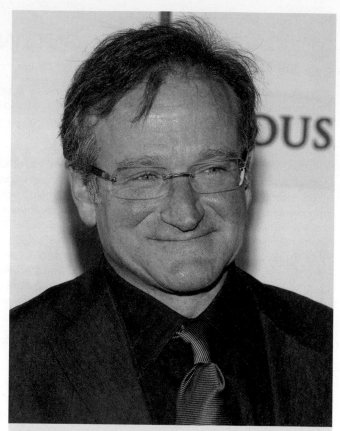

Suicide symptoms are not always obvious. Even "funny, life of the party" people may be struggling inwardly. It was only after his suicide in August 2014 that Robin Williams's struggles with severe depression became widely known.

If someone you know threatens suicide or displays warning signs, get involved—ask questions and seek help. Specific actions you can take include:[85]

- **Monitor the warning signals.** Keep an eye on the person or see that someone else is present. Don't leave the person alone.
- **Take threats seriously.** Don't brush them off as "cries for attention." Act now.
- **Let the person know how much you care.** State that you are there to help. Listen to them. Let them know help is available.
- **Ask directly.** Ask "Are you thinking of hurting or killing yourself?" Don't be judgmental. Let them share their thoughts.
- **Take action.** Remove any firearms or objects that could be used for suicide from the area.
- **Help the person think about alternatives to suicide.** Offer to go for help along with the person. Call your local suicide hotline, and use all available community and campus resources.
- **Tell the person's spouse, partner, parents, siblings, or counselor.** Do not keep suspicions to yourself. Don't let a suicidal friend talk you into keeping your discussions confidential. If your friend succeeds in a suicide attempt, you may blame yourself.

## LO 5 | SEEKING PROFESSIONAL HELP

Explain the different types of treatment options and professional services available to those experiencing mental health problems.

A physical ailment will readily send most of us to the nearest health professional, but many view seeking help for psychological problems as an admission of personal failure. Although estimates show that 20 percent of adults have some kind of mental disorder, only 6 to 7 percent of adults use mental health counseling services.[86] In fact, 40 percent of adults with severe mental illness such as schizophrenia or bipolar disorder received no treatment in the past year.[87]

Consider seeking help if:

- You feel out of control.
- You experience wild mood swings or inappropriate emotional responses to normal stimuli.
- Your fears or feelings of guilt frequently distract your attention.
- You begin to withdraw from others.
- You have hallucinations.
- You feel inadequate or worthless or that life is not worth living.
- Your daily life seems to be a series of repeated crises.
- You are considering suicide.
- You turn to drugs or alcohol to escape your problems.

Low-cost or free counseling sessions or support groups are often available on college campuses to help students deal with all types of issues, including mental illness. Investigate options on your campus.

## Mental Illness Stigma

**Stigmas** are negative perceptions about groups of people or certain situations or conditions. Common stigmas about people with mental illness are that they are dangerous, irresponsible, require constant care, or that they "just need to get over it." In truth, only 3 to 5 percent of all violent acts are attributed to people with serious mental illness. It is no more likely for most people with mental health problems to be violent than it is for anyone else, even though the mentally ill are ten times more likely to become victims of violence. Most hold regular jobs, are productive members of society, and lead normal lives.[88]

# 1 IN 3

COLLEGE STUDENTS WITH A MENTAL ILLNESS IDENTIFY **STIGMA** AS THE BIGGEST BARRIER TO RECEIVING TREATMENT.

The stigma of mental illness often leads to feelings of shame, guilt, loss of self-esteem, and a sense of isolation and hopelessness. Many who have successfully managed their mental illness report that the stigma was more disabling at times than the illness itself.[89] Stigma may cause people who are struggling with a mental illness to hide their difficulties from friends, delay seeking treatment, or avoid care that could dramatically improve their symptoms and quality of life.

**WHAT DO YOU THINK?**

Do you notice a stigma associated with mental illness in your community?

- How often do you hear terms like "crazy" or "whacko" used to describe people who appear to have a mental health problem, or a situation in general? Why are such expressions harmful to others?
- Why do so many people hide their mental illnesses and/ or refuse to seek treatment? What can be done to reduce one's fear of mental illness disclosure?

## Getting Evaluated for Treatment

If you are considering treatment, schedule a complete evaluation first. Consult a credentialed health professional for a thorough examination, including:

1. A physical checkup, which will rule out thyroid disorders, viral infections, and anemia—all of which can result in depression-like symptoms—and a neurological check of coordination, reflexes, and balance to rule out brain disorders.
2. A psychiatric history, which will trace the course of the apparent disorder, genetic or family factors, and any past treatments.

> **stigma** Negative perception about a group of people or a certain situation or condition.

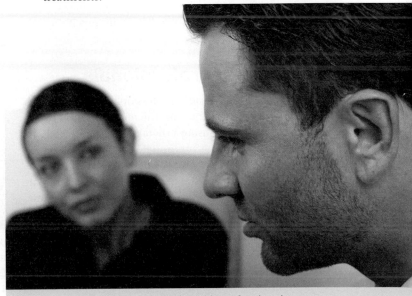

When you begin seeing a mental health professional, you enter into a relationship with that person, and just as with any person, you will connect better with some therapists than others. If one doesn't "feel right," trust your instincts and look for someone else.

## TABLE 2.1 | Mental Health Professionals

| What Are They Called? | What Kind of Training Do They Have? | What Kind of Therapy Do They Do? | Professional Association |
|---|---|---|---|
| Psychiatrist | Medical doctor degree (MD), followed by 4 years of mental health training | Can prescribe medications and may have admitting privileges at a local hospital | American Psychiatric Association www.psych.org |
| Psychologist | Doctoral degree in counseling or clinical psychology (PhD), plus several years of supervised practice to earn license | Various types, such as cognitive-behavioral therapy and specialties including family or sexual counseling | American Psychological Association www.apa.org |
| Clinical/psychiatric social worker | Master's degree in social work (MSW), followed by 2 years of experience in a clinical setting to earn license | May be trained in certain specialties, such as substance abuse counseling or child counseling | National Association of Social Workers www.socialworkers.org |
| Counselor | Master's degree in counseling, psychology, educational psychology, or related human service; generally must complete at least 2 years of supervised practice to obtain a license | Many are trained to provide individual and group therapy; may specialize in one type of counseling, such as family, marital, relationship, children, or substance abuse | American Counseling Association www.counseling.org |
| Psychoanalyst | Postgraduate degree in psychology or psychiatry (PhD or MD), followed by 8 to 10 years of training in psychoanalysis, which includes undergoing analysis themselves | Based on the theories of Freud and others, focuses on patterns of thinking and behavior and recalling early traumas that block personal growth. Treatment lasts 5 to 10 years, with three to four sessions per week. | American Psychoanalytic Association www.apsa.org |
| Licensed marriage and family therapist (LMFT) | Master's or doctoral degree in psychology, social work, or counseling, specializing in family and interpersonal dynamics; generally must complete at least 2 years of supervised practice to obtain a license | Treats individuals or families who want relationship counseling. Treatment is often brief and focused on finding solutions to specific relational problems. | American Association for Marriage and Family Therapy www.aamft.org |

3. A mental status examination, which will assess thoughts, speaking processes, and memory, and will include an in-depth interview with tests for other psychiatric symptoms.

Once physical factors have been ruled out, you may decide to consult a professional who specializes in psychological health.

## Mental Health Professionals

Several types of mental health professionals are available; TABLE 2.1 provides information on the most common types of practitioners. When choosing a therapist, it is important to verify that he or she has the appropriate training and certification. The most important factor is whether you feel you can work with him or her. A qualified mental health professional should be willing to answer all your questions during an initial consultation. Questions to ask the therapist or yourself include:

- Can you interview the therapist before starting treatment? An initial meeting can help you determine whether this person will be a good fit.
- Do you like the therapist as a person? Can you talk to him or her comfortably?
- Is the therapist watching the clock or easily distracted? You should be the focus of the session.

- Does the therapist demonstrate professionalism? Be concerned if your therapist is frequently late or breaks appointments, suggests social interactions outside your therapy sessions, talks inappropriately about himself or herself, has questionable billing practices, or resists releasing you from therapy.
- Will the therapist help you set your own goals and timetables? A good professional should evaluate your general situation and help you set goals to work on between sessions.

Note that the use of the title *therapist* or *counselor* is not nationally regulated. Check credentials and make your choice carefully.

## What to Expect in Therapy

Before making an appointment, call for information and to briefly explain your needs. Ask about office hours, policies and procedures, fees, and insurance participation. Most of us have misconceptions about what therapy is and what it can do. The first visit serves as a sizing-up between you and the therapist. The therapist will record your history and details about the problem that has brought you to therapy. Answer honestly and do not be embarrassed to acknowledge your feelings. It is critical to the success of your treatment that you trust the therapist enough to be open and honest.

Do not expect the therapist to tell you what to do or how to behave. The responsibility for improved behavior lies with you. If after your first visit (or even after several visits), you feel you cannot work with this person, say so. You have the right to find a therapist with whom you feel comfortable.

## Treatment Models
Many different types of counseling exist, including psychodynamic therapy, interpersonal therapy, and cognitive-behavioral therapy.

*Psychodynamic therapy* focuses on the psychological roots of emotional suffering. It involves self-reflection, self-examination, and the use of the relationship between therapist and patient as a window into problematic relationship patterns in the patient's life. Its goal is not only to alleviate the most obvious symptoms, but also to help people lead healthier lives.[90]

*Interpersonal therapy* focuses on social roles and relationships. The patient works with a therapist to evaluate specific problem areas, such as conflicts with family and friends or significant life changes or transition. Although past experiences help inform the process, interpersonal therapy focuses mainly on improving relationships in the present.[91]

Treatment for mental disorders can include various cognitive-behavioral therapies. *Cognitive therapy* focuses on the impact of thoughts and ideas on feelings and behavior. It helps a person to look at life rationally and correct habitually pessimistic or faulty thinking patterns. *Behavioral therapy* focuses on what we do. Behavioral therapy uses the concepts of stimulus, response, and reinforcement to alter behavior patterns. With cognitive-behavioral therapy, you work with a mental health professional in a structured way, attending a limited number of sessions to become aware of inaccurate or negative thinking. Cognitive-behavioral therapy enables you to view challenging situations more clearly and respond to them more effectively. It can be very helpful for treating anxiety or depression.[92]

## Pharmacological Treatment

It is not uncommon for psychotherapeutic treatment to combine talk therapy with drug therapy.

**Psychotropic drugs**—medicines that alter chemicals in the brain and affect mood and behavior—require a doctor's prescription and have been approved by the U.S. Food and Drug Administration (FDA). Common side effects include dry mouth, headaches, nausea, sexual dysfunction, and weight gain, among others. Additionally, the FDA requires warnings for antidepressant medications, including labeling that warns of increased risks of suicidal thinking and behavior during initial treatment in adults aged 18 to 24.[93]

Potency, dosage, and side effects of drugs can vary greatly. It is vital to completely understand the risks and benefits of any prescribed medication. Likewise, your doctor needs to be notified as soon as possible of any adverse effects you may experience. With some drug therapies, such as antidepressants, you may not feel the therapeutic effects for several weeks, so patience is important. Finally, be sure to follow your doctor's recommendations for beginning or ending a course of any medication.

To avoid the side effects of psychoactive drugs, some patients choose complementary or alternative therapies such as St. John's wort or omega-3 fatty acids for depression and kava or acupuncture for anxiety. While the efficacy of these therapies is not yet conclusive, the National Coordinating Center for Integrative Medicine continues to invest in exploratory research. While some complementary and alternative medicine (CAM) therapies, such as mindfulness meditation—associated with structural changes in the brain that may reduce symptoms of both anxiety and depression—is unlikely to cause any harm, some therapies, like St. John's wort, can be life-threatening when combined with traditional depression medications.[94] Research is still needed on both traditional and CAM therapies for mental illness, making it essential to talk to a medical professional when considering any new treatment or change in treatment.

**SEE IT!** VIDEOS

When should you consider professional psychological help? Watch **Psychological Disorders** in the Study Area of MasteringHealth™

**psychotropic drugs** medicines that alter chemicals in the brain and affect mood and behavior such as antianxiety and antidepressants

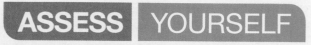

## How Psychologically Healthy Are You?

Being psychologically healthy requires both introspection and the willingness to work on areas that need improvement. Begin by completing the following assessment scale. Use it to determine how well each statement describes you. When you're finished, ask someone who is very close to you to take the same test and respond with his or her own perceptions of you.

| | Never | Rarely | Fairly frequently | Most of the time | All of the time |
|---|---|---|---|---|---|
| 1. My actions and interactions indicate that I am confident in my abilities. | 1 | 2 | 3 | 4 | 5 |
| 2. I am quick to blame others for things that go wrong in my life. | 1 | 2 | 3 | 4 | 5 |
| 3. I am spontaneous and like to have fun with others. | 1 | 2 | 3 | 4 | 5 |
| 4. I am able to give love and affection to others and show my feelings. | 1 | 2 | 3 | 4 | 5 |
| 5. I am able to receive love and signs of affection from others without feeling uneasy. | 1 | 2 | 3 | 4 | 5 |
| 6. I am generally positive and upbeat about things in my life. | 1 | 2 | 3 | 4 | 5 |
| 7. I am cynical and tend to be critical of others. | 1 | 2 | 3 | 4 | 5 |
| 8. I have a large group of people whom I consider to be good friends. | 1 | 2 | 3 | 4 | 5 |
| 9. I make time for others in my life. | 1 | 2 | 3 | 4 | 5 |
| 10. I take time each day for myself for quiet introspection, having fun, or just doing nothing. | 1 | 2 | 3 | 4 | 5 |
| 11. I am compulsive and competitive in my actions. | 1 | 2 | 3 | 4 | 5 |
| 12. I handle stress well and am seldom upset or stressed out by others. | 1 | 2 | 3 | 4 | 5 |
| 13. I try to look for the good in everyone and every situation before finding fault. | 1 | 2 | 3 | 4 | 5 |
| 14. I am comfortable meeting new people and interact well in social settings. | 1 | 2 | 3 | 4 | 5 |
| 15. I would rather stay in and watch TV or read than go out with friends or interact with others. | 1 | 2 | 3 | 4 | 5 |

| | Never | Rarely | Fairly frequently | Most of the time | All of the time |
|---|---|---|---|---|---|
| 16. I am flexible and can adapt to most situations, even if I don't like them. | 1 | 2 | 3 | 4 | 5 |
| 17. Nature, the environment, and other living things are important aspects of my life. | 1 | 2 | 3 | 4 | 5 |
| 18. I think before responding to my emotions. | 1 | 2 | 3 | 4 | 5 |
| 19. I tend to think of my own needs before those of others. | 1 | 2 | 3 | 4 | 5 |
| 20. I am consciously trying to be a better person. | 1 | 2 | 3 | 4 | 5 |
| 21. I like to plan ahead and set realistic goals for myself. | 1 | 2 | 3 | 4 | 5 |
| 22. I accept others for who they are. | 1 | 2 | 3 | 4 | 5 |
| 23. I value diversity and respect others' rights, regardless of culture, race, sexual orientation, religion, or other differences. | 1 | 2 | 3 | 4 | 5 |
| 24. I try to live each day as if it might be my last. | 1 | 2 | 3 | 4 | 5 |
| 25. I have a great deal of energy and appreciate the little things in life. | 1 | 2 | 3 | 4 | 5 |
| 26. I cope with stress in appropriate ways. | 1 | 2 | 3 | 4 | 5 |
| 27. I get enough sleep each day and seldom feel tired. | 1 | 2 | 3 | 4 | 5 |
| 28. I have healthy relationships with my family. | 1 | 2 | 3 | 4 | 5 |
| 29. I am confident that I can do most things if I put my mind to them. | 1 | 2 | 3 | 4 | 5 |
| 30. I respect others' opinions and believe that others should be free to express their opinions, even when they differ from my own. | 1 | 2 | 3 | 4 | 5 |

### Interpreting Your Scores

Look at items 2, 7, 11, 15, and 19. Add up your score for these five items and divide by 5. ____

Is your average for these items above or below 3? Did you score a 5 on any of these items? Do you need to work on any of these areas?

Now look at your scores for the remaining items (there should be 25 items). Total these scores and divide by 25. ____

Is your average above or below 3? On which items did you score a 5? Obviously you're doing well in these areas. Now remove these items from this grouping of 25 (scores of 5), and add up your scores for the remaining items. Then divide your total by the number of items included. Now what is your average? ____

Do the same for the scores completed by your friend or family member. Which scores, if any, are different, and how do they differ? Which areas do you need to work on? What actions can you take now to improve your ratings in these areas?

## YOUR PLAN FOR **CHANGE**

The **ASSESS YOURSELF** activity "How Psychologically Health Are You?" gives you the chance to look at various aspects of your psychological health and compare your self-assessment with a friend's perceptions. After considering these results, you can take steps to change behaviors that may be harmful.

**TODAY, YOU CAN:**

☐ Evaluate your behavior and identify patterns and specific things you are doing that negatively affect your psychological health. What can you change now? What can you change in the near future?

☐ Start a journal and list people you can rely on and trust in life. How do these individuals contribute to your overall life satisfaction? What can you do to make more room for those who contribute to your happiness?

**WITHIN THE NEXT TWO WEEKS, YOU CAN:**

☐ Visit your campus health center's website and find out about counseling services they offer. If you are feeling overwhelmed, depressed, or anxious, make an appointment with a counselor.

☐ Pay attention to negative thoughts that pop up throughout the day. Note times when you find yourself undermining your abilities and notice when you project negative attitudes. Bringing awareness to these thoughts gives you an opportunity to stop and reevaluate them. Try to block negative thoughts and focus on the positives in your life.

**BY THE END OF THE SEMESTER, YOU CAN:**

☐ Make a commitment to an ongoing practice aimed at improving your psychological health. Depending on your current situation, this could mean anything from seeing a counselor, taking time to be more supportive of people who enhance your life, or taking time to help others who are lonely, need help, or are facing challenges.

☐ Volunteer regularly with a local organization you care about. Focus your energy and gain satisfaction by helping to improve others' lives or the environment.

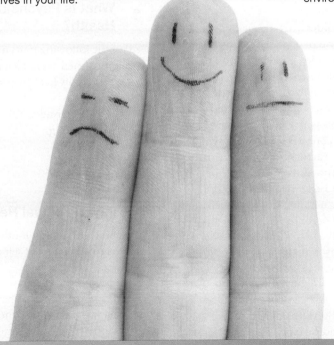

## CHAPTER REVIEW

To hear an MP3 Tutor Session, scan here or visit the Study Area in **MasteringHealth**.

### LO 1 What Is Psychological Health?

- Psychological health is a complex phenomenon involving mental, emotional, social, and spiritual dimensions.

### LO 2 Keys to Enhancing Psychological Health

- Developing self-esteem and self-efficacy, enhancing emotional intelligence, cultivating healthy personality traits, and pursuing happiness are key to enhancing psychological health. The mind-body connection is an important link in overall health and well-being.

### LO 3 When Psychological Health Deteriorates

- The college years are a high-risk time for developing disorders such as depression or anxiety because of high stress levels, pressures for grades, and financial problems, among others.
- Mood disorders include major depression, persistent depressive disorder, bipolar disorder, and seasonal affective disorder. Anxiety disorders include generalized anxiety disorder, panic disorders, and phobic disorders. People with OCD often have irrational concern about order, symmetry, or exactness, or have persistent intrusive thoughts.
- PTSD is caused by experiencing or witnessing a traumatic event, such as those that occur in war, natural disasters, or the loss of a loved one. Personality disorders include paranoid, narcissistic, and borderline personality disorders. Schizophrenia is often characterized by visual and auditory hallucinations, an altered sense of self, and radical changes in emotions, among others.

### LO 4 Suicide: Giving Up on Life

- Suicide is a result of negative psychological reactions to life. People intending to commit suicide often give warning signs of their intentions and can often be helped. Suicide prevention involves eliminating the conditions that may lead to attempts.

### LO 5 Seeking Professional Help

- Mental health professionals include psychiatrists, psychoanalysts, psychologists, social workers, and counselors/therapists. Many therapy methods exist, including psychodynamic, interpersonal, and cognitive-behavioral therapy.
- Treatment of mental disorders can combine talk therapy and drug therapy using psychotropic drugs, such as antidepressants.

## POP QUIZ

Visit **MasteringHealth** to personalize your study plan with Chapter Review Quizzes and Dynamic Study Modules.

### LO 1 What Is Psychological Health?

1. All of the following traits have been identified as characterizing psychologically healthy people *except*
   a. conscientiousness.
   b. understanding.
   c. openness.
   d. agreeableness.

### LO 2 Enhancing Psychological Health

2. A person with high self-esteem
   a. possesses feelings of self-respect and self-worth.
   b. believes he or she can successfully engage in a specific behavior.
   c. believes external influences shape one's psychological health.
   d. has a high altruistic capacity.

3. People who have experienced repeated failures at the same task may eventually give up and quit trying altogether. This pattern of behavior is termed
   a. post-traumatic stress disorder.
   b. learned helplessness.
   c. self-efficacy.
   d. introversion.

4. Subjective well-being includes all of the following components *except*
   a. psychological hardiness.
   b. satisfaction with present life.
   c. relative presence of positive emotions.
   d. relative absence of negative emotions.

### LO 3 When Psychological Health Deteriorates

5. Which statement below is *false*?
   a. One in five adults in the United States suffers from a diagnosable mental disorder in a given year.
   b. Mental disorders are the leading cause of disability in the United States.
   c. Dysthymia is an example of an anxiety disorder.
   d. Bipolar disorder can also be referred to as manic depression.

6. Which of the following statements is *not* correct?
   a. Seasonal depression and seasonal affective disorder are terms used interchangeably.
   b. Persistent depressive disorder is actually major depression that lasts a long time.
   c. Bipolar disorder has historically been referred to as manic depression.
   d. Many more women than men suffer from depression.

7. What is the most common mental health problem in the United States?
   a. Depression
   b. Anxiety disorders
   c. Alcohol dependence
   d. Schizophrenia

8. This disorder is characterized by a need to perform rituals over and over again; fear of dirt or contamination; or an unnatural concern with order, symmetry, and exactness.
   a. Personality disorder
   b. Obsessive-compulsive disorder
   c. Phobic disorder
   d. Post-traumatic stress disorder

## LO 4 | Suicide: Giving Up on Life

9. For 15- to 24-year-olds in the United States, suicide is the ___ leading cause of death.
   a. first
   b. second
   c. third
   d. fourth

## LO 5 | Seeking Professional Help

10. A person with a Ph.D. in counseling psychology and training in various types of therapy is a
    a. psychiatrist.
    b. psychologist.
    c. social worker.
    d. psychoanalyst.

*Answers to the Pop Quiz can be found on page A-1. If you answered a question incorrectly, review the section identified by the Learning Outcome. For even more study tools, visit MasteringHealth.*

# THINK ABOUT IT!

## LO 1 | What Is Psychological Health?

1. What is psychological health? What indicates that a person is or is not psychologically healthy? Why might the college environment provide a challenge to psychological health?

## LO 2 | Enhancing Psychological Health

2. Consider the factors that influence your overall level of psychological health. Which factors can you change? Which ones may be more difficult to change?

3. Which psychological dimensions do you need to work on? Which are most important to you, and why? What actions can you take today?

## LO 3 | When Psychological Health Deteriorates

4. What proportion of the student population suffers from some type of mental illness? What type of support networks exist on your campus?

5. What are the symptoms of major depression? Anxiety disorders? Panic attacks? What are risk factors for each and how are they treated?

## LO 4 | Suicide: Giving Up on Life

7. What are the warning signs of suicide? Why are some people more vulnerable to suicide than others? What could you do if you heard a classmate say to no one in particular that he was going to "do the world a favor and end it all"?

## LO 5 | Seeking Professional Help

8. Describe the various types of mental health professionals and types of therapies. If you felt depressed about breaking off a long-term relationship, which professional and which therapy do you think would be most beneficial to you?

# ACCESS YOUR HEALTH ON THE INTERNET

The following websites explore further topics related to psychological health. For links to the websites below, visit **MasteringHealth**.

*Active Minds.* Campus education and advocacy/volunteer organization formed to combat the stigma of mental illness, educate the campus community about mental health issues, encourage students who need help to seek it early, and prevent tragedies related to untreated mental illness. **www.activeminds.org**

*American Foundation for Suicide Prevention.* Provides resources for suicide prevention and support for family and friends of those who have committed suicide. Includes info on the National Suicide Prevention Hotline, 1-800-273-TALK (8255). **www.afsp.org**

*American Psychological Association Help Center.* Includes information on psychology at work, the mind-body connection, understanding depression, psychological responses to war, and other topics. **www.apa.org/helpcenter/wellness**

*National Alliance on Mental Illness.* Support and advocacy organization of families and friends of people with severe mental illnesses. **www.nami.org**

*National Institute of Mental Health (NIMH).* Provides an overview of mental health information and new research. **www.nimh.nih.gov**

*Helpguide.* Resources for improving mental and emotional health as well as specific information on topics such as self-injury, sleep, depressive disorders, and anxiety disorders. **www.helpguide.org**

# Cultivating Your Spiritual Health

A private area surrounded by nature can be an ideal spot for quiet contemplation and spiritual renewal.

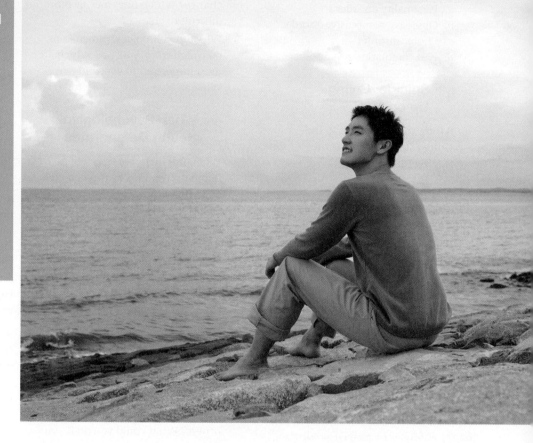

## LEARNING OUTCOMES

1 Define spirituality, describe its three facets, and distinguish between religion and spirituality.

2 Discuss the evidence that spiritual health has physical benefits, has psychological benefits, and lowers stress.

3 Describe three ways you can develop your spiritual health.

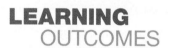

Lia's favorite spot on campus is the secluded Japanese garden on the south side of the library. Whether she's feeling stressed about exams or is mulling over an important decision, a few minutes alone in the garden always seem to help. Sometimes she sits quietly and watches the birds come and go. Sometimes she gets out her camera and photographs particularly brilliant blossoms. Often she simply rests, eyes closed, feeling the sun's warmth on her face, and lets her thoughts turn to gratitude for her health, her loving family, and her opportunity to be in college. However she spends it, her "garden break" leaves Lia feeling refreshed and refocused,

with greater confidence in her ability to tackle the challenges of her day.

Lia's desire to find a sense of purpose, meaning, and harmony in her life is shared by a majority of American college students, according to UCLA's Higher Education Research Institute (HERI).[1] Of the 153,015 students at 227 colleges and universities who were surveyed as they entered college in the fall of 2014, nearly 36 percent rated themselves as above average in spirituality.[2]

Spiritual health is one of six key dimensions of health (see Figure 1.4 on page 7 in Chapter 1). This chapter will look at what spiritual health is, as well as provide the tools for enhancing your own spiritual health.

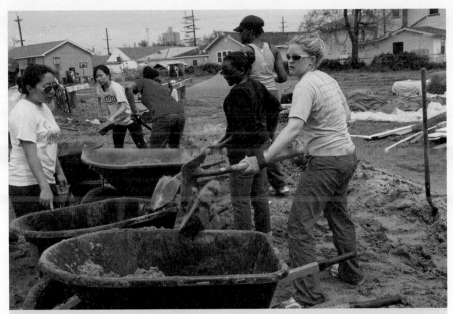

Spiritual and ethical concerns are important to most American college students. One of the ways students express their spirituality is by working to reduce suffering in the world; many contribute their time and skills to volunteer organizations, as these students are doing by working to build homes for Habitat for Humanity.

## LO 1 | WHAT IS SPIRITUALITY?

**Define spirituality, describe its three facets, and distinguish between religion and spirituality.**

From one day to the next, many of us attempt to satisfy our needs for belonging and self-esteem by acquiring material possessions, hanging with the "right crowd," and being the "best" at everything we do. But new "toys" and keeping up with others don't necessarily bring happiness or improve our sense of self-worth or well-being—nor do they protect us from life's ups and downs. Friends and family can disappoint; relationships can falter; and even the best-laid plans can fail. Buffeted by life, many of us begin seeking more answers; to grow and develop in a way that helps us

**HEAR IT! PODCASTS**

Want a study podcast for this chapter text? Download **Psychological Health: Being Mentally, Emotionally, and Spiritually Well,** available on **MasteringHealth™**

cope. With this seeking, our quest for spirituality begins.

But what is spirituality? Let's begin by exploring its root, *spirit,* which in many cultures refers to *breath,* or the force that animates life. When you're "inspired," your energy flows. You're not held back by doubts about the purpose or meaning of your work and life. Indeed, many definitions of spirituality incorporate this sense of transcendence, focused on an internal experience.

Harold G. Koenig, MD, one of the foremost researchers of spirituality and health, defines **spirituality** as the personal quest for understanding answers to ultimate questions about life, about meaning, and about our relationship with the sacred or transcendent.[3] The sacred or transcendent could be thought of as a higher power or being, or it could refer to the essential goodness of life, or our relationship with nature or forces we cannot explain. Many who become interested in spirituality seek out mentorship from a **spiritual teacher**, a person versed in the nature of spirituality and spiritual practice who can help people achieve a deeper recognition of what spirituality will mean to them. Spirituality may mean different things to

different people; however, there are often several common elements, including:

- Being aware of your impact on people, places, and events
- Actively searching for meaning in your life
- Finding a way to give back, knowing that service to others is a source of true happiness
- Understanding the interconnectedness of humanity, nature, and the universe and respecting all elements
- Nurturing loving relationships with yourself and others
- Living with intention, as if every day matters
- Developing a philosophy of life that guides your daily attitudes and decisions
- Accepting your limitations as well as your strengths

Essentially, spirituality is about learning to accept life on its own terms.

ACCORDING TO THE MOST RECENT STUDY OF FIRST-YEAR STUDENTS,

# 27.5%

OF STUDENTS MARKED "NONE" AS THEIR **RELIGIOUS PREFERENCE**, NEARLY DOUBLING THE 15.4% WHO INDICATED NO RELIGIOUS PREFERENCE IN 1971.

# Spirituality and Religion

Spirituality and religion are not the same thing. Religion is a set of rituals, beliefs, symbols, and practices intended to enable a feeling of connection to the holy or divine. It is possible to be spiritual and not religious and equally possible to be religious and not spiritual. In fact, while one global survey revealed that nearly 4 of 5 people worldwide are religiously affiliated, it also showed 16 percent (1.1 billion) are not affiliated, making them the third largest group surveyed.[4] Many people without religious affiliation still have certain religious or spiritual beliefs.[5] Thus, it's clear that religion does not have to be part of a spiritual person's life. **TABLE 1** identifies some characteristics that can help you distinguish religion and spirituality.

**values** Principles that influence our thoughts and emotions and guide the choices we make in our lives.

**conscious living** Adopting a more introspective, reflective way of looking at their purpose in life and the things that are most important to them and making intentional choices to their ideal self.

## Spirituality Integrates Three Facets

Brian Luke Seaward, a professor at the University of Northern Colorado and author of several books on spirituality and mind-body healing, identifies three facets of human existence that together constitute the core of human spirituality: relationships, values, and purpose in life (**FIGURE 1**).[6] Questions arising in these three domains prompt many of us to look for spiritual answers.

## Relationships

Have you ever wondered if someone you were attracted to is really right for you? Or, conversely, wondered if you should break off a long-term relationship? Have you ever wished you had more friends, or that you were a better friend to yourself? For many people,

| TABLE 1 | Characteristics Distinguishing Religion and Spirituality |
|---|---|
| **Religion** | **Spirituality** |
| Observable, measurable, objective | Less measurable, more subjective |
| Formal, orthodox, organized | Less formal, less orthodox, less systematic |
| Behavior-oriented, outward practices | Emotionally oriented, inwardly directed |
| Authoritarian in terms of behaviors | Not authoritarian, little accountability |
| Doctrine separating good from evil | Unifying, not doctrine oriented |

**Source:** National Center for Complementary and Alternative Medicine (NCCAM), "Prayer and Spirituality in Health: Ancient Practices, Modern Science," *CAM at the NIH* 12, no. 1 (2005): 1–4.

such questions and yearnings are natural triggers for spiritual growth: As we contemplate who we should choose as a life partner or how to mend a quarrel with a friend, we begin to foster our own inner wisdom. At the same time, healthy relationships are a sign of spiritual well-being. When we think well of ourselves, and consequently treat others with respect, honesty, integrity, and love, we are manifesting our spiritual health.

## Values

Our personal **values** are our principles—the set of fundamental rules by which we conduct our lives. It's what we stand for. When we attempt to clarify our values, and then live according to those values, we're moving closer to a life of integrity. Spiritual health is characterized by a strong personal value system.

## Meaningful Purpose in Life

What career do you plan to pursue? Do you hope to marry? Do you plan to have or adopt children? What things will make you feel happy and "complete"? How do these choices reflect what you hold as your purpose in life? At the end of your days, what would you want people to say about how you've lived your life and what your life has meant to others? Contemplating these questions fosters spiritual growth. People who are spiritually healthy seek **conscious living**, adopting a more introspective, reflective way of looking at their purpose in life and the things that are most important to them. They take a more thoughtful, deliberate approach to achieving their ideal self.

Picture in your mind someone you think has made the world a better place—whether someone close to you or someone like Gandhi, Martin Luther King, Jr., or Mother Theresa—people whose spiritual quest took on a life-size view of a better world and had a real purpose. Allow yourself to see your life as having its own mission and purpose.

## Spiritual Intelligence

Our relationships, values, and sense of purpose together contribute to our overall **spiritual intelligence (SI).** This term was

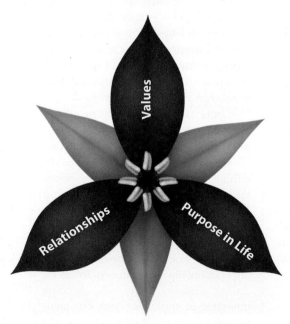

**FIGURE 1** **Three Facets of Spirituality** Most of us are prompted to explore our spirituality because of questions relating to our relationships, values, and purpose in life. At the same time, these three facets together constitute spiritual well-being.

→ **VIDEO TUTOR** Facets of Spirituality

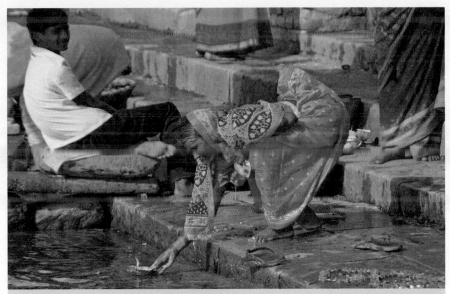

Spirituality and religion are not the same. Many people find that religious practices, for example, attending services or making offerings—such as the small lamp this Hindu woman is placing in the sacred Ganges River—help them to focus on their spirituality. However, religion does not have to be part of a spiritual person's life.

introduced by physicist and philosopher Danah Zohar, who defined it as "an ability to access higher meanings, values, abiding purposes, and unconscious aspects of the self."[7] Humility, the capacity to consider ideas that fall "outside the box," and tapping in to energies outside the ego all fit in her definition. SI allows us to utilize values, meanings, and purposes to be more creative and enrich our lives.

Since Zohar introduced the idea of SI, a number of psychologists, clerics, and even some business consultants have taken the liberty of expanding the definition of the term. For example, spiritual intelligence expert, Cindy Wigglesworth, explains that SI helps us find

compassion and wisdom to help guide us through life.[8] SI also helps us maintain our peaceful center. To find out your own spiritual IQ, see the **Assess Yourself** activity on page 69.

## LO 2 | THE BENEFITS OF SPIRITUAL HEALTH

Discuss the evidence that spiritual health has physical benefits, has psychological benefits, and lowers stress.

A broad range of large-scale surveys have documented the importance of the mind-body connection to human health and wellness.

## Physical Benefits

The emerging science of mind-body medicine is a research focus of the National Center for Complementary and Integrative Health (NCCIH) and an important objective of the organization's 2011–2015 Strategic Plan. One area under study is the association between spiritual health and general health. The NCCIH cites evidence that spirituality can have a positive influence on physical health and suggests that the connection may be due to improved

immune function, cardiovascular function, or a combination of physiological changes.[9] Increasing numbers of studies are examining the effect that certain spiritual practices, such as yoga, deep meditation, and prayer, have on the mind, body, social and emotional health, and behavior and how these practices may improve health and promote healthy behaviors.[10]

The National Cancer Institute (NCI) contends that when we get sick, spiritual or religious well-being may help restore health and improve quality of life by:[11]

- Decreasing anxiety, depression, anger, discomfort, and feelings of isolation
- Decreasing alcohol and drug abuse
- Decreasing blood pressure and the risk of heart disease
- Increasing the person's ability to cope with the effects of illness and with medical treatments
- Increasing feelings of hope and optimism, freedom from regret, satisfaction with life, and inner peace

Several studies show an association between spirituality and/or religion and a person's ability to cope with a variety of physical illnesses, including cancer.[12] For example, one study of people living with chronic pain and neurological conditions showed a benefit to using spiritual health and mind-body techniques,[13] as did another study of cardiac patients.[14] However, newer research has questioned the efficacy of many of these studies, citing small sample size and methodological issues.[15] Researchers have also looked into the overall association between religious and spiritual practices and mortality, and a review of over a decade of research studies indicated that individuals who incorporate weekly attendance at church or other organized religious settings may have a decreased risk of mortality, particularly from cardiovascular events.[16]

Another recent review of literature found being religious to be was strongly associated with positive habits for your

3 OUT OF 4

FIRST-YEAR COLLEGE STUDENTS REPORT THAT THEY ARE ACTIVELY "SEARCHING FOR **MEANING** AND PURPOSE IN LIFE."

**spiritual intelligence (SI)** The ability to access higher meanings, values, abiding purposes, and unconscious aspects of the self, a characteristic that helps us find a moral and ethical path to guide us through life.

health, including being less likely to smoke, less likely to drink to excess, and being more likely to get regular medical screenings. However, religiosity is only weakly related to biomarkers like blood pressure, immune factors, cardiac reactivity, and disease progression. Measures of spirituality, on the other hand, were related more strongly to those biomarkers.[17] More research is still necessary to determine health benefits of spirituality and religion.

## Psychological Benefits

Current research also suggests that spiritual health contributes to psychological health. For instance, the NCI and independent studies have found that spirituality reduces levels of anxiety and depression.[18] In the case of academic performance, spirituality may provide a protective factor against burnout. In a study of 259 medical students, each completed a survey asking questions intended to measure levels of burnout, spirituality, psychological distress, ability to cope, and general happiness. Results showed students with higher scores of spiritual exercise and well-being to be more satisfied with their lives than students scoring lower.[19]

When people undergo psychological trauma, the meaning of life can be severely challenged. Counselors work with trauma survivors to help them find meaning in their trauma, to change their ways of thinking, and move them toward involvement in meaningful life experiences. Psychologists at the U.S. Department of Veterans Affairs have done extensive clinical work with veterans who are experiencing *post-traumatic stress disorder (PTSD)* as a result of their combat service. An example of the value of spiritual or religious practice may be that, following trauma, powerful emotions like anger, rage, and wanting to get even may be softened by values like forgiveness or other spiritual beliefs and practices.[20]

People who have found a **spiritual community**—a group of people meeting together for the purpose of enriching and expanding their spirituality—also benefit from increased social support. For instance, participation in charitable organizations, religious groups, social gatherings, or spiritual learning experiences can help members avoid isolation. A community may include retired members who offer child care for working parents, support for those with addictions or mental health problems, shelter and food for the homeless, or transportation to medical appointments. Spiritually active members may volunteer or receive help from other volunteers, all of which may enhance feelings of self-worth, security, and belonging.

Additionally, the NCI cites stress reduction as one probable mechanism among spiritually healthy people for improved health and longevity and for better coping with illness.[21] **Chapter 3: Managing Stress and Coping with Life's Challenges,** goes into more detail on this topic.

## LO 3 | CULTIVATING YOUR SPIRITUAL HEALTH

**Describe three ways you can develop your spiritual health.**

Cultivating your spiritual side takes just as much work as becoming physically fit. Ways to develop your spiritual health include tuning in, training your body, expanding your mind, and reaching out.

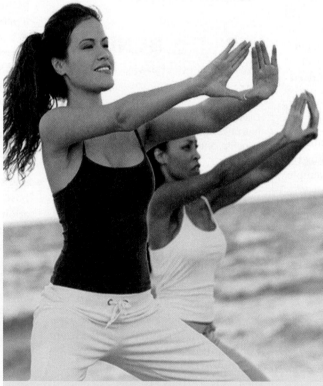

Spirituality is widely acknowledged to have a positive impact on health and wellness, from reductions in overall morbidity and mortality to improved abilities to cope with illness and stress. These students are using the movement techniques of tai chi to improve their spiritual health.

## Tune in to Yourself and Your Surroundings

Focusing on your spiritual health has been likened to tuning in on a radio: Inner wisdom is perpetually available to us, but if we fail to tune our "receiver," we won't be able to hear it through all the "static" of daily life. Fortunately, four ancient practices still in use today can help you tune in. These are *contemplation* (studying), *mindfulness* (observing), *meditation* (quieting), and *prayer* (communing with the divine).

### Contemplation

In a dictionary, the word *contemplation* means a study of something—whether a candle flame or a theory of quantum mechanics. In the domain of spirituality, **contemplation** refers to concentrating the mind on a spiritual or ethical question or subject, a view of the natural world, or an icon or other image representative of divinity. Most religious and spiritual traditions advocate engaging in the contemplation of gratitude, forgiveness, and unconditional love.

When practicing contemplation, it can be helpful to keep a journal to record any insights that arise, and journaling itself can be a form of contemplation. For example, you might want to make a list of 20 things in your life you are grateful for or write a letter of forgiveness for yourself or a loved one. You might also use your journal to record inspirational quotations that you encounter in your readings. Journaling can fill a larger role in spiritual health and development by providing a sense of overall calmness.

## Mindfulness

A practice of focused, nonjudgmental observation, **mindfulness** is the ability to be fully present in the moment (**FIGURE 2**). Being "tuned in" could mean being fully present while listening to a mournful song by Sam Smith, feeling incredibly happy to have great friends around you, or just enjoying a morning cup of coffee. In any case, mindfulness is an awareness of present-moment reality—a holistic sensation of being totally involved in the moment rather than focused on some worry or being on "autopilot."[22]

The range of opportunities to practice mindfulness is as infinite as the

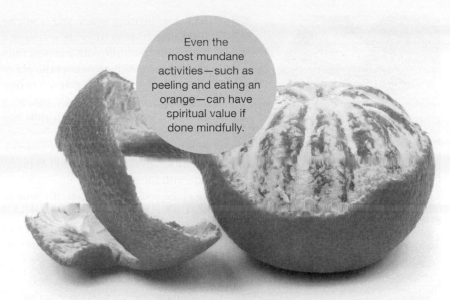

Even the most mundane activities—such as peeling and eating an orange—can have spiritual value if done mindfully.

moments of our lives. Living mindfully means allowing ourselves to be present in the current moment—to be wholly aware of what we are feeling in each moment.[23] For instance, the next time you are going to eat an orange, pay attention! What does it feel like to pierce the skin? How does it smell as you peel it? What does the rind really look like?

Pursuing almost any endeavor that requires close concentration can help you develop mindfulness. Even household activities such as cooking or cleaning can foster mindfulness—as long as you pay attention while you do them!

In this era of global environmental concerns, we can also cultivate mindfulness by paying attention to how our choices affect our world. Mindfulness of our environment calls on us to examine our values and behaviors as we share our Earth with all living creatures every moment of each day. It includes having a shared sense of responsibility for improving the world for future generations.

## Meditation

**Meditation** is a practice of cultivating a still or quiet mind. Although the precise details vary with different schools of meditation, the fundamental task is the same: to quiet the mind's noise (variously referred to as "chatter," "static," or "monkey mind").

**FIGURE 2** Qualities of Mindfulness

*now*
*here*
*focused*
*self-forgetful*
*non-judgmental*

Why would you want to cultivate stillness? For thousands of years, human beings of different cultures and traditions have found that achieving periods of meditative stillness each day enhances their spiritual health. Today, researchers are beginning to discover why. The NCCIH reports that researchers using brain-scanning techniques found experienced meditators to show a significantly increased level of *empathy*—the ability to understand and share another person's experience.[24] Similar research has shown that participants who practiced a specific form of meditation, known as *compassion-meditation*, further increased their levels of compassion toward others.[25] Studies also suggest that meditation improves the brain's ability to process information; reduces stress,

**mindfulness** Practice of purposeful, nonjudgmental observation in which we are fully present in the moment.

**meditation** Practice of concentrated focus upon a sound, object, visualization, the breath, movement, or attention itself in order to increase awareness of the present moment, reduce stress, promote relaxation, and enhance personal and spiritual growth.

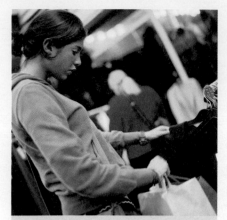

To be mindfully green requires us to ask ourselves some tough questions, such as What is my fair share? and How much do I really need?

anxiety, and depression; reduces insomnia; improves concentration; and decreases blood pressure.[26]

The physiological processes that produce these effects are only partially understood. One theory suggests meditation works by reducing the body's stress response. By practicing deep, calm contemplation, people who meditate seem to promote activity in the body's systems, leading to a sense of peacefulness and subjective well-being as well as to physical relaxation that may slow breathing, lower blood pressure, improve sleep, and reduce symptoms of digestive problems.[27]

New research has shown actual differences in the brain structures of experienced meditators compared to those with no history of meditation.[28] Other studies have shown meditation to boost gray matter density in parts of the brain critical to learning and memory and improved psychological and emotional health, compassion, and introspection.[29] At the same time, meditation may decrease gray matter areas of the brain known to play a key role in anxiety and stress.[30]

So how do you meditate? Detailed instructions are beyond the scope of this text, but most teachers suggest beginning by sitting in a quiet place

**prayer** Communication with a transcendent Presence.

**yoga** System of physical and mental training involving controlled breathing, physical postures (*asanas*), meditation, chanting, and other practices believed to cultivate unity with the *Atman*, or spiritual life principle of the universe.

with low lighting where you won't be interrupted. Many advocate assuming a "full lotus" position, with legs bent fully at the knees, each ankle over the opposite knee. If this is impossible or uncomfortable, you may want to assume a modified lotus position, with your legs simply crossed in front of you. Rest your hands on your knees, palms upward. Beginners usually find it easier to meditate with the eyes closed.

Once you're in position, it's time to start emptying your mind. The various schools of meditation teach different methods to achieve this. Some options include:

- **Mantra meditation.** Focus on a *mantra,* a single word such as *Om, Amen, Love,* or *God* and repeat this word silently. When a distracting thought arises, simply set it aside. It may help to imagine the thought as a leaf, and visualize placing it on a gently flowing stream. Do not fault yourself for becoming distracted. Simply notice the thought, release it, and return to your mantra.
- **Breath meditation.** Count each breath: Pay attention to each inhalation, the brief pause that follows, and the exhalation. Together, these equal one breath. When you have counted ten breaths, return to one. As with mantra meditation, release distractions as they arise, and return to following the breath.
- **Color meditation.** When your eyes are closed, you may perceive a field of color, such as a deep, restful blue. Focus on this color. Treat distractions as in other forms of meditation.

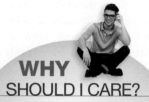

## WHY SHOULD I CARE?

Practicing meditation can improve concentration and your brain's ability to process information; it can also reduce stress, anxiety, and depression, all important factors when trying to manage your classes and handle daily demands.

- **Candle meditation.** With your eyes open, focus on the flame of a candle. Allow your eyes to soften as you meditate on this object. Treat distractions as in the other forms of meditation.

After several minutes of meditation, and with practice, you may come to experience a sensation sometimes described as "dropping down," in which you feel yourself release into the meditation. In this state, which can be likened to a wakeful sleep, distracting thoughts are far less likely to arise, and yet you may receive surprising insights.

Initially, try meditating for just 10 to 20 minutes, once or twice a day. In time, you can increase your sessions to 30 minutes or more. As you meditate for longer periods, you will likely find yourself feeling more rested and less stressed, and you may begin to experience the increased levels of empathy recorded among expert meditators.

### Prayer

In **prayer,** an individual focuses the mind in communication with a transcendent Presence. For many, prayer offers a sense of comfort, a sense that we are not alone. It can be the means of expressing concern for others, for admission of transgressions, for seeking forgiveness, and for renewing hope and purpose. Focusing on the things we are grateful for can move people to look to the future with hope and give them the strength to get through the most challenging times. Research has shown that spiritual practices can increase the ability to cope and decrease stress among cancer patients.[31]

## Train Your Body

For thousands of years, in regions throughout the world, spiritual seekers have pursued transcendence through physical means. One of the foremost examples is the practice of **yoga.**

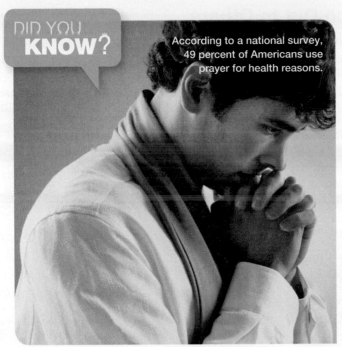

## Expand Your Mind

For many people, psychological counseling is a first step toward improving their spiritual health. Therapy helps you let go of past hurts, accept your limitations, manage stress and anger, reduce anxiety and depression, and take control of your life—all steps that can lead to spiritual growth. If you've never engaged in therapy, making the first appointment can feel daunting. Your campus health department can usually help by providing a referral. It is important to find a therapist who is open to the concepts described in this chapter.

Another practical way to expand your mind is to study the sacred texts of the world's major religions and spiritual practices. Libraries and bookstores are filled with volumes that explore the diverse approaches humans take to achieving spiritual fulfillment.

Finally, you can expand your awareness of different spiritual practices by

Although many in the West tend to picture yoga as having to do with a number of physical postures and some controlled breathing, more traditional forms tend to also emphasize chanting, meditation, and other techniques believed to encourage unity with the *Atman,* or spiritual life principle of the universe.

If you are interested in exploring yoga, sign up for a class on campus, at your local YMCA, or at a yoga center. Choose a form that seems right to you: Some, such as *hatha yoga,* focus on developing flexibility, deep breathing, and tranquility, whereas others, such as *ashtanga yoga,* are fast-paced and demanding and thus more focused on developing physical fitness. See Chapter 3 and Chapter 11 for more on various styles of yoga.

The Eastern meditative movement practices of tai chi or qigong can also increase physical activity and mental focus. With roots in Chinese medicine, both have been shown to have beneficial effects on bone health, stress, cardiopulmonary fitness, mood, balance, and quality of life.[32]

See Chapter 3 for more on tai chi and qigong.

Training your body to improve your spiritual health doesn't necessarily require you to engage in a formal practice. By energizing your body and sharpening your mental focus, jogging, biking, aerobics, dance, or any other regular exercise can contribute to your spiritual health. To transform exercise into a spiritual workout, begin by acknowledging gratitude for your body and its abilities, and throughout the session, maintain mindfulness of your breathing.

# 20.4 MILLION

U.S. ADULTS PRACTICE **YOGA**, ACCORDING TO A RECENT SURVEY BY *YOGA JOURNAL.*

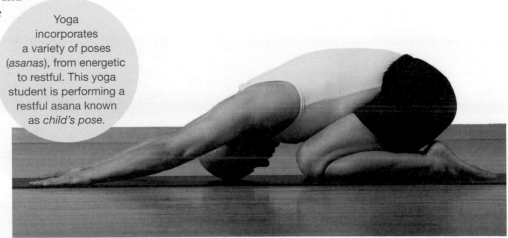

Yoga incorporates a variety of poses (*asanas*), from energetic to restful. This yoga student is performing a restful asana known as *child's pose.*

exploring on-campus meditation or service-oriented groups, taking classes in spiritual or religious subjects, attending religious meetings or services, attending public lectures, and checking out the websites of various spiritual and religious organizations. In each case, you can evaluate the messages and ideas you encounter and decide which practices or beliefs hold meaning for you.

**altruism** Giving of oneself out of genuine concern for others.

## Reach Out to Others

**Altruism,** the giving of oneself out of genuine concern for others, is a key aspect of a spiritually healthy lifestyle. Working for a nonprofit organization, volunteering time, donating money or other resources to a food bank or other program—even spending an afternoon picking up litter in your neighborhood—are all ways to serve others and simultaneously enhance your own spiritual and overall health. Researchers have referred to the benefits of volunteering as a "helpers high," a specific feeling connected with helping others.[33] About 50 percent of people who participated in one study reported feeling more energetic and stronger after helping others; many also said they felt more calm and less depressed, with a greater sense of self-worth.[34]

For more strategies to enhance your spiritual health by reaching out to others, refer to the **Skills for Behavior Change** box.

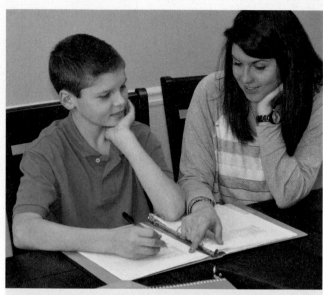

Volunteering can be a fun and fulfilling way to broaden your experience, connect with your community, and focus on your spiritual health.

# ASSESS | YOURSELF

## What's Your Spiritual IQ?

Many tools are available for assessing your SI. Although each differs significantly according to its target audience (therapy clients, business executives, church members, etc.), most share certain underlying principles reflected in the questionnaire below. Answer each question as follows:

0 = not at all true for me
1 = somewhat true for me
2 = very true for me

_____ 1. I frequently feel gratitude for the many blessings of my life.

_____ 2. I am often moved by the beauty of Earth, music, poetry, or other aspects of my daily life.

_____ 3. I readily express forgiveness toward those whose missteps have affected me.

_____ 4. I recognize in others qualities that are more important than their appearance and behaviors.

_____ 5. When I do poorly on an exam, lose an important game, or am rejected in a relationship, I am able to know that the experience does not define who I am.

_____ 6. When fear arises, I am able to know that I am eternally safe and loved.

_____ 7. I meditate or pray daily.

_____ 8. I frequently and fearlessly ponder the possibility of an afterlife.

_____ 9. I accept total responsibility for the choices that I have made in building my life.

_____ 10. I feel that I am on Earth for a unique and sacred reason.

### Scoring

The higher your score on this quiz, the higher your SI. To improve your score, apply the suggestions for spiritual practices from this chapter.

## YOUR PLAN FOR **CHANGE**

The **ASSESS YOURSELF** activity gives you the chance to evaluate your spiritual intelligence, and the text introduced you to some practices used successfully by millions over many generations to enhance their spiritual health. If you are interested in further cultivating your spirituality, consider some of the small but significant steps listed below.

**TODAY,** YOU CAN:

☐ Find a quiet spot, turn off your cell phone, close your eyes, and contemplate, meditate, or pray for 10 minutes. Or spend 10 minutes in quiet mindfulness of your surroundings.

☐ In a journal or on your computer, compose a list of at least ten things you are grateful for. Include people, pets, talents and abilities, achievements, places, foods … whatever comes to mind!

**WITHIN THE NEXT TWO WEEKS,** YOU CAN:

☐ Explore the options on campus for beginning psychotherapy, joining a spiritual or religious group, or volunteering with an organization working for positive change.

☐ Think of a person in your life with whom you have experienced conflict. Spend a few minutes contemplating forgiveness toward this person and then write a letter or e-mail apologizing for any offense and offering your forgiveness in return. Wait a day or two before deciding whether you are truly ready to send the message.

☐ Take a time out. Focus on the things around you;

the sounds and sights and smells. Take time to look at people as you pass them, say "hello" or merely nod indicating you notice their existence. Write down the things you noticed today that were beautiful or you never noticed before.

**BY THE END OF THE SEMESTER,** YOU CAN:

☐ Develop a list of several spiritual texts you would like to read during your break.

☐ Begin exploring options for volunteer work that would serve others and have meaning for you.

**S**kyrocketing tuition, roommates and friends who bug you, anxiety over fitting in, dating, pressure to get good grades, money, and worries about getting a job after graduation—they all lead to STRESS! In today's fast-paced, 24/7-connected world, stress can cause us to feel overwhelmed and zap our energy. It can also cause us to push ourselves to improve performance, bring excitement, and help us thrive.

Chronic stress inhibits normal functioning for prolonged periods and is a growing public health crisis among people of all ages. According to recent American Psychological Association studies, the health care system is not giving Americans the support they need to cope with stress and build healthy lifestyles. Key findings indicate that[1]

- Americans consistently report high stress levels (20% report extreme stress), and teenagers are reporting stress levels on par with adults.
- Adults aged 18-46 report the highest levels of stress overall, and the greatest increases in the last year.
- Only about half of all teens say they feel confident in their ability to handle personal problems.
- Biggest sources of stress for adults ages 18–32 are work, relationships, money, job stability. Individuals aged 67 and older are more likely to cite personal or family health concerns as a key source of stress.

# 39%

OF MILLENNIALS (AGES 18–33) SAY THEIR STRESS LEVELS HAVE **INCREASED** IN THE LAST YEAR, WITH 52% SAYING THEIR STRESS LEVELS KEEP THEM AWAKE AT NIGHT.

While key sources of stress are similar for men and women (money, work, the economy), huge gender differences exist in how people experience, report, and cope with stress. Both men and women report above average levels of stress, but women are more likely to report stress levels that are on the rise and more extreme than those of their male counterparts. Additionally, although men may recognize and report stress, they are much less likely to take action to reduce it.[2] Being "stressed out" can take a major toll on people at all ages and stages of life.

Is too much stress always a bad thing? Fortunately, the answer is no. How we react to real and perceived threats often is key to whether stressors are enabling or debilitating. Learning to assess our perceptions and to anticipate, avoid, and develop skills to reduce or better manage those stressors is key. The first step in controlling or reducing stress is to understand what stress is and how it affects the body.

## LO 1 | WHAT IS STRESS?

Define *stress* and examine its potential impact on health, relationships, and success in college and life.

Most current definitions of **stress** describe it as the mental and physical response and adaptation by our bodies to real or perceived change and challenges. A **stressor** is any real or perceived physical, social, or psychological event or stimulus that causes our bodies to react or respond. Several factors influence one's response to stressors, including *characteristics of the stressor* (How traumatic is it? Can you control it? Did it catch you by surprise? Has anything in your life experience prepared you for it?); *biological factors* (e.g., your age or gender, your health status, whether you've had enough sleep recently); and *past experiences* (e.g., things that have happened to you, their consequences, and how you felt or responded to the situation). Stressors may be *tangible*, such as a failing grade on a test, or *intangible,* such as the angst associated with meeting your significant other's parents for the first time. **Distress**, or negative stress, is more likely to occur when you are tired, under the influence of alcohol or other drugs, under pressure to do well, or coping with an illness, financial trouble, or relationship problems. *Change* can also be a major stressor.

Generally, positive stress is called **eustress.** Eustress presents the opportunity for personal growth and satisfaction and can actually improve health. Getting married, the

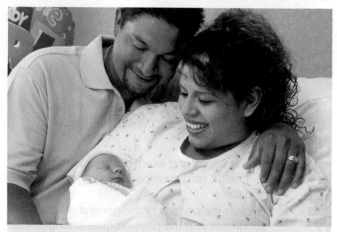

Not all stress is bad for you! Although events that cause prolonged *distress,* such as a natural disaster, can undermine your health, events that cause *eustress,* such as the birth of a child or the excitement of a new love can have positive effects on your growth and well-being. People usually live their lives to the fullest when they experience a moderate level of stress—just enough to keep them challenged and motivated—and deal with that stress in a productive manner. Just as too much stress can be detrimental to your health, too little stress can leave you stagnant and unfulfilled.

**stress** A series of mental and physiological responses and adaptations to a real or perceived threat to one's well-being.

**stressor** A physical, social, or psychological event or condition that upsets homeostasis and produces a stress response.

**distress** Stress that can have a detrimental effect on health; negative stress.

**eustress** Stress that presents opportunities for personal growth; positive stress.

excitement of a first date, or winning a major competition can give rise to the pleasurable rush associated with eustress.

There are several kinds of distress. The most common type, **acute stress**, comes from demands and pressures of the recent past and near future.[3] Usually, acute stress is intense, lasts for a short time, and disappears quickly without permanent damage to your health. Seeing someone you have a crush on could cause your heart to race and your muscles to tense while you appear cool, calm, and collected on the outside. The positive reaction to acute stress is that you rise to the occasion and put your most charming self forward. In contrast, anticipating a class presentation could cause shaking hands, nausea, headache, cramping, or diarrhea, along with a galloping heartbeat, stammering, and forgetfulness. **Episodic acute stress** is the state of regularly reacting with wild, acute stress to various situations. Individuals experiencing episodic acute stress may complain about all they have to do and focus on negative events that may or may not occur. These "awfulizers" are often reactive and anxious, constantly complaining about their lack of sleep and all they have to do—habits so much a part of them that they seem normal. Others may respond to stress with a "hyperactive, chirpy, happy-happy" persona that may also be a stress reaction.

Acute stress and episodic acute stress can both cause physical and emotional reactions, but they may or may not result in negative physical or emotional outcomes. In fact, they may serve as a form of self-protection. In contrast, **chronic stress** can linger indefinitely and wreak silent havoc on your body systems. Caregivers are especially vulnerable to prolonged physiological stress as they watch a loved one struggle with illness. Upon a loved one's eventual death, survivors may struggle to balance the need to process emotions with the need to stay caught up in classes, work, and everyday life.

Another type of stress, **traumatic stress**, is often a result of witnessing or experiencing events like major accidents, war, shootings, sexual violence, assault, or natural disasters. Effects of traumatic stress may be felt for years after the event and cause significant disability, potentially leading to posttraumatic stress disorder, or PTSD (see Chapter 2 for a discussion of PTSD).[4]

## LO 2 | YOUR BODY'S STRESS RESPONSE

Explain the phases of the general adaptation syndrome and the physiological changes that occur during them.

The body's physiological responses to stressors evolved to protect humans from harm. Thousands of years ago, if your ancestors didn't respond by fighting or fleeing, they might have been eaten by a saber-toothed tiger or killed by a marauding enemy clan. Today, when we face real or perceived threats, these same physiological responses kick into gear, but our instinctual reactions to fight, scream, or run must be held in check. While we learn culturally acceptable restraint, our bodies remain charged for battle—sometimes chronically. Over time, this vigilant, simmering stress response can lead to serious health problems.

## The General Adaptation Syndrome

When stress levels are low, the body is often in a state of **homeostasis,** or balance; all body systems are operating smoothly to maintain equilibrium. Stressors trigger a crisis-mode physiological response, after which the body attempts to return to homeostasis by means of an **adaptive response**. First characterized by Hans Selye in 1936, the internal fight to restore homeostasis in the face of a stressor is known as the **general adaptation syndrome (GAS)** (**FIGURE 3.1**). The GAS has three distinct phases: alarm, resistance, and exhaustion.[5]

**Alarm Phase** Suppose you are walking home after a night class on a dimly lit campus. You hear someone cough behind you and sense them approaching rapidly. You walk faster, only to hear the other person's footsteps quicken. Your senses go on high alert, your breathing quickens, your heart races, and you begin to perspire. In desperation you stop, rip off your backpack, and prepare to fling it at your would-be attacker. You turn around, arms flailing, and let out a blood-curdling yell. To your surprise, the would-be-attacker screeches back. It's just one of your classmates trying to stay close out of her own

**acute stress** The short-term physiological response to an immediate perceived threat.

**episodic acute stress** The state of regularly reacting with wild, acute stress about one thing or another.

**chronic stress** An ongoing state of physiological arousal in response to ongoing or numerous perceived threats.

**traumatic stress** A physiological and mental response that occurs for a prolonged period of time after a major accident, war, assault, natural disaster, or an event in which one may have been seriously hurt, killed, or witness to horrible things.

**homeostasis** A balanced physiological state in which all the body's systems function smoothly.

**adaptive response** The physiological adjustments the body makes in an attempt to restore homeostasis.

**general adaptation syndrome (GAS)** The pattern followed in the physiological response to stress, consisting of the alarm, resistance, and exhaustion phases.

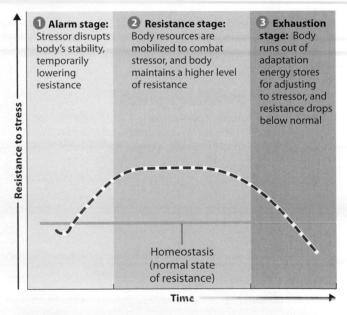

**FIGURE 3.1** The General Adaptation Syndrome (GAS) The GAS describes the body's method of coping with prolonged stress.

fear of being alone in the dark! You have just experienced the alarm phase of GAS. Also known as the **fight-or-flight response**, this physiological reaction is one of our most basic, innate survival instincts[6] (**FIGURE 3.2**).

When the mind perceives a real or imaginary stressor, the cerebral cortex, the region of the brain that interprets the nature of an event, triggers an **autonomic nervous system (ANS)** response that prepares the body for action. The ANS is the portion of the nervous system that regulates body functions that we do not normally consciously control, such as heart and glandular functions and breathing.

The ANS has two branches: sympathetic and parasympathetic. The **sympathetic nervous system** energizes the body for fight or flight by signaling the release of several key stress hormones, particularly epinephrine, norepeinephrine and cortisol. The **parasympathetic nervous system** slows systems stimulated by the stress response—in effect, it counteracts the actions of the sympathetic branch.

The sympathetic nervous system's responses to stress involves a series of biochemical exchanges between different parts of the body. The **hypothalamus**, a structure in the brain, functions as the control center of the sympathetic nervous system and determines the overall reaction to stressors. When the hypothalamus perceives that extra energy is needed to fight a stressor, it stimulates the adrenal glands, located near the top of the kidneys, to release the hormone **epinephrine**, also called *adrenaline*. Epinephrine more or less "kicks" the body into gear, causing more blood to be pumped with each beat of the heart, dilates the airways in the lungs to increase oxygen intake, increases breathing rate, stimulates the liver to release more glucose (which fuels muscular exertion), and dilates the pupils to

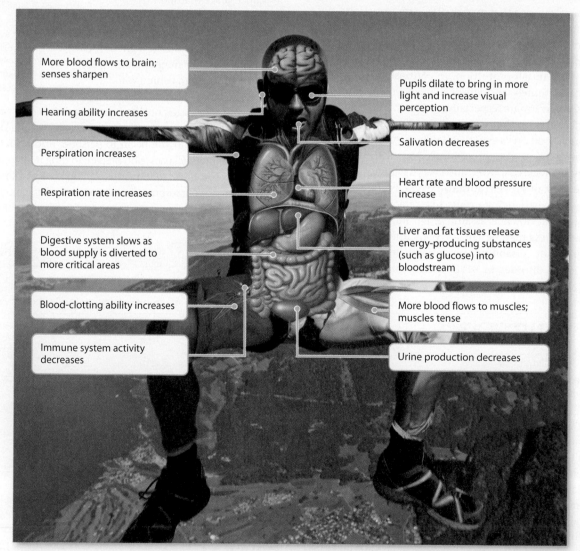

- More blood flows to brain; senses sharpen
- Hearing ability increases
- Perspiration increases
- Respiration rate increases
- Digestive system slows as blood supply is diverted to more critical areas
- Blood-clotting ability increases
- Immune system activity decreases
- Pupils dilate to bring in more light and increase visual perception
- Salivation decreases
- Heart rate and blood pressure increase
- Liver and fat tissues release energy-producing substances (such as glucose) into bloodstream
- More blood flows to muscles; muscles tense
- Urine production decreases

**FIGURE 3.2** **Fight-or-Flight: The Body's Acute Stress Response** Exposure to stress of any kind causes a complex series of involuntary physiological responses.

→ **VIDEO TUTOR**
Body's Stress Response

improve visual sensitivity. In addition to the fight-or-flight response, the alarm phase can trigger a longer-term reaction to stress. The hypothalamus uses chemical messages to trigger the pituitary gland within the brain to release a powerful hormone, *adrenocorticotropic hormone (ACTH)*. ACTH signals the adrenal glands to release **cortisol**, a key hormone that makes stored nutrients more readily available to meet energy demands. Finally, other parts of the brain and body release *endorphins*, which can relieve the pain and anxiety that a stressor may cause.

**Resistance Phase** In the resistance phase of the GAS, the body tries to return to homeostasis by resisting the alarm responses. However, because some perceived stressor still exists, the body does not achieve complete calm or rest. Instead, the body stays activated or aroused at a level that causes a higher metabolic rate in some organ tissues.

**Exhaustion Phase** In the exhaustion phase of the GAS, the hormones, chemicals, and systems that trigger and maintain the stress response are depleted, and the body returns to balance. You may feel tired or drained as your body returns to normal. In situations where stress is *chronic*, triggers may reverberate in the body, keeping body systems at a heightened arousal state. The prolonged effort to adapt to the stress response leads to **allostatic load**, or exhaustive wear and tear on the body. As the body adjusts to chronic unresolved stress, the adrenal glands continue to release cortisol, which remains in the bloodstream for longer periods of time as a result of slower metabolic responsiveness. Over time, cortisol can reduce **immunocompetence**—the ability of the immune system to respond to attack—as well as increase risk of diabetes, cardiovascular disease (CVD), and other chronic diseases.[7]

## Do Men and Women Respond Differently to Stress?

Ever since Walter Cannon's landmark studies in the 1930s, it's been thought that humans as well as many species of animals respond similarly to stressful events. However, newer research indicates that men and women may actually respond very differently to stressors. While men may be prone to fighting or fleeing, women may be more likely to "tend and befriend" by befriending the enemy or obtaining social support from others to ease stress-related reactions.[8] Many believe that neurotransmitter oxytocin is key to the *tend and befriend* female response to stress.[9] In a large study, those receiving a nasal spray containing oxytocin appeared more trusting than those in the placebo group. According

to a recent Australian study, a gene known as *SRY* may prime males to secrete more stress-related hormones and be more aggressive than women.[10] Other studies point to the fact that males and females may differ in their in stress responses based on the way they perceive stressful events.[11]

## LO 3 | PHYSICAL EFFECTS OF STRESS

Examine the physical health risks that may occur with chronic stress.

Researchers have only recently begun to untangle the complex web of responses that can take a toll on a person's physical, intellectual, and emotional well-being. Stress is often described as a "disease of prolonged arousal" that leads to a cascade of negative health effects. Some warning symptoms of prolonged stress are shown in **FIGURE 3.3**.

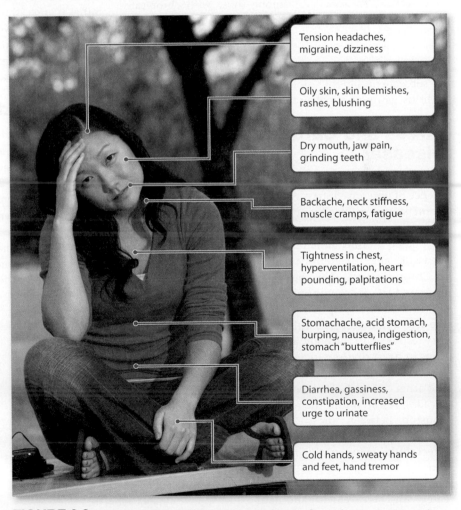

Tension headaches, migraine, dizziness

Oily skin, skin blemishes, rashes, blushing

Dry mouth, jaw pain, grinding teeth

Backache, neck stiffness, muscle cramps, fatigue

Tightness in chest, hyperventilation, heart pounding, palpitations

Stomachache, acid stomach, burping, nausea, indigestion, stomach "butterflies"

Diarrhea, gassiness, constipation, increased urge to urinate

Cold hands, sweaty hands and feet, hand tremor

**FIGURE 3.3** **Common Physical Symptoms of Stress** Sometimes you may not even notice how stressed you are until your body starts sending you signals. Do you frequently experience any of these physical symptoms of stress?

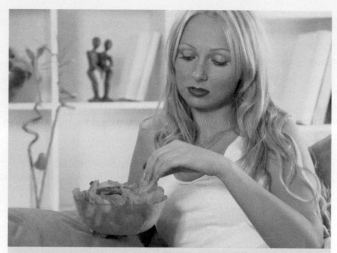
High stress levels may increase cortisol levels in the bloodstream, increasing hunger and encouraging stress eating.

The higher the levels of stress you experience and the longer that stress continues, the greater the likelihood of damage to your physical health.[12] A recent international study indicated a universal tendency toward negative health consequences among those with chronically high stress in their lives.[13] Specifically, the more traumatic life events a person experiences, the greater the risk of a wide range of subsequent illnesses, including cardiovascular diseases, arthritis, gastrointestinal disorders, and others.[14]

**psychoneuroimmunology (PNI)** The study of the interrelationship between mind and body on immune system functioning.

## Stress and Cardiovascular Disease

Perhaps the most studied and documented health consequence of unresolved stress is cardiovascular disease (CVD). A recent summary of accumulated knowledge indicates that chronic stress plays a significant role in heart rate problems, high blood pressure, atherosclerosis, as well as increased risk for a wide range of cardiovascular diseases.[15]

Chronic stress has been linked to increased arterial plaque buildup due to elevated cholesterol, hardening of the arteries, increases in inflammatory responses in the body, alterations in heart rhythm, increased and fluctuating blood pressures, and other CVD risks.[16] In recent decades, research into the relationship between stress and CVD contributors has shown direct links between the incidence and progression of CVD and stressors such as job strain, caregiving, bereavement, and natural disasters.[17] (For more on CVD, see Chapter 12.)

## Stress and Weight Gain

Are you a *"stress"* or *"emotional eater"*? Do you run for the refrigerator when you are under pressure or feeling anxious or down? If you think that when you are extremely stressed, you tend to eat more and gain weight, you didn't imagine it. Higher stress levels may increase cortisol levels in the bloodstream, which contributes to increased hunger and seems to activate fat-storing enzymes. Animal and human studies, including those in which subjects suffer from post-traumatic stress, seem to support the theory that cortisol plays a role in laying down extra belly fat and increasing eating behaviors.[18]

## Stress and Hair Loss: A Little Known Fact

Too much stress can lead to thinning hair, and even baldness, in men and women. The most common type of stress-induced hair loss is *telogen effluvium*. Often seen in individuals who have lost a loved one or experienced severe weight loss or other trauma, this condition pushes colonies of hair into a resting phase. Over time, hair begins to fall out. A similar stress-related condition known as *alopecia areata* occurs when stress triggers white blood cells to attack and destroy hair follicles, usually in patches.[19]

## Stress and Diabetes

Controlling stress levels is critical for preventing development of type 2 diabetes, as well as for successful short- and long-term diabetes management.[20] People under lots of stress often don't get enough sleep, don't eat well, and may drink or take other drugs to help them get through a stressful time. All of these behaviors can alter blood sugar levels and appear to increase the risks of type 2 diabetes.[21] Stress hormones may affect blood glucose levels directly.[22] (For more, see **Focus On: Minimizing Your Risk for Diabetes** beginning on page 386.)

## WHY SHOULD I CARE?

Compelling evidence links stress and immune system functioning. Exposure to academic stressors and self-reported stress are associated with increased upper respiratory tract infection among students. If you spend exam week in a state of high stress, sleeping too little and worrying a lot, chances are you will reduce your body's ability to fight off cold and flu viruses. Take time to de-stress, and you might avoid that bad cold.

## Stress and Digestive Problems

Digestive disorders are physical conditions for which causes are often unknown. It is widely assumed that an underlying illness, pathogen, injury, or inflammation is already present when stress triggers nausea, vomiting, stomach cramps and gut pain, or diarrhea. Although stress doesn't directly cause these symptoms, it is clearly related and may actually make your risk of having symptoms worse.[23] For example, people with depression or anxiety, or who feel tense, angry, or overwhelmed, are more susceptible to dehydration, inflammation, and other digestive problems.[24]

## Stress and Impaired Immunity

A growing area of scientific investigation known as **psycho-neuroimmunology (PNI)** analyzes the intricate relationship between the mind's response to stress and the immune system's ability to function effectively. Several recent research reviews suggest that too much stress over a long period can negatively affect various aspects of the cellular immune response. This increases risks for upper respiratory infections and certain chronic conditions, increases adverse fetal development and birth outcomes, and exacerbates problems for children and adults suffering from post-traumatic stress.[25] More prolonged stressors, such as the loss of a loved one, caregiving, living with a handicap, and unemployment, also have been shown to impair the natural immune response over time.[26]

## LO 4 | STRESS AND YOUR MENTAL HEALTH

**Examine the intellectual and psychological health risks that may occur due to high levels of stress.**

In a recent national survey of college students, over half (51.4 percent) of the respondents said that they felt overwhelmed by all that they had to do within the past 2 weeks, with a similar number reporting they felt exhausted.[27] Nearly 44 percent of students said they had experienced a larger than average amount of stress, and another 11 percent said they had experienced tremendous stress during the past year.[28] Not surprisingly, these same students rated stress as their number one impediment to academic performance. Stress can play a huge role in whether students stay in school, get good grades, and succeed on their career path. It can also wreak havoc on students' ability to concentrate, understand, and retain information.

## Stress, Memory, and Concentration

Although the exact ways stress affects grades and job performance are complex, new research provides possible clues. Animal studies suggest glucocorticoids—stress hormones released from the adrenal cortex—may affect cognitive functioning and overall mental health. In humans, memory is impaired when acute stress bombards the brain with hormones and neurotransmitters— affecting the way we think, make decisions, and respond in stressful situations.[29] Recent laboratory studies have linked prolonged exposure to cortisol to actual shrinking of the hippocampus, the brain's major memory center.[30] Other research indicates that prolonged exposure to high levels of stress hormones may actually predispose women, in particular, to Alzheimer's disease. More research is needed to determine the validity of these theories.[31]

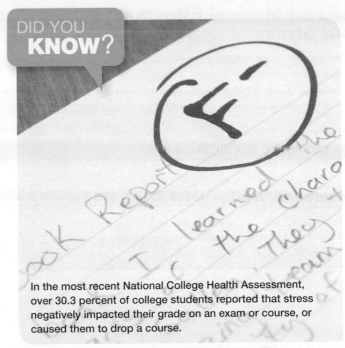

DID YOU **KNOW**?

In the most recent National College Health Assessment, over 30.3 percent of college students reported that stress negatively impacted their grade on an exam or course, or caused them to drop a course.

**Source:** Data are from American College Health Association, *American College Health Association–National College Health Assessment II (ACHA-NCHA II): Reference Group Data Report Spring 2014* (Hanover, MD: American College Health Association, 2014).

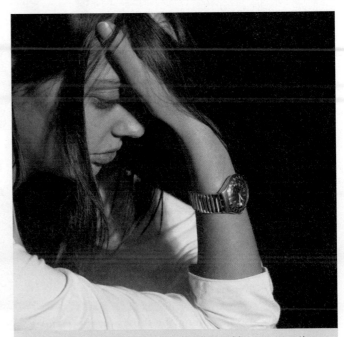

Stress and depression have complicated interconnections based on emotional, physiological, and biochemical processes. Prolonged stress can trigger depression in susceptible people, and prior periods of depression can leave individuals more susceptible to stress.

# Psychological Effects of Stress

Stress may be one of the single greatest contributors to mental disability and emotional dysfunction in industrialized nations. Studies have shown that rates of mental disorders, particularly depression and anxiety, are associated with various environmental stressors from childhood through adulthood, including violence and abuse, marital and relationship conflict, and poverty.[32]

## LO 5 | WHAT CAUSES STRESS?

**Discuss sources of stress and examine the unique stressors that affect young adults, particularly college students.**

On any given day, we all experience eustress and distress from a wide range of sources. The American Psychological Association conducts one of the most comprehensive studies examining sources of stress among various populations annually. The 2014 survey found that concerns over money, work, family responsibilities, and health were the biggest reported causes of stress for American adults (**FIGURE 3.4**).[33] College students, in particular, face stressors from internal sources, as well as external pressures to succeed in a competitive environment. Awareness of the sources of stress can do much to help you develop a plan to avoid, prevent, or control stressors.

## Psychosocial Stressors

*Psychosocial stressors* refer to the factors in our social and physical environments that cause us to experience stress. Key psychosocial stressors include adjustment to change, hassles, interpersonal relationships, academic and career pressures, frustrations and conflicts, overload, and stressful environments.

**Adjustment to Change** Any change to your routine can result in stress. Unfortunately, although your first days on campus can be exciting, they can also be among the most stressful you will face in your life. Moving away from home, trying to fit in and make new friends, adjusting to a new schedule, and learning to live with strangers in housing that is often lacking the comforts of home can all cause sleeplessness and anxiety and keep your body in a continual fight-or-flight mode.

**Hassles: Little Things That Bug You** A growing chorus of psychologists propose that the little stressors, frustrations, and petty annoyances, known collectively as *hassles,* can eventually be just as stressful and damaging to your physical and mental health as major life changes34 Put another way, cumulative hassles add up, increasing allostatic load and resulting in wear and tear on body systems. Listening to others monopolize class time, long lines, hunting for parking, loud music while you are trying to study, and a host of other irritants can push your buttons, triggering fight-or-flight responses. A lifetime of hassles can wreak havoc on the body, triggering mental health issues, high blood pressure, and other chronic health problems.35 In addition to life and work stressors, electronic devices pose increased stress load for many. See the **Tech & Health** box for more on technostress.

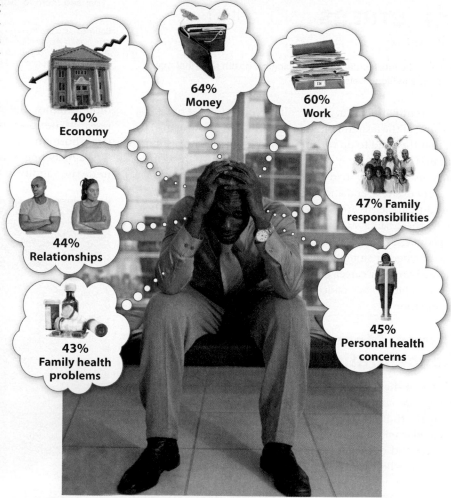

40% Economy

64% Money

60% Work

47% Family responsibilities

44% Relationships

45% Personal health concerns

43% Family health problems

**FIGURE 3.4**  What Do We Say Stresses Us?  The data above represents the percentage of American adults who reported each category as a very significant or somewhat significant source of stress in their lives. Money, work, family responsibilities, and health are the top stressors.

**Source:** Data from American Psychological Association, "Stress in America: Paying with Our Health," 2015, http://www.apa.org/news/press/releases/stress/2014/stress-report.pdf

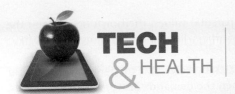

# TECH & HEALTH

# TECHNOSTRESS AND TAKING TIME TO UNPLUG

C an you disconnect totally from your smart phone or other device for a day, or would you nervously long to check it? If you are someone who is always connected and finds that even an hour unplugged in class is too much, you may need to reconsider your priorities. *High-frequency cell phone use* is on the rise, and with it comes a variety of problems. According to a new study, college students who can't keep their hands off their mobile devices are reporting higher levels of anxiety, less satisfaction with life, and lower grades than peers who use their devices less often. The average student surveyed spent nearly 5 hours per day using their cell phones for everything from calling and texting (over 77 messages/day), tweeting, checking Facebook, sending e-mails, gaming, and more. Surprised?

Today, the media has a veritable dictionary of words describing the potential negative effects of too much time on social media and other sites. *Technostress* refers to stress created by a dependence on technology and the constant state of connection, which can include a perceived obligation to respond, chat, or tweet. Some have likened this obsessive desire to check in, tweet, text, or "like" to a form of *technology addiction,* whereby individuals may check their phones 35–50 times on an average day, even waking in the night to respond. Such obsessive behavior can sap energy, lead to insomnia/sleep disorders, damage relationships and normal in-person

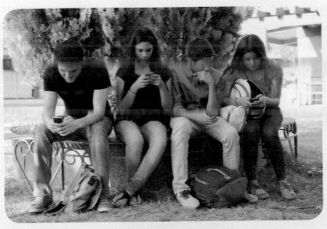

Technology may keep you in touch, but it can also add to your stress and take you away from real-world interactions.

relationships, as well as hurt grades. These negative consequences, known as *iDisorders* are on the rise, along with the surge in smart technology across the globe. If you find yourself in an unhealthy relationship with your smartphone or tablet, it may be time to unplug. Here are some tips that may help:

- **Schedule screen time.** Set time aside to check e-mail, text messages, and Twitter feeds, like once in the morning and once in the evening for no more than a half hour. Resist the urge to check if you're outside your set time frame. NO reading messages in the middle of the night!

- **Unfriend the annoying and offensive.** Lighten your load by focusing only on those who really matter to you and add to your day in a positive way.

- **Connect with your friends in real-time.** Socialize with friends in person

rather than spending hours commenting and scrolling through their Facebook pages.

- **Don't overshare.** Refrain from sharing intimate photos or details of your love life.

- **Power devices down.** Turn off all your devices completely (not just silent mode) when you're driving, in class, at work, in bed, having dinner with friends, or on vacation.

**Sources:** S. Deatherage, H. Servaty-Seib, and I. Aksoz, "Stress, Coping and the Internet Use of College Students," *Journal of American Health* 62, no. 1 (2014): 40–46; Y. Lee et al., "The Dark Side of Smartphone Usage: Psychological Traits, Compulsive Behavior and Technostress," *Computers in Human Behavior* 31 (2014): 373–81; A. Lepp, J. Barkley, and A. Karpinski, "The Relationship between Cell Phone Use, Academic Performance, Anxiety, and Satisfaction with Life in College Students," *Computers in Human Behavior* 31 (2014): 343–50; M. Salahan and A. Negahban, "Social Networking on Smartphones: When Mobile Phone Use Becomes Addictive," *Computers in Human Behavior* 29, no. 6 (2013): 2632–39; L. D. Rosen et al., "Is Facebook Creating 'iDisorders'? The Link between Clinical Symptoms of Psychiatric Disorders and Technology Use, Attitudes and Anxiety," *Computers in Human Behavior* 29, no. 3 (2013): 1243–54, Available at http://dx.doi.org/10.1016/j.chb.2012.11.012; NIH Medline Plus, "Avid Cellphone Use by College Kids Tied to Anxiety, Lower Grades," December 2013, www.nlm.nih.gov/;medlineplus/news/fullstory_143389.html; A. Lepp, T. Barkley, and A. Karpinski, "The Relationship between Cell Phone Use, Academic Performance, Anxiety and Satisfaction with Life in College Students," *Computers in Human Behavior* 31 (2014): 343–50.

## The Toll of Relationships

Let's face it, relationships can trigger some of the biggest fight-or-flight reactions of all. Although romantic relationships are the ones we often think of first, relationships with friends, family, and coworkers can be sources of struggle as easily as support. In addition, job insecurity, jobs with high demands and low control, jobs where there is conflict among coworkers and between workers and management, and jobs with unrelenting performance expectations increase the risks of a wide range of health problems.[36] Competition for rewards and systems that favor certain classes of employees or pit workers against one another are among the most stressful job situations.

## Academic and Financial Pressure

College and university students face a number of difficulties managing ever-increasing tuition, housing, and general expenses of

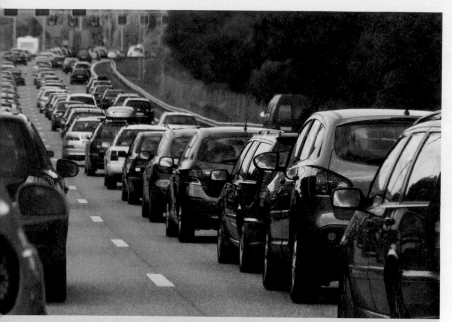

Traffic jams and noise pollution are examples of daily hassles that can add up and jeopardize our health.

among parental values, their own beliefs, and the beliefs of others different from themselves.

**Overload** We've all experienced times in our lives when the demands of work, responsibilities, deadlines, and relationships all seem to be pulling us underwater. **Overload** occurs when we are overextended and, try as we might, there are not enough hours in the day to do everything. Students suffering from overload may experience depression, sleeplessness, mood swings, frustration, anxiety, or a host of other symptoms. Binge drinking and high consumption of junk food—often coping strategies for stress overload—catch many in a downward spiral as their negative behaviors actually add to their stress load. Unrelenting stress and overload can lead to a state of physical and mental exhaustion known as **burnout**.

**Stressful Environments** For many students, living environment causes significant levels of stress. Perhaps you cannot afford safe, healthy housing, a bad roommate constantly makes life uncomfortable, or loud neighbors keep you up at night. Noise, pressure of people in crowded living situations, and

college life. Many must hold jobs to stay afloat, and some incur huge student loan debt. Finances surface as a major cause of stress for most students.[37] (For tips on how to head off some financial stressors before they start, see **Focus On: Improving Your Financial Health** on page 25.)

**Frustrations and Conflicts** Whenever there is a disparity between our goals (what we hope to obtain in life) and our behaviors (actions that may or may not lead to these goals), frustration can occur. Conflicts occur when we are forced to decide among competing motives, impulses, desires, and behaviors (for example, to party or study) or when we are forced to face pressures or demands that are incompatible with our own values and sense of importance (for example, get good grades or compete in college athletics). College students may face a variety of conflicts

**overload** A condition in which a person feels overly pressured by demands.

**burnout** A state of physical and mental exhaustion resulting from unrelenting stress.

# 55%
OF COLLEGE STUDENTS SAY THAT THEY HAVE EXPERIENCED MORE THAN AVERAGE TO TREMENDOUS LEVELS OF **STRESS** DURING THE LAST 12-MONTH PERIOD.

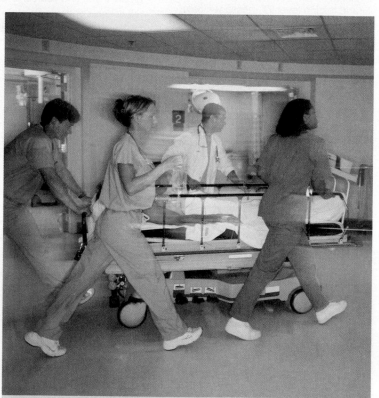

Certain jobs can be especially stressful, particularly those where the stakes are high and coworkers have little control over many outcomes. Individuals such as doctors and nurses face long work hours and a high-stakes work environment that make them especially prone to stress, overload, and burnout.

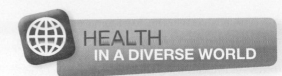
International students experience unique adjustment issues related to language barriers, cultural barriers, financial issues, and a lack of social support, among other challenges. Academic stress may pose a particular problem for the nearly 886,054 international students who left their native countries to study in the United States in 2013–2014. Accumulating evidence suggests that emotional support from others, on-campus socialization opportunities, and strong host networks are particularly effective ways for students to cope with stressful aculturation issues. Yet, many international students refrain from doing so because of cultural norms, feelings of shame, and the belief that seeking support is a sign of weakness that calls inappropriate attention to both the individual and the respective ethnic group. This reluctance, coupled with language barriers, cultural conflicts, loneliness, and the pressure to succeed, can lead international students to suffer significantly more stress-related illnesses than their American counterparts.

**Language barriers, cultural conflicts, racial prejudices, and a reluctance to seek social support all contribute to a significantly higher rate of stress-related illnesses among international students studying in the United States.**

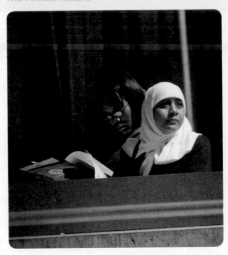

Many universities are responding to this extra stress by hosting stress management workshops each term that are geared toward the needs of international students and that encourage them to

share stress management techniques from their home countries. Both American and international students can help each other reduce stress with simple actions: Share companionship and communication, and lend a helping hand. To paraphrase a popular Hindu proverb: "Help thy neighbor's boat across and thine own boat will also reach the shore."

**Sources:** K. Cokley, et al. "An Examination of the Impact of Minority Status Stress and Imposter Feelings on the Mental Health of Diverse Ethnic Minority College Students," *Journal of Multicultural Counseling and Development* 41, no. 2 (2013): 82–93; P. Hoffman, *Examining Factors of Acculturative Stress on International Students as They Affect Utilization of Campus-Based Health and Counseling Services at Four-Year Public Universities in Ohio,* doctoral dissertation, Ohio State University, 2010; E. Gomez, A. Ursua, and C. R. Glass, "International Student Adjustment to College: Social Networks, Acculturation and Leisure," *Journal of Parks and Recreation* 32, no. 1 (2014), http://js.sagamorepub.com/jpra/article/view/2972; Institute of International Education, "Open Doors: Record Numbers of International Students in U.S. Higher Education," November 17, 2014, www.iie.org/Who-We-Are/News-and-Events/Press-Center/Press-Releases/2014/2014-11-17-Open-Doors-Data

---

uncertainties over food and housing can keep even the most resilient person on edge.

Natural disasters can cause tremendous stress initially and for years later. Typhoons and hurricanes, earthquakes and tsunamis, killer tornadoes, as well as human disasters such as the Gulf Oil Spill, terrorist attacks, and the devastation of war have disrupted millions of lives and damaged ecosystems. Even after the initial images of suffering pass and the crisis has subsided, shortages of vital resources such as gasoline, clean water, food, housing, health care, sewage disposal, and other necessities, as well as electricity outages and transportation problems, can wreak havoc in local communities and on campuses.

**Background distressors** in the environment, such as noise, air, and water pollution; allergy-aggravating pollen and dust; unsafe food; or

### WHAT DO YOU THINK?

Do you get stressed out by things in your home or school environment?

- Which environmental stressors bug you the most?
- When you encounter these environmental stressors, what actions do you take, if any?

environmental tobacco smoke can also be incredibly stressful. As with other challenges, our bodies respond to environmental distressors with the GAS. People who cannot escape background distressors may exist in a constant resistance phase.

**Bias and Discrimination** Racial and ethnic diversity of students, faculty members, and staff enriches everyone's educational experience on campus. It also challenges us to examine our personal attitudes, beliefs, and biases. Today's campuses include a diverse cultural base of vastly different life experiences, languages, and customs. Bias and discrimination based on race, ethnicity, religious affiliation, age, sexual orientation, or other "differences"—whether in viewpoints, appearance, behaviors, or backgrounds—can take the form of bigotry, insensitivity, harassment, hostility, or simply ignoring a person or group.[38] See **Health in a Diverse World** for more on stress and international students.

> **background distressors**
> Environmental stressors of which people are often unaware.

# LO 6 | INDIVIDUAL FACTORS THAT AFFECT YOUR STRESS RESPONSE

Explain key individual factors that may influence whether or not a person is able to cope with stressors

Although stress can come from the environment and external sources, it can also be a result of internal or individual factors; the "baggage" that we carry with us from a lifetime of real and perceived experiences. Low self-esteem, negative appraisal, lack of self-compassion, fears and anxiety, narcissistic tendencies, and other learned behaviors and coping mechanisms can increase stress levels.

## Appraisal

A lot of times, our **appraisal** of life's demands, not the demands themselves, result in experiences of stress. Appraisal is defined as the interpretation and evaluation of information provided to the brain by the senses. As new information becomes available, appraisal helps us recognize stressors, evaluate them based on past experiences and emotions, and decide whether we can cope. When you feel that the stressors of life are overwhelming and you lack control, you are more likely to feel strain and distress.

**appraisal** The interpretation and evaluation of information provided to the brain by the senses.

**suicidal ideation** A desire to die and thoughts about suicide.

**hostility** The cognitive, affective, and behavioral tendencies toward anger, distrust, and cynicism.

## Self-Esteem and Self-Efficacy

Recall that *self-esteem* refers to your sense of self-worth; how you judge yourself in comparison to others. Research with adolescents and young adults indicates that high stress and low self-esteem significantly predict **suicidal ideation**, a desire to die and thoughts about suicide. Fortunately, research has shown that you can improve your ability to cope with stress by increasing self-esteem.[39] (In Chapter 2 we discussed several ways to develop and maintain self-esteem.)

While a healthy dose of self-esteem has long been regarded as necessary for mental health, new research also points to a potential dark side to self-esteem: the feeling that it's unacceptable to be *average*.[40] Critics of the self-esteem movement point to the fact that today's college students have the highest level of

narcissism ever recorded and that the quest to have thousands of "friends" on Facebook or huge twitter followings can be huge stressors.[41] Environments where individuals are always compared to others as indicators of self-worth may in fact contribute to more elitism, more bullying in a quest for power, more prejudice between groups, and a host of other negative self-esteem behaviors.

Research has shown that people with high levels of confidence in their skills and ability to cope with life's challenges tend to feel more in control of stressful situations and, as such, report fewer stress effects.[42] Self-efficacy is considered one of the most important personality traits that influences psychological and physiological stress responses.[43] Developing self-efficacy is also vital to coping with and overcoming academic pressures and worries.[44] High test anxiety has been shown to account for up to 15 percent of the variance in student performance on exams.[45] By learning to handle test anxiety, research suggests that your confidence may increase and test scores will improve, leading to improved performance overall.[46] Tips on how to deal with test-taking anxiety and build your testing self-efficacy, can be found in the **Skills for Behavior Change** box. (For more on self-efficacy, see Chapters 1 and 2.)

## Type A and Type B Personalities

It should come as no surprise that personality can have an impact on whether you are happy and socially well-adjusted or sad and socially isolated. But personality may also be a critical factor in stress levels, as well as in your risk for CVD, cancer, and other chronic and infectious diseases.

In 1974, physicians Meyer Friedman and Ray Rosenman published a book indicating that Type A individuals had a greatly increased risk of heart disease due to increased physiological reactivity and prolonged activation of the stress response, including increased heart rate and blood pressure.[47] *Type A* personalities have historically been defined as hard-driving, competitive, time-driven perfectionists. In contrast, *Type B* personalities are described as being relaxed, noncompetitive, and more tolerant of others.

Today, most researchers recognize that none of us are wholly Type A or Type B; we may exhibit either type in selected situations. In addition, recent research indicates that not all Type A people experience negative health consequences; in fact, some Type A individuals thrive on their supercharged lifestyles. Often Type A's who exhibit a "toxic core," that is,

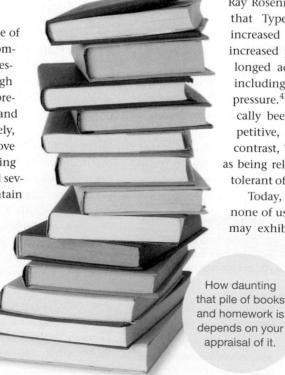

How daunting that pile of books and homework is depends on your appraisal of it.

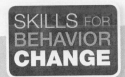

## SKILLS FOR BEHAVIOR CHANGE

### OVERCOMING TEST-TAKING ANXIETY

Testing well is a skill needed in college and beyond. Try these tips on your next exam.

**Before the Exam**

▶ Manage your study time. Keep up with reading during the term. Make sure your preparation for the test is a review rather than an initial reading of material. Don't wait until the last minute to cram. At least 1 week before your test, start studying for a set amount of time each day. Do a limited review the night before, get a good night's sleep, and arrive for the exam early.

▶ Think about how much time you might need to answer different types of test questions. If you know how much time will be available for the test, make a general strategy for using the time that you can and quickly refine at the beginning of the test.

▶ Eat a balanced meal before the exam. Avoid sugar and rich or heavy foods, as well as foods that might upset your stomach. You want to feel your best.

▶ Wear a watch to class on the day of the test, in case there is no clock.

**During the Exam**

▶ Manage your time during the test. Look at how many questions there are and what each is worth. Prioritize the high-point questions, allow a certain amount of time for each, and make sure that you leave some time for the rest. Hold to this schedule.

▶ Slow down and pay attention. Focus on one question at a time. Check off each part of multipart questions to make sure your answers are complete.

who have disproportionate amounts of anger, distrust, and a cynical, glass-half-empty approach to life—a set of characteristics referred to as **hostility**—are at increased risk for heart disease.[48]

## Type C and Type D Personalities

In addition to CVD, personality types have often been linked to increased risk for a variety of other illnesses. A type commonly discussed is the *Type C* personality, characterized as stoic, with a tendency to stuff feelings down and conform to the wishes of others. Preliminary research suggests that Type C individuals may be more susceptible to illnesses such as asthma, multiple sclerosis, autoimmune disorders, and cancer; however, more research is necessary to support this relationship.[49]

A more recently identified personality type is *Type D* (distressed), which is characterized by a tendency toward excessive negative worry, irritability, gloom, and social inhibition. Several recent studies have indicated that Type D people may be up to eight times more likely to die of a heart attack or sudden death.[50]

## Psychological Hardiness

While several internal factors seem to predispose individuals to excess stress; others seem to be protective and reduce stress. According to psychologist Susanne Kobasa, **psychological hardiness** is the key to reducing self-imposed stress associated with Type A behavior.[51] Psychologically, hardy people are characterized by *control, commitment,* and willingness to embrace *challenge.* People with a sense of *control* are able to accept responsibility for their behaviors and work to change situations they discover to be debilitating. People with a sense of *commitment* have healthy self-esteem and know their purpose in life. Those who embrace *challenge* see change as a stimulating opportunity for personal growth.

## Psychological Resilience

Today the concept of hardiness has evolved to include a person's ability to cope with stress and adversity.[52] As such, it has become common for people to think of this general hardiness concept in terms of **psychological resilience**. Essentially, resilience refers to our capacity to maintain or regain psychological well-being in the face of challenge.[53] Resilient individuals are able to respond well to adversity as they often have resources and supportive social networks reflective of good overall mental health and social development.[54]

**psychological hardiness** A personality trait characterized by control, commitment, and the embrace of challenge.

**psychological resilience** The capacity to maintain or regain psychological well-being in the face of adversity, trauma, tragedy, threats, or significant sources of stress.

**shift and persist** A strategy of reframing appraisals of current stressors and focusing on a meaningful future that protects a person from the negative effects of too much stress.

## Shift and Persist

Some young people who face extreme poverty, abuse, and unspeakable living conditions as they grow up seem to thrive, despite bleak conditions. Why? An emerging body of sociological research proposes that in the midst of extreme, persistent adversity, young people—often with the help of positive role models in their lives—are able to reframe appraisals of current stressors more positively (*shifting*), while *persisting* in focusing on the future. This outlook enables people to endure the present by adapting, holding on to meaningful things in their lives, and staying optimistic and positive. These "**shift and persist**" strategies are among the most recently identified factors that protect against the negative effects of stress in our lives.[55]

## LO 7 | MANAGING STRESS IN COLLEGE

Explore stress-management and stress-reduction strategies, ways you can cope more effectively with stress, and ways you can enrich your life experiences to protect against the effects of stress.

College students thrive under a certain amount of stress; however, excessive stress can leave them overwhelmed and unable to cope. Recent studies of college students indicate that the emotional health self-rating of first-year college students compared to their peers is at an all-time low, with increasing numbers frequently feeling overwhelmed. Students spend more time studying and less time socializing with friends, and nearly 10 percent report that they are frequently depressed.[56] In contrast, sophomores and juniors reported fewer problems with these issues, and seniors reported the fewest problems. This may indicate students' progressive emotional growth through experience, maturity, increased awareness of support services, and more social connections.[57]

Although you can't eliminate all life stressors, you can train yourself to recognize the events that cause stress and to

**coping** Managing events or conditions to lessen the physical or psychological effects of excess stress.

**stress inoculation** Stress-management technique in which a person consciously anticipates and prepares for potential stressors.

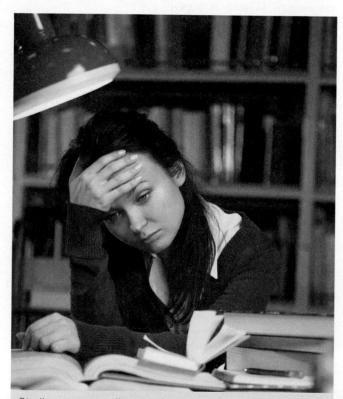
Studies suggest college students are more stressed out than other groups—the combination of new environment, peer and parent pressures, and juggling the demands of work, school, and a social life likely contribute to this phenomenon.

# ONLY ABOUT 10%

OF ADULTS REPORT TAKING ANY **ACTION** TO REDUCE THEIR STRESS LEVELS. TEENS REPORT STRIKINGLY SIMILAR RESULTS.

anticipate your reactions to them. **Coping** is the act of managing events or conditions to lessen the physical or psychological effects of excess stress.[58] One of the most effective ways to combat stressors is to build coping strategies and skills, known collectively as *stress-management techniques*.

## Practicing Mental Work to Reduce Stress

Stress management isn't something that just happens. It calls for getting a handle on what is going on in your life, taking a careful look at yourself, and coming up with a personal plan of action. Because your perceptions are often part of the problem, assessing your self-talk, beliefs, and actions are good first steps. Why are you so stressed? How much of it is due to perception rather than reality? What's a realistic plan of action for you? Think about your situation and map out a strategy for change. The tools in this section will help you.

### Assess Your Stressors and Solve Problems

Assessing what is really going on in your life is an important first step to solving problems and reducing your stress. Here's how:

- Start a journal. Track your worries and the factors that seem to trigger stress every day for 1 week. Think about when your stress is greatest, who is around you, and how you respond.
- Examine the causes. Which are tangible? Intangible?
- Consider the consequences of doing nothing versus taking action.
- List your options, including ones that you may not like very much.
- Outline an action plan, and then *act*. Remember that even little things can sometimes make a big difference and that you shouldn't expect immediate results.
- After you act, evaluate. How did you do? How do you feel about your actions? How can you change to achieve better outcomes?

One useful way of coping with your stressors is to consciously anticipate and prepare for specific ones, a technique known as **stress inoculation**. For example, if speaking in front of a class scares you, practice in front of friends or a video camera to prevent freezing up on the day of the presentation.

**Change the Way You Think and Talk to Yourself** Several types of negative self-talk exist, but among the most common are *pessimism,* or focusing on the negative; *perfectionism,* or expecting superhuman standards, "*should-ing,*" or reprimanding yourself for things that you should have done; *blaming* yourself or others for circumstances and events; and *dichotomous thinking,* in which everything is either black or white (good or bad). To combat negative self-talk, we must first become aware of it, then stop it, and finally replace the negative thoughts with positive ones—a process called **cognitive restructuring**. Once you realize that some of your thoughts may be negative, irrational, or overreactive, interrupt this self-talk by saying, "Stop" (under your breath or aloud), and make a conscious effort to think positively. See the **Skills for Behavior Change** box for other suggestions of ways to rethink your thinking habits.

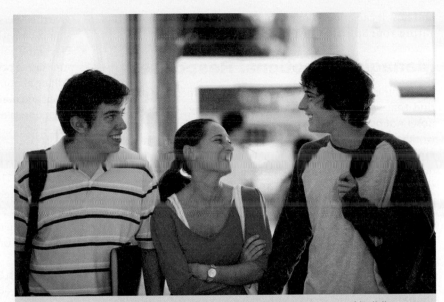
Spending time socializing face-to-face can be an important part of building a support network and reducing your stress level.

## Developing a Support Network

As you plan a stress-management program, remember the importance of social networks and social bonds. Friendships are important for inoculating yourself against harmful stressors. Studies of college students have demonstrated the importance of social support in *buffering* individuals from the effects of stress.[59]

Family members and friends can be a steady base of support when the pressures of life seem overwhelming. Additionally, most colleges and universities offer counseling services at no cost for short-term crises. Clergy, instructors, and residence hall supervisors also may be excellent resources.

In order to have a healthy social support network, we have to invest time and energy. Cultivate and nurture the relationships that matter: those built on trust, mutual acceptance and understanding, honesty, and genuine caring. If you want others to be there for you to help you cope with life's stressors, you need to be there for them. Spend more time in face-to-face interactions.

## Cultivating Your Spiritual Side

One of the most important factors in reducing stress in your life is taking the time and making the commitment to cultivate your spiritual side: finding your purpose in life and living your days more fully. Spiritual health and spiritual practices can be vital components of your support system, often linking you to a community of like-minded individuals and giving you perspective on the things that truly matter in your life. (For information on spirituality

**WHAT DO YOU THINK?**

Who are the biggest supporters in your life?

- Would you characterize them as stressed out or well-adjusted?
- Could you follow their lead if they are more relaxed?
- What tips would you give them if they're stressed?

**cognitive restructuring** The modification of thoughts, ideas, and beliefs that contribute to stress.

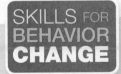

**SKILLS FOR BEHAVIOR CHANGE**

### RETHINK YOUR THINKING HABITS

▶ Reframe a distressing event from a positive perspective. For example, if you feel frustrated that you aren't the best in every class, change your perspective on the issue to highlight your strengths.

▶ Tolerate mistakes. Rather than getting upset by mishaps, evaluate what happened and learn from it. Take yourself less seriously.

▶ Break the worry habit. If you are preoccupied with what-ifs and worst-case scenarios, the following suggestions can help slow the worry drain:

  ■ If you must worry, create a 20-minute "worry period" when you can journal or talk about it each day. After that, block the worry if it pops up again.

  ■ Try to focus on what is going right, rather than what *might* go wrong.

  ■ Learn to accept what you cannot change. Each of us must learn to live with some uncertainty.

  ■ Seek help. Talk with a trusted friend or family member or make an appointment with a counselor.

and how it can affect your overall health, see **Focus On: Cultivating Your Spiritual Health,** beginning on page 60.)

# Managing Emotional Responses

Have you ever gotten all worked up about something only to find that your perceptions were totally wrong? We often get upset not by realities, but by our faulty perceptions. Social networking sites and e-mails are often perfect places for reading meaning into things that are said and perceiving issues that don't exist. Interactions where body language, voice intonation, and opportunities for clarification are present are much better for interpreting true meanings than are cryptic texts or e-mails.

Stress management requires examining your emotional responses. With any emotional response to a stressor, you are responsible for the emotion and the resulting behaviors. Learning to tell the difference between normal emotions and emotions based on irrational beliefs or expressed and interpreted in an over-the-top manner can help you stop the emotion or express it in a healthy and appropriate way.

## Fight the Anger Urge
Major sources of anger include (1) perceived *threats* to self or others we care about; (2) *reactions to injustice,* such as unfair actions, policies, or behaviors; (3) *fear,* which leads to negative responses; (4) *faulty emotional reasoning,* or misinterpretation of normal events; (5) *low frustration tolerance,* often fueled by stress, drugs, lack of sleep, and other factors; (6) *unreasonable expectations* about ourselves and others; and (7) *people rating,* or applying derogatory ratings to others.

There are three main approaches to dealing with anger: *expressing it, suppressing it,* or *calming it.* You may be surprised to find out that expressing anger is probably the healthiest thing to do in the long run, if you express anger in an assertive rather than an aggressive way. There are several strategies you can use to keep aggressive reactions at bay.[60]

- **Identify your anger style.** Do you express anger passively or actively? Do you hold anger in, or do you explode?
- **Learn to recognize patterns in your anger responses and how to de-escalate them.** For 1 week, keep track of everything that angers you or keeps you stewing. What thoughts or feelings lead up to your boiling point? Explore ways to interrupt patterns of anger, such as counting to 10, getting a drink of water, or taking some deep breaths.
- **Find the right words to de-escalate conflict.** When conflict arises, be respectful and state your needs or feelings rather than shooting zingers at the other person. Avoid "you always" or "you never" and instead say, "I feel _____ when you _____" or "I would really appreciate it if you could _____." If you find yourself continually revved up for battle, consider taking a class or workshop on assertiveness training or anger management.
- **Plan ahead.** Explore options to minimize your exposure to anger-provoking situations, such as traffic jams.
- **Vent to your friends.** Find a few close friends you trust and who can be honest with you. Allow them to listen and give their perspectives on things, but don't wear down your supporter with continual rants.
- **Develop realistic expectations of yourself and others.** Are your expectations of yourself and others realistic? Try talking about your feelings with those involved at a time when you are calm.
- **Turn complaints into requests.** When frustrated or angry with someone, try reworking the problem into a request. Instead of screaming and pounding on the wall because your neighbors are blaring music at 2:00 A.M., talk with them. Think about the words you will use, and try to reach an agreement that works for everyone.
- **Leave past anger in the past.** Learn to resolve issues and not bring them up over and over. Let it go. If you can't, seek the counsel of a professional to learn how.

## Learn to Laugh, Be Joyful, and Cry
Have you ever noticed that you feel better after a belly laugh or a good cry? Adages such as "laughter is the best medicine" and "smile and the world smiles with you" didn't come from nowhere. Humans have long recognized that actions like smiling, laughing, singing, and dancing can elevate our moods, relieve stress, and improve our relationships. Learning to take yourself less seriously is a good starting place.

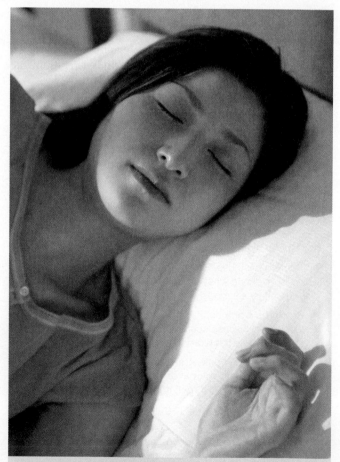

Taking care of your physical health—through quality sleep, sufficient exercise, and healthful nutrition—is a crucial component of stress management.

# HAPPINESS AND FLOURISHING
*New Strategies to Reduce Stress*

For decades, noted psychologist Martin Seligman has conducted research focused on *positive psychology* and *authentic happiness*. His work has been the framework for a new way of looking at life with a more "glass half full" perspective. His theories have carried over into new movements to help us find happiness in the face of adversity, with research supporting the idea that people who are optimistic and happier have fewer mental and physical problems. Today, Seligman takes happiness a step further, focusing on the concept of "flourishing," which consists of *positive emotion, engagement, relationships, meaning,* and *accomplishments* (PERMA). With these elements in your life, positive psychologists believe that you will flourish in all aspects of life, avoid stress, and be healthier.

- **Positive Emotion.** Share highs of the day rather than lows. Be active in complimenting others, verbalize their strengths, laugh, show appreciation, be kind. When you start to assess people in the negative, find something *good* about them. Ditch the negative thoughts!
- **Engagement.** Practice mindfulness. See, hear, touch, feel—experience your present. Live and notice the moments, rather than focusing on the past or the future. Make time for things that bring you joy, and remember to be good to others.

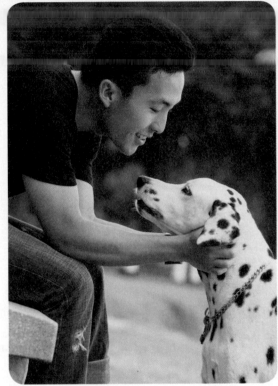

Four-legged friends can be great stress relievers as they allow you to focus on something besides yourself and can add laughter to your life.

- **Relationships.** Listen and ask questions. Connect in *person*. Look people in the eyes. Empower others to see their strengths. Hug freely. Be honest and sincere. Check in to show that you care. Acknowledge that people matter.
- **Meaning.** Think about how you would like to be remembered. Show appreciation. Give to others, and show your emotions. Renew and refresh continually. Read and explore new things.

Learn about different cultures and history. Work to help others. Improve the world. Cherish the environment.

- **Achievement.** What are the steps to achieving your goals? Try new things; don't be afraid to fail. View change as opportunity. Celebrate accomplishments. Acknowledge the good things that others do. Remember the little things that are important in your day. Give praise, and be unselfish in your support to others.

While flourishing offers an expanded approach to individual and community well-being, another group has developed the Action for Happiness movement—a ten-step set of recommendations designed to provide momentum for actions that will lead to a more positive society. Among these ten keys to happier living are the following recommendations:

- Do things for others.
- Connect with people.
- Take care of your body.
- Notice the world around you.
- Keep learning new things.
- Have goals to look forward to.
- Find ways to bounce back.
- Take a positive approach.
- Be comfortable with who you are.
- Be part of something bigger.

**Sources:** M. E. Seligman, *Flourishing: A Visionary New Understanding of Happiness and Well-Being* (New York: Free Press/Simon and Schuster, 2011); M. E. P. Seligman, *Authentic Happiness: Using the New Positive Psychology to Realize Your Potential for Lasting Fulfillment* (New York: Free Press/Simon & Schuster, 2002); Action for Happiness, "10 Keys To Happier Living," Accessed January 30, 2015, www.actionforhappiness .org/10-keys-to-happier-living

Crying can have similar positive physiological effects in relieving tension. Several preliminary studies indicate that laughter and joy may increase endorphin levels, increase oxygen levels in the blood, decrease stress levels, relieve pain, help in recovery from cardiovascular disease, improve relationships, and even reduce risks of chronic disease; however, the evidence for *long-term* effects must be validated through larger, more rigorous studies.[61] For ideas on how to find more joy and laughter in your daily life, see the **Health Headlines** box.

## Taking Physical Action

Are you often feeling sluggish and ready to nap? Or, are you feeling wired, restless, and ready to explode? Either could be the result of too much stress.

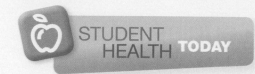
# *FENG SHUI* FOR STRESS RELIEF

Today, many space designers are trying to create peaceful "me caves" for reducing the stress of harried lives. One strategy, known as *feng shui* (translation "wind and water"), is part of an ancient Chinese art designed to restore balance of *chi* and create peace and harmony with help from the built environment. There are several feng shui tips for reducing stress in your bedroom area:

- **De-clutter.** Get rid of any extra "things" in your space. Pick up and put things away each day.
- **Paint.** Use peaceful and welcoming colors. Coordinate linens and tapestry colors to enhance warmth.

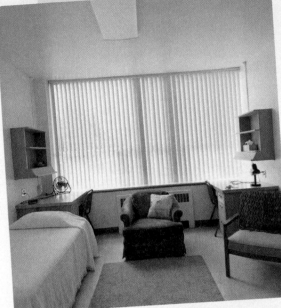

Keeping your room clear of clutter and well organized using feng shui techniques can reduce stress.

- **Relocate.** Your bed should never be in line with the door; nightstands should be balanced on either side of bed, and mirrors should *never* reflect the bed.
- **Shut out the world.** Use shades that allow you to darken or dim the room.
- **Beautify.** Include things that make you feel peaceful.
- **Invest.** Get a set of soft sheets, duvet covers, and blankets. Plump and soften pillows.
- **Refresh.** Open windows to remove stale odors. If needed, use relaxing fragrances such as lavender.
- **Block.** If you can't get rid of a desk covered in work, use a curtain to keep things out of sight. Put your phone away, and *relax*.

**Get Enough Exercise** Remember that the human stress response is intended to end in physical activity. Exercise "burns off" existing stress hormones by directing them toward their intended metabolic function.[62] Exercise can also help combat stress by raising levels of endorphins—mood-elevating, painkilling hormones—in the bloodstream, increasing energy, reducing hostility, and improving mental alertness. Still, according to a recent meta-analysis of stress and exercise research, those who would benefit most—particularly sedentary, overweight individuals—are more likely to eat when they are stressed and less likely to exercise. Motivating people unready to exercise for health and stress relief is a major challenge that could reap huge rewards.[63] (For more on the beneficial effects of exercise, see Chapter 11.)

**sympathomimetics** Food substances that can produce stresslike physiological responses.

**procrastinate** To intentionally put off doing something.

**Get Enough Sleep** Adequate amounts of sleep allow you to refresh your vital energy, cope with multiple stressors more effectively, and be productive when you need to be. In fact, sleep is one of the biggest stress busters of them all. (These benefits and others are discussed in much more depth in **Focus On: Improving Your Sleep** beginning on page 98.)

**Eat Healthfully** It is clear that eating a balanced, healthy diet can stress-proof you in ways that are not fully understood. It is also known that undereating, overeating, and eating the wrong kinds of foods can create distress in the body. In particular, avoid **sympathomimetics**, substances in foods that produce (or mimic) stresslike responses, such as caffeine. (For more information about the benefits of sound nutrition, see Chapter 9.)

## Managing Your Time

Ever put off writing a paper until the night before it was due? We all **procrastinate**, or voluntarily delay some task despite expecting to be worse off for the delay. Procrastination can result in academic difficulties, financial problems, relationship problems, and a multitude of stress-related ailments.

How can you avoid the temptation to procrastinate? According to recent research, setting clear "implementation intentions," a series of goals to accomplish toward a specific end, is key.[64] Having a plan that includes specific deadlines (and rewards for meeting deadlines) can help you stay on task. Another strategy is to get started early and set a personal end date that is well ahead of the deadline.

Keep a journal for 2 days to become aware of how you spend your time. Write down your activities every day—everything from going to class to doing your laundry to texting your friends—and the amount of time you spend doing each. What can you do to make better use of your time? Use the following time-management tips in your stress-management program:

- **Do one thing at a time.** Don't multitask. Instead of watching TV, doing laundry, and writing your term paper all at once, pick one and stay focused.
- **Clean off your desk.** Sort your desk, tossing unnecessary paper and mail and filing the important papers in labeled folders. (For more on organizing to de-stress, see the **Student Health Today** box.)
- **Prioritize your tasks.** Make a daily "to do" list and stick to it. Categorize the things you must do today, the things that must eventually get done, and the things that it would be nice to do. Consider the "nice to do" items only if you finish the others (or if they include something fun).
- **Find a clean, comfortable place to work, and avoid interruptions.** Schedule uninterrupted time for work. Don't answer the phone; close your door and post a "Do Not Disturb" sign; or go to a quiet room in the library or student union.
- **Reward yourself for work completed.** When you finish a task, do something nice for yourself. Rest breaks give you time to recharge.
- **Work when you're at your best.** If you're a morning person, study and write papers in the morning, and take breaks when you start to slow down.
- **Break overwhelming tasks into small pieces, and allocate a certain amount of time to each.** If you are floundering in a task, move on and come back to it when you're refreshed.
- **Remember that time is precious.** Many people learn to value their time only when they face a terminal illness. Try to value each day. If you have trouble saying no to people and projects that steal your time, see the **Skills for Behavior Change** box for some suggestions.

## Consider Downshifting

Today's lifestyles are hectic, and stress often comes from trying to keep up. Many people are questioning whether "having it all" is worth it, and are working to simplify their lives. This trend has been labeled **downshifting**, or

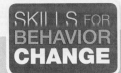

### SKILLS FOR BEHAVIOR CHANGE

## LEARN TO SAY NO AND MEAN IT!

Is your calendar so full you barely have time to breathe? When you are asked to do something you don't really want to do or are overextended, practice the following tips to avoid overcommitment:

▶ **Be sympathetic, but firm.** Explain that although you think it's a great cause or idea, you can't participate right now. Don't waver if they persist or pressure you.

▶ **Don't say you want to think about it and will get back to them.** This only leads to more forceful requests later.

▶ **Don't give in to guilt.** Stick to your guns. Remember you don't owe anyone your time.

▶ **Even if something sounds good, avoid spontaneous "yes" responses.** Make a rule that you will take at least a day to think about committing your time.

▶ **Schedule time for yourself first.** If you don't have time for the things you love to do, stop and prioritize your activities. Don't let your time be sucked up by things that you really don't want to do.

*voluntary simplicity*. Moving out of the big city and into smaller homes in smaller towns, giving up high-stress jobs for ones you enjoy, house decluttering, and making other life changes is part of downshifting.

Deciding what is most important in life, cutting down on "things" and considering your environmental footprint are part of downshifting. When you contemplate any form of downshift—or perhaps even start your career this way—it's important to move slowly and have a plan.

> **downshifting** Taking a step back and simplifying a lifestyle that is hectic, packed with pressure and stress, and focused on trying to keep up; also known as *voluntary simplicity*.

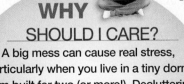

## WHY SHOULD I CARE?

A big mess can cause real stress, particularly when you live in a tiny dorm room built for two (or more!). Decluttering and throwing out garbage will not only help with stress, but it may also keep you from having to find a new roommate! It can also help your grades by allowing you to study with fewer distractions. How could you improve your study space to be more conducive to college success?

## Relaxation Techniques for Stress Management

Relaxation techniques to reduce stress have been practiced for centuries and offer opportunities for calming your nervous energy and coping with life's challenges. Some common techniques include yoga, qigong, tai chi, deep breathing, meditation, visualization, progressive muscle relaxation, massage therapy, biofeedback, and hypnosis. Newer forms of relaxation may be found in the latest technology; see the **Tech & Health** box on the next page for more information.

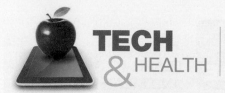

# TECH & HEALTH | APPS FOR THE RELAXATION RESPONSE

Looking for a way to relax that you can carry with you? Check out the following apps to help you de-stress.

- **Stress Check** (Free: Android, iPhone, iPod), www.azumio.com/apps/stress-check

    This nifty app has a stress gauge and heart monitor onboard. Just put your finger over your phone's camera lens, and the app will pick up your heart rate and give you readouts.

- **Nature Sounds Relax and Sleep** (Free: Android), https://play.google.com/store/apps/details?id=com.zodinplex.naturesound&hl=en

    Sounds of nature to help you relax and sleep. Select sounds that calm you, like the ocean, rain, and other sounds to help you unwind when stress keeps you awake.

- **Pocket Yoga Version 4.1.0** (Modest cost: iPhone), http://pocket-sports.com

    With three different practices designed by experienced instructors, three different levels of difficulty, and three different session durations, you can tailor the app to your needs. Both visual and voice-over instructions are included.

- **Breathe2Relax** (Modest Cost Android, iPhone, iPod, iPad), https://play.google.com/store/apps/details?id=com.meditationoasis.Breathe2&hl=en

    This relaxation tool uses guided information to help you learn and practice diaphragmatic breathing.

- **Relax and Rest Guided Meditation** (modest cost, iPhone and Android), www.amazon.com/Meditation Oasis-Relax-Rest-Meditations/dp/B0052OSTOS, itunes.apple.com/us/app/relax-rest-guided

    Guided meditations involving breathing awareness, deep meditation, and whole body meditation.

This is just a sample of the broad array of stress management and relaxation apps. And remember, technology cuts both ways. It can be a stressor if you let it. But you can also use it to help yourself deal with hassles, stressors, and beat stress.

## Yoga

Yoga is an ancient practice that combines meditation, stretching, and breathing exercises designed to relax, refresh, and rejuvenate. It began about 5,000 years ago in India and has been evolving ever since. Approximately 21 million Americans practice yoga regularly.[65] The majority of those into yoga are women between the ages of 18 and 44 who want to improve their fitness and flexibility levels, find stress relief and improve overall health

*Classical yoga* is the ancestor of nearly all modern forms of yoga. Breathing, poses, and verbal mantras are often part of classical yoga. Of the many branches of classical yoga, *Hatha yoga* is the most well-known; it is body focused, involving the practice of breath control and *asanas*—held postures and choreographed movements that enhance strength and flexibility. (Several other forms of yoga are discussed in Chapter 11.) Recent research shows increased evidence of benefits of Hatha yoga in reducing inflammation, boosting mood, increasing relaxation, and reducing stress among those who practice regularly.[66] Although studies have shown yoga to have similar benefits in treating insomnia and PTSD, reducing anxiety, lowering heart rate and blood pressure, improving fitness and flexibility, reducing pain, and other benefits, much of this research is still in its infancy and could benefit from more rigorous investigation. (See **Focus On: Cultivating Your Spiritual Health,** starting on page 60, for additional information on yoga.)

## Qigong and Tai Chi

*Qigong* (pronounced "chee-kong"), one of the fastest-growing, most widely accepted forms of mind-body health exercise, is used by some of the country's largest health care organizations, particularly for people suffering from chronic pain or stress. An ancient Chinese practice, Qigong involves awareness and control of vital body energy known as *qi* (or *chi*, pronounced "chee"). A complex system of internal pathways called *meridians* are believed to carry *qi* throughout your body. If *qi* becomes stagnant or blocked, you'll feel sluggish or powerless. Qigong incorporates a series of flowing movements, breath techniques, mental visualization exercises, and vocalizations of healing sounds that are designed to restore balance and integrate and refresh the mind and body.

Another popular form of mind-body exercise is *tai chi* (pronounced "ty-chee"), often described as "meditation in motion." Originally developed in China over 2,000 years ago, this graceful form of exercise began as a form of self-defense. Tai chi is noncompetitive, self-paced, and involves a defined series of postures or movements done in a slow, graceful manner. Each movement or posture flows into the next without pause. Tai chi has been widely practiced in China for centuries and is now becoming increasingly popular around the world, both as a basic exercise program and as a key

**SEE IT! VIDEOS**

Looking for ways to relax and reduce stress? Watch **Generation Stress: Tips for Millenials to Reduce Stress** in the Study Area of **MasteringHealth™**

component of stress reduction and balance and flexibility programs. Research demonstrating the effectiveness of these benefits is only in it's infancy.

**Diaphragmatic or Deep Breathing** Typically, we breathe using only our upper chest and thoracic region. Simply stated, diaphragmatic breathing is deep breathing that maximally fills the lungs by involving the movement of the diaphragm and lower abdomen. This technique is commonly used in yoga exercises and in other meditative practices. Try the diaphragmatic breathing exercise in **FIGURE 3.5** right now and see whether you feel more relaxed!

**Meditation** There are many different forms of **meditation**. Most involve sitting quietly for 15 to 20 minutes, focusing your thoughts, blocking the "noise" in your life, controlling breathing, and ultimately, relaxing. Practiced by Eastern religions for centuries, meditation is believed to be an important form of introspection and personal renewal. When used as an aide in de-stressing, it is believed to calm the physiological responses of stress and has been reported to reduce risks of illness. According to a recent review of key *randomized controlled trials (RCTs)* by the American Heart Association, one form of meditation, *transcendental meditation (TM)*, appeared to be most effective in lowering blood pressure, overall mortality, and CVD events. Other forms of meditation appeared to have little or no effect on these health risks.[67] More rigorous, controlled research must be done to better understand potential benefits of meditation. (Meditation and other aspects of spiritual health are discussed in detail in **Focus On: Cultivating Your Spiritual Health** beginning on page 60.) Meditation can be performed alone or in a group. Many colleges and universities offer classes on how to meditate. Check with your campus wellness center.

**Visualization** Often our thoughts and imagination provoke distress by conjuring up worst-case scenarios. Our imagination, however, can also be tapped to reduce stress. In **visualization**, you use your imagination to create calming mental scenes. The choice of mental images is unlimited, but natural settings such as ocean beaches, deep forests, and mountain lakes often conjure up soothing sights, sounds, and smells. These sensory experiences can replace

**meditation** A relaxation technique that involves deep breathing and concentration.

**visualization** The creation of mental images to promote relaxation.

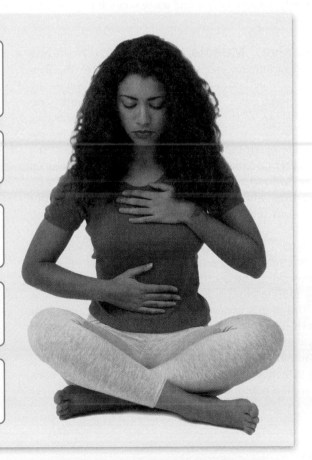

1. Assume a natural, comfortable position either sitting up straight with your head, neck, and shoulders relaxed, or lying on your back with your knees bent and your head supported. Close your eyes and loosen binding clothes.

2. In order to feel your abdomen moving as you breathe, place one hand on your upper chest and the other just below your rib cage.

3. Breathe in slowly and deeply through your nose. Feel your stomach expanding into your hand. The hand on your chest should move as little as possible.

4. Exhale slowly through your mouth. Feel the fall of your stomach away from your hand. Again, the hand on your chest should move as little as possible.

5. Concentrate on the act of breathing. Shut out external noise. Focus on inhaling and exhaling, the route the air is following, and the rise and fall of your stomach.

**FIGURE 3.5 Diaphragmatic Breathing** This exercise will help you learn to breathe deeply as a way to relieve stress. Practice this for 5 to 10 minutes several times a day, and soon diaphragmatic breathing will become natural for you.

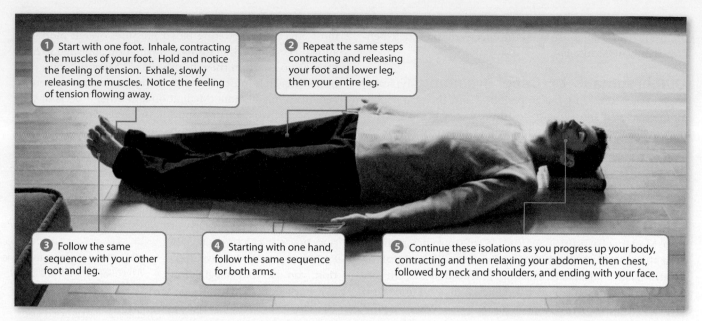

① Start with one foot. Inhale, contracting the muscles of your foot. Hold and notice the feeling of tension. Exhale, slowly releasing the muscles. Notice the feeling of tension flowing away.

② Repeat the same steps contracting and releasing your foot and lower leg, then your entire leg.

③ Follow the same sequence with your other foot and leg.

④ Starting with one hand, follow the same sequence for both arms.

⑤ Continue these isolations as you progress up your body, contracting and then relaxing your abdomen, then chest, followed by neck and shoulders, and ending with your face.

**FIGURE 3.6** **Progressive Muscle Relaxation** Sit or lie down in a comfortable position and follow the steps described to increase your awareness of tension in your body and your ability to release it.

stressful stimuli with peaceful or pleasurable thoughts. Think of a place that is "quieting" for you. Try to imagine yourself there, sitting quietly. Breathe deeply and allow yourself to be in that space/moment.

## Progressive Muscle Relaxation

Progressive muscle relaxation involves teaching awareness of the feeling of tension and release by systematically focusing on areas of the body; contracting and relaxing different muscle groups while breathing in deeply and slowly exhaling. The standard pattern is to begin with the feet and work your way up your body, contracting and releasing as you go (**FIGURE 3.6**). With practice, you can quickly identify tension in your body and consciously release that tension to calm yourself.

**biofeedback** A technique using a machine to self-monitor physical responses to stress.

## Massage Therapy

Massage not only feels great, it is also an excellent way to relax. Techniques vary from deep-tissue massage to the gentler acupressure, use of hot rocks on tense muscle groups, and a wide range of other techniques. Although a variety of studies have been carried out to assess the health effects of massage, much of this research is poorly controlled, lacks sufficient sample size, and results are preliminary or conflicting. However, there is a growing body of evidence indicating that massage may ease back pain, as well as potentially increase quality of life for cancer patients, as well as those with HIV/AIDS and depression.[68] Though promising, this research is in its infancy. (**Focus On: Understanding Complementary and Alternative Medicine,** starting on page 494, provides more information about the benefits of massage and other body-based methods such as acupressure and shiatsu.)

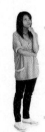

WHICH **PATH** WOULD YOU TAKE **?**

Scan the QR code to see how different stress management choices YOU make today can affect your health tomorrow.

## Biofeedback

Biofeedback is a technique in which a person learns to use the mind to consciously control bodily functions, such as heart rate, body temperature, and breathing rate. Using devices from those as simple as stress dots that change color with body temperature variation to sophisticated electrical sensors, individuals learn to listen to their bodies and make necessary adjustments, such as relaxing certain muscles, changing breathing, or concentrating to slow heart rate and relax. Eventually, individuals develop the ability to recognize and lower stress responses without machines and can practice it anywhere.

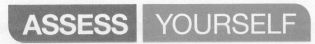

# How Stressed Are You?

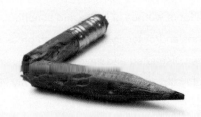

**LIVE IT!** ASSESS YOURSELF
An interactive version of this assessment is available online in **MasteringHealth**™

Let's face it: Some periods in life, including your college years, can be especially stressful! Learning to "chill" starts with an honest examination of your life experiences and your reactions to stressful situations. Respond to each section, assigning points as directed. Total the points from each section, then add them and compare them to the life-stressor scale.

## 1 Recent History

In the last year, how many of the following major life events have you experienced? (Give yourself **five points** for each event you experienced; if you experienced an event more than once, give yourself **ten points,** etc.)

1. Death of a close family member or friend     _____

2. Ending a relationship (whether by choice or not)     _____

3. Major financial upset jeopardizing your ability to stay in college     _____

4. Major move, leaving friends, family, and/or your past life behind     _____

5. Serious illness (you)     _____

6. Serious illness (of someone you're close with)     _____

7. Marriage or entering a new relationship     _____

8. Loss of a beloved pet     _____

9. Involved in a legal dispute or issue     _____

10. Involved in a hostile, violent, or threatening relationship     _____

Total _____

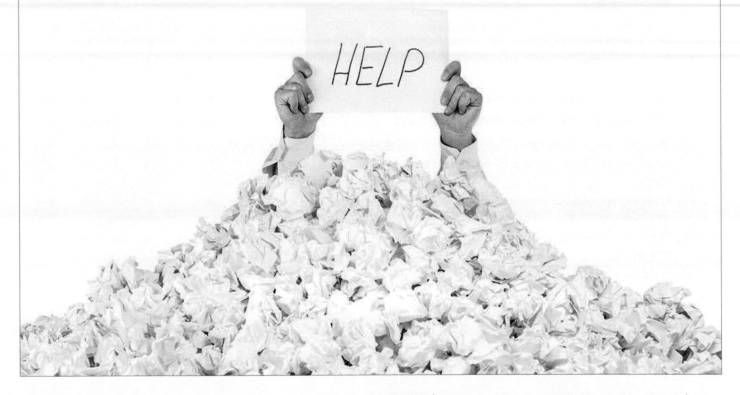

# 2 Self-Reflection

For each of the following, indicate where you are on the scale of 0 to 5.

| | | Strongly Disagree | | | | | Strongly Agree |
|---|---|---|---|---|---|---|---|
| 1. | I have a lot of worries at home and at school. | 0 | 1 | 2 | 3 | 4 | 5 |
| 2. | My friends and/or family put too much pressure on me. | 0 | 1 | 2 | 3 | 4 | 5 |
| 3. | I am often distracted and have trouble focusing on schoolwork. | 0 | 1 | 2 | 3 | 4 | 5 |
| 4. | I am highly disorganized and tend to do my schoolwork at the last minute. | 0 | 1 | 2 | 3 | 4 | 5 |
| 5. | My life seems to have far too many crisis situations. | 0 | 1 | 2 | 3 | 4 | 5 |
| 6. | Most of my time is spent sitting; I don't get much exercise. | 0 | 1 | 2 | 3 | 4 | 5 |
| 7. | I don't have enough control in decisions that affect my life. | 0 | 1 | 2 | 3 | 4 | 5 |
| 8. | I wake up most days feeling tired/like I need a lot more sleep. | 0 | 1 | 2 | 3 | 4 | 5 |
| 9. | I often have feelings that I am alone and that I don't fit in very well. | 0 | 1 | 2 | 3 | 4 | 5 |
| 10. | I don't have many friends or people I can share my feelings or thoughts with. | 0 | 1 | 2 | 3 | 4 | 5 |
| 11. | I am uncomfortable in my body, and I wish I could change how I look. | 0 | 1 | 2 | 3 | 4 | 5 |
| 12. | I am very anxious about my major and whether I will get a good job after I graduate. | 0 | 1 | 2 | 3 | 4 | 5 |
| 13. | If I have to wait in a restaurant or in lines, I quickly become irritated and upset. | 0 | 1 | 2 | 3 | 4 | 5 |
| 14. | I have to win or be the best in activities or in classes or I get upset with myself. | 0 | 1 | 2 | 3 | 4 | 5 |
| 15. | I am bothered by world events and am cynical and angry about how people behave. | 0 | 1 | 2 | 3 | 4 | 5 |
| 16. | I have too much to do, and there are never enough hours in the day. | 0 | 1 | 2 | 3 | 4 | 5 |
| 17. | I feel uneasy when I am caught up on my work and am relaxing or doing nothing. | 0 | 1 | 2 | 3 | 4 | 5 |
| 18. | I sleep with my cell phone near my bed and often check messages/tweets/texts during the night. | 0 | 1 | 2 | 3 | 4 | 5 |
| 19. | I enjoy time alone but find that I seldom get enough alone time each day. | 0 | 1 | 2 | 3 | 4 | 5 |
| 20. | I worry about whether or not others like me. | 0 | 1 | 2 | 3 | 4 | 5 |
| 21. | I am struggling in my classes and worry about failing. | 0 | 1 | 2 | 3 | 4 | 5 |
| 22. | My relationship with my family is not very loving and supportive. | 0 | 1 | 2 | 3 | 4 | 5 |
| 23. | When I watch people, I tend to be critical and think negatively about them. | 0 | 1 | 2 | 3 | 4 | 5 |
| 24. | I believe that people are inherently selfish and untrustworthy, and I am careful around them. | 0 | 1 | 2 | 3 | 4 | 5 |
| 25. | Life is basically unfair, and most of the time there is little I can do to change it. | 0 | 1 | 2 | 3 | 4 | 5 |
| 26. | I give more than I get in relationships with people. | 0 | 1 | 2 | 3 | 4 | 5 |
| 27. | I tend to believe that what I do is often not good enough or that I should do better. | 0 | 1 | 2 | 3 | 4 | 5 |
| 28. | My friends would describe me as highly stressed and quick to react with anger and/or frustration. | 0 | 1 | 2 | 3 | 4 | 5 |

| | Strongly Disagree | | | | | Strongly Agree |
|---|---|---|---|---|---|---|
| 29. My friends are always telling me I "need a vacation to relax." | 0 | 1 | 2 | 3 | 4 | 5 |
| 30. Overall, the quality of my life right now isn't all that great. | 0 | 1 | 2 | 3 | 4 | 5 |
| | | | | | Total | _____ |

## Scoring

### Total your points from sections 1 and 2.

Although the following scores are not meant to be diagnostic, they do serve as an indicator of potential problem areas. If your scores are:

0–50, your stress levels are low, but it is worth examining areas where you did score points and taking action to reduce your stress levels.

51–100, you may need to reduce certain stresses in your life. Long-term stress and pressure from your stresses can be counterproductive. Consider what you can do to change your perceptions of things, your behaviors, or your environment.

100–150, you are probably pretty stressed. Examine what your major stressors are and come up with a plan for reducing your stress levels right now. Don't delay or blow this off because it could lead to significant stress-related problems, affecting your grades, your social life, and your future!

151–200, you are carrying high stress, and if you don't make changes, you could be heading for some serious difficulties. Find a counselor on campus to talk with about some of the major issues you identified above as causing stress. Try to get more sleep and exercise, and find time to relax. Surround yourself with people who are supportive of you and make you feel safe and competent.

## YOUR PLAN FOR **CHANGE**

The **ASSESS YOURSELF** activity gave you the chance to look at your sources of chronic stress, identify major stressors that you experienced in the last year, and see how you typically respond to stress. Now that you are aware of these patterns, you can focus on developing behaviors that lead to reduced stress.

**TODAY,** YOU CAN:

☐ Practice one new stress-management technique. For example, you could spend 10 minutes doing a deep-breathing exercise or find a good spot on campus to meditate.

☐ In a journal, write down stressful events or symptoms of stress that you experience. Try to focus on intense emotional experiences and explore how they affect you.

**WITHIN THE NEXT TWO WEEKS,** YOU CAN:

☐ Attend a class or workshop in yoga, tai chi, qigong, meditation, or some other stress-relieving activity. Look for beginner classes offered on campus or in your community.

☐ Make a list of the papers, projects, and tests that you have over the coming semester and create a schedule for them. Break projects and term papers into small, manageable tasks with a plan for completing each. Be realistic about how much time you'll need to get these tasks done.

☐ Chart your day. Keep track of how much time you spend on Facebook, Twitter, or surfing the Internet, and how much you spend on school-work, exercise, and watching TV. Set time aside for you, but limit your nonproductive time each day.

**BY THE END OF THE SEMESTER,** YOU CAN:

☐ Keep track of the money you spend and where it goes. If your spending is out of control, your credit cards and savings will quickly be depleted, adding to your stress levels. Track your daily spending. Establish a realistic budget for fun versus necessities and stick to it.

☐ Find some form of exercise you can do regularly. You may consider joining a gym or just arranging regular "walk dates" or bike rides with your friends. Try to exercise at least 30 minutes every day, making sure that strength training is part of this regimen. (See Chapter 11 for more information about physical fitness.)

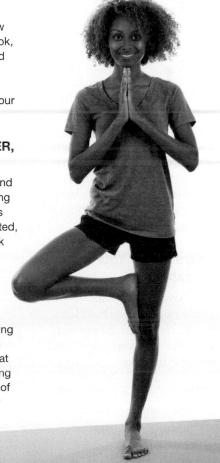

## CHAPTER REVIEW

To hear an MP3 Tutor Session, scan here or visit the Study Area in **MasteringHealth**.

### LO 1 | What Is Stress?

■ Stress is an inevitable part of our lives. *Eustress* refers to stress associated with positive events; *distress* refers to stress associated with negative events. Both forms can have a negative physiological impact on your health.

### LO 2 | Body Responses to Stress

■ The alarm, resistance, and exhaustion phases of the general adaptation syndrome (GAS) involve physiological responses to both real and imagined stressors and cause complex hormonal reactions.

### LO 3 | Physical Effects of Stress

■ Undue stress for extended periods of time can compromise the immune system and result in serious health consequences. Stress has been linked to numerous health problems, including cardiovascular disease, weight gain, hair loss, diabetes, digestive problems, and increased susceptibility to infectious diseases. *Psychoneuroimmunology* is the science that analyzes the relationship between the mind's reaction to stress and the function of the immune system.

### LO 4 | Stress and Your Mental Health

■ Stress can have negative impacts on your intellectual and psychological health, including impaired memory, poor concentration, depression, anxiety, and other disorders.

### LO 5 | What Causes Stress?

■ Psychosocial and physical sources of stress include change, hassles, relationships, academic and financial pressure, frustrations and conflict, overload, bias/discrimination, and environmental stressors

### LO 6 | Individual Factors that Affect Your Stress Response

■ Some sources of stress are internal and are related to appraisal, self-esteem, self-efficacy, personality types, hardiness, resilience, and shift and persist factors.

### LO 7 | Managing Stress in College

■ College and the transition to independent adulthood can be especially stressful. Managing stress begins with learning coping skills. Managing emotional responses, taking mental or physical action, developing a support network, cultivating spirituality, downshifting, learning time management, managing finances, or learning relaxation techniques—will help you better cope with stress in the long run.

## POP QUIZ

Visit **MasteringHealth** to personalize your study plan with Chapter Review Quizzes and Dynamic Study Modules.

### LO 1 | What Is Stress?

1. Even though Andre experienced stress when he graduated from college and moved to a new city, he viewed these changes as an opportunity for growth. What is Andre's stress called?
   a. Strain
   b. Distress
   c. Eustress
   d. Adaptive response

### LO 2 | Body Responses to Stress

2. In which stage of the general adaptation syndrome does the fight-or-flight response occur?
   a. Exhaustion stage
   b. Alarm stage
   c. Resistance stage
   d. Response stage

3. The branch of the autonomic nervous system that is responsible for energizing the body for either fight or flight and for triggering many other stress responses is the
   a. central nervous system.
   b. parasympathetic nervous system.
   c. sympathetic nervous system.
   d. endocrine system.

### LO 3 | Physical Effects of Stress

4. The area of scientific investigation that analyzes the relationship between the mind's response to stress and the immune system's ability to function effectively is called
   a. psychoneuroimmunology.
   b. immunocompetence.
   c. psychoimmunology.
   d. psychology.

### LO 4 | Stress and Your Mental Health

5. When Jesse encounters a stressful situation, he adapts well and tends to bounce back easily, even though the same situation may derail others. What protective factor is Jesse exhibiting to deal with stress?
   a. Cognitive restructuring
   b. Type A personality
   c. High self-esteem
   d. Psychological resilience

### LO 5 | What Causes Stress?

6. Losing your keys is an example of what psychosocial source of stress?
   a. Pressure
   b. Inconsistent behaviors
   c. Hassles
   d. Conflict

7. A state of physical and mental exhaustion caused by excessive stress is called
   a. conflict.
   b. overload.
   c. hassles.
   d. burnout.

### LO 6 | Individual Factors That Affect Your Stress Response

8. Which of the following is an accurate example of a reinforcing factor?
   a. Being raised in a home where parents prioritized taking time for themselves to relax/renew on a regular basis
   b. Having an inexpensive fitness facility and pool within a couple of blocks of your home
   c. Rewarding yourself with a bike ride with friends after you finished a tough term paper
   d. Being close in proximity to a large number of fast-food chains

### LO 7 | Managing Stress in College

9. Which of the following is the best strategy to avoid test-taking anxiety on an exam?
   a. Do the majority of your studying the night before the exam so it is fresh in your mind.
   b. Plan ahead and study over a period of time for the exam with a limited, yet thorough, review the night before.
   c. Drink a caffeinated beverage right before the exam because sympathomimetics are known to reduce stress.
   d. Go through the exam as quickly as possible so you don't dwell on potential mistakes.

10. After 5 years of 70-hour work weeks, Tom decided to leave his high-paying, high-stress law firm and lead a simpler lifestyle. What is this trend called?
    a. Adaptation
    b. Conflict resolution
    c. Burnout reduction
    d. Downshifting

*Answers to the Pop Quiz questions can be found on page A-1. If you answered a question incorrectly, review the section identified by the Learning Outcome. For even more study tools, visit MasteringHealth.*

# THINK ABOUT IT!

### LO 1 | What Is Stress?

1. Define stress. What are some examples of scenarios where you might feel distress? Eustress?

### LO 2 | Body Responses to Stress

2. Describe the alarm, resistance, and exhaustion phases of the general adaptation syndrome and the body's physiological response to stress. Does stress lead to more irritability or emotionality, or does irritability or emotionality lead to stress? Provide examples.

### LO 3 | Physical Effects of Stress

3. What are some of the health risks that result from chronic stress? How does the study of psychoneuroimmunology link stress and illness?

### LO 4 | Stress and Your Mental Health

4. Why might stress and the occurrence of mental disorders be correlated?

### LO 5 | What Causes Stress?

5. Why are the college years often high-stress for many? What factors increase stress risks?

### LO 6 | Individual Factors That Affect Your Stress Response

6. What predisposing, reinforcing and enabling factors influence your ability to cope with stress?

### LO 7 | Managing Stress in College

7. What are three important actions you can take right now to help manage your stressors?

8. How does anger affect the body? Discuss the steps you can take to manage your own anger and help your friends control theirs.

9. How much of a procrastinator are you? What sorts of situations make you the most likely to be a "procrastinator?" What could you do to reduce the likelihood of procrastinating in these situations?

# ACCESS YOUR HEALTH ON THE INTERNET

Visit **MasteringHealth** for links to the websites and RSS feeds.

The following websites explore further topics and issues related to personal health.

*American College Counseling Association.* The website of the professional organization for college counselors offers useful links and articles. **www.collegecounseling.org**

*American College Health Association.* This site provides yearly information and data from the National College Health Assessment survey, which covers stress, anxiety and other health issues for students. **www.acha.org**

*American Psychological Association.* Here you can find current information and research on stress and stress-related conditions as well as an annual survey. **www.apa.org**

*Higher Education Research Institute.* This organization provides annual surveys of first-year and senior college students that cover academic, financial, and health-related issues and problems. **www.heri.ucla.edu**

*National Institute of Mental Health.* A resource for information on all aspects of mental health, including the effects of stress. **www.nimh.nih.gov**

# Improving Your Sleep

Today's college students are largely a sleep-deprived bunch—and their health and success in college may be in jeopardy as a result.

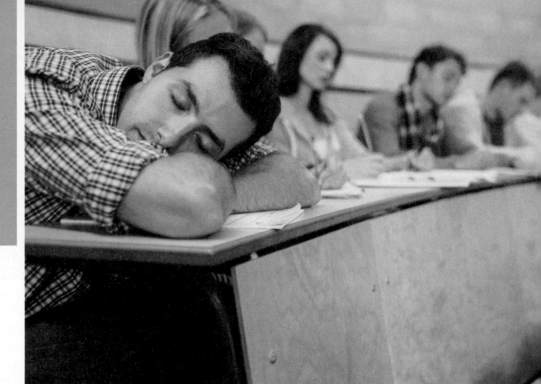

## LEARNING OUTCOMES

1 Describe the problem of sleep deprivation in the United States.

2 Explain why we need sleep and what happens if we don't get enough, including potential physical, emotional, social, and safety threats to health.

3 Explain the processes of sleep, including circadian rhythms, non-REM (NREM) sleep, REM sleep, and sleep needs.

4 Explore what you can do to make sure you get enough sleep.

5 Describe the common sleep disorders insomnia, sleep apnea, restless legs syndrome, and narcolepsy, and what can be done to prevent or treat them.

Nearly every night, we leave our waking world and slide into a series of sleep stages, punctuated by changes in heart rate, respiration rate, blood pressure, and other bodily processes. We all need sleep—the stages and changes that allow the body to repair, restore, and refresh itself. Between 50 and 70 million adults in the United States don't get the sleep they need due to sleep or wakefulness disorders.[1]

Inadequate sleep, which is linked with a variety of health problems, isn't just an American problem. Sleep deprivation is believed to affect the quality of life of 45 percent of the world's population, and those numbers are on the increase.[2] **FIGURE 1** compares average nightly sleep times across a number of countries.

## LO 1 | SLEEPLESS IN AMERICA

Describe the problem of sleep deprivation in the United States.

In a recent survey from the American College Health Association (ACHA), only 11.9 percent of students reported getting enough sleep to feel well rested in the morning 6 or more days a week.[3] Nearly 61 percent of students aged 18 to 29 say they often stay awake late and

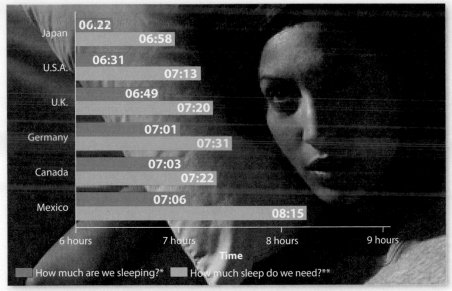

| Country | How much are we sleeping?* | How much sleep do we need?** |
|---|---|---|
| Japan | 06:22 | 06:58 |
| U.S.A. | 06:31 | 07:13 |
| U.K. | 06:49 | 07:20 |
| Germany | 07:01 | 07:31 |
| Canada | 07:03 | 07:22 |
| Mexico | 07:06 | 08:15 |

6 hours    7 hours    8 hours    9 hours

**Time**

■ How much are we sleeping?*    ■ How much sleep do we need?**

  * Represents workdays. All slept an average of 45 minutes more on weekends.
** Represents the number of hours needed for respondents to function at their best the next day (self-reported).

**FIGURE 1** International Sleep Statistics

**Source:** Data from National Sleep Foundation, *2013 International Sleep Poll: Summary of Findings* (Arlington, VA: National Sleep Foundation, 2014), Available at http://sleepfoundation.org/sites/default/files/RPT495a.pdf

get up early, resulting in **sleep deprivation,** a condition that occurs when sleep is insufficient for a given age. Lack of sleep leads to **somnolence**—drowsiness, sluggishness, and lack of mental alertness that can affect daily performance.[4] Sleep deficiencies have been linked to a host of student issues, including poor academic performance, weight gain, increased alcohol abuse, accidents, daytime drowsiness, relationship issues, depression, and other problems.[5]

The sleepiest members of the U.S. population are people aged 13 to 29, with people aged 30 to 64 reporting they are less sleepy than their younger counterparts.[6] Approximately 20 percent of the U.S. population suffers from a condition known as **excessive daytime sleepiness** or **excessive sleepiness**—a major compulsion to sleep, along with persistent sluggishness and fatigue, that can cause individuals to nod off at inopportune times and interfere with most aspects of life.[7]

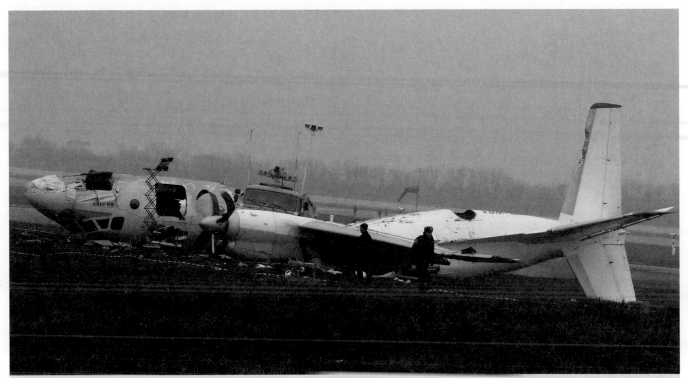

People we trust for transportation suffer from on-the-job sleepiness at alarming rates. Over 26 percent of train operators and 23 percent of pilots admit to sleepiness on the job in the last week. Twenty percent of pilots, 18 percent of train operators, and 14 percent of truck drivers report making a serious error or having a "near miss" while at work.

**Source:** Data from National Sleep Foundation, "Sleepy Pilots, Train Operators and Drivers," March 2012, www.sleepfoundation.org

As many as 1 million traffic accidents and up to 7,500 deaths each year are due to impaired driving.[8] Since over 41 percent of all adults admit to nodding off or falling asleep while driving at least once in their lifetime, accident numbers may be underestimated.[9]

## Why So Sleep Deprived?

Several factors can lead to sleep deprivation:

- **Shift work.** Changing shifts or shifts that are outside the normal 9 to 5 work schedule can disrupt biological clocks and lead to sleeplessness, insomnia and a host of other problems.[10] Drowsy workers are also more likely to have on-the-job accidents, be depressed, miss work, and have motor vehicle accidents when commuting.[11]
- **Long haul driving.** Sleep deprivation is common among truckers, particularly those who drive commercially over 60 hours per week and drive alone.[12]
- **Drugs and medications.** As noted on warning labels, prescription, over-the-counter, and illicit drugs can lead to excessive sleepiness. Antihistamines, anxiety and insomnia drugs, Parkinson's medications, antidepressants, certain blood pressure and antinausea drugs, muscle relaxants, as well as alcohol and marijuana, are among key culprits.
- **Sleep habits.** Burning the candle at both ends, exercising before bed, and hours of time on smartphones or tablets can lead to excess sleepiness.
- **Gender.** Women have twice the sleep difficulties of men, believed due to hormonal factors, pain syndromes, and psychological issues such as anxiety and depression.[13]
- **Sleep disorders.** Numerous studies point to sleep disorders such as sleep apnea as major risks for excessive daytime sleepiness and subsequent automobile accidents.[14]

## Wired and Tired

The average 18- to 34-year-old college student has up to seven tech devices (including TVs) and may be using a smartphone from 1 to 4 hours each day![15] In fact, according to recent research, technology invades the bedrooms of millions, with over 90 percent of respondents reporting using electronic devices before bed and during the night.[16] See the **Skills for Behavior Change** box for more on safeguarding your sleep against blue lights.

# 61%

OF STUDENTS SAY THEY FELT TIRED, DRAGGED OUT, OR **SLEEPY** FOR 3 OR MORE DAYS IN THE PAST WEEK.

## LO **2** | THE **IMPORTANCE** OF SLEEP

Explain why we need sleep and what happens if we don't get enough, including potential physical, emotional, social, and safety threats to health.

Sleep helps maintain your physical health, affects your ability to function, and promotes your psychological health. It achieves these results by serving at least two biological purposes:

- **It restores you both physically and mentally.** Certain reparative chemicals are released while you sleep. There is also evidence that during sleep the brain is cleared of daily minutiae, learning is synthesized, and memories are consolidated.
- **It conserves body energy.** When you sleep, your core body temperature and the rate at which you burn calories drop. This leaves you with more energy to perform activities throughout your waking hours.

## Sleep and Health

Sleep has beneficial effects on most body systems. That's why, when you consistently don't get a good night's rest, your body doesn't function as well, and you become more vulnerable to a

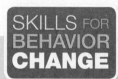

## SKILLS FOR BEHAVIOR CHANGE

### DITCH BLUE LIGHT DEVICES

Researchers in a recent study assessing biological changes associated with using blue light devices like tablets or smartphones showed significant decreases in *melatonin*, a hormone that helps people fall asleep. While sleepless nights are an initial threat, long-term melatonin drops may increase risks of diabetes, certain types of cancer, and migraines among others.

Here are a few ways to avoid the melatonin-draining effects of blue light on your sleep and health:

▶ Stick to small screens, and keep them far away from your eyes.

▶ Dim your screen and home lights as dusk settles in.

▶ Purchase amber-tinted glasses that block blue light.

▶ Allow yourself only an hour or two of screen time after dark.

**Sources:** A. M Chang et al., "Evening Use of Light-Emitting eReaders Negatively Affects Sleep, Circadian Timing, and Next-Morning Alertness," *Proceedings of the National Academy of Sciences* (2014): 201418490; S. L. Chellappa et al., "Acute Exposure to Evening Blue-Enriched Light Impacts on Human Sleep," *Journal of Sleep Research* 22, no. 5 (2013): 573-80; G. Gaggiaoni et al., "Neuroimaging, Cognition, Light and Circadian Rhythms," *Frontiers in Systems Neuroscience* 8 (2014): 126, doi: 10.3389/fnsys.2014.00126; A. Haim and A. Zubidat, "LED light between Nobel Prize and cancer risk factor," *Chronobiology International*, Early Online: 1–3, (2015), Informa Healthcare USA, Inc., DOI: 10.3109/07420528.2015.1027901

wide variety of health problems.[17] Researchers are only just beginning to explore the physical benefits of sleep. The following is a brief summary of the physical benefits of sleep.

- **Sleep helps maintain your immune system.** The common cold, strep throat, flu, mononucleosis, cold sores, and a variety of other ailments are more common when your immune system is depressed. If you aren't getting enough sleep, immune response is weakened. In fact, poor sleep quality and shorter sleep duration increase susceptibility to diseases like the common cold.[18] Other studies have shown that sleep disruption, particularly when circadian rhythms are disturbed repeatedly, disrupts overall immune function.[19] In contrast, adolescents getting more than 9 hours of sleep per night showed improvements in markers of immune functioning.[20]

- **Sleep helps reduce your risk for cardiovascular disease.** Several studies have indicated that high blood pressure is more common in people who get fewer than 7 hours of sleep a night.[21] Newer research points to a strong association between short-duration

sleep and increased risk of developing and/or dying from cardiovascular disease.[22]

- **Sleep contributes to a healthy metabolism.** Chemical reactions in your body's cells break down food and synthesize compounds that the body needs. The sum of all these reactions is called *metabolism*. Several recent studies suggest that sleep contributes to healthy metabolism and possibly a healthy body weight. In fact, those who sleep less than 5 hours per night have a 40 percent higher risk of developing obesity than those sleeping 7 to 8 hours per night.[23] Sleeping less is associated with eating more—particularly high-fat, high-protein foods—and exercising less.[24] There is evidence that sleep deficiencies, particularly sleep disorders such as sleep apnea, can increase the risk of *type 2 diabetes*, a disorder of glucose metabolism.[25]

- **Sleep contributes to neurological functioning.** There are parts of the brain, including the cerebral cortex—which is important for consciousness—that only truly rest during sleep.[26] Restricting sleep can cause a wide range of neurological problems, including lapses of attention, slowed or poor memory, reduced cognitive ability, difficulty in concentrating, and a tendency for your thinking to get "stuck in a rut."[27] Your ability not only to remember facts, but also to integrate them, make meaningful

generalizations about them, and consolidate what you've learned into lasting memories requires adequate sleep time.[28] College students who pull all-nighters, as well as students who are short sleepers, have significantly lower overall grade-point averages compared with classmates who get adequate sleep.[29]

- **Sleep improves motor tasks, particularly driving.** Sleep also has a restorative effect on motor function, that is, the ability to perform tasks such as shooting a basket, playing a musical instrument, or driving a car. Motor function is affected by sleep throughout the life span among otherwise healthy individuals.[30] Some researchers contend that a night without sleep impairs your motor skills and reaction time as much as if you were driving drunk.[31] A recent survey found that, in the last month, nearly one third of drivers drove when they couldn't keep their eyes open.[32] Drivers under the age of 26 are the most likely of any age group to report falling asleep at the wheel within the last year, and men of all ages are more likely to fall asleep than are women.[33] Data from the National Highway Traffic Safety Administration (NHTSA) indicate that sleepy drivers are involved in 2 percent of all fatal crashes; however, other sources estimate these figures may be considerably higher, ranging from 15 to 33 percent.[34]

- **Sleep plays a role in stress management and mental health.** The relationship between sleep and stress is highly complex: Stress can cause or contribute to sleep problems, and sleep problems can cause or increase your level of stress! The same is true of depression and anxiety disorders: Reduced or poor-quality sleep can trigger these disorders, but it's also a common symptom resulting from them. Nondepressed individuals who suffer from chronic insomnia have over twice the risk of developing depression.[35]

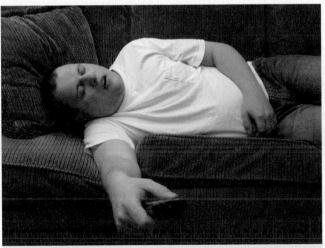

Obesity is a significant risk for diabetic-related excessive daytime sleepiness, as well as a variety of sleep disorders.

# 21%

OF STUDENTS SAY
THAT SLEEP PROBLEMS
HAVE AFFECTED THEIR
**ACADEMIC** PERFORMANCE.

## LO 3 | THE PROCESSES OF SLEEP

Explain the processes of sleep, including circadian rhythms, NREM sleep, REM sleep, and sleep needs.

If you've ever taken a flight that crossed two or more time zones, you've probably experienced *jet lag,* a feeling that your body's "internal clock" is out of sync with the hours of daylight and darkness at your destination. Jet lag happens because the new day/night

> **circadian rhythm** The 24-hour cycle by which you are accustomed to going to sleep, waking up, and performing habitual behaviors.
>
> **melatonin** A hormone that affects sleep cycles, increasing drowsiness.
>
> **REM sleep** A period of sleep characterized by brain-wave activity similar to that seen in wakefulness; rapid eye movement and dreaming occur during REM sleep.
>
> **non-REM (NREM) sleep** A period of restful sleep dominated by slow brain waves; during non-REM sleep, rapid eye movement is rare.

pattern disrupts the 24-hour biological clock by which you are accustomed to going to sleep, waking up, and performing habitual behaviors throughout your day. This cycle, known as your **circadian rhythm,** is regulated by a master clock that coordinates the activity of nerve cells, protein, and genes. The hypothalamus and a tiny gland in your brain called the *pineal body,* responsible for the drowsiness-inducing hormone called **melatonin,** are key to these cyclical rhythms.[36]

Sleep researchers generally distinguish between two primary sleep stages. During **REM sleep,** rapid eye movement and dreams occur, and brain-wave activity appears similar to that which occurs when you are awake. **Non-REM (NREM) sleep,** in contrast, is the period of restful sleep with slowed brain activity that does *not* include rapid eye movement. During the night, you alternate between periods of NREM and REM sleep, repeating one full cycle about once every 90 minutes.[37] Overall, you spend about 75 percent of each night in NREM sleep and 25 percent in REM (**FIGURE 2**).

## Non-REM Sleep

During non-REM (NREM) sleep, the body rests. Both your body temperature and your energy use drop; sensation is dulled; and your brain waves, heart rate, and breathing slow. In contrast, digestive processes speed up, and your body stores nutrients. During NREM sleep—also called *slow-wave sleep*—you do not typically dream. Four

**SEE IT!** VIDEOS
How you can avoid nodding off behind the wheel? Watch **Dozing and Driving,** available on **MasteringHealth**™

distinct stages of NREM sleep have been distinguished by their characteristic brain-wave patterns.

*Stage 1* is the lightest stage of sleep, lasts only a few minutes, and involves the transition between waking and sleep. Your brain begins to produces *theta waves* (slow brain waves), and you may experience sensations of falling with quick, jerky muscle reactions. During *stage 2,* your eyes close, body movement slows, and you disengage from your environment. During *stages 3* and *4,* a sleeper's brain generates slow, large-amplitude *delta waves.* Blood pressure drops, your heart rate and respiration slow considerably, and you enter deep sleep. Human growth hormone is released, signaling the body to repair worn tissues. Speech and movement are rare during the final stage (but sometimes people sleepwalk, cook, clean, or drive, particularly those on certain sleep medications!).

## REM Sleep

Dreaming takes place primarily during REM sleep. On an electroencephalogram (EEG)—a test detecting electrical activity in your brain—REM sleeper's brain-wave activity is almost indistinguishable from that of someone wide awake, and the brain's energy use is higher than that of a person performing a difficult math

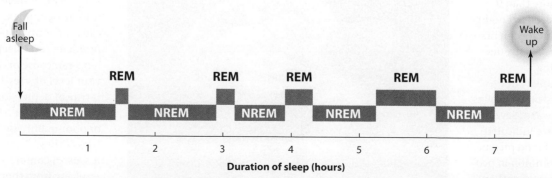

FIGURE 2 caption:
**FIGURE 2** **The Nightly Sleep Cycle** As the number of hours you sleep increases, your brain spends more and more time in REM sleep. Thus, sleeping for too few hours could mean you're depriving yourself primarily of needed REM sleep.

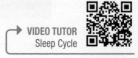

VIDEO TUTOR
Sleep Cycle

problem![38] Your muscles, on the other hand, are paralyzed during REM sleep: You may dream that you're rock climbing, but your body is incapable of movement. Almost the only exceptions are your respiratory muscles, which allow you to breathe, and the tiny muscles of your eyes, which move your eyes rapidly as if you were following the scenario of your dream. This *rapid eye movement* gives REM sleep its name.

Research indicates that deep phases of slow-wave sleep consolidate and organize the day's information, while REM sleep stabilizes consolidated memory.[39] Without adequate slow-wave sleep and REM sleep, your short-term memory may suffer.

## Your Sleep Needs

Researchers find that most people need between 7 and 8 hours of sleep per day, on average.[40] But sleep needs vary from person to person, and your gender, health, and lifestyle will also affect how much rest your body demands.

Not only do sleep needs vary, but sleep patterns also change over the life span. Newborns need 16 to 18 hours of sleep daily, and teens and younger adults need 8 to 9 hours per night, slightly more than the adult average. Older adults may experience sleep difficwulties that result in fewer hours of rest per night owing to health conditions, pain, and the need to use the bathroom more frequently.[41]

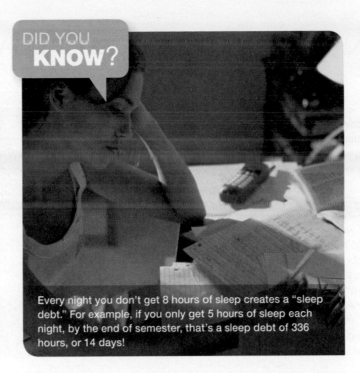

Every night you don't get 8 hours of sleep creates a "sleep debt." For example, if you only get 5 hours of sleep each night, by the end of semester, that's a sleep debt of 336 hours, or 14 days!

Research has consistently shown that sleep deprivation and disorders contribute significantly to premature death and disability from a variety of conditions, including cardiovascular disease, cancer, depression, obesity, and diabetes in older adults. However, a recent study of healthy undergraduate males indicated that short sleep cycles resulted in significant prolonged elevations in heart rate and diastolic pressure recovery after exposure to stressful stimuli as compared to those with longer sleep cycles.[42] Many scientists believe that diabetes, obesity, and other metabolic disorders may be linked with biological clock activity.[43] In general, those who get adequate sleep live longer and enjoy more quality days than those who don't.[44]

### Sleep Debt

In addition to your body's physiological need, consider your current **sleep debt.** That's the total number of hours of missed sleep you're carrying around with you. Let's say that last week you managed just 5 hours of sleep a night Monday through Thursday. Even if you get 7 to 8 hours a night Friday through Sunday, your unresolved sleep debt of 8 to 12 hours will leave you feeling tired and groggy when you start the week again. That means you need *more than* 8 hours a night for the next several nights to "catch up."

The good news is that you *can* catch up if you go about it sensibly. Whittle away at that sleep debt by sleeping 9 hours a night throughout your break—then start the new term resolved to sleep 7 to 8 hours a night.

### Napping

Speaking of catching up, do naps count? Although naps can't entirely cancel out a significant sleep debt, they can improve your mood, alertness, and performance. Regular naps may also improve immune functioning and help ward off infections.[45] It's best to nap in the early to midafternoon, when the pineal body in your brain releases a small amount of melatonin and your body experiences a natural dip in its circadian rhythm. Never nap in the late afternoon, as it could interfere with your ability to fall asleep that night. Keep your naps short, because a nap of more than 30 minutes can leave you in a state of **sleep inertia,** which is characterized by cognitive impairment, grogginess, queasiness, and a disoriented feeling.

### LO 4 | GETTING A GOOD NIGHT'S SLEEP

Explore what you can do to make sure you get enough sleep.

Do you need a jolt of caffeine to get started in the morning? Do you find it hard to stay awake in class? Have you ever nodded off behind the wheel? These are all signs of inadequate or poor-quality sleep. To find out whether

**sleep debt** The difference between the number of hours of sleep an individual needed in a given time period and the number of hours he or she actually slept.

**sleep inertia** A state characterized by cognitive impairment, grogginess, and disorientation that is experienced upon rising from short sleep or an overly long nap.

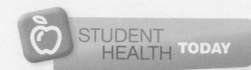

# CAFFEINE, SLEEP, AND YOUR HEALTH

Caffeine has long been recognized for its ability to increase vigilance and alertness and decrease sleepiness when you want to stay awake. Drink too much caffeine and you could end up wide awake when you want desperately to sleep.

A recent study indicated that effects of caffeine can last 5.5 to 7.7 hours or more—depending on how "stiff" your coffee or energy drink really is. An ever-increasing body of research points to risk of cardiac irregularities, psychological problems, and neurological side effects, including headaches and migraines from high-caffeine drinks, particularly energy drinks. Excess consumption of caffeine can severely disrupt circadian cycles, leading to the inability to fall asleep and stay asleep. Consuming caffeinated beverages up to 8 hours before bedtime can have a significant effect on sleep!

**Sources:** N. Olson, "Caffeine Consumption Habits and Perceptions among University of New Hampshire Students," 2013, http://scholars.unh.edu/cgi/viewcontent.cgi?article=1102&context=honors; A. Aubrey, "Young Adults Swapping Soda for the Super Buzz of Coffee," January 14, 2013, www.npr.org/blogs/thesalt/2013/01/14/169161207/young-adults-swapping-soda-for-the-super-buzz-of-coffee; M. Drici et al., "Cardiac Safety of So-Called 'Energy Drinks,'" *European Heart Journal* 35 (2014); H. Whiteman, Medical News Today, "Rising Energy Drink Consumption May Pose a Threat to Public Health, Says WHO," October 15, 2014, www.medicalnewstoday.com/articles/283929; J. J. Breda et al., "Energy Drink Consumption in Europe: A Review of the Risks, Adverse Health Effects and Policy Options," *Frontiers in Public Health* 2 (2014), doi:10:3389/fpubh.2014.00134

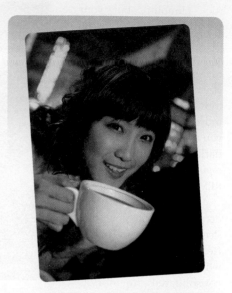

you're sleep deprived, take the **Assess Yourself** questionnaire on page 108.

The following tips can help you get a more restful night's sleep.

- **Let there be light.** According to Kelly Brown, MD, at the Vanderbilt Sleep Disorders Center, light is the best tool for reigning in your internal clock. Light travels through the retina and regulates melatonin, slowing its production in daylight and encouraging it in darkness, helping to regulate the sleep cycle.[46] While exposure to natural light outdoors is best, opening shades and turning on lights indoors on dark winter days can help.
- **Stay active.** According to recent polls, people who engage in vigorous exercise during the day appear to sleep best overall.[47] There was no significant difference in sleepiness or quality of sleep between those who exercised less than 4 hours before bedtime and those who exercised more than 4 hours before bedtime.
- **Sleep tight.** Don't let a lumpy or pancake pillow, scratchy or pilled sheets, or a threadbare blanket keep you from sleeping soundly. Invest in a good mattress. And make your bed in the morning and air out your room; cool sheets and bedding and a lavender-scented room have been shown to be calming and help you sleep better.[48]
- **Create a sleep "cave."** As bedtime approaches, keep your bedroom quiet, cool, and dark. If your living area is noisy from roommates or neighbors, wear earplugs or get an electronic device that produces "white noise." Turn down the thermostat or, on hot nights, run an electric fan. If you can't block out the light, wear an eye mask.
- **Condition yourself into better sleep.** Go to bed and get up at the same time each day. Establish a bedtime ritual that signals to your body that it's time for sleep. For instance, listen to a quiet song, practice meditation and deep breathing exercises, take a warm shower, or read something that lets you quietly wind down.
- **Make your bedroom a mental escape.** Don't stew about things you can't fix right now. Clear your mind of worries and frustrations, and allow your body to unwind.
- **Don't get revved by emotional upheavals.** Avoid late-night phone calls, texts, or e-mails that can end up in arguments, disappointments, and other emotional stressors. If something does jazz you up before bed, journal about it briefly, then promise yourself that you'll make time the next day to explore your feelings more deeply.
- **Don't toss and turn.** If you're not asleep after 20 minutes, get up. Turn on a low light, read something relaxing, or listen to some gentle music. Once you feel sleepy, go back to bed.
- **Avoid foods and drinks that keep you awake.** Drinking liquids may contribute to **nocturia**, or overactive bladder, meaning you have to get up several times during the night. Large meals, nicotine, energy drinks, caffeine, and alcohol close to bedtime can also affect your ability to sleep. See **Student Health Today** for more on the effects of caffeine on your sleep (and health).
- **Don't take nonprescribed sleeping pills or nighttime pain medications.** Casual use of over-the-counter sleeping aids can interfere with your brain's natural progression through the healthy stages of sleep.

**nocturia** Frequent urination at night caused by an overactive bladder.

| | Day 1 | Day 2 | Day 3 |
|---|---|---|---|
| **Fill out in morning** | | | |
| Bedtime | 11 pm | 11:30 pm | |
| Wake time | 7:30 am | 8:30 am | |
| Time to fall asleep | 45 min | 30 min | |
| Awakenings (how many and how long?) | 2 times<br>1 hour | 1 time<br>45 min | |
| Total sleep time | 6.75 hrs | 7.75 hrs | |
| Feeling at waking (refreshed, groggy, etc.) | Still tired | Energized | |
| **Fill out at bedtime** | | | |
| Exercise (what, when, how long?) | Jog at 2 pm<br>30 min | Soccer practice<br>at 4 pm; 2 hrs | |
| Naps (when, where, how long?) | 4 pm, my bed<br>30 min | 2 pm, library<br>1 hour | |
| Caffeine (what, when, how much?) | 2 cups coffee<br>at 8 am | 1 latte at 10 am;<br>1 soda at 9 pm | |
| Alcohol (what, when, how much?) | 1 beer at<br>8 pm | None | |
| Evening snacks (what, when, how much?) | Bag of popcorn<br>at 10 pm | Chips and<br>soda at 9 pm | |
| Medications (what, when, how much?) | None | None | |
| Feelings (happiness, anxiety, major cause, etc.) | Stressed<br>about paper | Worried<br>about sister | |
| Activities 1 hour before bed (what and how long?) | Wrote paper | Watched TV | |

**FIGURE 3** Sample Sleep Diary Using a sleep diary can help you and your health care provider discover behavioral factors that might be contributing to your sleep problem.

## LO 5 | SLEEP DISORDERS

Describe the common sleep disorders insomnia, sleep apnea, restless legs syndrome, and narcolepsy, and what can be done to prevent or treat them.

As many as 70 million U.S. adults suffer from sleep-related disorders.[49] Although over 4 percent of college students report regularly suffering from insomnia and 2.1 percent have diagnosed sleep disorders, the exact number receiving treatment is unknown.[50] Nearly 27 percent of students say they have had sleep difficulties in the last year that were traumatic or difficult to handle.[51] If you're following the advice in this chapter and still aren't sleeping well, visit your health care provider. To aid in diagnosis, you will probably be asked to keep a sleep diary like the one in **FIGURE 3**. You may also be referred to a sleep disorders center for an overnight clinical **sleep study.** While you are asleep in the sleep center, sensors and electrodes record data that can help a sleep specialist and your doctor diagnose and treat your sleep problem.

The American Academy of Sleep Medicine identifies more than 80 sleep disorders. The most common disorders in adults are *insomnia, sleep apnea, restless legs syndrome,* and *narcolepsy.*

## Insomnia

**Insomnia**—difficulty in falling asleep, frequent arousals during sleep, or early morning awakening—is the most common sleep complaint. Young adults aged 18 to 29 experience the most insomnia, with 68 percent reporting symptoms.[52] Somewhat fewer adults (59%) aged 30 to 64 experience regular symptoms, and only 44 percent of those

**sleep study** A clinical assessment of sleep in which the patient is monitored while spending the night in a sleep disorders center.

**insomnia** A disorder characterized by difficulty in falling asleep quickly, frequent arousals during sleep, or early morning awakening.

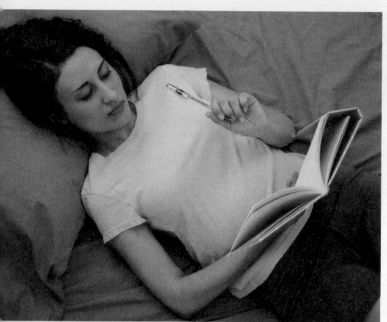

If a worry keeps you awake, jot it down in a journal. You'll be better prepared to handle it in the morning after a good night's sleep.

over age 65 have regular symptoms.[53] Adults with children in the household tend to report more insomnia symptoms than those without children.[54] Approximately 10 to 15 percent of Americans have experienced chronic insomnia that lasts longer than a month.[55] About 4 percent of college students are being treated for insomnia.[56]

## Symptoms and Causes of Insomnia

Symptoms of insomnia include difficulty falling asleep, waking up frequently during the night, difficulty returning to sleep, waking up too early in the morning, unrefreshing sleep, daytime sleepiness, and irritability. Sometimes insomnia is related to stress and worry. In other cases it may be related to disrupted circadian rhythms. Insomnia can also occur as a side effect from taking certain medications. Left untreated, long-term insomnia may be associated with depression, drug and alcohol use, and heart disease.[57]

## Treatment for Insomnia

Because of the close connection between behavior and insomnia,

---

**sleep apnea** A disorder in which breathing is briefly and repeatedly interrupted during sleep.

---

cognitive behavioral therapy is often part of treatment. A cognitive behavioral therapist assists a patient in identifying thought and behavioral patterns that contribute to the inability to fall asleep. Sometimes, hormonal changes or issues with the gastrointestinal tract or bladder may be an underlying cause. Excess stress is also a key factor in insomnia.

In some cases of insomnia, *hypnotic* or *sedative* medications may be prescribed. Over 4 percent of adults aged 20 and over use prescription sleep aids.[58] These drugs induce sleep, and some may help relieve anxiety. However, some have undesirable side effects ranging from daytime sleepiness and hallucinations to sleepwalking and other strange nighttime behaviors. Antidepressants are also commonly prescribed for insomnia.

Relaxation strategies, including yoga and meditation, can be helpful in preparing the body to sleep. Exercise, done early in the day, can also help reduce stress and promote deeper sleep. Talk to a health professional if insomnia is unresolved in spite of your best efforts to make changes.

## Sleep Apnea

**Sleep apnea** is a disorder in which breathing is briefly and repeatedly interrupted during sleep.[59] *Apnea* refers to a breathing pause that lasts at least 10 seconds. Sleep apnea affects more than 18 million Americans, or 1 in every 15 people.[60]

## Symptoms and Causes of Sleep Apnea

There are two major types of sleep apnea: central and obstructive. *Central sleep apnea* occurs when the brain fails to tell the respiratory muscles to initiate breathing. Consumption of alcohol, certain illegal drugs, and certain medications can contribute to central sleep apnea.

*Obstructive sleep apnea (OSA)* is more common and occurs when air cannot move in and out of a person's nose or mouth, even though the body tries to breathe. Typically, OSA occurs when a person's throat muscles and tongue relax during sleep and block the airways, causing snorting, snoring, and gagging. These sounds occur because falling oxygen saturation levels in the blood stimulate the body's autonomic nervous system to trigger inhalation, often via a sudden gasp of breath. This response may wake the person, preventing deep sleep and causing the person to wake in the morning feeling like he or she hasn't slept.

People who are overweight often have sagging internal throat tissue, putting them at higher risk for sleep apnea. In addition to overweight, other risk factors include smoking and alcohol use, being age 40 or older, and ethnicity—sleep apnea occurs at higher rates in African Americans, Pacific Islanders, and Hispanics.[61] Anatomical risk factors for OSA can include a small upper airway (or large tongue, tonsils, or uvula), a recessed chin, small jaw or a large overbite, and a large neck size. Genetics may also play a role.[62]

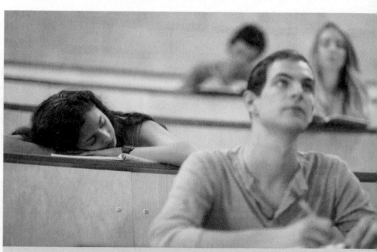

There are more than 80 different clinical sleep disorders, and it is estimated that 50 to 70 million Americans—children and adults—suffer from one.

OSA is associated with higher risk for chronic high blood pressure, irregular heartbeats, heart attack, and stroke. Apnea-associated sleeplessness may also increase the risk of type 2 diabetes, immune system deficiencies, and a host of other problems.[63]

## Treatment for Sleep Apnea

The most commonly prescribed therapy for OSA is *continuous positive airway pressure (CPAP)*, which consists of an airflow device, long tube, and mask (see **FIGURE 4**). People with sleep apnea wear this mask during sleep, and air is forced into the nose to keep the airway open.

Other methods for treating OSA include dental appliances, which reposition the lower jaw and tongue, and surgery to remove tissue in the upper airway. In general, these approaches are most helpful for mild disease or heavy snoring. Lifestyle changes, which may include losing weight, avoiding alcohol, and quitting smoking, are often effective ways of reducing symptoms of OSA.

# Restless Legs Syndrome

**Restless legs syndrome (RLS)** is a neurological disorder characterized by unpleasant sensations in the legs when at rest combined with an uncontrollable urge to move in an effort to relieve these feelings. These sensations range in severity from mildly uncomfortable to painful. Some researchers estimate that RLS affects over 10 percent of the U.S. population, with increasing diagnosis in all age groups.[64]

## Symptoms and Causes of RLS

Restless legs syndrome sensations are often described as burning, creeping, or tugging, or like insects crawling inside the legs. In general, symptoms are more pronounced in the evening or at night. Lying down or trying to relax activates the symptoms, so people with RLS often have difficulty falling and staying asleep.

In most cases, the cause of RLS is unknown. A family history of the condition is seen in approximately 50 percent of cases, suggesting some genetic link. In other cases, RLS appears to be related to other conditions, including Parkinson's disease, kidney failure, diabetes, peripheral neuropathy, and anemia. Pregnancy or hormonal changes can worsen symptoms.[65]

## Treatment of RLS

If there is an underlying condition, treatment of that condition may provide relief. Other treatment options include use of prescribed medications, decreasing tobacco and alcohol use, and applying heat to the legs. For some people, relaxation techniques or stretching exercises can alleviate symptoms.

# Narcolepsy

**Narcolepsy** is a neurological disorder caused by the brain's inability to properly regulate sleep–wake cycles. The result is excessive, intrusive sleepiness and daytime sleep attacks. Narcolepsy occurs in about 1 of every 3,000 people.[66] Narcolepsy is not rare, but it is an underrecognized and underdiagnosed condition.

## Symptoms and Causes of Narcolepsy

Narcolepsy is characterized by overwhelming and uncontrollable sleepiness during the day. Narcoleptics are prone to falling asleep at inappropriate times and places—in class, at work, while driving or eating, or even midconversation.

**restless legs syndrome (RLS)** A neurological disorder characterized by an overwhelming urge to move the legs when they are at rest.

**narcolepsy** A neurological disorder that causes people to fall asleep involuntarily during the day.

These sleep attacks can last from a few seconds to several minutes. Other symptoms include *cataplexy* (the sudden loss of voluntary muscle tone, often triggered by emotional stimuli), hallucinations during sleep onset or upon awakening, and brief episodes of paralysis during sleep–wake transitions.

In most cases narcolepsy appears to be caused by a deficiency of sleep-regulating chemicals in the brain. Genetics may also play a role.[67] Other factors, including having another sleep disorder, using certain medications, or having a mental disorder or substance abuse disorder may also be factors.

## Treatment for Narcolepsy

Narcolepsy is commonly treated with medications that improve alertness, and antidepressants may be prescribed to treat cataplexy, hallucinations, and sleep paralysis. Behavioral therapy can help narcoleptics cope with their condition. Some lifestyle changes, such as scheduling brief naps during the day or eating smaller meals on a regular schedule may be helpful.

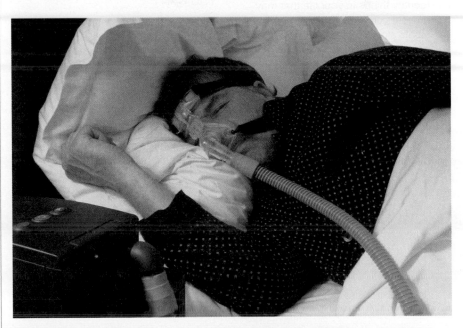

**FIGURE 4** **Continuous Positive Airway Pressure (CPAP) Device** People with sleep apnea can get a better night's sleep by wearing a CPAP device. A gentle stream of air flows continuously into the nose through a tube connected to a mask, helping keep the sleeper's airway open.

Read each statement below, then circle True or False according to whether or not it applies to you in the current school term.

1. I sometimes doze off in my morning classes.  True  False

2. I sometimes doze off in my last class of the day.  True  False

3. I go through most of the day feeling tired.  True  False

4. I feel drowsy when I'm a passenger in a bus or car.  True  False

5. I often fall asleep while reading or studying.  True  False

6. I often fall asleep at the computer or watching TV.  True  False

7. It usually takes me a long time to fall asleep.  True  False

8. My roommate tells me I snore.  True  False

9. I wake up frequently throughout the night.  True  False

10. I have fallen asleep while driving.  True  False

If you answer True more than once, you may be sleep deprived. Try the strategies in this chapter for getting more or better quality sleep, but if you still experience sleepiness, see your health care provider.

## YOUR PLAN FOR CHANGE

Here are some steps you can take to improve your sleep, starting tonight.

**TODAY,** YOU CAN:

☐ Identify things in your life that may prevent you from getting a good nights sleep. Develop a plan. What can you do differently starting today?

☐ Write a list of personal Do's and Don'ts. For instance: Do turn off your cell phone after 11 P.M. Don't drink anything with caffeine after 3 P.M.

**WITHIN THE NEXT TWO WEEKS,** YOU CAN:

☐ Keep a sleep diary, noting not only how many hours of sleep you get each night, but also how you feel and function the next day.

☐ Arrange your room to promote restful sleep. Keep it quiet, cool, dark, and comfortable.

☐ Visit your campus health center for more information about getting a good night's sleep.

**BY THE END OF THE SEMESTER,** YOU CAN:

☐ Establish a regular sleep schedule. Get in the habit of going to bed and waking up at the same time, even on weekends.

☐ Create a ritual, such as stretching, meditation, reading something light, or listening to music, that you follow each night to help your body ease from the activity of the day into restful sleep.

☐ If you are still having difficulty sleeping, contact your health care provider.

# STUDY PLAN

Customize your study plan—and master your health! in the Study Area of MasteringHealth™

## CHAPTER REVIEW

 To head an MP3 Tutor Session, scan here or visit the Study Area in **MasteringHealth**.

**LO 1 | Sleepless in America**

- Sleep deprivation, or insufficient sleep is a major problem in America, affecting 50 to 70 million adults overall and nearly 60 percent of students, resulting in major problems with excessive daytime sleepiness.

**LO 2 | The Importance of Sleep**

- Sleep serves as a mental and physical restorer, helps conserve energy, reduces risks of CVD and other chronic ailments, aides in healthy metabolism and neurological functioning, improves motor tasks, and helps manage stress.

**LO 3 | The Processes of Sleep**

- The sleep cycle is regulated by a biological clock known as circadian rhythms. Melatonin is the hormone that regulates the sleep cycle.
- REM and NREM sleep occur throughout the night; NREM sleep is slow-wave, restful sleep, while REM sleep mimics wakened states.
- How much sleep you need varies by age throughout the lifespan.

**LO 4 | Getting a Good Night's Sleep**

- Staying active, paying attention to your sleep environment, improving sleep hygiene, avoiding emotional upset as well as food and drink prior to sleep are all important to a good nights sleep.

**LO 5 | Sleep Disorders**

- Major sleep disorders include insomnia, sleep apnea, restless leg syndrome, and narcolepsy, each with varying symptoms, causes, prevention, and treatment options.

## POP QUIZ

Visit **MasteringHealth** to personalize your study plan with Chapter Review Quizzes and Dynamic Study Modules.

**LO 1 | Sleepless in America**

1. About how many American adults are sleep deprived?
   a. Between 50 and 70 million
   b. Between 30 and 50 million
   c. Between 10 and 30 million
   d. Between 70 and 90 million

**LO 2 | The Importance of Sleep**

2. Which of the following age groups is reportedly most likely to fall asleep at the wheel?
   a. Over 53
   b. Over 34
   c. Under 26
   d. Under 18

**LO 3 | The Processes of Sleep**

3. Which of the following occurs when your body's circadian rhythm becomes out of sink with daylight hours?
   a. Jet lag
   b. REM sleep
   c. NREM sleep
   d. Somnolence

**LO 4 | Getting a Good Night's Sleep**

4. Which of the following is *not* recommended if you want to get a good nights sleep?
   a. Getting adequate exposure to light; particularly sunlight during the day.
   b. Exercising each day
   c. Paying careful attention to your sleep environment, including clean scents and cool temperatures
   d. Consume lots of fluids and foods that make you feel sleepy/full just prior to sleeping.

**LO 5 | Sleep Disorders**

5. Which sleep disorder involves difficulty falling asleep, waking up during the night, and/or difficulty falling back asleep?
   a. Obstructive sleep apnea
   b. Narcolepsy
   c. Restless leg syndrome
   d. Insomnia

*Answers to the Pop Quiz questions can be found on page A-1. If you answered a question incorrectly, review the section identified by the Learning Outcome. For even more study tools, visit MasteringHealth.*

# 4 Preventing Violence and Injury

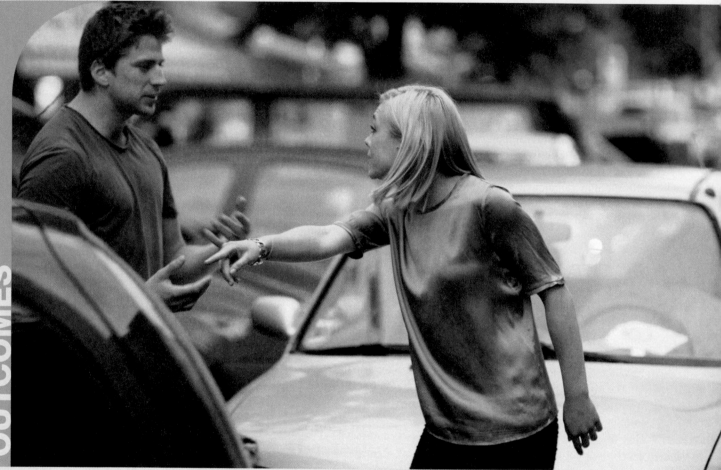

1 Differentiate between intentional and unintentional injuries and discuss the prevalence of violence in American society and on college campuses.

2 Identify societal and personal factors that contribute to violence in American society.

3 Discuss the prevalence, types, and common causes of interpersonal and collective acts of violence, including homicide, hate crimes, gang violence, and terrorism; describe intimate partner violence and the cycle of IPV.

4 Describe types of and social contributors to sexual victimization, and discuss efforts to prevent and respond to sexual victimization.

5 Articulate personal and community strategies for preventing violence.

6 Describe precautions to take to minimize the risk and effect of unintentional injuries.

*Fear follows crime, and is its punishment.*
—Voltaire, 1694–1778[1]

**V**iolence permeates today's world news. Terrorist activities, including bombings, beheadings, rapes, and government takeovers, stream into our homes 24/7. Nationally, homicide, rape, abuse, neglect, hate crimes, shootings, animal abuse, and other victimizations fill our local news channels, prompting some to wonder if there is any good news out there. We watch, we listen, and we shudder, wondering where it will all lead—and who will become the next victim.

Put into perspective, violence has always been part of human existence. Throughout history, humans have sought to dominate others, achieve religious or political power, or grab land and resources. A key difference today is that we are much more aware of the violence occurring around us. We can now watch horrendous acts play out across the world from the safety of our own televisions, computers, and mobile devices.

Are all forms of violence growing worse, as the media would have us believe? Which kinds of violence are college students particularly vulnerable to? Are we destined to be victims living in fear, or are there things each of us can do to change the course of violence in society? Where do we start?

## LO 1 | **WHAT** IS VIOLENCE?

Differentiate between intentional and unintentional injuries and discuss the prevalence of violence in American society and on college campuses.

Before we can discuss the extent of violence, it's important to understand what the word *violence* means. The World Health Organization (WHO) defines **violence** as *"the intentional use of physical force or power, threatened or actual, against oneself, another person, or a group or community that results in or has a high likelihood of resulting in injury, death, psychological harm, maldevelopment or deprivation."*[2] Today, most experts realize that emotional and psychological forms of violence can be as devastating as physical blows to the body.

The U.S. Public Health Service historically categorized violence resulting in injuries into two categories: intentional injuries or unintentional injuries. **Intentional injuries** are those committed with intent to harm and typically include assaults, homicides, self-inflicted injuries, and suicides. **Unintentional injuries**, on the other hand, are those committed without intent to harm, such as motor vehicle crashes, fires, and drownings.

So, why devote a chapter to violence and injury in an introductory health text for college and university students? The answer is simple: Young adults are disproportionately affected by violence and injury. Unintentional injuries, particularly from motor vehicle crashes, are the number one cause of death among 15- to 44-year-olds in the United States today, where suicide and homicide are the second and third leading causes of death in 15- to 34-year-olds.[3]

## Violence Overview

Each year, over 1.3 million people globally die from some form of violence.[4] People in the 15 to 44 age group, particularly males, are at most risk for death by violence; however, untold millions, particularly women and children, suffer in silence, bearing lifelong physical and emotional scars. Post-traumatic stress disorder (PTSD), depression, anxiety, substance abuse, and difficulties holding jobs or forming lasting relationships are just some of the emotional consequences victims may experience.[5] Patterns of violence vary significantly among countries, with lower income countries often experiencing higher rates of violence than those with higher income.[6]

Violence has been a part of the American landscape since colonial times. However, it wasn't until the 1980s that the U.S. Public Health Service identified violence as a leading cause of death and disability and gave it chronic disease status, indicating that it was a pervasive threat to society. Statistics from the Federal Bureau of Investigation (FBI) have shown that, after steadily increasing from 1973 to 2006, rates of overall crime and major types of violent crime have been slowly decreasing in recent years. At the same time, the Bureau of Justice Statistics reported a significant increase in violence in 2012.[7]

> **violence** A set of behaviors that produces injuries, as well as the outcomes of these behaviors (the injuries themselves).
>
> **intentional injuries** Injury, death, or psychological harm inflicted with the intent to harm.
>
> **unintentional injuries** Injury, death, or psychological harm caused unintentionally or without premeditation.

How do we determine crime rates each year? Historically, we use two measures for violence in the United States: the FBI's *Uniform Crime Reporting (UCR) Program* and the Bureau of Justice Statistics *National Crime Victimization Survey (NCVS)*. While the FBI's UCR collects data on violent crimes involving force or threat actually *reported* to law enforcement agencies, the Bureau of Justice Statistics collects self-reported information on crimes through twice-yearly surveys of nearly 160,000 people in 90,000 homes. In these surveys, people recount incidents of crime they experienced and whether they reported them to police. Analysts then make estimates about national crime based on extrapolated data.[8] Because of their different data collection methods, you may see conflicting media reports about crime rates rising or falling, as happened in 2012. In 2013, the FBI and Bureau of Justice statistics reported similar declines in rates of violent crime.[9] See **FIGURE 4.1** for the percent change of violent crimes reported in 2013 and **FIGURE 4.2** for the frequency of different types of crimes.

Whether total rates of crime are up or down in a given year, there are huge disparities in crime rates based on race, sex, age, socioeconomic status, location, crime type, and other factors. Additionally, over 50 percent of violent victimizations are not reported to the police.[10] Rates of nonreporting are even higher for some offenses such as rape. If those nonreports suddenly become reported crimes, we might have a very different profile.[11] Although you may never be a direct victim of crime—those who live in fear of being victimized, are afraid to go out for a walk or run at night, or avoid international travel or mass transit because of terrorist threats—are already indirectly affected.

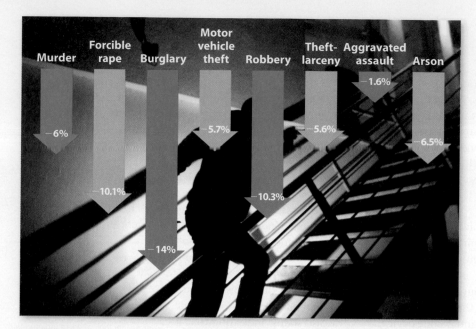

**FIGURE 4.1** Changing Crime Rates (percent) FBI statistics show reported violent crimes decreasing in early 2014. Although numbers of violent crimes reported to police have decreased in recent years, surveys of Americans indicate that overall crime rates have increased in the last 2 years, particularly as identity theft, burglaries, theft, simple assaults, and other crimes have increased.

**Source:** FBI, "Preliminary Semiannual Uniform Crime Report, January–June 2014," accessed June, 2015, https://www.fbi.gov/about-us/cjis/ucr/crime-in-the-u.s/2014/preliminary-semiannual-uniform-crime-report-january-june-2014

## Violence on U.S. Campuses

A spate of campus violence in recent years has caused increased concern among Americans. Whether discussing the deadliest mass shooting in U.S. history at Virginia Tech in 2007 or reports of rapes, hate crimes, and other violations on campuses across the country, it is clear that campus violence is real and not likely to go away without a concerted effort. Pressure

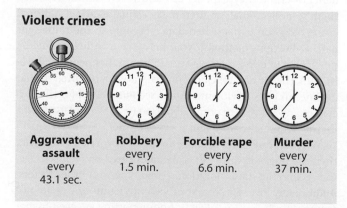

**Violent crimes**

| Aggravated assault | Robbery | Forcible rape | Murder |
|---|---|---|---|
| every 43.1 sec. | every 1.5 min. | every 6.6 min. | every 37 min. |

**FIGURE 4.2** Crime Clock The crime clock represents the annual ratio of crime to fixed time intervals. The crime clock should not be taken to imply a regularity in the commission of crime.

**Source:** Adapted from Federal Bureau of Investigation, "Crime in the United States, 2013," Accessed February 2015, www.fbi.gov/about-us/cjis/ucr/crime-in-the-u.s/2013/crime-in-the-u.s.-2013/offenses-known-to-law-enforcement/browse-by/national-data

from legislators, parents, and alumni has moved the campus safety issue front and center on the national stage. Calls for enforcement of zero violence tolerance policies on campuses that receive federal funding, major improvements in record keeping, improved victim assistance and support, and swift punishment for offenders have all been recommended.

Relationship violence is one of the most prevalent problems on campus. In the most recent American College Health Association survey, 10.5 percent of women and 6.3 percent of men reported being emotionally abused in the past 12 months by a significant other.[12] Almost 6.5 percent of women and 2.8 percent of men reported being stalked, and 2 percent of women and 1.7 percent of men reported being involved in a physically abusive relationship. Nearly 1 percent of men and 1.7 percent women reported being in a sexually abusive relationship.[13] Only 30 percent of women indicate they feel safe on campus after dark. Even fewer—22.5 percent—feel safe in surrounding campus communities.[14] The statistics on reported campus violence represent only a glimpse of the big picture. It is believed that fewer than 25 percent of campus crimes in general are reported to *any* authority.[15] Even though as many as 20 to 25 percent of college women will be raped or sexually assaulted before they graduate, 95 percent of these women never report these crimes.[16]

Why would students not report crimes? Typical reasons include concerns over privacy, fear of retaliation, embarrassment or shame, lack of support, perception that the crime was too minor or they were somehow at fault, a history of inaction by campuses in response to reports, or uncertainty that it was a crime.

## LO 2 | FACTORS CONTRIBUTING TO VIOLENCE

Identify societal and personal factors that contribute to violence in American society.

Several social, community, relationship, and individual factors increase the likelihood of violent acts. Key risk factors include the following:[17]

■ **Poverty.** Low socioeconomic status can create a hopeless environment—one in which some people view violence as the only way to obtain what they want.[18]

- **Unemployment.** Financial strain, losing or fear of losing a job, economic downturns, and living in economically depressed areas can increase rates and severity of violence.[19]
- **Societal factors.** Policies and programs that seek to remove inequality/disparity and discourage discrimination decrease risks; social and cultural norms that support male dominance over women and violence as a means of settling problems increase risks.[20]
- **Religious beliefs and differences.** Extreme religious beliefs can lead people to think violence against others is justified.
- **Political differences.** Civil unrest and political differences have historically been triggers for violent acts.
- **Breakdowns in the criminal justice system.** Overcrowded prisons, lenient sentences, early releases, and inadequate availability of mental health services can encourage repeat offenses and future violence.
- **Stress, depression, or other mental health issues.** People who are in crisis, depressed, or under stress are more apt to be highly reactive, strike out at others, display anger, or act irrationally.[21]

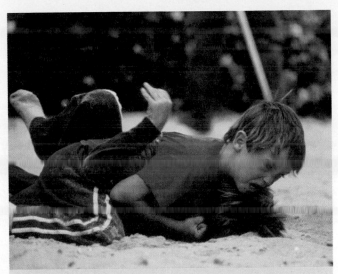

Most adults learn to control outbursts of anger in a rational manner. However, some people act out their aggressive tendencies in much the same way they did as children—with anger and violence that are a form of self-assertion or a response to frustration.

## What Makes Some Individuals Prone to Violence?

In addition to the broad, societal-based factors that contribute to crime, personal factors can also increase risks for violence. Emerging evidence suggests that family and home environment may be the greatest contributors to eventual violent behavior among family members.[22] Key predictors of aggressive behavior include anger and irrational beliefs, genetic predispositions toward anger, and the influence of coercive and contagious peers.[23]

### Aggression and Anger
*Aggressive* behavior is often a key aspect of violent interactions. **Primary aggression** is goal-directed, hostile self-assertion that is destructive in nature. **Reactive aggression** is more often part of an emotional reaction brought about by frustrating life experiences. Whether aggression is reactive or primary, it is most likely to flare up in times of acute stress.

Anger is a well-known catalyst for violence. Anger typically occurs when there is a *triggering event* or a person has learned that acting out in angry ways can get him or her what he or she wants. Anger tends to be an active, attack-oriented emotion in which people feel powerful and in control for a short period.[24]

People who anger quickly often have a low tolerance for frustration. The cause may be genetic or physiological; there is evidence that some people are born with strong tendencies toward anger.[25]

Typically, anger-prone people come from families that are disruptive, chaotic, and unskilled in emotional expression and where anger, domestic violence, and abuse occur regularly.[26] Those who have been bullied in school may also be prone to react with violence in future situations.[27]

**primary aggression** Goal-directed, hostile self-assertion that is destructive in nature.

**reactive aggression** Hostile emotional reaction brought about by frustrating life experiences.

### Substance Abuse
Alcohol and drug abuse are often catalysts for violence at all levels of society, both nationally and internationally.[28] Consumption of alcohol precedes over half of all violent crimes and is a major factor in domestic violence at all levels. In a recent meta-analysis of nearly 30,000 homicides, 48 percent of offenders were under the influence of alcohol and 37 percent were intoxicated.[29] Men who are heavier drinkers and more frequently drink to intoxication are the most likely to be perpetrators of sexual violence.[30] Alcohol abuse, particularly binge drinking, is associated with physical victimization among males and sexual victimization among females on campuses.[31] People treated for alcohol abuse also have 10 times greater risk of suicide than those not requiring treatment; in fact, 30–40 percent of suicides and suicide attempts are among problem drinkers.[32]

**WHAT DO YOU THINK?**

Why do you think rates of violence in the United States are so much higher than those of other developed nations, such as Great Britain and Japan?

- What factor do you think is the single greatest cause of violence?
- What could be done to reduce risk from this factor?

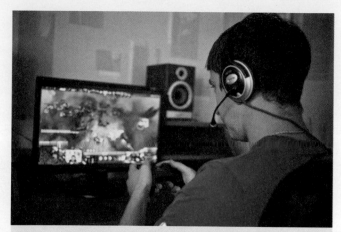

Arguably, Americans today—especially children—are exposed to more depictions of violence than ever before, but research has not shown a clear link between a person's exposure to violent media and his or her propensity to engage in violent acts.

## How Much Impact Do the Media Have?

Although the media are often blamed for having a major role in the escalation of violence, this association has been challenged continuously. Increasing numbers of professional organizations have indicated that exposure to media violence is a risk factor for aggression, desensitization toward violence, and lack of sympathy for victims, particularly in youth.[33] However, much of this research has been called into question for methodological problems such as poor measures of violence and aggression, biased subject selection, sample size, and the fact that many studies report perceptions of violence by physicians and others rather than documented evidence from the field.[34]

Critics also point to the declining rates of violent crime over recent decades despite the explosive increases in violent video games in our digital, age, as well as declining trends in bullying, physical fighting, and weapon carrying in youth during that same period.[35] A recent review of 25 years of research indicates that claims of a strong relationship between violent video games and aggression are not supported by current studies.[36] Other researchers continue to point out that exposure to violent videos has neither long- nor short-term effects of either positive or negative behaviors.[37]

> **interpersonal violence** Violence inflicted against one individual by another or by a small group of others.
>
> **collective violence** Violence committed by groups of individuals.
>
> **homicide** Death that results from intent to injure or kill.

While some continue to believe that exposure to violent media somehow numbs people to humanity, allows people to commit violence without empathy or regret, or even triggers violent events, critics of these theories abound.[38] More research is needed to fully understand the role that violent media may play in violent behavior.

## LO 3 | INTERPERSONAL AND COLLECTIVE VIOLENCE

Discuss the prevalence, types, and common causes of interpersonal and collective acts of violence, including homicide, hate crimes, gang violence, and terrorism; describe intimate partner violence and the cycle of IPV.

**Interpersonal violence** refers to violence between individuals such as families, friends, intimate partners, and others in the community.[39] It includes intentionally using "physical force or power, threatened or actual," to inflict harm on an individual that results in injury, death, or psychological harm.[40] Homicide and hate crimes fit into this category, as do domestic violence and sexual victimization. **Collective violence** is violence perpetrated by groups against other groups and includes violent acts related to political, governmental, religious, cultural, or social clashes.[41] Gang violence and terrorism are two forms of collective violence that have become major threats in recent years.

### WHY SHOULD I CARE?

The amount you drink tonight can directly affect your chances of becoming a victim of injury or assault. College students are particularly at risk for crimes committed under the influence of alcohol, including assault, rape, and intimate partner violence, but understanding the impact of alcohol in escalating potentially violent situations can help you stay out of harm's way.

### Homicide

**Homicide,** defined as murder or nonnegligent manslaughter (killing another human), is the fifteenth leading cause of death in the United States, the second leading cause of death for persons aged 15 to 24, and is among the top five leading causes of death for ages 1 to 44.[42] It accounted for over 14,000 deaths in the United States in 2013, the majority of which were caused by firearms.[43] (See the **Health Headlines** box for a discussion of the role of guns in United States homicide rates.) Nearly 44 percent of all homicides occur among people who know one another, like family members, friends, acquaintances, significant others, neighbors, and coworkers.[44]

In spite of media sensationalism that may lead you to think otherwise, overall homicide rates in the United States have

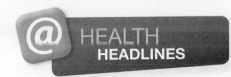

# BRINGING THE GUN DEBATE TO CAMPUS

On average, each year in the United States 100,000 people are shot. Over 31,000 of them die, and of those who survive, many experience significant physical and emotional repercussions. Some facts about guns and gun violence include the following:

- Handguns are consistently responsible for more murders than any other type of weapon.
- Today, 35 percent of American homes have a gun on the premises, with nearly 300 million privately owned guns registered—and millions more that are unregistered and/or illegal.
- Firearms are the weapons most often used in attacks on American campuses. The most common reason for an incident is "related to an intimate relationship," followed by "retaliation for a specific action."
- The presence of a gun in the home triples the risk of a homicide in that location and increases suicide risk more than five times.

What factors contribute to gun deaths in the United States? Gun critics argue that large numbers of guns in the United States as well as relatively lax gun-control laws are the culprits. However, gun-rights advocates say that the problem lies not with guns, but with the people who own them, and point to countries such as Canada, with similar numbers of guns as in the United States, but with much lower gun-related crime rates.

High-profile shootings at schools and other public places have brought the gun debate to campuses. The National Conference on State Legislatures reported that while 50 states allow citizens to carry concealed weapons, only 20 allow concealed weapons on campus. But in 23 other states, the decision to ban

or allow concealed carry weapons on campuses is made by each institution. Seven states allow concealed weapons in postsecondary public education campuses. Proponents argue that there is no evidence that legally allowing guns on campus would increase the risk of campus violence. Early in 2015, gun advocates are making the case for carrying by saying that doing so would prevent rape and sexual assault of women. What do you think?

**Sources:** National Conference of State Legislators (NCSL), Guns on Campus: Overview," February 23, 2015, www.ncsl.org/research/education/guns-on -campus-overview.aspx; D. Drysdale, W. Modzeleski, and A. Simons, *Campus Attacks: Targeted Violence Affecting Institutions of Higher Learning* (Washington DC; United States Secret Service, United States Department of Education, and the Federal Bureau of Investigation, 2010); Brady Campaign to Prevent Gun Violence, "Facts: Gun Violence," Revised 2010, www .bradycampaign.org; A. Schwartz, "A Bid for Guns on Campus to Deter Rape," *New York Times*, February 18, 2015, www.nytimes.com/2015/02/19/us/in-bid -to-allow-guns-on-campus-weapons-are-linked-to -fighting-sexual-assault.html?_r=0

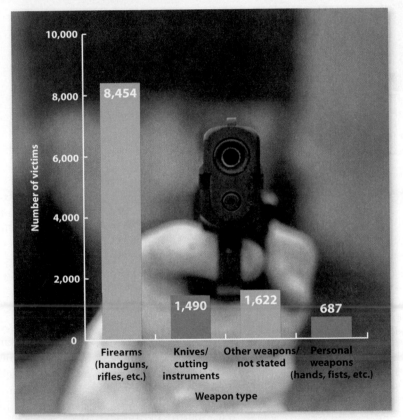

Homicide in the United States by Weapon Type, 2013. Sixty-seven percent of murders in the United States are committed using firearms, far outweighing all other weapons combined.

**Source:** Data from U.S. Department of Justice, Federal Bureau of Investigation, *Crime in the United States, 2013*, "Murder," Table 20, www.fbi.gov/about-us/cjis/ucr/crime-in-the -u.s/2013/crime-in-the-u.s.-2013/tables/table-20/table_20_murder_by_state_types_of _weapons_2013.xls

---

declined by nearly half (49%), falling from 9.3 homicides per 100,000 U.S. residents in 1992 to 4.7 in 2011.[45] Although young adults (particularly males) aged 18 to 24 have the highest homicide rates of any age group, their rates have also gone down over 22 percent in the last 10 years.[46] Men have a murder rate 3.6 times higher than do women.[47] Rates also vary across races, with the average homicide rate 6.3 times higher among blacks than whites.[48]

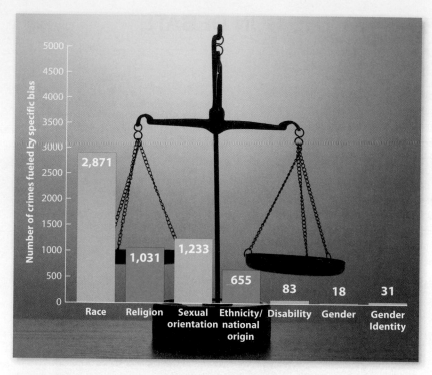

**FIGURE 4.3** Bias-Motivated Crimes, Single-Bias Incidence, 2013

**Source:** Data from Federal Bureau of Investigation, "Hate Crime Statistics, 2013," Table 1, 2013, www.fbi.gov

## Hate and Bias-Motivated Crimes

A **hate crime** is a crime committed against a person, property, or group of people that is motivated by the offender's bias against a race, religion, disability, sexual orientation, gender/gender identity, or ethnicity. Reports of hate crimes have declined to 5,928 reported incidents in 2013, according to the FBI (**FIGURE 4.3**).[49] In sharp contrast, when a representative sample of Americans completed the anonymous Bureau of Justice Statistics National Crime Victimization Survey, an estimated 294,000 violent and property hate crimes occurred in 2012![50] Fear of retaliation keeps many hate crimes hidden. While 60 percent of hate crimes may never be reported, only about one fourth of those reported are reported by victims themselves.[51]

*Bias-motivated crime*, sometimes referred to as **ethnoviolence**, describes violence based on prejudice and discrimination among ethnic groups in the larger society. **Prejudice** is an irrational attitude of hostility directed against an individual; a group; a race; or the supposed characteristics of an individual, group, or race. **Discrimination** constitutes actions that deny equal treatment or opportunities to a group of people, often based on prejudice.

Common reasons given to explain bias-motivated and hate crimes include (1) *thrill seeking* by multiple offenders through a group attack; (2) *feeling threatened* that others will take their jobs or property or beset them in some way; (3) *retaliating* for some real or perceived insult or slight; and (4) *fearing the unknown or differences*. For other people, hate crimes are a part of their mission in life, either due to religious zeal, lack of understanding, or distorted moral beliefs.

Campuses have responded to reports of hate crimes by offering courses that emphasize diversity, zero tolerance for violations, training faculty to recognize possible offenses and act appropriately, and developing policies that strictly enforce punishment for hate crimes.

## Gang Violence

Gang violence is increasing in many regions of the world; U.S. communities face escalating threats from gang networks engaged in drug trafficking, sex trafficking, shootings, beatings, thefts, carjackings, and the killing of innocent victims caught in the crossfire. Currently, there are over 33,000 gangs in the United States, with membership in excess of 1.4 million.[52] The vast majority are street gangs, (88%), followed by prison gangs (9.5%) and outlaw motorcycle gangs (2.5%).[53] Gangs are believed to be responsible for 48 percent of U.S. violent crime overall, and in some locations, as much as 90 percent.[54]

Why do young people join gangs? Often, gangs give members a sense of self-worth, companionship, security, and excitement. In other cases, gangs provide economic security through drug sales, prostitution, and other types of criminal activity. Friendships with delinquent peers, lack of parental monitoring, negative life events, and alcohol and drug use appear to increase risks for gang affiliation. Other risk factors include low self-esteem, academic problems, low socioeconomic status, alienation from family and society, a history of family violence, and living in gang-controlled neighborhoods.[55]

## Terrorism

Terrorist attacks around the world reveal the vulnerability of all nations to domestic and international threats. Effects on our economy, travel restrictions, additional security measures, and military buildups are but a few of the examples of how terrorist threats have affected our lives. As defined in the U.S. Code of Federal Regulations, **terrorism** is the "unlawful use of force or violence against persons or property to

**hate crime** Crime targeted against a particular societal group and motivated by bias against that group.

**ethnoviolence** Violence directed at persons affiliated with a particular ethnic group.

**prejudice** A negative evaluation of an entire group of people that is typically based on unfavorable and often wrong ideas about the group.

**discrimination** Actions that deny equal treatment or opportunities to a group, often based on prejudice.

**terrorism** Unlawful use of force or violence against persons or property to intimidate or coerce a government, civilian population, or any segment thereof in furtherance of political or social objectives.

intimate or coerce a government, the civilian population, or any segment thereof in furtherance of political or social objectives."[56] Increasingly, the Internet and social media are being used for recruitment and radicalization of youth throughout the world. Efforts to counteract such activities are underway by several major groups in the United States and internationally.[57]

Over the past decade, the Centers for Disease Control and Prevention (CDC) established the *Emergency Preparedness and Response Division*. This group monitors potential public health problems, such as bioterrorism, chemical emergencies, radiation emergencies, national disasters, and severe weather; develops plans for mobilizing communities in the case of emergency; and provides information about terrorist threats. Preparing yourself for emergency situations can help you cope in the event actual problems with communication lines, food supplies, power, or water occur.

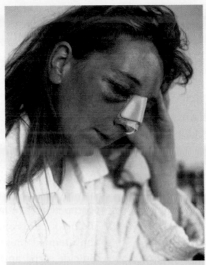

People who stay with their abusers may do so because they are dependent on the abuser, because they fear the abuser, or even because they love the abuser. In some cultures, women may not be free to leave an abusive relationship because of restrictive laws, religious beliefs, or social mores.

## Intimate Partner Violence

**Domestic violence** has historically referred to the use of force to control and maintain power over another person in the home environment—whether emotional abuse, verbal abuse, threats of physical harm, or physical violence. It can occur between parent and child, between siblings or other family members, or more commonly, between spouses or intimate partners. Although still used, the term *domestic violence* is slowly being replaced by more specific categories of violence—violence that may or may not occur in the home.

**Intimate partner violence (IPV)** includes physical, sexual, or psychological harm done by a boyfriend, girlfriend, or current or former spouse. Over the course of a year, millions of women and men are victims of rape, physical and psychological abuse, stalking, and other offenses performed by an intimate partner. Homicide committed by a current or former intimate partner is the leading cause of death of pregnant women in the United States.[58] In addition, 74 percent of all murder-suicides in the United States involve an intimate partner; 90 percent are carried out by a male with a gun.[59]

Psychological aggression in the form of constant criticism, verbal attacks, displays of explosive anger meant to intimidate, and controlling behavior are commonly seen in intimate partner abuse. Psychological abusers seek to intimidate and debase their partners, thereby gaining control over the

**SEE IT!** VIDEOS

Should strangers step in to prevent partner abuse? Watch **Will Anyone Confront Abusive Boyfriend?** available on MasteringHealth™

partner and relationship. Stress, mental health issues, economic uncertainty/frustration, jealousy, issues of power/control and gender roles, and issues with self-esteem are among common reasons given for IPV.[60] Victims are more likely to report depression, difficulty in intimate relationships, frequent headaches, chronic pain, difficulty sleeping, activity limitations, poor physical health, irritable bowel syndrome, and other health problems.[61]

**The Cycle of IPV** Have you ever heard of a woman repeatedly beaten by her partner and wondered, "Why doesn't she just leave him?" There are many reasons some women find it difficult to break ties with abusers. Some women, particularly those with small children, are financially dependent on their partners. Others fear retaliation against themselves or their children. Some hope the situation will change with time, and others stay because cultural or religious beliefs forbid divorce. Still others love the abusive partner and are concerned about what will happen if they leave.

In the 1970s, psychologist Lenore Walker developed a theory called the *cycle of violence* that explained predictable, repetitive patterns of psychological and/or physical abuse that seemed to occur in abusive relationships. The cycle consisted of three major phases:[62]

1. **Tension building.** Prior to the overtly abusive act, tension building includes breakdowns in communication, anger, psychological aggression, growing tension, and fear.
2. **Incident of acute battering.** When the acute attack is over, he may respond with shock and denial about his own behavior or blame her for making him do it.
3. **Remorse/reconciliation.** During a "honeymoon" period, the batterer may be kind, loving, and apologetic, swearing that he will work to change his behavior.

Walker's initial work was criticized by some for its lack of scientific rigor and for what appeared to be a simplified approach to a complex problem. In her most recent book, *The Battered Woman Syndrome*, Walker's conclusions were based on improved quantitative analysis, reviews of recent research, and an extensive list of experts in the field of violence.[63] Today, *battered woman syndrome* is considered to be a subgrouping of PTSD.[64]

**domestic violence** The use of force to control and maintain power over another person in the home environment, including both actual harm and the threat of harm.

**intimate partner violence (IPV)** Describes physical, sexual, or psychological harm by a current or former partner or spouse.

# Child Abuse and Neglect

**Child maltreatment** is defined as any act or series of acts of commission or omission by a parent or caregiver that results in harm, potential for harm, or threat of harm to a child.[65] **Child abuse** refers to *acts of commission,* which are deliberate or intentional words or actions that cause harm, potential harm, or threat of harm to a child. The abuse may be sexual, psychological, physical, or a combination. **Neglect** is an *act of omission,* meaning a failure to provide for a child's basic physical, emotional, or education tion needs or to protect a child from harm or potential harm. Although exact figures for child abuse are difficult to obtain, in 2014 an estimated 3 million cases of child abuse were reported, involving the alleged maltreatment of approximately 6 million children. As alarming as current reports may seem, of greater concern are reports that few of the reported physical or sexual abuse cases are investigated by social services–even in the higher income countries of the world. Reporting and investigating of psychological/emotional abuse is completed in fewer than 10 percent of cases.[66] **FIGURE 4.4** shows the rates of abuse among children in different age groups.

It is important to remember that child abuse occurs at every socioeconomic level, across ethnic and cultural lines, within all religions, and at all levels of education. Not all violence

**child maltreatment** Any act or series of acts of commission or omission by a parent or caregiver that results in harm, potential for harm, or threat of harm to a child.

**child abuse** Deliberate or intentional words or actions that cause harm, potential for harm, or threat of harm to a child.

**neglect** Failure to provide a child's basic needs such as food, clothing, shelter, and medical care.

# 1 IN 3

WOMEN AND 1 IN 10 MEN HAVE BEEN VICTIMS OF INTIMATE PARTNER **VIOLENCE** IN THE FORM OF RAPE, STALKING, OR PHYSICAL VIOLENCE IN THEIR LIFETIMES.

against children is physical. Health can be severely affected by psychological violence—assaults on personality, character, competence, independence, or general dignity as a human being. Victims of child abuse have a higher risk of depression, unintended pregnancy, sexually transmitted diseases (STIs), suicide, drug and alcohol abuse, and an overall lowered life expectancy, particularly among those repeatedly victimized.[67]

## Elder Abuse

By 2030, the number of people in the United States over the age of 65 will exceed 71 million—nearly double their number in 2000. Each year, hundreds of thousands of adults over the age of 60, particularly women, are abused, neglected, or financially exploited. Tragically, fewer than 1 in 20 cases of physical or sexual abuse are reported.[68] Many victims fail to report abuse because they are embarrassed or because they don't want the abuser to get in trouble or retaliate by putting them in a nursing home or escalating the abuse. Some do not report due to feeling guilty because someone has to take care of them. Others suffer from dementia and may not be aware of the abuse. A variety of social services focus on protecting our seniors, just as we endeavor to protect other vulnerable populations.

## LO 4 | SEXUAL VICTIMIZATION

Describe types of and social contributors to sexual victimization, and discuss efforts to prevent and respond to sexual victimization.

The term *sexual victimization* refers to any situation where an individual is coerced or forced to comply with or endure another's sexual acts or overtures. It can run the gamut from harassment to stalking to assault and rape by perpetrators known or unknown to the victim. It can even include sexual coercion and rape by spouses within the confines of marriage. Fear, sexual avoidance, sleeplessness, anxiety, and depression are just a few of the long-term consequences for victims.[69]

**FIGURE 4.4**  Child Abuse and Neglect Victims by Age, 2013

**Source:** U.S. Department of Health and Human Services, Administration for Children and Families, Administration on Children, Youth and Families, Children's Bureau, 2015, Child Maltreatment 2013, Table 3-5, www.acf.hhs.gov/programs/cb/research-data-technology/statistics-research/child-maltreatment

## Sexual Assault and Rape

**Sexual assault** is any act in which one person is sexually intimate with another person without that person's consent. This may range from simple touching to forceful penetration and may include, for example, ignoring indications that intimacy is not wanted, threatening force or other negative consequences, and actually using force.

Considered the most extreme form of sexual assault, **rape** is defined as penetration without the victim's consent. Incidents of rape generally fall into one of two types—aggravated or simple. An **aggravated rape** is any rape involving one or multiple attackers, strangers, weapons, or physical beatings. A **simple rape** is a rape perpetrated by one person, whom the victim knows, and does not involve a physical beating or use of a weapon. Most rapes are classified as simple rape, but that terminology should not be taken to mean that a simple rape is any less violent or criminal. The FBI identifies rape as the second ranked type of violent crime, trailing only murder.[70]

Nearly 1 in 5 women and 1 in 59 men in the United States have been raped at some time in their lives, with nearly 80 percent of female rape victims experiencing their first rape before the age of 25.[71] More than one fourth of male rape victims were raped before they were 10 years old.[72]

By most indicators, reported cases of rape appear to have declined in the United States since the early 1990s, even as reports of other forms of sexual assault have increased. This decline is thought to be due to shifts in public awareness and attitudes about rape, combined with tougher crime policies, improved DNA testing, major educational campaigns, and media attention. These changes enforce the idea that rape is a violent crime and should be treated as such. However, numerous sources indicate that rape is among one of the most underreported crimes; a recent report to the U.S. Senate says that fewer than 5 percent of campus rapes are ever reported to the police.[73]

**Acquaintance Rape** The terms *date rape* and *acquaintance rape* have been used interchangeably in the past. However, most experts now believe that the term *date rape* is inappropriate because it implies a consensual interaction in an arranged setting and may, in fact, minimize the crime of rape when it occurs. Today, **acquaintance rape** refers to any rape in which the rapist is known to the victim. Acquaintance rape is more common when drugs or alcohol have been consumed by the offender or victim; this makes the campus party environment a high-risk venue for young college women and men.[74] Alcohol is frequently involved in acquaintance rape, as are a growing number of rape-facilitating drugs such as gamma-hydroxybutyrate (GHB), ketamine, and Rohypnol.

GHB is one of the most common drugs used in rape cases. Intended for treating narcolepsy, it is quick acting and has a depressant affect, causing motor impairment and confusion/sleepiness. *Ketamine* is a drug used by veterinarians as an anesthetic. It can cause motor dysfunction and memory loss, making it difficult even for an awake person to fight back. *Rohypnol,* also known as a "roofie," is a strong sedative and muscle relaxant that puts victims in a deep sleep. Legal forms of the original drug make drinks cloudy in appearance; however, there are many forms on the illegal market.

If you're going out, be aware of your drink and your surroundings. Go with a group of people you know and trust, and be cautious if anyone offers you an unsealed beverage. If you feel incredibly tired or clumsy after drinking a relatively small amount, get to a safe place as soon as possible. The **Skills for Behavior Change** box on the next page identifies more practical tips for preventing dating violence.

**Rape on U.S. Campuses** Rape and sexual assault on campus are not new phenomena, even though such crimes on campus have been chronically underreported.[75] By some estimates, between 20 and 25 percent of college women have experienced an attempted or completed rape in college.[76]

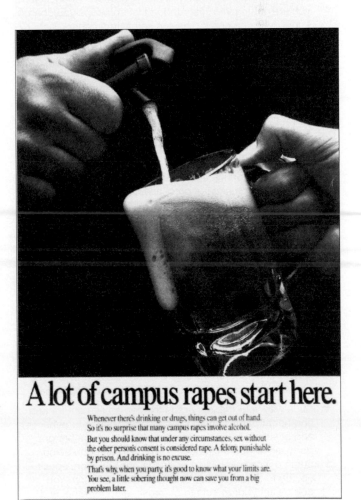

# A lot of campus rapes start here.

Whenever there's drinking or drugs, things can get out of hand. So it's no surprise that many campus rapes involve alcohol.

But you should know that under any circumstances, sex without the other person's consent is considered rape. A felony, punishable by prison. And drinking is no excuse.

That's why, when you party, it's good to know what your limits are. You see, a little sobering thought now can save you from a big problem later.

Acquaintance rape is particularly common on college campuses, where alcohol and drug use can impair young people's judgment and self-control.

→ **VIDEO TUTOR**
Acquaintance
Rape on Campus

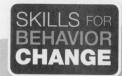

## REDUCING YOUR RISK OF DATING VIOLENCE: TIPS FOR WOMEN AND MEN

Remember that if a romantic partner truly cares for you and respects you, that person will respect your wishes and feelings. Here are some tips for dealing with sexual pressure or unwanted advances when dating and socializing:

▶ Prior to your date, think about your values, and set personal boundaries before you walk out the door. Have a plan for staying safe and stick to it.

▶ Get consent for sexual activity. Educate yourself on what YES and NO really mean and don't make assumptions, especially in situations involving drugs or alcohol. Ask yourself, "Is this worth my reputation, or is this worth having a sexual assault or rape charge and being prosecuted?" Ignorance is no excuse for illegal actions.

▶ Do not go off to a special room, car, or bedroom at a party where there is heavy drinking. Stay with friends. If you are getting intoxicated, don't let someone you don't know drive you home. There is safety in numbers, particularly if you stay in full view of others.

▶ Set limits. Practice what you will say to friends if they pressure you into actions that you would not normally engage in, or if your date pressures you in an uncomfortable direction. If the situation feels like it is getting out of control, or someone is really coming on to you, change the dialogue. Be firm and say you are uncomfortable. Say "no" directly, loudly, and firmly. Don't worry about hurting feelings.

▶ Don't accept drinks that you haven't had total control over from the minute of purchase. Don't leave drinks unattended.

▶ Remember that acts you might not think of as serious could get you into a lot of trouble. Forced heavy kissing, touching, and pressing flesh are all grounds for charges of assault.

▶ Pay attention to your date's actions. If there is too much teasing, if there is encouragement to drink more and more, if there is a tendency to keep you from staying with your friends, or if you sense unusual pressure, it may mean trouble. Trust your intuition.

▶ Go out in groups when dating someone new. If you know the person, make sure they understand where you are coming from in terms of unwanted sexual advances.

▶ Stick with your friends. Agree to keep an eye out for one another at parties and have a plan for leaving together and checking in with each other. Never leave a bar or party alone with a stranger. If you see someone being put into a compromising or dangerous situation, speak up. Try to steer the situation in another direction. You don't want your friends to be prosecuted for rape, and you don't want your friends to be victimized.

## OVER 20%

OF UNDERGRADUATE WOMEN HAVE BEEN SEXUALLY **ASSAULTED** ONE OR MORE TIMES DURING THEIR UNDERGRADUATE YEARS.

In 1990, Congress passed the *Clery Act,* requiring institutions to collect and report sexual crimes on their campuses. As part of Clery Act, three main areas were to be addressed or the institutions would lose federal aid: (1) victim's rights, (2) disciplinary procedures, and (3) educational programs.

Under further fire for failure to respond to student victimization on campus, Congress passed the *Campus Sexual Assault Victim's Bill of Rights,* known as the *Ramstad Act,* in 1992. The act gave victims the right to call in off-campus authorities to investigate serious campus crimes and required universities to develop educational programs and notify students of available counseling.

In 2013, under pressure from President Obama and in response to a detailed report from Senator Claire McCaskill about the existing risks to students on American campuses, the *Campus Sexual Violence Elimination Act* passed and was fully implemented by October 1, 2014.[77] As part of the act, intimate partner violence, dating violence, sexual assault, and stalking cases must be reported on annual campus crime reports. Notification procedures, options for victims and accused perpetrators, and consequences—including loss of federal support if schools don't conduct campus climate surveys and assess their prevention activities—are all part of the new act provisions.[78]

In 2014, the State of California became the first in the nation to implement a *"yes means yes"* law, changing the definition of sexual consent to require "an affirmative, conscious, and voluntary agreement to engage in sexual activity."[79] If one party is unable to give consent due to intoxication or other factors, the perpetrator could be prosecuted for sexual assault. Beyond changing definitions, the law also requires schools who receive funding from the state to develop policies around numerous situations related to sexual assault.[80]

**Marital Rape** Although its legal definition varies within the United States, *marital rape* can be any unwanted intercourse or penetration (vaginal, anal, or oral) obtained by force, threat of force, or when the spouse is unable to consent. This problem has undoubtedly existed since the origin of marriage as an institution, and it is noteworthy that marital rape did not become a crime in all 50 states until 1993. Even more noteworthy is the fact that several states still allow "marital exemptions" from prosecution, meaning that the judicial system may treat it as a lesser crime.[81]

Although research in this area is scarce, it has been estimated that 10 to 14 percent of married women are raped by their husbands in the United States.[82] About one third of women report having had "unwanted sex" with their partner.[83] In general, women under the age of 25 and those from lower socioeconomic groups are at highest risk of marital rape.[84]

## Social Contributors to Sexual Assault and Rape

Certain societal assumptions and traditions can promote sexual violence, including the following:

- **Trivialization.** Many people think that rape committed by a husband or intimate partner doesn't count as rape.
- **Blaming the victim.** In spite of efforts to combat this type of thinking, many believe that a scantily clad woman "asks" for sexual advances.
- **Pressure to be macho.** Males are taught from a young age that showing emotions is a sign of weakness. This portrayal often depicts men as aggressive and predatory and females as passive targets.
- **Male socialization.** Many still believe ideas like "sowing wild oats" and "boys will be boys" are merely a normal part of male development. Women are often *objectified* (treated as sexual objects) in the media, which contributes to the idea that it's natural for men to be predatory.
- **Male misperceptions.** With media implying that sex is the focus of life, it's not surprising that some men believe that when a woman says no, she is really asking to be seduced. Later, these same men may be surprised when the woman says she was raped.
- **Situational factors.** Dates in which the male makes all the decisions, pays for everything, and generally controls the entire situation are more likely to end in an aggressive sexual scenario. Alcohol and other drugs increase the risk and severity of assaults.

### What to Do if Rape Occurs

If you are a rape victim, report the attack. Follow these steps:

- Call 9-1-1.
- Do not bathe, shower, douche, clean up, or touch anything the attacker may have touched.
- Save the clothes you were wearing, and do not launder them. They will be needed as evidence. Bring a clean change of clothes to the clinic or hospital.
- Contact the rape assistance hotline in your area, and ask for advice on counseling if you need additional help.

A recent report indicates that over 58 percent of college students say they wouldn't know what to do to help a victim of dating abuse or sexual assault.[85] If someone you know is assaulted, here's how you can help:

- Believe the rape victim. Don't ask questions that may appear to imply that she/he is at a fault in any way for the assault or that they were somehow looking for this to happen.
- Encourage the victim to see a doctor immediately, because she/he may have medical needs but feel too embarrassed to seek help. Offer to go along with him or her.
- Encourage the victim to report the crime to the police.

- Be understanding, and let the person know you will be there if she/he needs help or to talk.
- Recognize that this is an emotional recovery and it may take time for the person to bounce back.
- Encourage the person to seek counseling.

## Sexual Harassment

**Sexual harassment** typically involves unwelcome advances, verbal or physical harassment, or requests for favors of a sexual nature. Still, it doesn't have to be sexual in nature.[86] It can include offensive remarks about a person's sex or remarks by either sex directed at individuals or groups because of their gender or sexual orientation.

> **sexual harassment** Any form of unwanted sexual attention related to any condition of employment, education, or performance evaluation.

Faculty, students, and employees on U.S. campuses are protected from sexual harassment and other sexual offenses under *Title IX of the Education Amendment of 1972* Act, which prohibits discrimination based on sex in all education programs or activities that receive federal funds. Although these policies are in place, several factors keep individuals from reporting violations, including lack of awareness about what constitutes sexual harassment.

Often people think of harassment as involving only faculty members or persons in power, where sex is used to exhibit control of a situation. However, peers and members of the same sex can harass one another too. Sexual harassment may include unwanted touching; unwarranted sex-related comments, or subtle pressure for sexual favors; deliberate or repeated humiliation or intimidation based on sex; and

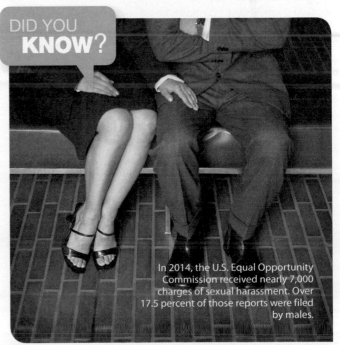

DID YOU **KNOW**?

In 2014, the U.S. Equal Opportunity Commission received nearly 7,000 charges of sexual harassment. Over 17.5 percent of those reports were filed by males.

**Source:** Data are from U.S. Equal Employment Opportunity Commission, "Charges Alleging Sexual Harassment, FY 2010–2014)," 2014, www.eeoc.gov

gratuitous comments, jokes, questions, or remarks about clothing or bodies, sexuality, or past sexual relationships.

Today, violations of Title IX amendments exist on many campuses; in fact, the U.S. Department of Education has a long list of campuses in violation of the Title IX provisions because of reported sexual violations.[87] Colleges and universities are scrambling to improve educational programs, monitoring, reporting, and enforcement of Title IX provisions.

If you feel you are being harassed, the most important thing you can do is be assertive:

- **Tell the harasser to stop.** Be clear and direct. Tell the person if it continues that you will report it. If the harassing is via phone or Internet, block the person.
- **Document the harassment.** Make a record of each incident. If the harassment becomes intolerable, a record of exactly what occurred (and when and where) will help make your case. Save copies of all communication from the harasser.
- **Try to make sure you aren't alone in the harasser's presence.** Witnesses to harassment can ensure appropriate validation of the event.
- **Complain to a higher authority.** Talk to legal authorities or your instructor, adviser, or counseling center psychologist about what happened.
- **Remember that you have not done anything wrong.** You will likely feel awful after being harassed (especially if you have to complain to superiors). However, feel proud that you are not keeping silent.

## Stalking and Cyberstalking

**Stalking** can be defined as a course of conduct directed at a specific person that would cause a reasonable person to feel fear. This may include repeated visual or physical proximity, nonconsensual written or verbal communication, and implied or explicit threats.[88] Stalking that occurs online is referred to as **cyberstalking**.

More than 1 in 4 victims report being stalked through the use of some form of technology.[89] The most common stalking behaviors included unwanted phone calls and messages, spreading rumors, spying on the victim, and showing up at the same places as the victim without having a reason to be there. Over 15 percent of women and nearly 6 percent of men have been a victim of stalking during their lifetimes.[90] The vast

**stalking** Willful, repeated, and malicious following, harassing, or threatening of another person.

**cyberstalking** Stalking that occurs online.

## WHAT DO YOU THINK?

**What policies does your school have regarding consensual relationships between faculty members and students?**

- Should consenting adults have the right to become intimate or interact socially, regardless of their positions within a school system or workplace?
- What are the potential dangers of such interactions? Are such interactions ever okay?

majority of stalkers are persons involved in relationship breakups or are other dating acquaintances; fewer than 10 percent of stalkers are strangers to their victims.[91] Adults between the ages of 18 and 24 experience the highest rates of stalking. Like sexual harassment, stalking is an underreported crime. Often students do not think a stalking incident is serious enough to report, or they worry that the police will not take it seriously.

## Child Sexual Abuse

Sexual abuse of children by adults or older children includes sexually suggestive conversations; inappropriate kissing; touching; petting; oral, anal, or vaginal intercourse; and other kinds of sexual interaction. Recent studies indicate that the rates of sexual abuse in children range from 3 to 32 percent of all children, with girls being at greater risk than young boys, even though young boys are abused in significant numbers.[92]

Most experts believe that as high as these numbers are, the shroud of secrecy surrounding child sexual abuse makes it very likely the number of actual cases is grossly underestimated. Ninety percent of child sexual abuse victims know their perpetrator, with nearly 70 percent of children abused by family members, usually an adult male.[93]

People who were abused as children bear spiritual, psychological, and/or physical scars. Children who experience sexual abuse are at increased risk for anxiety disorders, depression, eating disorders, PTSD, and suicide attempts.[94] Youth who have been sexually abused are more likely to experience teen pregnancy, more likely to abuse their own children, and much more likely to have problems with alcohol abuse or drug addiction.[95]

## LO 5 | PREVENTING VIOLENCE

Articulate personal and community strategies for preventing violence.

It is far better to prevent a violent act than to recover from it. Both individuals and communities can play important roles in preventing violence and intentional injuries.

## Self-Defense against Personal Assault and Rape

Assault can occur no matter what preventive actions you take, but commonsense self-defense tactics can lower the risk. Self-defense is a process that includes increasing your awareness, developing self-protective skills, taking reasonable precautions, and having the judgment necessary to respond quickly to changing situations. It is important to know ways to avoid and extract yourself from potentially dangerous situations.

**SEE IT! VIDEOS**

What are the repercussions of sexual assault? Watch **Sexual Assaults on College Campuses: 95 Colleges Under Federal Investigation** in the Study Area of **MasteringHealth**

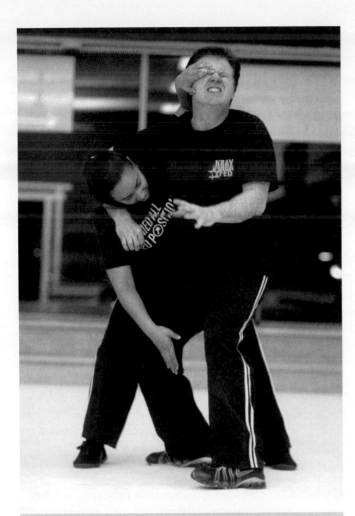

College campuses often offer safety workshops and self-defense classes to arm students with the physical and mental skills that may help them repel or deter an assailant.

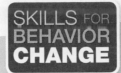

## SKILLS FOR BEHAVIOR CHANGE

## STAY SAFE ON ALL FRONTS

**Follow these tips to protect yourself from assault.**

### Outside Alone

▶ Carry a cell phone and keep it turned on, but stay off it. Be aware of what is happening around you.

▶ If you are being followed, don't go home. Head for a location where there are other people. If you decide to run, run fast and scream loudly to attract attention.

▶ Vary your routes. Stay close to other people.

▶ Park in lighted areas; avoid dark areas where someone could hide.

▶ Carry pepper spray or other deterrents. Consider using your campus escort service.

▶ Tell others where you are going and when you expect to be back.

### In Your Car

▶ Lock your doors. Do not open your doors or windows to strangers.

▶ If someone hits your car, drive to the nearest gas station or other public place if you are able. Call the police or road service for help, and stay in your car until help arrives.

▶ If a car appears to be following you, do not drive home. Drive to the nearest police station.

### In Your Home

▶ Install dead bolts on all doors and locks on all windows. Make sure the locks work, and don't leave a spare key outside.

▶ Lock doors when at home, even during the day. Close blinds and drapes whenever you are away and in the evening when you are home.

▶ Rent apartments that require a security code or clearance to gain entry, and avoid easily accessible apartments, such as first-floor units. When you move into a new residence, pay a locksmith to change the keys and locks.

▶ Don't let repair people in without asking for identification, and have someone else with you when repairs are being made.

▶ Keep a cell phone near your bed and call 9-1-1 in emergencies. Buy phones that have E911 locators so that emergency personnel can find you even when you can't respond or don't know where you are.

▶ If you return home to find your residence has been broken into, don't enter. Call the police. If you encounter an intruder, it is better to give up money or valuables than to resist

---

Most attacks by unknown assailants are planned in advance. Many rapists use certain ploys to initiate their attacks. Examples include asking for help, offering help, staging a deliberate "accident" such as bumping into you, or posing as a police officer or other authority figure. Sexual assault frequently begins with a casual, friendly conversation.

The **Skills for Behavior Change** box describes some steps you can take to reduce your risk of being assaulted. In addition, trust your intuition. Be assertive and direct to someone who is getting out of line or becoming threatening—this may convince a would-be attacker to back off. Don't try to be nice, and don't fear making a scene. Use the following tips to let a potential assailant know that you are prepared to defend yourself:

■ **Speak in a strong voice.** State, "Leave me alone!" rather than, "Will you please leave me alone?" Sound like you mean it.

■ **Maintain eye contact.** This keeps you aware of the person's movements and conveys an aura of strength and confidence.

■ **Stand up straight, act confident, and remain alert.** Walk as though you own the sidewalk.

If you are attacked, act immediately. Draw attention to yourself and your assailant. Scream "Fire!" as loudly as you can. Passersby are much more likely to help if they hear the word *fire* rather than just a scream.

## Campus-Wide Responses to Violence

Many college administrators have been proactive in establishing violence prevention policies, programs, and services. Campuses are conducting emergency response drills and reviewing the effectiveness of emergency messaging systems, including mobile phone alert systems. The REVERSE 9-1-1 system uses database and geographic information system (GIS) mapping technologies to notify campus police and community members in the event of problems, and other systems allow administrators to send out alerts in text, voice, e-mail, or instant message format. Some schools program the phone numbers, photographs, and basic student information for all incoming first-year students into a university security system so that in the event of a threat, students need only hit a button on their phones, whereupon campus police will be notified and tracking devices will pinpoint their location.

There are many changes that can be made to the campus environment to improve safety. Campus lighting, parking lot

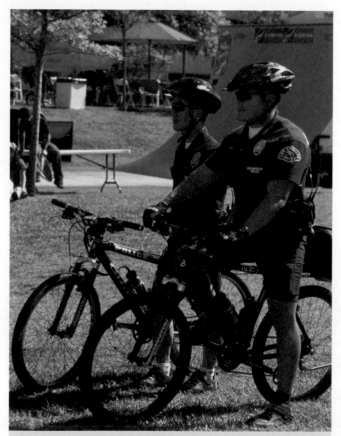

The presence and visibility of campus law enforcement have increased in recent years.

security, emergency call boxes, removal of overgrown shrubbery, safe ride programs, and stepped-up security are increasingly on the radar of campus safety personnel. Buildings can be designed with better lighting and enhanced security features, and security cameras can be installed in hallways, classrooms, and public places.

Campus law enforcement has changed over the years by increasing both its numbers and its authority to prosecute student offenders. Campus police are responsible for emergency responses, and they have the power to enforce laws with students in the same way they are handled in the general community. In fact, many campuses now hire state troopers or local law enforcement officers to deal with campus issues rather than maintain a separate police staff.

## Community Strategies for Preventing Violence

There are many steps you can take to ensure your personal safety; however, it is also necessary to address the issues of violence and safety at a community level. Strategies recommended by the CDC's injury response initiatives include the following:

- Develop and enforce policies and laws that prevent violence.
- Develop skills-based educational programs that teach the basics of interpersonal communication, elements of healthy relationships, anger management, conflict resolution, appropriate assertiveness, stress management, and other health-based behaviors.
- Involve families, schools, community programs, athletics, music, faith-based organizations, and other community groups in providing experiences that help young people to develop self-esteem and self-efficacy.
- Promote tolerance and acceptance and establish and enforce policies that forbid discrimination. Offer diversity training and mandate involvement.
- Improve community services focused on family planning, mental health services, day care and respite care, and alcohol and substance abuse prevention.
- Make sure walking trails, parking lots, and other public areas are well lit, unobstructed, and patrolled regularly to reduce threats.
- Improve community-based support and treatment for victims and ensure that individuals have choices available when trying to stop violence in their lives.

## LO 6 | UNINTENTIONAL INJURIES

Describe precautions to take to minimize the risk and effect of unintentional injuries.

Unintentional injuries occur without planning or intention to harm. How big a problem is unintentional injury? In 2013, intentional injury became the fourth leading cause of

## SEE IT! VIDEOS

Are you at risk of falling asleep at the wheel? Watch **Dozing and Driving: 1 in 24 Asleep at Wheel**, available on **MasteringHealth**™

death overall in America, surpassing stroke for the first time.[96] For Americans aged 15 to 44, unintentional injuries are the leading cause of death, killing over 42,000 people in the prime of life.[97] Only recently did unintentional drug overdose overtake motor vehicle accidents (MVAs) as the number one cause of unintentional death.[98] Other causes of significant unintentional mortalities each year include falls, drownings, and fires.

## Motor Vehicle Safety

In 2013, 32,719 Americans of all ages died and 2.3 million more were injured in MVAs reported by police.[99] Factors within your control—impaired driving via alcohol and other drugs, distracted driving via phone and text, speeding, and vehicle safety issues such as failure to wear a helmet or your seat belt—contribute to the great majority of MVAs.[100]

### Impaired Driving
In 2013, nearly one third of all motor vehicle fatalities involved a drunk or alcohol-impaired driver.[101] Of these, nearly one fourth had a previous history of license suspension or revocation for drunk driving.[102] The age group with the highest percentage of alcohol-impaired drivers involved in fatal crashes is people age 21 through 24.[103]

Although alcohol is the primary cause of **impaired driving**, other substances and situations are also responsible. For example, use of drugs other than alcohol, including marijuana, cocaine, and prescription medications, is a significant cause of MVA injury and death.[104] A recent study of fatal crashes in Colorado shows increases in the number of fatal crashes since the legalization of marijuana.[105] Sleep is also a major factor in fatal crashes. Many researchers contend that driving while sleep deprived is as dangerous as driving drunk. Drowsy driving causes an estimated 5,000 to 6,000 fatal MVAs each year.[106]

### Distracted Driving
Four types of activities constitute **distracted driving**: looking at something other than the road, hearing something not related to driving, manipulating something other than the steering wheel, and thinking about something other than driving.[107] In 2013, over 3,300 Americans died—10 percent of all fatal crashes—and over 420,000 were injured in distraction-affected crashes.[108]

Although there's no conclusive evidence identifying the forms of distraction most likely to contribute to MVAs, the behaviors of greatest concern are texting and talking on a cell phone. Overall, 31 percent of U.S. drivers age 18 to 64 report texting while driving, and 69 percent report that they talk on their cell phone while driving.[109] Texting is particularly deadly: Highway safety experts estimate that the average time a person's eyes are off the road while texting is about 5 seconds. At 55 mph, that's the equivalent of driving the length of a football field blindfolded.[110] As of March 2015, 44 states ban text messaging for all drivers, and 14 states ban all handheld cell phone use of any kind while driving.[111] See the **Points of View** box on the next page for more on the debate surrounding bans on cell phone use while driving.

### Vehicle Safety Issues
Wearing a safety belt cuts your risk of death or serious injury in a crash by almost half.[112] In 2012, 52 percent of the passenger vehicle occupants killed in traffic crashes were unrestrained.[113] Buckle up, and insist any passengers do the same. If you're

**impaired driving** Driving under the influence of alcohol or other drugs.

**distracted driving** Driving while performing any nondriving activity that has the potential to distract someone from the primary task of driving and increase the risk of crashing.

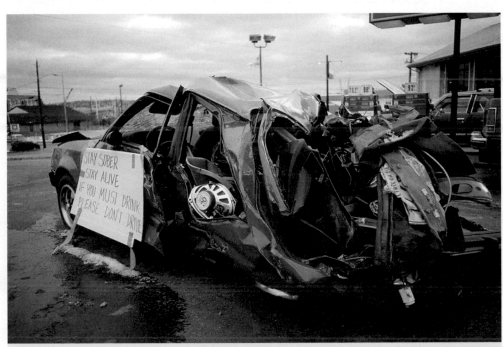

Driving under the influence of alcohol greatly increases the risk of being involved in a motor vehicle crash. Of all drivers between the ages of 21 and 24 involved in fatal crashes, nearly 1 out of 3 was legally drunk.

**Source:** NHTSA, "Traffic Safety Facts 2012 Data: Alcohol-Impaired Driving," DOT HS 811 870, December 2013, www-nrd.nhtsa.dot.gov/Pubs/811870.pdf

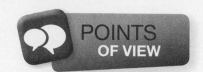
# Banning Phone Use While Driving
## *Good Idea or Going Too Far?*

Okay, 'fess up: How often in recent history have you chatted on the phone while driving, tried to read a text message, or switched the music on your iPhone? For many of us, that answer is more than once. In fact, texting drivers make up 31 percent of drivers aged 18 to 64. In addition, 69 percent of all drivers report talking on their cell phones regularly while driving. The problem is that in 2011, 3,331 people were killed and an estimated 387,000 were injured in crashes that were reported to involve distracted driving.

Forty-three states ban texting while driving, and 12 states ban the use of handheld phones completely but allow hands-free phone calls. All laws are primary enforcement, meaning that an officer may cite a driver for handheld use without any other traffic offenses. Are these laws necessary to protect American drivers, passengers, cyclists, and pedestrians, or do they go too far?

### Arguments in Favor of Banning Cell Phone Use while Driving

- Laws against driving under the influence of alcohol or other drugs and laws mandating seat belt use have saved millions of lives. Cell phone bans could do the same.
- Drivers who use handheld devices are three times as likely to get into crashes than those who do not use them. Headset cell phone use is not substantially safer than handheld use.

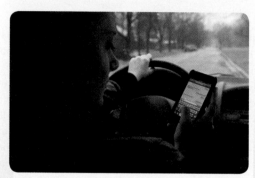

### Arguments Opposing Banning Cell Phone Use while Driving

- Talking with passengers, eating, working a GPS device, putting on makeup, and changing the radio station are also shown to greatly increase the chance of accidents. Why ban cell phone use without banning the other activities?
- These laws are difficult to enforce and spend tax dollars that might be better spent improving traffic safety in other ways.

## WHERE DO YOU STAND?

- What are your own state's laws regarding cell phone use? If it is against the law in your state, do you obey the rules?

- Do you think cell phone use while driving should be banned? If so, all forms or only certain things like texting? Why?

- Do you personally think that other driving distractions are as dangerous as cell phone use? Is it possible to avoid getting distracted while driving?

**Sources:** U.S. Centers for Disease Control and Prevention, "Distracted Driving," 2014, www.cdc.gov/Motorvehiclesafety/Distracted_Driving; Governors Highway Safety Association, "Cell Phone and Texting Laws," May 2014, www.ghsa.org; National Highway Traffic Safety Administration, "What Is Distracted Driving? Key Facts and Statistics," 2014, www.distraction.gov/content/get-the-facts/facts-and-statistics.html; M. Reardon, "Study: Distractions, Not Phones, Cause Car Crashes" in CNET.com *Signal Strength*, January 29, 2010, http://news.cnet.com

---

transporting an infant or child in your vehicle, follow state laws governing use and location of age-appropriate safety seats. In addition to seat belts, buying larger vehicles or those with the highest crash safety ratings, those with side and knee airbags, antilock brakes, traction and stability controls, impact-absorbing crumple zones, strong compartment and roof supports, as well as automatic braking for impending frontal crashes and blind spot assistance, all make good sense if you are trying to keep yourself and loved ones safe on the road. Lastly, if you ride a motorcycle, wear a helmet. Motorcycle drivers in states where helmets weren't required have 11 times the rate of death of those in helmeted states.[114]

**Risk-Management Driving** Although you can't control what other drivers are doing, you can reduce your risk of injury in an MVA by practicing risk-management driving techniques. These include the following:

- Don't use electronic devices while driving. Avoid talking on a cell phone while driving, even if the phone is hands free.
- Don't drink and drive—take a taxi or arrange for someone to be the designated driver.
- Don't drive when tired, highly emotional, or highly stressed.
- Never tailgate. The rear bumper of the car ahead of you should be at least 3 seconds worth of distance away, making

# 96%

OF COLLEGE STUDENTS SURVEYED REPORTED THAT THEY MOSTLY OR ALWAYS WEAR A **SEAT BELT** WHEN DRIVING OR RIDING IN A CAR.

stopping safely possible. Increase the distance when visibility is reduced, speed is increased, or roads are slick.

- Scan the road ahead of you and to both sides.
- Drive with your low-beam headlights on, *day and night,* to make your car more visible to other drivers.
- Drive defensively. Be on the alert for unsignaled lane changes, sudden braking, or other unexpected maneuvers.
- Obey all traffic laws.
- Always wear a seat belt, whether you're the driver or the passenger.

Even the most careful drivers may find themselves having to avoid an accident at some time in their lives. See the **Skills for Behavior Change** box for tips on how to reduce your risk of injury in an accident.

## Cycling Safety

The National Highway and Traffic Safety Administration (NHTSA) reports that, in 2012, 726 people died in cycling accidents, and 49,000 were injured.[115] Most fatal collisions occur at nonintersections (60 percent) between the hours of 4 P.M. and midnight. The average age of cyclists killed in traffic accidents is 43 years, with 88 percent of victims being male.[116] Alcohol also plays a significant role in bicycle deaths and injuries: In 2012, 28 percent of cyclists killed were legally drunk, and in 37 percent of all fatal accidents between motor vehicles and bicycles, either the driver or the cyclist was drunk.[117]

All cyclists should wear a properly fitted bicycle helmet every time they ride (**FIGURE 4.5**). In addition to wearing a helmet approved by the American National Standards Institute (ANSI) or the Snell Memorial Foundation, cyclists should consider the following suggestions:

- Watch the road and listen for traffic sounds! Never listen to an MP3 player or talk on a cell phone while cycling.

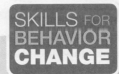
- Don't drink and ride.
- Follow all traffic laws, signs, and signals.
- Ride with the flow of traffic.
- Wear light or brightly colored reflective clothing that is easily seen at dawn, dusk, and during full daylight.
- Avoid riding after dark. If you must ride at night, use a front light and a red reflector or flashing rear light, as well as reflective tape or other markings on your bike and clothing.
- Use proper hand signals.
- Keep your bicycle in good condition.
- Use bike paths whenever possible.
- Stop at stop signs and traffic lights.

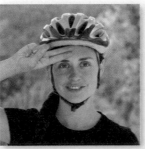 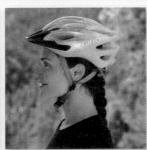 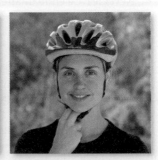

**①** The helmet should sit level on your head and low on your forehead—one or two finger-widths above your eyebrows.

**②** The sliders on the side straps should be adjusted to form a "V" shape under, and slightly in front of, your ears. Lock the sliders if possible.

**③** The chin strap buckle should be centered under your chin. Tighten the strap until it is snug, so that no more than two fingers fit under the strap.

**FIGURE 4.5** Fitting a Bicycle Helmet
Proper fit for helmets is an essential part of staying safe. Invest in a high-quality helmet and make sure it is fit properly.

 **VIDEO TUTOR** Biking Safety

## Stay Safe in the Water

About ten Americans die every day from drowning, making it the fifth leading cause of unintentional injury death among Americans of all ages. Males make up nearly 80 percent of all people who die from drowning.[118] African Americans are significantly more likely to die of drowning than white populations.[119] Many near drownings result in brain damage, leading to memory loss, learning disabilities, and permanent physical disability.[120]

**Drowning Risk Factors** Lack of swimming ability, lack of barriers around unsupervised swimming areas, lack of skilled supervision around water locations, failure to wear life jackets, temperature extremes that cause hypothermia, riptides and other hazardous conditions, seizure disorders, and excess alcohol use all increase drowning risk. In fact, the vast majority of adults who drown are not wearing life jackets (88 percent) and are under the influence of alcohol (70 percent).[121]

Most drownings occur during water recreation—either in backyard pools or natural water locations where people congregate to have fun. Often parents or lifeguards are not present, and people unexpectedly find themselves in dangerous situations. Many victims are strong swimmers, but can't get out of dangerous waters quickly enough. To be safe, take the following precautions around water:

- Learn how to swim. It is never too late.
- Learn CPR. When seconds can mean the difference between life and death, you want to be ready and able to save a loved one's life.
- Don't drink alcohol or take other drugs before or while swimming.
- Never swim alone, even if you are a skilled swimmer. Tell others where you are going.
- Pay attention to water temperature. Hypothermia can cause you to become disoriented and weak very quickly.
- Never leave a child unattended, even in extremely shallow water. Keep gates and barriers to backyard pools locked at all times.
- Before entering the water, check the depth. Most neck and back injuries result from diving into water that is too shallow.
- Never swim in a river with currents too swift for easy, relaxed swimming.
- Watch riptide warnings and beach conditions. If you are caught in a rip current, swim parallel to the shore. Once you are free of the current, swim toward the shore.

**Boating** In 2013, the U.S. Coast Guard received reports of 2,620 injured boaters and 560 deaths.[122] About 77 percent of these boating fatalities were drownings, and among those who drowned, 84 percent were not wearing a **personal flotation device**—that is, a lifejacket.[123]

Although operator inattention, inexperience, excessive speed, and mechanical failure also contributed to these deaths, alcohol consumption was the leading factor.[124] The U.S. Coast Guard and every state have "Boating under the Influence" (BUI) laws that carry stringent penalties for violation, including fines, license revocation, and even jail time.[125]

To stay safe when boating, the American Boating Association recommends sharing your plans for your outing, checking the weather ahead of time, making sure your boat is in good condition and has the proper safety equipment, and carrying an emergency radio and cell phone.[126] In addition, make sure you have enough life jackets for all who are on board, put on your life jacket before setting out, and wear it at all times while on the water. Don't drink alcohol before you leave, and don't bring any aboard.

If going on a snorkeling, diving, sailing, or other venture, check the qualifications and safety record of the company you are using. Make sure they have life jackets for everyone, have emergency rafts and radios easily accessible, and have wet or dry suits for trips to frigid waters. Also, don't sign up for trips where boat operators "party" with their passengers.

## Safety at Home

Injuries within the home typically occur in the form of poisonings, falls, or burns. Some populations, such as the elderly, are particularly vulnerable. However, older adults are not the only victims; each year, thousands of young adults, teens, and children are brought to hospital emergency rooms for treatment of such injuries.

**Prevent Poisoning** A **poison** is any substance that is harmful to your body when ingested, inhaled, injected, or absorbed through the skin. Any substance can be poisonous if too much is taken; however, nine out of ten poisoning deaths now result from drug overdose.[127] The drugs most commonly involved in these deaths and injuries are prescription medications—whether or not they were prescribed for the victim.[128] Over-the-counter (OTC) drugs are also commonly implicated in overdose incidents. These include cough syrup and sleep medications, as well as aspirin and other pain relievers.

In 2012, the 57 poison control centers in the United States logged more than 2.2 million calls for assistance with a poisoning.[129] The safety tips below were adapted from the American Association of Poison Control Centers:[130]

- Read and follow all usage and warning labels before taking medications or working with chemicals, including household products.
- Never share or sell your prescription drugs. Don't take prescriptions meant for others.
- Never take more than one medication at the same time without the approval of your health care provider. Also follow medication guidelines for alcohol consumption.
- Never mix household products together, as combinations of products can give off toxic fumes.

**personal flotation device** A device worn to provide buoyancy and keep the wearer, conscious or unconscious, afloat with the nose and mouth out of the water; also known as a life jacket.

**poison** Any substance harmful to the body when ingested, inhaled, injected, or absorbed through the skin.

- When working with chemicals, wear a protective mask and make sure the area in which you are working is well ventilated. Wear gloves and other protective clothing if there is any possibility of skin contact and eyeglasses or an eye guard if splashing could occur.
- Program the national poison control number, 1-800-222-1222, into your cell phone. The line is open 24 hours a day, 7 days a week.

**Avoid Falls** Falls are the third most common cause of death from unintentional injury, and a very common source of injury in the home. About 20 to 30 percent of people who fall suffer moderate to severe injury, such as bruises, a fracture, a dislocation, or a head injury. In fact, falls are the most common cause of traumatic brain injury.[131] Observe the following measures to reduce your risk of falls:

- Keep the floor and the stairs clear from all objects.
- Avoid using small scatter rugs and mats, which can slide out from under your feet. Use rubberized liners or strips to secure large rugs to the floor.
- Train your pets to stay away from your feet.
- Install slip-proof mats, treads, or decals in showers and tubs and on the stairs.
- If you need to reach something in a high cupboard or closet, or to change a ceiling light, use an appropriate step stool or short ladder.

**Reduce Your Risk of Fire** In 2011 more than 3,414 Americans died in a fire.[132] Although fire-related deaths are less common on college campuses in the United States, a total of 85 fatal fires have occurred on campuses over the past 15 years, claiming the lives of 122 students and staff.[133] The primary causes of fires in campus housing are cooking, use of candles, careless disposal of smoking materials, faulty wiring, and arson.[134] However, impaired judgment from alcohol consumption is also considered a major contributor to campus

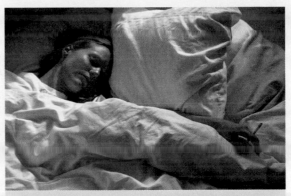

Smoking is the number one cause of fire-related deaths. If you fall asleep with a lit cigarette, bedding and clothing can quickly ignite. If you can't quit, take it outside.

**Source:** U.S. Fire Administration, "U.S. fire statistics," March 2015, www.usfa.fema.gov/data/statistics.

fires and fire deaths, in part because of delays in responding, calling 9-1-1, and evacuating.[135]

Tips to prevent fires include the following:

- Extinguish all cigarettes in ashtrays before bed, and never smoke in bed!
- Set lamps and candles away from curtains, linens, paper, and other combustibles. Never leave candles unattended or burning while you sleep.
- In the kitchen, keep hot pads and kitchen cloths away from stove burners; avoid reaching over hot pans. Use caution when lighting barbecue grills.
- Avoid overloading electrical circuits with appliances and cords.
- Have the proper fire extinguishers ready in case of fire, and replace batteries in smoke alarms and test them periodically.

How often are you at risk for sustaining an intentional or unintentional injury? Answer the questions below to find out.

## 1 Relationship Risk

How often does your partner:

|  | Never | Sometimes | Often |
|---|---|---|---|
| 1. Criticize you for your appearance (weight, dress, hair, etc.)? | ○ | ○ | ○ |
| 2. Embarrass you in front of others by putting you down? | ○ | ○ | ○ |
| 3. Blame you or others for his or her mistakes? | ○ | ○ | ○ |
| 4. Curse at you, shout at you, say mean things, insult, or mock you? | ○ | ○ | ○ |
| 5. Demonstrate uncontrollable anger? | ○ | ○ | ○ |
| 6. Criticize your friends, family, or others who are close to you? | ○ | ○ | ○ |
| 7. Threaten to leave you if you don't behave in a certain way? | ○ | ○ | ○ |
| 8. Manipulate you to prevent you from spending time with friends or family? | ○ | ○ | ○ |
| 9. Express jealousy, distrust, and anger when you spend time with other people? | ○ | ○ | ○ |
| 10. Make threats to harm others you care about, including pets? | ○ | ○ | ○ |
| 11. Control your telephone calls, monitor your messages and where you go, or read your e-mail without permission? | ○ | ○ | ○ |
| 12. Punch, hit, slap, or kick you? | ○ | ○ | ○ |
| 13. Force you to perform sexual acts that make you uncomfortable or embarrassed? | ○ | ○ | ○ |
| 14. Threaten to kill himself or herself if you leave? | ○ | ○ | ○ |

## 2 Risk for Assault or Rape

How often do you:

|  | Never | Sometimes | Often |
|---|---|---|---|
| 1. Leave your drink unattended while you get up to dance or go to the bathroom? | ○ | ○ | ○ |
| 2. Accept drinks from strangers while out at a bar or party? | ○ | ○ | ○ |
| 3. Leave parties with people you barely know or just met? | ○ | ○ | ○ |
| 4. Walk alone in poorly lit or unfamiliar places? | ○ | ○ | ○ |
| 5. Open the door to strangers? | ○ | ○ | ○ |
| 6. Leave your car or home door unlocked? | ○ | ○ | ○ |
| 7. Talk on your cell phone, oblivious to your surroundings? | ○ | ○ | ○ |

## 3 Risk for Vehicular Injuries

How often do you:

|  | Never | Sometimes | Often |
|---|---|---|---|
| 1. Drive after you have had one or two drinks? | ○ | ○ | ○ |
| 2. Drive after you have had three or more drinks? | ○ | ○ | ○ |
| 3. Drive when you are sleepy/extremely tired? | ○ | ○ | ○ |
| 4. Drive while you are extremely upset? | ○ | ○ | ○ |
| 5. Drive while using and holding your cell phone? | ○ | ○ | ○ |
| 6. Drive or ride in a car while not wearing a seat belt? | ○ | ○ | ○ |
| 7. Drive faster than the speed limit? | ○ | ○ | ○ |
| 8. Accept rides from friends who have been drinking? | ○ | ○ | ○ |

## 4 Online Safety

How often do you:

|  | Never | Sometimes | Often |
|---|---|---|---|
| 1. Give out your name or address on the Internet? | ○ | ○ | ○ |
| 2. Put personal identifying information on your blog, Facebook, or other websites? | ○ | ○ | ○ |
| 3. Post personal pictures, travel/vacation plans, and other private material on social networking sites? | ○ | ○ | ○ |
| 4. Date people you meet online? | ○ | ○ | ○ |
| 5. Use a shared or public computer to check e-mail without clearing the browser cache? | ○ | ○ | ○ |

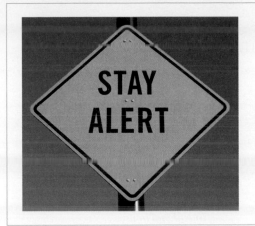

## Analyzing Your Responses

Look at your responses to the list of questions in each of these sections. Part 1 focused on relationships—if you answered "sometimes" or "often" to several of these questions, you may need to evaluate your situation. In Parts 2 through 4, if you answered "often" to any question, you may need to take action to ensure that you stay safe.

# YOUR PLAN FOR **CHANGE**

The **ASSESS YOURSELF** activity gave you the chance to consider symptoms of abuse in your relationships and signs of unsafe behavior in other realms of your life. Now that you are aware of these signs and symptoms, you can work on changing behaviors to reduce your risk.

**TODAY,** YOU CAN:

☐ Pay attention as you walk your normal route around campus and think about whether you are taking the safest route. Is it well lit? Do you walk in areas that receive little foot traffic? Are there any emergency phone boxes along your route? Does campus security patrol the area? If part of your route seems unsafe, look around for alternate routes. Vary your route when possible.

☐ Look at your residence's safety features. Is there a secure lock, dead bolt, or keycard entry system on all outer doors? Can windows be shut and locked? Is there a working smoke alarm in every room and hallway? Are the outside areas well lit? If you live in a dorm or apartment building, is there a security guard at the main entrance? If you notice any potential safety hazards, report them to your landlord or campus residential life administrator right away.

**WITHIN THE NEXT TWO WEEKS,** YOU CAN:

☐ If you are worried about potentially abusive behavior in a partner or in a friend's partner, visit the campus counseling center and ask about resources on campus or in your community to help you deal with potential relationship abuse. Consider talking to a counselor about your concerns or sitting in on a support group.

☐ Next time you go out to a bar or a party, set limits for yourself in order to avoid putting yourself in a dangerous or compromising position. Decide ahead of time on the number of drinks you will have, arrange with a friend to look out for each other during the party, and be sure you have a reliable, safe way of getting home.

**BY THE END OF THE SEMESTER,** YOU CAN:

☐ Sign up for a self-defense or violence prevention class or workshop.

☐ Get involved in an on-campus or community group dedicated to promoting safety. You might want to attend a meeting of an antiviolence group, join in a Take Back the Night rally, or volunteer at a local rape crisis center or battered women's shelter.

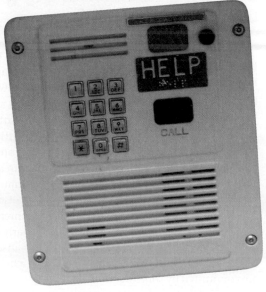

## CHAPTER REVIEW

To head an MP3 Tutor Session, scan here or visit the Study Area in MasteringHealth.

### LO 1 | What Is Violence?

- Violence continues to be a major problem in the United States today. Intentional injuries result from actions committed with the intent to do harm; unintentional injuries are committed without intent to harm. Violence affects everyone in society—from the direct victims, to children and families who witness it, to those who modify their behaviors because they are fearful.

### LO 2 | Factors Contributing to Violence

- Factors that lead to violence include poverty or economic difficulties, unemployment, parental and family influences, cultural beliefs, discrimination or oppression, religious or political differences, breakdowns in the criminal justice system, and stress. Anger and substance abuse can contribute to violence and aggression.

### LO 3 | Interpersonal and Collective Violence

- Interpersonal violence includes homicide, hate crimes, intimate partner violence, and elder abuse, among others. Victims of these crimes often suffer long-term emotional, social, and physical consequences. Forms of collective violence, including gang violence and terrorism, result in fear, anxiety, and issues of discrimination.

### LO 4 | Sexual Victimization

- Most sexual victimization crimes are committed by someone the victim already knows and includes unwanted touching, stalking, harassment, rape, and child sexual abuse.

### LO 5 | Preventing Violence

- To reduce the risk of becoming a victim of violence, recognize how to protect yourself and your friends, know where to turn for help, and have honest, straightforward dialogue about sexual matters in dating situations. Alcohol moderation is another key factor in reducing your risks. Campuses have stepped up educational programs, increased support for victims, increased surveillance, and provided clear messages about victim rights and consequences for offenders. They have also mandated campus climate surveys so they will better understand what is happening on campus before problems exist. With increasing reports of violence on campus, national attention has sharply focused what we can do to change a culture of violence. Preventing violence on a community level means prioritizing mental and emotional health, providing services to people in trouble, alcohol and drug abuse prevention, and providing behavioral skills training.

### LO 6 | Unintentional Injuries

- Unintentional injuries, particularly motor vehicle injuries, continue to be a leading cause of death for people aged 15 to 44. Impaired driving, drowsy driving, and distracted driving are key contributors to vehicular deaths and injuries. To avoid unintentional injuries, focus on personal protection and pay attention to threats.
- Injuries from bicycles, drownings, poisonings, falls, and fires pose threats for people of all ages, particularly the very young and old Americans. They also impact young adults who are impaired or not using commonsense safety practices. Young males are at significantly greater risk of unintentional injury than young females.

## POP QUIZ

Visit MasteringHealth to personalize your study plan with Chapter Review Quizzes and Dynamic Study Modules.

### LO 1 | What Is Violence?

1. _____ is an example of an *intentional injury*.
   a. A car accident
   b. Murder
   c. Accidental drowning
   d. Cycling collision

### LO 2 | Factors Contributing to Violence

2. An emotional reaction brought about by frustrating life experience is called
   a. reactive aggression.
   b. primary aggression.
   c. secondary aggression.
   d. tertiary aggression.

### LO 3 | Interpersonal and Collective Violence

3. Which of the following is *not* a common explanation for bias-motivated crimes?
   a. Fear of the unknown
   b. Self-defense
   c. Thrill seeking
   d. Retaliation for a perceived slight

4. Which of the following is an example of collective violence?
   a. Sexual assault
   b. Homicide
   c. Domestic violence
   d. Terrorism

5. Psychologist Lenore Walker developed a theory known as the
   a. aggression cycle.
   b. sexual harassment cycle.
   c. cycle of child abuse.
   d. cycle of violence.

### LO 4 | Sexual Victimization

6. When Jane began a new job with all male coworkers, her supervisor told her that he enjoyed having

an attractive woman in the workplace, and he winked at her. His comment constitutes
   a. poor judgment, but not a problem if Jane likes compliments.
   b. sexual assault.
   c. sexual harassment.
   d. sexual battering.

7. Rape by a person known to the victim that does not involve a physical beating or use of a weapon is called
   a. simple rape.
   b. sexual assault.
   c. simple assault.
   d. aggravated rape.

8. Which of the following is an example of stalking?
   a. Making intimate and personal sexually charged comments to another person
   b. Repeated visual or physical seeking out of another person
   c. An unwelcome sexual conduct by the perpetrator
   d. Sexual abuse upon a child

## LO 5 | Preventing Violence

9. Which of the following is a tip to protect yourself from assault?
   a. If a car is following you, drive home, go in, and lock your doors.
   b. If you get home and find your residence has been broken into, go inside, assess damages, and call the police.
   c. Talk or text on your phone when you're outside alone to look busy.
   d. If you're going somewhere alone, tell others where you are going and when you expect to be back.

## LO 6 | Unintentional Injuries

10. What is the leading cause of death for persons aged 15 to 44 in the United States?
    a. Homicide
    b. Heart disease/CVD
    c. Unintentional injury
    d. Suicide

Answers to the Pop Quiz can be found on page A-1. If you answered a question incorrectly, review the section identified by the Learning Outcome. For even more study tools, visit MasteringHealth.

# THINK ABOUT IT!

## LO 1 | What Is Violence?

1. What forms of violence do you think are most significant or prevalent in the United States today? Why?

2. What type of violence is most common on your campus? How do you think campus violence affects students at your school? Are there differences in how men and women respond to news that there has been a rape or violent assault on campus? If so, why?

## LO 2 | Factors Contributing to Violence

3. Why do some people develop into violent or abusive adults and others become pacifists or peaceful adults? What key factors influence violent offenders to be violent?

## LO 3 | Interpersonal and Collective Violence

4. Have you been affected by acts of terrorism or gang violence? What strategies can you take to discourage collective violence, as an individual and as a community?

## LO 4 | Sexual Victimization

5. Have you known anyone personally who has been sexually assaulted on campus? What actions were taken to help him or her cope with the assault? What campus services, if any, were used?

## LO 5 | Preventing Violence

6. What are some everyday decisions you can make to minimize your risk of becoming a victim of violence? How can you be a good

friend to someone who has become a victim of violence?

7. Is your campus safe? What steps has your campus administration and community taken to reduce levels of campus-wide violence?

## LO 6 | Unintentional Injuries

8. Think about an unintentional injury that affected you. What led up to it? What could have been done to prevent it? How much control did you have over the situation and how much was it affected by others?

# ACCESS YOUR HEALTH ON THE INTERNET

Visit **MasteringHealth** for links to the websites and RSS feeds.

The following websites explore further topics and issues related to personal health.

*Not Alone.* This site houses the report of the White House Task Force to Protect Students from Sexual Assault and recommendations for reporting, responding, and preventing future assaults. Detailed recommendations and action plans are presented. **www.whitehouse.gov/sites/default/files/docs/report_0.pdf**

*Men Can Stop Rape.* Practical suggestions for men interested in helping to protect women from sexual predators and assault are provided on this site. **www.mencanstoprape.org**

*National Center for Injury Prevention and Control.* The Web-based Injury Statistics Query and Reporting System (WISQARS) database of this CDC section provides statistics and information on fatal and nonfatal injuries, both intentional and unintentional. **www.cdc.gov/injury**

*National Sexual Violence Resource Center.* This is an excellent resource for victims of sexual violence. **www.nsvrc.org**

# 5 Connecting and Communicating in the Modern World

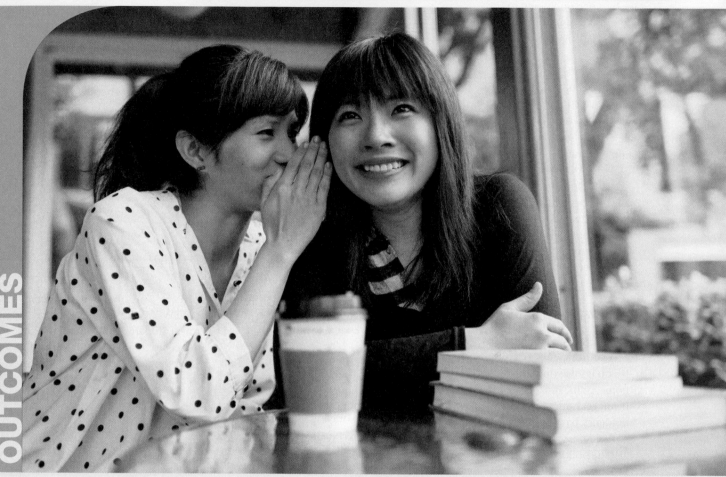

1. Discuss the purpose and common forms of intimate relationships.

2. Describe the types of social support available and the impact of social networks on health status.

3. Discuss ways to improve communication skills and interpersonal interactions, particularly in the digital environment.

4. Identify the characteristics of successful relationships, including how to overcome common conflicts, and discuss how to cope when relationships end.

5. Compare and contrast the types of committed relationships and lifestyle choices.

Humans are social beings—we have a basic need to belong and to feel loved, accepted, and wanted. We can't thrive without relating to and interacting with others. Strong connections to others reduce depression, build our immune systems, improve sleep, and strengthen our resolve.[1] In fact, people with positive, fulfilling relationships with spouses, family members, friends, and coworkers are 50 percent more likely to survive over time than people with poor relationships.[2] However, having a healthy social life is not a given, even for people who regularly interact with many others. A person can feel lonely, even in a crowd, because loneliness does not result from being physically alone; it is caused by feeling disconnected from others.[3] In this chapter, we examine the vital role relationships play in our lives and the communication skills necessary to create and maintain them.

## LO 1 | INTIMATE CONNECTIONS

Discuss the purpose and common forms of intimate relationships.

We all need people in our lives who affirm who we are and provide **intimate connectedness**.[4] These **intimate relationships** often include four characteristics: *behavioral interdependence, need fulfillment, emotional attachment,* and *emotional availability.* Each of these characteristics may be related to interactions with family, close friends, and romantic partners.

*Behavioral interdependence* refers to the mutual impact that people have on each other as their lives intertwine. What one person does influences what the other person wants to do and can do. Behavioral interdependence usually becomes stronger over time, to the point that each person would feel a great void if the other were gone.

Intimate relationships are also a means of *need fulfillment.* Through relationships with others, we fulfill our needs for:

- Intimacy—someone with whom we can share our feelings freely.
- Social integration—someone with whom we can share worries and concerns.
- Nurturance—someone we can take care of and who will take care of us.
- Assistance—someone to help us in times of need.
- Affirmation—someone who will reassure us of our own worth.

In mutually rewarding intimate relationships, partners and friends meet each other's needs. They disclose feelings, share confidences, and provide support and reassurance. Each person comes away feeling better for the interaction and validated by the other person.

In addition to behavioral interdependence and need fulfillment, intimate relationships involve strong bonds of *emotional attachment,* or feelings of love. When we hear the word *intimate,* we often think of a sexual relationship. Although sex can play an important role in emotional attachment to a romantic partner, relationships can be intimate without being sexual; for example, two people can be emotionally intimate (share feelings) or spiritually intimate (share spiritual beliefs and practices) without being sexually intimate.

*Emotional availability,* the ability to give to and receive emotionally from others without fear of being hurt or rejected, is the fourth characteristic of intimate relationships. At times, it is healthy to limit our emotional availability. For example, after a painful breakup, we may decide not to jump into another relationship immediately, or we may decide to talk about it only with close friends. Holding back can offer time for introspection, healing, and for considering lessons learned. Some people who have experienced intense trauma find it difficult to ever be fully available emotionally, which can limit their ability to experience intimate relationships.[5]

## Relating to Yourself

You have probably heard the old saying that you must love yourself before you can love someone else. What does this mean, exactly? Learning how you function emotionally and how to nurture yourself through all life's situations is a lifelong task. You should certainly not postpone intimate connections with others until you achieve this state. However, a certain level of individual maturity will help you maintain relationships.

Two personal qualities that are especially important to any good relationship are *accountability* and *self-nurturance.* **Accountability** means that you recognize responsibility for your own choices and actions. You don't hold others responsible for positive or negative experiences. **Self-nurturance** means developing individual potential through a balanced and realistic appreciation of self-worth and ability. To make good choices in life, a person must balance many physical and emotional needs—sleeping, eating, exercising, working, relaxing, and socializing. When the balance is disrupted, self-nurturing people are patient with themselves as they put things back on course. Learning to live in a balanced and healthy way is a lifelong process. Individuals who are on a path of accountability and self-nurturance have a much better chance of achieving this balance and maintaining satisfying relationships with others.

Important factors that affect your ability to nurture yourself and maintain healthy relationships with others include the way you define yourself (*self-concept*) and the way you evaluate yourself (*self-esteem*). Your self-concept is like a mental mirror that reflects how you view your physical features, emotional states, talents, likes and dislikes, values, and roles. A person might define herself as an activist, a mother, an honor student, an athlete, or a musician. As we've discussed in earlier chapters, how you feel about yourself or evaluate yourself constitutes your self-esteem.

**intimate connectedness** A relationship that makes you feel who you are is affirmed.

**intimate relationships** Relationships with family members, friends, and romantic partners, characterized by behavioral interdependence, need fulfillment, emotional attachment, and emotional availability.

**accountability** Accepting responsibility for personal decisions, choices, and actions.

**self-nurturance** Developing individual potential through a balanced and realistic appreciation of self-worth and ability.

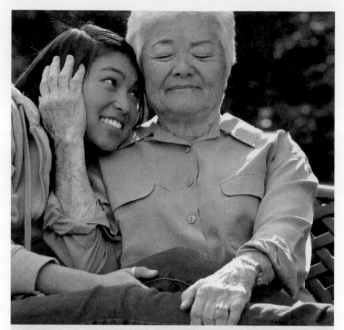

We may be accustomed to hearing "intimacy" used to describe romantic or sexual relationships, but intimate relationships can take many forms. The emotional bonds that characterize intimate relationships often span the generations and help individuals gain insight and understanding into each other's worlds.

Your perception and acceptance of yourself influences your relationship choices. If you feel unattractive, insecure, or inferior to others, you may choose not to interact with other people or to avoid social events. You may even unconsciously seek out individuals who confirm your negative view of yourself by treating you poorly. Conversely, if you are secure about your unique characteristics and talents, that positive self-concept will make it easier to form relationships with people who support and nurture you and to interact with a variety of people in a healthy, balanced way.

## Family Relationships

A family is a recognizable group of people with roles, tasks, boundaries, and personalities whose central focus is to protect, care for, love, and socialize with one another. Because the family is a dynamic institution that changes as society changes, the definition of *family* changes over time. Historically, most families have been made up of people related by blood, marriage or long-term committed relationships, or adoption. Today, however, many groups of people are recognized and function as family units. Although there is no "best" family type, we do know that a healthy family's key roles and tasks include nurturance and support. Healthy families foster a sense of security and feelings of belonging that are central to growth and development.

During the childhood years, families provide our most significant relationships. It is from our **family of origin**, the people present in our household during our first years of life, that we initially learn about feelings, problem solving, love, intimacy, and

**family of origin** People present in the household during a child's first years of life—usually parents and siblings.

gender roles. We learn to negotiate relationships and have opportunities to communicate effectively, develop attitudes and values, and explore spiritual belief systems. It is not uncommon when we establish relationships outside the family to rely on these initial experiences and on skills modeled by our family of origin.

## Friendships

Friendships are often the first relationships we form outside our immediate families. Establishing and maintaining strong friendships may be a good predictor of your success in establishing romantic relationships, as both require shared interests and values, mutual acceptance, trust, understanding, respect, and self-confidence.

Developing meaningful friendships is more than merely "friending" someone on Facebook. Getting to know someone well requires time, effort, and commitment. But the effort is worth it—a good friend can be a trustworthy companion, someone who respects your strengths and accepts your weaknesses, someone who can share your joys and your sorrows, and someone you can count on for support.

## Romantic Relationships

At some point, most people choose to enter an intimate romantic and sexual relationship with another person. Beyond the characteristics of friendship, romantic relationships typically include the following characteristics related to passion and caring:

- **Fascination.** Lovers tend to pay attention to the other person even when they should be involved in other activities. They are preoccupied with the other and want to think about, talk to, and be with the other.
- **Exclusivity.** Lovers have a special relationship that usually precludes having the same kind of relationship with a third party. The love relationship often takes priority over all others.
- **Sexual desire.** Lovers desire physical intimacy and want to touch, hold, and engage in sexual activities with the other.
- **Giving the utmost.** Lovers care enough to give the utmost when the other is in need, sometimes to the point of extreme sacrifice.
- **Being a champion or advocate.** Lovers actively champion each other's interests and attempt to ensure that the other succeeds.

### Theories of Love
There is no single definition of *love*, and the word may mean different things to different people, depending on cultural values, age, gender, and situation. Although we may not know how to put our feelings into words, we know it when the "lightning bolt" of love strikes.

Several theories related to how and why love develops have been proposed. In his classic triangular theory of love, psychologist Robert Sternberg proposed the following three key components to loving relationships (**FIGURE 5.1**):[6]

- **Intimacy.** The emotional component, which involves closeness, sharing, and mutual support.
- **Passion.** The motivational component, which includes lust, attraction, and sexual arousal.

- **Commitment.** The cognitive component, which includes the decision to be open to love in the short term and commitment to the relationship in the long term.

According to Sternberg, the quality of a love relationship is related to the level of intimacy, passion, and commitment each person brings to the relationship over time. He suggests that relationships including two or more of those components are more likely to endure than those that include only one. He uses the term **consummate love** to describe a combination of intimacy, passion, and commitment—an ideal and deep form of love that is, unfortunately, all too rare.[7]

Quite different from Sternberg's approach are theories of love and attraction based on brain circuitry and chemistry. Anthropologist Helen Fisher, among others, hypothesizes that attraction and falling in love follow a fairly predictable pattern based on (1) *imprinting,* in which our evolutionary patterns, genetic predispositions, and past experiences trigger a romantic reaction; (2) *attraction,* in which neurochemicals produce feelings of euphoria and elation; (3) *attachment,* in which endorphins (natural opiates) cause lovers to feel peaceful, secure, and calm; and (4) *production of a cuddle chemical;* that is, the brain secretes the hormone oxytocin, which stimulates sensations during love-making and elicits feelings of satisfaction and attachment.[8]

According to Fisher's theory, lovers who claim to be swept away by passion may not be far from the truth. A love-smitten person's endocrine system secretes chemical substances such as dopamine, norepinephrine, and phenylethylamine (PEA)—chemical cousins of amphetamines.[9] Attraction may in fact be a "natural high"; however, this passion "buzz" loses effectiveness over time as the body builds up a tolerance. Fisher speculates that some people become attraction junkies, seeking out the intoxication of new love much as a drug user seeks a chemical high.

## Choosing a Romantic Partner
*Attraction Theory* suggests that more than just chemical and psychological processes influence who a person falls in love with. This theory suggests proximity, similarities, reciprocity, and physical attraction also play strong roles.[10] *Proximity* is being in the same place at the same time. When you are out and about in the community, it is more likely that an interaction will occur than if you stay at home. And if you meet a person while at work, at the dog park, or at a religious event, it is likely that you may share interests. While physical proximity is important, with the growth of Internet dating sites, it has become easier to meet people outside your geographic proximity.

> **consummate love** A relationship that combines intimacy, compassion, and commitment.

You also choose a partner based on *similarities* (in attitudes, values, intellect, interests, education, and socioeconomic status); the old adage that "opposites attract" usually isn't true, at least not in the long run. If your potential partner expresses interest, you may react with mutual regard—*reciprocity.* The more you express interest, the safer it is for someone else to reciprocate, continuing the cycle and strengthening the connection.

A final factor that plays a significant role in selecting a partner is *physical attraction.* Attraction is a complex notion, influenced by social, biological, and cultural factors.[11] People seem to seek out "similarly attractive" partners, meaning more attractive people seek out more attractive partners and vice versa; however, as relationships evolve, status and personality become more important and the importance of personal appearance diminishes.[12]

## LO 2 | THE **VALUE** OF RELATIONSHIPS

Discuss the types of social support available and the impact of social networks on health status.

Historically, research examining the benefits of intimate relationships has focused on marriage; however, recent studies report that all types of close relationships are good for our health.[13] The benefits range from a decreased likelihood of catching a cold, to a faster recovery from stressful tasks, to a longer life span. On the flip side, those with poor social connections—lonely people—have decreased immune function, higher blood pressure, and higher rates of depression, pain, and fatigue.[14] Having weak ties to a community or a small number of friends can be as harmful to your overall health as alcohol abuse or smoking roughly a pack of cigarettes per day.[15]

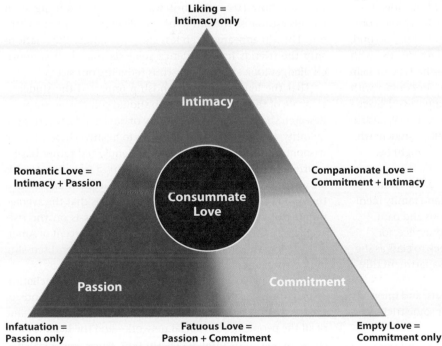

**FIGURE 5.1** Sternberg's Triangular Theory of Love According to Sternberg's model, three elements—intimacy, passion, and commitment—existing alone or in combination, form different types of love. The most complete, ideal type of love in the model is consummate love, which combines balanced amounts of all three elements.

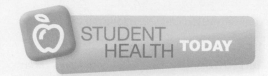
# HOOKING UP
## The New Norm or Nothing New?

"Hooking up" is a vague term often used to describe sexual encounters, from kissing to intercourse, without the expectation of commitment. While the media often report about the new "hookup culture" on campus, research tells a different story. Longitudinal data tells us that young adults' sexual behavior hasn't changed much in the past few decades. College students are not having more sex or a greater number of partners than their counterparts 20 or 30 years ago. Today's college students are more likely to describe their sex partner as a "friend" than in the past, but today's college students are still twice as likely to have sex with a romantic partner than with a hookup.

While hook-up behavior may not be as pervasive as some think, college students should understand the risks involved:

1. **Recognize the role of emotions in sex.** Sternberg's Triangle of Love would place hooking up in the "infatuation" category, passion with no commitment or intimacy, far from Sternberg's picture of "ideal." Additionally, according to Fisher, attraction and sex create a chemical reaction in the brain that fosters an emotional response, even if we say, "It's just about the sex."

2. **Recognize the role of alcohol in hooking up.** In a recent study of college hookups, students reported that they were more likely to hook up if they had been drinking alcohol. Among participants who consumed alcohol prior to their last hookup, 31 percent of females and 28 percent of males indicated that they would likely not have hooked up with their partners had alcohol not been involved.

3. **Recognize the risk of unintended pregnancy and STIs.** In one study, only 70 percent of students reported condom use during their last hookup. Reduced inhibitions due to alcohol plus a lack of communication with a new partner increase the risk of unprotected sex and thus the risk for unintended pregnancy and STIs.

**Sources:** M. A. Monto and A. G. Carey, "A New Standard of Sexual Behavior? Are Claims Associated with the "Hookup Culture" Supported by General Social Survey Data?," *Journal of Sex Research* 56, no. 6 (2014): 605–15; R. L. Fielder, K. B. Carey, and M. P. Carey, "Are Hookups Replacing Romantic Relationships? A Longitudinal Study of First-Year Female College Students," *Journal of Adolescent Health* 52, no. 5 (2012): 657–59; J. M. Bearak, "Casual Contraception in Casual Sex: Life-Cycle Change in Undergraduates' Sexual Behavior in Hookups," *Social Forces* 93, no. 2 (2014): 483–513.

---

**social support** Help we receive from people in our social network in the form of emotional, instrumental, informational, and appraisal support.

**social network** People you know who can provide social support when needed.

**social capital** Collective value of all the people in your social network and the likelihood of those people providing social support when you need it.

Why do relationships make us healthier? First, we tend to mimic our friends' habits, especially with diet and exercise; studies show that we eat healthier if our friends do (and we are more likely to become obese if our friends do).[16] Second, friends often provide us with **social support**—the type of help we receive from our contact with others. Social support is delivered in four forms: emotional, instrumental, informational, and appraisal.[17] For a college student who breaks her leg playing basketball, social support might be:

- **Emotional support.** Displays of caring, love, trust, and empathy; for example, when close friends and family members provide a listening ear about frustrations and pain.
- **Instrumental support.** Concrete help and service; for example, a roommate carrying her backpack to class as she learns to use her crutches and keeping the apartment tidy so she doesn't trip.
- **Informational support.** Advice, suggestions, and information, for example, when an aunt shows her some tricks to better navigate on crutches.
- **Appraisal support.** Information that is useful for self-evaluation, for example, when her high school coach reminds her of how she bounced back when she sprained her ankle in high school, encouraging an accurate assessment of her current situation.

Another theory suggests that having friends can change your perspective of how challenging a task is. In one clever study, a group of students were taken to the foot of a steep hill and fitted with a heavy backpack. They were then told to estimate how steep the hill was. Students standing with friends estimated the hill to be less steep than students without. The hill appeared even less steep the longer the relationship the friends had. Evidence suggests that with support, challenges look easier to us—thus reducing our stress.[18]

That the length of the friendship impacted the students' estimate of the difficulty of climb should come as no surprise. Research shows that it is the quality of our friendships, not the quantity, that matters when it comes to health. There's a lot of wisdom in Al Capone's quip about friends, "I'd rather have 4 quarters than 100 pennies." He was right, a few close friends are worth far more to our health than 100 acquaintances—or a thousand Facebook friends. The good news is that the average number of confidants reported by Americans is on the rise, averaging a little over two per person; sadly, 9 percent of Americans report they have no one they can turn to for discussing important matters.[19]

Besides our closest relationships, we all have a constellation of neighbors, relatives, classmates, coworkers, and friends of friends that make up our **social network**. The collective value of all the people in your social network—and the likelihood of those people providing social support when you need it—determines your **social capital**. The more social capital we have, the happier and healthier we are.[20]

To build social capital, we can both strengthen our existing ties and widen our existing network. John Cacioppo, a leading

What factors do you consider most important in a potential partner?

- Are any absolute musts?
- Does what you believe to be important in a relationship differ from what your parents might feel is important?

researcher on loneliness, describes these actions as building relational connectedness and collective connectedness.[21]

**Relational connectedness** comes from mutually rewarding face-to-face contact. We deepen our relational connectedness each time we interact positively with people in our social network, strengthening our ties and increasing the likelihood of someone coming to our aid when asked.

**Collective connectedness,** on the other hand, comes from the feeling that you are part of a group beyond yourself. It manifests itself in feelings like trust, having a sense of community, as well as in actions like voting and volunteering. The groups you belong to deepen your collective connectedness and can expand your social network. People find collective connectedness in many ways: cheering for the same sports team, volunteering together, or worshipping at the same temple. The important thing is feeling that you are a part of something, even when you might not have intimate ties to the group.

Collective connectedness appears to be on the rise. Seventy-four percent of Americans now belong to a sports league, worship community, charitable organization, or another type of local group. Additionally, 12 percent more Americans report knowing their neighbors by name than just a few years ago. Some believe this increase is due to economic changes, encouraging Americans to turn to neighbors and community groups for social support during harder times.[22] No matter the reason, feeling connected to your community is connected to improved health.

Developing these relationships is hard but important work, bolstered by our ability to communicate well with those in our social network.

## LO 3 | BUILDING COMMUNICATION SKILLS

Discuss ways to improve communication skills and interpersonal interactions, particularly in the digital environment.

From the moment of birth, we struggle to be understood. We flail our arms, cry, scream, smile, frown, and make sounds and gestures to attract attention or to communicate our wants or needs. By adulthood, each of us has developed a unique way of communicating through gestures, words, expressions, and body language. No two people communicate exactly the same way or have the same need for connecting with others, yet we all need to connect.

Different cultures have different ways of expressing feelings and using body language. Members of some cultures gesture broadly; others maintain a closed body posture. Some are offended by direct eye contact; others welcome a steady gaze. Men and women also tend to have different styles of communication, largely dictated by culture and socialization (see the

**Health in a Diverse World** box on page 140).

Although people differ in the ways they communicate, this doesn't mean that one gender, culture, or group is better at communication than another. We have to be willing to accept differences and work to keep lines of communication open and fluid. Remaining interested, actively engaging in interaction, and being open and willing to exchange ideas and thoughts are all things we can typically learn with practice. By understanding how to deliver and interpret information, we can enhance our relationships.

## Learning Appropriate Self-Disclosure

Sharing personal information with others is called **self-disclosure.** If you are willing to share personal information with others, they will likely share personal information with you. Likewise, if you want to learn more about someone, you have to be willing to share some of your personal background and interests with that person. Self-disclosure is not only storytelling or sharing secrets; it is also sharing emotions about what you are currently experiencing in life and providing any information about the past that is relevant to the other person's understanding of your current reactions.

**relational connectedness** Mutually rewarding face-to-face contacts.

**collective connectedness** Feeling that you are part of a community or group.

**self-disclosure** Sharing feelings or personal information with others.

Self-disclosure can be a double-edged sword because there is risk in divulging personal insights and feelings. If you sense that sharing feelings and personal thoughts will result in a closer relationship, you will likely take such a risk. But if you believe that the disclosure may result in rejection or alienation, you may not open up so easily. If the confidentiality of previously shared information has been violated, you may hesitate to be as open in the future. However, the risk in not disclosing yourself to others is a lack of intimacy in relationships.[23]

If self-disclosure is a key element in creating healthy communication, but fear is a barrier to that process, what can be done? The following suggestions can help:

- **Get to know yourself.** Remember that your *self* includes your feelings, beliefs, thoughts, and concerns. The more you know about yourself, the more likely you will be able to share yourself with others.
- **Become more accepting of yourself.** No one is perfect or has to be.
- **Be willing to talk about sex.** The U.S. culture puts many taboos on discussions of sex, so it's no wonder we find it hard to disclose our sexual past to those with whom we are sexually intimate. However, the threats of unintended

**SEE IT!** VIDEOS
Meet Elise and learn about her project: 100 Dates of Summer. Watch **One Woman's Journey Through 100 Dates** in the Study Area of **MasteringHealth™**

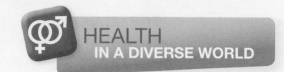
There are some gender-specific communication patterns and behaviors that are obvious to the casual observer (see graphic). However, according to Dr. Cynthia Burggraf Torppa at Ohio State University, the bigger difference is the way in which men and women interpret or process the same message. She indicates that women are more sensitive to interpersonal meanings "between the lines," and men are more sensitive to subtle messages about status or social hierarchy. Recognizing these differences and how they make us unique is a good first step in avoiding unnecessary frustrations and miscommunications.

**Sources:** C. Burggraf Torppa, Family and Consumer Sciences, Ohio State University Extension, "Gender Issues: Communication Differences in Interpersonal Relationships," 2010, http://ohioline.osu.edu/flm02/pdf/fs04.pdf, J. Wood, *Gendered Lives. Communication, Gender, and Culture*, 10th ed. (Belmont, CA: Cengage, 2013).

▶ VIDEO TUTOR
Gender Differences in Communication

## Women

**FACIAL EXPRESSIONS**
• Smile and nod more often
• Maintain better eye contact

**SPEECH PATTERNS**
• Higher pitched, softer voices
• Use approximately 5 speech tones
• May sound more emotional
• Make more tentative statements
• Interrupt less often

**BODY LANGUAGE**
• Take up less space
• Gesture toward the body
• Lean forward when listening
• More gentle when touching others
• More feedback via body language

**BEHAVIORAL DIFFERENCES**
• Express intimate feelings more readily
• More likely to ask for help
• Apologize more frequently
• Talk is primarily a means of rapport, establishing connections, and negotiating relationships

## Men

**FACIAL EXPRESSIONS**
• Frown more often
• Often avoid eye contact

**SPEECH PATTERNS**
• Lower pitched, louder voices
• Use approximately 3 speech tones
• May sound more abrupt
• Make more direct statements
• More likely to interrupt

**BODY LANGUAGE**
• Occupy more space
• Gesture away from the body
• Lean back when listening
• More forceful gestures
• Less feedback via body language

**BEHAVIORAL DIFFERENCES**
• Have more difficulty in expressing intimate feelings
• Less likely to ask for help
• Apologize less often
• Talk is primarily a means of preserving independence and negotiating and maintaining status

pregnancy and sexually transmitted infections make it important for partners to discuss sexual history.
■ **Choose a safe context for self-disclosure.** When and where you make such disclosures and to whom may greatly influence the response you receive. Choose a setting where you feel safe to let yourself be heard.

■ **Be thoughtful about self-disclosure via social media.** Self-disclosure can be an effective method of building intimacy with another person, but not with large groups. Sharing too much information or information that is too personal on Facebook or Twitter may cause you to feel vulnerable or embarrassed later.

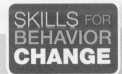

## SKILLS FOR BEHAVIOR CHANGE

### LEARNING TO REALLY LISTEN

To become a better listener, practice the following skills on a daily basis:

▶ To avoid distractions, turn off the TV, shut your laptop lid, and put your phone away.

▶ Be present in the moment. Good listeners participate and acknowledge what the other person is saying through nonverbal cues such as nodding or smiling and asking questions at appropriate times.

▶ Ask for clarification. If you aren't sure what the speaker means, say that you don't completely understand or paraphrase what you think you heard.

▶ Control that deadly desire to interrupt. Try taking a deep breath for 2 seconds, then hold your breath for another second, and really listen to what is being said as you slowly exhale.

▶ Resist the temptation to "set the other person straight."

▶ Focus on the speaker. Hold back the temptation to launch into a story of your own experience in a similar situation.

## Becoming a Better Listener

Listening is a vital part of interpersonal communication. Good listening skills enhance our relationships, improve our grasp of information, and allow us to more effectively interpret what others say. We listen best when (1) we believe that the message is somehow important and relevant to us; (2) the speaker holds our attention through humor, dramatic effect, or other techniques; and (3) we are in the mood to listen (free of distractions and worries). See the **Skills for Behavior Change** box for suggestions on improving your listening skills.

**The Three Basic Listening Modes** There are three main ways in which we listen:

■ *Competitive listening* happens when we are more interested in explaining our own point of view than in understanding someone else's.[24]

■ *Passive listening* occurs when we are listening but not providing either verbal or nonverbal feedback to the speaker. The speaker may feel unsure if the message is being received.[25]

■ *Active listening* is when we not only hear the words, but also are trying to understand what is really being said. The listener confirms understanding by restating

or paraphrasing the speaker's message before responding. By actively listening, we show genuine interest in what the other person is thinking and feeling.[26]

## Using Nonverbal Communication

Understanding what someone is saying usually involves more than listening and speaking. Often, what is not said may actually speak louder than any words could. Rolling the eyes, looking at the floor or ceiling rather than maintaining eye contact, body movements and hand gestures—all these nonverbal clues influence the way we interpret messages. **Nonverbal communication** includes all unwritten and unspoken messages, both intentional and unintentional, including touch, gestures, interpersonal space, body language, tone of voice, and facial expressions.[27] Ideally, our nonverbal communication matches and supports our verbal communication, but this is

> **nonverbal communication** Unwritten and unspoken messages, both intentional and unintentional.

not always the case. Research shows that when verbal and nonverbal communication doesn't match, we are more likely to believe the nonverbal cues.[28] This is one reason it is important to be aware of the nonverbal cues we use regularly and to understand how others might interpret them.

While facial expressions like smiling are believed to have near universal meaning, other facial expressions and most body language is culturally specific.[29] A gesture of agreement or approval in one culture can be offensive in another. To communicate as effectively as possible, it is important to recognize and use appropriate nonverbal cues that support and help clarify your verbal messages. Awareness and practice of your verbal and nonverbal communication will help you better understand others.

## Connecting Digitally: Too Much of a Good Thing?

You may have noticed a few pages ago that, in the definition of *relational connectedness*, Dr. Cacioppo specifically describes the contact as "face-to-face." Does Facetime count? Is oxytocin—the hormone that make us feel happy when we interact with friends in person—released when we receive a Snap? Or when we comment on a friend's Facebook post?

While preliminary research shows some similarities, we don't really know yet. We do know that digital communication is different from face-to-face communication in many ways. Digital communication often lacks the nonverbal cues that make face-to-face communication so rich. With no accompanying tone of voice, eye roll, or smile, interpreting text-based communication can be challenging.

On the flip side, digital communication allows us to have a more diverse social network

### WHY SHOULD I CARE?

Why is developing communication skills so important? Unless you decide to be a hermit, there is hardly a career or life path you might choose that won't require communicating and cooperating with others. Develop good communication skills now, and you'll be poised for success.

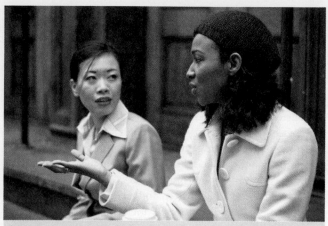

One way to communicate better is to pay attention to your body language. Much of our message is conveyed by nonverbal cues. Laughing, smiling, and gesturing all help convey meaning and assure your partner that you are actively engaged in the conversation.

and easily keep in touch over long distances.[30] According to some reports, Americans spend more time on social networking sites (SNSs) that any other online activity.[31] These connections seem to strengthen our social networks, as frequent Facebook users report 9 percent more close core ties than other Internet users.[32] Frequent Facebook users also score higher in social support, specifically in emotional and instrumental support. The boost is significant too—it is about half the total support you would expect from being married.[33]

While some worry that SNS users are becoming more socially isolated and have weaker social ties, according to Pew Research, SNS users actually have larger social networks, both on- and offline.[34] The more frequently someone uses SNSs, the larger that person's network tends to be and the more close ties he or she has.[35] Facebook actually seems to "support intimacy, rather than undermine it."[36] Thus, the concerns that the use of social networking sites is limiting our social networks or weakening our bonds are likely unfounded.[37]

Still, there can always be too much of a good thing. While social networking sites can be sources of connection and social support, some users experience envy of the activities and lifestyles of their friends. When Facebook or SnapChat is used as a way to size yourself up against others, it leads to increased reports of depression.[38] Remember, people often show a curated image of themselves; it is not always an accurate representation of their lives. And regardless, the number of likes or followers you have is not a reflection of your worth as a person.

Another concern is addiction. While one study found that the average person checks his or her phone 150 times a day,[39] still others estimate college students spend at least 7 hours a day on their cellphones.[40] About 60 percent of college students admit to possibly being addicted to using their phone, feeling agitated when separated from it.[41]

The lack of nonverbal communication in text-based digital communication can lead to confusion and misunderstanding.[42] Some experts are concerned that, over time, reduced exposure to nonverbal communication may reduce people's ability to read facial expressions—impacting their in-person communication

## SKILLS FOR BEHAVIOR CHANGE

## SOCIAL MEDIA MEANNESS

It's not your imagination; people are more rude online than in person.

▶ Three in four people report that they have witnessed an argument on social media.

▶ Three in five people report someone is rude to them on social media more than once a month.

▶ Virtual arguments have caused one in five people to stop being friends with or unfriend someone.

Why does technology seem to bring out the worst in people? Psychologists often call anonymity and invisibility the culprits for this lack of restraint. When people feel anonymous, they are more willing to say things they normally wouldn't. And even when we aren't anonymous, impulse control is reduced because we can respond or vent immediately.

Perhaps another reason is that we can't see the person when commenting. At the University of Haifa in Israel, a group of researchers tested this hypothesis, asking 71 pairs of unacquainted college students to use Instant Messenger to debate an issue. Pairs chatted under different conditions, some shared personal info, some could see the person's body, and some were asked to look directly into the other person's eyes onscreen. More than any other condition, whether or not participants had to make eye contact with each other predicted how poorly they treated each other. In the absence of eye contact, subjects were 200 percent more likely to be impolite. The lead researcher, Noam Lapidot-Lefler, suggests that "seeing a partner's eyes helps you understand the other person's feelings, the signals that the person is trying to send you"—something that often gets lost in the anonymity of the online environment.

What can you do when people are rude or are trolling you?

▶ Try not to respond emotionally. Don't type anything you wouldn't say to the person's face.

▶ When you are angry, press "pause," not "send." Take a while to think about your response.

▶ Watch your words. Re-read your response and think about how your words may be interpreted without the benefit of tone of voice or other nonverbal cues.

▶ End the conversation. If you want to respond without continuing the rudeness, you can thank the person for giving you their thoughts, ask to meet to talk about it in person, or "agree to disagree."

What has been your experience with social media rudeness? Would you end a relationship because of online behavior? Do you have any unresolved feelings over online conversations that didn't provide closure? What could you do to have better online manners?

**Sources:** A. Moscaritolo, "Surprise, People Are Rude on Social Media," *PC Magazine*, April 11, 2013, www.pcmag.com/article2/0,2817,2417664,00.asp; D. Archer, "Rude Technology," *Psychology Today*, September 27, 2014, www.psychologytoday.com/blog/reading-between-the-headlines/201409/rude-technology; M. W. Moyer, "Eye Contact Quells Online Hostility," *Scientific American*, August 2, 2012, www.scientificamerican.com/article/rudeness-on-the-internet/; R. A. Clay, "That's Just Rude," *APA Monitor on Psychology*, November 2013, www.apa.org/monitor/2013/11/rude.aspx

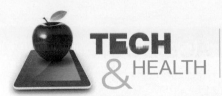

# TECH & HEALTH | LOVE IN THE TIME OF TWITTER

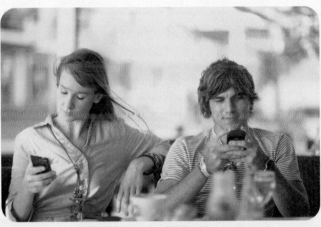

Technology has revolutionized our access to information and the ways we communicate. Couples can meet on Tinder, keep in constant contact via texting, and inform the world of their relationship highs and lows via Facebook and Twitter. With all these tools available, it can be easy to share **TMI** (too much information). Ilana Gershon, author of *The Breakup 2.0: Disconnecting over New Media*, suggests we currently lack standard etiquette for the use of new media in relationships. At its best, social media can bring people closer together; at its worst, it can be used intentionally or unintentionally to embarrass or hurt. Consider the following suggestions to safeguard yourself:

## When meeting:

- If you join a dating site, be honest about yourself; state your own interests and characteristics fairly, including things that you think might be less attractive than stereotypes and cultural norms dictate.

- If you meet someone online and want to meet in person, put safety first! Plan something brief, preferably during daylight hours. Meet in a public place, like a coffee shop. Do not meet with anyone who wants to keep the time and location a secret. Tell a friend or family member the details

of when and where you are meeting and any information you have on the person you are meeting.

## While dating:

- Discuss limits with your partner on the type of information you each want shared online. Agree to share only within those limits.

- Recognize that constant electronic updates throughout the day can leave little to share when you are together. Save some information for face-to-face talks!

- Sober up before you click "submit." Things that seem funny under the influence may not seem funny the next morning.

- Remember that the Internet is forever. Once a picture or a post is sent, it can never be completely erased.

Never post anything that would embarrass someone if it was seen by a family member or potential employer.

- Respect your partner's privacy. Logging onto his or her e-mail or Facebook account to look at private messages is a breach of trust.

- Know that the GPS in a phone can be used to track your location, and cell phone spyware can be installed that allows e-mail and texts to be read from another device. If you think you may be a victim of "cyberstalking" by a current or former partner, get a new phone or ask the phone company to reinstall the phone's operating system to wipe out the software.

## If breaking up:

- Do not break up with someone via text/e-mail/tweet/Facebook/chat. People deserve the respect of a more personal breakup.

- Upon breaking up, be sure to change any passwords you may have confided in your partner. The temptation to use those for ill may be too strong to resist.

**Source:** I. Gershon, *The Breakup 2.0: Disconnecting over New Media* (Ithaca, NY: Cornell University Press, 2012).

skills.[43] See the **Skills for Behavior Change** box for more on the impact of facial expressions on how we communicate.

A final concern is "technology rewiring the brain." It is important to note that rewiring isn't necessarily a bad thing; activities like learning a second language can also rewire the brain. However, technology does train the brain to attend to information in a different way than reading does. To describe how, Nicholas Carr, author of the *New York Times* Best Seller, *The Shallows: What the Internet Is Doing to Our Brains,* speaks of the difference between scuba diving and jet skiing. He says reading a book is like scuba diving; the diver is submerged in a focused, slow-paced setting, and as a result, is required to focus on the limited information that is available to her. In contrast, using the Internet is like jet skiing, where the jet skier skims along the

surface of the water at top speed, with many things to look at, only able to focus on any one thing for a second.[44] While this change in the way we receive information appears to reduce our attention span and focus, at the same time, it strengthens our ability to scan information rapidly and efficiently.

Today, there are more questions than answers about technology's impact on society in general, and on communication specifically. The bottom line is that real hugs and kisses cannot be replaced by typing XOXO, and the lack of accompanying nonverbal communication with most digital communication can create confusion and conflict due to a lack of clarity. While technology allows us to be more connected than during any other time in history, we must be sure to use digital communication as a complement to other ways of communicating—not a replacement.

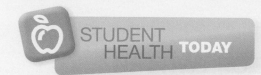
# LIFE IS AN OPEN (FACE)BOOK

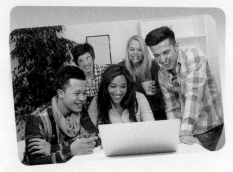

Headlines like "Justin Bieber Caught Telling Racist Joke" and "Caitlyn Jenner's Transition" confirm that celebrities have no expectation of privacy in a world where nearly everyone has a camera phone and an Internet connection. But headlines such as "Gay Students Accidentally Outed to Parents via Facebook" remind us that we cannot expect complete privacy either. We are just one photo tag away from a family member or potential employer seeing us in less than flattering circumstances or knowing information we'd prefer kept quiet.

"Social media screening," the practice of searching out all possible information on a prospective employee is practiced by about a third of employers. Increasingly, job applicants are being asked to share their Facebook pages to see if they are a good fit for a job! Mostly they want to see if job candidates present themselves professionally, are a good fit for company culture, have good communication skills, or are lying about their qualifications. Employers also report looking for inappropriate photos or evidence of drug or alcohol abuse.

If you are concerned about your privacy, make sure your publicly available information is what you want prospective employers, family, and other people to see. Tighten your privacy settings and untag yourself in photos you don't want people to see. Due to cached sites and reposts, you can't erase everything, so you may need to prepare an explanation for past posts, photos, and other information. As our "private" lives get more public all the time, we may have to accept that what we do in private always has the potential to become public knowledge.

**Sources:** L. Dearden, "Justin Bieber in Trouble Again: Singer Caught on Video Repeating N-word in Racist Joke," *The Independent*, February 27, 2015, www.independent.co.uk/news/people/justin-bieber-caught-on-video-repeating-nword-in-racist-joke-9467828.html; H. Cristomo, "Is Bruce Jenner Transitioning into a Woman?," *Kicker Daily News*, February 6, 2015, http://kickerdaily.com/is-bruce-jenner-transitioning-into-a-woman/; G. Fowler, "When the Most Personal Secrets Get Outed on Facebook," *The Wall Street Journal*, October 13, 2012, http://online.wsj.com; J. Smith, How Social Media Can Help (or Hurt) You in your Job Search," *Forbes*, January 10, 2013, www.forbes.com/sites/jacquelynsmith/2013/01/10/how-to-use-social-media-to-make-sales-2/

## Managing Conflict through Communication

A **conflict** is an emotional state that arises when the behavior of one person interferes with that of another. Conflict is inevitable whenever people live or work together. Not all conflict is bad; in fact, airing feelings and coming to resolution over differences can sometimes strengthen relationships. **Conflict resolution** and successful conflict management form a systematic approach to resolving differences fairly and constructively, rather than allowing them to fester. The goal of conflict resolution is to solve differences peacefully and creatively.

Here are some strategies for conflict resolution:

1. **Identify the problem or issue.** Talk with each other to clarify exactly what the conflict is. Try to understand both sides. In this first stage, you must say what you want and listen to what the other person wants. Focus on using "I" messages and avoid "you" messages. Be an active listener: Repeat what the other person has said and ask questions for clarification.

2. **Generate several possible solutions.** Base your search for solutions on the goals and interests identified in the first step. Come up with several different alternatives, and avoid evaluating any of them until you have finished brainstorming.

3. **Evaluate the alternative solutions.** Narrow solutions to one or two that seem to work for both parties. Be honest with each other about a solution that feels unsatisfactory, but also be open to compromise.

4. **Decide on the best solution.** Choose a solution that is acceptable to both parties. You both need to be committed to the decision for it to be effective.

5. **Implement the solution.** Discuss how the decision will be carried out. Establish who is responsible to do what and when. The solution stands a better chance of working if you agree on how it will be implemented.

6. **Follow up.** Evaluate whether the solution is working. Check in with the other person to see how he or she feels about it. Are you satisfied with the way the solution is working out? If something is not working as planned, or if circumstances have changed, discuss revising the plan. Remember that both parties must agree to any changes to the plan, as they did with the original idea.

**conflict** Emotional state that arises when opinions differ or the behavior of one person interferes with the behavior of another.

**conflict resolution** Concerted effort by all parties to constructively resolve differences or points of contention.

## LO 4 | RELATIONSHIPS: FOR BETTER AND WORSE

Identify the characteristics of successful relationships, including how to overcome common conflicts, and discuss how to cope when relationships end.

Success in a relationship is often defined by whether a couple stays together and remains close over the years. Learning to communicate, respecting each other, and sharing a genuine fondness are crucial. Many social scientists agree that the happiest committed relationships are flexible enough to allow partners to grow throughout their lives.

# Characteristics of Healthy Relationships

Satisfying and stable relationships are based on good communication, intimacy, friendship, and other factors. A key ingredient is *trust,* the degree to which each partner feels he or she can rely on the integrity of the other. Without trust, intimacy will not develop, and the relationship will likely fail. Trust includes three fundamental elements:

- Predictability—the ability to predict your partner's behavior based on past actions.

- Dependability—the ability to rely on your partner to emotionally support you in all situations, particularly those in which you feel threatened or hurt.
- Faith—belief in your partner having positive intentions and behavior.

What does a healthy relationship look and feel like? Healthy and unhealthy relationships are contrasted in FIGURE 5.2. Answering some basic questions can also help you determine if a relationship is working.

- Do you love and care for yourself to the same extent that you did before the relationship? Can you be yourself in the relationship?
- Is there genuine caring and goodwill? Do you share interests, values, and opinions? Is there mutual respect for differences?

| In an unhealthy relationship... | In a healthy relationship... |
|---|---|
| You care for and focus on another person only and neglect yourself or you focus only on yourself and neglect the other person. | You both love and take care of yourselves before and while in a relationship. |
| One of you feels pressure to change to meet the other person's standards and is afraid to disagree or voice ideas. | You respect each other's individuality, embrace your differences, and allow each other to "be yourselves." |
| One of you has to justify what you do, where you go, and people you see. | You both do things with friends and family and have activities independent of each other. |
| One of you makes all the decisions and controls everything without listening to the other's input. | You discuss things with each other, allow for differences of opinion, and compromise equally. |
| One of you feels unheard and is unable to communicate what you want. | You express and listen to each other's feelings, needs, and desires. |
| You lie to each other and find yourself making excuses for the other person. | You both trust and are honest with yourselves and with each other. |
| You don't have any personal space and have to share everything with the other person. | You respect each other's need for privacy. |
| Your partner keeps his or her sexual history a secret or hides a sexually transmitted infection from you, or you do not disclose your history to your partner. | You share sexual histories and information about sexual health with each other. |
| One of you is scared of asking the other to use protection or has refused the other's requests for safer sex. | You both practice safer sex methods. |
| One of you has forced or coerced the other to have sex. | You both respect sexual boundaries and are able to say no to sex. |
| One of you yells and hits, shoves, or throws things at the other in an argument. | You resolve conflicts in a rational, peaceful, and mutually agreed upon way. |
| You feel stifled, trapped, and stagnant. You are unable to escape the pressures of the relationship. | You both have room for positive growth, and you both learn more about each other as you develop and mature. |

**FIGURE 5.2** Healthy versus Unhealthy Relationships

**Source:** Advocates for Youth, Washington, DC, 2006, www.advocatesforyouth.org. Copyright © 2000. Used with permission.

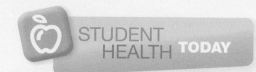
We know technology like dating sites can help couples meet, and texting can help people get to know each other better, but what about after a relationship begins? Does technology help or hurt? Two University of Nevada–Las Vegas researchers attempted to find out by interviewing 410 college students about the good and bad of technology in relationships.

**The Good:** Not surprisingly, text messaging was highly praised for its ability to keep couples in constant contact. People also reported using the Internet to search for information to improve their relationship, on topics from relationship building to sexual positions. Couples appreciated that they could make their relationship public, both by setting a status to "in a relationship," as well as posting pictures that their friends could see. Using technology as a way to manage conflict was also a common theme. People reported it was easier to use text messaging to apologize, to test the waters after a fight, and to argue slowly and more clearly.

**The Bad:** Texting sometimes seemed impersonal and detached, especially sexting. The presence of phones made people feel they did not always have the full attention of their partner. Trust was also an issue. People were concerned with who else their partner might be in contact with—that a phone is "another outlet for infidelity." Finally, the lack of nonverbal cues made it harder to interpret messages, creating opportunities for misunderstanding and for information to be taken out of context.

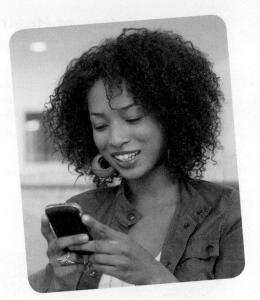

**Source:** K. Herlein and K. Ancheta, "Advantages and Disadvantages of Technology in Relationships: Findings from an Open-Ended Survey," *Qualitative Report* 19, no. 22 (2014): 1–11, Available at www .nova.edu/ssss/QR/QR19/hertlein22.pdf.

- Is there mutual encouragement? Do you support each other unconditionally?
- Do you trust each other? Are you honest with each other? Can you comfortably express your feelings, opinions, and needs?
- Is there room in your relationship for growth as you both evolve and mature?

Relationships are nurtured by consistent communication, actions, and self-reflection. Poor communication can weaken bonds and create mistrust. We all need to reflect periodically on how we typically relate to others through our words and actions. Have we been honest, direct, and fair in our conversations? Have we listened to others' thoughts, wants, and needs? Have we behaved in ways consistent with our words, values, and beliefs?

Breakdowns in relationships often begin with a change in communication, however subtle. Either partner may stop listening and cease to be emotionally present for the other. In turn, the other feels ignored, unappreciated, or unwanted. Unresolved conflicts increase, and unresolved anger can cause problems in sexual relations, which can further increase communication difficulties. New communication technologies add a whole new dimension (see the **Student Health Today** box for more on pros and cons).

College students, particularly those who are socially isolated and far from family and hometown friends, may be particularly vulnerable to staying in unhealthy relationships. They may become emotionally dependent on a partner. Mutual obligations, such as shared rental, financial, or transportation arrangements, and sometimes childcare, can complicate a decision to end a bad relationship. It's also easy to mistake sexual advances for physical attraction or love. Without a strong social network to validate feelings or share concerns, a student can feel stuck in an unhealthy relationship.

Honesty and verbal affection are usually positive aspects of a relationship. In a troubled relationship, however, they can be used to cover up irresponsible or hurtful behavior. Saying "at least I was honest" is not an acceptable substitute for acting in a trustworthy way, and claiming "but I really do love you" is not a license for being inconsiderate or hurtful.

## Confronting Couples Issues

Couples seeking a long-term relationship must confront a number of issues that can either enhance or diminish their chances of success. These issues can involve jealousy, sharing power and responsibility, and communication about unmet expectations.

**Jealousy** Jealousy is a negative reaction evoked by a real or imagined relationship involving one's partner and another person. Contrary to what many people believe, jealousy is not

**jealousy** Aversive reaction evoked by a real or imagined relationship involving a person's partner and a third person.

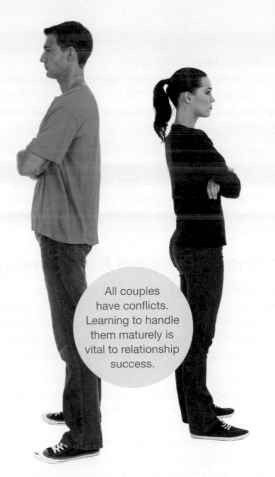

All couples have conflicts. Learning to handle them maturely is vital to relationship success.

38%

OF SINGLE ADULTS WHO ARE LOOKING FOR A PARTNER HAVE USED AN ONLINE OR MOBILE **DATING APP**—66% HAVE GONE ON A DATE WITH A MATCH.

Although a certain amount of jealousy can be expected in any loving relationship, it doesn't have to threaten the relationship as long as partners communicate openly about it.[45]

### Sharing Power and Responsibilities

Power can be defined as the ability to make and implement decisions. Historically, men have been the primary wage earners and, consequently, had decision-making power. Women exerted much influence, but ultimately, they needed a man's income for survival. As increasing numbers of women have entered the workforce and generated their own financial resources, the power dynamics between women and men have shifted considerably. The increase in the divorce rate in the past century was partly due to working women gaining the ability to support themselves rather than stay in difficult or abusive relationships solely for financial reasons.

Where gender roles and tasks were rigid in the past, modern society has very few gender-specific roles. Both women and men work, care for children, drive, run businesses, manage family finances, and perform equally well in the tasks of daily living. Rather than taking on traditional female and male roles, many couples find it makes more sense to divide tasks on the basis of schedule, convenience, and preference. However, while many women work as many hours outside the home as men, the division is of labor at home is rarely equal. The Bureau of Labor Statistics estimates that on a typical day, 49 percent of women do household chores like laundry, where the same is true of only 19 percent of men; over two thirds of women prepare food or clean up afterward, while less than half of men share those tasks.[46] Over time, if couples can't communicate how they feel about sharing power and responsibility and arrive at an equitable solution, the relationship is likely to suffer.

### Unmet Expectations

We all have expectations of ourselves and our partners—how we will spend our time and our money, how we will express love and intimacy, and how we will grow together as a couple. Expectations are an extension of our values, beliefs, hopes, and dreams for the future. When communicated and agreed upon, these expectations help relationships thrive. If we are unable to communicate our expectations, we set ourselves up for disappointment and hurt. Partners in healthy relationships can communicate wants and needs and have honest discussions when things aren't going as expected.

a sign of intense devotion. Instead, jealousy often indicates underlying problems, such as insecurity or possessiveness—significant barriers to a healthy relationship. Often, jealousy is rooted past experiences of deception or loss. Other causes of jealousy typically include the following:

- **Overdependence on the relationship.** People who have few social ties and rely exclusively on their partners tend to be overly fearful of losing them.
- **Severity of the threat.** People may feel uneasy if someone with good looks or a great personality appears to be interested in their partner.
- **High value on sexual exclusivity.** People who believe that sexual exclusivity is a crucial indicator of love are more likely to become jealous.
- **Low self-esteem.** People who think poorly of themselves are more likely to fear that someone else will gain their partner's affection.
- **Fear of losing control.** Some people need to feel in control of every situation. Feeling that they may be losing control over a partner can cause jealousy.

In both men and women, jealousy is also related to believing it would be difficult to find another relationship if the current one ends.

**power** Ability to make and implement decisions.

### WHAT DO **YOU** THINK?

Have you ever been jealous or had a jealous partner?

- Can you identify what actions or events caused you to feel this way?
- Did you have actual facts to support your feelings, or was your response based on suspicions?

# When and Why Relationships End

Relationships end for many reasons, including illness, financial concerns, career problems, and personality conflicts. Many people enter a relationship with certain expectations about how they and their partner will behave. Failure to communicate these beliefs can lead to resentment and disappointment. Differences in sexual needs may also contribute to the demise of a relationship. Under stress, communication and cooperation between partners can break down. Conflict, negative interactions, and a general lack of respect between partners can erode even the most loving relationship.

What behaviors signal trouble? Based on 35 years of research and couples therapy, therapist John Gottman has identified four behavior patterns in couples that predict future divorce with 85 percent or better accuracy.

- **Criticism.** Phrasing complaints in terms of a partner's defect; for example: "You never talk about anyone but yourself. You are self-centered."

- **Defensiveness.** Righteous indignation as a form of self-protection; for example: "It's not my fault we missed the flight; you always make us late."
- **Stonewalling.** Withdrawing emotionally from a given interaction; for example: The listener seems to ignore the speaker as she speaks, giving no indication that the speaker was heard.
- **Contempt.** Talking down to a person; for example: "How could you be so stupid?"[47]

Of these, contempt is the biggest predictor of divorce. While these behaviors do not guarantee that an individual couple will divorce, they are "red flags" for relationships at high risk for failure.

## Coping with Failed Relationships

No relationship comes with a guarantee. Losing love is as much a part of life as falling in love. That being said, uncoupling can be very painful. Whenever we risk getting close to another person, we also risk getting hurt if things don't work out. Consider the following tips for coping with a failed relationship:[48]

- **Acknowledge that you've gone through a rough spot.** You may feel grief, loneliness, rejection, anger, guilt, relief, sadness, or all of these. Seek out trusted friends and, if needed, professional help.
- **Let go of negative thought patterns and habits.** Engage in activities that make you happy. Take a walk, read, listen to music, go to the movies or a concert, spend time with fun friends, volunteer with a community organization, or write in a journal. Find your joy!

## LO 5 | MARRIAGE, PARTNERING, AND SINGLEHOOD

Compare and contrast the types of committed relationships and lifestyle choices.

Commitment in a relationship means that one intends to act over time in a way that perpetuates the well-being of the other person, oneself, and the relationship. Polls show that the vast majority of Americans strive to develop a committed relationship whether in the form of marriage, cohabitation, or partnerships.[49] Still, many Americans choose to remain single.

## Marriage

In many societies, traditional committed relationships take the form of marriage. In the United States, marriage means entering into a legal agreement that includes shared finances, property, and often the responsibility for raising children. Many Americans also view marriage as a religious sacrament that emphasizes certain rights and obligations for each spouse. Marriage is socially sanctioned and highly celebrated in American culture, so there are numerous incentives for couples to formalize their relationship in this way.

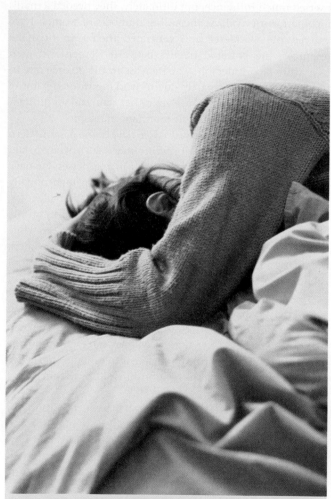

It may feel as if there is no end to the sorrow, anger, and guilt that often accompany a difficult breakup, but time is a miraculous healer. Acknowledging your feelings and finding healthful ways to express them will help you deal with the end of a romantic relationship.

Historically, close to 90 percent of Americans married at least once during their lifetime,[50] and at any given time, about 50 percent of U.S. adults are married (**FIGURE 5.3**). However, in recent years Americans have become less likely to marry. Since 1960, the annual number of marriages has steadily declined.[51] This decrease may be due to a delay of first marriages, as well as a substitution of cohabitation for marriage. In 1960, the median age for first marriage was 23 years for men and 20 years for women; today, the median age for first marriage has risen to 29 years for men and 27 years for women.[52]

Divorce rates in the United States have been high for multiple decades. Some estimates indicate that approximately 50 percent of first marriages end in divorce, with even higher divorce rates for second and third marriages.[53] Other studies, however, suggest the divorce rate is only 30 percent and that it has been declining since the early 1980s.[54] This decrease is related to an increase in the number of couples who cohabit instead of marry, an increase in the age at which persons first marry, and a higher level of education among those who are marrying.[55] The risk of divorce is lower for college-educated people marrying for the first time; it is lower still for people who wait to marry until their midtwenties and who haven't lived with multiple partners prior to marriage.[56]

Many Americans believe that marriage involves **monogamy**, or exclusive sexual involvement with one partner.

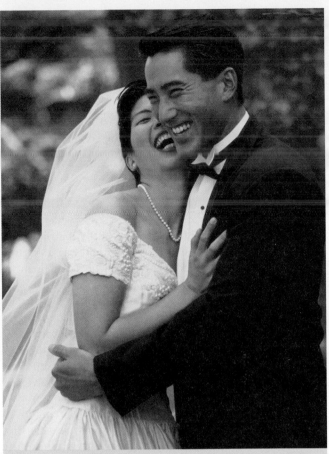

For many, weddings or commitment ceremonies serve as the ultimate symbol of a long-term, exclusive relationship between two people.

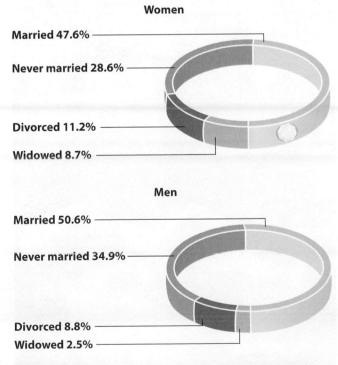

**Women**

Married 47.6%

Never married 28.6%

Divorced 11.2%

Widowed 8.7%

**Men**

Married 50.6%

Never married 34.9%

Divorced 8.8%

Widowed 2.5%

**FIGURE 5.3** Marital Status of the U.S. Population by Sex
**Note:** The figure does not list the percentages for married men and women with a spouse absent and separated.

**Source:** U.S. Census Bureau, "Table A1, Marital Status of People 15 Years and Over, by Age, Sex Personal Earnings, Race, and Hispanic Origin: 2014," America's Families and Living Arrangements, 2014, www.census.gov

However, the lifetime pattern for many Americans appears to be **serial monogamy**, which means a person has a monogamous sexual relationship with one partner before moving on to another monogamous relationship.[57] A small number of couples choose an **open relationship** (or open marriage), in which partners agree that there may be sexual involvement outside their relationship.

A healthy marriage provides emotional support by combining the benefits of friendship with a loving committed relationship. It also provides stability for both the couple and for those involved in their lives. Considerable research indicates that married people live longer, feel happier, remain mentally alert longer, and suffer fewer physical and mental health problems.[58] A new study by the National Bureau of Economic Research confirms the long-lasting benefits of marriage, indicating that friendship is the critical element of these benefits. It should be noted, however, that these benefits are also enjoyed by *unmarried* romantic partners who live together.[59] On the other hand, being in an unhealthy marriage can be worse for psychological well-being than staying single.[60]

**monogamy** Exclusive sexual involvement with one partner.

**serial monogamy** Series of monogamous sexual relationships.

**open relationship** A relationship in which partners agree that sexual involvement can occur outside the relationship.

# 73%

Couples in healthy marriages have less stress, which in turn contributes to better overall health. A healthy marriage contributes to lower stress levels in three important ways: less risky personal behaviors, expanded support networks, and financial stability.

Risky personal behaviors, including smoking and heavy alcohol use, are lower in married adults. They are about half as likely to be smokers as are cohabitating, divorced, separated, or widowed adults.[61] They are also less likely to be heavy drinkers and more likely to get sufficient sleep compared to divorced adults.[62] While it may be that marriage causes the improved behaviors, it may also be that people who engage in healthier behaviors are just more likely to get married. One negative health indicator for married men is body weight. Married men are far more likely than never-married men to be overweight. Married women, however, are less likely than divorced women to be overweight or obese.[63] Marriage additionally provides the possibility for integration into an existing social network of family and friends to provide assistance and help couples cope when stressors inevitably arise. Finally, marriage is strongly related to economic well-being, which can impact both health status and stress levels.

> **cohabitation** Intimate partners living together without being married.
>
> **common-law marriage** Cohabitation lasting a designated period of time (usually 7 years) that is considered legally binding in some states.

## Cohabitation

**Cohabitation** is a relationship in which two unmarried people with an intimate connection live together in the same household. For a variety of reasons, more Americans are choosing cohabitation. In some states, cohabitation that lasts a designated number of years (usually 7) legally constitutes a **common-law marriage** for purposes of purchasing real estate and sharing other financial obligations.

Cohabitation can offer many of the same benefits as marriage: love, sex, companionship, and the opportunity to know a partner better over time. In addition to emotional and physical benefits, some people may live together for practical reasons, such as the opportunity to share bills and housing costs. Over the past 20 years, there has been a large increase in the number of persons who have cohabited. In fact, the majority of young couples now live together before marriage; it is more

and more common for cohabitation to be the first coresidential partnership for young adults.[64] On average, the first cohabitation before marriage for people over age 20 lasts about 18 months, with about 40 percent of couples transitioning into marriage within 3 years.[65]

Cohabitation before marriage has been a controversial issue for decades. While some voiced moral objections, other concerns were related to higher divorce rates among couples who cohabited before marriage. However, according to recent research based on more than 7,000 respondents to the National Survey of Family Growth, cohabitation before marriage is no longer a predictor for divorce.[66]

While cohabitation can serve as a prelude to marriage for some people, for others, it is a permanent alternative to marriage. The most likely to cohabit include those of lower socioeconomic status, those who are less religious, people who have been divorced, and those who have experienced parental divorce or high levels of parental conflict during childhood.[67] Although cohabitation has advantages, it also has drawbacks. Perhaps the greatest disadvantage is the lack of societal validation for the relationship, especially if the couple subsequently has children. Many cohabitants must deal with pressure to marry from parents and friends, difficulties in obtaining insurance and tax benefits, and legal issues over property.

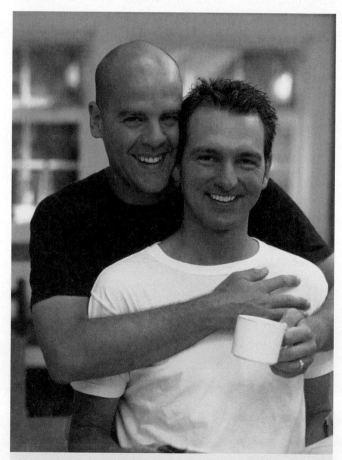

Most adults want to form committed, lasting relationships regardless of their sexual orientation.

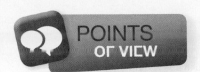

# The End of the Defense of Marriage Act

## POINTS OF VIEW

The federal Defense of Marriage Act (DOMA), enacted in 1996, was a law defining marriage as a legal union exclusively between one man and one woman and establishing that no state must recognize the relationship between persons of the same sex as a marriage, even if the relationship is considered a marriage in another state. DOMA also denied same-sex couples federal protections and benefits that heterosexual couples enjoy, such as social security benefits, health insurance benefits, and hospital visitation rights. However, in a historic decision on June 26, 2015, the Supreme Court ruled that same-sex marriage is a constitutional right, ending DOMA and paving the way for greater acceptance of same-sex marriages. While considered a victory by many, the Supreme Court decision was not without controversy. Some common arguments include:

### Arguments for the Supreme Court's legalization of same-sex marriage:

- The U.S. Constitution guarantees equal rights for all U.S. citizens; thus, having unequal marriage rights is a form of discrimination.
- The U.S. Constitution requires each state to give "full faith and credit" to the laws of other states, including states' obligations to honor marriages validated in other states and districts.
- Civil unions and domestic partnerships do not offer all of the benefits of marriage, and they vary greatly from state to state.

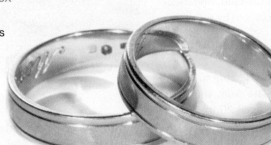

### Arguments against the Supreme Court's legalization of same-sex marriage:

- Marriage is largely a religious institution, and many religious groups are opposed to the idea of same-sex marriage.
  - A change of this magnitude should have been decided by legislative action at the state level, not judicial action at the federal level.
- Allowing same-sex couples to marry undermines the institution of marriage itself.

## WHERE DO YOU STAND?

- What person(s) or institution(s) should define marriage?

- Do you think the Supreme Court was correct in ruling on the constitutionality of same-sex marriage or should individual states have decided one-by-one?

- Are you aware of the rights, responsibilities, and protections granted to married couples by the federal government?

# Gay and Lesbian Marriage and Partnerships

The 2013 American Community Survey identified an estimated 726,600 same-sex couples in the United States, 35 percent of whom are legally married.[68] Whether they are gay or straight, male or female, most adults want intimate, committed relationships. Lesbians and gay men seek the same things in primary relationships that heterosexual partners do: love, friendship, communication, validation, companionship, and a sense of stability.

In addition to facing the same challenges to successful relationships as heterosexual couples, lesbian and gay couples often face discrimination and difficulties dealing with social, religious, and legal issues. For lesbian and gay couples, obtaining the same level of marriage benefits such as tax deductions,

power-of-attorney rights, partner health insurance, and child custody rights has been a longstanding challenge. Now, however, with the 5-to-4 Supreme Court ruling in the Obergefell v. Hodges case[69], same-sex marriage is legal in all 50 states (see the **Points of View** box for more on this topic).

This was a long hoped-for decision for many same-sex couples across the country, especially those in the 13 states yet to legalize same-sex marriage. Supreme Court Justice Anthony Kennedy, the deciding vote in the decision, said the Court's decision was based on the acknowledgement of four fundamental principles: that marriage is inherent to the concept of individual autonomy, that it is of unparalleled importance to committed couples, that it is crucial for safeguarding the rights of the children of couples in committed relationships, and that marriage has long been a keystone of social order.[70]

In explanation of his opinion, Justice Kennedy stated, "It would misunderstand these men and women to say they disrespect the idea of marriage. Their plea is that they do respect it, respect it so deeply that they seek to find its fulfillment for themselves. Their hope is not to be condemned to live in loneliness, excluded from one of civilization's oldest institutions. They ask for equal dignity in the eyes of the law. The Constitution grants them that right."[71]

With this victory a new era begins for same-sex couples, although challenges remain. Within days of the ruling, the Texas Attorney General said state workers could refuse to grant marriage licenses to same-sex couples if doing so violates their religious beliefs and three months after the ruling a county clerk in Kentucky went to jail rather than issue marriage licenses to same-sex couples.[72] These rebuttals indicate that while same-sex marriage is now the law of the land, homosexual couples still face challenges in being accepted by some.

## Staying Single

Increasing numbers of adults of all ages are electing to marry later or to remain single. According to data from the most recent U.S. Census, 57 percent of women aged 20 to 34 had never been married. Likewise, men in this age group postponed marriage in increasing numbers, with 67 percent remaining unmarried.[73]

Singles clubs, social outings arranged by communities and religious groups, extended family environments, and many

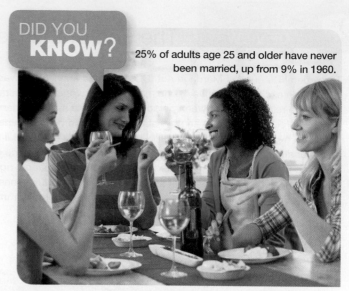

**DID YOU KNOW?**

25% of adults age 25 and older have never been married, up from 9% in 1960.

**Source:** K. Parker, W. Wang, and M. Rohol, "Record Share of Americans Have Never Married," Pew Research (2014), www.pewsocialtrends.org/files/2014/09/2014-09-24_Never-Married-Americans.pdf

social services support the single lifestyle. Many singles live rich, rewarding lives and maintain a large network of close friends and family. Although sexual intimacy may or may not be present, the intimacy achieved through other interactions with loved ones is a key aspect of the single lifestyle.

# ASSESS | YOURSELF

## How Well Do You Communicate?

How do you think you rate as a communicator? How do you think others might rate you? Are you generally someone who expresses his or her thoughts easily, or are you more apt to say nothing for fear of saying the wrong thing? Read the following scenarios and indicate how each describes you, based on the following rating scale.

5 = Would describe me *all* or *nearly all* of the time
3 = Would describe me *sometimes*, but it would be a struggle for me
1 = Would describe me *never* or *almost never*

1. In a roomful of mostly strangers, you find it easy to mingle and strike up conversations with just about anyone in the room.

2. Someone you respect is very critical/hateful about someone that you like a lot. You are comfortable speaking up and saying you disagree and why you feel this way.

3. Someone in your class is not doing her part on a group project, and her work is substandard. You can be direct and tell her the work isn't acceptable.

4. One of your friends asks you to let him look at your class assignment because he hasn't had time to do his. You know that he skips class regularly and seems to never do his own work, so you politely tell him no.

5. You realize that the person you are dating is not right for you and you are probably not right for him or her. When he or she blurts out, "I love you," you say, "I'm sorry, but I don't have those same feelings for you."

6. Your instructor asks you to give a speech at a state conference, discussing health problems faced by students on campus. You tell the instructor that you'd love to do it and begin planning what you will say.

7. You don't want to go out drinking at a party on Friday night, even though all of your good friends are going to go. When asked what time they should pick you up, you tell them you appreciate the offer, but you really don't want to go.

8. Your best friend, Bill, is in an abusive relationship with his girlfriend, Molly. You tell him that you think he might benefit by visiting the campus counseling center.

9. Students in your class have done poorly on a recent exam and believe that the test was unfair. You volunteer to be the spokesperson and talk with the instructor, telling her what the class thinks of the exam.

10. You see someone you are really attracted to. You walk up to him or her at a party and strike up a conversation with the intention of asking him or her out on a date.

## How Did You Do?

The higher your score on the above scenarios (the more 5s you have), the more likely it is that you are a direct and clear communicator. Are there areas that you rated as 3 or as 1? Why do you think you have difficulties in these situations? How might you best communicate in these situations to achieve the results you want? Any time you have to communicate with others about difficult topics, it is best to speak and listen carefully, keep the other person's feelings in mind, and show respect for the individual. Try to think about what you might say ahead of time so that you are prepared to speak.

## YOUR PLAN FOR CHANGE

The ASSESS YOURSELF activity gave you the chance to look at how you communicate. Now that you have considered your responses, you can take steps toward becoming a better communicator and improving your relationships.

**TODAY, YOU CAN:**

☐ Call a friend you haven't talked to in a while or arrange to meet a new acquaintance for coffee to get to know each other better.

☐ Start a journal for keeping track of communication and relationship issues that arise. Look for trends and think about ways you can change your behavior to address them.

**WITHIN THE NEXT TWO WEEKS, YOU CAN:**

☐ Spend some time letting the people you care about know how important they are to you and how you appreciate the social support they provide.

☐ If there is someone with whom you have a conflict, arrange a time to talk about the issues. Be sure to meet in a neutral setting away from distractions.

**BY THE END OF THE SEMESTER, YOU CAN:**

☐ Practice being an active listener and notice when your mind wanders while you are listening to someone.

☐ Think about the ways you communicate with a sexual partner. Consider removing yourself from an unhappy relationship or improving communication with a partner to reach a satisfying relationship.

## CHAPTER REVIEW

 To hear an MP3 Tutor Session, scan here or visit the Study Area in **MasteringHealth**.

### LO 1 | Intimate Connections

- Characteristics of intimate relationships include behavioral interdependence, need fulfillment, emotional attachment, and emotional availability. Relationships help us fulfill our needs for intimacy, social integration, nurturance, assistance, and affirmation. Family, friends, and romantic partners provide the most common opportunities for intimacy. Each relationship may include healthy and unhealthy characteristics that can affect daily functioning.

### LO 2 | The Value of Relationships

- All types of relationships can bolster our health. Social support, in the form of emotional, instrumental, informational, and appraisal support, helps to reduce our stress and strengthen our resolve.
- In addition to our need for feeling close to family and friends, collective connectedness, the feeling of being part of a group, widens our social network and increases our social capital.

### LO 3 | Building Communication Skills

- To improve our communication with others, we need to develop our skills related to self-disclosure, listening effectively, conveying and interpreting nonverbal communication, and managing and resolving conflicts.
- Digital communication allows us to keep in contact like at no other time in history, but there are concerns about its relationship to envy, addiction, a lack of nonverbal cues, and impact on the brain.

### LO 4 | Relationships: For Better and Worse

- There are many strategies for building better relationships. Examining one's own behaviors to determine what to change and how to change is an important ingredient of success. Characteristics of successful relationships include good communication, intimacy, friendship, and trust.
- Factors that can cause problems in romantic relationships include breakdowns in communication, erosion of mutual respect, jealousy, difficulty sharing power and responsibilities, and unmet expectations. Before relationships fail, warning signs often appear. By recognizing these signs and taking action to change behaviors, partners may save and enhance their relationship.

### LO 5 | Partnering and Singlehood

- For most people, commitment is an important part of a successful relationship. Types of committed relationships include marriage, partnership, and cohabitation. Success in committed relationships requires understanding the elements of a good relationship.
- Remaining single is more common than ever before. Most single people lead healthy, happy, and well-adjusted lives.

## POP QUIZ

Visit **MasteringHealth** to personalize your study plan with Chapter Review Quizzes and Dynamic Study Modules.

### LO 1 | Intimate Connections

1. Intimate relationships fulfill our psychological need for someone to listen to our worries and concerns. This is known as our need for
   a. dependence.
   b. social integration.
   c. enjoyment.
   d. spontaneity.

2. According to anthropologist Helen Fisher, attraction and falling in love follow a pattern based on
   a. lust, attraction, and attachment.
   b. intimacy, passion, and commitment.
   c. imprinting, attraction, attachment, and the production of a cuddle chemical.
   d. fascination, exclusiveness, sexual desire, giving the utmost, and being a champion.

### LO 2 | The Value of Relationships

3. When Neil received a midterm report saying he had a D in his chemistry course, Mariah told him about the tutors available. This is an example of
   a. appraisal support.
   b. emotional support.
   c. informational support.
   d. instrumental support.

4. The power of all the people who could come to your aid with their resources is your
   a. social support.
   b. social potential.
   c. social network.
   d. social capital.

### LO 3 | Building Communication Skills

5. Sharika sits quietly while listening to her sister, not providing her with any nonverbal feedback as she speaks. This is an example of:
   a. competitive listening.
   b. passive listening.
   c. active listening.
   d. reflective listening.

6. The goal of conflict resolution is to
   a. constructively resolve points of contention.
   b. declare a winner and a loser.
   c. ensure that couples argue as little as possible.
   d. set a time limit on discussion of difficult issues.

## LO 4 | Relationships: For Better and Worse

7. Predictability, dependability, and faith are three fundamental elements of
   a. trust.
   b. friendship.
   c. attraction.
   d. attachment.

8. All of the following are typical causes of jealousy *except*
   a. overdependence on the relationship.
   b. low self-esteem.
   c. a past relationship that involved deception.
   d. belief that relationships can easily be replaced.

## LO 5 | Partnering and Singlehood

9. A relationship in which two unmarried people with an intimate connection share the same household is known as
   a. monogamy.
   b. cohabitation.
   c. common-law household.
   d. civil union.

10. Sofia is 30 years old, and she decides to stay single rather than get married. Which of the following is *true* regarding Sofia's decision?
    a. Sofia needs to seek out sexual intimacy to stay content throughout life.
    b. Sofia is unique as staying single is becoming less common.
    c. Sofia is in the minority of women ages 20 to 34, as most are married.
    d. Sofia can obtain intimacy through relationships with family and friends.

*Answers can be found on page A-1. If you answered a question incorrectly, review the section identified by the Learning Outcome. For even more study tools, visit MasteringHealth.*

## THINK ABOUT IT!

### LO 1 | Intimate Relationships

1. What are the characteristics of intimate relationships? What are behavioral interdependence, need fulfillment, emotional attachment, and emotional availability, and why is each important in relationship development?

2. What problems can form barriers to intimacy? What actions can you take to reduce or remove these barriers?

### LO 2 | The Value of Relationships

3. What are the four types of social support? What are examples of social support you give and receive in your life?

4. How can people increase the social capital in their lives? How does social capital impact health status?

### LO 3 | Building Communication Skills

5. What is nonverbal communication, and why is it important to develop skills in this area? Give examples of some things you do to communicate without words.

6. Why might Facebook users report more social support in their lives? How can Facebook affect social capital?

### LO 4 | Relationships: for Better and Worse

7. What are common elements of good relationships? What are some warning signs of trouble? What actions can you take to improve your own interpersonal relationships?

8. How can you tell the difference between a love relationship and one that is based primarily on attraction? What characteristics do love relationships share?

9. What are some of the common warning signs that a relationship is going to fail? What are some actions people can take to change behaviors to save or even enhance a troubled relationship?

### LO 5 | Partnering and Singlehood

10. What are the different types of committed relationships? How are they different? What does it take for any kind of committed relationship to succeed?

11. Name some common misconceptions about people who choose to remain single. Why might people hold those opinions?

## ACCESS YOUR HEALTH ON THE INTERNET

The following websites explore further topics and issues related to personal health. For links to the websites below, visit MasteringHealth.

*National Center for Health Statistics.* This division of the Centers for Disease Control and Prevention has up-to-date statistics on trends in marriage, divorce, and cohabitation. **www.cdc.gov/nchs**

*The Gottman Institute.* This organization helps couples directly and provides training to therapists. The website includes research information, self-help tips for relationship building, and a relationship quiz. **www.gottman.com**

*The National Gay and Lesbian Task Force.* This organization works toward lesbian, gay, bisexual, and transgender (LGBT) equality and provides research and policy analysis to create social change. **www.thetaskforce.org**

*National Healthy Marriage Resource Center.* A clearinghouse for news and research related to healthy marriages. **www.healthymarriageinfo.org**

*The Hotline.* This site provides information about domestic violence, including how to recognize abuse and how to get help in your local area. Phone support is available 24/7 at 1-800-799-SAFE (7233). **www.thehotline.org**

# Understanding Your Sexuality

Your understanding of gender roles, your contact with people of various gender identities or sexual orientations, and your own degree of emotional maturity can all affect your sense of sexual identity.

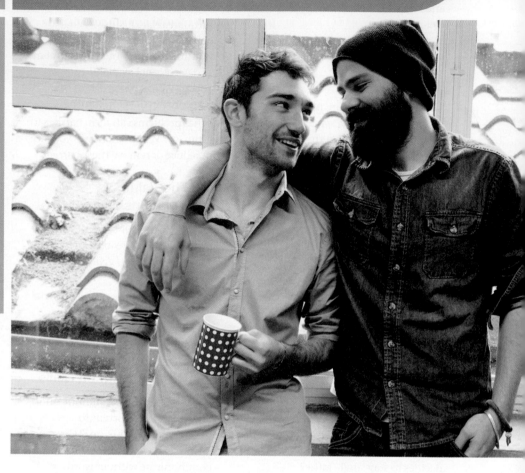

## LEARNING OUTCOMES

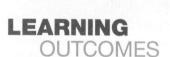

1 Define *sexual identity* and discuss its major components, including biology, gender identity, gender roles, and sexual orientation.

2 Identify the primary structures of male and female reproductive anatomy and explain the functions of each.

3 List and describe the stages of the human sexual response and classify types of sexual dysfunctions.

4 Explain the options available for the expression of one's sexuality and discuss the components of healthy and responsible sexuality.

**H**uman sexuality is complex and involves physical health, personal values, and interpersonal relationships, as well as cultural traditions, social norms, new technologies, and changing political agendas. **Sexuality** is much more than sexual feelings or intercourse. Rather, it includes all the thoughts, feelings, and behaviors associated with being male or female, experiencing attraction, being in love, and being in relationships that include sexual intimacy. Having a comprehensive understanding of your sexuality will help you make responsible and satisfying decisions about your behaviors and your interpersonal relationships.

## LO 1 | YOUR SEXUAL IDENTITY

Define *sexual identity* and discuss its major components, including biology, gender identity, gender roles, and sexual orientation.

**Sexual identity,** the recognition and acknowledgment of oneself as a sexual being, is determined by a complex

---

**sexuality** Thoughts, feelings, and behaviors associated with being male or female, experiencing attraction, being in love, and being in relationships that include sexual intimacy.

**sexual identity** Recognition of oneself as a sexual being; a composite of biological sex characteristics, gender identity, gender roles, and sexual orientation.

interaction of genetic, physiological, environmental, and social factors. The beginning of sexual identity occurs at conception with the combining of chromosomes that determine sex. All eggs carry an X sex chromosome; sperm may carry either an X or a Y chromosome. If a sperm carrying an X chromosome fertilizes an egg, the resulting combination of sex chromosomes (XX) provides the blueprint to produce a female. If a sperm carrying a Y chromosome fertilizes an egg, the XY combination produces a male.

Sometimes chromosomes are added, lost, or rearranged in this process and the sex of a baby is not clear, a condition known as **intersexuality.** *Disorders of sexual development (DSDs)* is a less confusing term that has been recommended to refer to intersex conditions. While the exact number of babies born with a DSD each year is unknown, estimates range from 1 in 1,500 to 1 in 4,500 births.[1]

The genetic instructions included in the sex chromosomes lead to the differential development of male and female **gonads** (reproductive organs) at about the eighth week of fetal life. Once the male gonads (testes) and the female gonads (ovaries) develop, they play a key role in all future sexual development through the production of sex hormones. The primary female sex hormones are estrogen and progesterone. The primary male sex hormone is testosterone. The release of testosterone in a maturing fetus stimulates the development of a penis and other male genitals. If no testosterone is produced, female genitals form.

At the time of **puberty,** sex hormones again play major roles in development. Hormones released by the **pituitary gland,** called *gonadotropins,* stimulate the testes and ovaries to make appropriate sex hormones. The increase of estrogen production in females and testosterone production in males leads to the development of **secondary sex**

## SEE IT! VIDEOS

What terms are used in talking about gender and sexuality? Watch **Transgender Terms: Breaking Down Definitions and Dos & Don'ts** in the Study Area of

**MasteringHealth™**

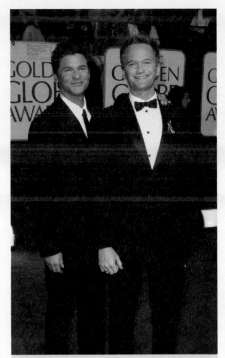

The presence of gay and lesbian celebrities in the media—such as actor Neil Patrick Harris and his husband David Burtka—contributes to the increasing acceptance of gay relationships in everyday life.

**characteristics.** Male secondary sex characteristics include deepening of the voice, development of facial and body hair, and growth of the skeleton and musculature. Female secondary sex characteristics include growth of the breasts, widening of the hips, and the development of pubic and underarm hair.

In addition to a person's biological status as a male or female, another important component of sexual identity is gender. **Gender** refers to characteristics and actions typically associated with men or women (masculine or feminine) as defined by the culture in which one lives. **Gender roles** are the behaviors and activities we use to express masculinity or femininity in ways that conform to society's expectations. Our sense of masculine and feminine traits is largely a result of socialization during our childhood.

For some, gender roles can be confining when they lead to stereotyping. Bounds established by *gender role stereotypes* can make it difficult to express one's true sexual identity. In the United States, common masculine gender role stereotypes include being independent, aggressive, logical, and in control of emotions, whereas common feminine gender role stereotypes include being passive, nurturing, intuitive, sensitive, and emotional. **Androgyny** refers to the combination of traditional masculine and feminine traits in a single person. Androgynous people do not always follow traditional gender roles but instead choose behaviors based on a given situation.

**Gender identity** is a person's sense or awareness of being masculine or feminine. A person's gender identity does not always match his or her biological sex; this is called being **transgender.** There is a broad spectrum of expression among transgender persons, reflecting different degrees of dissatisfaction with their sexual anatomy. Some transgender persons are very comfortable with their bodies, content to dress only as the other gender (*cross-dressing*). At the other end of the spectrum are **transsexuals,** who feel trapped in their bodies and may opt for therapeutic interventions, such as sex reassignment surgery; distress about incongruity between a person's biological sex and gender identity is called **gender dysphoria**.

---

**intersexuality** Not exhibiting exclusively male or female sex characteristics; also known as disorders of sexual development (DSD).

**gonads** The reproductive organs that produce germ cells and sex hormones in a man (testes) or woman (ovaries).

**puberty** The period of sexual maturation.

**pituitary gland** The endocrine gland in the brain controlling the release of hormones from the gonads.

**secondary sex characteristics** Characteristics associated with sex but not directly related to reproduction, such as vocal pitch, amount of body hair, breasts, and location of fat deposits.

**gender** The characteristics and actions associated with being feminine or masculine as defined by the society or culture in which one lives.

**gender roles** Expression of maleness or femaleness in everyday life that conform to society's expectations.

**androgyny** Combination of traditional masculine and feminine traits in a single person.

**gender identity** Personal sense or awareness of being masculine or feminine, a male or a female.

**transgender** Having a gender identity that does not match one's biological sex.

**transsexual** A person who is psychologically of one sex but physically of the other.

**gender dysphoria** Distress associated with assigned sex and gender.

**sexual orientation** A person's enduring emotional, romantic, sexual, or affectionate attraction to other persons.

**heterosexual** Experiencing primary attraction to and preference for sexual activity with people of the other sex.

**homosexual** Experiencing primary attraction to and preference for sexual activity with people of the same sex.

**bisexual** Experiencing attraction to and preference for sexual activity with people of both sexes.

**gay** Sexual orientation involving primary attraction to people of the same sex; usually but not always applies to men attracted to men.

**lesbian** Sexual orientation involving attraction of women to other women.

**sexual prejudice** Negative attitudes and hostile actions directed at those with a different sexual orientation.

**vulva** Region that consists of the female's external genitalia.

## Sexual Orientation

**Sexual orientation** refers to a person's enduring emotional, romantic, or sexual attraction to others. You may be primarily attracted to members of the opposite sex (**heterosexual**), the same sex (**homosexual**), or both sexes (**bisexual**). Many homosexuals prefer the terms **gay**, queer, or **lesbian** to describe their sexual orientation. *Gay* and *queer*

can apply to both men and women, but *lesbian* refers specifically to women.

Gay and bisexual people are often targets of **sexual prejudice**—negative attitudes and hostile actions directed at members of a particular social group. Hate crimes, discrimination, and hostility toward sexual minorities are evidence of ongoing sexual prejudice.[2] According to the Department of Justice, bias related to sexual orientation is the motivation for 21 percent of all hate crimes in the United States.[3]

Most researchers today agree that sexual orientation is best understood using a model that incorporates biological, psychological, and socio-environmental factors. Biological explanations focus on research into genetics, hormones, and differences in brain anatomy. Psychological and socio-environmental explanations examine parent-child interactions, sex roles, and early sexual and interpersonal interactions. Collectively, this growing body of research suggests that the origins of homosexuality, like heterosexuality, are complex.[4] To diminish the complexity of sexual orientation to "a choice" is a clear misrepresentation of current research. Homosexuals do not "choose" their sexual orientation any more than heterosexuals do.

LO **2**
# REPRODUCTIVE
## ANATOMY AND PHYSIOLOGY

Identify the primary structures of male and female reproductive anatomy and explain the functions of each.

Understanding the functions of the female and male reproductive systems will help you derive pleasure and satisfaction from your sexual relationships, be sensitive to your partner's wants and needs, and make responsible choices regarding your own sexual health.

## Female Reproductive Anatomy and Physiology

The female reproductive system includes two major groups of structures, the external genitals and the internal organs (**FIGURE 1**). The external female genitals are collectively known as the **vulva** and include all structures that are outwardly visible: the mons pubis, the labia minora and majora, the clitoris, the urethral and vaginal openings,

**External Anatomy**

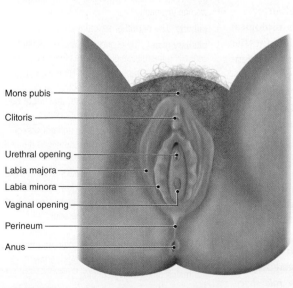

Mons pubis
Clitoris
Urethral opening
Labia majora
Labia minora
Vaginal opening
Perineum
Anus

**Internal Organs**

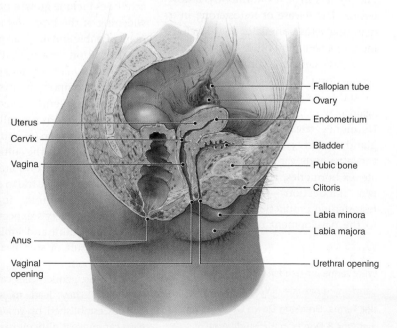

Fallopian tube
Ovary
Endometrium
Bladder
Pubic bone
Clitoris
Labia minora
Labia majora
Urethral opening

Uterus
Cervix
Vagina
Anus
Vaginal opening

**FIGURE 1** Female Reproductive System

and the vestibule of the vagina and its glands. The **mons pubis** is a pad of fatty tissue covering and protecting the pubic bone; after the onset of puberty, it becomes covered with coarse hair. The **labia majora** are folds of skin and erectile tissue that enclose the urethral and vaginal openings; the **labia minora,** or inner lips, are folds of mucous membrane found just inside the labia majora.

The **clitoris** is located at the upper end of the labia minora and beneath the mons pubis; its only known function is to provide sexual pleasure. Directly below the clitoris is the urethral opening through which urine is expelled from the body. Below the urethral opening is the vaginal opening. In some women, the vaginal opening is covered by a thin membrane called the **hymen**. It is a myth that an intact hymen is proof of virginity, as the hymen is not present in all women and is sometimes stretched or torn by physical activity.

The internal female genitals include the vagina, uterus, fallopian tubes, and ovaries. The **vagina** is a muscular, tubular organ that serves as a passageway from the uterus to the outside of the body. It allows menstrual flow to exit the uterus during a woman's monthly cycle, receives the penis during intercourse, and serves as the birth canal during childbirth. The **uterus (womb)** is a hollow, muscular, pear-shaped organ. Hormones acting on the inner lining of the uterus (the **endometrium**) either prepare the uterus for implantation and development of a fertilized egg or signal that no fertilization has taken place by deteriorating and becoming menstrual flow.

The lower end of the uterus, the **cervix,** extends down into the vagina. The **ovaries,** almond-sized organs

## SEE IT! VIDEOS

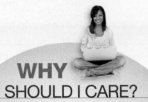

## WHY SHOULD I CARE?

It is more difficult to please a partner sexually or to describe to a partner how to please you if you don't understand basic sexual anatomy. For example, the clitoris in females is very responsive to touch, and when stimulated, often leads to orgasm. The urethral opening located nearby is not. You should know the difference.

suspended on either side of the uterus, have two main functions: producing hormones (estrogen, progesterone, and small amounts of testosterone) and serving as the reservoir for immature eggs. All the eggs a woman will ever have are present in her ovaries at birth. Eggs mature and are released from the ovaries in response to hormone levels. Extending from the upper end of the uterus are two thin, flexible tubes called the **fallopian tubes.** The fallopian tubes, which do not actually touch the ovaries, capture eggs as they are released from the ovaries during ovulation, and they are the site where sperm and egg meet and fertilization takes place. The fallopian tubes then serve as the passageway to the uterus, where the fertilized egg becomes implanted and development continues.

## The Menstrual Cycle

With the onset of puberty, the female reproductive system matures, and the development of secondary sex characteristics transforms young girls into young women. The first sign of puberty is the beginning of breast development, which generally occurs around age 10.[5] Around age 9½ to 11½, the **hypothalamus** receives the message to begin secreting *gonadotropin-releasing hormone (GnRH)*. The release of GnRH in turn signals the pituitary gland to release two hormones, *follicle-stimulating hormone*

*(FSH)* and *luteinizing hormone (LH)*, which signal the ovaries to start producing **estrogens** and **progesterone.** Estrogens regulate the menstrual cycle, and increased estrogen levels assist in the development of female secondary sex characteristics. Progesterone helps the endometrium to develop in preparation for nourishing a fertilized egg and helps maintain pregnancy.

The normal age range for the onset of the first menstrual period, termed **menarche,** is 10 to 18 years, with the average age falling between 12 and 13 years.[6] The average menstrual cycle lasts 28 days and consists of three phases: the proliferative phase, the

**mons pubis** Fatty tissue covering the pubic bone in females; in physically mature women, the mons is covered with coarse hair.

**labia majora** "Outer lips," or folds of tissue covering the female sexual organs.

**labia minora** "Inner lips," or folds of tissue just inside the labia majora.

**clitoris** A pea-sized nodule of tissue located at the top of the labia minora; central to sexual arousal and pleasure in women.

**hymen** Thin tissue covering the vaginal opening in some women.

**vagina** The passage in females leading from the vulva into the uterus.

**uterus (womb)** Hollow, muscular, pear-shaped organ whose function is to contain the developing fetus.

**endometrium** Soft, spongy matter that makes up the uterine lining.

**cervix** Lower end of the uterus that opens into the vagina.

**ovaries** Almond-size organs that house developing eggs and produce hormones.

**fallopian tubes** Tubes that extend from near the ovaries to the uterus; site of fertilization and passageway for fertilized eggs.

**hypothalamus** An area of the brain located near the pituitary gland; works in conjunction with the pituitary gland to control reproductive functions.

**estrogens** Hormones secreted by the ovaries, which control the menstrual cycle and assist in the development of female secondary sex characteristics.

**progesterone** Hormone secreted by the ovaries; helps the endometrium develop and helps maintain pregnancy.

**menarche** The first menstrual period.

**ovarian follicles** Areas within the ovary in which individual eggs develop.

**graafian follicle** Mature ovarian follicle that contains a fully developed ovum, or egg.

**ovum** A single mature egg cell.

**ovulation** The point of the menstrual cycle at which a mature egg ruptures through the ovarian wall.

**corpus luteum** A body of cells that forms from the remains of the graafian follicle following ovulation; it secretes estrogen and progesterone during the second half of the menstrual cycle.

**premenstrual syndrome (PMS)** Comprises the mood changes and physical symptoms that occur in some women during the 1 or 2 weeks prior to menstruation.

**premenstrual dysphoric disorder (PMDD)** Collective name for a group of negative symptoms similar to but more severe than PMS.

**dysmenorrhea** Condition of pain or discomfort in the lower abdomen just before or during menstruation.

**prostaglandin** Hormone-like substance associated with muscle contractions and inflammation.

secretory phase, and the menstrual phase (**FIGURE 2**).

The *proliferative phase* begins with the end of menstruation, when hypothalamus senses very low blood levels of estrogen and progesterone. In response, it increases its secretions of GnRH, which in turn triggers the pituitary gland to release FSH. FSH signals several **ovarian follicles** to begin maturing. While the follicles mature, they begin producing estrogen, which in turn signals the endometrium to proliferate. High estrogen levels signal the pituitary gland to slow down FSH production and increase release of LH. Under the influence of LH, the mature ovarian follicle (known as a **graafian follicle**) ruptures and releases a mature **ovum** (plural: *ova*), a single mature egg cell, near a fallopian tube (around day 14). This is the process of **ovulation.**

The phase following ovulation is called the *secretory phase.* The ruptured graafian follicle, which remains in the ovary, is transformed into the **corpus luteum** and begins secreting large amounts of estrogen and progesterone. These hormone secretions peak around day 20 or 21 of the average cycle and cause the endometrium to thicken. If fertilization and implantation take place, cells surrounding the developing embryo release a hormone called *human chorionic gonadotropin*

*(HCG),* increasing estrogen and progesterone secretions that maintain the endometrium and signal the pituitary not to start a new menstrual cycle.

If no implantation occurs, the hypothalamus responds by signaling the pituitary gland to stop producing FSH and LH, thus causing the levels of progesterone in the blood to peak. The corpus luteum begins to decompose, leading to rapid declines in estrogen and progesterone levels. Without these hormones, the endometrium is sloughed off in the menstrual flow, and this begins the *menstrual phase*. The low estrogen levels of the menstrual phase signal the hypothalamus to release GnRH, which acts on the pituitary gland to secrete FSH, and the cycle begins again.

## Menstrual Problems

**Premenstrual syndrome (PMS)** is a term used for a collection of physical, emotional, and behavioral symptoms that many women experience 7 to 14 days prior to their menstrual period. The most common symptoms are tender breasts, bloating, food cravings, fatigue, irritability, and depression. It is estimated that 85 percent of menstruating women experience at least one symptom of PMS each month.[7] For the majority of women, these disappear as their period begins, but for a small subset of women (5 to 8 percent),

symptoms are severe enough to affect their daily routines and activities to the point of being disabling. This severe form of PMS has its own diagnostic category in the *Diagnostic and Statistical Manual of Mental Disorders,* fifth edition (*DSM-5*), **premenstrual dysphoric disorder (PMDD),** with symptoms that include severe depression, hopelessness, anger, anxiety, low self-esteem, difficulty concentrating, irritability, and tension.[8]

There are several natural approaches to managing PMS that can also help PMDD. These strategies include eating healthy carbohydrates (grains, fruits, and vegetables), reducing caffeine and salt intake, exercising regularly, and taking measures to reduce stress. Recent investigation into methods of controlling the severe emotional swings has led to the use of antidepressants for treating PMDD, primarily selective serotonin reuptake inhibitors (SSRIs; e.g., Prozac, Paxil, and Zoloft).[9]

**Dysmenorrhea** is a medical term for menstrual cramps, the pain or discomfort in the lower abdomen that many women experience just before or during menstruation. Along with cramps, some women can experience nausea and vomiting, loose stools, sweating, and dizziness. Menstrual cramps can be classified as primary or secondary dysmenorrhea. Primary dysmenorrhea doesn't involve any physical abnormality and

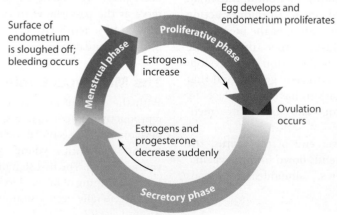

**FIGURE 2** The Three Phases of the Menstrual Cycle

**Source:** Rathus et al., Human Sexuality in a World of Diversity, 6th ed., © 2009. Figure "The Three Phases of the Menstrual Cycle," © 2005 Allyn & Bacon. Reproduced with permission of Pearson Education, Inc.

usually begins 6 months to a year after a woman's first period, while secondary dysmenorrhea has an underlying physical cause such as endometriosis or uterine fibroids.[10] You can reduce the discomfort of primary dysmenorrhea by using over-the-counter nonsteroidal anti-inflammatory drugs (NSAIDS) such as aspirin, ibuprofen (Advil or Motrin), or naproxen (Aleve). Other self-care strategies such as soaking in a hot bath or using a heating pad on your abdomen may also ease your cramps. For severe cramping, your health care provider may recommend a low-dose oral contraceptive to prevent ovulation. Without ovulation, there are fewer **prostaglandins** to trigger muscle contractions, thus reducing the severity of the cramps caused by the muscle contractions. Managing secondary dysmenorrhea involves treating the underlying cause.

*Toxic shock syndrome (TSS),* although rare, is still something women should be aware of. It is caused by a bacterial infection facilitated by the use of a tampon, diaphragm, or contraceptive sponge (see Chapter 6). Symptoms occur during a woman's period or a few days afterward and are sometimes hard to recognize because they mimic the flu. They include sudden high fever, vomiting, diarrhea, dizziness, fainting, or a rash that looks like sunburn. Proper treatment usually ensures recovery in 2 to 3 weeks.

## Menopause

Just as menarche signals the beginning of a woman's reproductive years, **menopause**—the permanent cessation of menstruation—signals the end. *Perimenopause* refers to the 4 to 6 years preceding menopause when hormonal changes take place and menstrual cycles and flow can become irregular. Menopause generally occurs between the ages of 45 and 55; the average age is 51 in the United States.[11] Menopausal changes result in decreased estrogen levels, producing troublesome symptoms in some women. Decreased vaginal lubrication, hot flashes, night sweats, headaches, dizziness, and joint pain have all been associated with the onset of menopause.

Synthetic forms of estrogen and progesterone have long been prescribed as **hormone replacement therapy** (HRT) to relieve menopausal symptoms and reduce the risk of heart disease and osteoporosis. (The National Institutes of Health prefers use of the term *menopausal hormone therapy*, because hormone therapy is not a replacement and does not restore the physiology of youth.) Results from the Women's Health Initiative (WHI), a large-scale study by the National Institutes of Health, suggest that hormone therapy using synthetic hormones may actually do more harm than good. In fact, the

**menopause** The permanent cessation of menstruation, generally occurring between the ages of 40 and 60.

**hormone replacement therapy (menopausal hormone therapy)** Use of synthetic or animal estrogens and progesterone to compensate for decreases in estrogens in a woman's body during menopause.

WHI terminated research studies on synthetic hormone use ahead of schedule due to concerns about participants' increased risk of breast cancer, heart attack, stroke, blood clots, and other health problems.[12] New data, however, indicate that these risks may have been related to the age at which women began treatment and the form (pill or patch) utilized.[13] Conflicting research highlights the need to discuss the risks and benefits of menopausal hormone therapy with a health care provider to make an informed decision.

## Male Reproductive Anatomy and Physiology

The structures of the male reproductive system are divided into external and internal genitals (**FIGURE 3**). The external genitals are the penis and the scrotum. The internal male genitals include the testes, epididymides, vasa deferentia, ejaculatory ducts, urethra, and

**External Anatomy**

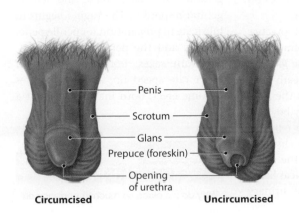

Circumcised      Uncircumcised

- Penis
- Scrotum
- Glans
- Prepuce (foreskin)
- Opening of urethra

**Internal Organs**

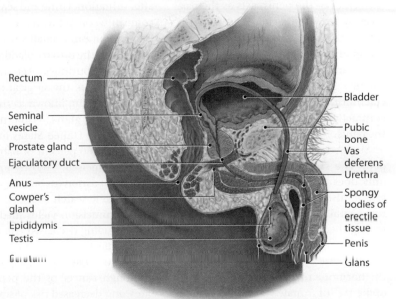

- Rectum
- Seminal vesicle
- Prostate gland
- Ejaculatory duct
- Anus
- Cowper's gland
- Epididymis
- Testis
- Scrotum
- Bladder
- Pubic bone
- Vas deferens
- Urethra
- Spongy bodies of erectile tissue
- Penis
- Glans

**FIGURE 3** Male Reproductive System

**penis** Male sexual organ that releases sperm into the vagina.

**ejaculation** The propulsion of semen from the penis.

**scrotum** External sac of tissue that encloses the testes.

**testes** Male sex organs that manufacture sperm and produce hormones.

**testosterone** The male sex hormone manufactured in the testes.

**sperm** Cell manufactured by male sex organs that combines with the female's ovum in fertilization.

**epididymis** The duct system where sperm mature and are stored.

**vas deferens** A tube that transports sperm from the epididymis to the ejaculatory duct.

**seminal vesicles** Glandular ducts that secrete nutrients for the semen.

**semen** Fluid containing sperm and nutrients that increase sperm viability and neutralize vaginal acid.

**prostate gland** Gland that secretes chemicals that help sperm fertilize an ovum and provides neutralizing fluids into the semen.

**Cowper's glands** Glands in the male reproductive system that secrete a fluid that lubricates the urethra and neutralizes any acid remaining in the urethra after urination.

**glans** Head of the penis.

**vasocongestion** The engorgement of the genital organs with blood.

other structures—the seminal vesicles, the prostate gland, and the Cowper's glands—that secrete components that, with sperm, make up semen. These three structures are sometimes referred to as the *accessory glands.*

The **penis** is the organ that deposits sperm in the vagina during intercourse. The urethra, a tube that passes through the center of the penis, acts as the passageway for both semen and urine to exit the body. During sexual arousal, the spongy tissue in the penis fills with blood, making the organ stiff (erect). Further sexual excitement leads to **ejaculation,** a series of rapid, spasmodic contractions that propel semen out of the penis.

Situated outside the body behind the penis is a sac called the **scrotum.** Not only does the scrotum protect the testes, it also maintains ideal temperature—vital to sperm production—by raising them closer to the body or lowering them. The **testes** (singular: *testis*) manufacture sperm and **testosterone,** the hormone responsible for the development of male secondary sex characteristics.

The development of **sperm** is called *spermatogenesis.* Like the maturation of eggs in the female, this process is governed by the pituitary gland. Follicle-stimulating hormone is secreted into the bloodstream to stimulate the testes to manufacture sperm. Immature sperm are released into a comma-shaped structure on the back of each testis called the **epididymis** (plural: *epididymides*), where they ripen and reach full maturity.

Each epididymis contains coiled tubules that gradually straighten out to become the **vas deferens** (plural: *vasa deferentia*). These make up the tubular transportation system whose sole function is to store and move sperm. Along the way, the **seminal vesicles** provide sperm with nutrients and other fluids that compose **semen.**

The vasa deferentia eventually connect each epididymis to the ejaculatory ducts, which pass through the prostate gland and empty into the urethra. The **prostate gland** contributes more fluids to the semen, including chemicals that help the sperm fertilize an ovum and neutralize the acidic environment of the vagina to make it more conducive to sperm motility (ability to move) and potency (potential for fertilizing an ovum). Just below the prostate gland are two pea-shaped nodules called the **Cowper's glands.** The Cowper's glands secrete a preejaculate fluid that lubricates the urethra and neutralizes any acid that may remain in the urethra after urination. Urine and semen do not come into contact with each other; during ejaculation, a small valve closes off the tube to the urinary bladder.

Debate continues over the practice of *circumcision,* the surgical removal of the fold of skin, known as the *foreskin,* covering the **glans.** While nearly universal in the United States in the past, only about 60 percent of baby boys are now circumcised,[14] mostly for religious or cultural reasons or because of hygiene concerns. Research supports the claim that circumcision yields medical benefits, including decreased risk of urinary tract infections in the first year, decreased risk of penile cancer (although cancer of the penis is very rare), and decreased risk of sexual transmission of human papillomavirus

(HPV) and human immunodeficiency virus (HIV).[15] Strong arguments against circumcision include a lack of medical necessity, a possible reduction in sexual sensitivity, and the possibility of bleeding, infection, and surgical complications. The American Academy of Pediatrics recently took a stand on the issue stating that scientific evidence shows potential medical benefits of newborn male circumcision but that the evidence is not currently strong enough to recommend routine circumcision.[16]

## LO 3 | HUMAN SEXUAL RESPONSE

List and describe the stages of the human sexual response and classify types of sexual dysfunctions.

Sexual response is a physiological process that generally follows a pattern. Sexual responses in both men and women are somewhat arbitrarily divided into four stages: excitement/ arousal, plateau, orgasm, and resolution. Regardless of the type of sexual activity (stimulation by a partner or self-stimulation), the response stages are the same; however, researchers agree that each individual has a personal response pattern that may or may not exactly conform to these phases.

During the first stage, *excitement/ arousal,* **vasocongestion** (increased blood flow that causes swelling in the genitals) stimulates male and female genital responses. The vagina begins to lubricate in preparation for penile penetration, and the penis becomes erect. For both sexes, both breathing and heart rate speed up, and the nipples become erect; both may also exhibit a "sex flush," or light blush all over their bodies.

During the *plateau phase,* the initial responses continue and intensify. The penis secretes a few drops of preejaculatory fluid, which may contain sperm, and the testicles are drawn closer to the body. The uterus rises and the vagina swells with increased blood flow. To avoid being directly stimulated by the penis, the clitoris then retracts under the clitoral hood.

During the *orgasmic phase,* vasocongestion and muscle tensions reach their peak, and rhythmic contractions occur through the genital regions. In women, these contractions are centered in the uterus, outer vagina, and anal sphincter. In men, the contractions occur in two stages. First, contractions within the prostate gland begin propelling semen through the urethra. In the second stage, the muscles of the pelvic floor, urethra, and anal sphincter contract. Semen usually, but not always, is ejaculated from the penis. In both sexes, spasms in other major muscle groups also occur, particularly in the buttocks and abdomen. Feet and hands may also contract, and facial features often contort.

Muscle tension and vasocongestion subside in the *resolution phase,* as the genital organs return to their prearousal states. Both sexes usually experience deep feelings of well-being and profound relaxation. Some men experience a refractory period, from a few minutes to several hours—tending to lengthen with age—during which systems are incapable of subsequent arousal. Women do not have true refractory periods the way men do; however, sensitivity, fatigue, and other factors may cause disinterest in sex after one or multiple orgasms. Men and women experience the same stages in the sexual response cycle; however, the length of time spent in any one stage varies. Thus, one partner may be in the plateau phase while the other is in the excitement or orgasmic phase. Sexual pleasure and satisfaction are also possible without orgasm or intercourse. Expressing sexual feelings for another person involves many pleasurable activities, of which intercourse and orgasm are only a part.

## TABLE 5.1 | Types of Sexual Dysfunction

| Desire Disorders | Description |
|---|---|
| Inhibited sexual desire | Lack of interest in sexual activity |
| Sexual aversion disorder | Phobias (fears) or anxiety about sexual contact |
| **Arousal Disorders** | |
| Erectile dysfunction | Inability to achieve or maintain an erection |
| Female sexual arousal disorder | Inability to remain sexually aroused |
| **Orgasmic Disorders** | |
| Premature ejaculation | Reaching orgasm rapidly or prematurely |
| Delayed ejaculation | Difficulty reaching orgasm despite normal desire and stimulation |
| Female orgasmic disorder | Inability to have an orgasm or difficulty or delay in reaching orgasm |
| **Pain Disorders** | |
| Dyspareunia | Pain during or after sex |
| Vaginismus | Forceful contraction of the vaginal muscles that prevents penetration from occurring |

## Sexual Dysfunction

Research indicates that *sexual dysfunction,* the term used to describe problems that can hinder sexual functioning, is quite common. Sexual dysfunction can be divided into four major categories: desire disorders, arousal disorders, orgasmic disorders, and pain disorders (see **TABLE 1**)—all of which can be treated successfully.

People should not feel embarrassed about sexual dysfunction. The reproductive system can malfunction just as any other body system can. If you experience a problem with sexual function, an important first step is to seek out a qualified health care provider to investigate the possible causes. Causes can be varied and overlapping and commonly include biological/medical factors; substance-induced factors (recreational, over-the-counter, or prescription drug use); psychological factors (stress, performance pressure);

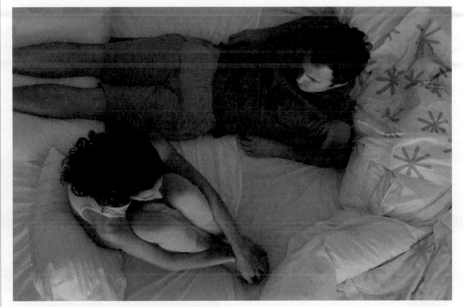

Sexual disorders can have both physical and psychological roots and can occur as a result of stress, fatigue, depression, or anxiety. They frequently have a physiological origin, such as overall poor health, chronic disease, or the use of alcohol or drugs.

→ **VIDEO TUTOR**
Male and Female Sexual Response

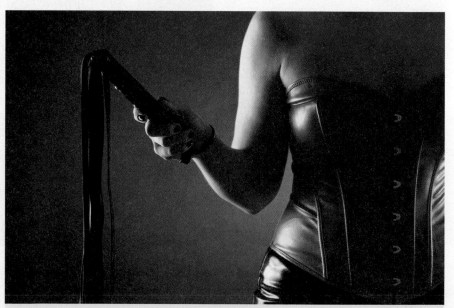

## WHAT DO **YOU** THINK?

Why do we find it so difficult to discuss sexual dysfunction?

- Do you think it is more difficult for men or for women to talk about dysfunction? Why?

and factors related to social context (relationship tensions, poor communication).[17]

## LO **4** | SEXUAL EXPRESSION AND BEHAVIOR

Explain the options available for the expression of one's sexuality and discuss the components of healthy and responsible sexuality.

Finding healthy ways to express your sexuality is an important part of developing sexual maturity. How do we know which sexual behaviors are considered appropriate or normal? What or whose criteria should we use? Every society sets standards and attempts to normalize sexual behavior. Rather than making blanket judgments about what society considers "normal," we might ask the following questions:[18]

- Is a sexual behavior healthy and fulfilling for a particular person?
- Is it safe?
- Does it lead to the exploitation of others?
- Does it take place between responsible, consenting adults?

In this way, we can view behavior along a continuum that takes into account the wide range of desires and behaviors. As you read about the options for sexual expression in the sections ahead, use these questions to explore your feelings about what is normal for you.

**celibacy** Avoidance of any sexual activities (complete) or sexual activities with others (partial).

**abstinence** Avoidance of intercourse.

**autoerotic behaviors** Sexual self-stimulation.

**sexual fantasies** Sexually arousing thoughts and dreams.

**masturbation** Self-stimulation of genitals.

## Options for Sexual Expression

The range of human sexual expression is virtually infinite. What you find enjoyable may not be an option for someone else. The ways you choose to meet your sexual needs today may be very different from what they were 2 weeks ago or will be 2 years from now. Accepting yourself as a sexual person with individual desires and preferences is the first step in achieving sexual satisfaction.

### Celibacy and Abstinence

While celibacy and abstinence are related terms, they aren't synonymous. **Celibacy** can refer to abstention from all sexual activities whatsoever, including masturbation (complete celibacy), or abstention from sexual activities with another person (partial celibacy). Some individuals choose celibacy for religious or moral reasons. Others may be celibate for a period of time because of illness, a breakup, or lack of an acceptable partner. For some, celibacy is a lonely, agonizing state, but others find it an opportunity for introspection, values assessment, and personal growth.

**Abstinence** usually refers to the avoidance of intercourse: oral, vaginal, or anal. People who are abstinent may engage in other sexual behaviors, such

74%

OF COLLEGE STUDENTS REPORT HAVING HAD ONE OR FEWER SEX **PARTNERS** IN THE PAST 12 MONTHS.

as kissing, touching, or masturbation. While no good estimates of celibacy exist, about 30 percent of college students report being abstinent (no oral, vaginal, or anal sex) in the past year.[19]

### Autoerotic Behaviors

**Autoerotic behaviors** involve sexual self-stimulation. The two most common are sexual fantasy and masturbation.

**Sexual fantasies** are sexually arousing thoughts and dreams. Fantasies may reflect real-life experiences, forbidden desires, or the opportunity to practice new or anticipated sexual experiences. The fact that you may fantasize about a particular sexual experience does not mean that you want to, or have to, act out that experience. Sexual fantasies are just that—fantasy.

**Masturbation** is self-stimulation of the genitals. Although many people feel uncomfortable discussing masturbation,

As with any other human behavior, the idea of "normal" sexual behavior varies from person to person and from society to society, usually along a spectrum of perceived acceptability or appropriateness.

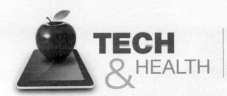

## CONSENSUAL TEXTS

Actress Jennifer Lawrence was livid. "I can't even describe to anybody what it feels like to have my naked body shoot across the world like a news flash against my will. It just makes me feel like a piece of meat." Photos on her phone, in various states of nudity, were hacked from the cloud and posted online. "I didn't tell you that you could look at my naked body," she said. She worried it would impact her career. She was mad that her friends looked at the pictures. She said she would rather give back the money from the *Hunger Games* than tell her dad about the pictures.

But wait, this wasn't a case of paparazzi stalking her and secretly taking a picture. She willingly shot those selfies and sent them to her boyfriend. What she didn't consent to was the pictures being shared with the world.

What can we take from Ms. Lawrence's story? One, once a photo has been taken, we have limited control over its future. Two, "consent," a concept we usually associate with sexual activity, may apply to sexting, too.

A few months after the photos were hacked, Ms. Lawrence posed nude with a boa constrictor for the same magazine where the quotes above were published. So when she said, "I didn't tell you that you could look at my naked body," was her concern less about *naked* and more about *I didn't tell you that you could*? Was her concern really about consent?

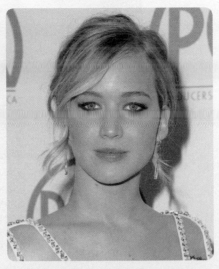

**Once a photo of us is taken, we sometimes have limited control over what happens next.**

According to popular video-blogger and sex educator Laci Green, there are three times consent can never be truly given: when a person is underage, drunk, or under pressure from a person is power. Perhaps we need to consider similar rules for texting.

1. Never take or send a sexy image of a person under 18. It is illegal.

2. When you are under the influence, you may regret any pictures you post. Wait to sober up before posting.

3. If you feel pressured to send a pic to someone, don't. While the vast majority of people report no negative outcomes of sexting, people who felt pressured to send the sext were more likely to have a negative outcome.

Perhaps the same rule we use for sex, "Yes means yes," could be applied to sharing photos too. Did the person who willingly sent you this photo say you could share it? Yes? Then go ahead. No? Then it was meant for you only; keep it that way.

Think about it:

Do you engage in any sexting activity that could cause you future hurt or embarrassment? Do males and females face the same threat of embarrassment from shared photos or videos? Why or why not? If you receive a sexy photo from a person you barely know, what is your responsibility to protect his/her privacy?

**Sources:** S. Kashner, "Both Huntress and Prey," *Vanity Fair* 56, no. 11, November 2014, Available at www.vanityfair.com/hollywood/2014/10/jennifer-lawrence-photo-hacking-privacy; K. Smith, "Girl Meets Boa," *Vanity Fair* 57 no. 3, March 2015; L. Green, "Wanna Have Sex: Consent 101," Video, www.youtube.com/watch?v=TD2EooMhqRI, March 2014; E. Englander, "Low Risk Associated with Most Teenage Sexting: A Study of 617 18-Year-Olds," *MARC Research Reports,* paper 6, 2012, Available at: http://vc.bridgew.edu/marc_reports/6

---

it is a common sexual practice across the life span. Masturbation is a natural pleasure-seeking behavior in infants and children. It is a valuable and important means for adolescents, as well as adults, to explore sexual feelings and responsiveness. In one survey of college students, 68 percent of women and 93 percent of men reported that they have masturbated.[20] Masturbation does not have to be a solitary activity. When separated physically, many couples use technology to connect sexually (see the **Tech & Health** box).

### Kissing and Erotic Touching

Kissing and erotic touching are two very common forms of nonverbal sexual communication. Both men and women have **erogenous zones**, areas of the body that when touched lead to sexual arousal. Erogenous zones may include genital as well as nongenital areas, such as the earlobes, mouth, nipples, and inner thighs. Almost any area of the body can be conditioned to respond erotically to touch. Spending time with your partner to explore and learn about

his or her erogenous areas is another pleasurable, safe, and satisfying means of sexual expression.

Both men and women can be sexually aroused and achieve orgasm through manual stimulation (masturbation) of the genitals by a partner. For many women, orgasm is more likely to be achieved through manual stimulation than through intercourse. *Sex toys*

**erogenous zones** Areas of the body of both men and women that, when touched, lead to sexual arousal.

include a wide variety of objects that can be used for sexual stimulation alone or with a partner. They can be used both to enhance the sexual experience and also as therapeutic devices to help with issues such as orgasmic difficulty and erectile dysfunction.

## Oral-Genital Stimulation

**Cunnilingus** refers to oral stimulation of a woman's genitals and **fellatio** to oral stimulation of a man's genitals. Many partners find oral-genital stimulation intensely pleasurable. In the most recent National College Health Assessment (NCHA), 45.5 percent of college students reported having oral sex in the past month.[21] Remember, HIV (human immunodeficiency virus) and other sexually transmitted infections (STIs) can be transmitted via unprotected oral-genital sex, just as they can through intercourse. Use of an appropriate barrier device (dental dam for cunnilingus and condom for fellatio) is strongly recommended if either partner's disease status is unknown.

## Vaginal Intercourse

The term *intercourse* generally refers to **vaginal intercourse** (*coitus,* or insertion of the penis into the vagina), which is the most frequently practiced form of sexual expression. In the latest NCHA survey, 49.2 percent of college students reported having vaginal intercourse in the past month.[22] Coitus can involve a variety of positions, including the missionary position (man on top facing the woman), woman on top, side by side, or man behind (rear entry). It is essential to protect yourself from unintended pregnancy and STIs during vaginal intercourse. (See Chapter 6 for information on contraceptives and Chapter 13 for information on safer sex.)

---

**cunnilingus** Oral stimulation of a woman's genitals.

**fellatio** Oral stimulation of a man's genitals.

**vaginal intercourse** The insertion of the penis into the vagina.

**anal intercourse** The insertion of the penis into the anus.

**variant sexual behavior** A sexual behavior that most people do not engage in.

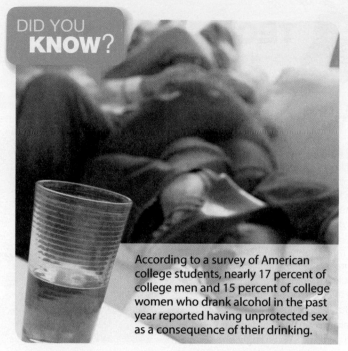

According to a survey of American college students, nearly 17 percent of college men and 15 percent of college women who drank alcohol in the past year reported having unprotected sex as a consequence of their drinking.

**Source:** Data from American College Health Association, *American College Health Association—National College Health Assessment II (ACHA-NCHA II): Reference Group Data Report, Spring 2014* (Hanover, MD: American College Health Association, 2014).

## Anal Stimulation and Intercourse

The anal area is highly sensitive to touch, and some people find pleasure in the stimulation of this area by mouth, fingers, or with sex toys. **Anal intercourse** is the insertion of the penis into the anus. Research indicates that 5.2 percent of college-aged men and women have had anal sex in the past month.[23] Note that condom use is especially important with anal intercourse, as the delicate tissues of the anus are more likely to tear than are vaginal tissues, significantly increasing the risk of transmission of HIV and other STIs. Also, anything inserted into the anus (fingers, penis, or toys) should not then be inserted directly into the vagina without cleaning, as bacteria commonly found in the anus can cause vaginal infections.

## Variant Sexual Behavior

Although attitudes toward sexuality have changed radically over time, some behaviors are still considered to be outside the norm. People who study sexuality prefer the neutral term **variant sexual behavior** to describe less common sexual activities, such as group sex, swinging (partner swapping), fetishism (using inanimate objects to heighten sexual arousal), and BDSM (a catch-all term for bondage, discipline, domination, submission, sadism, and masochism). These activities are all legal when they involve consenting adults.

Some variant sexual behaviors can be harmful to the individual, to others, or to both, and are illegal in most circumstances. These include exhibitionism (exposing one's genitals to strangers in public places), voyeurism (observing other people for sexual gratification without their consent), and pedophilia (any sexual activity involving a minor).

## Drugs and Sex

Because psychoactive drugs affect the body's entire physiological functioning, it is only logical that they also affect sexual behavior. Promises of increased pleasure make drugs very tempting to people seeking greater sexual satisfaction. But if drugs are necessary to increase sexual feelings, it is likely that partners are being dishonest about their feelings for each other. Good sex should not depend on chemical substances. Alcohol is notorious for reducing inhibitions and promoting feelings of well-being and desirability. At the same time, alcohol inhibits sexual response; thus, the mind may be willing, but not the body. A common danger associated with the use of drugs during sex is the tendency to blame alcohol or drugs for negative behavior or unsafe or undesired sexual activity.

An increasing number of young men have begun experimenting with the recreational use of drugs intended to treat erectile dysfunction (e.g., Viagra); however, one study indicated that the drugs may have confidence-lowering effects that actually diminish sexual performance and satisfaction.[24] For those who think the drugs work, they probably have only a placebo effect in men with normal erections, and combining them with other drugs, such as ketamine, amyl nitrate (poppers), or methamphetamine can lead to potentially fatal drug interactions. In particular, when combined with amyl nitrate, these drugs can lead to a sudden drop in blood pressure and possible cardiac arrest.[25]

"Date rape" drugs such as Rohypnol or gamma-hydroxybutyrate (GHB) have been a growing concern in recent decades. (See more details on these drugs in Chapters 4 and 7.) On college campuses, they are most often introduced to an unsuspecting woman through alcoholic drinks, often rendering her unconscious and vulnerable to rape. It is important to note that while Rohypnol and GHB are dangerous, alcohol is far more commonly associated with sexual assault than are "date rape" drugs.[26]

# Responsible and Satisfying Sexual Behavior

Healthy sexuality is a product of assimilating information and building skills, of exploring values and beliefs, and of making responsible and informed choices. Knowledge of yourself and your body, along with your ability to communicate effectively, will play a large part in determining the enjoyment and meaningfulness of sexual activity for you and your partner.

Healthy and responsible sexuality includes the following:

- **Good communication as the foundation.** Open and honest communication with your partner is the basis for establishing respect, trust, and intimacy. Can you share your thoughts and emotions freely with your partner? Do you talk about being sexually active and what that means? Can you share your sexual history with your partner? Do you discuss contraception and disease prevention? Are you able to communicate what you like and don't like?

- **Acknowledging that you are a sexual person.** People who can see and accept themselves as sexual beings are more likely to make informed decisions and take responsible actions. If you see yourself as a potentially sexual person, you will plan ahead for contraception and disease prevention. If you are comfortable being a sexually active person, you will not need or want your sexual experiences clouded by alcohol or other drug use. If you choose not to be sexually active, you do so consciously, as a personal decision.

- **Understanding sexual structures and their functions.** If you understand how the human body works, sexual pleasure and response will not be mysterious events. You will be better able to pleasure yourself and communicate to your partner how best to pleasure you. You will understand how pregnancy and STIs can be prevented. You will be able to recognize sexual dysfunction and take responsible actions to address the problem.

- **Accepting and embracing your gender identity and your sexual orientation.** "Being comfortable in your own skin" is an old saying that is particularly relevant when it comes to sexuality. It is difficult to feel sexually satisfied if you are conflicted about your gender identity or sexual orientation. You should explore and address questions and feelings you may have.

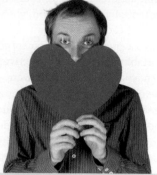

## What Are Your Attitudes about Sexual Differences?

Sexuality and sexual differences can be uncomfortable or difficult topics for many people. To complete this assessment, think about your attitudes regarding sexual differences and indicate how comfortable you would be in the following situations.

| | Completely Comfortable | | | | Not at All Comfortable |
|---|---|---|---|---|---|
| 1. Your close same-sex friend reveals to you his preference for same-sex partners. | 1 | 2 | 3 | 4 | 5 |
| 2. Your roommate tells you that she likes sexual encounters that involve three or more partners at one time. | 1 | 2 | 3 | 4 | 5 |
| 3. Your sister tells you that she would like to have a sex-change operation. | 1 | 2 | 3 | 4 | 5 |
| 4. Your 85-year-old grandfather reveals that he is sexually active with his 85-year-old girlfriend. | 1 | 2 | 3 | 4 | 5 |
| 5. A male friend reveals that, although he is primarily heterosexual, he occasionally has sex with men. | 1 | 2 | 3 | 4 | 5 |
| 6. Your lab partner, who looks and acts like a man, reveals that he is transgender. | 1 | 2 | 3 | 4 | 5 |
| 7. Your blind date tells you that he occasionally likes to engage in BDSM sexual play. | 1 | 2 | 3 | 4 | 5 |
| 8. Two women from your health class invite you to attend their commitment ceremony. | 1 | 2 | 3 | 4 | 5 |
| 9. Your cousin reveals that she has made a personal commitment not to engage in sexual activity until marriage. | 1 | 2 | 3 | 4 | 5 |
| 10. The person with whom you are romantically involved asks you to tell him your sexual fantasies. | 1 | 2 | 3 | 4 | 5 |
| 11. Your divorced mother reveals that she is dating a man who is 20 years younger than she is. | 1 | 2 | 3 | 4 | 5 |
| 12. Your partner says he would like to try anal sex. | 1 | 2 | 3 | 4 | 5 |
| 13. Your roommate believes it is important to be a virgin until marriage but engages in oral sex with her partner. | 1 | 2 | 3 | 4 | 5 |
| 14. Two of your classmates invite you over for "porn" night. | 1 | 2 | 3 | 4 | 5 |
| 15. Your best friend confides in you that he couldn't get an erection the last time he wanted to have intercourse. | 1 | 2 | 3 | 4 | 5 |
| 16. You walk in on your partner as he is trying on one of your dresses and heels. | 1 | 2 | 3 | 4 | 5 |
| 17. You go out dancing with friends at a gay bar and run into two women from your residence hall. | 1 | 2 | 3 | 4 | 5 |
| 18. Your sister and her husband share with you that their first child was born with a DSD. | 1 | 2 | 3 | 4 | 5 |
| 19. A same-sex acquaintance hits on you at a party. | 1 | 2 | 3 | 4 | 5 |
| 20. Your housemate asks how often you masturbate and if you own a vibrator. | 1 | 2 | 3 | 4 | 5 |

# YOUR PLAN FOR **CHANGE**

If you were surprised or unhappy with any of your responses to the **Assess Yourself** activity, consider ways to change the attitudes you want to work on.

**TODAY,** YOU CAN:

☐ Review your responses to the questionnaire and think about attitudes you would like to change. Evaluate your behavior and identify patterns and specific things you are doing. What can you change now? What can you change in the near future?

☐ Think about the level of sexual prejudice on campus. Consider joining or starting a group such as the Gay-Straight Alliance that works against sexual prejudice.

**WITHIN THE NEXT TWO WEEKS,** YOU CAN:

☐ Establish a time to sit down with the person with whom you are having a sexual relationship and have an honest and open discussion about sex. Before the discussion, think about what you would like to talk about and how you will bring it up. Are there sexual issues between you that need to be addressed? Are both you and your partner satisfied with the nature of your sexual relationship?

☐ Take steps to be more responsible about your sexuality. If you have had unprotected sex, make an appointment to be tested for STIs. If you have found yourself without contraception, stop by a drugstore and purchase several packages of condoms. If you feel your sexual decision making is sometimes impaired by drugs or alcohol, set goals to limit and control your use of these substances.

**BY THE END OF THE SEMESTER,** YOU CAN:

☐ Develop a greater understanding of and tolerance for people with different sexual values and lifestyles. Learn about different viewpoints by doing research, attending meetings on campus, or getting to know sexually diverse people.

☐ Expand your sense of gender identity. Consider taking a class or workshop in an activity or subject area that you traditionally associate with the opposite gender. Volunteer with a group that focuses on issues relating to the opposite gender.

## CHAPTER REVIEW

To hear an MP3 Tutor Session, scan here or visit the Study Area in **MasteringHealth.**

### LO 1 | Your Sexual Identity

■ Sexual identity is determined by a complex interaction of genetic, physiological, environmental, and social factors. Biological sex, gender identity, gender roles, and sexual orientation all are blended into our sexual identity. Sexual orientation refers to a person's enduring emotional, romantic, sexual, or affectionate attraction to others.

### LO 2 | Reproductive Anatomy and Physiology

■ The major structures of female reproductive anatomy include the mons pubis, labia minora and majora, clitoris, vagina, uterus cervix, fallopian tubes, and ovaries. The major structures of male reproductive anatomy are the penis, scrotum, testes, epididymides, vasa deferentia, ejaculatory ducts, urethra, and the accessory glands (seminal vesicles, prostate gland, and Cowper's glands).

### LO 3 | Human Sexual Response

■ Physiologically, both males and females experience four stages of sexual response: excitement/arousal, plateau, orgasm, and resolution.
■ Sexual dysfunctions can be categorized into four classes: desire disorders, arousal disorders, orgasmic disorders, and pain disorders. Stress, relationship issues, lack of exercise, smoking, alcohol and drug use, and other lifestyle choices can lead to sexual dysfunction.

### LO 4 | Sexual Expression and Behavior

■ People can express themselves sexually in a variety of ways, including celibacy, autoerotic behaviors, kissing and erotic touch, manual stimulation, oral-genital stimulation, vaginal intercourse, and anal intercourse. Variant sexual behaviors are those that are less common.
■ Alcohol and other psychoactive drugs can affect sexual behavior. Drug use can decrease inhibitions and lead people to engage in undesired or unsafe sexual activity.
■ Responsible and satisfying sexuality involves good communication, acknowledging yourself as a sexual being, understanding sexual structures and functions, and accepting your gender identity and sexual orientation.

## POP QUIZ

Visit **MasteringHealth** to personalize your study plan with Chapter Review Quizzes and Dynamic Study Modules.

### LO 1 | Your Sexual Identity

1. Your personal inner sense of masculinity or femininity is known as your
   a. sexual identity.
   b. sexual orientation.
   c. gender identity.
   d. gender.

### LO 2 | Reproductive Anatomy and Physiology

2. The most sensitive or erotic spot in the female genital region is the
   a. mons pubis.
   b. clitoris.
   c. vagina.
   d. labia.

### LO 3 | Human Sexual Response

3. Which of the following is *true* regarding the first stage of the human sexual response?
   a. In men, testes become completely engorged.
   b. In men and women, the rectal sphincter contracts.
   c. In men, the Cowper's gland may release fluid containing sperm.
   d. In men and women, vasocongestion occurs.

### LO 4 | Sexual Expression and Behavior

4. What is the effect of alcohol on sex?
   a. It promotes feelings of aversion.
   b. It promotes greater sexual satisfaction.
   c. It inhibits sexual response.
   d. It inhibits pregnancy.

*Answers to the Pop Quiz questions can be found on page A-1. If you answered a question incorrectly, review the section identified by the Learning Outcome. For even more study tools, visit MasteringHealth.*

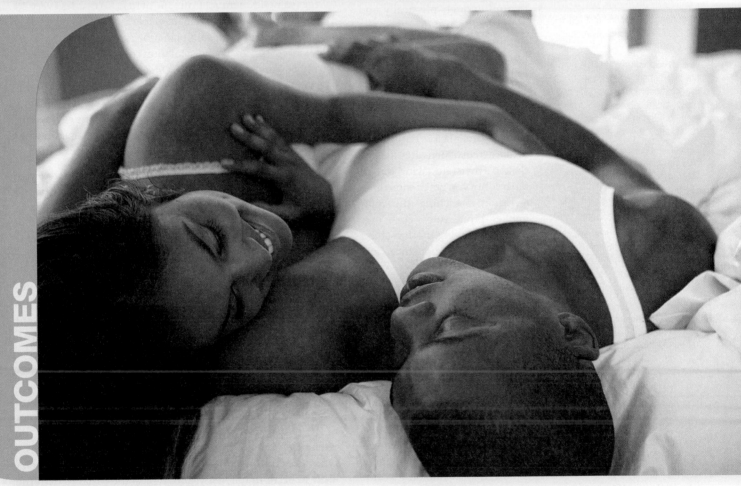

# 6 Considering Your Reproductive Choices

171

Today, we not only understand the intimate details of reproduction, but also possess technologies that can control or enhance our **fertility**. Along with information and technological advances comes choice, which goes hand in hand with responsibility. Choosing whether and when to have children is one of our greatest responsibilities. Children transform people's lives. They require a lifelong personal commitment of love and nurturing. Before having children, a person should ask: Am I mature enough physically and emotionally, and do I have the resources to care for another human being for the next 18 years?

One measure of maturity is the ability to discuss reproduction and birth control with your sexual partner before engaging in sexual activity. Men often assume their partners are taking care of birth control. Women sometimes feel that broaching the topic implies promiscuity. Both may feel that bringing up the subject interferes with romance and spontaneity.

Too often, neither partner brings up the topic, resulting in unprotected sex. In a recent survey, only 59 percent of college women and 54 percent of college men reported having used a method of contraception the last time they had vaginal intercourse.[1] Ambivalence toward contraception has serious consequences, as 51 percent of all pregnancies in the United States —more than 3 million a year— are unintended, and the highest rates are among women ages 18 to 24.[2]

Discussing this topic with your health care provider or your sexual partner will be easier if you understand human reproduction and contraception and honestly consider your attitudes toward these matters. Here we discuss information to consider as you contemplate your own sexual and reproductive choices.

**fertility** A person's ability to reproduce.

**contraception** Methods of preventing conception.

**conception** Fertilization of an ovum by a sperm.

**birth control** Methods that reduce the likelihood of conception or childbirth.

**perfect-use failure rate** The number of pregnancies (per 100 users) likely to occur in the first year of use of a particular birth control method if the method is used consistently and correctly.

**typical-use failure rate** The number of pregnancies (per 100 users) likely to occur in the first year of use of a particular birth control method if the method's use is not consistent or always correct.

**barrier method** Contraceptive methods that block the meeting of egg and sperm by means of a physical barrier (such as condom), a chemical barrier (such as spermicide), or both.

**hormonal methods** Contraceptive methods that introduce synthetic hormones into a woman's system to prevent ovulation, thicken cervical mucus, or prevent a fertilized egg from implanting.

**intrauterine methods** Contraceptive methods that insert a device into the uterus to either introduce synthetic hormones or interfere with sperm movement or egg fertilization.

**behavioral methods** Temporary or permanent abstinence or planning intercourse in accordance with fertility patterns.

**permanent methods** Surgically altering a man's or woman's reproductive system to permanently prevent pregnancy.

## HEAR IT! PODCASTS

Want a study podcast for this chapter? Download **Birth Control, Pregnancy, and Childbirth: Managing Your Fertility** available on **MasteringHealth**™

## LO 1 | BASIC PRINCIPLES OF BIRTH CONTROL

Explain the process of conception and describe how the effectiveness of contraception is measured.

The term **contraception** refers to methods of preventing conception. **Conception** occurs when a sperm fertilizes an egg. This usually takes place in a woman's fallopian tube. The following conditions are necessary for conception:

1. **A viable egg.** A sexually mature woman will release one egg (sometimes more) from one of her two ovaries every 28 days, on average. Eggs remain viable for 24 to 36 hours after their release into the fallopian tube.
2. **A viable sperm.** Each ejaculation contains between 200 and 500 million sperm cells. Once sperm reach the fallopian tubes, they survive an average of 48 to 72 hours—and can survive up to a week.
3. **Access to the egg by the sperm.** To reach the egg, sperm must travel up the vagina, through the cervical opening into the uterus, and from there, to the fallopian tubes.

Contraceptive methods prevent conception by interfering with one of these three conditions. While the terms contraceptives and **birth control** are commonly used interchangeably, contraceptives refer to devices, behaviors, or drugs that prevent conception, while birth control includes any method reducing the likelihood of pregnancy or childbirth, including contraceptives, contragestion (e.g., the morning-after pill), and abortion.

Without contraceptives, 85 percent of sexually active women would become pregnant within 1 year.[3] Society has searched for a simple, infallible, and risk-free way to prevent pregnancy since people first associated sexual activity with pregnancy. Outside of abstinence, we have not yet found one.

To evaluate the effectiveness of a particular contraceptive method, you must be familiar with two concepts: perfect-use failure rate and typical-use failure rate. **Perfect-use failure rate** refers to the number of pregnancies that are likely to occur in the first year of use (per 100 users of the method) if the method is used absolutely perfectly—without any error. The **typical-use failure rate** refers to the number of pregnancies likely to occur in the first year of typical use—that is, with the normal number of errors, memory lapses, and incorrect or incomplete use. The typical-use failure rate is always higher. Since it reflects how people actually use the method, it is more practical in helping people make informed decisions about contraceptive methods.

Present methods of contraception fall into several categories. **Barrier methods** block the egg and sperm from joining. **Hormonal methods** prevent ovulation, thicken cervical mucus, or prevent a fertilized egg from implanting. **Intrauterine methods** interfere with sperm movement and egg fertilization. **Behavioral methods** may involve temporary or permanent abstinence or planning intercourse around fertility patterns. **Permanent methods** surgically block the sperm's ability to fertilize the egg. Contraceptive methods could also be categorized by whether they are available with or without a visit to a health care provider or by the length of time it takes fertility to return after ending use.

Some contraceptive methods can also protect, to some degree, against **sexually transmitted infections (STIs)**.

TABLE 6.1 summarizes the failure rates, STI protection, frequency of use, and cost of various contraceptive methods.

**sexually transmitted infections (STIs)** Infectious diseases caused by pathogens transmitted through some form of sexual contact.

## TABLE 6.1 | Failure Rates, STI Protection, Frequency of Use, and Costs of Contraceptive Methods

| Method | Failure Rate: Typical Use | Failure Rate: Perfect Use | STI/HIV Protection | Frequency of Use | Cost |
|---|---|---|---|---|---|
| Continuous abstinence | 0 | 0 | Yes | N/A | None |
| Nexplanon | 0.05 | 0.05 | No | Inserted every 3 years | $0–$800/exam, device, and insertion; $100–$300 for removal |
| Male sterilization | 0.15 | 0.1 | No | Done once | $0–$1,000/interview, counseling, examination, operation, and follow-up sperm count |
| Female sterilization | 0.5 | 0.5 | No | Done once | $0–$6,000/interview, counseling, examination, operation, and follow-up |
| **IUD (intrauterine device)** | | | | | |
| ParaGard (copper T) | 0.8 | 0.6 | No | Inserted every 12 years | $0–$1,000/exam, insertion, and follow-up visit |
| Mirena/Skyla/Liletta | 0.2 | 0.2 | No | Inserted every 3–5 years | $0–$1,000/exam, insertion, and follow-up visit |
| Depo-Provera | 6 | 0.2 | No | Injected every 12 weeks | $0–$150/3-month injection; $0–$250 for initial exam |
| Oral contraceptives (combined pill and progestin-only pill) | 9 | 0.3 | No | Take daily | $0–$50 monthly pill pack at drugstores, often less at clinics; check for family planning programs in your student health center, $0–$250 for initial exam |
| Xulane patch | 9 | 0.3 | No | Applied weekly | $0–$80/month at drugstores; often less at clinics, $0–$250 for initial exam |
| NuvaRing | 9 | 0.3 | No | Inserted every 4 weeks | $0–$80/month at drugstores, often less at clinics; $0–$250 for initial exam |
| **Cervical cap (FemCap) (with spermicidal cream or jelly)** | | | | | |
| Women who have never given birth | 14 | 4 | No | Used every time | $0–$75 for cap; $0–$200 for initial exam; $0–$17/supplies of spermicide jelly or cream |
| Women who have given birth | 32 | No data | No | Used every time | |
| Male condom (without spermicides) | 18 | 2 | Some | Used every time | $1.00 and up/condom—some family planning or student health centers give them away or charge very little. Available in drugstores, family planning clinics, some supermarkets, and from vending machines |
| Diaphragm (with spermicidal cream or jelly) | 12 | 6 | No | Used every time | $0–$75 for diaphragm; $0–$250 for initial exam; $0–$17/supplies of spermicide jelly or cream |
| **Today Sponge** | | | | | |
| Women who have never given birth | 12 | 9 | No | Used every time | $0–$15/package of three sponges. Available at family planning centers, drugstores, online, and in some supermarkets |
| Women who have given birth | 24 | 20 | No | Used every time | |
| Female condom (without spermicides) | 21 | 5 | Some | Used every time | $2–$4/condom. Available at family planning centers, drugstores, and in some supermarkets |

Continued on next page

| Method | Failure Rate: Typical Use | Failure Rate: Perfect Use | STI/HIV Protection | Frequency of Use | Cost |
|---|---|---|---|---|---|
| Fertility awareness–based methods | 24 | 0.04–5.0 | No | Followed every month | $10–$12 for temperature kits. Charts and classes often free in health centers and churches |
| Withdrawal | 22 | 4 | No | Used every time | None |
| Spermicides (foams, creams, gels, vaginal suppositories, and vaginal film) | 28 | 18 | No | Used every time | $8/applicator kits of foam and gel ($4–$8 refills). Film and suppositories are priced similarly. Available at family planning clinics, drugstores, and some supermarkets |
| No method | 85 | 85 | No | N/A | None |
| Emergency contraceptive pill | Treatment initiated within 72–120 hours after unprotected intercourse reduces the risk of pregnancy by 75%–89% (with no protection against STIs). Costs depend on what services are needed: $30–$65 for over-the-counter pills. | | | | |

**Note:** "Failure Rate" refers to the number of unintended pregnancies per 100 women during the first year of use. "Typical Use" refers to failure rates for men and women whose use is not consistent or always correct. "Perfect Use" refers to failure rates for those whose use is consistent and always correct. Some family planning clinics charge for services and supplies on a sliding scale according to income. Cost varies based on insurance coverage.

**Sources:** Adapted from R. Hatcher et al., *Contraceptive Technology*, 20th rev. ed. (New York: Ardent Media, 2011); R. Hatcher et al., *Contraceptive Technology*, 19th rev. ed. Copyright © 2007 Contraceptive Technology Communications, Inc. Reprinted by permission of Ardent Media, LLC; Planned Parenthood, "Birth Control," 2014, www.plannedparenthood.org.

## LO 2 | **BARRIER** METHODS

Compare and contrast the advantages, disadvantages, and effectiveness of different barrier methods in preventing pregnancy and sexually transmitted infections.

Barrier methods work on the simple principle of preventing sperm from ever reaching the egg by use of a physical or chemical barrier. Some barrier methods prevent semen from contacting the woman's body, and others prevent sperm from going past the cervix. Many barrier methods contain or are used in combination with a substance that kills sperm.

## Male Condom

The **male condom** is a thin sheath designed to cover the erect penis and prevent semen from entering the vagina. Most male condoms are made of latex, although condoms made of polyurethane, polyisoprene, or lambskin are available. While lambskin condoms can prevent pregnancy, they are not effective protection against HIV and STIs. Condoms come in a wide variety of styles and may be purchased in pharmacies, supermarkets, some public bathrooms, and many health clinics. A new condom must be used for each act of vaginal, oral, or anal intercourse.

A condom must be rolled onto the penis before the penis touches the vagina, and it must be held in place when removing the penis from the vagina after ejaculation to prevent slippage (see **FIGURE 6.1**). Uncircumcised

**male condom** Single-use sheath of thin latex or other material designed to fit over an erect penis and to catch semen upon ejaculation.

**spermicide** Substance designed to kill sperm.

males should retract the foreskin slightly before putting on a condom. In condoms without a reservoir tip, a ½-inch space should be left to catch the ejaculate. To do so, the user can pinch the tip to remove air while unrolling the condom down the shaft of the penis.

Condoms come with or without lubrication. If desired, users can lubricate their own condoms with contraceptive foams, creams, and jellies or other water-based lubricants. Never use products such as baby oil, cooking oils, petroleum jelly, vaginal yeast infection medications, or body lotion with a condom. These products contain substances that will cause the latex to disintegrate.

Condoms are available with or without **spermicide**. Recent research indicates that the most commonly used spermicide, nonoxynol-9 (N-9), can cause irritation and increase the likelihood of infection, including HIV infection, when used multiple times per day.[4] The current recommendation is that users purchase condoms without spermicide and lubricate the condom themselves with water-based lubricants. Of course, the use of condoms with N-9 is safer than using no condom at all.

# 99%

OF U.S. WOMEN WHO HAVE EVER BEEN SEXUALLY ACTIVE REPORT HAVING USED AT LEAST ONE FORM OF **BIRTH CONTROL**.

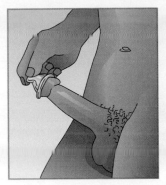

**1** Pinch the air out of the top half-inch of the condom to allow room for semen.

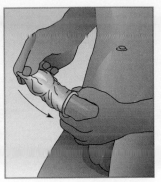

**2** Holding the tip of the condom with one hand, use the other hand to unroll it onto the penis.

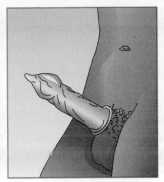

**3** Unroll the condom all the way to the base of the penis, smoothing out any air bubbles.

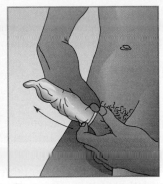

**4** After ejaculation, hold the condom around the base until the penis is totally withdrawn to avoid spilling any semen.

**FIGURE 6.1** How to Use a Male Condom

▶ **VIDEO TUTOR**
Choosing Contraception

Condom options are seemingly endless. If a couple is unhappy with one type, they should try another. Couples should note that not all condoms are labeled for contraceptive and STI-prevention purposes. Some novelty condoms, such as flavored, glow-in-the-dark, or ticklers, may only be for pleasure enhancement, so be sure check the label.

Condoms are less effective and more likely to break during intercourse if they are old or improperly stored. To maintain effectiveness, store them in a cool place (not in a wallet or glove compartment). Lightly squeeze the package before opening to feel that air is trapped inside and the package has not been punctured. Discard all condoms that have passed their expiration date.

## DID YOU KNOW?

Condoms have been protecting people for millennia. The ancient Egyptians used linen sheaths and animal intestines as condoms back in 1220 BC. The oldest evidence of condom use in Europe is said to come from cave paintings at the Grotte des Combarelles in France, dating from AD 100–200!

**Advantages** The condom is the only temporary means of birth control available for men, and latex, polyurethane, and polyisoprene condoms are the only barriers that effectively prevent the spread of some STIs and HIV. Many people choose condoms because they are inexpensive and readily available without a prescription, and their use is limited to times of sexual activity, with no negative health effects. Some men find condoms help them stay erect longer or help prevent premature ejaculation.

**Disadvantages** There is considerable potential for user error with the condom; as a result, the typical-use failure rate of condoms is 18 percent.[5] Improper use of a condom can lead to breakage, leakage, or slippage, potentially exposing the users to STI transmission or unintended pregnancy. Even when used perfectly, a condom doesn't protect against STIs that may have external areas of infection (e.g., herpes).

For some people, a condom ruins the spontaneity of sex because stopping to put it on may break the mood. Others report that condoms decrease sensation. These perceptions contribute to improper use or avoidance of condoms altogether. Partners who put on a condom as part of foreplay are generally more successful with this form of birth control. Also, as a new condom is required for each act of intercourse, users can find it difficult to always have a condom available when needed.

## Female Condom

The **female condom** is a single-use, soft, lubricated, loose-fitting sheath meant for internal vaginal use. The newest, improved version, called FC2, is made from nitrile rather than polyurethane. The sheath has a flexible ring at each end. One ring lies inside the sheath to serve as an insertion mechanism and hold the condom in place over the cervix. The other ring remains outside the

> **female condom** Single-use nitrile sheath for internal use during vaginal intercourse to catch semen upon ejaculation.

vagina once the condom is inserted and protects the labia and the base of the penis from exposure to STIs. **FIGURE 6.2** shows the proper use of the female condom.

**Advantages** Used consistently and correctly, female condoms can help prevent the spread of HIV and other STIs, including those transmitted by external genital contact (e.g., herpes). The female condom can be inserted in advance, so its use doesn't have to interrupt lovemaking. Some women choose the female condom because it gives them more personal control over pregnancy prevention and STI protection or because they cannot rely on their partner to use a male condom. Because the nitrile material is thin and pliable, there is less loss of sensation with the female condom than there is with the latex male condom. The female condom is relatively inexpensive, readily available without a prescription, and causes no negative health effects.

**Disadvantages** As with the male condom, there is potential for user error with the female condom, including possible slipping or leaking, both of which could lead to STI transmission or an unintended pregnancy. Because of the potential problems, the typical-use failure rate of the female condom is 21 percent.[6] Some people dislike using the female condom because they feel it is disruptive, odd looking, or difficult to use. Some women have reported external or vaginal irritation from use. As with the male condom, a new condom is required for each act of intercourse, so users may not always have one available when needed. Male and female condoms should never be used simultaneously.

## Jellies, Creams, Foams, Suppositories, and Film

Like condoms, some other barrier methods—jellies, creams, foams, suppositories, sponges, and film—do not require a prescription. They are referred to as spermicides—substances designed to kill sperm. The active ingredient in most of them is nonoxynol-9 (N-9).

*Jellies and creams* are packaged in tubes, and *foams* are available in aerosol cans. All have applicators designed for insertion into the vagina. They must be inserted far enough to cover the cervix, thus providing both a chemical barrier that kills sperm and a physical barrier that keeps sperm from an egg. Jellies and creams usually need to be inserted at least 10 minutes before intercourse and remain effective for about 1 hour after insertion.

> **vaginal contraceptive film** A thin film infused with spermicidal gel that is inserted into the vagina so that it covers the cervix.

*Suppositories* are waxy capsules inserted deep into the vagina, where they melt. They must be inserted 10 to 20 minutes before intercourse, but no longer than 1 hour prior to intercourse, or they lose their effectiveness. An additional suppository or other spermicide must be inserted for each act of intercourse.

**Vaginal contraceptive film** is another method of spermicide delivery. A thin film infused with spermicidal gel is

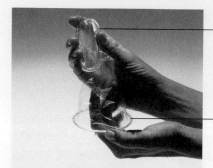

Inner ring is used for insertion and to help hold the sheath in place during intercourse.

Outer ring covers the area around the opening of the vagina.

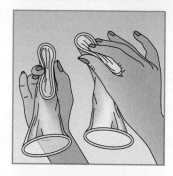

**❶** Grasp the flexible inner ring at the closed end of the condom, and squeeze it between your thumb and second or middle finger so it becomes long and narrow.

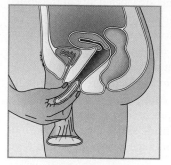

**❷** Choose a comfortable position for insertion: squatting, with one leg raised, or sitting or lying down. While squeezing the ring, insert the closed end of the condom into your vagina.

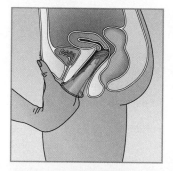

**❸** Placing your index finger inside of the condom, gently push the inner ring up as far as it will go. Be sure the sheath is not twisted. The outer ring should remain outside of the vagina.

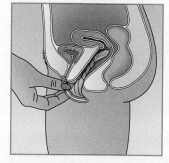

**❹** During intercourse, be sure that the penis is not entering on the side, between the sheath and the vaginal wall. When removing the condom, twist the outer ring so that no semen leaks out.

**FIGURE 6.2** How to Use a Female Condom

inserted into the vagina so that it covers the cervix 15 minutes before intercourse. The film dissolves into a spermicidal gel that is effective for up to 3 hours. A new film must be inserted for each act of intercourse.

**Advantages** Like condoms, spermicides are inexpensive, do not require a prescription or pelvic examination, and are readily available. They are simple to use, and their use is limited to the time of sexual activity.

**Disadvantages** Spermicides are most effective when used in conjunction with another barrier method; used alone their typical-use failure rate is 28 percent.[7] Spermicides can be messy and must be reapplied for each act of intercourse. Some experience irritation or allergic reactions to spermicides, and recent studies indicate that while spermicides containing N-9 are effective at preventing pregnancy, they are not effective in preventing transmission of HIV, chlamydia, or gonorrhea.[8] Frequent use (multiple times a day) of N-9 spermicides has been shown to cause irritation and breaks in the mucous layer or skin of the genital tract, creating a point of entry for viruses and bacteria that cause disease. Spermicides containing N-9 have also been associated with increased risk of urinary tract infection.[9] Contragel, sold in Europe, and Amphora, currently undergoing testing in the United States, use lactic acid to create an environment hostile to sperm. These and others will, it is hoped, provide future N-9 alternatives.

# Diaphragm with Spermicidal Jelly or Cream

Invented in the mid-nineteenth century, the **diaphragm** was the first widely used birth control method for women. The device is a soft, shallow cup made of thin latex rubber. Its flexible, rubber-coated metal ring is designed to fit snugly behind the pubic bone in front of the cervix and over the back of the cervix on the other side so it blocks access to the uterus. Where most diaphragms come in different sizes and must be fitted by

a trained health care provider, the U.S. Food and Drug Administration (FDA) approved a new one-size-fits-most diaphragm, Caya, for over-the-counter sale in the United States. It will likely appear in stores in 2015.

Spermicidal cream or jelly must be applied to the inside of the diaphragm before it is inserted, up to 6 hours before intercourse. The diaphragm holds the spermicide in place, creating a physical and chemical barrier against sperm; without spermicide, the diaphragm is ineffective (**FIGURE 6.3**). Although the diaphragm can be left in place for multiple acts of intercourse, additional spermicide must be applied each time. The diaphragm must then stay in place for 6 to 8 hours after intercourse. After removal, diaphragms should be cleaned, inspected for damage, and stored safely.

**Advantages** Diaphragms have a lower typical-use failure rate (12%) than other barrier methods.[10] After initial prescription and fitting, the only ongoing expense is spermicide. Because the diaphragm can be inserted up to 6 hours in advance, some users find it less disruptive than other barrier methods. Partners do not report being able to feel the diaphragm during intercourse.

**Disadvantages** The diaphragm does require a visit to a health care provider. Also, some women find inserting a diaphragm awkward at first. When inserted incorrectly, diaphragms are much less effective. It is also possible for a diaphragm to slip out of place, be difficult to remove, or require refitting by a health care provider (e.g., following a pregnancy or significant weight gain or loss). Like other barrier methods, supplies must be kept on hand as additional spermicide is required for each act of intercourse. The device cannot be used during the menstrual period or for longer than 48 hours because of the risk of **toxic shock syndrome (TSS)**.

> **diaphragm** Latex, cup-shaped device designed to cover the cervix and block access to the uterus; should always be used with spermicide.
>
> **toxic shock syndrome (TSS)** Rare, potentially life-threatening disease that occurs when specific bacterial toxins multiply and spread to the bloodstream, most commonly through improper use of tampons, diaphragms, or cervical caps.

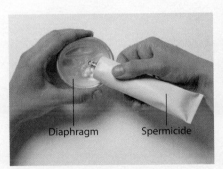

❶ Place spermicidal jelly or cream inside the diaphragm and all around the rim.

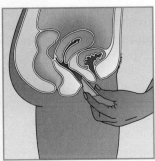

❷ Fold the diaphragm in half and insert dome-side down (spermicide-side up) into the vagina, pushing it along the back wall as far as it will go.

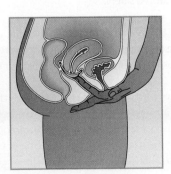

❸ Position the diaphragm with the cervix completely covered and the front rim tucked up against your pubic bone; you should be able to feel your cervix through the rubber dome.

**FIGURE 6.3** Proper Use and Placement of a Diaphragm

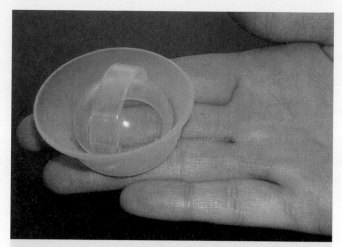

FemCap is used in conjunction with spermicide and is positioned to cover the cervix. It is shaped like a sailor's cap and has a loop to aid in removal.

## Cervical Cap with Spermicidal Jelly or Cream

One of the oldest methods used to prevent pregnancy, early **cervical caps** were made from beeswax, silver, or copper. The only cervical cap available in the United States, the *FemCap*, is a clear silicone cup that fits snugly over the entire cervix and has a ring on the back to assist with removal. It comes in three sizes and must be fitted by a health care provider. The FemCap is designed for use with spermicidal jelly or cream. It is held in place by suction created during application and works by blocking sperm from the uterus. The FemCap can be inserted up to 6 hours prior to intercourse. The device must be left in place for 6 to 8 hours after sex, using additional spermicide for any additional intercourse. After removal, the cervical cap should be cleaned, inspected for damage, and stored safely.

**cervical cap** Small cup made of silicone that is designed to fit snugly over the entire cervix; should always be used with spermicide.

**contraceptive sponge** Contraceptive device containing nonoxynol-9 and made of polyurethane foam that fits over the cervix to create a barrier against sperm.

**Advantages** With a typical-use failure rate of 14%,[11] cervical caps are reasonably effective. They are relatively inexpensive, as the only ongoing cost is the spermicide, and they last for 2 years.

Some users find FemCap less disruptive than other barrier methods because it can be inserted up to 6 hours prior to intercourse and used for multiple acts of intercourse. Because the FemCap is made of surgical-grade silicone, it is suitable for people allergic to latex.

**Disadvantages** The FemCap is somewhat more difficult to insert than a diaphragm because of its smaller size. Like a diaphragm, it requires an initial fitting by a physician and may require subsequent refitting if a woman's cervix size changes (e.g., after giving birth). Because the FemCap can become dislodged during intercourse, placement must be periodically checked. The device cannot be used during the menstrual period or for longer than 48 hours because of the risk of TSS. Some women report unpleasant vaginal odors after use. Like other barrier methods, users must keep a supply of spermicidal cream or jelly on hand.

## Contraceptive Sponge

The **contraceptive sponge** (sold in the United States as the *Today Sponge*) is a small, round pillow of polyurethane foam with a loop on the back to assist with removal and a dimple on the front to help it fit closely to the cervix. Prior to insertion, the sponge must be moistened with water to activate the infused spermicide. It is then folded and inserted deep into the vagina, where it fits over the cervix and creates a barrier against sperm. Protection begins immediately upon insertion and lasts for up to 24 hours. There is no need to reapply spermicide or insert a new sponge for any subsequent acts of intercourse within the same 24-hour period; it must be left in place for at least 6 hours after the last intercourse. After use, it is thrown away.

**Advantages** The main advantage of the sponge is convenience, because it does not require a trip to a health care provider for fitting. The sponge allows for more spontaneity than some other barrier methods because protection begins immediately upon insertion and lasts for 24 hours without reapplication of spermicide for additional intercourse.

**Disadvantages** The sponge is similarly effective as the diaphragm for women who have never given birth (12% typical-use failure rate), but less effective for women who have previously given birth (24% typical-use failure rate).[12] Allergic reactions are more common with the sponge than with other barrier methods. Should the vaginal lining become irritated, the risk of yeast infections and other STIs may increase. The sponge should not be used during menstruation. Some cases of TSS have been reported in women using the sponge, thus

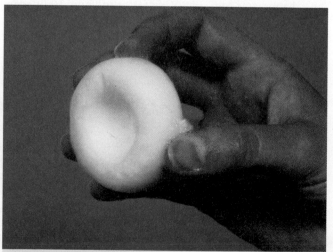

The Today Sponge is a barrier method infused with spermicide. It is a round pillow of polyurethane foam with a loop to assist with removal.

the same precautions should be taken as with the diaphragm and cervical cap. Some women find the sponge difficult or messy to remove. Finally, the sponge is infused with nonoxynol-9, thus users should be aware of related risks.

## LO 3 | HORMONAL METHODS

Compare the advantages, risks, and effectiveness of different hormonal methods in preventing pregnancy.

The term *hormonal contraception* refers to birth control that contains synthetic estrogen, progestin (synthetic progesterone), or both—similar to the hormones estrogen and progesterone that a woman's ovaries produce naturally for the process of ovulation and the menstrual cycle. Synthetic estrogen works to prevent the ovaries from releasing an egg. If no egg is released, there is nothing to be fertilized by the sperm and pregnancy cannot occur. Progestin thickens the cervical mucus, which hinders the movement of the sperm, inhibits the egg's ability to travel through the fallopian tubes, and suppresses the sperm's ability to unite with the egg. Progestin also thins the uterine lining, making it unlikely for a fertilized egg to implant in the uterine wall.

## Oral Contraceptives

**Oral contraceptive** pills were first marketed in the United States in 1960. Today, oral contraceptives are the most commonly used birth control method among college women.[13] Birth control pills are highly effective at preventing pregnancy (91% with typical use).[14] It is easier for a motivated user to approach perfect use with hormonal methods than with barrier contraceptives, as most errors are due to user error, not method failure.

Much of the pill's popularity is due to its convenience and ability to be used discreetly. Users tend like the fact that the pill doesn't interrupt lovemaking, potentially leading to greater sexual enjoyment.

The greatest disadvantage of oral contraceptives is that they must be taken every day at the same time, without fail. If a woman misses a pill, she should use a backup method of contraception for the remainder of that cycle. After discontinuing use of the pill, return of fertility may be delayed, but the pill is not known to cause infertility. Other drawbacks are that the pill does not protect against HIV and STIs, and its effectiveness may be affected by certain medications, including St. John's wort and the antibiotic rifampin, as well as some treatments for seizures, HIV, and yeast infections.

More than 40 brands of pills exist, fitting into two categories: combination pills and progestin-only pills.

## Combination Pills

Combination pills work through the combined effects of synthetic estrogen and progestin and are taken in a cycle. At the end of each 3-week cycle, the user stops taking pills or takes placebo pills for 1 week. The resultant drop in hormone level causes the uterine lining to shed, and the user will have a menstrual

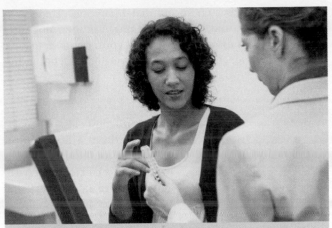

Studies show that college-age women are most familiar with the birth control pill and the male condom; talk to your health care provider about other options available to you and your partner.

period, usually within 1 to 3 days. Menstrual flow is generally lighter than it is for women who don't use the pill, because the hormones in the pill prevent thick endometrial buildup.

Several newer brands of combination pills have *extended cycles*, such as the 91-day *Seasonale* and *Seasonique*. A woman using this regimen takes active pills for 12 weeks, followed by 1 week of placebos. On this cycle, women can expect a menstrual period every 3 months. *Lybrel*, another extended-cycle pill, supplies an active dose of hormones every day for 365 days, eliminating menstruation completely during use. While the idea of not having a period for a year may be unsettling, there is no known physiological need for a woman to have a monthly period, and there are no known risks associated with avoidance.

**Advantages** In addition to effectively preventing pregnancy, the combination pill may lessen menstrual difficulties, such as cramps and premenstrual syndrome (PMS) and lower the risk of several health conditions, including endometrial and ovarian cancers, noncancerous breast disease, osteoporosis, ovarian cysts, pelvic inflammatory disease (PID), and iron-deficiency anemia.[15]

Many different brands of combination pills are on the market, some of which contain progestins that offer additional benefits, such as reducing acne, minimizing fluid retention, or relieving cramps. Users of extended-cycle pills also like that they don't need to remember when to stop or start a cycle of pills or when to use placebos. Less-expensive generic versions are available for many brands of combination pills, but not extended-cycle pills.

> **oral contraceptives** Pills containing synthetic hormones that prevent ovulation by regulating hormones.

**Disadvantages** Although estrogen in combination pills is associated with increased risk of several serious health problems among older women, the risk is low for most healthy, nonsmoking women under 35. Problems include increased risk for blood clots and higher risk for increased blood pressure, thrombotic stroke, and myocardial infarction. These risks increase with age and cigarette smoking. Early warning signs of complications associated with oral contraceptives include severe abdominal, chest, or leg pain; severe headache; and/or eye problems.[16]

Different brands of pills have varying minor side effects. Some of the most common are spotting between periods, breast tenderness, moodiness, and nausea. With most pills, side effects clear up within a few months. Other, less common side effects include acne, hair loss or growth, and a change in sexual desire. With so many brands available, most women who wish to use the pill are able to find one without unpleasant side effects.

**Xulane** Patch that releases hormones similar to those in oral contraceptives; each patch is worn for 1 week.

## Progestin-Only Pills

Progestin-only pills (or minipills) contain small doses of progestin and no estrogen. These pills are available in 28-day packs of active pills (menstruation usually occurs during the fourth week even though the active dose continues through the entire month). Ovulation may occur, but the progestin prevents pregnancy by thickening cervical mucus and interfering with implantation of a fertilized egg. Progestin-only pills are a good choice for women who are at high risk for estrogen-related side effects or who cannot take estrogen-containing pills because of diabetes, high blood pressure, or other cardiovascular conditions. They also can be used safely by women who are older than age 35 and by women who are currently breast-feeding.

**Advantages** Like combination pills, progestin-only pills are highly effective at preventing pregnancy: 91 percent with typical use.[17] Progestin-only pills share many of the health benefits of combination pills, but unlike combination pills, they carry no estrogen-related cardiovascular risks. Also, some of the typical side effects of combination pills, including nausea and breast tenderness, usually do not occur with progestin-only pills. With progestin-only pills, women's menstrual periods generally become lighter or stop altogether.

**Disadvantages** Because of the lower dose of hormones in progestin-only pills, it is especially important to take them at the same time each day. If a woman takes a pill 3 or more hours later than usual, she will need to use a backup method of contraception for the next 48 hours.[18] The most common side effect of progestin-only pills is irregular menstrual bleeding or spotting. Less common side effects include mood changes, changes in sex drive, and headaches.

## Contraceptive Skin Patch

**Xulane** (a generic form of Ortho Evra, which is being removed from the market) is a square transdermal (through the skin) adhesive patch less than 2 inches wide, as thin as a plastic strip bandage. It is worn for 1 week and replaced on the same day of the week for 3 consecutive weeks; during the fourth week, no patch is worn. Xulane works by delivering continuous levels of estrogen and progestin into the bloodstream. The patch can be worn on the buttocks, abdomen, upper torso (front or back, excluding the breasts), or upper outer arm. It should not be used by women over age 35 who smoke cigarettes and is less effective in women who weigh more than 198 pounds.[19]

**Advantages** Xulane is anticipated to have the same level of effectiveness with typical use (91%) as the brand-name patch Ortho Evra.[20] Women who choose to use the patch often do so because they find it easier to remember to replace it weekly than to take a daily pill. Xulane is not yet shown to, but likely offers, similar potential health benefits as combination pills (reduction in risk of certain cancers and diseases, lessening of PMS symptoms, etc.). Like other hormonal methods, the patch regulates a woman's menstrual cycle. Because the user only has to think about her birth control once a week, it may increase convenience and spontaneity.

**Disadvantages** Using the patch requires an initial exam by a physician and prescription, weekly patch changes, and the ongoing expense of patch purchases. A backup method is required during the first week of use. Similar to other hormonal birth control methods, the patch offers no protection against HIV or other STIs. Some women experience minor side effects like those associated with combination pills. Rarely, women report the patch falling off or irritation at the site of application. The estrogen in the patch is associated with cardiovascular risks, particularly in women who smoke and women over the age of 35. Amid evidence that the patch may increase the risk of life-threatening blood clots, the FDA mandated an additional warning label explaining that patch use exposes women to about 60 percent more estrogen than a typical combination pill.[21] There may be some delay in return of fertility with the patch, especially if a woman had irregular menstrual cycles before beginning use. As with oral contraceptives, some medications can make Xulane less effective.

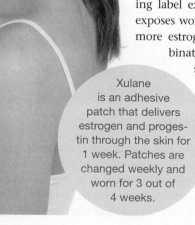

Xulane is an adhesive patch that delivers estrogen and progestin through the skin for 1 week. Patches are changed weekly and worn for 3 out of 4 weeks.

# Vaginal Contraceptive Ring

**NuvaRing** is a soft, flexible plastic hormonal contraceptive ring about 2 inches in diameter. The user inserts the ring into the vagina, leaves it in place for 3 weeks, then removes it for 1 week, during which she will have a menstrual period. Once the ring is inserted, it releases a steady flow of estrogen and progestin.

**Advantages** The ring is 91 percent effective with typical use.[22] Advantages of NuvaRing include lower risk of user error, as there is no pill to take daily or patch to change weekly, no need to be fitted by a health care provider, and rapid return of fertility when use is stopped. It also exposes the user to a lower dosage of estrogen than do the patch and some combination pills, and may have fewer estrogen-related side effects. It likely offers some of the same potential health benefits as combination pills, and regulates the menstrual cycle.

**Disadvantages** NuvaRing requires an initial exam and prescription, monthly ring changes, and the ongoing expense of purchasing the ring (there is currently no generic version). A backup method must be used during the first week, and the ring provides no protection against STIs. Like combination pills, the ring poses potentially serious health risks for some women. Possible side effects unique to the ring include increased vaginal discharge and vaginal irritation or infection. Oil-based vaginal medicines to treat yeast infections cannot be used when the ring is in place, and a diaphragm or cervical cap cannot be used as a backup method for contraception. Some medications can make NuvaRing less effective.

# Contraceptive Injections

**Depo-Provera** (injected intramuscularly) and the newer **Depo-subQ Provera** (injected just below the skin in a lower dose) are long-acting progestins injected every 3 months by a health care provider. Both prevent ovulation, thicken cervical mucus, and thin the uterine lining, all of which prevent pregnancy.

**Advantages** Depo-Provera and Depo-subQ Provera take effect within 24 hours of the first shot, so there is usually no need for a backup method. There is little room for user error as a health care provider administers the injection every 3 months. With typical use it has a 6 percent failure rate.[23] With continued use, a woman's menstrual periods become lighter and may eventually cease. There are no estrogen-related health risks associated with Depo-Provera and Depo-subQ Provera, and it offers the same potential health benefits as progestin-only

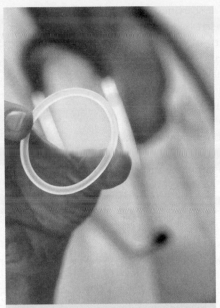

NuvaRing is inserted into the vagina, where it releases estrogen and progestin for 3 weeks.

pills. Unlike estrogen-containing hormonal methods, this method can be used by women who are breast-feeding.

**Disadvantages** Using Depo-Provera or Depo-subQ Provera requires an initial exam and prescription, then a follow-up visit every 3 months to have the shot administered. It offers no protection against STIs. The main disadvantage of this method is irregular bleeding, which can be troublesome at first, but within a year, most women are amenorrheic (have no menstrual periods). Weight gain is commonly reported. Prolonged use of Depo-Provera has been linked to loss of bone density.[24] Other possible side effects include dizziness, nervousness, and headache. Unlike other methods of contraception, this method cannot be stopped immediately if problems arise, and the drug and its side effects may linger for up to 6 months after the last shot. A disadvantage for women who want to get pregnant is that fertility may not return for up to 1 year after the final injection. Some medications can make contraceptive injections less effective.

# Contraceptive Implants

A single-rod implantable contraceptive, **Nexplanon** (formerly called **Implanon**) is a small, soft plastic capsule (about the size of a matchstick) that is inserted just beneath the skin on the inner side of a woman's upper underarm by a health care provider. Nexplanon continually releases a low, steady dose of progestin for up to 3 years, suppressing ovulation during that time.

**Advantages** After insertion, Nexplanon is generally not visible, making it a discreet method of birth control. Its main advantages are being highly effective, with less than a 1 percent typical-use failure rate, allowing no user error, and only needing to be replaced every 3 years.[25] It has benefits similar to other progestin-only forms of contraception, including the lightening or cessation of menstrual periods, the lack of estrogen-related side effects, and safety for use by breast-feeding women. Fertility usually returns quickly after removal of the implant.

**NuvaRing** Soft, flexible ring inserted into the vagina that releases hormones similar to those in oral contraceptives; each ring is worn for 3 weeks.

**Depo-Provera, Depo-subQ Provera** Injectable method of birth control that lasts for 3 months.

**Nexplanon (Implanon)** A plastic capsule inserted in a woman's upper arm that releases a low dose of progestin to prevent pregnancy.

**Disadvantages** Insertion and removal of Nexplanon must be performed by a health care provider. There is a higher initial cost for this method, if it is not covered by insurance. Potential minor side effects include irritation, allergic reaction, and swelling or scarring around the area of insertion, and there is a possibility of infection or complications with removal. Nexplanon may be less effective in women who are overweight.[26] As with other progestin-only contraceptives, users can experience irregular bleeding and less frequent reports of changes in sex drive, mood changes, or risks to the ovaries. Nexplanon offers no protection against STIs, and it may require a backup method during the first week of use.

## LO 4 | INTRAUTERINE CONTRACEPTIVES

Describe the effectiveness, advantages, and disadvantages of intrauterine contraceptives.

The **intrauterine device (IUD)** is a small plastic, flexible device, with a nylon string attached. It is placed in the uterus through the cervix and provides protection from pregnancy for 3 to 12 years. The exact mechanism by which it works is not clearly understood, but researchers believe that IUDs affect the way sperm and eggs move, thereby preventing fertilization, and/or affect the lining of the uterus to prevent a fertilized ovum from implanting.

The IUD was once extremely popular in the United States; however, in the 1970s most brands were removed from the market because of serious complications, such as pelvic inflammatory disease and infertility. Redesigned for safe use, the IUD is again very popular with women around the world and is experiencing a resurgence of popularity among U.S. women.[27]

## ParaGard, Mirena, Skyla, and Liletta

Four IUDs are currently available in the United States. *Para-Gard* is a T-shaped plastic device with copper around the shaft. It does not contain any hormones and can be left in place for 12 years. *Mirena,* is effective for 5 years and releases small amounts of progestin. *Skyla,* is a lower dose and smaller-sized version of Mirena. It was tested with and is designed for women who have not yet had a baby, and it is effective for 3 years. Newest to the market is *Liletta,* effective for 3 years, and designed to be a more affordable choice.

A health care provider must insert an IUD. One or two strings extend from the IUD into the vagina so the user can periodically check to make sure that the device is in place. While IUDs were initially not recommended for women who had never had a baby, the American Congress of Obstetricians and Gynecologists supports their use for women of all ages.[28]

**Advantages** The IUD is a safe, discreet, and highly effective method with a typical-use failure rate of less than 1 percent.[29] It is effective immediately and needs to be replaced only every 3 to 12 years. ParaGard has the benefit of containing no hormones and so has none of the potential negative

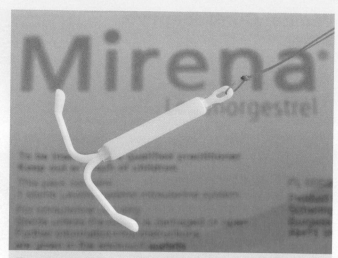

The Mirena IUD is a flexible plastic device inserted by a health care provider into a woman's uterus, where it releases progestin for up to 5 years.

health impacts of hormonal contraceptives. Skyla, Mirena, and Liletta, on the other hand, likely offer some of the same potential health benefits as other progestin-only methods. All four IUDs can be used by breast-feeding women. With Mirena and Skyla, periods become lighter or stop completely. IUDs are fully reversible; after removal, there is usually no delay in return of fertility. There is no need to keep supplies on hand or remember to pick up a pill or apply a patch. A health care provider can remove the IUD at any time.

**Disadvantages** Disadvantages of IUDs include possible discomfort during insertion and removal, the cost of insertion, and potential complications. Also, the IUD does not protect against HIV and STIs. In some women, Paraguard can cause heavy menstrual flow and severe cramps for the first few months; other negative side effects of Paraguard include acne, headaches, mood changes, uterine cramps, and backache, which seem to occur most often in women who have never been pregnant and go away after the first few months.

## LO 5 | BEHAVIORAL METHODS

Explain how behavioral methods of contraception work and compare their effectiveness to other methods of birth control.

Some methods of contraception rely on one or both partners altering their sexual behavior. In general, these methods require more self-control, diligence, and commitment, making them more prone to user error than hormonal and barrier methods.

## Withdrawal

**Withdrawal,** also called *coitus interruptus,* involves removing the penis from the vagina just before ejaculation. In the 2014 *American College Health Association's National College Health Assessment (ACHA-NCHA),* 29 percent of respondents reported that withdrawal was the method of birth control (or one of the methods) they used the last time they had sexual intercourse.[30] This statistic is startlingly high, considering the high risk of both pregnancy (22% failure rate with typical use) and STI transmission associated with this method of birth control.[31]

## Advantages and Disadvantages

Withdrawal is unreliable, even with "perfect" use, because there are a half-million sperm in just the drop of preejaculate fluid released *before* ejaculation. Timing withdrawal is also difficult, and males concentrating on accurate timing may not be able to relax and enjoy intercourse. Withdrawal offers no protection against STIs and requires a high degree of self-control, experience, and trust.

## Abstinence and "Outercourse"

Strictly defined, *abstinence* means avoiding oral, vaginal, and anal sex. This definition would allow one to engage in forms of sexual intimacy such as massage, kissing, and masturbation. Couples who go beyond fondling and kissing to activities such as oral sex and mutual masturbation, but not vaginal or anal sex, are sometimes said to be engaging in "outercourse."

## Advantages and Disadvantages

Abstinence is the only method of avoiding pregnancy that is 100 percent effective. It is also the only method that is 100 percent effective against transmitting and contracting STIs. Like abstinence, outercourse can be 100 percent effective for birth control as long as the male does not ejaculate near the vaginal opening. Unlike abstinence, however, outercourse is not 100 percent effective against STIs. Oral-genital contact can transmit disease, although the practice can be made safer by using a condom on the penis or a latex barrier, such as a dental dam, over the vulva. Both abstinence and outercourse require discipline and commitment for couples to sustain over long periods of time. Thirty percent of college students report being abstinent for the past 12 months. Thirty-one percent report having never engaged in vaginal sex, 27 percent never in oral sex, and 76 percent never in anal sex.[32]

## Fertility Awareness Methods

**Fertility awareness methods (FAMs)** of birth control, sometimes referred to as periodic abstinence, natural family planning, or the "rhythm" method, rely on altering sexual behavior during certain times of the month (**FIGURE 6.4**).

Fertility awareness methods are rooted in an understanding of basic physiology. A released ovum can survive about 36 hours after ovulation, and sperm can live for about 7 days in the reproductive tract. These techniques require observing female fertile periods and abstaining from sexual intercourse (or any penis-vagina contact) during the times which a sperm and egg could meet. Some of the more common forms include the following:

- **Cervical mucus method.** This method requires women to examine the consistency and color of their normal vaginal secretions. Prior to ovulation, vaginal mucus becomes slippery, thin, and stretchy, and normal vaginal secretions may increase. To prevent pregnancy, partners must avoid sexual activity involving penis-vagina contact while this mucus is present and for several days afterward.

- **Body temperature method.** This method relies on the fact that a woman's basal (resting) body temperature rises between 0.4 and 0.8 degrees after ovulation has occurred. For this method to be effective, a woman must chart her temperature for several months to learn to recognize her body's temperature fluctuations. To prevent pregnancy, partners must abstain from penis-vagina contact before the temperature rise until several days after the temperature rise is observed.

- **Calendar method.** This method requires the woman to record the exact number of days in her menstrual cycle. Because few women menstruate with complete regularity, this method involves keeping a record of the

> **fertility awareness methods (FAMs)** Several types of birth control that require alteration of sexual behavior rather than chemical or physical intervention in the reproductive process.

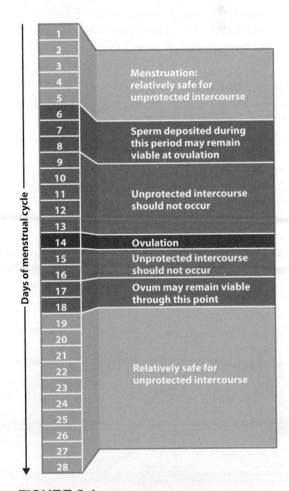

**FIGURE 6.4** **The Fertility Cycle** Fertility awareness methods (FAMs) can combine the use of a calendar, the cervical mucus method, and body temperature measurements to identify the fertile period. It is important to remember that most women do not have a consistent 28-day cycle.

menstrual cycle for 12 months, during which time some other method of birth control must be used. This method assumes that ovulation occurs during the midpoint of the cycle. To prevent pregnancy, the couple must abstain from penis-vagina contact during the fertile time.

**Advantages and Disadvantages** Fertility awareness methods are the only forms of birth control that comply with certain religious teachings, including those of the Roman Catholic Church. They don't require a medical visit or prescription, and there are no negative health effects. The effectiveness of FAMs depends on diligence, commitment, and self-discipline; they have a 24 percent failure rate with typical use.[33] Women who attempt to use these methods without proper training run a high risk of unintended pregnancy; anyone interested in using them is advised to take a class. Free classes are often offered by health centers and churches, and there is only minimal expense for supplies. These methods offer no STI protection, and they may not work for women with irregular menstrual cycles.

**emergency contraceptive pills (ECPs)** Drugs taken within 3 to 5 days after unprotected intercourse to prevent pregnancy.

**sterilization** Permanent fertility control achieved through surgical procedures.

**tubal ligation** Sterilization of a woman that involves cutting and tying off or cauterizing the fallopian tubes.

## LO 6 | EMERGENCY CONTRACEPTION

Describe emergency contraception and how it is used.

Emergency contraception is the use of a contraceptive to prevent pregnancy after unprotected intercourse, a sexual assault, or the failure of another birth control method. Combination estrogen-progestin pills and progestin-only pills are two common types of **emergency contraceptive pills (ECPs)**, sometimes referred to as "morning-after pills." ECPs contain the same type of hormones as regular birth control pills and are used after unprotected intercourse, but before a woman misses her period. A woman taking ECPs does so to prevent pregnancy; the method will not work if she is already pregnant, nor will it harm an existing pregnancy.

Multiple types of ECPs are available in the United States without a prescription. They must be taken within 72 hours (3 days) of intercourse. The FDA has more recently approved *ella,* which is available only by prescription, and can prevent pregnancy when taken up to 120 hours (5 days) after unprotected intercourse. ECPs use the same hormones that other hormonal contraceptives do and prevent pregnancy in the same way: by delaying or inhibiting ovulation, inhibiting fertilization, or blocking implantation of a fertilized egg, depending on the phase of the woman's menstrual cycle. When taken within 24 hours, ECPs reduce the risk of pregnancy by up to 95 percent; when taken 2 to 5 days later, ECPs reduce the risk of pregnancy by 88 percent.[34]

In the past, only people 17 and older could purchase emergency contraceptives, and it was only available by asking a pharmacist for it because it was kept behind the pharmacy counter. Today, anyone of any age can purchase ECPs, and it is kept on the regular store shelves, usually near other family planning supplies. According to a recent national survey, 1 in 10 sexually active college students reported using (or their partner using) emergency contraception within the past year.[35] Although ECPs are no substitute for taking proper precautions before having sex (such as using a condom), widespread availability of emergency contraception has the potential to significantly reduce the rates of unintended pregnancies and abortions, particularly among young women.

## LO 7 | PERMANENT METHODS OF BIRTH CONTROL

Describe permanent methods of birth control and discuss their advantages and disadvantages.

In the United States, **sterilization** has become the second leading method of contraception for women of all ages and the leading method of contraception among women over age 35.[36] Because sterilization is permanent, anyone considering it should think through possibilities such as divorce and remarriage or a future improvement in financial status that might make pregnancy realistic or desirable.

### Female Sterilization

One method of sterilization for women is **tubal ligation,** a surgical procedure in which the fallopian tubes are cut or tied shut to block the sperm's access to released eggs (see **FIGURE 6.5**). The operation is usually done laparoscopically (via a half-inch incision in the abdomen) on an outpatient basis. The procedure usually takes less than an hour, is performed under local or general anesthesia, and the patient is usually allowed to return home within a short time. A tubal ligation does not affect ovarian and uterine function. The woman's menstrual cycle continues; released eggs simply disintegrate and are absorbed by the lymphatic system.

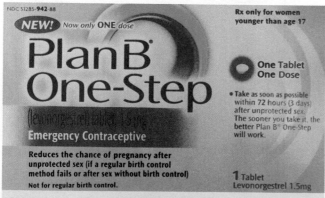

Emergency contraceptive pills contain hormones and are used after an act of unprotected intercourse. When taken within 72 hours of unprotected intercourse, ECPs reduce the risk of pregnancy by up to 95 percent.

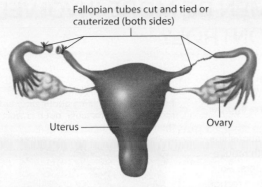

**FIGURE 6.5** Female Sterilization: Tubal Ligation In a tubal ligation, both fallopian tubes are cut and tied or sealed shut.

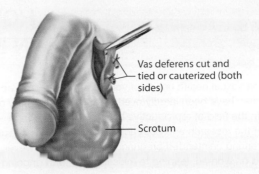

**FIGURE 6.6** Male Sterilization: Vasectomy In a vasectomy, the surgeon makes an incision in the scrotum, then locates and cuts the vasa deferentia, either sealing or tying both sides shut.

A newer sterilization procedure, *Essure*, involves the placement of small microcoils into the fallopian tubes via the vagina. The entire procedure takes about 35 minutes and can be performed in a physician's office, usually under local anesthetic. Once in place, the metallic microcoils expand to the shape of the fallopian tubes. The coils promote the growth of scar tissue around the coils and lead to a blockage in the fallopian tubes. Like traditional forms of tubal ligation, Essure is permanent. It is recommended for women who cannot have a tubal ligation because of chronic health conditions such as obesity or heart disease.

*Adiana* is another minimally invasive method of blocking a woman's fallopian tubes. A soft silicone insert about the size of a grain of rice is placed into each fallopian tube. Scar tissue begins to grow on and around the insert and eventually blocks the fallopian tubes. The insertion can be performed in a physician's office in about 15 minutes, usually under local anesthetic.

A **hysterectomy**, or removal of the uterus, is a method of sterilization requiring major surgery. It is usually done only when a woman's uterus is diseased or damaged, not as a primary means of female sterilization.

**Advantages** The main advantage to female sterilization is that it is highly effective (less than a 1% failure rate) and permanent.[37] After the one-time expense of the procedure, there is no other cost or ongoing action required. Sterilization has no negative effect on a woman's sex drive. A potential advantage of the Essure and Adiana methods is that they do not require an incision. These methods require no use of hormones, are discreet, and require no ongoing purchase or thought about supplies, thus allowing sex with full spontaneity.

**Disadvantages** As with any surgery, there are risks involved with a tubal ligation. Although rare, possible complications include infection, pulmonary embolism, hemorrhage, anesthesia complications, and ectopic pregnancy. Essure and Adiana do not require an incision, so the immediate risks are lower; however, because these are relatively new techniques, the long-term risks are unknown. Sterilization offers no protection against STIs, and it is initially expensive if not covered by your insurance plan. Sterilization is not effective immediately. A

backup method of birth control is needed for 3 months. While the permanent nature of this method is considered an advantage, people need to seriously consider if they may want children later, if circumstances were to change either financially or with a new partner. While female sterilization can be reversed in some instances, it should be considered permanent.

## Male Sterilization

Sterilization in men is less complicated than it is in women. A **vasectomy** is frequently done on an outpatient basis, using a local anesthetic (see **FIGURE 6.6**). This procedure involves making a small incision in the side of the scrotum to expose a vas deferens, cutting the vas deferens and either tying off or cauterizing the ends, then repeating the procedure on the other side.

Many men are reluctant to consider sterilization because they fear the operation will affect their sexual performance or sex drive. However, a vasectomy in no way affects sexual response. The testes continue to produce sperm, but the sperm can no longer enter the ejaculatory duct. Any sperm that are manufactured disintegrate and are absorbed into the lymphatic system. Because sperm constitute only a small part of the semen (about 2%), the amount of ejaculate is not changed significantly.

**Advantages** A vasectomy is a highly effective and permanent means of preventing pregnancy; typical failure rates are less than 1 percent. A vasectomy is a fairly simple outpatient procedure requiring minimal recovery time, and after the one-time expense, there is no other cost or ongoing action required. It is discreet, uses no hormones, allows for spontaneity, and is one of the few methods that allow men to be in charge of fertility. Of course, men don't necessarily have to make permanent body alterations to be more involved with birth control choices. See **Student Health Today** on the next page for more.

**Disadvantages** Male sterilization offers no protection against STI transmission. Also, a vasectomy is not immediately effective in preventing

**hysterectomy** Surgical removal of the uterus.

**vasectomy** Male sterilization procedure that involves cutting and tying off the vasa deferentia.

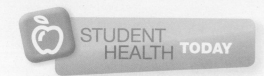

The sexual health needs of young men have been largely overlooked in the field of reproductive health. Most of the research and outreach related to preventing unintended pregnancy is focused on women, leading to missed opportunities to emphasize the importance of shared responsibility for sexual health.

There are many reasons for the disparity: Men seek health care less often; it is sometimes incorrectly assumed that men are not interested in sexual health issues; and since women carry the baby, they are often seen as having a bigger stake in pregnancy prevention. Male contraceptive methods are also more medically challenging, as you need to suppress up to 500,000 sperm per ejaculation, only one of which is needed for fertilization—as opposed to one egg per month in women.

However, healthy sexual relationships and ongoing reproductive health require that both partners be stakeholders. So, how can men be more involved in responsible sexual decision making?

- Initiate discussions with your partner about contraception and your sexual health histories.
- Take an active role in discussing and deciding what type of contraception is best for you and your partner.
- Buy and use condoms every time you have sex.

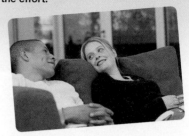

Don't let embarrassment put your health at risk! Talking about safer sex may be uncomfortable, but it is worth the effort.

- Help pay for contraceptive costs.
- If an unintended pregnancy occurs, share in the responsibility and decision making about the best way to handle the situation.

pregnancy. Because sperm are stored in other areas of the reproductive system besides the vasa deferentia, couples must use alternative birth control methods for at least 1 month after the vasectomy. A physician will do a semen analysis to determine when unprotected intercourse can take place. As with any surgery, there are some risks involved with a vasectomy. In a small percentage of cases, serious complications occur, such as formation of a blood clot in the scrotum, infection, or inflammatory reactions. Very infrequently, the vasa deferentia may create a new path, cancelling out the procedure. Sterilization is initially expensive if not covered by your insurance plan. While the permanent nature of this method is considered an advantage, people need to seriously consider if they may want children later if their circumstances change. While vasectomies can be reversed in some instances, the procedure is costly and not guaranteed to work.

## LO 8 | CHOOSING A METHOD OF CONTRACEPTION

List and explain factors that you should consider when choosing a method of contraception.

With all the options available, how does a person or a couple decide what method of contraception is best? Take some time to research the various methods, ask questions of your health care provider, and be honest with yourself about your own preferences. TABLE 6.2 lists the most popular forms of contraception among sexually active college students. Questions to ask yourself and discuss with your partner are included below.

- How comfortable would I be using a particular method? If you aren't at ease with a method, you may not use it consistently, and it probably will not be a reliable choice for you. Consider your own comfort level with touching your body or whether the method may cause discomfort for you or your partner.
- Will this method be convenient for me and my partner? Some methods require more effort than others. Be honest with yourself about how likely you are to use the method consistently. Are you willing to interrupt lovemaking, to abstain from sex during certain times of the month, or to take a pill at the same time every day?
- Am I at risk for the transmission of STIs? If you have multiple sex partners or are uncertain about the sexual history or disease status of your current sex partner, then you are at risk of contracting HIV or other STIs. Next to abstinence, condoms (male and female) are the best defense against STIs and HIV.
- Do I want to have a biological child in the future? If you are unsure about your plans for future childbearing, you should use a temporary birth control method rather than a permanent one such as sterilization. If you know you want to have children in the future, consider how soon that will be, as some methods, such as Depo-Provera, will cause a delay in return to fertility.

### WHAT DO YOU THINK?

Who do you think is responsible for deciding which method of contraception should be used in a sexual relationship?

- What are some examples of good opportunities for you and your partner to discuss contraceptives?
- What do you think are the biggest barriers in our society to the use of condoms?

| Method | Male | Female | Total |
|---|---|---|---|
| Male condom | 67% | 60% | 62% |
| Birth control pills (monthly or extended cycle) | 64% | 61% | 62% |
| Withdrawal | 27% | 30% | 29% |
| Intrauterine device | 7% | 8% | 7% |
| Fertility awareness (calendar, mucus, basal body temperature) | 5% | 7% | 6% |
| NuvaRing/ring | 4% | 4% | 4% |
| Depo-Provera/shots | 4% | 3% | 4% |
| Spermicide (foam, jelly, cream) | 5% | 3% | 3% |
| Nexplanon/implant | 3% | 3% | 3% |
| Sterilization | 2% | 2% | 2% |
| Xulane/patch | 1% | 1% | 1% |
| Female condom | 1% | 1% | 1% |
| Diaphragm/cervical cap | 1% | 0% | .4% |
| Sponge | 1% | 0% | .3% |

**Note:** Survey respondents could select more than one method.

**Source:** Data from American College Health Association, *American College Health Association—National College Health Assessment II: Reference Group Data, Spring 2014* (Hanover, MD: American College Health Association, 2014.)

- **How would an unplanned pregnancy affect my life?** If an unplanned pregnancy would be a potentially devastating event for you or would have a serious impact on your plans for the future, then you should choose a highly effective birth control method. If, however, you are in a stable relationship, have a reliable source of income, are planning to have children in the future, and would embrace a pregnancy should it occur now, then you may be comfortable with a less reliable method.

- **What are my religious and moral values?** If your beliefs prevent you from considering other birth control methods, FAMs are a good option. When both partners are motivated to use these methods, they can be successful at preventing unintended pregnancy. If you are considering this option, sign up for a class to get specific training for using the method effectively.

- **How much will the birth control method cost?** Some contraceptive methods involve an initial outlay of money and few continuing costs (e.g., sterilization, IUD), whereas others are fairly inexpensive but must be purchased repeatedly (e.g., condoms, spermicides, monthly pills). You should consider whether a method will be cost-effective for you in the long run. Remember that any prescription methods require routine checkups, which may involve some cost to you. Be sure to check your health

insurance to determine if the Affordable Care Act's requirement to cover "preventive services" makes hormonal contraceptives available to you at no cost. (See **Money & Health** on the next page for more information.) The provision lets a number of women upgrade their method of birth control to a more reliable (and more expensive) hormonal method or IUD for no extra cost. Your local family planning clinic or campus health center may offer low-cost options.

- **Do I have any health factors that could limit my choice?** Hormonal birth control methods can pose potential health risks to women with certain preexisting conditions, such as high blood pressure, a history of stroke or blood clots, liver disease, migraines, or diabetes. In addition, women who smoke or are over age 35 are at risk from complications of combination hormonal contraceptives. Breast feeding women can use progestin-only methods, but should avoid methods containing estrogen. Men and women with latex allergies can use barrier methods made of polyurethane, polyisoprene, silicone, or other materials, rather than latex condoms.

- **Are there any additional benefits I'd like from my contraceptive?** Hormonal birth control methods may have desirable secondary effects, such as the reduction of acne or the lessening of premenstrual symptoms. Some hormonal birth control methods have been associated

**WHY SHOULD I CARE?**
Even if you use another method for contraception, it's a good idea to also use a condom for protection against STIs. You don't want to get an STI—not only can they be unpleasant right now, but some STIs can stay with you for life, causing lasting harm to your health and your fertility, not to mention wreaking havoc on your love life!

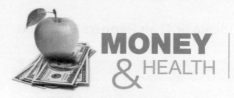

# MONEY & HEALTH | HEALTH CARE REFORM AND CONTRACEPTIVES

The Patient Protection and Affordable Care Act requires new private health insurance plans to cover "preventive services" with no co-payments or deductibles. Preventive services include birth control, yearly "wellness visits" (physical exams), breast-feeding counseling and supplies, and screening for domestic violence and sexually transmitted infections. Abortions are not included, but emergency contraception is.

Family planning experts anticipate that in coming years the law will significantly impact unintended pregnancy and abortion rates in two ways. One, women who have been unable to afford birth control will now have access. Half of all young adult women report having been unable to afford birth control consistently at some point, and when women have to choose between paying the heat bill and paying for birth control, birth control usually loses. Two, this coverage will enable women to "upgrade" their birth control to a more reliable method. Women who would prefer to use an IUD or implant to reduce the risk of "user error," but have been unable to because of the high upfront costs (up to

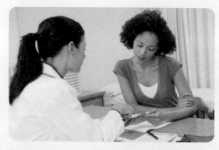

$1,000), will now be able to get one. The CHOICE study offered ACA-like benefits in St. Louis, Missouri, in advance of the implementation of the Affordable Care Act, and researchers found significant reductions in unplanned pregnancies, first abortions, and repeat abortions when women were given their choice of birth control method at no cost.

The law requires insurance companies to cover all contraceptive methods that have been approved by the FDA, but there are a few exceptions you might encounter:

1. This birth control benefit applies to all new plans. "New plan" doesn't mean you have to switch plans, it just means that the plan has changed since the passing of the health care law. Plans that have not

made changes do not have to comply with the law.

2. If your insurance is provided by a religious organization, it does not have to comply.

3. Insurance companies must cover all types of contraceptive methods, but not all brands. This may mean that while many oral contraceptives are covered, your brand may not be.

If your insurance plan doesn't seem to be following the law, contact The National Women's Law Center. They will help you figure it out for free. Call the toll-free hotline (1-866-745-5487), email CoverHer@nwlc.org, or visit CoverHer.org to get started.

**Sources:** U.S. Centers for Medicaid and Medicare Services, "What Are My Birth Control Benefits?," Accessed May 2014, www.healthcare.gov/what-are-my-birth-control-benefits/; Planned Parenthood, "Key Facts on Birth Control Coverage," 2014, www.plannedparenthood.org/files/PPFA/Myth_V_Fact_on_Birth_Control_coverage.pdf; A. Raphel, The Shorenstein Center, "The Affordable Care Act, Contraceptives, Abortion and Unintended-Pregnancy Rates," September 24, 2013, http://journalistsresource.org/studies/government/health-care/unintended-pregnancies-free-contraception#; National Women's Law Center, "CoverHer," Accessed April 2015, www.coverher.org

with reduced risks of certain cancers. Extended-cycle pills and some progestin-only methods cause menstrual periods to be less frequent or to stop altogether, which some women find desirable. Condoms carry the added health benefit of protecting against STIs.

## LO 9 | ABORTION

Summarize the political issues surrounding abortion and the various types of abortion procedures.

Women obtain abortions for a variety of reasons. The vast majority of abortions occur because of unintended pregnancies, as even the best birth control methods can fail.[38] In addition, some pregnancies are terminated because they are a consequence of rape or incest. Other reasons commonly cited are not being ready financially or emotionally to care for a child.[39] When an unintended pregnancy does occur, a woman

**abortion** Termination of a pregnancy by expulsion or removal of an embryo or fetus from the uterus.

must decide whether to terminate the pregnancy, carry to term and keep the baby, or carry to term and give the baby up for adoption. This is a personal decision that each woman must make based on her personal beliefs, values, and resources and after carefully considering all alternatives.

In 1973, the landmark U.S. Supreme Court decision in *Roe v. Wade* stated that the "right to privacy . . . founded on the Fourteenth Amendment's concept of personal liberty . . . is broad enough to encompass a woman's decision whether or not to terminate her pregnancy."[40] The decision maintained that during the first trimester of pregnancy a woman and her health care provider have the right to terminate the pregnancy through **abortion** without legal restrictions. It allowed individual states to set conditions for second-trimester abortions. Third-trimester abortions were ruled illegal unless the mother's life or health was in danger. Prior to the legalization of abortions, women wishing to terminate a pregnancy had to travel to a country where the procedure was legal, consult an illegal abortionist, or perform their own abortions. These procedures sometimes led to infertility from internal scarring or death from hemorrhage or infection.

# 47%

OF AMERICANS DESCRIBE THEMSELVES AS "**PRO-CHOICE**," 46% AS "**PRO-LIFE**."

## The Abortion Debate

Abortion is a highly charged and politically thorny issue in American society. In a recent national poll, 53 percent of people reported that *Roe v. Wade* should be kept in place, 29 percent felt it should be overturned, and 18 percent had no opinion.[41] Pro-choice individuals feel that it is a woman's right to make decisions about her own body and health, including the decision to continue or terminate a pregnancy. On the other side of the issue, pro-life individuals believe that the embryo or fetus is a human being with rights that must be protected.

In the 40 years since *Roe v. Wade* legalized abortion nationwide, hundreds of laws have been passed at the state and federal level to narrow or expand its limits. In 2014 alone, 26 new abortion-related laws were passed in the United States, most of which focused on regulation of abortion providers or facilities, limitations on provision of medication abortions, or bans on private insurance coverage of abortion.[42] These types of laws make abortions more difficult and costly to provide, consequently reducing the number of clinics and providers willing and able to provide abortion services. Thus, while abortion remains legal in all 50 states, for many women, due to difficulty accessing abortion services, abortion availability is severely limited.

## Emotional Aspects of Abortion

The best scientific evidence available indicates that among adult women who have an unplanned pregnancy, the risk of mental health problems is no greater if they have an abortion than if they deliver a baby. Although a variety of feelings such as regret, guilt, sadness, relief, and happiness are normal, no evidence has shown that an abortion causes long-term negative mental health outcomes.[43] Researchers have found that the best predictor of a woman's emotional well-being following an abortion was her emotional well-being prior to the procedure.[44] The factors that place a woman at higher risk for negative psychological responses following an abortion include the following: perception of stigma, need for secrecy, low levels of social support for the abortion decision, prior history of mental health issues, low self-esteem, and avoidance and denial coping strategies.[45]

## Methods of Abortion

The choice of abortion procedure is determined by how many weeks the woman has been pregnant. Length of pregnancy is calculated from the first day of her last menstrual period.

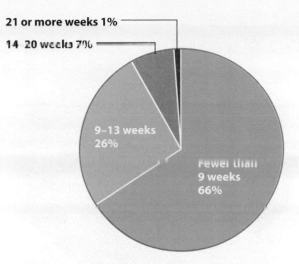

**FIGURE 6.7**  When Women Have Abortions (in weeks from the last menstrual period)

**Source:** K. Pazol et al., "Abortion Surveillance—United States 2011," *Surveillance Summaries* 63, no. SS11 (2014): 1–41.

**Surgical Abortions** The majority of abortions performed in the United States today are surgical. If performed during the first trimester, abortion presents a relatively low health risk to the mother. About 89 percent of abortions occur during the first 12 weeks of pregnancy (see **FIGURE 6.7**).[46] The most commonly used method of first-trimester abortion is **suction curettage**, also called vacuum aspiration or dilation and curettage (D&C) (**FIGURE 6.8**). The vast majority of abortions in the United States are done using this procedure, which is usually performed under local anesthesia. The cervix is dilated with instruments or by placing laminaria, a sterile seaweed product, in the cervical canal. The laminaria is left in place for a few hours or overnight and slowly dilates the cervix. After the laminaria is removed, a long tube is inserted through the cervix and into the uterus, and gentle suction removes fetal tissue from the uterine walls.

Pregnancies that progress into the second trimester (after week 12) are usually terminated through **dilation and evacuation (D&E)**. For this procedure, the cervix is dilated for 1 to 2 days, and a combination of instruments and vacuum aspiration is used to scrape and suck fetal tissue from the uterus. The D&E can be performed on an outpatient basis (usually in a physician's office), usually under general anesthesia. This procedure may cause moderate to severe uterine cramping and blood loss. After a D&E, a return visit to the clinic is an important follow-up.

Abortions during the third trimester are very rare (fewer than 2% of abortions in the United States).[47] When they are performed, a D&E is the most commonly utilized procedure. The much debated, **intact dilation and extraction (D&X)**,

> **suction curettage** Abortion technique that uses gentle suction to remove fetal tissue from the uterus; also called vacuum aspiration or dilation and curettage (D&C).
>
> **dilation and evacuation (D&E)** Abortion technique that uses a combination of instruments and vacuum aspiration.
>
> **intact dilation and extraction (D&X)** Late-term abortion procedure in which the body of the fetus is extracted up to the head and then the contents of the cranium are aspirated.

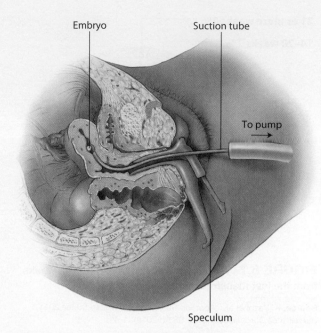

Embryo     Suction tube

To pump

Speculum

**FIGURE 6.8** **Suction Curettage Abortion** This procedure, in which a long tube with gentle suction is used to remove fetal tissue from the uterine walls, can be performed until the twelfth week of pregnancy.

often referred to as "partial birth abortion," is no longer legal in the United States.

The risks associated with surgical abortion include infection, incomplete abortion (when parts of the placenta remain in the uterus), excessive bleeding, and cervical and uterine trauma. Follow-up and attention to danger signs decrease the chances of long-term problems.

The mortality rate for women undergoing first-trimester abortions in the United States averages 1 death per every 1 million procedures at 8 or fewer weeks. The risk of death increases with the length of pregnancy. At 16 to 20 weeks, the mortality rate is 1 per 29,000; at 21 weeks or more, it increases to 1 per 11,000.[48] This higher rate later in the pregnancy is due to the increased risk of uterine perforation, bleeding, infection, and incomplete abortion; these complications occur because the uterine wall becomes thinner as the pregnancy progresses.

**Medical Abortions** Unlike surgical abortions, a **medical abortion** (also called medication abortion) is performed without entering the uterus. Mifepristone, formerly known as RU-486 and currently sold in the United States under the brand name Mifeprex, is a steroid hormone that induces abortion by blocking the action of progesterone, the hormone produced by the ovaries and placenta that maintains the uterine lining. As a result, the lining and embryo are expelled from the uterus, terminating the pregnancy. Medical abortions must be performed early in the pregnancy, no later than 9 weeks after a woman's last menstrual period.

**medical abortion** Termination of a pregnancy during the first 9 weeks using hormonal medications that cause the embryo to be expelled from the uterus.

Mifepristone's nickname, "the abortion pill," may imply an easy process; however, this treatment actually involves more steps than a suction curettage abortion, which takes approximately 15 minutes followed by a physical recovery of about 1 day. With mifepristone, an initial visit to the clinic involves a physical exam and a dose of mifepristone and antibiotics, which may cause minor side effects such as nausea, headaches, weakness, and fatigue. The patient returns 2 to 3 days later for a dose of prostaglandins (misoprostol), which causes uterine contractions that expel the fertilized egg. The patient is required to stay under observation at the clinic for 4 hours and to make a follow-up visit within 2 weeks.[49]

More than 99 percent of women who use mifepristone early in pregnancy will experience a complete abortion.[50] The side effects are similar to those reported during heavy menstruation and include cramping, minor pain, and nausea. Less than 1 percent have more serious outcomes requiring a blood transfusion because of severe bleeding or the administration of intravenous antibiotics.[51]

## LO 10 | PREGNANCY

Discuss key issues to consider when planning a pregnancy, describe the process of pregnancy and fetal development, and explain the importance of prenatal care.

Pregnancy is an important event in a woman's life, and in the life of her partner. The actions taken before as well as behaviors engaged in during pregnancy can significantly affect the health of both infant and mother.

## Planning for Pregnancy and Parenthood

Today, sexually active people are able to choose if and when they want to have children. As you approach the decision of whether or not to have children, or when to do so, take the time to evaluate your emotions, finances, and physical health.

**Emotional Health** First and foremost, consider why you may want to have a child. To fulfill an inner need to carry on the family? To share love? To give your parents grandchildren? To have a close tie or friendship? Then, consider the responsibilities involved with becoming a parent. Are you ready to make all the sacrifices necessary to bear and raise a child? Can you care for this new human being in a loving and nurturing manner? Do you have a strong social support system? This emotional preparation for parenthood can be as important as the physical preparation.

**Financial Evaluation** Finances are another important consideration. Can you afford to give your child the life you would like him or her to enjoy? The U.S. Department of Agriculture estimates that it will cost an average of $241,080 to raise a child born today to age 18, not including college tuition.[52]

It is important to check whether your medical insurance provides maternity benefits. If not, you can expect to pay, on average, $18,000 for a normal delivery and up to $28,000 for a cesarean section, including prenatal care.[53] Both partners should investigate their employers' policies concerning parental leave, including length of leave available and conditions for returning to work.

## Maternal Age

The average age at which a woman has her first child has been creeping up (from 21 in 1970 to almost 26 today), so a woman who becomes pregnant after age 35 has plenty of company.[54] Although births to women in their twenties are declining, the rate of first births to women between the ages of 30 and 39 is the highest reported in four decades, and births to women over 39 have continued to increase slightly over the years.[55]

Statistically, the chances of having a baby with birth defects rise after the age of 35. Researchers believe this is due to a decline in the quality of eggs after this age. Two specific age-related risks are **Down syndrome** and miscarriage. The risk of miscarriage nearly doubles for women 35 to 45 compared to women under 35.[56] Another concern is that a woman's fertility begins to decline as she ages. A gradual decline in fertility begins around age 32 and fertility decreases more rapidly after age 37 because of the reduction in the number and quality of eggs in the ovaries.[57] While some risks increase with age, many doctors note that older mothers bring some advantages to their pregnancies: They tend to follow medical advice during pregnancy more thoroughly, are more mature psychologically, better prepared financially, and generally more ready to care for an infant than are some younger women.

## Physical Health: Maternal Health

The birth of a healthy baby depends in part on the mother's **preconception care.** The fetus is most susceptible to developing certain problems in the first 4 to 10 weeks after conception, before prenatal care is normally initiated. Since many women don't realize they are pregnant until later, they often can't reduce health risks unless intervention had begun before conception.[58] Maternal factors that can affect a fetus or infant include drug use (illicit, prescription, or over-the-counter), alcohol consumption, tobacco use, or obesity. To promote preconception health, get the best medical care you can, practice healthy behaviors, build a strong support network, and encourage safe environments at home and at work.[59]

Nutrition counseling is an important part of preconception care. Among the many important nutrition issues is folic acid (folate) intake. When consumed the month before conception and during early pregnancy, folate reduces the risk of spina bifida, a congenital birth defect resulting from failure of the spinal column to close. A woman also needs to make sure her immunizations are up-to-date before becoming pregnant. If, for example, she has never had rubella (German measles), a woman needs to be immunized prior to becoming pregnant. A rubella infection can kill the fetus or cause blindness or hearing disorders in the infant.

## Physical Health: Paternal Health

Fathers-to-be are recommended to practice the same healthy habits as mothers-to-be because, by one route or another, dozens of chemicals studied so far (from occupational exposures to by-products of cigarette smoke) appear to harm sperm.[60] A fathers' age may also play a role; recent research shows a relationship between older fathers and autism, ADHD, bipolar disorder, and schizophrenia.[61]

# The Process of Pregnancy

The process of pregnancy begins the moment a sperm fertilizes an ovum in the fallopian tubes. From there, the single fertilized cell, now called a *zygote,* multiplies and becomes a sphere-shaped cluster of cells called a *blastocyst* that travels toward the uterus, a journey that may take 3 to 4 days. Upon arrival, the embryo burrows into the thick, spongy endometrium (implantation) and is nourished from this carefully prepared lining.

## Pregnancy Testing

A pregnancy test scheduled with your health care provider or at a local family planning clinic will confirm a pregnancy. Women who wish to know immediately can purchase home pregnancy test kits sold over-the-counter in drugstores. A positive test is based on the secretion of **human chorionic gonadotropin (HCG),** which is found in the woman's urine.

Home pregnancy tests vary, but some can be used as early as a week after conception and many are 99 percent reliable.[62] If the test is done too early in the pregnancy, it may show a false negative. Other causes of false negatives are unclean testing devices, ingestion of certain drugs, and vaginal or urinary tract infections. Blood tests administered and analyzed in a doctor's office are more accurate than home urine tests.

**Down syndrome** A genetic disorder caused by the presence of an extra chromosome that results in mental disabilities and distinctive physical characteristics.

**preconception care** Medical care received prior to becoming pregnant that helps a woman assess and address potential health issues.

**human chorionic gonadotropin (HCG)** Hormone detectable in blood or urine samples of a mother within the first few weeks of pregnancy.

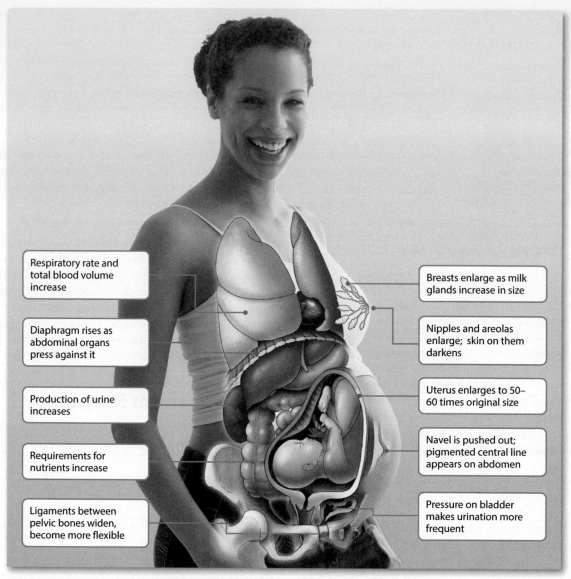

**FIGURE 6.9** Changes in a Woman's Body during Pregnancy

The labels in the figure read:

- Respiratory rate and total blood volume increase
- Diaphragm rises as abdominal organs press against it
- Production of urine increases
- Requirements for nutrients increase
- Ligaments between pelvic bones widen, become more flexible
- Breasts enlarge as milk glands increase in size
- Nipples and areolas enlarge; skin on them darkens
- Uterus enlarges to 50–60 times original size
- Navel is pushed out; pigmented central line appears on abdomen
- Pressure on bladder makes urination more frequent

## Early Signs of Pregnancy

A woman's body undergoes substantial changes during a pregnancy (**FIGURE 6.9**). The first sign of pregnancy is usually a missed menstrual period (although some women "spot" in early pregnancy, which may be mistaken for a period). Other signs include breast tenderness, emotional upset, extreme fatigue, sleeplessness, nausea, and vomiting (especially in the morning).

Pregnancy typically lasts 40 weeks and is divided into three phases, or **trimesters,** of approximately 3 months each. The due date is calculated from the expectant mother's last menstrual period.

## The First Trimester

During the first trimester, few noticeable changes occur in the mother's body. She may urinate more frequently and experience morning sickness, swollen breasts, or undue fatigue. These symptoms may not be frequent or severe, so women often do not realize they are pregnant right away. During the first 2 months after conception, the **embryo** differentiates and develops its various organ systems, beginning with the nervous and circulatory systems. At the start of the third month, the embryo is called a **fetus,** indicating that all organ systems are in place. For the rest of the pregnancy, growth and refinement occur in each body system so that at birth they can function independently, yet in coordination with all the others. The photos in **FIGURE 6.10** illustrate physical changes during fetal development.

## The Second Trimester

At the beginning of the second trimester, the fourth through sixth months of pregnancy, physical changes in the mother become more visible. Her breasts swell and her waistline thickens. During this time, the fetus makes greater demands on the mother's body. In

**trimester** A 3-month segment of pregnancy.

**embryo** Fertilized egg from conception through the eighth week of development.

**fetus** Developing human from the ninth week until birth.

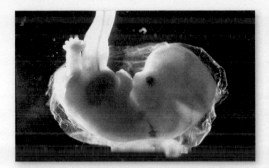

**a** A human embryo during the first trimester. The embryonic period lasts from the third to the eighth week of development. By the end of the embryonic period, all organs have formed.

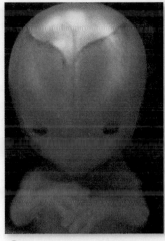

**b** A human fetus during the second trimester. Growth during the fetal period is very rapid.

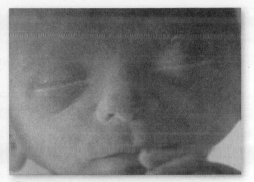

**c** A human fetus during the third trimester. By the end of the fetal period, the growth rate of the head has slowed relative to the growth rate of the rest of the body.

**FIGURE 6.10** Fetoscopic Photographs Showing Development in the First, Second, and Third Trimesters of Pregnancy

particular, the **placenta,** the network of blood vessels that carries nutrients and oxygen to the fetus and fetal waste products to the mother, becomes well established.

### The Third Trimester

The end of the sixth month through the ninth mark the third trimester. This is the period of greatest fetal growth. The growing fetus depends entirely on its mother for nutrition and must receive large amounts of calcium, iron, and protein from the mother's diet. Although the fetus may survive if it is born during the seventh month, it needs the layer of fat it acquires during the eighth month and time for the organs (especially the respiratory and digestive organs) to develop fully. Infants born prematurely usually require intensive medical care.

### Prenatal Care

A successful pregnancy depends on a mother who takes good care of herself and her fetus. Good nutrition and exercise; avoiding drugs, alcohol, and other harmful substances; and regular medical checkups from the beginning of pregnancy are all essential. Early detection of fetal abnormalities, identification of high-risk mothers and infants, and screening for possible complications are the major purposes of prenatal care.

Ideally, a woman should begin prenatal appointments in the first trimester. On the first visit, the practitioner should obtain a complete medical history of the mother and her family and note any hereditary conditions that could put a woman or her fetus at risk. Regular checkups to measure weight gain and blood pressure and to monitor the fetus's size and position should continue throughout the pregnancy.

**placenta** Network of blood vessels connected to the umbilical cord that transports oxygen and nutrients to a developing fetus and carries away fetal wastes.

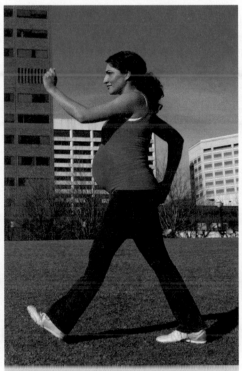

A doctor-approved exercise program during pregnancy can help control weight, make delivery easier, and have a healthy effect on the fetus.

### Nutrition and Exercise

Despite "eating for two," pregnant woman only need about 300 additional calories a day. Special attention should be paid to getting enough folic acid (found in dark leafy greens, citrus fruits, and beans), iron (dried fruits, meats, legumes, liver, egg yolks), calcium (nonfat or low-fat dairy products and some canned fish), and fluids. While vitamin supplements can correct some deficiencies, there is no substitute for a well-balanced diet. Babies born to poorly nourished mothers run high risks of substandard mental and physical development.

Weight gain during pregnancy helps nourish a growing baby. For a woman of normal weight before pregnancy, the recommended gain during pregnancy is 25 to 35 pounds.[63] For overweight women, weight gain of 15 to 25 pounds is recommended, and for obese women, 11 to 20 pounds is recommended. Underweight women should gain 28 to 40 pounds, and women carrying twins should gain about 35 to 45 pounds. Gaining too much or too little weight can lead to complications. With higher weight gains, women may develop gestational diabetes, hypertension, or increased risk of delivery complications. Gaining too little increases the chance of a low birth weight baby.

As in all other stages of life, exercise is an important factor in overall health during pregnancy. Regular exercise is recommended for pregnant women; however, they should consult with their health care provider before starting any exercise program. Exercise can help control weight, make labor easier, and help with a faster recovery due to increased strength and endurance. Women can usually maintain their customary level of activity during most of the pregnancy, although there are some cautions: pregnant women should avoid exercise that puts them at risk of falling or having an abdominal injury, and in the third trimester, exercises that involve lying on the back should be avoided as they can restrict blood flow to the uterus.

### Avoiding Drugs, Alcohol, Tobacco, and Other Teratogens

A woman should consult with a health care provider regarding the safety of any drugs she might use during pregnancy. Even too much of common over-the-counter medications such as aspirin can damage a developing fetus. During the first 3 months of pregnancy, the fetus is especially subject to the **teratogenic** (birth defect–causing) effects of drugs, environmental chemicals, X-rays, or diseases. The fetus can also develop an addiction to or tolerance for drugs that the mother is using.

Maternal consumption of alcohol is detrimental to a growing fetus. Birth defects associated with **fetal alcohol syndrome (FAS)** include developmental disabilities, neural and cardiac impairments, and cranial and facial deformities. The exact amount of alcohol that causes FAS is not known; therefore, the American Congress of Obstetricians and Gynecologists recommends completely avoiding alcohol during pregnancy.[64]

Women who smoke during pregnancy have a greater chance of miscarriage, complications, premature births, low birth weight infants, stillbirth, and infant mortality specifically due to sudden infant death syndrome.[65] Smoking restricts the blood supply to the developing fetus and thus limits oxygen and nutrition delivery and waste removal. Tobacco use also appears to be a significant factor in the development of cleft lip and palate.[66]

A pregnant woman should avoid exposure to X-rays, toxic chemicals, heavy metals, pesticides, gases, and other hazardous compounds. She should also avoid cleaning litter boxes, if possible, because cat feces can contain organisms that cause **toxoplasmosis.** If a pregnant woman contracts this disease, the baby may be stillborn or suffer mental disabilities or other birth defects.

**Prenatal Testing and Screening** Modern technology enables medical practitioners to detect health defects in a fetus as early as the fourteenth to eighteenth weeks of pregnancy. One common test is **ultrasonography** or **ultrasound,** which uses high-frequency sound waves to create a *sonogram,* or visual image, of the fetus in the uterus. The sonogram is used to determine the fetus's size and position, which can help to safely deliver the infant. Sonograms can also detect birth defects in the nervous and digestive systems.

**Chorionic villus sampling (CVS)** involves snipping tissue from the developing fetal sac. Chorionic villus sampling can be used at 10 to 12 weeks of pregnancy. This is an attractive option for couples who are at high risk for having a baby with Down syndrome or a debilitating hereditary disease.

The **triple marker screen** (often called the TMS or AFT [alpha-fetoprotein] test) is a commonly used maternal blood test that is optimally conducted between the sixteenth and eighteenth weeks of pregnancy. The TMS is a screening test, not a diagnostic tool; it can detect susceptibility for a birth defect or genetic abnormality, but it is not meant to confirm a diagnosis of any condition. A *quad screen test* (or AFP-plus test), which screens for an additional protein in maternal blood, is more accurate than the triple marker screen. Even more precise is the *integrated screen,* which uses the quad screen, plus results from an earlier blood test, plus ultrasound, to screen for abnormalities.

**Amniocentesis** is a common testing procedure that is strongly recommended for women over age 35. This test involves inserting a long needle through the mother's abdominal and uterine walls into the **amniotic sac,** the protective pouch surrounding the fetus. The needle draws out 3 to 4 teaspoons of fluid, which is analyzed for genetic information about the baby. Amniocentesis can be performed between weeks 14 and 18.

If any of these tests reveals a serious birth defect, parents are advised to undergo genetic counseling. In the case of a chromosomal abnormality such as Down syndrome, the parents are usually offered the option of a therapeutic abortion. Some parents choose this option; others research the condition and decide to continue the pregnancy.

### LO 11 | CHILDBIRTH

Explain the basic stages of childbirth and complications that can arise during pregnancy, labor, and delivery.

Prospective parents need to make several key decisions before the baby is born. These include where to have the baby,

---

**teratogenic** Causing birth defects; may refer to drugs, environmental chemicals, radiation, or diseases.

**fetal alcohol syndrome (FAS)** Pattern of birth defects, learning, and behavioral problems in a child caused by the mother's alcohol consumption during pregnancy.

**toxoplasmosis** Disease caused by an organism found in cat feces that, when contracted by a pregnant woman, may result in stillbirth or birth defects.

**ultrasonography (ultrasound)** Common prenatal test that uses sound waves to create a visual image of a developing fetus.

**chorionic villus sampling (CVS)** Prenatal test that involves snipping tissue from the fetal sac to be analyzed for genetic defects.

**triple marker screen (TMS)** Common maternal blood test that can be used to identify certain birth defects and genetic abnormalities in a fetus.

**amniocentesis** Medical test in which a small amount of fluid is drawn from the amniotic sac to test for Down syndrome and other genetic abnormalities.

**amniotic sac** Protective pouch surrounding the fetus.

whether to use pain medication during labor and delivery, which childbirth method to choose, and whether to breast-feed or use formula. Answering these questions in advance will help to smooth the passage into parenthood.

## Labor and Delivery

During the final weeks preceding delivery, the baby normally shifts to a head-down position, and the cervix begins to dilate (widen). The junction of the pubic bones loosens to permit expansion of the pelvic girdle during birth. The exact mechanisms that initiate labor are unknown. A change in the hormones in the fetus and mother cause strong uterine contractions to occur, signaling the beginning of labor. Another common early signal is the breaking of the amniotic sac, which causes a rush of fluid from the vagina (commonly referred to as "water breaking").

The birth process has three stages, shown in **FIGURE 6.11**, which can last from several hours to more than a day. In some cases, toward the end of the second stage, the attending health care provider may perform an *episiotomy,* a straight incision in the mother's perineum (the area between the vulva and the anus) to prevent the baby's head from tearing vaginal tissues and to speed the baby's exit from the vagina. After delivery, the attending provider assesses the baby's overall condition, clears the baby's mucus-filled breathing passages, and ties and severs the umbilical cord. The mother's uterus continues to contract in the third stage of labor until the placenta is expelled.

**Managing Labor** Pain medication given to the mother during labor can cause sluggish responses in the newborn and other complications. For this reason, some women choose a drug-free labor and delivery—but it is important to keep a flexible attitude about pain relief, because each labor is different. One person is not a "success" for delivering without medication or another a "failure" for using medical measures.

The Lamaze method is the most popular technique of childbirth preparation in the United States. It discourages the use of pain medication. Prelabor classes teach the mother to control her pain through special breathing patterns, focusing exercises, and relaxation. The partner (or labor coach) assists by giving emotional support, physical comfort, and coaching for proper breath control during contractions.

**Cesarean Section (C-Section)** If labor lasts too long or if a baby is in physiological distress or is about to exit the uterus any way but headfirst, a **cesarean section (C-section)** may be necessary. This surgical procedure involves making an incision across the mother's abdomen and through the uterus to remove the baby. A C-section may also be performed if labor is extremely difficult, maternal blood pressure falls rapidly, the placenta separates from the uterus too soon, the mother has diabetes, or other problems occur. Risks are the same as for any major abdominal surgery, and recovery from birth takes considerably longer after a C-section.

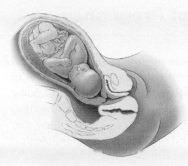

**1** **Stage I: Dilation of the cervix** Contractions in the abdomen and lower back push the baby downward, putting pressure on the cervix and dilating it. The first stage of labor may last from a couple of hours to more than a day for a first birth, but it is usually much shorter during subsequent births.

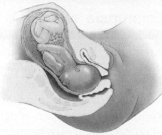

**2** **End of Stage I: Transition** The cervix becomes fully dilated, and the baby's head begins to move into the vagina (birth canal). Contractions usually come quickly during transition, which generally lasts 30 minutes or less.

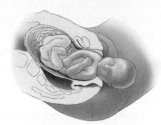

**3** **Stage II: Expulsion** Once the cervix has become fully dilated, contractions become rhythmic, strong, and more intense as the uterus pushes the baby headfirst through the birth canal. The expulsion stage lasts 1 to 4 hours and concludes when the infant is finally pushed out of the mother's body.

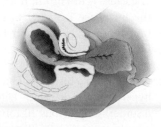

**4** **Stage III: Delivery of the placenta** In the third stage, the placenta detaches from the uterus and is expelled through the birth canal. This stage is usually completed within 30 minutes after delivery.

**FIGURE 6.11** **The Birth Process** The entire process of labor and delivery usually takes from 2 to 36 hours. Labor is generally longer for a woman's first delivery and shorter for subsequent births.

The rate of delivery by C-section in the United States has increased from 5 percent in the mid-1960s to 32 percent in 2013.[67] Although this procedure is necessary in certain cases, some doctors and critics, including the Centers for Disease Control and Prevention (CDC), feel that C-sections are performed too frequently in this country. Natural birth advocates suggest that hospitals, driven by profits and worried about malpractice, are too quick to intervene in the birth process. Some doctors say that the increase is due to maternal demand: busy mothers want to schedule their deliveries.[68]

**cesarean section (C-section)** Surgical birthing procedure in which a baby is removed through an incision made in the mother's abdominal wall and uterus.

# Complications of Pregnancy and Childbirth

Pregnancy carries the risk for potential complications and problems that can interfere with the proper development of the fetus or threaten the health of the mother and child. Some complications may result from a preexisting health condition of the mother, such as diabetes or an STI, and others can develop during pregnancy and may result from physiological problems, genetic abnormalities, or exposure to teratogens.

## Preeclampsia and Eclampsia

Preeclampsia is a condition characterized by high blood pressure, protein in the urine, and edema (fluid retention), which usually causes swelling of the hands and face. Symptoms may include sudden weight gain, headache, nausea or vomiting, changes in vision, racing pulse, mental confusion, and stomach or right shoulder pain. If preeclampsia is not treated, it can cause strokes and seizures, a condition called *eclampsia*. Potential problems can include liver and kidney damage, internal bleeding, poor fetal growth, and fetal and maternal death.

Preeclampsia tends to occur in the late second or third trimester. The cause is unknown; however, the incidence is higher in first-time mothers; women over 40 or under 18 years of age; women carrying multiple fetuses; and women with a history of chronic hypertension, diabetes, kidney disorder, or previous history of preeclampsia. Family history of preeclampsia is also a risk factor. Treatment for preeclampsia ranges from bed rest and monitoring for mild cases to hospitalization and close monitoring for more severe cases.

> **preeclampsia** Pregnancy complication characterized by high blood pressure, protein in the urine, and edema.
>
> **miscarriage** Loss of the fetus before it is viable; also called *spontaneous abortion*.
>
> **ectopic pregnancy** Dangerous condition that results from the implantation of a fertilized egg outside the uterus, usually in a fallopian tube.
>
> **stillbirth** Death of a fetus after the twentieth week of pregnancy but before delivery.
>
> **postpartum depression** Mood disorder experienced by women who have given birth; involves depression, fatigue, and other symptoms and may last for weeks or months.

## Miscarriage

Even when a woman does everything "right," not every pregnancy ends in delivery. In fact, in the United States, between 15 to 20 percent of known pregnancies end in **miscarriage** (also referred to as *spontaneous abortion*).[69] Most miscarriages occur during the first trimester.

Reasons for miscarriage vary. In some cases, the fertilized egg has failed to divide correctly. In others, genetic abnormalities, maternal illness, or infections are responsible. Maternal hormonal imbalance may also cause a miscarriage, as may a weak cervix, toxic chemicals in the environment, or physical trauma to the mother. In most cases, the cause is not known.

## Ectopic Pregnancy

The implantation of a fertilized egg outside the uterus, usually in the fallopian tube or occasionally in the pelvic cavity, is called an **ectopic pregnancy**. Because these structures are not capable of expanding and nourishing a developing fetus, the pregnancy must be terminated surgically or a miscarriage will occur. If an ectopic pregnancy progresses undiagnosed and untreated, the fallopian tube will rupture, which puts the woman at great risk of hemorrhage, peritonitis (infection in the abdomen), and even death. Ectopic pregnancy occurs in about 2 percent of pregnancies in North America and is a leading cause of maternal mortality in the first trimester.[70]

## Stillbirth

**Stillbirth** is the death of a fetus *after* the twentieth week of pregnancy but before delivery. A stillborn baby is born dead, often for no apparent reason. Each year in the United States, there is about 1 stillbirth in every 160 births.[71] Birth defects, placental problems, poor fetal growth, infections, and umbilical cord accidents are known contributing factors.

# The Postpartum Period

The postpartum period lasts 6 weeks after delivery. During this period, many women experience fluctuating emotions. Many new mothers experience what is called the "baby blues," characterized by periods of sadness, anxiety, headache, sleep disturbances, and irritability. About 1 in 7 new mothers experience **postpartum depression**, a more disabling syndrome characterized by mood swings, lack of energy, crying, guilt, and depression any time within the first year after childbirth.

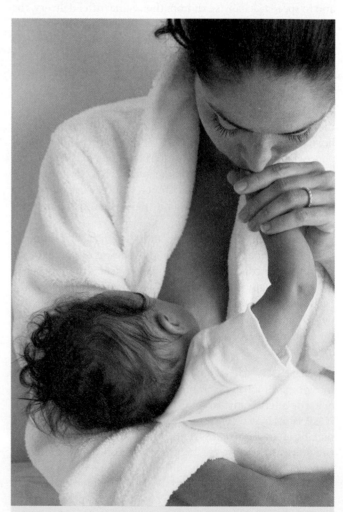

In addition to its numerous health benefits, breast-feeding enhances the development of intimate bonds between mother and child.

Mothers who experience postpartum depression should seek professional treatment. Counseling is the most common type of treatment, but sometimes medication is recommended.[72]

## Breast-Feeding

Although the new mother's milk will not begin to flow for 2 or more days after delivery, her breasts secrete a yellow fluid called *colostrum* beginning immediately after birth. Because colostrum contains vital antibodies to help fight infection and boost the baby's immune system, all newborns should be allowed to suckle.

The American Academy of Pediatrics strongly recommends that infants be exclusively breast-fed for 6 months and breast-fed as a supplement until 12 months of age. Scientific findings indicate there are many advantages to breast-feeding. Breast milk is perfectly matched to babies' nutritional needs as they grow. Breast-fed babies have fewer illnesses and a much lower hospitalization rate because breast milk contains maternal antibodies and immunological cells that stimulate the infant's immune system. When breast-fed babies do get sick, they recover more quickly. They are also less likely to be obese later in life than are babies fed formula, and they have fewer allergies. They may even be more intelligent: A recent study found that the longer a baby was breast-fed, the higher the IQ in adulthood.[73] Breast-feeding also has the added benefit of helping mothers lose weight after birth because the production of milk burns hundreds of calories a day. Breast-feeding also causes the hormone oxytocin to be released, which makes the uterus return to its normal size faster.

Breast milk is not the only way to nourish a baby. Some women are unable or unwilling to breast-feed; women with certain medical conditions or taking certain medications are advised not to breast-feed. Prepared formulas can provide nourishment that allows a baby to grow and thrive. Both feeding methods can supply the physical and emotional closeness essential to the parent-child relationship.

## Infant Mortality

After birth, infant death can be caused by birth defects, low birth weight, injuries, or unknown causes. In the United States, the unexpected death of a child under 1 year of age, for no apparent reason, is called **sudden infant death syndrome (SIDS)**. SIDS is responsible for about 2,500 deaths a year.[74] It is the leading cause of death for children age 1 month to 1 year and most commonly occurs in babies less than 6 months old.[75] It is not a specific disease; rather, it is ruled a cause of death after all other possibilities are ruled out. A SIDS death is sudden and silent; death occurs quickly, often during sleep, with no signs of suffering. The exact cause of SIDS is unknown, but a few risk factors are known. For example, babies placed to sleep on their stomachs are more likely to die from SIDS than those placed on their backs, as are babies who are placed on or covered by soft bedding; however, breast-feeding and avoiding exposure to tobacco smoke are known protective factors.[76]

## LO 12 | INFERTILITY

Review primary causes of and possible solutions for infertility.

An estimated 1 in 10 American couples experiences **infertility**, usually defined as the inability to conceive after trying for a year or more.[77] Although the focus is often on women, in about one third of cases, infertility is due to a cause involving only the male partner, and in another third of cases, infertility is due to causes involving both partners or an unknown origin.[78] Because of this, it is important for both partners to be medically evaluated.

**SEE IT!** VIDEOS

Looking for a new breakthrough in infertility treatment? Watch **New Pill to Help Women Get Pregnant Soon to Be Available Over the Counter** in the Study Area of MasteringHealth™

## Causes in Women

The most common cause for female infertility is *polycystic ovary syndrome (PCOS)*. A woman's ovaries have follicles, which are tiny, fluid-filled sacs that hold the eggs. When an egg is mature, the follicle breaks open to release the egg so it can travel to the fallopian tubes for fertilization. In women with PCOS, immature follicles bunch together to form large cysts or lumps. The eggs mature within the bunched follicles, but the follicles don't break open to release them. As a result, women with PCOS often don't have menstrual periods, or they have periods infrequently. Researchers estimate that 5 to 10 percent of women of childbearing age—as many as 5 million women in the United States—have PCOS.[79] Although obesity doesn't cause infertility, it is a risk factor for PCOS. It also increases the level of estrogen in the body and can cause ovulatory disorders, both of which interfere with getting pregnant.[80] In some women, the ovaries stop functioning before natural menopause, a condition called *premature ovarian failure*. Other causes of infertility include **endometriosis**. With this very painful disorder, parts of the lining of the uterus implant outside the uterus, blocking the fallopian tubes.

**Pelvic inflammatory disease (PID)** is a serious infection that scars the fallopian tubes and blocks sperm migration. Infection-causing bacteria (chlamydia or gonorrhea) can invade the fallopian tubes, causing normal tissue to turn into scar tissue. This scar tissue blocks or interrupts the normal movement of eggs into the uterus. About 1 in 10 women with PID becomes infertile, and if a woman has multiple episodes of PID, her chance of becoming infertile increases.[81]

## Causes in Men

Among men, the single largest fertility problem is **low sperm count**.[82] Although only one viable sperm is needed for fertilization, research has shown that all the other sperm in the ejaculate aid in the fertilization process. There are normally 60 to 80 million sperm per milliliter of semen. When the count drops below 20 million, fertility declines.

Low sperm count may be attributable to environmental factors

**sudden infant death syndrome (SIDS)** Sudden death of an infant under 1 year of age for no apparent reason.

**infertility** Inability to conceive after a year or more of trying.

**endometriosis** Disorder in which endometrial tissue establishes itself outside the uterus.

**pelvic inflammatory disease (PID)** Inflammation of the female genital tract that may cause scarring or blockage of the fallopian tubes, resulting in infertility.

**low sperm count** Sperm count below 20 million sperm per milliliter of semen.

(such as exposure of the scrotum to intense heat or cold, radiation, certain chemicals, or altitude), being overweight, or wearing excessively tight underwear or clothing. Other factors, such as the mumps virus, can damage the cells that make sperm, or varicocele (enlarged veins on a man's testicle) can heat the testicles and damage the sperm.[83]

## Infertility Treatments

Medical procedures can identify the cause of infertility in about 90 percent of cases.[84] Once the cause has been determined and an appropriate treatment has been instituted, the chances of becoming pregnant range from 30 to 70 percent, depending on the reason for infertility.[85]

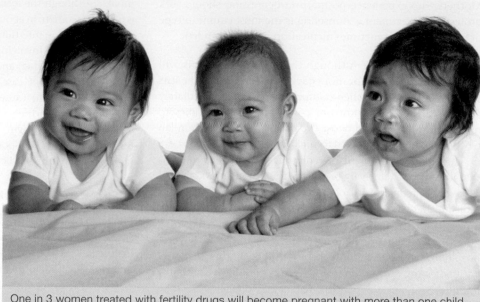

One in 3 women treated with fertility drugs will become pregnant with more than one child.

**Source:** American Society for Reproductive Medicine, "Fertility Drugs and the Risk for Multiple Births," Accessed March 2015, www.asrm.org/uploadedFiles/ASRM_Content/Resources/Patient_Resources/Fact_Sheets_and_Info _Booklets/fertilitydrugs_multiplebirths.pdf

**Fertility Drugs** Fertility drugs stimulate ovulation in women who are not ovulating. Of women who use these drugs, 60 to 80 percent will begin to ovulate; of those who ovulate, about half will conceive.[86] Fertility drugs can have many side effects, including headaches, depression, fatigue, fluid retention, and abnormal uterine bleeding. Women using fertility drugs are also at increased risk of developing multiple ovarian cysts and liver damage. The drugs sometimes trigger the release of more than one egg. As many as 1 in 3 women treated with fertility drugs will become pregnant with more than one child.[87]

**Alternative Insemination and Assisted Reproductive Technology** Another treatment option is **alternative insemination** (also known as *artificial insemination*) of a woman with her partner's sperm. The couple may also choose insemination by an anonymous donor through a sperm bank. Donated sperm are medically screened, classified according to the donor's physical characteristics (such as hair and eye color), and then frozen for future use.

Assisted reproductive technology (ART) includes several different medical procedures. The most common is **in vitro fertilization (IVF)**. During IVF, eggs and sperm are mixed in a laboratory dish to fertilize, and some of the fertilized eggs (zygotes) are then transferred to the woman's uterus.

**alternative insemination** Fertilization procedure accomplished by depositing semen from a partner or donor into a woman's vagina via a thin tube.

**in vitro fertilization (IVF)** Fertilization of an egg in a nutrient medium and subsequent transfer back to the mother's body.

## Surrogate Motherhood

Infertile couples who still cannot conceive after treatment may choose to live without children, or they may decide to pursue surrogate motherhood or adoption. With surrogacy, a woman is hired to carry another person's pregnancy to term, at which point the intended parents gain custody. In traditional surrogacy, the gestational carrier is also the biological mother of the child. In gestational surrogacy, the surrogate is not the biological mother; instead an embryo is created via IVF using the couple's own (or donor) egg and sperm. In the United States, an estimated 750 children a year are born via surrogates.[88]

## Adoption

Adoption provides a way for individuals and couples who may not be able to have a biological child to form a legal parental relationship with a child who needs a home. As such, it benefits children whose birth parents are unable or unwilling to raise them and provides adults who are unable to conceive or carry a pregnancy to term a means to create a family. Approximately 2 percent of U.S. children are adopted.[89]

There are two types of adoption: *confidential* and *open*. In confidential adoption, the birth parents and the adoptive parents never know each other. Adoptive parents are given only basic information about the birth parents, such as medical background that they need to care for the child. In open adoption, birth parents and adoptive parents know some information about each other. There are different levels of openness. Both parties must agree to this plan, and it is not available in every state.

Increasingly, couples are choosing to adopt children from other countries. In 2013, U.S. families adopted more than 5,000 foreign-born children.[90] The cost of overseas adoption varies widely, but can cost more than $30,000, including agency fees, dossier and immigration-processing fees, travel, and court costs.[91] Some families find it beneficial to serve as foster parents prior to deciding to adopt, and others choose to adopt older children from the foster system in the United States rather than wait for an infant placed through international adoption.

## Are You Comfortable with Your Contraception?

These questions will help you assess whether your current method of contraception or one you may consider using in the future will be effective for you. Answering yes to any of these questions predicts potential problems. If you have more than a few yes responses, consider talking to a health care provider, counselor, partner, or friend to decide whether to use this method or how to use it so that it will really be effective.

Method of contraception you use now or are considering:

_____

|   | | Yes | No |
|---|---|---|---|
| 1. | Have I or my partner ever become pregnant while using this method? | Y | N |
| 2. | Am I afraid of using this method? | Y | N |
| 3. | Would I really rather not use this method? | Y | N |
| 4. | Will I have trouble remembering to use this method? | Y | N |
| 5. | Will I have trouble using this method correctly? | Y | N |
| 6. | Does this method make menstrual periods longer or more painful for me or my partner? | Y | N |
| 7. | Does this method cost more than I can afford? | Y | N |
| 8. | Could this method cause serious complications? | Y | N |
| 9. | Am I, or is my partner, opposed to this method because of any religious or moral beliefs? | Y | N |
| 10. | Will using this method embarrass me or my partner? | Y | N |
| 11. | Will I enjoy intercourse less because of this method? | Y | N |
| 12. | Am I at risk of being exposed to HIV or other sexually transmitted infections if I use this method? | Y | N |

Total number of yes answers: _____

**Source:** Adapted from R. A. Hatcher et al., *Contraceptive Technology*, 19th revised ed. Copyright © 2007. Reprinted by permission of Ardent Media, Inc.

## YOUR PLAN FOR CHANGE

The **ASSESS YOURSELF** activity gave you the chance to assess your comfort and confidence with a contraceptive method you are using now or may use in the future. Depending on the results of the assessment, you may consider changing your birth control method.

**TODAY,** YOU CAN:

☐ Visit your local drugstore and study the forms of contraception that are available without a prescription. Think about those you would consider using and why.

☐ If you are not currently using any contraception or are not in a sexual relationship now, but might be in the future, purchase a package of condoms (or pick up free samples from your campus health center) to keep on hand just in case.

**WITHIN THE NEXT TWO WEEKS,** YOU CAN:

☐ Make an appointment for a checkup with your health care provider. Be sure to ask him or her any questions you have about contraception.

☐ Sit down with your partner and discuss contraception. Talk about how your current method is working for both of you, if the effectiveness level of the method you are using is high enough, and if you aren't using birth control consistently, what you can do together to improve.

**BY THE END OF THE SEMESTER,** YOU CAN:

☐ Periodically reevaluate whether your new or continued contraception is still effective for you. Review your experiences, and take note of any consistent problems you may have encountered.

☐ Always keep a backup form of contraception on hand. Check this supply periodically and throw out and replace any supplies that have expired.

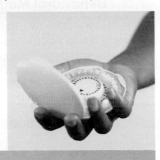

## CHAPTER REVIEW

To hear an MP3 Tutor Session, scan here or visit the Study Area in **MasteringHealth**.

### LO 1 | Basic Principles of Birth Control

- Contraception, commonly called birth control, prevents conception, the fertilization of an egg by sperm. Types of contraception include barrier, hormonal, intrauterine, behavioral, and permanent methods.

### LO 2 | Barrier Methods

- Latex, polyurethane, or polyisoprene male condoms and nitrile female condoms, when used correctly for oral sex or intercourse, provide the most effective protection of preventing sexually transmitted infections (STIs) and HIV. Other barrier contraceptive methods include spermicides, the diaphragm, the cervical cap, and the contraceptive sponge.

### LO 3 | Hormonal Methods

- Oral contraceptives, Xulane, NuvaRing, Depo-Provera, and Nexplanon are examples of hormonal contraceptives containing synthetic estrogen and/or progestin.

### LO 4 | Intrauterine Contraceptives

- Intrauterine devices are small devices that can be placed in the uterus through the cervix and provide contraception for 3 to 12 years.

### LO 5 | Behavioral Methods

- Fertility awareness methods rely on altering sexual practices to avoid pregnancy, as do abstinence, outercourse, and withdrawal.

### LO 6 | Emergency Contraception

- Emergency contraception may be used up to 5 days after unprotected intercourse or the failure of another contraceptive method.

### LO 7 | Permanent Methods

- While most methods of contraception are reversible, sterilization should be considered permanent.

### LO 8 | Choosing a Method of Contraception

- Choosing a method of contraception involves taking time to research the various options, asking questions of your health care provider, being honest with yourself, and having open conversations with potential partners.

### LO 9 | Abortion

- Abortion is legal in the United States, but strongly opposed by many Americans. Abortion methods include suction curettage, dilation and evacuation (D&E), and medical abortions.

### LO 10 | Pregnancy

- Prospective parents must consider emotional health, maternal and paternal health, and financial resources. Full-term pregnancy has three trimesters. Prenatal care includes a complete physical exam within the first trimester, follow-up checkups throughout the pregnancy, healthy nutrition and exercise, and avoidance of all substances that could have teratogenic effects on the fetus. Prenatal tests, including ultrasonography, chorionic villus sampling, triple marker screen, and amniocentesis, can be used to detect birth defects.

### LO 11 | Childbirth

- Childbirth occurs in three stages. Partners should jointly choose a labor method early in the pregnancy to be better prepared when labor occurs. Possible complications of pregnancy and childbirth include preeclampsia and eclampsia, miscarriage, ectopic pregnancy, and stillbirth.

### LO 12 | Infertility

- Infertility in women may be caused by polycystic ovary syndrome (PCOS), pelvic inflammatory disease (PID), or endometriosis. In men, it may be caused by low sperm count. Treatments may include fertility drugs, alternative insemination, in vitro fertilization (IVF), assisted reproductive technology (ART), embryo transfer, and embryo adoption programs. Surrogate motherhood and adoption are also options.

## POP QUIZ

Visit **MasteringHealth** to personalize your study plan with Chapter Review Quizzes and Dynamic Study Modules.

### LO 1 | Basic Principles of Birth Control

1. What is meant by the *failure rate* of contraceptive use?
   a. The number of times a woman fails to get pregnant when she wanted to
   b. The number of times a woman gets pregnant when she did not want to
   c. The number of pregnancies that occur in women using a particular method of birth control
   d. The number of times a couple fails to use birth control

### LO 2 | Barrier Methods

2. Which type of lubricant could you safely use with a latex condom?
   a. Coconut oil
   b. Water-based lubricant
   c. Body lotion
   d. Petroleum jelly

### LO 3 | Hormonal Methods

3. Hormonal birth control methods contain estrogen and/or
   a. oxytocin.
   b. testosterone.
   c. cortisol.
   d. progestin.

## LO 4 | Intrauterine Contraceptives

1. An IUD is placed in a woman's
   a. fallopian tube.
   b. ovary.
   c. uterus.
   d. vagina.

## LO 5 | Behavioral Methods

5. Mariana and David want to practice a method of avoiding pregnancy that is 100 percent effective. What method would you recommend?
   a. abstinence
   b. calendar method
   c. NuvaRing
   d. condoms

## LO 6 | Emergency Contraception

6. Emergency contraception is up to 88 percent effective when used within how many days of unprotected intercourse?
   a. 1
   b. 2–5
   c. 5–7
   d. 7–14

## LO 7 | Permanent Methods

7. Benjamin wants to be sterilized. The male sterilization process his health care provider will perform is called
   a. suction curettage.
   b. tubal ligation.
   c. hysterectomy.
   d. vasectomy.

## LO 8 | Choosing a Method of Contraception

8. Emily wants to use a contraception method that also protects against STIs. Her best option is
   a. Xulane.
   b. condoms.
   c. a contraceptive sponge.
   d. an IUD.

## LO 9 | Abortion

9. What is the most commonly used method of first-trimester abortion?
   a. Suction curettage
   b. Dilation and evacuation (D&E)
   c. Medical abortion
   d. Induction abortion

## LO 10 | Pregnancy

10. What is the recommended pregnancy weight gain for a woman who is at a healthy weight before pregnancy?
    a. 15 to 20 pounds
    b. 20 to 30 pounds
    c. 25 to 35 pounds
    d. 30 to 45 pounds

## LO 11 | Childbirth

11. In an ectopic pregnancy, the fertilized egg implants in the woman's
    a. fallopian tube.
    b. uterus.
    c. vagina.
    d. ovaries.

## LO 12 | Infertility

12. The number of American couples who experience infertility is
    a. 1 in 10.
    b. 1 in 24.
    c. 1 in 60.
    d. 1 in 100.

*Answers to the Pop Quiz can be found on page A-1. If you answered a question incorrectly, review the section identified by the Learning Outcome. For even more study tools, visit MasteringHealth.*

# THINK ABOUT IT!

## LO 1 | Basic Principles of Birth Control

1. How, in general, do contraceptives work? What is the difference between *perfect use* and typical-use failure rates? Which do you think is a better predictor of effectiveness?

## LO 2 | Barrier Methods

2. What are the options for barrier birth control methods? What are their major advantages and disadvantages?

## LO 3 | Hormonal Methods

3. What benefits can hormonal methods of birth control provide beyond preventing pregnancy? How could a person go about deciding which of the many hormonal methods to try?

## LO 4 | Intrauterine Contraceptives

4. How quickly does fertility return after the removal of an IUD? Can women who have not yet had a child use an IUD? What are some benefits of not having to think about birth control for 3–12 years?

## LO 5 | Behavioral Methods

5. Do your religious views impact your sexual behavior or choice of birth control methods? If so, how do they impact your family planning decisions?

## LO 6 | Emergency Contraception

6. Can you imagine using ECPs if you had a contraceptive failure? What do you think about ECPs being available to people of all ages without a prescription?

## LO 7 | Permanent Methods

7. Do you think there should an age limit on surgical methods so people don't give up their fertility too early? How do you think you will decide when you done having children?

## LO 8 | Choosing a Method of Contraception

8. List the most effective contraceptive methods. What are their drawbacks? What medical conditions would keep a person from using each one? Which methods do you think would be most effective for you? Why?

## LO 9 | Abortion

9. What are the various methods of abortion? What are the two opposing viewpoints concerning abortion? What is *Roe v. Wade,* and what impact has it had on the abortion debate in the United States?

## LO 10 | Pregnancy

10. Discuss the growth of the fetus through the three trimesters. What medical checkups or tests should be done during each trimester?

## LO 11 | Childbirth

11. What are some of the complications that can occur during pregnancy and childbirth? What actions can we take to prevent these complications?

## LO 12 | Infertility

12. If you and your partner are unable to have children, what alternative methods of conception would you consider? Would you consider adoption?

## ACCESS YOUR HEALTH ON THE INTERNET

Use the following websites to further explore topics and issues related to reproductive health. For links to the websites below, visit **MasteringHealth**.

*Guttmacher Institute.* This is a nonprofit organization focused on sexual and reproductive health research, policy analysis, and public education. **www.guttmacher.org**

*Association of Reproductive Health Professionals.* This organization was originally founded by Alan Guttmacher as the educational arm of Planned Parenthood. Now an independent organization, it provides education for health care professionals and the general public. The *Patient Resources* portion of the website includes information on various methods of birth control and an interactive tool to help you choose a method that will work for you. **www.arhp.org**

*Planned Parenthood.* This site offers a range of up-to-date information on sexual health issues, such as birth control, the decision of when and whether to have a child, sexually transmitted infections, abortion, and safer sex. **www.plannedparenthood.org**

*Bedsider.* This easy to read and humorous website offers up-to-date and thorough information on contraceptives. **www.bedsider.org**

*The American Pregnancy Association.* This is a national organization offering a wealth of resources to promote reproductive and pregnancy wellness. The website includes educational materials and information on the latest research. **www.americanpregnancy.org**

*Sexuality Information and Education Council of the United States.* Information, guidelines, and materials for the advancement of sexuality education are all found here. The site advocates the right of individuals to make responsible sexual choices. **www.siecus.org**

*International Council on Infertility Information Dissemination.* This site includes current research and information on infertility. **www.inciid.org**

# 7 Recognizing and Avoiding Addiction and Drug Abuse

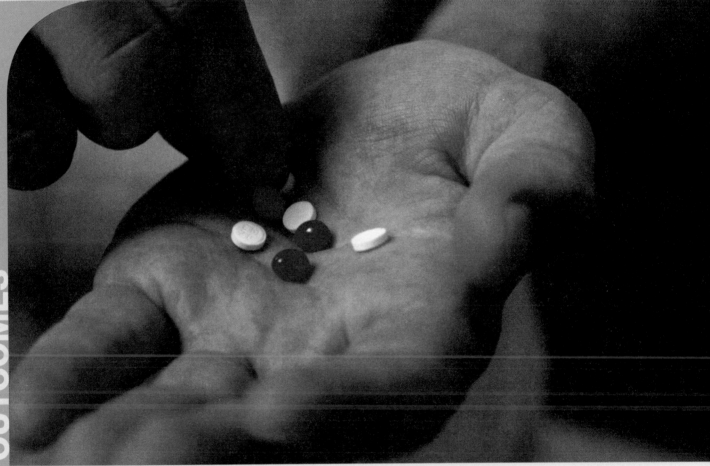

## LEARNING OUTCOMES

1 Identify the symptoms of addiction, explain the difference between addiction and habit, and discuss the impact of addiction on friends and family.

2 Describe types of process addictions, such as gambling disorder, exercise addiction, technology addictions, and compulsive buying disorder.

3 Identify the six categories of drugs and distinguish between drug misuse and drug abuse.

4 Discuss the issues of drug misuse and abuse in the United States, including the misuse and abuse of over-the-counter drugs and prescription drugs, the prevalence of drug use on college campuses, and risk factors for drug abuse.

5 Discuss the use and abuse of stimulants, cannabis, narcotics, depressants, hallucinogens, inhalants, and anabolic steroids.

6 Discuss treatment and recovery options for addicts, and discuss public health approaches to preventing drug abuse and reducing the impact of addiction on our society.

These days it's easy to find high-profile cases of compulsive and destructive behavior. Stories of celebrities and politicians struggling with addictions to alcohol, drugs, gambling, and sex are splashed in the headlines and profiled on television news programs. But millions of everyday people throughout the world are staging their own battles with addiction as well. In this chapter, we will examine addictions to common activities such as eating, gambling, and shopping, as well as specific drugs that are addictive and commonly abused. (Alcohol and tobacco are discussed in detail in Chapter 8.)

## LO 1 | WHAT IS ADDICTION?

Identify the symptoms of addiction, explain the difference between addiction and habit, and discuss the impact of addiction on friends and family.

**Addiction** is defined as continued involvement with a substance or activity despite its ongoing negative consequences. It is classified by the American Psychiatric Association (APA) as a mental disorder. Addictive behaviors initially provide a sense of pleasure or stability that is difficult for some individuals to achieve in other ways. Once they feel that unusual "high," they often seek that feeling again and again. Eventually, the individual needs to consume the addictive substance or enact the behavior to feel normal.

To be addictive, a substance or behavior must have the potential to produce positive mood changes, such as euphoria, anxiety reduction, or pain reduction. The danger develops when people come to depend on these substances or behaviors to feel normal or function on a daily basis. Signs of addiction become apparent when people continue to use the substance despite knowing the harm that it causes to themselves and others.

People with **physiological dependence** to a substance, such as an addictive drug, experience **tolerance** when increased amounts of the drug are required to achieve the desired effect. They also experience **withdrawal,** a series of temporary physical and psychological symptoms that occurs when substance use stops. Tolerance and withdrawal are important criteria for determining whether or not someone is addicted.

**Psychological dependence** can also play an important role in addiction, which explains why behaviors not related to the use of drugs, such as gambling or shopping, can lead to

**addiction** Continued involvement with a substance or activity despite ongoing negative consequences.

**physiological dependence** The adaptive state of brain and body processes that occurs with regular addictive behavior and results in withdrawal if the addictive behavior stops.

**tolerance** Phenomenon in which progressively larger doses of a drug or more intense involvement in a behavior are needed to produce the desired effects.

**withdrawal** A series of temporary physical and psychological symptoms that occur when an addict abruptly abstains from an addictive chemical or behavior.

**psychological dependence** Dependency of the mind on a substance or behavior, which can lead to psychological withdrawal symptoms, such as anxiety, irritability, or cravings.

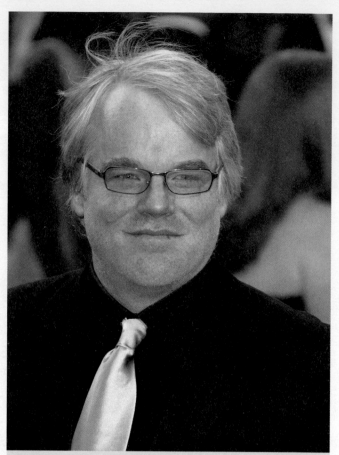

Addiction affects all kinds of people. Academy Award–winning actor Philip Seymour Hoffman, widely respected for his work, was found dead in his New York apartment with a needle in his arm. A mix of cocaine, heroin, and other drugs ultimately proved fatal.

dependence and addiction. Some researchers believe that compulsive behaviors, such as overeating, overexercising, and gambling, may produce the same feelings of euphoria as an addictive drug, along with a strong desire to repeat the behavior and a craving for the behavior when it stops. In fact, psychological and physiological dependence are so intertwined that it is not really possible to separate the two. Although the mechanism is not well understood, all forms of addiction probably reflect dysfunction of certain biochemical systems in the brain.[1]

## The Process of Addiction

Our brains are wired to ensure that we will repeat life-sustaining activities by associating those activities with reward or pleasure. We all engage in potentially addictive behaviors to some extent because some behaviors that are

**HEAR IT!** PODCASTS

Want a study podcast for this chapter? Download **Licit and Illicit Drugs: Use, Misuse, and Abuse,** available on MasteringHealth™

essential to our survival are also highly reinforcing, such as eating, drinking, and sex. At some point along the continuum, however, some individuals are not able to engage in these behaviors moderately, and they become addicted.

Addiction has five common characteristics: (1) **compulsion,** which is characterized by **obsession,** or excessive preoccupation, with the behavior and an overwhelming need to perform it; (2) **loss of control,** or the inability to predict reliably whether any isolated occurrence of the behavior will be healthy or damaging; (3) **negative consequences,** such as physical damage, legal trouble, financial problems, academic failure, or family dissolution, which do not occur with healthy involvement in any behavior; (4) **denial,** the inability to perceive that the behavior is self-destructive; and (5) **inability to abstain.** These five components are present in all addictions, whether chemical or behavioral.[2]

Addiction is a process that evolves over time. It begins when a person repeatedly seeks the illusion of relief to avoid unpleasant feelings or situations. This pattern is known as *nurturing through avoidance* and is a maladaptive way of taking care of emotional needs. As a person increasingly depends on the addictive behavior, there is a corresponding deterioration in relationships with family, friends, and coworkers; in performance at work or school; and in personal life. Eventually, addicts do not find the addictive behavior pleasurable but consider it preferable to the unhappy realities they are seeking to escape. **FIGURE 7.1** illustrates the cycle of psychological addiction. Later in the chapter, we'll discuss the physiological processes involved in addiction.

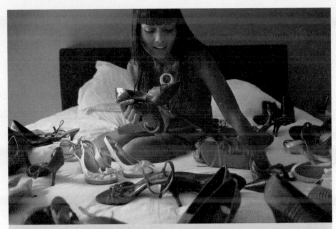

Once a person recognizes and decides to change a habit, it can usually be broken. With an addiction, however, the sense of compulsion is so strong that the behavior can't be controlled. For example, you may like to shop or spend time online hunting for bargains, but it isn't considered an addiction unless you have lost control over where and when you shop, and how much you spend.

## Habit versus Addiction

How do we distinguish between a harmless habit and an addiction? Addiction involves elements of **habit,** a repeated behavior in which the repetition may be unconscious. A habit can be annoying, but it can be broken without too much discomfort by becoming aware of its presence and choosing not to do it. Addiction also involves repetition of a behavior, but the repetition occurs by compulsion, and considerable discomfort is experienced if the behavior is not performed.

To understand addiction, we must look beyond the amount and frequency of the behavior. What happens when a person is involved in the behavior is far more meaningful than the time spent doing it. For example, someone who drinks only rarely and then engages in a night of heavy drinking may experience personality changes, blackouts (drug-induced amnesia), and other negative consequences (e.g., failing a test, missing appointments, getting into a fight) that would never have occurred otherwise. On the other hand, someone who has a few martinis every evening may never do anything out of character while under the influence of alcohol

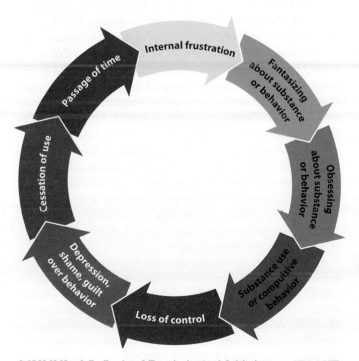

**FIGURE 7.1** Cycle of Psychological Addiction

**Source:** Adapted from Recovery Connection, Cycle of Addiction, 2012, www .recoveryconnection.org/cycle-of-addiction.

 **VIDEO TUTOR** Addiction Cycle

**compulsion** Preoccupation with a behavior and an overwhelming need to perform it.

**obsession** Excessive preoccupation with an addictive substance or behavior.

**loss of control** Inability to predict reliably whether a particular instance of involvement with an addictive substance or behavior will be healthy or damaging.

**negative consequences** Physical damage, legal trouble, financial ruin, academic failure, family dissolution, and other severe problems that do not occur with healthy involvement in any behavior.

**denial** Inability to perceive or accurately interpret the self-destructive effects of an addictive behavior.

**inability to abstain** Failure to avoid drug use over a sustained period of time.

**habit** A repeated behavior in which the repetition may be unconscious.

**codependence** A self-defeating relationship pattern in which a person helps or encourages addictive behavior in another.

**enabler** A person who knowingly or unknowingly protects an addict from the consequences of the addict's behavior.

**process addiction** A condition in which a person is dependent on (addicted to) some mood-altering behavior or process, such as gambling, buying, or exercise.

**gambling disorder** A set of behaviors including preoccupation with gambling, unsuccessful efforts to cut back or quit, using gambling to escape problems, and lying to family members to conceal the extent of involvement with gambling.

but may become irritable, manipulative, and aggressive without those regular drinks. Alcohol appears to perform a function (mood control) for both of these people that they should be able to perform for themselves, without the aid of chemicals. Needing a chemical to perform a normal function is a possible sign of addiction.

## Addiction Affects Family and Friends

The family and friends of an addicted person also suffer many negative consequences. Often they struggle with **codependence,** a self-defeating relationship pattern in which a person is controlled by an addict's addictive behavior.

Addicts can actually influence the development of a form of codependency in those around them. Codependency is the addiction to a supportive role in a relationship. A codependent person will often put his or her needs aside to take care of the addict. They find it hard to set healthy boundaries and often live in a chaotic, crisis-oriented mode.

Family and friends can play an important role in getting an addict to seek treatment. They are most helpful when they refuse to be enablers. **Enablers** are people who knowingly or unknowingly protect addicts from the natural consequences of their behavior. If they don't have to deal with the consequences, addicts cannot see the self-destructive nature of their behavior and will therefore continue it. Enabling is rarely conscious or intentional.

### WHAT DO YOU THINK?

Why might friends and family members become enablers and codependents of people engaging in destructive behaviors?

- Have you ever confronted someone you were concerned about? If so, was the confrontation successful?
- What tips would you give someone who wants to confront a loved one about an addiction?

## LO 2 | ADDICTIVE BEHAVIORS

Describe types of process addictions, such as gambling disorder, exercise addiction, technology addictions, and compulsive buying disorder.

The chemicals in drugs are not the only sources of addiction. People can form equally destructive addictions to certain behaviors. A **process addiction** is driven by the pathological pursuit of a reward or relief by an individual. Research about the brain's reward system suggests that, to the brain, a reward is a reward, meaning behaviors can be as addictive as drugs or other substances.[3] The altered or elevated mood is pleasurable to the addict, and he or she learns over time that a certain pattern of behavior leads to that pleasurable feeling. An addict feels a severe compulsion to engage in an activity repeatedly, even at the expense of physical, mental, relational, or financial well-being. Examples of process addictions include gambling disorder, compulsive buying disorder, exercise addiction, and technology addictions.

## Gambling Disorder

Gambling is a form of recreation and entertainment for millions of Americans. Most people who gamble do so casually and moderately to experience the excitement of anticipating a win. In the United States, between 6 and 8 million people meet the criteria for having a gambling addiction; still many others are directly or indirectly impacted by the gambling behavior of friends or relatives.[4] The APA, which previously used the term *pathological gambling,* now uses the term **gambling disorder** and recognizes it as an addictive disorder. According to the APA's *Diagnostic and Statistical Manual of Mental Disorders,* 5th edition (*DSM-5*), characteristic behaviors associated with gambling disorder include a preoccupation with gambling, unsuccessful efforts to cut back or quit, gambling when feeling distressed, and lying to family members to conceal the extent of gambling.[5]

There is strong evidence that disordered gambling has a biological component. A study of individuals with gambling disorder found the participants to have decreased blood flow to a key section of the brain's reward system.[6] It is thought that individuals with gambling disorder, like people who abuse drugs, compensate for this deficiency in their brain's reward system by overdoing it and getting hooked.[7] Most individuals with a gambling disorder seek excitement even more than money. They place increasingly larger bets to obtain the desired level of excitement. Like drug addicts, they live from fix to fix. Their subjective cravings can be as intense as those of drug abusers; they show tolerance in their need to increase the amount of their bets; and they experience highs rivaling those brought on by drugs. Up to half of those with gambling disorder show withdrawal symptoms similar to those of a mild form of drug withdrawal, including sleep disturbance, sweating, irritability, and craving.

Legal gambling age can vary by state and often depends on the type of gambling. For example, in Wisconsin you can gamble at age 18 regardless of the type of gambling you choose, while in New York can bet on horses at 18, but you must be 21 years of age to gamble in a casino.

Over the years, college students have gained easier access to gambling opportunities than ever before. The percentage of college students who gamble—about 75 percent (legally or illegally)—is consistent with these growing opportunities. About 18 percent of those students reported gambling once a week or more.[8] Regardless, with the advent of online gambling, televised poker tournaments, and a growing number of casinos, scratch tickets, lotteries, and sports-betting networks, there are many opportunities for college students to gamble. Students at most risk for problem gambling are males, African American, and those with lower socioeconomic status. It is estimated that

6 percent of college students in the United States have a serious gambling problem that can result in psychological difficulties, debt, and failing grades.[9]

## Compulsive Buying Disorder

In the United States today, many people use shopping as a way to make themselves feel better. But people who regularly engage in "retail therapy" in excess, running credit cards to the limit, may have **compulsive buying disorder.** Compulsive buyers are preoccupied with shopping and spending and exercise little control over their impulses to buy. Compulsive buying is estimated to afflict up to 5 percent of adults.[10] The vast majority of compulsive buyers are women.

Compulsive buying has many of the same characteristics as alcoholism, gambling, and other addictions. Symptoms that signal that a person has crossed the line into compulsive buying include preoccupation with shopping and spending, buying more than one of the same item, shopping for longer periods than intended, repeatedly buying much more than he or she needs or can afford, and buying to the point that it interferes with social activities or work and creates financial problems (e.g., indebtedness or bankruptcy). Compulsive buying frequently results in psychological distress, such as depression and feelings of guilt, as well as conflict with friends and between couples.[11]

## Exercise Addiction

Generally speaking, most Americans get too little physical activity, not too much. But exercise, when taken to extremes, can become addictive because of its powerful mood-enhancing effects. One indication of exercise addiction's prevalence is that a large portion of Americans with the eating disorders anorexia nervosa and bulimia nervosa use exercise to purge instead of, or in addition to, self-induced vomiting.[12] **Exercise addicts** use exercise compulsively to try to meet needs—for nurturance, intimacy, self-esteem, and self-competency—that an object or activity cannot truly meet. Consequently, addictive or compulsive exercise results in negative consequences similar to those found in other addictions: alienation of family and friends, injuries from overdoing it, and a craving for more. Warning signs of exercise addiction include only exercising by yourself; adhering to a rigid workout plan; working out longer than 2 hours daily, repeatedly; exercising through illness or injury; becoming fixated on burning calories or losing weight; cancelling social plans, skipping work or missing class to exercise; or working out beyond the point of pain.[13]

**SEE IT! VIDEOS**

How do you battle compulsive shopping? Watch **Woman's Shopping Addiction Revealed,** available on **MasteringHealth™**

### WHY SHOULD I CARE?

Addictions of any kind limit your ability to make good decisions and maintain your focus, making it hard for you to meet your full potential as a student and as a member of the community. A seemingly harmless habit may actually be progressing into an addiction that prevents you from attending classes, meeting new people, or participating in other activities that you might find enjoyable.

## Technology Addictions

Have you ever opened your Web browser to quickly check something and an hour later found yourself still checking your Facebook page? Do you have friends who seem more concerned with texting or surfing the Internet than with eating, going out, studying, or having a face-to-face conversation? These attitudes and behaviors are not unusual; many experts suggest that technology addiction is real and can present serious problems for those addicted. An estimated 1 in 8 Internet users will likely experience **internet addiction.**[14] Younger people are more likely to be addicted to the Internet than are middle-aged users.[15] Approximately 12 percent of college students report that Internet use and computer games have interfered with their academic performance.[16] To read about the experiences of students taking part in an "unplug from technology day," see the **Tech & Health** box on the next page.

Some online activities, such as gaming and cybersex, seem to be more compelling and potentially addictive than others. Internet addicts typically exhibit symptoms such as general disregard for their health, sleep deprivation, neglecting family and friends, lack of physical activity, euphoria when online, lower grades in school, and poor job performance. Internet addicts may feel moody or uncomfortable when they are not online. They may be using their behavior to compensate for loneliness, marital or work problems, a poor social life, or financial problems.

While process addictions are becoming more commonly recognized in society, drug addiction still garners most of the public attention.

**compulsive buying disorder** A preoccupation with shopping and spending accompanied by little control over the impulse to buy.

**exercise addict** A person who always works out alone, following the same rigid pattern; exercises for more than 2 hours daily, repeatedly, and when sick or injured; focuses on weight loss or calories burned; exercises to the point of pain and beyond; and skips work, class, or social activities for workouts.

**Internet addiction** Compulsive use of the computer, PDA, cell phone, or other form of technology to access the Internet for activities such as e-mail, games, shopping, and blogging.

**drugs** Nonfood, nonnutritional substances that are intended to affect the structure or function of the mind or body through chemical action.

## LO 3 | WHAT IS A DRUG?

Identify the six categories of drugs and distinguish between drug misuse and drug abuse.

**Drugs** are substances other than food that are intended to affect the structure or function of the mind or the body through chemical action. Many drugs have large benefits; however, the potential for addiction is great for even the most therapeutic substances due to their potent effects on the brain.

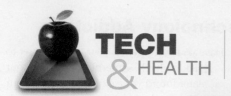

# TECH & HEALTH

# MOBILE DEVICES, MEDIA, AND THE INTERNET *Could You Unplug?*

If someone asked you to give up your mobile devices, media, and the Internet for 24 hours, how hard would it be? Judging from the results of a study with participants hailing from 37 different countries on six continents—extremely hard! All students followed the same assignment: give up Internet, newspapers, magazines, TV, radio, phones, iPods/MP3 players, movies, Facebook, chat, Twitter, video games, and any other form of electronic or social media for 24 hours.

Students around the world repeatedly used the term addiction to speak about their dependence on media and likened their reactions to feelings of a drug withdrawal. "Media is my drug; without it I was lost," said one student from the UK. A student from the United States noted: "I was itching, like a crackhead, because I could not use my phone." A student from Argentina observed: *"Sometimes I felt 'dead,'"* and a student from Slovakia simply noted: *"I felt sad, lonely, and depressed."*

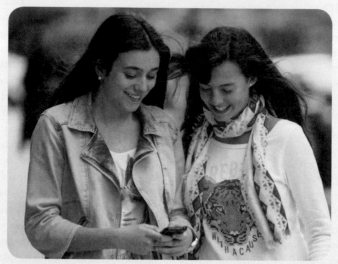

**As the world goes wireless, many of us are increasingly attached to our cell phones, laptops, and tablet computers.**

Students also reported that media—especially their mobile phones—have virtually become an extension of themselves. Going without media, therefore, made it seem like they had lost part of themselves.

Despite the withdrawal symptoms, many students found there were definite benefits to being unplugged for 24 hours. Some students found they had more time to talk, listen, and share with others. Students also reported feeling liberated. They took time to do things they normally would not do, such as visiting relatives, playing board games, or having face-to-face conversations.

How do you "unplug" from texting and Twitter for 24 hours (or more) without the anxiety of ignoring your friends online? Smartphone and computer apps can actually help! Available apps can post automatic status updates to Facebook and Twitter, send you reminders before scheduled technology breaks, or temporarily lock out your access to the Internet for a set interval. Here are a few suggested apps:

- **Off time.** http://Offtime.co//
- **Unplug and Reconnect.** (Free: Android) www.unplugreconnect.com
- **Unplug** www.weareunplugged.com

**Source:** Adapted from The World Unplugged, "Going 24 Hours Without Media," 2011, http://theworldunplugged.wordpress.com

---

**Drug misuse** involves using a drug for a purpose for which it was not intended. For example, taking a friend's high-powered prescription painkiller for your headache is a misuse of that drug. This is not too far removed from **drug abuse,** or the excessive use of any drug, and may cause serious harm.

Drug misuse and abuse are problems of staggering proportions in our society. Approximately 9 percent of Americans report being current (defined as use during the past month) users of illicit drugs.[17] By senior year in high school, 49 percent of Americans report having used illicit drugs in their lifetime.[18] Approximately 14 percent of high school students have taken prescription drugs without a doctor's supervision.[19]

Recently, the overall rate of drug use in the United States rose to its highest level in almost a decade, mostly driven by an increase in the use of marijuana.[20] Drug abuse costs taxpayers more than $193 billion annually in health care costs, public costs related to crime, and lost productivity.[21] It's impossible to put a dollar amount on the pain, suffering, and dysfunction that drugs cause in our everyday lives.

## How Drugs Affect the Brain

Pleasure, which scientists call *reward,* is a powerful biological force for survival. If you do something that feels pleasurable, the brain is wired in such a way that you tend to want to do it again. Life-sustaining activities, such as eating, activate a circuit of specialized nerve cells devoted to producing and regulating pleasure. One important set of these nerve cells, which uses a chemical **neurotransmitter** called *dopamine,* sits at the

**drug misuse** Use of a drug for a purpose for which it was not intended.

**drug abuse** Excessive use of a drug.

**neurotransmitter** A chemical that relays messages between nerve cells or from nerve cells to other body cells.

very top of the brain stem. These dopamine-containing neurons relay messages about pleasure through their nerve fibers to nerve cells in the limbic system, structures in the brain regulating emotions. Still other fibers connect to a related part of the frontal region of the cerebral cortex, the area of the brain that plays a key role in memory, perception, thought, and consciousness. Thus, this "pleasure circuit," known as the *mesolimbic dopamine system*, spans the survival-oriented brain stem, the emotional limbic system, and the thinking frontal cerebral cortex.

All drugs that are addicting—in fact, all addictive substances and behaviors—can activate the brain's pleasure circuit. Drug addiction is a biological, pathological process that alters the way in which the pleasure center, as well as other parts of the brain, functions. Almost all **psychoactive drugs** (those that change the way the brain works) do so by affecting chemical neurotransmission by enhancing it, suppressing it, or interfering with it. Some drugs, such as heroin and LSD, mimic the effects of a natural neurotransmitter. Others, such as PCP, block receptors and thereby prevent neuronal messages from getting through. Still others, such as cocaine, block the *reuptake* of neurotransmitters by neurons, thus increasing the concentration of the neurotransmitters in the synaptic gap, the space between individual neurons (**FIGURE 7.2**). Finally, some drugs, such as methamphetamine, cause neurotransmitters to be released in greater amounts than is normal.

## Routes of Drug Administration

*Route of administration* refers to the way in which a given drug is taken into the body. The most common method is by swallowing a tablet, capsule, or liquid (**oral ingestion**). Drugs taken in this manner don't reach the bloodstream as quickly as do drugs introduced to the body by other means. A drug taken orally may not reach the bloodstream for as long as 30 minutes.

Drugs can also enter the body through the respiratory tract via sniffing, snorting, smoking, or inhaling (**inhalation**). Drugs that are inhaled and absorbed by the lungs travel the most rapidly compared to all the routes of drug administration.

Another rapid form of drug administration is by **injection** directly into the bloodstream (intravenously), muscles (intramuscularly), or just under the skin (subcutaneously). Intravenous injection, which involves inserting a hypodermic needle directly into a vein, is the most common method of injection for drug users owing to the rapid speed (within seconds in most cases) with which a drug's effect is felt. It is also the most dangerous method of administration

**psychoactive drugs** Drugs that affect brain chemistry and have the potential to alter mood or behavior.

**oral ingestion** Intake of drugs through the mouth.

**inhalation** The introduction of drugs through the respiratory tract.

**injection** The introduction of drugs into the body via a hypodermic needle.

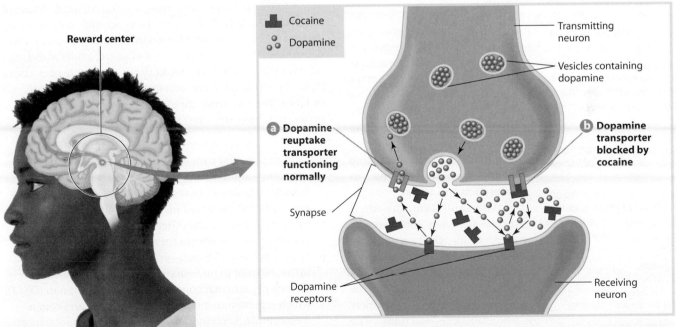

**FIGURE 7.2** The Action of Cocaine at Dopamine Receptors in the Brain

(a) In normal neural communication, dopamine is released into the synapse between neurons. It binds temporarily to dopamine receptors on the receiving neuron and then is recycled back into the transmitting neuron by a transporter. (b) When cocaine molecules are present, they attach to the dopamine transporter and block the recycling process. Excess dopamine remains active in the synaptic gaps between neurons, creating feelings of excitement and euphoria.

→ **VIDEO TUTOR**
Psychoactive Drugs
Acting on the Brain

**Source:** Adapted from *NIDA Research Report—Cocaine Abuse and Addiction*, NIH Publication no. 10-4166, (Bethesda, MD: National Institute of Drug Addiction Rev. 2010), Available at, www.drugabuse.gov

because of the risk of damaging blood vessels and contracting HIV (human immunodeficiency virus) and hepatitis B.

Drugs can also be absorbed through the skin or tissue lining (**transdermal**)—the nicotine patch is a common example of a drug that is administered in this manner—or through the mucous membranes, such as those in the nose (snorting) or in the vagina or anus (**suppositories**). Suppositories are typically mixed with a waxy medium that melts at body temperature, releasing the drug into the bloodstream.

Using a needle to inject drugs poses health threats beyond the effects of the drug.

## Drug Interactions

**Polydrug use**—taking several medications, vitamins, recreational drugs, or illegal drugs simultaneously—can lead to dangerous health problems. Alcohol in particular frequently has dangerous interactions with other drugs. Hazardous interactions include synergism, inhibition, antagonism, intolerance, and cross-tolerance.

**Synergism,** also called *potentiation*, is an interaction of two or more drugs in which the effects of the individual drugs are multiplied beyond what would normally be expected if they were taken alone. You might think of synergism as 2 + 2 = 10. A synergistic reaction can be very dangerous and even deadly.

**Antagonism,** although usually less serious than synergism, can also produce unwanted and unpleasant effects. In an antagonistic reaction, drugs work at the same receptor site so that one drug blocks the action of the other. The blocking drug occupies the receptor site and prevents the other drug from attaching, thus altering its absorption and action.

With **inhibition,** the effects of one drug are eliminated or reduced by the presence of another drug at the receptor site, while **intolerance** occurs when drugs combine in the body to produce extremely uncomfortable reactions. The drug Antabuse, used to help alcoholics give up alcohol, works by producing this type of interaction.

**Cross-tolerance** occurs when a person develops a physiological tolerance to one drug that also increases the body's tolerance to other substances that act similarly on the body.

**transdermal** The introduction of drugs through the skin.

**suppositories** Mixtures of drugs and a waxy medium designed to melt at body temperature after being inserted into the anus or vagina.

**polydrug use** Use of multiple medications, vitamins, recreational drugs, or illicit drugs simultaneously.

**synergism** Interaction of two or more drugs that produces more profound effects than would be expected if the drugs were taken separately; also called *potentiation*.

**antagonism** A type of interaction in which two or more drugs work at the same receptor site so that one blocks the action of the other.

**inhibition** A drug interaction in which the effects of one drug are eliminated or reduced by the presence of another drug at the same receptor site.

**intolerance** A type of interaction in which two or more drugs produce extremely uncomfortable reactions.

**cross-tolerance** Development of a tolerance to one drug that reduces the effects of another, similar drug.

Discuss the issues of drug misuse and abuse in the United States, including the misuse and abuse of over-the-counter drugs and prescription drugs, the prevalence of drug use on college campuses, and risk factors for drug abuse.

Although drug abuse is usually referred to in connection with illicit psychoactive drugs, many people also abuse and misuse prescription, over-the-counter (OTC), and recreational drugs. In this section, we discuss these drug-related behaviors and focus, in particular, on college students' drug use.

## Abuse of Over-the-Counter Drugs

Over-the-counter medications come in many different forms, including pills, liquids, nasal sprays, and topical creams. Although many people assume that no harm can come from legal nonprescription drugs, OTC medications can be abused, with resultant health complications and potential addiction. People who appear to be most vulnerable to abusing OTC drugs are teenagers, young adults, and people over the age of 65.

OTC drug abuse can involve taking more than the recommended dosage, combining it with other drugs, or taking it over a longer period of time than is recommended. Abuse of and addiction to OTC drugs can be accidental. A person may develop tolerance from continued use, creating an unintended dependence. However, teenagers and young adults sometimes intentionally abuse OTC medications in search of a cheap high—by drinking large amounts of cough medicine, for instance. The following are a few types of OTC drugs that are subject to misuse and abuse:

- **Caffeine pills and energy drinks.** Energy drinks, OTC caffeine pills, and pain relievers containing caffeine are commonly abused for the energy boost they provide. Caffeine in large doses can result in tremors/shaking, restlessness and edginess, insomnia, dehydration, panic attacks, heart irregularities, and other symptoms. We'll look more closely at caffeine later in the chapter.
- **Cold medicines (cough syrups and tablets).** There are many different ingredients in cough and cold medicines, but one of particular concern is dextromethorphan (DXM), which is present in many types of OTC cold and cough medications. As many as 4 percent of high school seniors report taking drugs containing DXM to get high.[22] Large doses of products containing DXM can cause hallucinations, loss of motor control, and "out-of-body" (dissociative) sensations. In combination with alcohol or other drugs, large doses can be deadly. Some states have passed laws limiting the amount of products containing DXM that a person can purchase or prohibiting sale to individuals under age 18.[23]
- **Diet pills.** Some teens use diet pills as a way of getting high, whereas other people use these drugs in an attempt to lose

weight. Diet pills often contain a stimulant such as caffeine or an herbal ingredient claimed to promote weight loss, such as *Hoodia gordonii*. Although they can sometimes cause serious side effects, many diet pills are marketed as dietary supplements and so are regulated by the Food and Drug Administration (FDA) as "food," not as "drugs." This means their manufacturers may make unsubstantiated claims of effectiveness or use untested and unsafe ingredients.

## Nonmedical Use or Abuse of Prescription Drugs

In the United States today, the abuse of prescription medications is at an all-time high. Only marijuana is more widely abused.[24] Individuals abuse prescription medications because they are an easily accessible and inexpensive means of altering a user's mental and physical state. Some people also have the mistaken idea that prescription drugs are a "safer high." The latest data available indicate that approximately 6.5 million Americans aged 12 and older used prescription drugs for nonmedical reasons in the past month.[25]

Over-the-counter cough syrup is frequently abused by young people seeking a high from the ingredient DXM.

Prescription drug abuse is particularly common among teenagers and young adults. In 2013, 3 percent of teenagers age 12 to 17 and 5 percent of people 18 to 25 reported abusing prescription drugs in the past month.[26] Often these drugs are taken from friends or family members who have prescriptions. The problem may be getting worse, with nearly 15 percent of twelfth graders reporting abuse of prescription drugs by the time they graduate from high school.[27]

### College Students and Prescription Drug Abuse

Prescription drug abuse among college students has increased dramatically over the past decade. Because drugs are prescribed by doctors and approved by the FDA, many college students seem to perceive prescription drugs as safer and more socially acceptable than illicit drugs, or they believe prescription drugs will enhance their well-being or performance. However, nothing could be further from the truth when these drugs are misused.

According to the 2013 *American College Health Association–National College Health Assessment,* the illicit use of prescription drugs is a growing trend on campuses. The report shows 14 percent of surveyed students reported illegally using prescription drugs in the last year, compared to 13.5 percent in 2008.[28] Students who illegally use prescription drugs are also more likely to use other illegal drugs and binge drink.[29]

The most commonly abused prescription drugs on college campuses are painkillers (e.g., OxyContin and Vicodin). Approximately 6 percent of students report using painkillers that were not prescribed to them in the past 12 months. Of those reporting use, 7 percent were men and 6 percent women.[30]

Also of particular concern on college campuses is the increased abuse of stimulant drugs such as Adderall and Ritalin, which are intended to treat attention-deficit/hyperactivity disorder (ADHD). Students primarily report using ADHD drugs for academic gain. Approximately 8 percent of students report using stimulants that were not prescribed to them in the past 12 months.[31] According to a recent study, friends with prescriptions were the most commonly reported source of prescription stimulants, and most students obtained their drugs for free or at a cost of $1 to $5.[32] Users generally believed that the drugs were beneficial, despite frequent reports of adverse reactions. The most commonly reported adverse effects were sleeping difficulties, irritability, and reduced appetite.

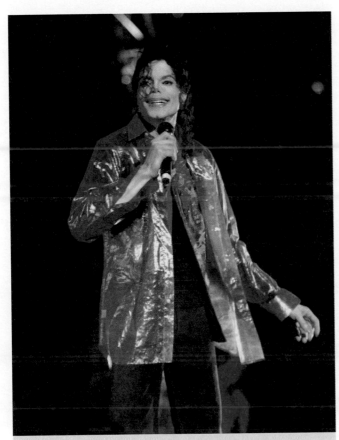

Abusing prescription drugs is no safer than abusing illicit drugs, as tragically demonstrated by the 2010 death of pop star Michael Jackson, whose death ultimately stemmed from his abuse of numerous prescription medications.

# 6.2%

OF COLLEGE STUDENTS REPORT HAVING ABUSED PRESCRIPTION **PAINKILLERS** SUCH AS CODEINE, VICODIN, AND OXYCONTIN IN THE PAST YEAR.

## Use and Abuse of Illicit Drugs

The problem of illicit (illegal) drug use touches us all. We may use illicit substances ourselves, watch someone we love struggle with drug abuse, or become the victim of a drug-related crime. At the very least, we pay increasing taxes for law enforcement and drug rehabilitation. When our coworkers use drugs, the effectiveness of our own work is diminished.

Illicit drug users span all age groups, genders, ethnicities, occupations, and socioeconomic groups. The good news about illicit drug use is that it peaked at around 25 million users between 1979 and 1986, then declined until 1992, and has since remained stable around 24 million users per year.[33] Among youth, however, illicit drug use, notably of marijuana, has been rising in recent years.[34]

**Illicit Drug Use on Campus** Illicit drug use has seen a resurgence on college campuses in recent years. Even so, it is not the norm. Close to 50 percent of college-aged students nationwide have tried an illicit drug at some point; the vast majority of them reported using marijuana (see **TABLE 7.1**).[35] Daily use of marijuana is at its highest point since 1989. Cocaine use is down sharply, but LSD use has more than doubled.[36]

College administrators, staff, and faculty are concerned about the link between substance abuse and poor academic performance, depression, anxiety, suicide, property damage, vandalism, fights, serious medical problems, and death. Students who use marijuana and/or other illicit drugs are at increased risk for disruptions in college attendance.[37] A longer-term consequence of illicit drug use among college students is a significantly increased chance of unemployment after college. The most recent research shows that 10 percent of people who were persistent drug

### WHY SHOULD I CARE?

You may think drugs are helping you relax, improving your concentration, or enhancing your social enjoyment, but those effects are transient—and often illusory—and they are nothing compared to the many negative effects those same drugs can have on your life and health. Sooner or later, drug misuse and abuse is likely to catch up with you and cause problems—be they academic, social, career, legal, financial, or health related. Are a few moments of excitement really worth a lifetime of trouble?

## TABLE 7.1 | 30-Day Drug Use Prevalence, Full-Time College Students vs. Respondents 1–4 Years beyond High School

| | Full-Time College (%) | Others (%) |
|---|---|---|
| Any illicit drug | 22.5 | 27.2 |
| Any illicit drug other than marijuana | 8.2 | 10.5 |
| Marijuana | 20.6 | 25.8 |
| Inhalants | 0.1 | 0.3 |
| Hallucinogens | 1.0 | 1.7 |
| LSD | 0.4 | 0.8 |
| Hallucinogens other than LSD | 0.8 | 1.1 |
| Ecstasy (methylene-dioxymethamphetamine, MDMA) | 0.8 | 1.4 |
| Cocaine | 0.9 | 2.6 |
| Crack | 0.3 | 0.2 |
| Other cocaine | 0.9 | 2.0 |
| Heroin | 0.2 | 0.3 |
| Narcotics other than heroin | 1.5 | 4.1 |
| Amphetamines, adjusted | 5.3 | 4.1 |
| Crystal methamphetamine | * | 0.2 |
| Sedatives (barbiturates) | 0.9 | 1.8 |
| Tranquilizers | 1.2 | 1.9 |
| Alcohol | 63.1 | 57.2 |
| Been drunk | 40.2 | 33.6 |
| Flavored alcoholic beverage | 29.1 | 27.0 |
| Cigarettes | 14.0 | 28.1 |
| Approximate weighted N = | 1,090 | 790 |

*Indicates prevalence less than 0.05%.

**Source:** L. D. Johnston et al., *Monitoring the Future National Survey Results on Drug Use, 1975–2013, Volume 2, College Students and Adults Ages 19–50* (Ann Arbor, MI: Institute for Social Research, The University of Michigan, 2014), Available at http://monitoringthefuture.org/new.html

users during college experienced unemployment after college compared with 1.7 percent of students who did not use drugs and 4.8 percent of those who used drugs sporadically.[38]

## Why Do Some College Students Use Drugs?

Research has identified the following factors in a student's life that increase the risk of substance abuse; the more factors, the greater the risk.

- **Positive expectations.** As mentioned previously, some students take drugs such as Adderall and Ritalin believing that the drugs will help their ability to study. But the vast majority of students say they take drugs in order to relax, reduce stress, and forget problems.

- **Genetics and family history.** Genetics and family history play a significant role in the risk for developing an addiction.
- **Substance use in high school.** Two-thirds of college students who use illicit drugs began doing so in high school.[39]
- **Curiosity.** College students are learning a lot about themselves, both personally and professionally. Sometimes, that journey of self-discovery includes experimenting with different mind-altering substances.
- **Social Norms.** College students often overestimate the amount of drug use on campus. Surveys conducted on college campuses found students perceived that 84 percent of their peers used marijuana within the last 30 days, when actually 18 percent had.
- **Sorority and fraternity membership.** Being a member of a sorority or fraternity increases the likelihood of abusing alcohol and drugs.[40] A few factors that may contribute to more drinking and use of drugs in sororities and fraternities include group living, hazing or initiation rituals, lack of supervision, and social pressure.[41]
- **Stress.** For some students under academic and social stress, seemingly easy relief comes in the form of drugs or alcohol.

## Why *Don't* Some College Students Use Drugs?

Many protective factors can influence a student to avoid drugs. Some of the most commonly reported include the following:[42]

- **Parental attitudes and behavior.** Students who say they are more influenced by their parents' concerns or expectations drink less, use marijuana less, and smoke significantly less than do students who are less influenced by parents.

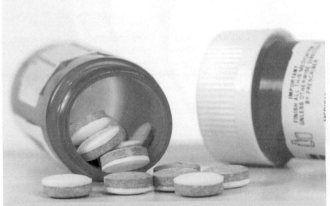

Painkillers such as OxyContin, Percocet, Percodan, Vicodin, and others are highly addictive. If they are taken daily for several weeks, that is enough time for addiction to develop. OxyContin, in particular, can be a highly addictive and dangerous narcotic when abused.

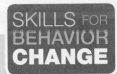

## SKILLS FOR BEHAVIOR CHANGE

### RESPONDING TO AN OFFER OF DRUGS

No matter what your experience has been up until now, it is likely that you will be invited to use drugs at some point in your life. Here are some questions to consider *before* you find yourself in a situation in which you have the opportunity or feel pressure to use illicit drugs:

- ▶ Why am I considering trying drugs? Am I trying to fit in or impress my friends? What does this say about my friends if I need to take drugs to impress them? Are my friends really looking out for what is best for me?
- ▶ Am I using this drug to cope or feel different? Am I depressed?
- ▶ What could taking drugs cost me? Will this cost me my career if I am caught using? Could using drugs prevent me from getting a job?
- ▶ What are the long-term consequences of using this drug?
- ▶ What will this cost me in terms of my friendships and family? How would my close family and friends respond if they knew I was using drugs?

Even when you make the decision not to use drugs, it can be difficult to say no gracefully. Some good ways to turn down an offer:

- ▶ "Thanks, but I've got a big test (game, meeting) tomorrow morning."
- ▶ "I've already got a great buzz right now. I really don't need anything more."
- ▶ "I don't like how (insert drug name here) makes me feel."
- ▶ "I'm driving tonight. So I'm not using."
- ▶ "I want to go for a run in the morning."
- ▶ "No."

- **Religion and spirituality.** The greater a student's level of religiosity (hours in prayer, attendance at services), the less likely he or she is to drink, smoke, or use other drugs.
- **Student engagement.** The more a student is involved in the learning process and extracurricular activities, the less likely he or she is to binge drink, use marijuana, or abuse prescription drugs.
- **College athletics.** College athletes drink at higher rates than do nonathletes, but are less likely to use illicit drugs.
- **Healthy social network.** Having a wide range of friends and supports to help cope with the challenges of life is a well-known protective factor against many negative behaviors, including drug use.

To prepare yourself for a possible offer of drugs on campus and to be ready to make the decision that is best for *you*, see the **Skills for Behavior Change** box.

Discuss the use and abuse of stimulants, cannabis, narcotics, depressants, hallucinogens, inhalants, and anabolic steroids.

Hundreds of drugs are subject to abuse—some are legal, such as recreational drugs and prescription medications, whereas many others are illegal and classified as "controlled substances." For general purposes, drugs can be divided into the following categories: *stimulants, cannabis products (cannabinoids) including marijuana, narcotics, depressants, hallucinogens, inhalants,* and

**stimulants** Drugs that increase activity of the central nervous system.

*anabolic steroids* . These categories are discussed in subsequent sections; **TABLE 7.2** summarizes the categorization, uses, and effects of various drugs of abuse, both legal and illicit.

## Stimulants

A **stimulant** is a drug that increases activity of the central nervous system. Its effects usually involve increased activity, anxiety, and agitation; users often seem jittery or nervous while high. Commonly used illegal stimulants include cocaine, amphetamines, and methamphetamine. Legal stimulants include caffeine and nicotine (see Chapter 8 for a discussion of nicotine, the addictive substance in tobacco products).

## TABLE **7.2** | Drugs of Abuse: Uses and Effects

| Category | Drugs | Trade or Street Names | Dependence | Usual Method | Possible Effects | Overdose Effects | Withdrawal Syndrome |
|---|---|---|---|---|---|---|---|
| **Stimulants** | Cocaine | Coke, Flake, Snow, Crack, *Coca, Blanca, Perico* | *Physical*: Possible *Psychological*: High *Tolerance*: Yes | Snorted, smoked, injected | Increased alertness, excitation, euphoria, increased pulse rate and blood pressure, insomnia, loss of appetite | Agitation, increased body temperature, hallucinations, convulsions, possible death | Apathy, long periods of sleep, irritability, depression, disorientation |
| | Amphetamine, methamphetamine | Crank, Ice, Cristal, Crystal Meth, Speed, Adderall, Dexedrine | *Physical*: Possible *Psychological*: High *Tolerance*: Yes | Oral, injected, smoked | | | |
| | Methylphenidate | Ritalin (Illy's), Concerta, Focalin, Metadate | *Physical*: Possible *Psychological*: High *Tolerance*: Yes | Oral, injected, snorted, smoked | | | |
| **Cannabis** | Marijuana | Pot, Grass, Sinsemilla, Blunts, *Mota, Yerba* | *Physical*: Possible *Psychological*: High *Tolerance*: Yes | Oral, smoked | Euphoria, relaxed inhibitions, increased appetite, disorientation | Fatigue, paranoia, possible psychosis | Hyperactivity, decreased appetite, insomnia |
| | Hashish, hashish oil | Hash, hash oil | *Physical*: Unknown *Psychological*: Moderate *Tolerance*: Yes | Smoked, oral | | | |
| **Narcotics** | Heroin | Diamorphine, Horse, Smack, Black tar, *Chiva* | *Physical*: High *Psychological*: High *Tolerance*: Yes | Injected, snorted, smoked | Euphoria, drowsiness, respiratory depression, constricted pupils, nausea | Slow and shallow breathing, clammy skin, convulsions, coma, possible death | Watery eyes, runny nose, yawning, loss of appetite, irritability, tremors, panic, cramps, nausea, chills and sweating |
| | Morphine | MS-Contin, Roxanol | *Physical*: High *Psychological*: High *Tolerance*: Yes | Oral, injected | | | |
| | Hydrocodone, oxycodone | Vicodin, OxyContin, Percocet, Percodan | *Physical*: High *Psychological*: High *Tolerance*: Yes | Oral | | | |
| | Codeine | Acetaminophen w/Codeine, Tylenol w/Codeine | *Physical*: Moderate *Psychological*: Moderate *Tolerance*: Yes | Oral, injected | | | |

Continued on next page

TABLE **7.2** | Drugs of Abuse: Uses and Effects (Continued)

| Category | Drugs | Trade or Street Names | Dependence | Usual Method | Possible Effects | Overdose Effects | Withdrawal Syndrome |
|---|---|---|---|---|---|---|---|
| **Depressants** | Gamma-hydroxybu-tyrate | GHB, Liquid Ecstasy, Liquid X | *Physical:* Moderate *Psychological:* Moderate *Tolerance:* Yes | Oral | Slurred speech, disorientation, drunken behavior without odor of alcohol, impaired memory of events, interacts with alcohol | Shallow respiration, clammy skin, dilated pupils, weak and rapid pulse, coma, possible death | Anxiety, insomnia, tremors, delirium, convulsions, possible death |
| | Benzodiaz-epines | Valium, Xanax, Halcion, Ativan, Rohypnol (Roofies, R-2), Klonopin | *Physical:* Moderate *Psychological:* Moderate *Tolerance:* Yes | Oral, injected | | | |
| | Other depres-sants | Ambien, Sonata, Barbiturates, Methaqualone (Quaalude) | *Physical:* Moderate *Psychological:* Moderate *Tolerance:* Yes | Oral | | | |
| **Hallucinogens** | Methylene-dioxym-etham-phetamine (MDMA), analogs | Ecstasy, XTC, Adam, MDA (Love Drug), MDEA (Eve) | *Physical:* None *Psychological:* Moderate *Tolerance:* Yes | Oral, snorted, smoked | Heightened senses, teeth grinding, dehydration | Increased body temperature, electrolyte imbalance, cardiac arrest | Muscle aches, drowsiness, depression, acne |
| | LSD | Acid, Microdot, Sunshine, Boomers | *Physical:* None *Psychological:* Unknown *Tolerance:* Yes | Oral | Hallucinations, altered perception of time and distance | Longer, more intense "trips" | None |
| | Phency-clidine, analogs | PCP, Angel Dust, Hog, Ketamine (Special K) | *Physical:* Possible *Psychological:* High *Tolerance:* Yes | Smoked, oral, injected, snorted | | Unable to direct movement, feel pain, or remember | Drug-seeking behavior |
| | Other hal-lucinogens | Psilocybe mushrooms, mescaline, peyote, Dex-tromethorphan | *Physical:* None *Psychological:* None *Tolerance:* Possible | Oral | | | |
| **Inhalants** | Amyl and butyl nitrite | Pearls, Poppers, Rush, Locker Room | *Physical:* Unknown *Psychological:* Unknown *Tolerance:* No | Inhaled | Flushing, hypotension, headache | Methemo-globinemia | Agitation |
| | Nitrous oxide | Laughing gas, Balloons, Whippets | *Physical:* Unknown *Psychological:* Low *Tolerance:* No | Inhaled | Impaired memory, slurred speech, drunken behavior, slow-onset vitamin deficiency, organ damage | Vomiting, respiratory depression, loss of con-sciousness, possible death | Trembling, anxiety, insomnia, vitamin deficiency, confusion, hallucinations, convulsions |
| | Other inhalants | Adhesives, spray paint, hairspray, lighter fluid | *Physical:* Unknown *Psychological:* High *Tolerance:* No | Inhaled | | | |
| **Anabolic Ster-oids** | Testoster-one | Depo testoster-one, Sustanon, Sten, Cypt | *Physical:* Unknown *Psychological:* Unknown *Tolerance:* Unknown | Injected | Virilization, edema, tes-ticular atrophy, gynecomastia, acne, aggressive behavior | Unknown | Possible depression |
| | Other anabolic steroids | Parabolan, Winstrol, Equi-pose, Anadrol, Dianabol | *Physical:* Unknown *Psychological:* Yes *Tolerance:* Unknown | Oral, injected | | | |

**Source:** Adapted from U.S. Department of Justice Drug Enforcement Administration, "DEA Drug Fact Sheets," 2011, www.justice.gov

## Cocaine

A white crystalline powder derived from the leaves of the South American coca shrub (not related to cocoa plants), *cocaine* ("coke") has been described as one of the most powerful naturally occurring stimulants.

Cocaine can be taken in several ways, including snorting, smoking, and injecting. The powdered form is snorted through the nose, which can damage mucous membranes and cause sinusitis. It can destroy the user's sense of smell, and occasionally it even eats a hole through the septum. When snorted, the drug enters the bloodstream through the lungs in less than 1 minute and reaches the brain in less than 3 minutes. It binds at receptor sites in the central nervous system, producing an intense high that disappears quickly, leaving a powerful craving for more.

Cocaine alkaloid, or *freebase,* is obtained from removing the hydrochloride salt from cocaine powder. *Freebasing* refers to smoking freebase by placing it at the end of a pipe and holding a flame near it to produce a vapor, which is then inhaled. *Crack* is identical pharmacologically to freebase, but the hydrochloride salt is still present and is processed with baking soda and water. It is a cheap, widely available drug that is smokable and very potent. Crack is commonly smoked in the same manner as freebase. Because crack is such a pure drug, it takes little time to achieve the desired high, and a crack user can become addicted quickly.

> **amphetamines** A large and varied group of synthetic agents that stimulate the central nervous system.

Some cocaine users occasionally inject the drug intravenously, which introduces large amounts into the body rapidly, creating a brief, intense high, and a subsequent crash. Injecting users place themselves at risk not only for contracting HIV and hepatitis (a severe liver disease) through shared needles, but also for skin infections, vein damage, inflamed arteries, and infection of the heart lining.

Cocaine is both an anesthetic and a central nervous system stimulant. In tiny doses, it can slow the heart rate. In larger doses, the physical effects are dramatic: increased heart rate and blood pressure, loss of appetite that can lead to dramatic weight loss, convulsions, muscle twitching, irregular heartbeat, and even death from overdose. Other effects of cocaine include temporary relief of depression, decreased fatigue, talkativeness, increased alertness, and heightened self-confidence. However, as the dose increases, users become irritable and apprehensive, and their behavior may turn paranoid or violent.

## Amphetamines

The **amphetamines** include a large and varied group of synthetic agents that stimulate the central nervous system. Small doses of amphetamines improve alertness, lessen fatigue, and generally elevate mood. With repeated use, however, physical and psychological dependence develops. Sleep patterns are affected (insomnia); heart rate, breathing rate, and blood pressure increase; and restlessness, anxiety, appetite suppression, and vision problems are common. High doses over long time periods can produce hallucinations, delusions, and disorganized behavior.

Certain types of amphetamines or amphetamine-like drugs are used for medicinal purposes. As discussed earlier, drugs prescribed to treat ADHD are stimulants and are increasingly abused on campus.

## Methamphetamine

An increasingly common form of amphetamine, *methamphetamine* (commonly called "meth") is a potent, long-acting, inexpensive drug that is highly addictive. In the short term, methamphetamine produces increased physical activity, alertness, euphoria, rapid breathing, increased body temperature, insomnia, tremors, anxiety, confusion, and decreased appetite. Over 595,000 Americans are regular users of methamphetamine, and it is believed that more than 12 million Americans have tried it.[43] In 2013, about 1 percent of high school seniors reported using methamphetamine in their lifetime.[44] The rate of methamphetamine use may be increasing because it is relatively easy to make. Recipes often include common OTC ingredients such as ephedrine and pseudoephedrine.

Methamphetamine can be snorted, smoked, injected, or orally ingested. When snorted, the effects can be felt in 3 to 5 minutes; if orally ingested, effects occur within 15 to 20 minutes. The pleasurable effects of methamphetamine are typically an intense rush lasting only a few minutes when snorted; in contrast, smoking the drug can produce a high lasting more than 8 hours. Users often experience tolerance after the first use, making methamphetamine highly addictive.

Methamphetamine increases the release of and blocks the reuptake of the neurotransmitter dopamine, leading to high levels of the chemical in the brain (refer back to Figure 7.2). This action occurs rapidly and produces the intense euphoria, or "rush," that many users feel. Over time, meth destroys dopamine receptors, making it impossible to feel pleasure. Researchers have now established that due to the destruction of dopamine receptors, people who abuse methamphetamine (or cocaine) are at increased risk for developing Parkinson's disease later in life.[45]

Other long-term effects of methamphetamine can include severe weight loss, cardiovascular damage, increased risk of heart attack and stroke, hallucinations, extensive tooth decay and tooth loss ("meth mouth"), violence, paranoia, psychotic

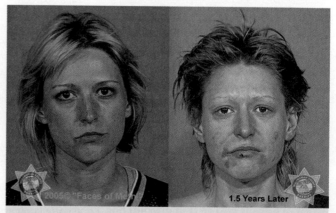

1.5 Years Later

The physical consequences of methamphetamine use are often dramatic. The photo at left shows a person before she began using methamphetamine. The photo at right shows the same person after just 1.5 years of methamphetamine use.

behavior, and even death. Chronic methamphetamine abusers often demonstrate severe structural and functional changes in areas of the brain associated with emotion and memory, which may account for many of the emotional and cognitive problems observed in chronic methamphetamine abusers. Some of these changes persist after the methamphetamine abuse has stopped. Other changes reverse after sustained periods of abstinence from methamphetamine, lasting typically longer than a year, but problems can remain.[46]

Meth users are at increased risk for transmission of HIV, hepatitis B and C, and other sexually transmitted diseases. Meth can alter judgment, increase libido, and lessen inhibitions, leading users to engage in unsafe behaviors, including risky sexual behavior. Among meth users who inject the drug, HIV and other infectious diseases can be spread through sharing of contaminated needles, syringes, and other injection equipment that is used by more than one person.

## Bath Salts

"Bath salts" is one of the latest additions to the growing list of items people are using to get high. The new designer drug is synthetic powder sold legally online and in corner stores and truck stops. The powder substance is sold in a packet with a disclaimer "not for human consumption." It is not subject to FDA regulation; however, some of the substances used in making bath salts were made illegal in 2012. These packages contain various amphetamine or cocaine-like substances such as methylene-dioxypyrovalerone (MPDV), mephedrone, and pyrovalerone. The powder can be smoked, snorted, injected, and wrapped in pieces of paper and ingested or "bombed." These chemicals cannot be detected by routine drug screening, making them attractive for misuse.[47]

Effects include intense stimulation, alertness, euphoria, elevated mood, and pleasurable rush. Users may describe feelings of closeness, sociability, and moderate sexual arousal. Other symptoms can include tremor, shortness of breath, and loss of appetite. Changes in body temperature regulation are accompanied by hot flashes and sweating, with bleeding from the nose and throat from ulcerations when snorted.[48]

This drug also can have significant effects on the cardiovascular system, resulting in rapid heart rate, increased blood pressure, and chest pain. Psychiatric effects at higher doses consist of anxiety, agitation, hallucinations, paranoia, and erratic behavior. Depression and suicide have also been reported as a result of use. While withdrawal symptoms are reported as minimal, users often have described a strong craving for the drug.[49]

## Caffeine

Unlike cocaine and methamphetamine, **caffeine** is a legal stimulant. More than 85 percent of Americans drink at least one caffeinated beverage per day.[50] Ninety-six percent of beverage caffeine consumed is from coffee, soft drinks, and tea.[51] Beverages like energy drinks, chocolate drinks, and energy shots represent only a small portion of overall caffeine intakes.[52] One of the many reasons coffee, tea, soft drinks, chocolate, and other caffeine-containing products are loved is for their wake-up effects. Caffeine may be commonplace, but excessive consumption is associated with addiction and certain health problems.

> **caffeine** A stimulant drug that is legal in the United States and found in many coffees, teas, chocolates, energy drinks, and certain medications.

Caffeine is derived from the chemical family called *xanthines*, which are found in plant products such as coffee, tea, and chocolate. The xanthines are mild central nervous system stimulants that enhance mental alertness, reduce feelings of fatigue, and increase heart muscle contractions, oxygen consumption, metabolism, and urinary output. A person feels these effects within 15 to 45 minutes of ingesting a caffeinated product. It takes 4 to 6 hours for the body to metabolize half of the caffeine ingested, so, depending on the amount of caffeine taken in, it may continue to exert effects for a day or longer. **FIGURE 7.3** compares the caffeine content of various products.

As the effects of caffeine wear off, frequent users may feel let down—mentally or physically depressed, tired, and weak. To counteract this, they commonly choose to drink another cup of coffee or tea, or another soda. Habitually engaging in this practice leads to tolerance and psychological dependence. Symptoms of excessive caffeine consumption include chronic insomnia, jitters, irritability, nervousness, anxiety, and involuntary muscle twitches. Withdrawing from caffeine may compound the effects and produce severe headaches, fatigue, and

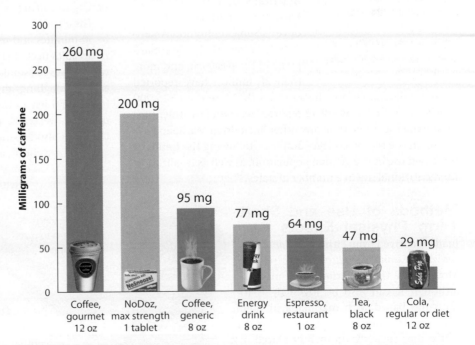

**FIGURE 7.3** Caffeine Content Comparison

**Source:** Data from USDA National Nutrient Database for Standard Reference, Release 25 (2012), www.ars.usda.gov

nausea. Because caffeine meets the requirements for addiction—tolerance, psychological dependence, and withdrawal symptoms—it can be classified as addictive.

Long-term caffeine use has been suspected of being linked to several serious health problems. However, no strong evidence exists to suggest that moderate caffeine use (less than 300 mg daily, or approximately three cups of regular coffee) produces harmful effects in healthy, nonpregnant people. For most people, caffeine poses few health risks and may actually have some benefits, such as lower risk of depression among women, a lower risk of prostate cancer among men, and lower risk of stroke among both men and women.[53]

**Khat** Khat is a stimulant drug used for centuries by people in East Africa and the Arabian peninsula.[54] Like chewing tobacco, the young leaves of the *Catha edulis* shrub are typically chewed and held in the cheek, releasing the plant's stimulants.[55] One Khat's active ingredients, cathinone, is a Schedule 1 drug, because its mind-altering properties.[56] Chewing khat leaves increases arousal and alertness. It is also reported to induce a state of euphoria. Using khat compulsively can lead to paranoia, manic behavior, and hallucinations.

# Marijuana and Other Cannabinoids

Although archaeological evidence documents the use of **marijuana** ("grass," "weed," or "pot") as far back as 6,000 years, the drug did not become popular in the United States until the 1960s. Today marijuana is the most commonly used illicit drug in the United States. Approximately 48 percent of Americans over the age of 12 have tried marijuana at least once.[57] Some 33 million Americans have reported using marijuana in the past year, and more than 20 million have reported using marijuana within the past month. More than 845,000 Americans over the age of 12 reported receiving treatment for marijuana use, more than any other illicit drug. Marijuana use is also on the rise on college campuses, following the trends of increased use in the general population, as well as legalization for recreational use in a number of states.[58]

**marijuana** Chopped leaves and flowers of *Cannabis indica* or *Cannabis sativa* plants (hemp); a psychoactive stimulant.

**tetrahydrocannabinol (THC)** The chemical name for the active ingredient in marijuana.

## Methods of Use and Short-Term Physical Effects
Marijuana is derived from either the *Cannabis sativa* or *Cannabis indica* (hemp) plant. Most of the time, marijuana is smoked, although it can also be ingested, as in brownies baked with marijuana in them. When marijuana is smoked, it is usually rolled into cigarettes (joints) or placed in a pipe or water pipe (bong).

**Tetrahydrocannabinol** (THC) is the psychoactive substance in marijuana and

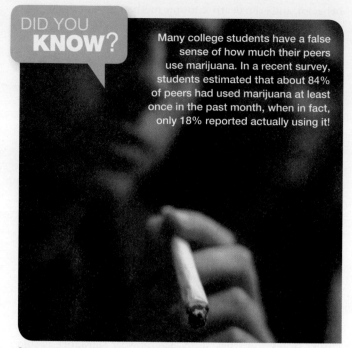

**Source:** Data are from American College Health Association, *American College Health Association—National College Health Assessment II: Reference Group Data Report, Spring 2014* (Hanover, MD: American College Health Association, 2014).

the key to determining how powerful a high it will produce. More potent forms of the drug can contain up to 27 percent THC, but most average 15 percent.[59] *Hashish,* a potent cannabis preparation derived mainly from the plant's thick, sticky resin, contains high THC concentrations. Hash oil, a substance produced by percolating a solvent such as ether through dried marijuana to extract the THC, is a tar-like liquid that may contain up to 300 mg of THC in a dose.

The effects of smoking marijuana are generally felt within 10 to 30 minutes and usually wear off within 3 hours. The most noticeable effect of THC is the dilation of the eyes' blood vessels, which gives the smoker bloodshot eyes. Marijuana smokers also exhibit coughing; dry mouth and throat ("cotton mouth"); increased thirst and appetite; lowered blood pressure; and mild muscular weakness, primarily exhibited in drooping eyelids. Users can also experience severe anxiety, panic, paranoia, and psychosis, and may have intensified reactions to various stimuli; colors, sounds, and the speed at which things move may seem altered. High doses of hashish may produce vivid visual hallucinations.

One common way of smoking marijuana is to use a pipe.

## Marijuana and Driving
Marijuana use presents clear hazards for drivers of motor vehicles and others on the road with them. The drug substantially reduces a driver's ability to react and make quick decisions. Perceptual and other performance deficits resulting from marijuana use may persist for some time after the high subsides. Users who attempt to drive, fly, or operate heavy machinery often fail to recognize their impairment.

# 9.9 MILLION

PEOPLE REPORTED **DRIVING** UNDER THE INFLUENCE OF ILLICIT DRUGS IN THE PAST YEAR.

Recent research indicates you are two and a half times more likely to be involved in a motor vehicle accident if you drive under the influence of marijuana.[60] Combining even a low dose of marijuana and alcohol enhances the impairing effects of both drugs.

## Effects of Chronic Marijuana Use
Marijuana smoke contains 50 to 70 percent more carcinogenic hydrocarbons than appear in tobacco smoke. Because marijuana smokers typically inhale more deeply and hold the smoke in their lungs longer than do tobacco smokers, the lungs are exposed to more carcinogens. Likewise, effects from irritation (e.g., cough, excessive phlegm, and increased lung infections) similar to those experienced by tobacco smokers can occur.[61] Lung conditions such as chronic bronchitis, emphysema, and other lung disorders are also associated with smoking marijuana. Furthermore, the tar from cannabis contains higher levels of carcinogens than does tobacco smoke.

Frequent and/or long-term marijuana use may significantly increase a man's risk of developing testicular cancer. The risk was particularly elevated (about twice that of those who never smoked marijuana) for those who used marijuana at least weekly or who had long-term exposure to the substance beginning in adolescence.[62]

The link between marijuana and common mental health disorders is somewhat conflicting. While marijuana may ease the symptoms of depression, depression may actually worsen once the positive effects wear off.[63] Marijuana users are more likely to suffer from depression and depressive symptoms than nonusers, with risk increasing for people using both marijuana and alcohol.[64]

Some research suggests that frequent or heavy use of marijuana during adolescence may be associated developing anxiety disorders in young adulthood.[65] Additionally, research shows that frequent cannabis use in teenagers predicts both depression and anxiety later in life, with the highest risk among daily users.[66] Certain personality disorders, interpersonal violence, and suicidal ideation are also correlated with marijuana use. In general, the younger marijuana use started, the greater the risk of eventually developing a mental health disorder.

Other risks associated with marijuana use include suppression of the immune system, blood pressure changes, and impaired memory function. Recent studies suggest that pregnant women who smoke marijuana may have children who have subtle brain changes that can cause difficulties with problem-solving skills, memory, and attention and can more than double the risk of giving birth prematurely.[67]

**Marijuana as Medicine** Although classified as a dangerous drug by the U.S. government, marijuana has been legalized for medicinal uses in 23 states and the District of Columbia, and is known to have several medical purposes. It helps control such side effects as the severe nausea and vomiting produced by chemotherapy, the chemical treatment for cancer. It improves appetite and forestalls the loss of lean muscle mass associated with AIDS-wasting syndrome. Marijuana reduces the muscle pain and spasticity caused by diseases such as multiple sclerosis. Opponents of medical marijuana argue that there are FDA-approved drugs that are just as effective in treating the same conditions, and that the potential side effects of marijuana make it inappropriate for FDA approval. Although several states have legalized marijuana for medicinal and/or recreational purposes, its legal status continues to be hotly debated (see the **Point of View** box on the next page).

## Synthetic Marijuana (Spice or K2)
Also known as K2 or "Spice," synthetic marijuana is used to describe a diverse family of herbal blends marketed under many names, including K2, fake marijuana, Yucatan Fire, Skunk, Moon Rocks, and others. These products contain dried, shredded plant material and one or more synthetic cannabinoids, with results that mimic marijuana intoxication but with longer duration and poor detection on urine drug screens. K2 is sold legally as herbal blend incense. However, Spice is smoked by people to gain effects similar to marijuana, hashish, and other forms of cannabis.[68]

Spice is used by nearly 1 in 10 college students and is more commonly used by males and first- and second-year college students. Students who reported using Spice were more likely to have smoked cigarettes, marijuana, and hookahs. It is also gaining more attention among high school seniors, with reports that 1 in every 9, or 11.3 percent, of high school seniors are using this drug.[69]

The most common way of smoking Spice is smoked by rolling it in papers (as with marijuana or handmade tobacco cigarettes).[70] Sometimes it is mixed with marijuana. Some users also make it as an herbal tea for drinking.[71] People smoking Spice may experience several adverse health effects such as hallucinations, severe agitation, extremely elevated heart rate and blood pressure, coma, suicide attempts, and drug dependence, which is not common among cannabis users.[72] Emergency departments are also reporting a significant increase in the numbers of people being treated for Spice use.[73]

**depressants** Drugs that slow down the activity of the central nervous and muscular systems and cause sleepiness or calmness.

## Depressants

Whereas central nervous system stimulants increase muscular and nervous system activity, **depressants** have the opposite effect. These drugs slow down neuromuscular activity and cause sleepiness or calmness. If the dose is high enough, brain function can stop, causing death. Alcohol is the most widely used central nervous system depressant. (For details on alcohol's effect on the body, see Chapter 8). Other forms include benzodiazepines, barbiturates, and GHB.

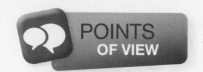
# Marijuana

Currently, 23 states and the District of Columbia have chosen to legalize marijuana for medicinal use, and voters in Washington, Colorado, Oregon, and Alaska recently passed ballot initiatives to legalize marijuana for recreational use. The arguments for and against the legalization of marijuana have been very strong over the past few decades. Below are some of the major points from both sides.

### Arguments for Legalization

- There are medical benefits for individuals dealing with cancer and other chronic diseases.
- Legalizing marijuana and taxing its sale would bring in revenue for the government.
- Legal government and U.S. Food and Drug Administration (FDA) oversight would allow for standardization of marijuana growth and production and could promote more responsible cultivation methods.
- Legalizing marijuana will result in more effective law enforcement and criminal justice since police officers will have more time and money to pursue criminals for other, more serious crimes.
- Having legal outlets for drugs such as marijuana may reduce illegal drug trafficking from off-shore criminal elements and reduce the risk of harmful drug additives.

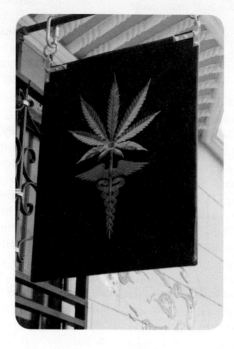

### Arguments against Legalization

- Some individuals believe that it is morally wrong to consume marijuana.
- Research indicates that marijuana use impacts young users the most in the long term.
- Research has found that those who used marijuana heavily as teenagers lose an average of 8 IQ points that are not recovered with quitting or aging.
- Marijuana use can cause or worsen respiratory symptoms or conditions such as bronchitis, alter mood and judgment, damage the immune system, and impair short-term memory and motor coordination. These side effects make it inappropriate for FDA approval.
- Marijuana is known to be addictive; approximately 9 percent of people who experiment with marijuana become addicted.
- Legalization could make marijuana more available to children and teenagers.

## WHERE DO YOU STAND?

- Do you think marijuana should be legalized by the federal government? What potential problems do you think this would create or solve?

- What criteria do you think should be used to determine the legality of a particular substance? Who should make those determinations?

- What are your feelings on drug laws in general—do you think they should be more or less prohibitive? What sort of policies would you propose to protect individuals and their rights?

**Sources:** National Institute on Drug Abuse, "DrugFacts: Is Marijuana Medicine?," July 2014, www.drugabuse.gov; DrugRehab.us, "Pros and Cons of Legalizing Recreational Marijuana," April 2014, www.drugrehab.us/news/pros-cons-legalizing-recreational-marijuana; N. Volkow et al., "Adverse Health Effects of Marijuana Use," *The New England Journal of Medicine*, 370 (2014): 2219–27.

---

**benzodiazepines** A class of central nervous system depressant drugs with sedative, hypnotic, and muscle relaxant effects; also called *tranquilizers*.

**barbiturates** Drugs that depress the central nervous system, have sedative and hypnotic effects, and are less safe than benzodiazepines.

## Benzodiazepines and Barbiturates A *sedative* drug promotes mental calmness and reduces anxiety, whereas a *hypnotic* drug promotes sleep or drowsiness. The most common sedative-hypnotic drugs are **benzodiazepines,** more commonly known as *tranquilizers*. These include prescription drugs such as Valium, Ativan, and Xanax. Benzodiazepines are most commonly prescribed for tension, muscular strain, sleep problems, anxiety, panic attacks, and alcohol withdrawal. **Barbiturates** are sedative-hypnotic drugs such as Amytal and Seconal. Today, benzodiazepines have largely replaced barbiturates, which were used medically in the past for relieving tension and inducing relaxation and sleep.

Sedative-hypnotics have a synergistic effect when combined with alcohol, another central nervous system depressant.

Taken together, these drugs can lead to respiratory failure and death. All sedative or hypnotic drugs can produce physical and psychological dependence in several weeks. A complication specific to sedatives is cross-tolerance, which occurs when users develop tolerance for one sedative or become dependent on it and develop tolerance for others as well. Withdrawal from sedative or hypnotic drugs may range from mild discomfort to severe symptoms, depending on the degree of dependence.

### Rohypnol
One benzodiazepine of concern is Rohypnol, a potent tranquilizer similar in nature to Valium but many times stronger. The drug produces a sedative effect, amnesia, muscle relaxation, and slowed psychomotor responses. The most publicized "date rape" drug, Rohypnol has gained notoriety as a growing problem on college campuses. The drug has been added to punch and other drinks at parties, where it is reportedly given to a woman in hopes of incapacitating her so she is unable to resist sexual assault. (See Chapter 4 for more on drug-facilitated rape.)

### GHB
*Gamma-hydroxybutyrate (GHB)* is a central nervous system depressant known to have euphoric, sedative, and anabolic (bodybuilding) effects. It was originally sold over the counter to bodybuilders to help reduce body fat and build muscle. Concerns about GHB led the FDA to ban OTC sales in 1992, and GHB is now a Schedule I drug. (Schedule I drugs are classified as having a high potential for abuse, with no currently accepted medical use in the United States).[74] GHB is an odorless, tasteless fluid. Like Rohypnol, GHB has been slipped into drinks without being detected, resulting in loss of memory, unconsciousness, amnesia, and even death. Other dangerous side effects include nausea, vomiting, seizures, hallucinations, coma, and respiratory distress.

## Opioids (Narcotics)

**Opioids** cause drowsiness, relieve pain, and produce euphoria. Also called *narcotics,* opioids are derived from the parent drug **opium**, a dark, resinous substance made from the milky juice of the opium poppy seedpod, and they are all highly addictive. Opium and heroin are both illegal in the United States, but some opioids are available by prescription for medical purposes: Morphine is sometimes prescribed for severe pain, and codeine is found in prescription cough syrups and other painkillers. Several prescription drugs, including Vicodin, Percodan, OxyContin, Demerol, and Dilaudid, contain synthetic opioids.

Opium is extracted from opium poppy seedpods like this one.

### Physical Effects of Opioids
Opioids are powerful depressants of the central nervous system. In addition to relieving pain, these drugs lower heart rate, respiration, and blood pressure. Side effects include weakness, dizziness, nausea, vomiting, euphoria, decreased sex drive, visual disturbances, and lack of coordination.

The human body's physiology could be said to encourage opioid addiction. Opioid-like hormones called **endorphins** are manufactured in the body and have multiple receptor sites, particularly in the central nervous system. When endorphins attach themselves at these points, they create feelings of painless well-being; medical researchers refer to them as "the body's own opioids." When endorphin levels are high, people feel euphoric. The same euphoria occurs when opioids or related chemicals are active at the endorphin receptor sites. Of all the opioids, heroin has the greatest notoriety as an addictive drug. While the following section discusses the progression of heroin addiction, addiction to any opioid follows a similar path.

**opioids** Drugs that induce sleep, relieve pain, and produce euphoria; includes derivatives of opium and synthetics with similar chemical properties; also called *narcotics.*

**opium** The parent drug of the opioids; made from the seedpod resin of the opium poppy.

**endorphins** Opioid-like hormones that are manufactured in the human body and contribute to natural feelings of well-being.

### Heroin
*Heroin* is a white powder derived from morphine. *Black tar heroin* is a sticky, dark brown, foul-smelling form of heroin that is relatively pure and inexpensive. Once considered a cure for morphine dependence, heroin was later discovered to be even more addictive and potent than morphine. Today heroin has no medical use.

Heroin is a depressant that produces drowsiness and a dreamy, mentally slow feeling. It can cause drastic mood swings, with euphoric highs followed by depressive lows. Heroin slows respiration and urinary output and constricts the pupils of the eyes. Symptoms of tolerance and withdrawal can appear within 3 weeks of first use.

In 2013, 681,000 Americans reported using heroin in the past year, a considerable increase since 2002.[75] Once predominant in urban areas, heroin use is becoming increasingly common in suburban and rural communities, particularly among white men and women.[76] There has also been an increasing number of deaths due to heroin overdose.[77] This trend appears to be driven largely by 18- to 25-year-olds, among whom there have been the largest increases. This younger age group may be more likely to purchase heroin since it is both cheaper and generally easier to obtain than prescription opioids.[78]

While heroin is usually injected intravenously ("mainlined"), the contemporary version of heroin is so potent that users can get high by snorting or smoking the drug. This has attracted a more affluent group of users who may not want to inject, for reasons such as the increased risk of contracting diseases like HIV. Still, it is estimated that within 2 to 3 weeks of beginning snorting or smoking, the majority of users experience an increase in tolerance and begin injecting their heroin.

Many users describe the rush they feel when injecting themselves as intensely pleasurable, whereas others report unpredictable and unpleasant side effects. The temporary nature of the rush contributes to the drug's high potential for addiction—many addicts shoot up four or five times a day. Mainlining can cause veins to scar and eventually collapse. Once a vein has collapsed, it can no longer be used to introduce heroin into the bloodstream. Addicts become expert at locating new veins to use: in the feet, the legs, the temples, under the tongue, or in the groin.

Heroin addicts experience a distinct pattern of withdrawal. Symptoms of withdrawal include intense desire for the drug, sleep disturbance, dilated pupils, loss of appetite, irritability, goose bumps, and muscle tremors. The most difficult time in the withdrawal process occurs 24 to 72 hours following last use. All of the preceding symptoms continue, along with nausea, abdominal cramps, restlessness, insomnia, vomiting, diarrhea, extreme anxiety, hot and cold flashes, elevated blood pressure, and rapid heartbeat and respiration. Once the peak of withdrawal has passed, all these symptoms begin to subside.

# Hallucinogens

**Hallucinogens,** or *psychedelics,* are substances that are capable of creating auditory or visual hallucinations and unusual changes in mood, thoughts, and feelings. The major receptor sites for most of these drugs are in the reticular formation (located in the brain stem at the upper end of the spinal cord), which is responsible for interpreting outside stimuli before allowing these signals to travel to other parts of the brain. When a hallucinogen is present at a reticular formation site, messages become scrambled, and the user may see wavy walls instead of straight ones or may "smell" colors and "hear" tastes. This mixing of sensory messages is known as *synesthesia.* Users may also become less inhibited or recall events long buried in the subconscious mind. The most widely recognized hallucinogens are LSD, Ecstasy, PCP, mescaline, psilocybin, and ketamine. All are illegal and carry severe penalties for manufacture, possession, transportation, or sale.

**hallucinogens** Substances capable of creating auditory or visual distortions and unusual changes in mood, thoughts, and feelings.

**LSD** First synthesized in the late 1930s by Swiss chemist Albert Hoffman, *lysergic acid diethylamide* (*LSD*) received media attention in the 1960s when young people used the drug to "turn on, tune in, drop out." In 1970, federal authorities placed LSD on the list of controlled substances (Schedule I). Today, this dangerous psychedelic drug, known alternately as "acid," has been making a comeback. It is estimated that 9.4 percent of Americans aged 12 or older have used LSD at least once in their lifetime.[79] A national survey of college students showed that less than 1 percent had used the drug in their lives.[80]

The most common and most popular form of LSD is blotter acid—small squares of blotter-like paper that have been impregnated with a liquid LSD mixture. The blotter is swallowed or chewed briefly. LSD also comes in tiny thin squares of gelatin called *windowpane* and in tablets called *microdots,* which are less than an eighth of an inch across (it would take ten or more to equal the size of an aspirin tablet).

One of the most powerful drugs known to science, LSD can produce strong effects in doses as low as 20 micrograms (μg). (To give you an idea of how small a dose this is, the average postage stamp weighs approximately 60,000 μg.) The potency of a typical dose currently ranges from 20 to 80 μg, compared to 150 to 300 μg commonly used in the 1960s.

Depending on the quantity users have eaten, LSD usually takes 20 to 60 minutes to take effect, and can last 6 to 8 hours. For many people there is also a period (2 to 6 hours) where it becomes difficult to sleep, and everyday reality is noticeably different. The psychological effects of LSD vary. Euphoria is the common psychological state produced by the drug, but dysphoria (a sense of evil and foreboding) may also be experienced. LSD also distorts ordinary perceptions, such as the movement of stationary objects, as well as auditory or visual hallucinations. In addition, the drug shortens attention span, causing the mind to wander. Thoughts may be interposed and juxtaposed, so the user experiences several different thoughts simultaneously. Users become introspective, and suppressed memories may surface, often taking on bizarre symbolism. Many more effects are possible,

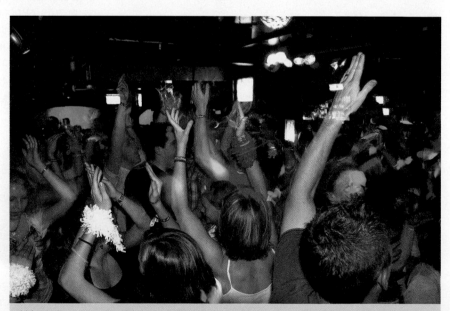

Although users may think so-called club drugs (such as Ecstasy, GHB, and ketamine) are harmless, research has shown that they can produce hallucinations, paranoia, amnesia, dangerous increases in heart rate and blood pressure, coma, and, in some cases, death.

including decreased aggressiveness and enhanced sensory experiences.

In addition to its psychedelic effects, LSD produces several physical effects, including increased heart rate, elevated blood pressure and temperature, goose bumps (roughened skin), increased reflex speeds, muscle tremors and twitches, perspiration, increased salivation, chills, headaches, and mild nausea. Because the drug also stimulates uterine muscle contractions, it can lead to premature labor and miscarriage in pregnant women. Research into long-term effects has been inconclusive.

Although there is no evidence that LSD creates physical dependence, it may create psychological dependence. Many LSD users become depressed for 1 or 2 days following a trip and turn to the drug to relieve this depression. The result is a cycle of LSD use to relieve post-LSD depression, which often leads to psychological addiction.

### Ecstasy

Ecstasy is the most common street name for the drug *methylene-dioxymethamphetamine (MDMA),* a synthetic compound with both stimulant and mildly hallucinogenic effects. It is one of the most well-known **club drugs** or "designer drugs," a term applied to synthetic analogs of existing illicit drugs popular at nightclubs and all-night parties. Ecstasy creates feelings of extreme euphoria, openness and warmth; an increased willingness to communicate; feelings of love and empathy; increased awareness; and heightened appreciation for music. Young people may use Ecstasy initially to improve their mood or get energized. Ecstasy can enhance the sensory experience and distort perceptions, but it does not create visual hallucinations. Effects begin within 20 to 90 minutes and can last for 3 to 5 hours.

Some of the risks associated with Ecstasy use are similar to those of other stimulants. Because of the nature of the drug, Ecstasy users are at greater risk of inappropriate or unintended emotional bonding and have a tendency to say things they might feel uncomfortable about later. Physical consequences of Ecstasy use may include mild to extreme jaw clenching; tongue and cheek chewing; short-term memory loss or confusion; increased body temperature; and increased heart rate and blood pressure. Combined with alcohol, Ecstasy can be extremely dangerous and sometimes fatal. As the effects of Ecstasy wear off, the user can experience mild depression, fatigue, and a hangover that can last from days to weeks. Chronic use appears to damage the brain's ability to think and to regulate emotion, memory, sleep, and pain. Some studies indicate that the drug may cause long-lasting neurotoxic effects by damaging brain cells that produce serotonin.[81]

MDMA in powder or crystal form—called "Molly," short for molecule—has become a popular festival drug. Unlike Ecstasy, which tends to be laced with ingredients like caffeine or methamphetamine, Molly is considered pure MDMA. Still, many powders sold as Molly contain zero actual MDMA. Some typical side effects of using Molly include grinding ones teeth, becoming dehydrated, feeling anxious, having trouble sleeping, fever, and losing one's appetite, as well as uncontrollable seizures, elevated blood pressure, high body temperature, and depression.[82]

### PCP (Phencyclidine)

The synthetic substance *phencyclidine (PCP)* was originally developed as a dissociative anesthetic—patients administered this drug could keep their eyes open, apparently remain conscious, and feel no pain during a medical procedure. Afterward, they would experience amnesia for the time that the drug was in their system. Such a drug had obvious advantages as an anesthetic, but its unpredictability and drastic effects (postoperative delirium, confusion, and agitation) caused it to be withdrawn from the legal market.

On the illegal market, PCP is a white, crystalline powder that users often sprinkle onto marijuana cigarettes. It is dangerous and unpredictable regardless of the method of administration. The effects of PCP depend on the dose. A dose as small as 5 mg will produce effects similar to those of strong central nervous system depressants—slurred speech, impaired coordination, reduced sensitivity to pain, and reduced heart and respiratory rate. Doses between 5 and 10 mg cause fever, salivation, nausea, vomiting, and total loss of sensitivity to pain. Doses greater than 10 mg result in a drastic drop in blood pressure, coma, muscular rigidity, violent outbursts, and possible convulsions and death.

**club drugs** Synthetic analogs that produce similar effects of existing drugs.

Psychologically, PCP may produce either euphoria or dysphoria. It also is known to produce hallucinations as well as delusions and overall delirium. Some users experience a prolonged state of "nothingness." The long-term effects of PCP use are unknown.

### Mescaline

Mescaline is one of hundreds of chemicals derived from the peyote cactus, a small, button-like plant that grows in the southwestern United States and in Latin America. Natives of these regions have long used the dried peyote "buttons" for religious purposes. It is both a powerful hallucinogen and a central nervous system stimulant.

Users typically swallow 10 to 12 buttons. They taste bitter and generally induce immediate nausea or vomiting. Long-time users claim that the nausea becomes less noticeable with frequent use. Those who are able to keep the drug down begin to feel the effects within 30 to 90 minutes, when mescaline reaches maximum concentration in the brain. Effects may persist for up to 9 or 10 hours.

Mescaline comes from "buttons" of the peyote cactus, like this one.

Products sold on the street as mescaline are likely to be synthetic chemical relatives of the true drug. Street names of these products include DOM, STP, TMA, and MMDA. Any of these can be toxic in small quantities.

**Psilocybin** *Psilocybin* and *psilocin* are the active chemicals in a group of mushrooms sometimes called "magic mushrooms." *Psilocybe* mushrooms, which grow throughout the world, can be cultivated from spores or harvested wild. When consumed, these mushrooms can cause hallucinations. Because many mushrooms resemble the *Psilocybe* variety, people who harvest wild mushrooms for any purpose should be certain of what they are doing. Mushroom varieties can be easily misidentified, and mistakes can be fatal. Psilocybin is similar to LSD in its physical effects, which generally wear off in 4 to 6 hours.

Psilocybe mushrooms produce hallucinogenic effects when ingested.

**Ketamine** The liquid form of *ketamine* ("Special K") is used as an anesthetic in some hospitals and veterinary clinics. After stealing it from hospitals or medical suppliers, dealers typically dry the liquid (usually by cooking it) and grind the residue into powder. Special K causes hallucinations, because it inhibits the relay of sensory input; the brain fills the resulting void with visions, dreams, memories, and sensory distortions. The effects of ketamine are similar to those of PCP—confusion, agitation, aggression, and lack of coordination—but even less predictable. Aftereffects of ketamine are less severe than those of Ecstasy, so it has grown in popularity as a club drug.

**Salvia** Native to Southern Mexico, salvia is an herb from the mint family.[83] Its main active ingredient, salvinorin A, causes hallucinations by changing brain chemistry.[84] Although associated hallucinatory episodes have been described as intense, they are relatively short lasting, often beginning after a minute and fading after 30 minutes.[85] These brief, but extreme hallucinations often include changes in mood, body sensations, changes to visual perception, emotional swings, feeling detached, and an altered sense of self and reality.[86] Salvia's long-term effects have not been studied.

**inhalants** Chemical vapors that are sniffed or inhaled to produce highs.

**anabolic steroids** Artificial forms of the hormone testosterone that promote muscle growth and strength.

**ergogenic drugs** Substances believed to enhance athletic performance.

## Inhalants

**Inhalants** are chemicals whose vapors, when inhaled, can cause hallucinations and create intoxicating and euphoric effects. Not commonly recognized as drugs, inhalants are legal to purchase and widely available, but dangerous. They generally appeal to young people who can't afford or obtain illicit substances. Some misused products include rubber cement, model glue, paint thinner, aerosol sprays, lighter fluid, varnish, wax, spot removers, and gasoline. Most of these substances are sniffed or "huffed" by users in search of a quick, cheap high. Amyl nitrite, a vasodilator, and nitrous oxide ("laughing gas"), an anesthetic, are also sometimes abused.

Because they are inhaled, the volatile chemicals in these products reach the bloodstream within seconds. This characteristic, along with the fact that dosages are extremely difficult to control because everyone has unique lung and breathing capacities, makes inhalants particularly dangerous. The effects of inhalants usually last fewer than 15 minutes and resemble those of central nervous system depressants: dizziness, disorientation, impaired coordination, reduced judgment, and slowed reaction times. Combining inhalants with alcohol produces a synergistic effect and can cause severe liver damage.

An overdose of fumes from inhalants can cause unconsciousness. If the user's oxygen intake is reduced during the inhaling process, death can result within 5 minutes. *Sudden sniffing death* syndrome can be a fatal consequence, whether it's the user's first time or not. This syndrome can occur if a user inhales deeply and then participates in physical activity or is startled.

## Anabolic Steroids

**Anabolic steroids** are artificial forms of the male hormone testosterone that promote muscle growth and strength. Steroids are available in two forms: injectable solutions and pills. These **ergogenic drugs** are used primarily by people who believe the drugs will increase their strength, power, bulk (weight), speed, and athletic performance.

It was once estimated that up to 20 percent of college athletes used steroids. Now that stricter drug-testing policies have been instituted by the National Collegiate Athletic Association (NCAA), reported use of anabolic steroids among intercollegiate athletes has decreased. Currently, less than half of 1 percent of college athletes surveyed report use of anabolic steroids within the past 12 months.[87] It has been estimated that approximately 1 million adults have used anabolic steroids.[88] Among both adolescents and adults, steroid abuse is higher among men than it is among women. However, steroid abuse is growing most rapidly among young women.[89]

**Physical Effects of Steroids** Although their primary effects are not psychotropic, anabolic steroids can produce a state of euphoria and diminished fatigue in addition to increased bulk and power in both sexes. These qualities give steroids an addictive quality. When users stop, they can experience psychological withdrawal and sometimes severe depression, in some cases leading to suicide attempts. If untreated, depression associated with steroid withdrawal has been known to last for a year or more after steroid use stops.

Men and women who use steroids experience a variety of adverse effects, including mood swings (aggression and violence, sometimes known as "roid rage"), acne, liver tumors, elevated cholesterol levels, hypertension, kidney disease, and immune system disturbances. There is also a danger of transmitting HIV and hepatitis through shared needles. In women, large doses of anabolic steroids may trigger the development of masculine attributes such as lowered voice, increased facial and body hair, and male-pattern baldness; they may also result in an enlarged clitoris, smaller breasts, and changes in or absence of menstruation. When taken by healthy men, anabolic steroids shut down the body's production of testosterone, causing men's breasts to grow and testicles to atrophy.

**Steroid Use and Society** The Anabolic Steroids Control Act (ASCA) of 1990 makes it a crime to possess, prescribe, or distribute anabolic steroids for any use other than the treatment of specific diseases. Penalties for their illegal use include up to 5 years' imprisonment and a $250,000 fine for the first offense and up to 10 years' imprisonment and a $500,000 fine for subsequent offenses.

In recent years, high-profile athletes in sports such as cycling, track and field, swimming, and baseball have garnered media attention for suspected use of steroids or other banned performance-enhancing drugs. Six athletes were barred from the 2014 Winter Olympic Games for illegal drug use.

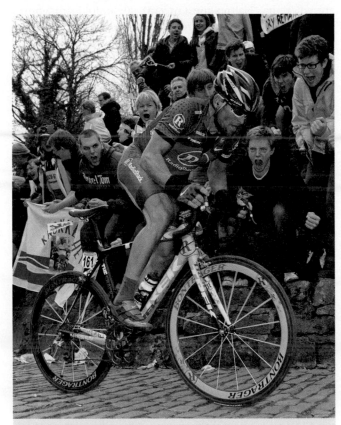

After being stripped of seven Tour de France titles in 2012 and an Olympic medal in 2013, cyclist Lance Armstrong publicly ended his years of denial and admitted to doping. He was banned from cycling for life and has been sued by the U.S. federal government and others for fraud.

### WHAT DO YOU THINK?

Do you believe an athlete's admission of steroid use invalidates his or her athletic achievements?

- How do you think professional athletes who have used steroids or other performance enhancers should be disciplined?

- If you are an athlete, have you ever considered using some type of ergogenic aid to improve your performance?

## LO 6 | TREATING AND REDUCING DRUG ABUSE

**Discuss treatment and recovery options for addicts, and discuss public health approaches to preventing drug abuse and reducing the impact of addiction on our society.**

An estimated 22.7 million Americans aged 12 or older needed treatment for an illicit drug or alcohol use problem in 2013. Of these, only 2.5 million—approximately 10.9 percent—received treatment.[90] This gap between needing and receiving treatment occurs because the most difficult step in the treatment and recovery process is for the substance abuser to admit that he or she is an addict. Admitting to addiction is difficult because of the power of *denial*—the inability to see the truth. Denial is the hallmark of addiction. It can be so powerful that a planned intervention is sometimes necessary to break down the addict's defenses against recognizing the problem.

Recovery from drug addiction or addiction to a behavior is a long-term process and frequently requires multiple episodes of treatment. The first step generally begins with abstinence—refraining from the behavior. **Detoxification** refers to an early abstinence period during which an addict adjusts physically and cognitively to being free from the addiction's influence. It occurs in virtually every recovering addict, and although it is uncomfortable for most addicts, it can be dangerous for some. This is primarily true for those addicted to chemicals, especially alcohol and heroin, and painkillers such as OxyContin. For these people, early abstinence may involve profound withdrawals that require medical supervision. Because of this, most inpatient treatment programs provide a pretreatment component of supervised detoxification to achieve abstinence safely before treatment begins.

> **detoxification** The process, which involves abstinence, of freeing a drug user from an intoxicating or addictive substance in the body or from dependence on such a substance.

### Treatment Approaches

*Outpatient behavioral treatment* encompasses a variety of programs for addicts who visit a clinic at regular intervals. Most

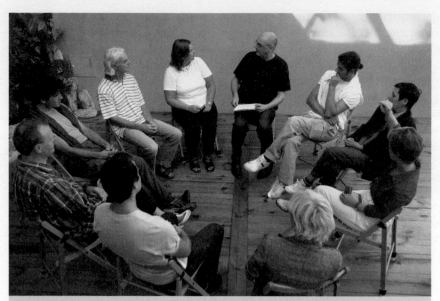

For most addicts, recovery is a long, difficult process—for some people it can be a lifelong journey. Therapy often takes the form of group meetings, such as those held by 12-step programs like Narcotics Anonymous.

of the programs involve individual or group drug counseling. *Residential treatment programs* can also be very effective, especially for those with more severe problems. Therapeutic communities (TCs) are highly structured programs in which addicts remain at a residence, typically for 6 to 12 months, with a focus on resocializing the addict to a drug-free lifestyle.

## 12-Step Programs
The first 12-step program was Alcoholics Anonymous (AA), begun in 1935 in Akron, Ohio. The 12-step program has since become the most widely used approach to dealing with not only alcoholism, but also with drug abuse and various other addictive or dysfunctional behaviors. There are more than 200 different recovery programs based on the program, including Narcotics Anonymous, Cocaine Anonymous, Crystal Meth Anonymous, Gamblers Anonymous, and Pills Anonymous.

The 12-step program is nonjudgmental and based on the idea that a program's only purpose is to work on personal recovery. Working the 12 steps includes admitting to having a serious problem, recognizing there is an outside power that could help, consciously relying on that power, admitting and listing character defects, seeking deliverance from defects, apologizing to those individuals one has harmed in the past, and helping others with the same problem. There is no membership cost, and the meetings are open to anyone who wishes to attend.

## Vaccines against Addictive Drugs
A promising new cocaine vaccine is in development. The vaccine does not eliminate the desire for cocaine; instead, it keeps the user from getting high by stimulating the immune system to attack the drug when it's taken. Clinical human trials are expected to begin soon. Vaccines against nicotine, heroin, and methamphetamine are also in development.

## Other Pharmacological Treatments
Methadone maintenance is one treatment available for people addicted to heroin or other opioids. Methadone, a synthetic narcotic, is chemically similar enough to opioids to control the tremors, chills, vomiting, diarrhea, and severe abdominal pains of withdrawal. Methadone dosage is decreased over a period of time until the addict is weaned off it.

Methadone maintenance is controversial because of the drug's own potential for addiction. Critics contend that the program merely substitutes one addiction for another. Proponents argue that people on methadone maintenance are less likely to engage in criminal activities to support their habits than heroin addicts are. For this reason, many methadone maintenance programs are financed by state or federal government and are available free of charge or at reduced cost.

A number of new drug therapies for opioid dependence are emerging. Naltrexone (Trexan), an opioid antagonist, has been approved as a treatment. While on naltrexone, recovering addicts do not have the compulsion to use heroin, and if they do use it, they don't get high, so there is no point in using the drug. Another new drug therapy, buprenorphine (Temgesic), is a mild, nonaddicting synthetic opioid; it works a lot like methadone by blocking withdrawal symptoms and heroin cravings. One of the advantages of buprenorphine is that it does not require addicts to go to a clinic/pharmacy to get take their medication; rather, it can be taken at home.

## Drug Treatment and Recovery for College Students

For college students who have developed substance or behavioral addictions, early intervention increases the likelihood of successful treatment. Depending on the severity of the abuse or dependence, college students undergoing drug treatment may be required to spend time away from school in a residential drug rehabilitation inpatient facility. The needs of college students seeking drug treatment in rehab do not differ greatly from other adult recovering addicts, but for best results, the community of addicts should include others of a similar age and educational background. Private therapy, group therapy, cognitive training, nutrition counseling, and health therapies can all be used to help with recovery. A growing number of colleges and universities offer special services to students who are recovering from alcohol and other drug addiction and want to stay in school without being exposed to excessive drinking or drug use.

## Addressing Drug Misuse and Abuse in the United States

Illegal drug use in the United States costs about $193 billion per year.[91] This estimate includes $11 billion in the cost of health care, $120 billion in lost productivity, and $61 billion in the cost of criminal investigation, prosecution, incarceration, and other associated criminal justice costs.[92] Americans are alarmed by the persistent problem of illegal drug use. Respondents in public opinion polls feel that the most important strategy for fighting drug abuse is educating young people. They also endorse strategies such as stricter border surveillance to reduce drug trafficking; longer prison sentences for drug dealers; increased government spending on prevention; antidrug law enforcement; and greater cooperation among government agencies, private groups, and individuals providing treatment assistance. To address safety concerns, many employers have instituted mandatory drug testing. Despite controversies over accuracy of urinalysis tests, this practice is becoming more common.

All of these approaches will probably help up to a point, but they do not offer a total solution to the problem. Drug abuse has been a part of human behavior for thousands of years, and it is not likely to disappear in the near future. For this reason, it is necessary to educate ourselves and to develop the self-discipline necessary to avoid dangerous drug dependence.

In general, researchers in the field of drug education agree that a multimodal approach is best. Young people should be taught the difference between drug use, misuse, and abuse. Factual information that is free of scare tactics must be presented; lecturing and moralizing have proven not to work.

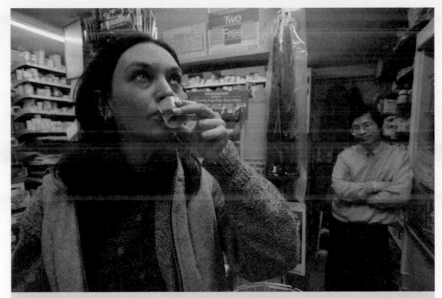

Methadone is a synthetic narcotic that blocks the effects of heroin withdrawal. Although it is still a narcotic and must be administered under the supervision of clinic or pharmacy staff, methadone allows many heroin addicts to lead somewhat normal lives.

**Harm Reduction Strategies** *Harm reduction* is a set of practical approaches to reducing negative consequences of drug use, incorporating a spectrum of strategies from safer use to abstinence. For example, needle exchange programs for injection drug users provide clean needles and syringes and bleach for cleaning needles; these efforts help reduce the number of HIV and hepatitis B cases. Harm reduction may also involve changing the legal sanctions associated with drug use, increasing the availability of treatment services to drug abusers, and/or attempting to change drug users' behavior through education. Harm reduction strategies meet drug users "where they're at," addressing conditions of use along with the use itself. This strategy recognizes that people always have and always will use drugs and, therefore, attempts to minimize the potential hazards associated with drug use rather than the use itself.

Answering the following questions will help you determine whether you have developed a drug problem:

| Yes | No | |
|---|---|---|
| ____ | ____ | 1. In the past year, have you found it significantly difficult to pay attention in class, at work, or at home? |
| ____ | ____ | 2. Have you ever felt you should cut down on your drug use? |
| ____ | ____ | 3. Have you had blackouts or flashbacks as a result of your drug use? |
| ____ | ____ | 4. Have people annoyed (irritated, angered, etc.) you by criticizing your drug use? |
| ____ | ____ | 5. Have you ever been arrested or in trouble with the law because of your drug use? |
| ____ | ____ | 6. Have you lost friends because of your drug use? |
| ____ | ____ | 7. Have you ever felt bad or guilty about your drug use? |
| ____ | ____ | 8. Have you ever thought you might have a drug problem? |

If you answered "yes" to *any* of the questions, you should consider talking to a counselor or health care provider either on campus at your health or counseling center.

**Source:** Adapted from U.S. Department of Health and Human Services, Substance Abuse and Mental Health Services Administration, Center for Substance Abuse Treatment, "Should You Talk to Someone About a Drug, Alcohol or Mental Health Problem?" 2011, www.samhsa.gov

## YOUR PLAN FOR **CHANGE**

The **ASSESS YOURSELF** activity describes signs of being controlled by drugs or having a drug problem. Depending on your results, you may need to change certain behaviors that may be detrimental to your health.

### TODAY, YOU CAN:

☐ Imagine a situation in which someone offers you a drug, and think of several different ways of refusing. Rehearse these scenarios in your head.

☐ Think about the drug use patterns among your social group. Are you ever uncomfortable with these people because of their drug use? Is it difficult to avoid using drugs when you are with them? If the answers are yes, begin exploring ways to expand your social circle.

### WITHIN THE NEXT TWO WEEKS, YOU CAN:

☐ Stop by your campus health center to find out about drug treatment programs or support groups they may have.

☐ If you are concerned about your own drug use or the drug use of a close friend, make an appointment with a counselor to talk about the issue.

### BY THE END OF THE SEMESTER, YOU CAN:

☐ Participate in clubs, activities, and social groups that do not rely on substance abuse for their amusement.

☐ If you have a drug problem, make a commitment to enter a treatment program. Acknowledge that you have a problem and that you need the assistance of others to help you overcome it.

# STUDY PLAN

Customize your study plan—and master your health!—in the Study Area of MasteringHealth™

## CHAPTER REVIEW

To hear an MP3 Tutor Session, scan here or visit the Study Area in **MasteringHealth**.

### LO **1** | What Is Addiction?

- Addiction is the continued involvement with a substance or activity despite ongoing negative consequences of that involvement. Addiction is behavior resulting from compulsion; without the behavior, the addict experiences withdrawal. In contrast, habits can be broken without much discomfort. All addictions share four common symptoms: compulsion, loss of control, negative consequences, and denial.
- Codependents are typically friends or family members who are controlled by an addict's behavior. Enablers are people who knowingly or unknowingly protect addicts from the consequences of their behavior.

### LO **2** | Addictive Behaviors

- Addictive behaviors include disordered gambling, compulsive buying, exercise addiction, and technology addiction.

### LO **3** | What Is a Drug?

- Drugs are substances other than food that are intended to affect the structure or function of the mind or the body through chemical action. Almost all psychoactive drugs affect neurotransmission in the brain.
- The six categories of drugs are prescription drugs, OTC drugs, recreational drugs, herbal preparations, illicit (illegal) drugs, and commercial drugs. Routes of administration include oral ingestion, inhalation, injection (intravenous, intramuscular, and subcutaneous), transdermal, and suppositories.

### LO **4** | Drug Misuse and Abuse

- OTC medications are drugs that do not require a prescription. Some OTC medications, including sleep aids,

cold medicines, and diet pills, can be addictive.
- Prescription drug abuse is at an all-time high, particularly among college students. Only marijuana is more commonly abused. The most commonly abused prescription drugs are opioids/narcotics, depressants, and stimulants.
- People from all walks of life use illicit drugs. Drug use declined from the mid-1980s to the early 1990s, but has remained steady since then. However, among young people, use of drugs has been rising in recent years.

### LO **5** | Common Drugs of Abuse

- Drugs of abuse (both legal and illegal) include stimulants; cannabis products, including marijuana; narcotics/depressants; hallucinogens; inhalants; and anabolic steroids. Each has its own set of risks and effects.

### LO **6** | Treating and Reducing Drug Abuse

- Treatment begins with abstinence from the drug or addictive behavior, usually instituted through intervention by close family, friends, or other loved ones. Treatment programs may be outpatient or residential and may include individual, group, or family therapy, as well as 12-step programs.
- The drug problem reaches everyone through crime and elevated health care costs. Public health and governmental approaches to the problem involve regulation, enforcement, education, and harm reduction.

## POP QUIZ

Visit **MasteringHealth** to personalize your study plan with Chapter Review Quizzes and Dynamic Study Modules.

### LO **1** | What Is Addiction?

1. Which of the following is not a characteristic of addiction?
   a. Denial
   b. Acknowledgment of self-destructive behavior
   c. Loss of control
   d. Obsession with a substance or behavior

### LO **2** | Addictive Behaviors

2. An example of a process addiction is
   a. a cocaine addiction.
   b. a gambling addiction.
   c. a marijuana addiction.
   d. a caffeine addiction.

### LO **3** | What Is a Drug?

3. Rebecca takes a number of medications for various conditions, including Prinivil (an antihypertensive drug), insulin (a diabetic medication), and Claritin (an antihistamine). This is an example of
   a. synergism.
   b. illegal drug use.
   c. polydrug use.
   d. antagonism.

4. Cross-tolerance occurs when
   a. drugs work at the same receptor site so that one blocks the action of the other.
   b. the effects of one drug are eliminated or reduced by the presence of another drug at the receptor site.
   c. a person develops a physiological tolerance to one drug and shows a similar tolerance to selected other drugs as a result.
   d. two or more drugs interact and the effects of the individual drugs are multiplied beyond what normally would be expected if they were taken alone.

### LO **4** | Drug Misuse and Abuse

5. The excessive use of any drug is called
   a. drug misuse.
   b. drug addiction.
   c. drug tolerance.
   d. drug abuse.

6. Which of the following is *not* an example of drug misuse?
   a. Developing tolerance to a drug
   b. Taking a friend's prescription medicine
   c. Taking medicine more often than is recommended
   d. Not following the instructions when taking a medicine

### LO 5 | Common Drugs of Abuse

7. Which of the following is classified as a stimulant?
   a. Methamphetamine
   b. Alcohol
   c. Marijuana
   d. LSD

8. The psychoactive drug mescaline is found in what plant?
   a. Mushrooms
   b. Peyote cactus
   c. Marijuana
   d. Belladonna

### LO 6 | Treating and Reducing Drug Abuse

9. Generally, the first step in a drug treatment program is
   a. cognitive therapy.
   b. behavioral therapy.
   c. resocialization.
   d. detoxification.

10. Which of the following is an example of a *harm reduction strategy*?
    a. Providing clean needles and syringes to a heroin user
    b. Using scare tactics to show the negative consequences of drug use
    c. Enforcing antidrug laws
    d. Favoring longer prison sentences for drug dealers

*Answers to the Pop Quiz can be found on page A-1. If you answered a question incorrectly, review the section identified by the Learning Outcome. For even more study tools, visit MasteringHealth.*

## THINK ABOUT IT!

### LO 1 | What Is Addiction?

1. Discuss how addiction affects family and friends. What role do family and friends play in helping the addict get help and maintain recovery?

### LO 2 | Addictive Behaviors

2. What differentiates a process (behavioral) addiction from a substance abuse addiction?

### LO 3 | What Is a Drug?

3. What is the current theory that explains how drugs work in the brain?

4. Explain the terms *synergism* and *antagonism*.

5. Why and how to drugs work? What are some of the different ways that different types of drugs interact with brain chemistry?

### LO 4 | Drug Misuse and Abuse

6. Do you think there is such a thing as responsible use of illicit drugs? Would you change any of the current laws governing drugs? How would you determine what is legitimate and illegitimate use?

7. Why do you think so many young people today are abusing prescription drugs? Do you perceive prescription drug abuse as being less dangerous or illegal than illicit drug use? Why? Do you think this is an accurate or biased perception?

### LO 5 | Common Drugs of Abuse

8. Why do you think many people today feel that marijuana use is not dangerous? What are the arguments in favor of legalizing marijuana? What are the arguments against legalization?

9. What accounts for the fact that some drugs are more addictive than others, chemically, culturally, and psychologically?

### LO 6 | Treating and Reducing Drug Abuse

10. What types of programs do you think would be effective in preventing drug abuse among high school and college students? How would programs for high school students differ from those for college students?

## ACCESS YOUR HEALTH ON THE INTERNET

The following websites explore further topics and issues related to personal health. For links to the websites below, visit the Study Area in MasteringHealth.

*Club Drugs.* The website provides science-based information about club drugs. **www.drugabuse.gov/drugs-abuse/club-drugs**

*Join Together.* An excellent site for the most current information related to substance abuse. Also includes information on alcohol and drug policy and provides advice on organizing and taking political action. **www.drugfree.org/join-together**

*National Institute on Drug Abuse (NIDA).* The home page of this U.S. government agency has information on the latest statistics and findings in drug research. **www.nida.nih.gov**

*Substance Abuse and Mental Health Services Administration (SAMHSA).* Outstanding resource for information about national surveys, ongoing research, and national drug interventions. **www.samhsa.gov**

*National Center for Responsible Gambling.* A resource for gambling information pertinent to college campuses. **www.collegegambling.org**

# 8 Drinking Alcohol Responsibly and Ending Tobacco Use

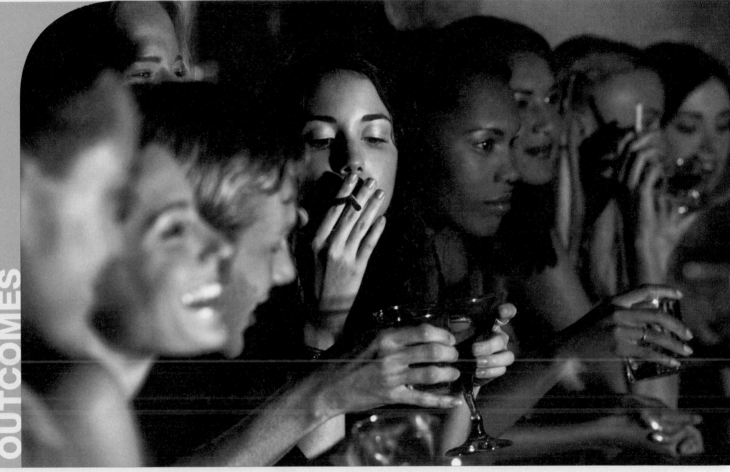

1 Explain the physiological and behavioral effects of alcohol, including absorption, metabolism, and blood alcohol concentration.

2 Identify short-term and long-term health risks associated with alcohol consumption.

3 Describe alcohol use patterns of college students, practical strategies for drinking responsibly, and ways to cope with campus and societal pressures to drink.

4 Describe alcohol use disorder, its risk factors, causes, and costs to society, and discuss options for treatment.

5 Discuss the rate of tobacco use in the United States in general and among college students in particular, and explain the social and political issues involved in tobacco use and prevention.

6 Identify different types of tobacco products, the chemicals they contain, and explain their effects on the body.

7 Describe the health risks and physical impact associated with using tobacco products, as well as with environmental tobacco smoke.

8 Describe methods and benefits of smoking cessation.

When many of us think of dangerous drugs, illegal substances such as heroin or cocaine often come to mind. But in reality, two socially accepted drugs—alcohol and tobacco—kill far more people. Annually, excessive use of alcohol is responsible for about 88,000 deaths—twice as many as illicit drugs[1]—and tobacco is the single largest preventable cause of death in the United States, claiming nearly 480,000 lives a year.[2]

# 88%

OF PEOPLE AGES 18 OR OLDER REPORT DRINKING **ALCOHOL** AT SOME POINT IN THEIR LIFETIME.

## LO 1 | ALCOHOL: AN OVERVIEW

Explain the physiological and behavioral effects of alcohol, including absorption, metabolism, and blood alcohol concentration.

Throughout history, humans have used alcohol for everything from social gatherings to religious ceremonies. The consumption of alcoholic beverages is interwoven with many traditions, and moderate use of alcohol can enhance celebrations or special times. Research shows that very low levels of alcohol consumption, particularly red wine, may actually lower some health risks in older adults.[3] While alcohol can sometimes play a positive role in some people's lives, it is first and foremost a chemical substance that affects physical and mental behavior. Alcohol is a drug; if not used responsibly, it can be dangerous.

An estimated half of Americans consume alcoholic beverages regularly, and about 21 percent abstain from drinking alcohol altogether.[4] Among those who drink, consumption patterns vary. More men are regular drinkers, and men typically drink more than do women. White drinkers are more likely to drink daily or nearly daily than are nonwhites. Abstainers are more likely to be women, Asian American or African American, and employed. Adults in poor families are more than twice as likely to be lifetime abstainers as adults in non-poor families.[5]

**ethyl alcohol (ethanol)** Addictive drug produced by fermentation that is the intoxicating substance in alcoholic beverages.

**fermentation** Process in which yeast organisms break down plant sugars to yield ethanol.

**distillation** Process in which alcohol vapors are condensed and mixed with water to make hard liquor.

**proof** Measure of the percentage of alcohol in a beverage; the proof is double the percentage of alcohol in the drink.

**standard drink** Amount of any beverage that contains about 14 grams of pure alcohol.

## The Chemistry and Potency of Alcohol

The intoxicating substance found in beer, wine, liquor, and liqueurs is **ethyl alcohol**, or **ethanol**. It is produced during a process called **fermentation**, in which yeast organisms break down plant sugars, yielding ethanol and carbon dioxide. For beer and wine, the process ends with fermentation. Hard liquor is produced through **distillation**, a process during which alcohol vapors are condensed and mixed with water to make the final product.

The **proof** of an alcoholic drink is a measure of the percentage of alcohol in the beverage—and therefore its strength. Alcohol percentage is half of the given proof. For example, 80 proof whiskey is 40 percent alcohol by volume, and 100 proof vodka is 50 percent alcohol by volume. Lower-proof drinks will produce fewer alcohol effects than the same amount of higher-proof drinks. Most wines are between 12 and 15 percent alcohol, and most beers are between 2 and 8 percent, depending on state laws and type of beer.

When discussing alcohol consumption, researchers usually talk in terms of "standard drinks." As defined by the National Institute on Alcohol Abuse and Alcoholism (NIAAA), a **standard drink** is any drink that contains about 14 grams of pure alcohol (about 0.6 fluid ounce or 1.2 tablespoons; see **FIGURE 8.1**). The actual size of a standard drink depends on

| Standard drink equivalent (and % alcohol) | Approximate number of standard drinks in: |
|---|---|
| Beer = 12 oz (~5% alcohol) | 12 oz = 1 <br> 16 oz = 1.3 <br> 22 oz = 2 <br> 40 oz = 3.3 |
| Malt liquor = 8.5 oz (~7% alcohol) | 12 oz = 1.5 <br> 16 oz = 2 <br> 22 oz = 2.5 <br> 40 oz = 4.5 |
| Table wine = 5 oz (~12% alcohol) | 750-mL (25-oz) bottle = 5 |
| 80 proof spirits (gin, vodka, etc.) = 1.5 oz (~40% alcohol) | mixed drink = 1 or more* <br> pint (16 oz) = 11 <br> fifth (25 oz) = 17 <br> 1.75 L (59 oz) = 39 |

**FIGURE 8.1** What Is a Standard Drink?
*****Note:** It can be difficult to estimate the number of standard drinks in a single mixed drink made with hard liquor. Depending on factors such as the type of spirits and the recipe, a mixed drink can contain from one to three or more standard drinks.

**Source:** Adapted from National Institute on Alcohol Abuse and Alcoholism, *Rethinking Drinking: Alcohol and Your Health,* NIH Publication no. 10-3770 (Bethesda, MD: National Institutes of Health, Revised 2010).

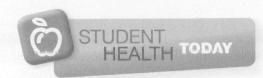

# ALCOHOL AND ENERGY DRINKS
## A Dangerous Mix

Energy drinks are aggressively marketed on college campuses, with manufacturers often giving away samples to promote them. The success of these products is based on claims that they provide a burst of energy from caffeine and other plant-based stimulants and vitamins. Thirty-four percent of 18- to 24-year-olds are regular energy drink consumers.

The alcohol industry has used the popularity of energy drinks to promote its own products, introducing premixed alcohol and energy drink products like Sparks, Rockstar 21, and Tilt. In addition, energy drink companies promote mixing energy drinks with alcohol products. Red Bull, for example, promotes a top drinks list suggesting "Jaegerbombs" and "Tucker Death mix."

Students often mix energy drinks with alcohol, and these drinks can be particularly dangerous. College men who use alcohol-mixed energy drinks score more highly on risk-taking measures. In a recent study, most college students had neutral or negative views of alcohol-mixed drinks.

Those who most frequently consume alcohol-mixed drinks had positive expectations, such as being able to party longer. Other reasons for alcohol-mixed drinks include "liking the taste" and wanting to drink something else.

Students also report not noticing the signs of intoxication (dizziness, fatigue, headache, or lack of coordination) when they had consumed alcohol-mixed energy drinks. Caffeine may delay the onset of normal sleepiness, increasing the amount of time a person would normally stay awake and drink. The caffeine in energy drinks also reduces the subjective feeling of drunkenness without actually reducing alcohol-related impairment.

Studies indicate that students who report drinking alcohol-mixed energy drinks are more likely to consume large amounts of alcohol, have unprotected sex or sex under the influence of alcohol or drugs, be hurt or injured, and meet criteria for alcohol dependency.

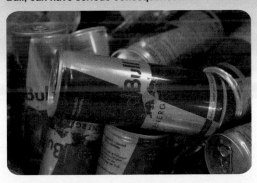

**Mixing alcohol with energy drinks, such as Red Bull, can have serious consequences.**

**Sources:** J. Verster et al., "Motives for Mixing Alcohol with Energy Drinks and Other Nonalcoholic Beverages and Consequences for Overall Alcohol Consumption," *International Journal of Internal Medicine* 7 (2014): 285–93; A. Peacock et al., "Patterns of Use and Motivations for Consuming Alcohol Mixed with Energy Drinks," *Psychology of Addictive Behaviors* 27, no. 1 (2013): 202–206; J. Howland et al., "Risks of Energy Drinks with Alcohol," *JAMA* 309, no. 3 (2013): 245–46; A. M. Arria et al., "Energy Drink Consumption and Increased Risk for Alcohol Dependence," *Alcoholism: Clinical and Experimental Research* 35, no. 2 (2011): 365–75; W. I. William et al., "Energy Drinks: Psychological Effects and Impact on Well-being and Quality of Life: A Literature Review," *Innovations in Clinical Neuroscience* 9, no. 1 (2012): 25–34.

---

the proof: A 12-ounce can of beer and a 1.5-ounce shot of vodka are both considered one standard drink because they contain the same amount of alcohol—about 0.6 fluid ounces. If you are estimating your blood alcohol concentration using standard drinks as a measure, you need to keep in mind the size of your drinks as well as their proof. For example, you may have bought only one beer at the ballpark last weekend, but if it came in a 22-ounce cup, you actually consumed two standard drinks.

## Absorption and Metabolism

Unlike the molecules found in most foods and drugs, alcohol molecules are sufficiently small and fat soluble to be absorbed throughout the entire gastrointestinal system. Approximately 20 percent of ingested alcohol diffuses through the stomach lining into the bloodstream, and nearly 80 percent passes through the lining of the upper third of the small intestine. A negligible amount of alcohol is absorbed through the lining of the mouth.

Several factors influence how quickly your body will absorb alcohol: the alcohol concentration in your drink, the amount of alcohol you consume, the amount of food in your stomach, your metabolism, your weight, your body mass index, and your mood. The higher the concentration of alcohol in your drink, the more rapidly it will be absorbed. As a rule, wine and beer are absorbed more slowly than distilled beverages. "Fizzy" alcoholic beverages—such as champagne and carbonated wines— are absorbed more rapidly than those containing no carbonation.

Carbonated beverages and drinks served with mixers cause the pyloric valve—which controls passage of stomach contents into the small intestine—to relax, thereby emptying stomach contents more rapidly into the small intestine. Because the greatest absorption of alcohol occurs in the small intestine, carbonated beverages increase the rate of absorption. In drinkers of high concentrations of alcohol, the pyloric valve can become stuck in the closed position—a condition called pylorospasm. During pylorospasm, alcohol becomes trapped in the stomach, causing irritation and often inducing vomiting. The **Student Health Today** box discusses the effects of mixing energy drinks with alcohol.

### HEAR IT! PODCASTS

Want a study podcast for this chapter? Download Alcohol, Tobacco, and Caffeine: Daily Pleasures, Daily Challenges on MasteringHealth™

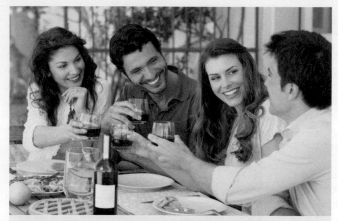

Eating while drinking slows the absorption of alcohol into your bloodstream. Other factors that influence how rapidly a person's body absorbs alcohol include gender, body weight, body composition, and mood.

The more alcohol you consume, the longer absorption takes. Alcohol also takes longer to absorb if there is food in your stomach, because the surface area exposed to alcohol is smaller, and because a full stomach retards the emptying of alcoholic beverages into the small intestine.

Mood is another factor in absorption. In fact, powerful moods like stress and tension are likely to cause the stomach to dump its contents into the small intestine rapidly, meaning alcohol is absorbed much faster when people are tense than when they are relaxed.

Once absorbed into the bloodstream, alcohol circulates throughout the body and is metabolized in the liver, where it is converted to *acetaldehyde*—a toxic chemical that can cause nausea and vomiting as well as long-term effects such as liver damage—by the enzyme *alcohol dehydrogenase.* It is then rapidly oxidized to *acetate,* converted to carbon dioxide and water, and eventually excreted from the body. A very small portion of alcohol is excreted unchanged by the kidneys, lungs, and skin.

Alcohol contains 7 calories (kcal) per gram (learn more about calories in Chapter 9). This means the average beer contains about 150 calories. Mixed drinks may contain more if combined with sugary soda or fruit juice. The body uses the calories in alcohol in the same way as those found in carbohydrates: for immediate energy or for storage as fat if not immediately needed.

**blood alcohol concentration (BAC)** The ratio of alcohol to total blood volume; the factor used to measure the physiological and behavioral effects of alcohol.

Alcohol breakdown occurs at a fairly constant rate of 0.5 ounce per hour (slightly less than one standard drink)—approximately equivalent to 12 ounces of 5 percent beer, 5 ounces of 12 percent wine, or 1.5 ounces of 40 percent (80 proof) liquor. Unmetabolized alcohol circulates in the bloodstream until enough time passes for the body to break it down.

## Blood Alcohol Concentration

**Blood alcohol concentration (BAC)** is the ratio of alcohol to total blood volume. It is the factor used to measure the physiological and behavioral effects of alcohol. Despite individual differences, alcohol produces some general behavioral effects, depending on BAC (see **FIGURE 8.2**).

At a BAC of 0.02 percent, a person feels slightly relaxed and in a good mood. At 0.05 percent, relaxation increases, there is some motor impairment, and a willingness to talk becomes apparent. At 0.08, the person feels euphoric, and there is further motor impairment. The legal limit for driving a motor vehicle is 0.08 percent BAC in all states and the District of Columbia. At 0.10 percent, the depressant effects of alcohol become apparent, drowsiness sets in, and motor skills are further impaired, followed by a loss of judgment. Thus, a driver may not be able to estimate distance or speed, and some drinkers may do things they wouldn't when sober. As BAC increases, the drinker suffers increasingly negative physiological and psychological effects.

A drinker's BAC depends on weight and percentage of body fat, the water content in body tissues, the concentration of

| Blood Alcohol Concentration (BAC) | Psychological and Physical Effects |
|---|---|
| **Not Impaired** | |
| **<0.01%** | Negligible |
| **Sometimes Impaired** | |
| **0.01–0.04%** | Slight muscle relaxation, mild euphoria, slight body warmth, increased sociability and talkativeness |
| **Usually Impaired** | |
| **0.05–0.07%** | Lowered alertness, impaired judgment, lowered inhibitions, exaggerated behavior, loss of small muscle control |
| **Always Impaired** | |
| **0.08–0.14%** | Slowed reaction time, poor muscle coordination, short-term memory loss, judgment impaired, inability to focus |
| **0.15–0.24%** | Blurred vision, lack of motor skills, sedation, slowed reactions, difficulty standing and walking, passing out |
| **0.25–0.34%** | Impaired consciousness, disorientation, loss of motor function, severely impaired or no reflexes, impaired circulation and respiration, uncontrolled urination, slurred speech, possible death |
| **0.35% and up** | Unconsciousness, coma, extremely slow heartbeat and respiration, unresponsiveness, probable death |

**FIGURE 8.2** The Psychological and Physical Effects of Alcohol

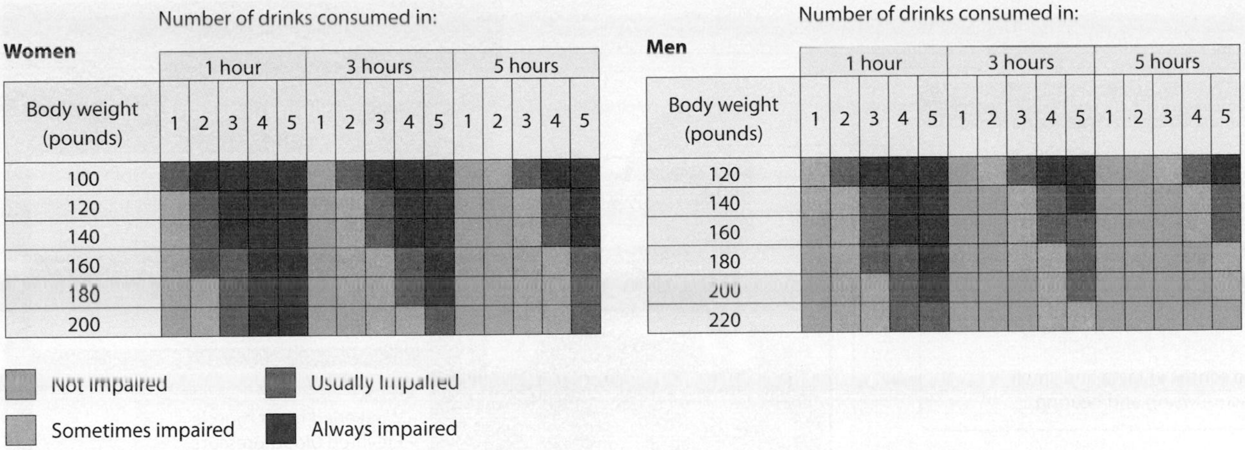

## FIGURE 8.3

Number of drinks consumed in:

**Women**

| Body weight (pounds) | 1 hour | | | | | 3 hours | | | | | 5 hours | | | | |
|---|---|---|---|---|---|---|---|---|---|---|---|---|---|---|---|
| | 1 | 2 | 3 | 4 | 5 | 1 | 2 | 3 | 4 | 5 | 1 | 2 | 3 | 4 | 5 |
| 100 | | | | | | | | | | | | | | | |
| 120 | | | | | | | | | | | | | | | |
| 140 | | | | | | | | | | | | | | | |
| 160 | | | | | | | | | | | | | | | |
| 180 | | | | | | | | | | | | | | | |
| 200 | | | | | | | | | | | | | | | |

Number of drinks consumed in:

**Men**

| Body weight (pounds) | 1 hour | | | | | 3 hours | | | | | 5 hours | | | | |
|---|---|---|---|---|---|---|---|---|---|---|---|---|---|---|---|
| | 1 | 2 | 3 | 4 | 5 | 1 | 2 | 3 | 4 | 5 | 1 | 2 | 3 | 4 | 5 |
| 120 | | | | | | | | | | | | | | | |
| 140 | | | | | | | | | | | | | | | |
| 160 | | | | | | | | | | | | | | | |
| 180 | | | | | | | | | | | | | | | |
| 200 | | | | | | | | | | | | | | | |
| 220 | | | | | | | | | | | | | | | |

■ Not impaired ■ Usually impaired
■ Sometimes impaired ■ Always impaired

**FIGURE 8.3** Approximate Blood Alcohol Concentration (BAC) and the Physiological and Behavioral Effects
Remember that there are many variables that can affect BAC, so this is only an estimate of what your BAC would be.

alcohol in the beverage consumed, the rate of consumption, and the volume of alcohol consumed. Heavier people have larger body surfaces through which to diffuse alcohol; therefore, they have lower concentrations of alcohol in their blood than do thin people after drinking the same amount. Alcohol does not diffuse as rapidly into body fat as into water, therefore alcohol concentration is higher in a person with more body fat. Because women tend to have more body fat and less water in their tissues than men of the same weight, they become more intoxicated after drinking the same amount of alcohol.

Body fat is not the only contributor to the differences in alcohol's effects on men and women. Compared to men, women have half as much *alcohol dehydrogenase,* the enzyme that breaks down alcohol in the stomach before it reaches the bloodstream and the brain. So if a man and a woman drink the same amount of alcohol, the woman's BAC will be approximately 30 percent higher than the man's. Hormonal differences can also play a role: Certain points in the menstrual cycle and the use of hormonal contraceptives likely contribute to longer periods of intoxication. **FIGURE 8.3** compares blood alcohol levels in men and women by weight and number of drinks consumed.

Both breath analysis (breathalyzer tests) and urinalysis are used to determine whether an individual is legally intoxicated, but blood tests are more accurate measures of BAC. An increasing number of states require blood tests for people suspected of driving while intoxicated. In some states, refusal to take the breath, urine, or blood test results in immediate revocation of a person's driver's license.

People can develop physical and psychological tolerance to the effects of alcohol through regular use. Over time, the nervous system adapts, requiring greater amounts of alcohol to produce the same physiological and psychological effects. Though BAC may be quite high, some individuals learn to modify their behavior to appear sober. This ability is called **learned behavioral tolerance**.

## LO 2 | ALCOHOL AND YOUR HEALTH

Identify short-term and long-term health risks associated with alcohol consumption.

The immediate and long-term effects of alcohol consumption can vary greatly (**FIGURE 8.4**). Whether or not you experience any immediate or long-term consequences depends on you as an individual, the amount of alcohol you consume, and your circumstances.

### Short-Term Effects of Alcohol Use

The most dramatic effects ethanol produce occur within the central nervous system (CNS). Alcohol depresses CNS functions, decreasing respiratory rate, pulse rate, and blood pressure. As CNS depression deepens, vital functions become noticeably affected. In extreme cases, coma and death can result.

Alcohol is a diuretic that increases urinary output. Although this effect might be expected to lead to automatic **dehydration,** the body actually retains water, most of it in the muscles or cerebral tissues. Because water is usually pulled out of the *cerebrospinal fluid* (fluid within the brain and spinal cord), drinkers may suffer symptoms that include "morning-after" headaches.

Alcohol irritates the gastrointestinal system and may cause indigestion and heartburn if consumed on an empty stomach. In addition, people who engage in brief drinking sprees of unusually high amounts of alcohol put themselves at risk for irregular heartbeat or even total loss of heart rhythm, which can disrupt blood flow and damage the heart muscle.

**learned behavioral tolerance** The ability of heavy drinkers to modify behavior so that they appear to be sober even when they have high BAC levels.

**dehydration** Loss of water from body tissues.

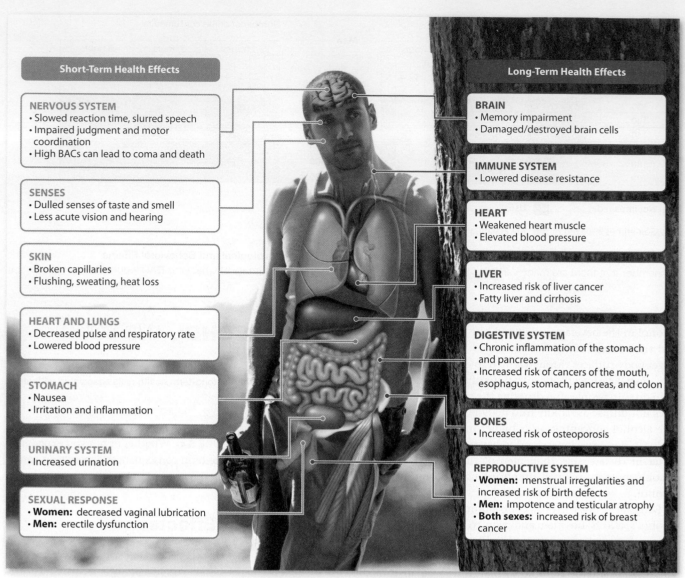

**Short-Term Health Effects**

**NERVOUS SYSTEM**
• Slowed reaction time, slurred speech
• Impaired judgment and motor coordination
• High BACs can lead to coma and death

**SENSES**
• Dulled senses of taste and smell
• Less acute vision and hearing

**SKIN**
• Broken capillaries
• Flushing, sweating, heat loss

**HEART AND LUNGS**
• Decreased pulse and respiratory rate
• Lowered blood pressure

**STOMACH**
• Nausea
• Irritation and inflammation

**URINARY SYSTEM**
• Increased urination

**SEXUAL RESPONSE**
• **Women:** decreased vaginal lubrication
• **Men:** erectile dysfunction

**Long-Term Health Effects**

**BRAIN**
• Memory impairment
• Damaged/destroyed brain cells

**IMMUNE SYSTEM**
• Lowered disease resistance

**HEART**
• Weakened heart muscle
• Elevated blood pressure

**LIVER**
• Increased risk of liver cancer
• Fatty liver and cirrhosis

**DIGESTIVE SYSTEM**
• Chronic inflammation of the stomach and pancreas
• Increased risk of cancers of the mouth, esophagus, stomach, pancreas, and colon

**BONES**
• Increased risk of osteoporosis

**REPRODUCTIVE SYSTEM**
• **Women:** menstrual irregularities and increased risk of birth defects
• **Men:** impotence and testicular atrophy
• **Both sexes:** increased risk of breast cancer

**FIGURE 8.4** Effects of Alcohol on the Body and Health

➤ **VIDEO TUTOR**
Long- and Short-Term Effects of Alcohol

### Hangover

A **hangover** is often experienced the morning after a drinking spree. Its symptoms include: headache, muscle aches, upset stomach, anxiety, depression, diarrhea, and thirst. Hangovers kick in for more than half of people after their blood alcohol content reaches 0.11. Approximately 20 to 25 percent of those who drink enough to get a hangover do not experience them.[6] Smoking while drinking may worsen hangovers. The more people smoke on the day they drink heavily, the more likely they'll have a hangover, and heavy drinking paired with heavy smoking leads to more intense hangovers.[7] **Congeners**, forms of alcohol that metabolize slower than ethanol and are more toxic, are thought to play a role in hangover development. The body metabolizes the congeners after the ethanol is gone from the system, and their toxic by-products may contribute to the hangover. Alcohol also upsets the water balance in the body, which results in excess urination, dehydration, and thirst the next day. Increased production of hydrochloric acid can irritate the stomach lining and cause nausea. Recovery from a hangover usually takes 12 hours. Bed rest, solid food, plenty of water, and aspirin or ibuprofen may help relieve a hangover's discomforts, but the only sure way to avoid one is to abstain from excessive alcohol use in the first place.

### Alcohol and Injuries

Alcohol use plays a significant role in the types of injuries people experience. Hospitalizations due to alcohol overdoses among 18- to 24-year-olds rose by 25 percent over a 10-year period, and about 30 percent of young adults hospitalized for overdoses involve excessive alcohol consumption.[8] Approximately 70 percent of fatal injuries

**hangover** Physiological reaction to excessive drinking, including headache, upset stomach, anxiety, depression, diarrhea, and thirst.

**congeners** Forms of alcohol that are metabolized more slowly than ethanol and produce toxic by-products.

during activities such as swimming and boating involve alcohol. A boat operator with a BAC over 0.1 is 16 times more likely to be killed in a boating accident than an operator with zero BAC.[9] Forty percent of fatal injuries due to house fires also involve alcohol.[10]

Alcohol use is also a key risk factor for suicide—playing a role in approximately one third of suicides in the United States.[11] Alcohol may increase suicide risk by increasing the intensity of depressive thoughts, lowering inhibitions to harm oneself, and interfering with the ability to assess future consequences of one's actions.[12]

**Alcohol and Sexual Decision Making** Because it lowers inhibitions, alcohol has a clear influence on one's ability to make good decisions about sex. Intoxicated people are less likely to use safer sex practices and are more likely to engage in high-risk sexual activity. About 1 in 5 college students reports engaging in sexual activity, including having sex with someone they just met and having unprotected sex, after drinking.[13] The chance of acquiring a sexually transmitted infection or experiencing unplanned pregnancy also increases as students drink more heavily.[14]

**Alcohol and Rape, Sexual Assault, and Dating Violence** In a recent survey, almost 20 percent of undergraduate women reported experiencing some type of sexual assault since entering college—with most incidents involving alcohol or unknowingly consuming a drug placed in their drinks.[15] Another study of college students showed heavy drinking to be associated with dating violence by men in their first year of college.[16] Among women, heavy drinking in their sophomore year predicted dating violence in their junior year. (For more on sexual assault, see Chapter 4.)

**Alcohol Poisoning** **Alcohol poisoning** (also known as **acute alcohol intoxication**) occurs much more frequently than people realize—and it can be fatal. Alcohol, used alone or with other drugs, is responsible for more toxic overdose deaths than any other substance.

The amount of alcohol that causes a person to lose consciousness—0.35% BAC for most (see Figure 8.4)—is dangerously close to the lethal dose. Death from alcohol poisoning can be caused by central nervous system and respiratory system depression or by inhaling vomit or fluid into the lungs. Alcohol depresses the nerves that control involuntary actions such as breathing and the gag reflex (which prevents choking). As BAC levels reach higher concentrations, eventually these functions can be completely suppressed. If a drinker becomes unconscious and vomits, there is a danger of asphyxiation through choking to death on one's own vomit.

Blood alcohol concentration can continue rising even after a drinker becomes unconscious, because alcohol in the stomach and intestine continues to empty into the bloodstream. Signs of alcohol poisoning include inability to be roused; a weak, rapid pulse; an unusual or irregular breathing pattern; and cool (possibly damp), pale, or bluish skin. If you are with someone who has been drinking heavily and exhibits these symptoms, or if you are unsure about the person's condition, call your local emergency number (9-1-1 in most areas) for immediate assistance.

# Drinking and Driving

Traffic accidents are the leading cause of accidental death for all age groups from 1 to 44 years old in the United States.[17] In the United States, adults drank too much and got behind the wheel approximately 112 million times in a year.[18] Alcohol-impaired drivers are involved in about 1 in 3 crash deaths, resulting in nearly 10,000 deaths a year—roughly one traffic fatality every 51 minutes.[19] Unfortunately, college students are overrepresented in alcohol-related crashes. A recent survey reported that 23 percent of college students have driven after drinking, and about 2 percent said they had driven after drinking five or more drinks in the past 30 days.[20]

> **alcohol poisoning (acute alcohol intoxication)** Potentially lethal BAC that inhibits the brain's ability to control consciousness, respiration, and heart rate; usually occurs as a result of drinking a large amount of alcohol in a short period of time.

Over the past 20 years, the percentage of intoxicated drivers involved in fatal crashes decreased for all age groups (**FIGURE 8.5**). Several factors probably contributed: laws that raised the drinking age to 21, stricter law enforcement, laws prohibiting anyone under 21 from driving with any detectable BAC, increased automobile safety, and educational programs designed to discourage drinking and driving. Furthermore, all states have zero-tolerance laws for driving while intoxicated, and the penalty is usually suspension of the driver's license.

Despite these measures, the risk of being involved in an alcohol-related automobile crash remains substantial. Laboratory and test track research shows that the vast majority of drivers are impaired even at 0.08 BAC with regard to critical driving tasks. The likelihood of a driver being involved in a

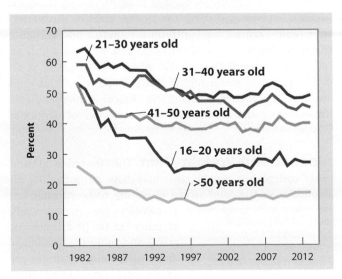

**FIGURE 8.5** Percentage of Fatally Injured Drivers with BACs Greater Than 0.08%, by Driver Age, 1982–2013

**Source:** Insurance Institute for Highway Safety, "Alcohol Impaired Driving 2013: Alcohol," Copyright 2015. Reprinted with permission.

ALCOHOL-RELATED **LIVER DISEASE** IS THE
PRIMARY CAUSE OF ALMOST

# 1 IN 3

LIVER TRANSPLANTS IN THE UNITED STATES.

fatal crash rises significantly with a BAC of 0.05 percent and even more rapidly after 0.08 percent.[21]

Alcohol-related fatal crashes occur more often at night than during the day, and the hours between 9:00 P.M. and 6:00 A.M. are the most dangerous. Sixty-eight percent of fatally injured drivers involved in nighttime single-vehicle crashes had BACs at or above 0.08 percent.[22] The risk of being involved in an alcohol-related crash increases not only with the time of day, but also with the day of the week; 25 percent of all fatal crashes during the week were alcohol related, compared with 46 percent on weekends.[23]

## Long-Term Effects of Alcohol

Alcohol is distributed throughout most of the body and may affect many organs and tissues. Problems associated with long-term, habitual use of alcohol include diseases of the nervous system, cardiovascular system, and liver, as well as some cancers.

### Effects on the Nervous System
The nervous system is especially sensitive to alcohol. Even people who drink moderately experience shrinkage in brain size and weight and a loss of some degree of intellectual ability.

Research suggests that developing brains in adolescents are much more prone to damage than previously thought. Alcohol appears to damage the frontal areas of the adolescent brain—crucial for controlling impulses and thinking through consequences of intended actions.[24] In addition, researchers suggest that people who begin drinking at an early age are at much higher risk of experiencing alcohol abuse or dependence, drinking five or more drinks per drinking occasion, and driving under the influence of alcohol at least weekly.[25]

### Alcohol and Weight Gain
The "freshman 15" and other college-year weight gains may have more to do with alcohol than the food served in dining halls. Alcohol has 7 calories per gram—nearly as much as fat (9 calories per gram)—and more than carbohydrates or protein (4 calories per gram)—and the calories from alcohol provide few nutrients. A standard drink contains 12 to 15 grams of alcohol, meaning a single drink can add about 100 empty calories to your daily intake. By drinking an extra 150 calories a day more than you need, you can gain 1 pound a month and up to 12 pounds a year.[26]

### Cardiovascular Effects
Alcohol affects the cardiovascular system in a number of ways. Numerous studies have associated light to moderate alcohol consumption (no more than two drinks a day) with a reduced risk of coronary artery disease.[27] Several mechanisms have been proposed to explain how this might happen. The strongest evidence points to an increase in high-density lipoprotein (HDL) cholesterol—"good" cholesterol—among moderate drinkers.[28] Alcohol's effects on blood clotting, insulin sensitivity, and inflammation are also thought to play a role in protecting against heart disease. However, alcohol consumption is not a preventive measure against heart disease—it causes many more hazards than benefits. Drinking too much alcohol contributes to high blood pressure and higher calorie intake, both of which are risk factors for cardiovascular disease.[29]

### Liver Disease
One result of heavy drinking is that the liver begins to store fat—a condition known as *fatty liver.* If there is insufficient time between drinking episodes, this fat cannot be transported to storage sites, and the fat-filled liver cells stop functioning. Continued drinking can cause a further stage of liver deterioration called *fibrosis,* in which the damaged area of the liver develops fibrous scar tissue. Cell function can be partially restored at this stage with proper nutrition and abstinence from alcohol. However, if the person continues to drink, **cirrhosis** of the liver results (**FIGURE 8.6**). Among the top ten causes of death in the United States, cirrhosis occurs as liver cells die and damage becomes permanent. **Alcoholic hepatitis** is another serious condition resulting from prolonged use of alcohol. A chronic inflammation of the liver develops, which may be fatal in itself or progress to cirrhosis.

### Cancer
Alcohol is considered a carcinogen. The repeated irritation caused by long-term use of alcohol has been linked to cancers of the esophagus, stomach, mouth, tongue, and liver. In one study, NIAAA scientists discovered a possible link between acetaldehyde and DNA damage that could help explain the connection between drinking and certain types of cancer.[30]

Substantial evidence suggests women who consume even low levels of alcohol (three to six drinks per week) have a higher risk of breast cancer than those who abstain, and the risk is even higher for women who consume more than two drinks per day.[31] Girls and young women who drink alcohol also increase their risk of benign (noncancerous) breast

**cirrhosis** The last stage of liver disease associated with chronic heavy use of alcohol, during which liver cells die and damage becomes permanent.

**alcoholic hepatitis** Condition resulting from prolonged use of alcohol, in which the liver is inflamed; can be fatal.

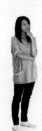

WHICH **PATH**
WOULD YOU TAKE **?**
Scan the QR code to see how different drinking choices YOU make today can affect your overall health tomorrow.

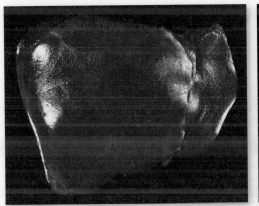
**a** A normal liver

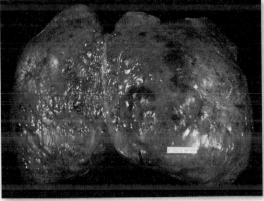
**b** A liver with cirrhosis

**FIGURE 8.6** Comparison of a Healthy Liver with a Cirrhotic Liver
In cirrhosis, healthy liver cells are replaced with scar tissue that interferes with the liver's ability to perform its many vital functions.

disease, which in turn increases the risk for developing breast cancer. In a recent study, girls and young women who drank 6 or 7 days a week were 5.5 times more likely to have benign breast disease than those who didn't drink or who had less than one drink per week.[32]

## Other Effects

Alcohol abuse is a major cause of chronic inflammation of the pancreas, the organ that produces digestive enzymes and insulin. Chronic alcohol abuse inhibits enzyme production, which further inhibits the absorption of nutrients. Drinking alcohol can block the absorption of calcium, a nutrient that strengthens bones. This should be of particular concern to women because of their risk for osteoporosis (see Chapter 14). Evidence also suggests that alcohol impairs the body's ability to recognize and fight foreign bodies, such as bacteria and viruses.

## Alcohol and Pregnancy

*Teratogenic* substances cause birth defects. Of the 30 known teratogens in the environment, alcohol is one of the most dangerous. If a woman ingests alcohol while pregnant, it will pass through the placenta and enter the growing fetus's bloodstream. A study found that more than 8.5 percent of children have been exposed to alcohol *in utero,* and 2.7 percent of pregnant women reported binge drinking.[33] Fetal development can be disrupted by alcohol at any point during a woman's pregnancy, even before she is aware that she is pregnant. When pregnant, no amount of alcohol is known to be safe to drink.[34] Alcohol consumed during the first trimester poses the greatest threat to organ development; exposure during the

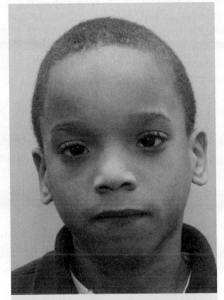
Characteristic facial features of FAS include a small, upturned nose with a low bridge and a thin upper lip.

last trimester, when the brain is developing rapidly, is most likely to affect CNS development.

A disorder called **fetal alcohol syndrome (FAS)** is associated with alcohol consumption during pregnancy. FAS is the third most common birth defect and the second leading cause of mental retardation in the United States, with an estimated incidence of 0.2 to 1.5 cases in every 1,000 live births.[35] It is the most common preventable cause of mental impairment in the Western world.[36]

**fetal alcohol syndrome (FAS)** Birth defect involving physical and mental impairment that results from the mother's alcohol consumption during pregnancy.

Among the symptoms of FAS are mental retardation; small head size; tremors; and abnormalities of the face, limbs, heart, and brain. Children with FAS may experience problems such as poor memory and impaired learning, reduced attention span, impulsive behavior, and poor problem-solving abilities, among others.

Some children may have fewer than the full physical or behavioral symptoms of FAS and may be diagnosed with disorders such as partial fetal alcohol syndrome (PFAS) or alcohol-related neurodevelopmental disorder (ARND); all of these disorders (including FAS) fall under the umbrella term *fetal alcohol spectrum disorders* (FASD). An estimated 40,000 infants in the United States are affected by FASD each year—more than those affected by spina bifida, Down syndrome, and muscular dystrophy combined.[37] Infants whose mothers habitually consumed more than 3 ounces of alcohol (approximately six drinks) in a short time period when pregnant are at high risk for FASD. Risk levels for babies whose mothers consume smaller amounts are uncertain. To avoid any chance of harming her fetus, any woman of childbearing age who is or may become pregnant is advised to refrain from consuming any amount of alcohol.

# LO 3 | ALCOHOL USE IN COLLEGE

Describe alcohol use patterns of college students, practical strategies for drinking responsibly, and ways to cope with campus and societal pressures to drink.

Alcohol is the most popular drug on college campuses: 67 percent of students report having consumed alcoholic beverages in the past 30 days (**FIGURE 8.7**).[38] Approximately 39 percent of all college students engage in **binge drinking**.[39] For a typical adult, this means consuming five or more drinks (men), or four or more drinks (women), in about 2 hours.[40] Students who drink only once a week are considered binge drinkers if they consume these amounts within 2 hours. On college campuses, the gap between men and women's alcohol consumption is closing. In 1992, 36 percent of men and 20 percent of women engaged in binge drinking one or more times per week; in 2012, 27 percent of men and 20 percent of women did so.[41]

College is a critical time to become aware of and responsible for drinking. Many students are away from home, often for the first time, and are excited by their newfound independence. For some students, this independence and the rite of passage into the college culture are symbolized by alcohol use. More than 80 percent of college students drink alcohol to celebrate their twenty-first birthday.[42] In a recent study, nearly half of students celebrating experienced at least one negative consequence of drinking alcohol (e.g., headache, feeling very sick to their stomach, etc.).[43]

The transition into college itself may put first-year students at risk for alcohol misuse. During high school, students who are college bound drink less than their classmates who aren't headed to college, and students who report a difficult transition to college are more likely to engage in high-risk drinking.[44] Many students say they drink to have fun, but may be coping with stress, boredom, or pressures created by academic and social demands. For other students, alcohol lowers inhibitions and is a way to manage social anxiety and shyness.

A significant number of students experience negative consequences as a result of their alcohol consumption (**FIGURE 8.8**). Nearly 2 percent reported having sex with someone without giving consent, and 0.6 percent reported having sex with someone without getting consent.[45] A recent study found students who played

> **binge drinking** A pattern of drinking alcohol that brings BAC to 0.08 gram-percent or above; corresponds to consuming five or more drinks (adult male) or four or more drinks (adult female) in 2 hours.

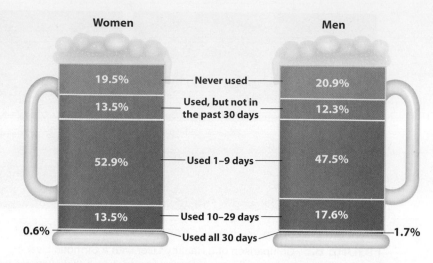

**Women** / **Men**

| | Women | | Men |
|---|---|---|---|
| Never used | 19.5% | | 20.9% |
| Used, but not in the past 30 days | 13.5% | | 12.3% |
| Used 1–9 days | 52.9% | | 47.5% |
| Used 10–29 days | 13.5% | | 17.6% |
| Used all 30 days | 0.6% | | 1.7% |

**FIGURE 8.7** College Students' Patterns of Alcohol Use in the Past 30 Days

**Source:** Data from American College Health Association, *American College Health Association—National College Health Assessment II: Reference Group Executive Summary, Spring 2014* (Hanover, MD: American College Health Association, 2014).

intramural sports, were in abusive relationships, had high levels of stress, belonged to a fraternity or sorority, or were depressed reported higher levels of drinking and negative consequences.[46]

Alcohol use among college students also has consequences related to academic performance.[47] Alcohol consumption

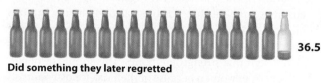 **36.5%**

**Did something they later regretted**

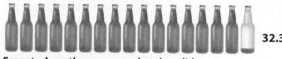 **32.3%**

**Forgot where they were or what they did**

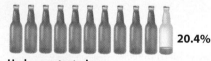 **20.4%**

**Had unprotected sex**

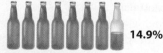 **14.9%**

**Physically injured self**

 **3.0%**

**Got in trouble with the police**

 **1.8%**

**Physically injured another person**

**FIGURE 8.8** Prevalence of Negative Consequences of Drinking among College Students, Past Year

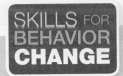

## SKILLS FOR BEHAVIOR CHANGE

### TIPS FOR DRINKING RESPONSIBLY

▶ Eat before and while you drink.

▶ Stay with the same group of friends the entire time you drink.

▶ Don't drink before the party.

▶ Avoid drinking if you are angry, anxious, or depressed.

▶ Have no more than one alcoholic drink per hour.

▶ Alternate between alcoholic and nonalcoholic drinks.

▶ Set limits on how much to have before you start drinking.

▶ Avoid drinking games.

▶ Don't drink and drive.

▶ Avoid parties where you can expect heavy drinking.

tends to disrupt sleep, particularly the second half of the night's sleep. These disruptive effects increase daytime sleepiness and decrease alertness, which can also negatively impacts students' academic performance.[48]

Fortunately, many college students report practicing protective behaviors when consuming alcohol to reduce the risk of negative consequences as a result of their alcohol use. The **Skills for Behavior Change** box provides some strategies for drinking responsibly.

## High-Risk Drinking and College Students

According to a recent study, 1,825 college students die each year because of alcohol-related unintentional injuries, including car accidents.[49] Consumption of alcohol is the number one cause of preventable death among undergraduate college students in the United States today.[50]

Although everyone who drinks is at some risk for alcohol-related problems, college students seem particularly vulnerable for the following reasons:

■ Alcohol exacerbates their already high risk for suicide, automobile crashes, and falls.

■ Many college and university students' customs and celebrations encourage certain dangerous practices and patterns of alcohol use.

■ The alcoholic beverage industry heavily targets university campuses.

■ Drink specials enable students to consume large amounts of alcohol cheaply.

■ College students are particularly vulnerable to peer influence.

■ College administrators often deny that alcohol problems exist on their campuses.

College students are also more likely than their non-collegiate peers to drink recklessly, play drinking games, and engage in other dangerous practices.[51] **Pre-gaming** (also called pre-loading or front-loading) involves planned heavy drinking, in a compressed time frame, usually in someone's home, apartment, or residence hall, prior to going out to a bar, party, or sporting event. In a recent study, 25 percent of students reported pre-gaming in the past month.[52] Pre-gamers have higher alcohol consumption during the evening and increased risk of negative consequences like blackouts, hangovers, passing out, and alcohol poisoning.[53]

> **pre-gaming** Drinking heavily at home before going out to an event or other location.

Two thirds of college students engage in drinking games that involve binge drinking.[54] Those who participate in drinking games are much less likely to monitor or regulate how much they are drinking and are at risk for extreme intoxication. Men more often than women participate in drinking games to consume larger amounts of alcohol,[55] and drinking games have been associated with alcohol-related injuries and deaths from alcohol poisoning.

Unfortunately, recent studies confirm what students have been experiencing for a long time—binge drinkers cause problems not only for themselves, but also for those around them. One study indicated that more than 696,000 students between the ages of 18 and 24 were assaulted by another student who had been drinking.[56] Significant evidence links campus rape to binge drinking. Although exact numbers are hard to find,

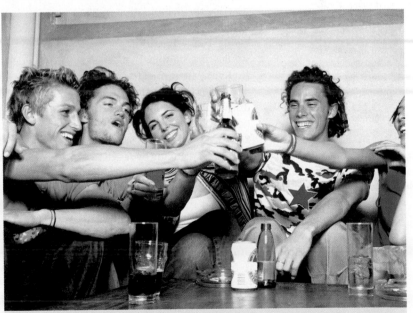

While about 64 percent of college students drink only occasionally, and 21.3 percent don't drink at all, college students have high rates of binge drinking Take control of when you drink and how much.

**Source:** American College Health Association, *American College Health Association—National College Health Assessment II (ACHA-NCHA II) Reference Group Data Report Spring 2013* (Linthicum, MD: American College Health Association, 2013).

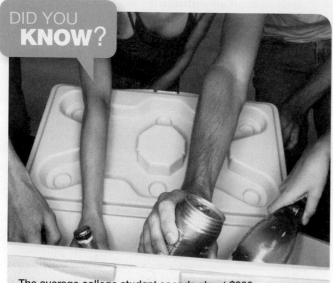

The average college student spends about $900 per year on alcohol—compared to spending an average of about $450 a year on books.

**Source:** Data from Phoenix House's Facts on Tap, "School Daze?," Accessed 2011, www.factsontap.org

estimates are that more than 97,000 U.S. students between the ages of 18 and 24 experience alcohol-related sexual assault or date rape each year.[57] Other students report sleep and study disruptions and vandalism of personal property.

Some people use extreme measures to control their eating and/or exercise excessively so that they can save calories, consume more alcohol, and become intoxicated faster.[58] "**Drunkorexia**" is a colloquialism used to describe the combination of two dangerous behaviors: disordered eating and heavy drinking. Early studies have found that college students who restrict the number of calories they consume prior to drinking are more likely to drink heavily.[59] One study found that 28 percent of women and 8 percent of men surveyed "saved" calories for drinking by restricting normal caloric intake.[60] The same study found 29 percent of those surveyed engaged in drunkorexia before all drinking occasions.[61] Similarly, another study found that highly physically active college students are more likely to binge drink than their nonactive peers.[62] Motivations for drunkorexia include preventing weight gain, getting drunk faster, and saving money that would be spent on food to buy alcohol. Potential risks of drunkorexia include blackouts, forced sexual activity, unintended sexual activity, and alcohol poisoning.

**drunkorexia** A colloquial term to describe the combination of disordered eating, excessive physical activity, and heavy alcohol consumption.

**alcohol use disorder** Refers to problem drinking so severe that at least two or more alcohol-related issues are present, such as engaging in risky behaviors, having problems at work or school, or issues with relationships.

## Efforts to Reduce Student Drinking

What are colleges currently doing to address the problem of drinking on campus? Programs that have proven particularly effective use cognitive-behavioral skills training with *motivational interviewing,* a nonjudgmental approach to working with students to change behavior. The NIAAA has recognized Brief Alcohol Screening and Intervention for College Students (BASICS) as an effective program for students who drink heavily and have experienced or are at risk for alcohol-related problems. A recent study found that both male and female students significantly decreased their alcohol consumption as a result of participation.[63] E-interventions—electronically based alcohol education interventions using text messages, e-mails, and podcasts—and Web interventions such as the Alcohol e-Check Up to Go (e-Chug) have shown promise in reducing alcohol-related problems among first-year students.

Web-based education for first-year students has become an increasingly important intervention. Because first-year students are at increased risk for alcohol-related problems, schools ensure that students are made aware of risks and effects of alcohol, as well as and campus resources available for dealing with issues with alcohol use.

WHAT DO YOU THINK?

Why do some college students drink excessive amounts of alcohol?

- Are there particular traditions or norms related to when and why students drink on your campus?

- Have you ever had your sleep or studies interrupted, or have you had to babysit a friend because he or she had been drinking?

## LO 4 | ABUSE AND DEPENDENCE

Describe alcohol use disorder, its risk factors, causes, and costs to society, and discuss options for treatment.

The new edition of the *Diagnostic and Statistical Manual of Mental Disorders (DSM-5)* has integrated alcohol abuse and alcohol dependence into a single disorder: **Alcohol use disorder (AUD).** Any person who meets two or more of the new criteria would receive a diagnosis of AUD. Severity of AUD falls along a spectrum from mild, to moderate, to severe, according to the number of criteria a person meets (**FIGURE 8.9**). For example if a student shares having a strong desire or craving to use alcohol and a high tolerance for alcohol with a counselor or clinician, he would meet the criteria for mild AUD.

## Identifying an Alcoholic

As with other addictions, craving, loss of control, tolerance, psychological dependence, and withdrawal symptoms must be present to qualify a drinker as an addict (see Chapter 7). Irresponsible and problem drinkers, such as people who get into fights or embarrass themselves or others when they drink, are not necessarily alcoholics. Alcoholics can be found at all socioeconomic levels and in all professions, ethnic groups, geographical locations, religions, and races. Data indicate that about 15 percent of people in the United States are problem drinkers, and about 5 to 10 percent of male drinkers and 3 to 5 percent of females would be diagnosed as alcohol dependent.[64]

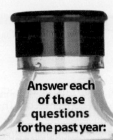

Answer each of these questions for the past year:

Do you ever drink more or for longer periods of time than you'd planned?

Do you have a strong desire to cut down, or are you unable to control your alcohol use?

At times, are you unable to think of anything other than your next drink?

Do you spend considerable time in activities related to drinking or recovering from drinking?

Have you reduced your involvement in pleasurable social, occupational, or recreational activities?

Have you neglected responsibilities at work, school, and/or at home?

Do you continue drinking despite knowing that physical/psychological problems are caused or exacerbated by your drinking? Or after a memory blackout?

Have you more than once physically endangered yourself during or after drinking?

Have you continued to use alcohol despite social or interpersonal problems caused or aggravated by use?

Do you meet the definition of having developed tolerance based on these criteria?
1) You need increasingly greater amounts of alcohol to get the same desired effect.
2) Over time, you experience fewer effects from alcohol when you drink the same amount.

Do you experience characteristic signs of alcohol withdrawal when you stop drinking or do you use another substance to relieve or avoid withdrawal?

If you answered yes to two or more of the questions, you are considered someone with an alcohol use disorder (AUD). The level of AUD is defined as: **mild:** 2–3 items; **moderate:** 4–5 items; and **severe:** 6 or more items.

**FIGURE 8.9** Alcohol Use Disorder (AUD) Criteria

**Source:** National Institutes of Health, *Alcohol Use Disorder: A Comparison between DSM-IV and DSM-5*, National Institute on Alcohol Abuse and Alcoholism NIH Publication No.13-7999, 2013, http://pubs.niaaa.nih.gov/publications/dsmfactsheet/dsmfact.htm

Recognizing and admitting the existence of an alcohol problem is often extremely difficult. Alcoholics often deny their problem with statements like, "I can stop any time I want to. I just don't want to right now." The fear of being labeled a "problem drinker" often prevents people from seeking help. People who recognize alcoholic behaviors in themselves may wish to seek professional help. (The **Skills for Behavior Change** box gives tips for cutting down on drinking.)

AUD is not uncommon among college students. In a survey of full-time college students, 1 in 4 experienced alcohol abuse or dependence in the past year.[65] College students at highest risk for AUD drank to facilitate socializing with peers or to have a good time, drank in a parked car, or drank to bolster their confidence to talk to or have sex with someone.[66] In a recent study, the progression to alcohol dependency based on college students' drinking patterns when they entered college indicated that 1.9 percent of nondrinkers, 4.3 percent of light drinkers, 12.8 percent of moderate drinkers, and 19 percent of heavy drinkers developed alcohol dependency.[67]

## The Causes of Alcohol Use Disorder

We know alcoholism is a disease with biological and social/environmental components, but we do not know what role each component plays.

**Biological and Family Factors** Research into the hereditary and environmental causes of alcoholism has found higher rates of alcoholism among children of alcoholics than in the general population. Alcoholism among individuals with a family history of alcoholism is about four to eight times more common than it is among individuals with no such family history.[68]

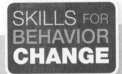 CUT DOWN ON YOUR DRINKING

If you have a severe drinking problem, alcoholism in your family, or other medical problems, you should stop drinking completely. If you need to cut down on your drinking, these steps can help you:

▶ If you suspect that you drink too much, talk with a counselor or a clinician at your student health center.

▶ Write your reasons for cutting down or stopping.

▶ Set a drinking limit. If you aren't sure what goal is right for you, talk with your counselor.

▶ Keep a diary of your drinking.

▶ Keep little or no alcohol at home.

▶ Drink slowly.

▶ Learn how to say no. Stay away from people who give you a hard time about not drinking.

▶ Stay active.

▶ Get support. Ask your family and friends to help you reach your goal. Talk to your counselor if you are having trouble cutting down.

▶ Avoid temptations. Watch out for people, places, or times that make you drink, even if you do not want to.

▶ Remember, don't give up!

**Source:** Adapted from National Institutes of Health, National Institute on Alcohol Abuse and Alcoholism, NIH Publication No. 13-3770, *Rethinking Drinking* (2010), http://pubs.niaaa.nih.gov/publications/RethinkingDrinking/Rethinking_Drinking.pdf

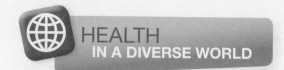
# GLOBAL HEALTH AND ALCOHOL USE

Alcohol consumption comes with many serious social and developmental issues, including violence, child neglect and abuse, and absenteeism in the workplace. Throughout the world, alcohol is a factor in 60 types of diseases and injuries and a component cause in 200 others. Almost 4 percent of all deaths worldwide are attributed to alcohol, greater than deaths caused by HIV/AIDS, violence, or tuberculosis. Worldwide, the impact of alcohol use is as follows:

- Alcohol use results in 3.3 million deaths each year.

- 7.6% of male deaths and 4.0% of female deaths worldwide are attributable to alcohol consumption.
- Early alcohol use (before the age of 14) is positively correlated with harmful behaviors later in life, including alcohol addiction and drunk driving.
- At the same level of alcohol consumption, men are more likely to become injured and women are more likely to experience negative health outcomes such as cancer (particularly breast cancer), cardiovascular disease, and gastrointestinal problems.

A large variation exists in adult per capita alcohol consumption. The highest consumption levels can be found in the developed world, including Europe and the Americas. Intermediate consumption levels can be found in regions of the Western Pacific and Africa. Low consumption levels can be found in Southeast Asia and the Eastern Mediterranean regions. Many factors, including culture, religion, economic development, and socioeconomic status, contribute to these differences.

**Source:** World Health Organization, "Global Status Report on Alcohol and Health," 2014, www.who.int/substance_abuse/publications/global_alcohol_report/en

---

Despite evidence of heredity's role, scientists do not yet understand the precise role of genes in increased risk for alcoholism, nor have they identified a specific "alcoholism" gene. Alcohol use disorders are between 50 percent and 60 percent heritable.[69] Anxiety and depression, by comparison, are around 20 to 40 percent heritable, respectively. Adoption studies have helped demonstrate a strong link between biological parents' substance use and their children's risk for addiction. Recently, scientists found a gene that, by controlling the way alcohol stimulates the brain to release dopamine, can trigger feelings of reward.[70] Alcohol gives individuals with the gene a stronger sense of reward from alcohol, making it more likely for them to be heavy drinkers. However, there is nothing deterministic about the genetic basis for addiction. Although no single gene causes addiction, multiple genes can affect the ability to develop addiction.

### Social and Cultural Factors

Some people begin drinking as a way to dull the pain of an acute loss or an emotional or social problem. Unfortunately, they become even sadder as the depressant effect of the drug begins to take its toll, sometimes causing them to antagonize friends and other social supports. Eventually, the drinker becomes physically dependent on the drug.

Family attitudes toward alcohol also seem to influence whether a person will develop a drinking problem. People raised in cultures where drinking is a part of religious or ceremonial activities or part of the family meal are less prone to alcohol dependence. In contrast, societies where alcohol purchase is carefully controlled and drinking is regarded as a rite of passage to adulthood appear to have greater tendency for abuse. The **Health in a Diverse World** box discusses some of the patterns of alcohol use and abuse around the world.

The amount of alcohol a person consumes seems to be directly related to the drinking habits of that individual's social group. A recent study found that those whose friends and relatives drank heavily were 50 percent more likely to drink heavily themselves.[71] The opposite is also true, that people with abstinent friends or family members were less likely to drink themselves. This finding has increased importance for individuals in treatment or who have been in treatment and their need to sever ties with heavy drinkers to maintain abstinence.

## Women and Alcoholism

Women tend to become alcoholics at later ages and after fewer years of heavy drinking than do men. Women also get addicted faster with less alcohol use. With greater risks for cirrhosis; excessive memory loss and shrinkage of the brain; heart disease; and cancers of the mouth, throat, esophagus, liver, and colon than male alcoholics, women suffer the consequences of alcoholism more profoundly.[72]

Highest risks for alcoholism occur among women who are unmarried but living with a partner, are in their twenties or early thirties, or have a husband or partner who drinks heavily. Other risk factors for women include a family history of drinking problems, pressure to drink from a peer or spouse, depression, and stress.

## Alcohol and Prescription Drug Abuse

When alcohol and prescription drugs are taken together, severe medical problems can result, including alcohol poisoning, unconsciousness, respiratory depression, and death.

The greatest risks from drug mixing occur when alcohol is mixed with prescription painkillers. Both drugs slow breathing rates in unique ways and inhibit the coughing reflex; when combined, they can stop breathing altogether. Alcohol also interacts with antianxiety medications, antipsychotics, antidepressants, sleep medications, and muscle relaxants, causing dizziness and drowsiness and making falls and unintentional injuries more likely. Prescription drugs most commonly combined with alcohol include opioids (e.g., Vicodin, OxyContin, Percocet), stimulants (e.g., Ritalin, Adderall, Concerta), sedative/anxiety medications (e.g., Ativan, Xanax), and sleeping medications (e.g., Ambien, Halcion).

## Costs to Society

Alcohol-related costs to American society are estimated to be well over $223.5 billion when health insurance, criminal justice, treatment, and lost productivity are considered.[73] Alcoholism is directly or indirectly responsible for over 25 percent of the nation's medical expenses and lost earnings.[74] A recent study estimated that underage drinking costs society $62 billion annually.[75] The largest costs were related to violence ($35 billion) and drunk-driving accidents (nearly $10 billion), followed by high-risk sex ($5 billion), property crime ($3 billion), and addiction treatment programs ($2.5 billion).[76] By dividing the cost of underage drinking by the estimated number of underage drinkers, the study estimated each underage drinker costs society an average of over $2,000 a year.[77]

## Treatment and Recovery

Only a very small percentage of alcoholics ever receive care in special treatment facilities. Numerous factors contribute to this low treatment utilization, including an inability or unwillingness to admit to an alcohol problem, the social stigma attached to alcoholism, potential loss of income, inability to pay for treatment, breakdowns in referral and delivery systems, and failure of the medical establishment to recognize and diagnose alcoholic symptoms.[78] Most drinkers who seek help have experienced a turning point when the person recognizes that alcohol controls his or her life.

Alcoholics who decide to quit drinking will experience *detoxification,* the process by which addicts end their dependence on a drug. Withdrawal symptoms include hyperexcitability, confusion, agitation, sleep disorders, convulsions, tremors, depression, headache, and seizures. For a small percentage of people, alcohol withdrawal results in a severe syndrome known as **delirium tremens (DTs)**, characterized by confusion, delusions, agitated behavior, and hallucinations.

The alcoholic who is ready for help has several avenues of treatment: psychologists and psychiatrists specializing in treatment, private treatment centers, hospitals specifically designed to treat alcoholics, community mental health facilities, and support groups such as **Alcoholics Anonymous (AA)**.

### Private Treatment Facilities

Upon admission to a private treatment facility, the patient receives a complete physical exam to determine whether underlying medical problems will interfere with treatment. Shortly after detoxification, alcoholics begin their treatment for psychological addiction. Most treatment facilities keep their patients from 3 to 6 weeks. Treatment at private centers can cost several thousand dollars, but some insurance programs or employers will assume most of this expense.

**Therapy** Several types of therapy are commonly used in alcoholism recovery programs. In family therapy, the person and family members examine the psychological reasons underlying the addiction and environmental factors enabling it. In individual and group therapy, alcoholics learn positive coping skills for situations that have regularly caused them to turn to alcohol.

While there are many recovery management strategies for adults, understanding an appropriate recovery support system for college students has received less attention. In particular, there has been a lack of campus-based services for recovering students. The high prevalence of alcohol and other drug use on college campuses makes attending college a threat to sobriety. However, many campuses recognize the need to create recovery-friendly space and supportive environments for students engaged in recovery. Common features of such programs include a designated campus meeting space, drug-free housing options, individual or group counseling, relapse prevention, and sober leisure activities; peer support and 12-step tenets are typically emphasized.[79]

**delirium tremens (DTs)** State of confusion, delusions, and agitation brought on by withdrawal from alcohol.

**Alcoholics Anonymous (AA)** Organization whose goal is to help alcoholics stop drinking; includes auxiliary branches such as Al-Anon and Alateen.

**Relapse** Success in recovery varies with the individual. Up to 70 percent of alcoholics relapse (resume drinking) within 1 year of treatment.[80] Treating an addiction requires more than getting the addict to stop using a substance; it also requires getting the person to break a pattern of behavior that has dominated his or her life. Many alcoholics refer to themselves as "recovering" rather than "cured."

People seeking to regain a healthy lifestyle must not only confront their addiction, but also guard against the tendency to relapse. For alcoholics, it is important to identify situations that could trigger a relapse, such as becoming angry or frustrated and being around others who drink. During the initial recovery period, it can help to join a support group, maintain stability (resisting the urge to move, travel, assume a new job, or make other drastic life changes), set aside time each day for reflection, and maintain a pattern of assuming responsibility for their own actions. To be effective, recovery programs must offer alcoholics ways to increase self-esteem and resume personal growth.

## LO 5 | TOBACCO USE IN THE UNITED STATES

Discuss the rate of tobacco use in the United States in general and among college students in particular, and explain the social and political issues involved in tobacco use and prevention.

In the United States, tobacco use is the single most preventable cause of death. Close to a half a million Americans die each year of tobacco-related diseases.[81] Moreover, another 16 million people will suffer from health disorders caused by tobacco. To date, tobacco is known to cause about 20 diseases, and about half of all regular smokers die of smoking-related diseases.[82]

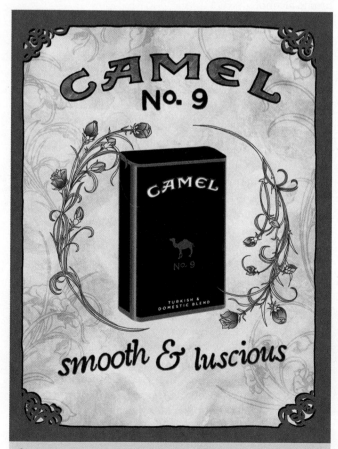

Cigarette companies have become adept at marketing to women using "glamorous" packaging and ad campaigns borrowed from cosmetics, perfume (such as the famous Chanel scents evoked by this Camel No. 9 brand), and the fashion industry.

TABLE **8.1** | Percentage of Population That Smokes (Age 18 and Older) among Select Groups in the United States

| | Percentage |
|---|---|
| United States overall | 18.7 |
| **Race** | |
| Asian | 9.6 |
| Black, non-Hispanic | 18.3 |
| Hispanic | 12.1 |
| Native American | 26.1 |
| White, non-Hispanic | 19.9 |
| Multiple race | 26.8 |
| **Age** | |
| 18–24 | 18.7 |
| 25–44 | 20.1 |
| 45–64 | 19.9 |
| 65+ | 8.8 |
| **Gender** | |
| Male | 20.5 |
| Female | 15.3 |
| **Education** | |
| Undergraduate degree | 9.1 |
| High School diploma | 22.0 |
| GED diploma | 41.4 |
| 12th grade, (no diploma) | 19.7 |
| Graduate degree | 5.6 |
| **Income Level** | |
| Below poverty level | 29.2 |
| At or above poverty level | 16.2 |
| **Sexual Orientation** | |
| Straight | 17.6 |
| Lesbian/Gay/Bisexual | 26.6 |

**Source:** Centers for Disease Control and Prevention, "Current Cigarette Smoking Among Adults—United States, 2005–2013," *Morbidity and Mortality Weekly* 63, no. 47 (2014): 1108–1112.

Approximately 70 million Americans age 12 and older report using tobacco products in the past month.[83] Declines in cigarette smoking over the past two decades have slowed compared with earlier periods. In 2012, 20.5 percent of men and 15.8 percent of women were current cigarette smokers. Adults 25 to 44 years old had the highest percentage of current cigarette smoking (22 percent), and the percentage continues to decrease with age, with 19.5 percent of adults 45 to 64 years old and 9 percent of adults aged 65 years and older reported to be current smokers.[84] **TABLE 8.1** shows the percentages of Americans who smoke by demographic group.

# Tobacco and Social Issues

The production and distribution of tobacco products involve many political and economic issues. Tobacco-growing states derive substantial income from tobacco production, and federal, state, and local governments benefit enormously from cigarette taxes.

## Advertising

The tobacco industry spends an estimated $01 million per day on advertising and promotional material.[85] With the number of smokers declining by about 1 million each year, the industry must actively recruit new smokers. Tobacco advertising encourages young people to begin smoking before they are old enough to understand the long-term health risks.[86] Of adult smokers, 90 percent started by age 21, and half became regular smokers by age 18. Tobacco companies target children and teens with tobacco products that are candy, fruit, or alcohol flavored, thus making them more palatable to young people.[87]

Advertisements in women's magazines imply that smoking is the key to financial success, thinness, independence, and social acceptance—and they have apparently been working. From the mid-1970s through the early 2000s, cigarette sales to women increased dramatically. Not coincidentally, by 1987 cigarette-induced lung cancer had surpassed breast cancer as the leading cancer killer among women and has remained the leading cancer killer among women in every year since.[88]

Women are not the only targets of gender-based cigarette advertisements. Men are depicted in locker rooms, charging over rugged terrain in off-road vehicles, or riding stallions in blatant appeals to masculinity. Minorities are also often targeted. Tobacco advertising, particularly of menthol cigarettes, is much more common in magazines aimed at African Americans, such as *Jet* and *Ebony*, than in similar magazines aimed at broader audiences, such as *Time* and *People*. Billboards and posters spreading the cigarette message have dotted the landscape in Hispanic communities for many years, especially in low-income areas. Tobacco companies also sponsor community-based events such as festivals and annual fairs.

## Financial Costs to Society

Estimated annual costs attributed to smoking in the United States are between $289 and $333 billion.[89] The economic burden of tobacco use totals more than $132 to $176 billion in direct medical expenditures and $156 billion in lost productivity. It is estimated that smoking-related health costs and productivity losses are $18.20 per pack of cigarettes sold.[90] These costs far exceed the tax revenues on the sale of tobacco products, even though the average cigarette tax in 2012 was $1.53 per pack and rising in some states.[91]

# College Students and Tobacco Use

College students are the targets of heavy tobacco marketing and advertising campaigns. The tobacco industry has set up aggressive marketing promotions at bars, music festivals, and other events specifically targeted at the 18- to 24-year-old age group. On top of targeted advertising, peer influence can prompt students to start smoking, and many colleges and universities still sell tobacco products in campus stores. However, cigarette smoking among U.S. college students has decreased in recent years (see **FIGURE 8.10**). In a 2014 study, about 12.6 percent of college students reported having smoked cigarettes in the past 30 days.[92] College men have slightly higher rates of smoking (15 percent) compared to women (10 percent).[93] Men also use more cigars and smokeless tobacco.[94]

See the **Points of View** box on the next page for a discussion of banning smoking on campuses.

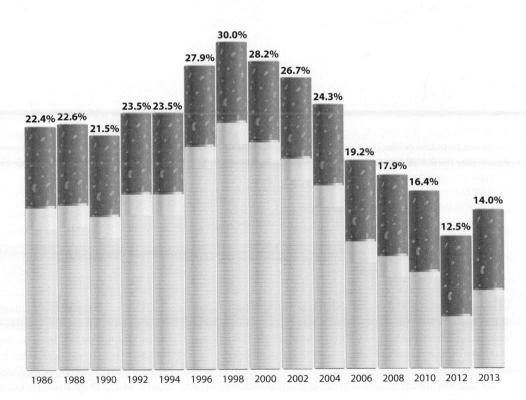

**FIGURE 8.10** Trends in Prevalence of Cigarette Smoking in the Past Month among College Students

**Source:** Data from L. D. Johnston et al., *Monitoring the Future National Survey Results on Drug Use, 1975–2013, Volume II: College Students and Adults Ages 19–55* (Ann Arbor, MI: Institute for Social Research, The University of Michigan, 2014).

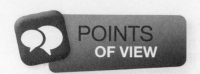
# Smoking on College & University Campuses
*Should It Be Banned?*

In recent years hundreds of campuses implemented all-out prohibitions or significant restrictions on tobacco use, with many more campuses pursuing becoming smoke-free. Currently there are an estimated 1,514 smoke-free campuses. Of these, 1,014 are completely free of tobacco and 587 more ban e-cigarettes anywhere on campus. The debate regarding tobacco-free (including the ban of e-cigarettes) campuses is contentious at many schools. Below are some of the major points for both sides of the question.

### Arguments for Banning Tobacco on Campuses

- The majority of college students— 4 out of 5—do not smoke.
- Two thirds of students and most employees prefer to attend classes held on a smoke-free campus.
- One in 5 students say they have experienced some immediate health impact from exposure to environmental tobacco smoke.
- Nonsmokers are 40 percent less likely to become smokers if they live in smoke-free dorms.
- Still very little is known about the harmful effects caused by exposure to e-cigarettes.
- Secondhand e-cigarette vapor contains nicotine, low levels of carcinogens, and ultrafine particles.

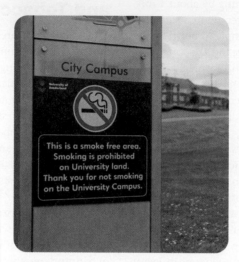

### Arguments against Banning Tobacco on Campuses

- There are so many other causes of potentially harmful fumes on campus—from diesel trucks, for example—that banning smoking wouldn't really affect the overall health and air quality on campus.
- The policy would be difficult if not impossible to enforce.
- Smokers forced outside to light up are possibly being put in danger at night or in other situations when they would have to leave residence halls.
- Smoking bans in public and private places violate the rights of smokers and encourage discriminatory treatment of people addicted to nicotine.

## WHERE DO YOU STAND?

- Is smoking on a college campus a threat to public health?
- Do you think that smokers have the right to smoke in dorms, in campus buildings, in adjacent parks, or in other public places on campus? Why or why not?

- How do you feel when you are walking across campus and someone is smoking close to you? Do you feel as though you could or should ask smokers to put out their cigarettes?

- Would banning smoking be discriminatory? A violation of individual rights? Should student smokers be singled out for exclusion on college campuses?

**Sources:** University of Michigan, National Tobacco Free Campus Initiative, http://sph.umich.edu; American Nonsmokers' Rights Foundation, Smoke-Free and Tobacco-Free U.S. and Tribal Colleges and Universities, January 1, 2015, U.S. Surgeon General's June 2012 webinar on tobacco-free college campuses.

**Why Do College Students Smoke?** Some of the reasons students smoke are to relax or to reduce stress. Smokers are more likely to have higher levels of perceived stress than nonsmokers. Students also smoke to fit in or because they are addicted.

For some students weight control is an important motivator, and fear of weight gain is a common reason for smoking relapse among those who quit. Students diagnosed or treated for depression are much more likely to use tobacco compared to students who are not.

**Social Smoking** Many college smokers identify themselves as "social smokers"—those who smoke only with people, rather than alone. Up to half of college smokers deny being smokers, even though they reported smoking in the past 30 days. Many students smoke in social situations where they also drink alcohol.[95] Like regular smokers, social smokers engage in more alcohol use, illicit drug use, and higher sexual risk-taking behaviors than do nonsmokers.[96] Even occasional smoking is not without risks of damaging health effects. Social smoking in college can lead to a complete dependence on nicotine and all the same health risks associated with smoking regularly.

## Tobacco Use and Prevention Policies

It has been more than 40 years since the U.S. government began warning that tobacco use was hazardous health. Despite all the education on the health hazards of tobacco use, health care spending and lost productivity associated with smoking costs between $289 and $333 billion each year.[97]

In 1998, the tobacco industry reached the Master Settlement Agreement with 46 states. The agreement requires tobacco companies to pay out more than $206 billion over 25 years. The agreement includes a variety of measures to support antismoking education and advertising and to fund research to determine effective smoking-cessation strategies. The agreement also curbs certain advertising and promotions directed at youth.

Unfortunately, most of the money designated for tobacco control and prevention at the state level has not been used for this purpose. Facing budget woes, many states have drastically cut spending on antismoking programs. In the few states that have spent the settlement money on smoking-cessation programs, there has been some reported success in decreasing cigarette use.[98] The Family Smoking Prevention and Tobacco Control Act of 2009 allows the U.S. Food and Drug Administration (FDA) to forbid tobacco advertising geared toward children, to lower the amount of nicotine in tobacco products, to ban sweetened cigarettes that appeal to young people, and to prohibit labels such as "light" and "low tar."[99] One of the most significant impacts of the law is that it requires more prominent health warnings on advertising of tobacco products. Smokeless tobacco ads now must contain a warning that fills 20 percent of the advertising space. The FDA attempted to require cigarette packages and advertising to have larger, graphical warnings depicting the negative consequences of smoking, but a federal judge declared the requirement unconstitutional in 2012.

## LO 6 | TOBACCO AND ITS EFFECTS

Identify different types of tobacco products, the chemicals they contain, and explain their effects on the body.

Smoking, the most common form of tobacco use, delivers a strong dose of nicotine, as well as 7,000 other chemical substances, including arsenic, formaldehyde, and ammonia, directly to the lungs. Among these chemicals are more than 69 known or suspected carcinogens.[100] Inhaling hot toxic gases exposes sensitive mucous membranes to irritating chemicals that weaken the tissues and contribute to cancers of the mouth, larynx, and throat. The heat from tobacco smoke is also harmful to tissues.

## Nicotine

The highly addictive chemical stimulant **nicotine** is the major psychoactive substance in all tobacco products. In its natural form, nicotine is a colorless liquid that turns brown upon exposure to air. When tobacco leaves are burned in a cigarette, pipe, or cigar, nicotine is released and inhaled into the lungs. Sucking or chewing tobacco releases nicotine into the saliva, and the nicotine is then absorbed through mucous membranes in the mouth. In a cigarette, nicotine is released when a mixture of nicotine, glycol, glycerin, and flavorings is vaporized into an aerosol ultimately inhaled by the smoker.

Nicotine is a powerful central nervous system stimulant producing a variety of physiological effects. In the cerebral cortex, it produces an aroused, alert mental state. Nicotine stimulates the adrenal glands, which increases the production of adrenaline. It also increases heart and respiratory rates, constricts blood vessels, and, in turn, increases blood pressure because the heart must work harder to pump blood through the narrowed vessels.

**nicotine** The primary stimulant chemical in tobacco products; nicotine is highly addictive.

**tar** Thick, brownish sludge condensed from particulate matter in smoked tobacco.

**carbon monoxide** Gas found in tobacco smoke that reduces the ability of blood to carry oxygen.

## Tar and Carbon Monoxide

Cigarette smoke is a complex mixture of chemicals and gases produced by the burning of tobacco and its additives. Particulate matter condenses in the lungs to form a thick, brownish sludge called **tar**, which contains various carcinogenic agents, such as benzopyrene, and chemical irritants, such as phenol. Phenol has the potential to combine with other chemicals that contribute to developing lung cancer.

In healthy lungs, millions of tiny hairlike projections (*cilia*) on the surfaces lining the upper respiratory passages sweep away foreign matter, which is expelled from the lungs by coughing. However, the cilia's cleansing function is impaired in smokers' lungs by nicotine, which paralyzes the cilia for up to 1 hour following a single cigarette. This allows tars and other solids in tobacco smoke to accumulate and irritate sensitive lung tissue. **FIGURE 8.11** illustrates how tobacco smoke damages the lungs.

Cigarette smoke also contains poisonous gases, the most dangerous of which is **carbon monoxide,** the deadly gas emitted in car exhaust. Carbon monoxide reduces the oxygen-carrying capacity of red blood cells by binding with the receptor sites for oxygen, causing oxygen deprivation in many body tissues. It is at least partly responsible for increased risk of heart attacks and strokes in smokers.

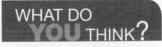

### WHAT DO YOU THINK?

Because nicotine is highly addictive, should it be regulated as a controlled substance?

- How could tobacco be regulated effectively?
- Should more resources be used for research into nicotine addiction? Why or why not?

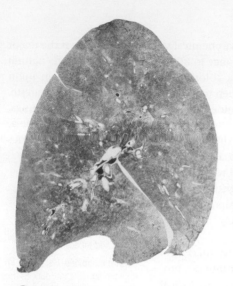

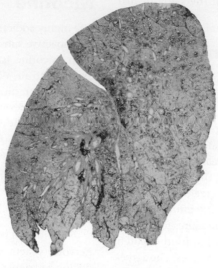

(a) A healthy lung

(b) A smoker's lung permeated with deposits of tar

**FIGURE 8.11** Lung Damage from Chemicals in Tobacco Smoke
Smoke particles irritate lung pathways, causing extra mucus production, and nicotine paralyzes the cilia that normally function to keep the lungs clear of excess mucus. The result is difficulty breathing, "smoker's cough," and chronic bronchitis. At the same time, tar collects within the alveoli (air sacs), ultimately causing their walls to break, leading to emphysema. Tar and other carcinogens in tobacco smoke also cause cellular mutations that lead to cancer.

## Tobacco Products

Tobacco comes in several forms. Cigarettes, cigars, pipes, and bidis are used for burning and inhaling tobacco. Smokeless tobacco is sniffed or placed in the mouth. Electronic cigarettes are an increasingly popular vehicle for nicotine, with their own health risks (see the **Health Headlines** box).

**Cigarettes** *Filtered cigarettes* are the most common form of tobacco available today. Almost all manufactured cigarettes have filters designed to reduce levels of gases such as hydrogen cyanide and carbon monoxide, but these products may actually deliver more hazardous gases to the user than do nonfiltered brands. Some smokers use low-tar and low-nicotine products as an excuse to smoke more cigarettes, but wind up exposing themselves to more harmful substances than they would with regular-strength cigarettes.

*Clove cigarettes* contain about 40 percent ground cloves (a spice) and about 60 percent tobacco. Many users mistakenly believe that these products are made entirely of ground cloves and that smoking them eliminates the risks associated with tobacco. In fact, clove cigarettes contain higher levels of tar and carbon monoxide than do regular cigarettes—and the numbing effect of eugenol, the active ingredient in cloves, allows smokers to inhale the smoke more deeply. The same effect is true of *menthol cigarettes:* The throat-numbing effect of the menthol allows for deeper inhalation.

## Tobacco Use Disorder

A recent study found about half of high school students had experimented with smoking.[101] Why do some people walk away from cigarettes while others get hooked? There are several possible reasons: Nicotine is a very addictive drug; people can become hooked on inhalation itself, and U.S. residents are bombarded with cigarette advertising.

Beginning smokers usually feel the effects of nicotine with their first puff. These symptoms, called **nicotine poisoning**, can include dizziness, light-headedness, rapid and erratic pulse, clammy skin, nausea, vomiting, and diarrhea. The unpleasant effects cease as tolerance to the chemical develops—almost immediately in new users, but by the second or third cigarette. In contrast, tolerance to most other drugs, such as alcohol, develops over a period of months or years. Regular smokers often no longer experience the "buzz" of smoking, but continue to smoke because quitting is difficult.

Smokers are not just physically dependent, they are also psychologically dependent. A pack-a-day smoker experiences 300 "hits," or **pairings**, a day. In pairing, an environmental cue triggers a craving for nicotine.[102] Simple pairings, such as drinking a cup of coffee, sitting in a car, finishing a meal, or sipping a beer, induce nicotine craving. The brain gets used to these pairings and cries out in displeasure when the association is missing.

**nicotine poisoning** Symptoms often experienced by beginning smokers, including dizziness, diarrhea, light-headedness, rapid and erratic pulse, clammy skin, nausea, and vomiting.

**pairing** An environmental cue that triggers nicotine cravings.

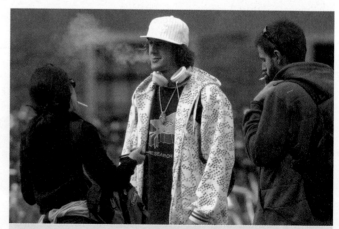

There is no "safe" amount of tobacco use—any exposure to smoke increases your risks for negative health effects. Even if you consider yourself "only" a social smoker, chances are you're on the road to dependence and a more frequent smoking habit.

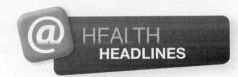

## E-CIGARETTES
### Health Risks and Concerns

Electronic cigarettes, also called e-cigarettes, are increasingly used worldwide, even though there is limited information on their health effects. In the United States, they are readily available in most states and on the Internet. A recent report from the Centers for Disease Control and Prevention (CDC) showed in 2013, over 250,000 junior high and high school students—who had never smoked cigarettes before—had tried e-cigarettes, triple the amount as in 2011. Adult use of e-cigarettes has also risen—to 8.5 percent in 2013, up from 3.3 percent in 2010.

Most e-cigarettes consist of a battery, a charger, an atomizer, and a cartridge containing nicotine and propylene glycol. When a smoker draws air through an e-cigarette, an airflow sensor activates the battery and heats the atomizer to vaporize the propylene glycol and nicotine. Upon inhalation, the aerosol vapor delivers a dose of nicotine into the lungs of the smoker, after which, residual aerosol is exhaled into the environment. Nothing is known, however, about the chemicals present in the aerosolized vapors emanating from e-cigarettes.

Although manufacturers claim that electronic cigarettes are a safe alternative to conventional cigarettes, the FDA analyzed samples of two popular brands and found variable amounts of nicotine and traces of toxic chemicals, including known cancer-causing substances (carcinogens). These carcinogens included an ingredient used in antifreeze and formaldehyde, which was present in higher amounts when higher-voltage charges are used. This prompted the FDA to issue a warning about potential health risks associated with electronic cigarettes. There is no quality control in the manufacturing of the product. Many e-cigarettes are manufactured in China under no controlled conditions.

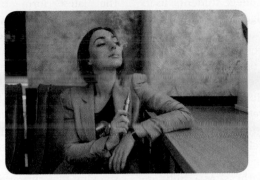

**Electronic cigarette, or e-cigarette.**

Furthermore, New York City, Chicago, and Los Angeles have banned e-cigarette use in public places. Many employers are struggling with employees wanting to "vape" indoors on break. Some corporations such as Exxon allow vaping, while Starbucks Corp. and Wal-Mart Stores, Inc. do not. UPS charges nonunion e-cigarette and tobacco users a higher price for their insurance premiums.

With various colors, fruity flavors, clever designs, and other options, e-cigarettes may hold too much appeal for young people, critics warn, offering an easy gateway to nicotine addiction.

Currently, e-cigarettes do not contain any health warnings comparable to FDA-approved nicotine-replacement products or conventional cigarettes. They are often marketed as a method to quit smoking, but health professionals recommend using FDA-approved medications and aids that have been shown to be safe and effective for this purpose. A recent study found no merit to the claim that e-cigarettes are better in terms of helping people quit smoking over the nicotine patch.

As e-cigarettes have increased in popularity, a new health risk has emerged for those who do not smoke. The CDC has reported a dramatic increases in calls

to poison control centers regarding e-cigarettes and liquid nicotine poisoning. Over 51 percent of these calls involved children under 5 years of age. The cartridges are not required to be childproof and feature flavors such as spearmint, banana, and bubble gum, making them appealing to children.

As a result, health professionals continue to urge for more action to regulate these products.

**Sources:** Centers for Disease Control and Prevention, "Smoking & Tobacco Use: Electronic Cigarettes," 2014, www.cdc.gov/tobacco/basic_information/e-cigarettes/youth-intentions/index.htm; CDC, "Key Findings: Trends in Awareness and Use of Electronic Cigarettes among U.S. Adults, 2010–2013, 2014, www.cdc.gov/tobacco/basic_information/e-cigarettes/adult-trends/index.htm; American Lung Association, "American Lung Association Statement on E-Cigarettes," March 2015, www.lung.org/stop-smoking/tobacco-control-advocacy/federal/e-cigarettes.html; U.S. Food and Drug Administration, "FDA and Public Health Experts Warn about Electronic Cigarettes," 2010, www.fda.gov/newsevents/newsroom/pressannouncements/ucm173222.htm; L. Dale, Mayo Clinic, "Electronic Cigarettes: A Safe Way to Light Up?," 2011, www.mayoclinic.com/health/electronic-cigarettes/AN02025; E. Sohn, Discovery News, "How Safe are E-Cigarettes?," 2011, www.news.discovery.com/human/e-cigarettes-health-nicotine-tobacco-110127.html; A. Norton, "Are E-Cigarettes Bad for Health?," 2012, www.huffingtonpost.com/2012/01/05/study-finds-e-cigarettes-_n_1187166.html; L. M. Dutra and S. A. Glanz, "Electronic Cigarettes and Conventional Cigarette Use among US Adolescents. A Cross-sectional Study," *JAMA Pediatrics*, March 06, 2014, doi:10.1001/jamapediatrics.2013.5488 (Epub ahead of print.); L. Weber et al., "E-Cigarette Rise Poses Quandary for Employers," *The Wall Street Journal*, January 16, 2014, 41-2; K. Chatham-Stephens et al., "Notes from the Field: Calls to Poison Centers for Exposures to Electronic Cigarettes—United States, September 2010-February 2014," *Morbidity and Mortality Weekly* 63, no. 13 (2014): 292–93; Centers for Disease Control and Prevention, "Youth and Tobacco Use," *Smoking and Tobacco Use*, February 2014, www.cdc.gov/tobacco/data_statistics/fact_sheets/youth_data/tobacco_use

**Cigars** Many people believe that cigars are safer than cigarettes, when in fact the opposite is true. Cigar smoke contains 23 poisons and 43 carcinogens. Most cigars contain as much nicotine as several cigarettes, and when cigar smokers inhale, nicotine is absorbed as rapidly as it is with cigarettes. For those who don't inhale, nicotine is still absorbed through the mucous membranes in the mouth.

Surprisingly, cigar use has increased by 233 percent in recent years; the sale of little cigars has increased approximately 65 percent.[103] Little cigars are roughly the same size

**bidis** Hand-rolled flavored cigarettes.

**chewing tobacco** Stringy form of tobacco that is placed in the mouth and then sucked or chewed.

**dipping** Placing a small amount of chewing tobacco between the lower lip and teeth for rapid nicotine absorption.

**snuff** A powdered form of tobacco that is sniffed and absorbed through the mucous membranes in the nose or placed inside the cheek and sucked.

and shape as cigarettes; come in packs of 20, as do cigarettes; can be flavored; and cost much less than cigarettes. In a recent study of college students, users of little cigars were more likely to be younger, male, black, and current cigarette, cigar, hookah, or marijuana smokers.[104] Users also tended to have a lower perception of harm, greater sensation-seeking behaviors, and higher perceived levels of stress.

### Bidis
Generally made in India or Southeast Asia, **bidis** are small, hand-rolled cigarettes that come in a variety of flavors, such as vanilla, chocolate, and cherry. They have become increasingly popular with college students because they are viewed to be safer and cheaper than cigarettes. However, they are far more toxic than cigarettes. Smoke from a bidi contains three times more carbon monoxide and nicotine and five times more tar than cigarettes.[105] The leaf wrappers are non-porous, which means that smokers must suck harder to inhale and inhale more to keep the bidi lit. During testing, it took an average of 28 puffs to smoke a bidi, compared to only 9 puffs for a regular cigarette.[106] This results in much more exposure to higher amounts of tar, nicotine, and carbon monoxide.

### Pipes and Hookahs
Pipes have had a long history of use throughout the world, including ritualistic and ceremonial use in many cultures. According to the National Cancer Institute and the American Cancer Society, pipe smoking carries risks similar to cigar smoking.[107]

Hookahs—a type of water pipe with a long hose for inhaling—originated in the Middle East, but has become particularly popular among young adults in the United States recently. While water pipes may cut down on the throat irritation users feel by cooling smoke before it is inhaled, they do not eliminate or filter out harmful substances.[108] In addition to the health risks associated with all tobacco products, risks associated with hookah use include the possibility of infectious disease transmission by sharing a pipe.

### Smokeless Tobacco
There are two types of smokeless tobacco: chewing tobacco and snuff.

**Chewing tobacco** comes in three forms—loose leaf, plug, or in a pouch—and contains tobacco leaves treated with molasses and other flavorings. The user "dips" the tobacco by placing a small amount between the lower lip and teeth to stimulate the flow of saliva and release the nicotine. **Dipping** rapidly releases nicotine into the bloodstream. Use of chewing tobacco by teenagers, especially white males, has increased in recent years.[109]

**Snuff** is a finely ground form of tobacco that can be inhaled, chewed, or placed against the gums. It comes in dry or moist powdered form or sachets (tea bag–like pouches). In 2009, "snus" became the latest form of smokeless tobacco to hit the market in the United States. Popular for more than 100 years in Sweden, these small sachets of tobacco are placed inside the cheek and sucked. Some people prefer snus to chewing tobacco because it doesn't require the user to spit frequently.

Smokeless tobacco is just as addictive as cigarettes and actually contains more nicotine—holding an average-sized dip or chew in the mouth for 30 minutes delivers as much nicotine as smoking four cigarettes. A two-can-a-week snuff user gets as much nicotine as a ten-pack-a-week smoker.

**SEE IT!** VIDEOS

What are the dangers of e-cigarettes for children? Watch **GMA Investigates Liquid Nicotine** in the Study Area of **MasteringHealth**™

## LO 7 | HEALTH HAZARDS OF TOBACCO PRODUCTS

Describe the health risks and physical impact associated with using tobacco products, as well as with environmental tobacco smoke.

Each day, tobacco contributes to approximately 1,200 deaths from cancer, cardiovascular disease, and respiratory disorders.[110] In addition, tobacco use can negatively impact the health of almost every system in your body. **FIGURE 8.12** summarizes some physiological and health effects of smoking.

### Cancer

Lung cancer is the leading cause of cancer deaths in the United States. The American Cancer Society estimates that tobacco smoking causes 90 percent of all cases of lung cancer in men

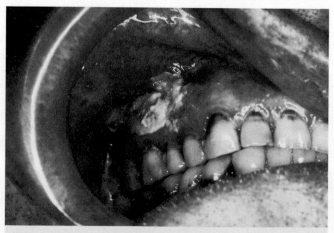

Leukoplakia can appear on the tongue or gums, as shown here.

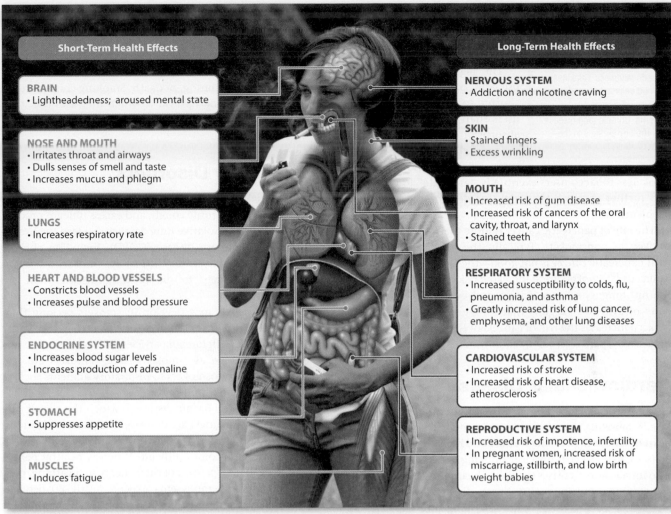

| Short-Term Health Effects | | Long-Term Health Effects |
|---|---|---|

**BRAIN**
• Lightheadedness; aroused mental state

**NOSE AND MOUTH**
• Irritates throat and airways
• Dulls senses of smell and taste
• Increases mucus and phlegm

**LUNGS**
• Increases respiratory rate

**HEART AND BLOOD VESSELS**
• Constricts blood vessels
• Increases pulse and blood pressure

**ENDOCRINE SYSTEM**
• Increases blood sugar levels
• Increases production of adrenaline

**STOMACH**
• Suppresses appetite

**MUSCLES**
• Induces fatigue

**NERVOUS SYSTEM**
• Addiction and nicotine craving

**SKIN**
• Stained fingers
• Excess wrinkling

**MOUTH**
• Increased risk of gum disease
• Increased risk of cancers of the oral cavity, throat, and larynx
• Stained teeth

**RESPIRATORY SYSTEM**
• Increased susceptibility to colds, flu, pneumonia, and asthma
• Greatly increased risk of lung cancer, emphysema, and other lung diseases

**CARDIOVASCULAR SYSTEM**
• Increased risk of stroke
• Increased risk of heart disease, atherosclerosis

**REPRODUCTIVE SYSTEM**
• Increased risk of impotence, infertility
• In pregnant women, increased risk of miscarriage, stillbirth, and low birth weight babies

**FIGURE 8.12**  Effects of Smoking on the Body and Health

→ **VIDEO TUTOR**
Long- and Short-Term Effects of Tobacco

and 78 percent in women.[111] There were an estimated 221,000 *new* cases of lung cancer in the United States in 2015 alone, and an estimated 158,040 Americans died from the disease in 2015.[112]

Lung cancer can take 10 to 30 years to develop, and the outlook for its victims is poor. Most lung cancer is not diagnosed until it is fairly widespread in the body; at that point, the 5-year survival rate is only 17 percent.[113] When a malignancy is diagnosed and recognized while still localized, the 5-year survival rate rises to 54 percent.

If you are a smoker, your risk of developing lung cancer depends on several factors. First, the amount you smoke per day is important. Someone who smokes two packs a day is 15 to 25 times more likely to develop lung cancer than a nonsmoker. Also, smoking as little as one cigar per day can double the risk of several cancers, including that of the oral cavity (lip, tongue, mouth, and throat), esophagus, larynx, and lungs. A second factor is when you started smoking; if you started in your teens, you have a greater chance of developing

lung cancer than do people who start later. And a third risk factor is if you inhale deeply when you smoke. Smokers are also more susceptible to the cancer-causing effects of exposure to other irritants, such as asbestos and radon, than are nonsmokers.

A major health risk of chewing tobacco is **leukoplakia,** a condition characterized by leathery white patches inside the mouth, produced by contact with irritants in tobacco juice. Approximately 1 out of 5 leukoplakias is either cancerous or precancerous on first sighting, eventually progressing to cancer if not treated.[114] There were over 45,780 cases of oral cancer diagnosed in 2015—the vast majority of which were caused by smokeless tobacco or cigarettes.[115] Smokeless tobacco users have significantly higher rates of oral cancer than nonusers. Warning signs include lumps in the jaw or neck; color changes or lumps inside the lips; white, smooth, or scaly patches in the

**leukoplakia** A condition characterized by leathery white patches inside the mouth; produced by contact with irritants in tobacco juice.

mouth, lips, or tongue; a red spot or sore on the lips or gums or inside the mouth that does not heal in 2 weeks; repeated bleeding in the mouth; and difficulty or abnormality in speaking or swallowing.

The lag time between first use and contracting cancer is shorter for smokeless tobacco users than for smokers because absorption through the gums is the most efficient route of nicotine administration. Many smokeless tobacco users eventually "graduate" to cigarettes and further increase their risk for developing additional problems.

**platelet adhesiveness** Stickiness of red blood cells associated with blood clots.

**emphysema** Chronic lung disease in which the tiny air sacs in the lungs are destroyed, making breathing difficult.

The rate of pancreatic cancer is more than twice as high for smokers as nonsmokers. Typically, the prognosis for people with pancreatic cancer is not good—the 5-year survival rate is 5 percent.[116] Smokers are at increased risk to develop cancers of the lip, tongue, salivary glands, and esophagus. A growing body of evidence suggests that long-term use of smokeless tobacco increases the risk of cancers of the larynx, esophagus, nasal cavity, pancreas, colon, kidney, and bladder.

## Cardiovascular Disease

Over a third of all tobacco-related deaths occur from heart disease.[117] Smoking cigarettes poses as great a risk for developing heart disease as high blood pressure and high cholesterol levels do (see Chapter 12). Daily cigar smoking, especially for people who inhale, also increases the risk of heart disease.[118]

Smoking contributes to heart disease by aging the arteries.[119] This occurs because smoking and exposure to environmental tobacco smoke (ETS) encourage and accelerate the buildup of fatty deposits (plaque) in the heart and major blood vessels (*atherosclerosis*). Smokers can experience a 50 percent increase in plaque accumulation in the arteries, compared with ex-smokers. Nonsmokers regularly exposed to ETS can have a 20 to 25 percent increase in plaque buildup.[120] For unknown reasons, smoking decreases blood levels of HDLs, the "good cholesterol" that helps protect against heart attacks.

Smoking also contributes to **platelet adhesiveness**, the sticking together of red blood cells associated with blood clots. The oxygen deprivation associated with smoking decreases the oxygen supplied to the heart and can weaken tissues. Smoking also contributes to irregular heart rhythms, which can trigger a heart attack. Both carbon monoxide and nicotine in cigarette smoke can precipitate angina attacks (pain spasms in the chest when the heart muscle does not get the blood supply it needs).

**WHY SHOULD I CARE?**

If the life-threatening health consequences aren't enough to make you give up smoking, consider the negative impact smoking can have on your social (and romantic!) life. Popular media may make smoking seem glamorous and sexy, but in reality, smoking makes your breath, hair, and clothing smell bad; it causes your skin to age prematurely; it yellows your teeth; and it can interfere with a man's ability to achieve and maintain an erection.

Smokers are two to four times as likely to suffer strokes as nonsmokers.[121] A stroke occurs when a small blood vessel in the brain bursts or is blocked by a blood clot, denying oxygen and nourishment to vital portions of the brain. Depending on the area of the brain affected, stroke can result in paralysis, loss of mental functioning, or death. Smoking contributes to strokes by raising blood pressure, which increases the stress on vessel walls, and platelet adhesiveness contributes to blood clot formation.

## Respiratory Disorders

Smoking quickly impairs the respiratory system in the form of breathlessness, chronic cough, and excess phlegm production. Over time, cumulative lung damage can lead to chronic obstructive pulmonary disease (COPD), including chronic bronchitis and emphysema. Ultimately, smokers are up to 25 times more likely to die of lung disease than are nonsmokers.[122]

*Chronic bronchitis* may develop in smokers because their inflamed lungs produce more mucus, which they constantly try to expel along with foreign particles. This results in the persistent cough known as "smoker's hack." Smokers are also more prone than nonsmokers to respiratory ailments such as influenza, pneumonia, and colds.

**Emphysema** is a chronic disease in which the alveoli (the tiny air sacs in the lungs) are destroyed, impairing the lungs' ability to obtain oxygen and remove carbon dioxide. As a result, breathing becomes difficult. Whereas healthy people expend only about 5 percent of their energy in breathing, people with advanced emphysema expend nearly 80 percent. Because the heart has to work harder to do even the simplest tasks, it may become enlarged, and death from heart damage may result. There is no known cure for emphysema, and the damage is irreversible. Approximately 80 percent of all cases are related to cigarette smoking.[123]

## Sexual Dysfunction and Fertility Problems

Despite attempts by tobacco advertisers to make smoking appear sexy, research shows it can actually cause impotence in men. Studies have found that male smokers are much more likely to experience erectile dysfunction than are nonsmokers.[124] Toxins in cigarette smoke damage blood vessels, reducing blood flow to the penis and leading to an inadequate erection. Impotence may indicate oncoming cardiovascular disease.

In women, smoking can lead to infertility and problems with pregnancy. Women who smoke increase their risk for infertility, ectopic pregnancy, miscarriage, and stillbirth. Smoking during pregnancy also increases risk of sudden infant death syndrome and the chances of the baby being born with a cleft lip or cleft palate.[125] Smoking during pregnancy increases the chance of premature birth and the risk of low birth weight (less than 5.5 pounds), increasing the likelihood of infant illness or death.[126]

## Unique Risks for Women

Today, 15.3 percent of women smoke, compared with 20.5 percent of men. Women who smoke are just as likely to die of cancer and other smoking-related diseases as men, and both active and passive smoking increase chances of breast cancer.[127] Accordingly, women smokers have assumed a much larger burden of smoking-related diseases than they did 40 years ago.

Higher rates of osteoporosis, depression, and thyroid-related diseases are just some of the risks that women who smoke take. Women who smoke (particularly those who also use oral contraceptives) are also at increased risk for blood clots, on top of heavier menstrual bleeding, longer duration of cramps, and less predictable length of menstrual cycle.

## Other Health Effects

Studies have shown tobacco use to be a serious risk factor in the development of gum disease.[128] In addition, smoking increases risk of macular degeneration, one of the most common causes of blindness in older adults. It also causes premature skin wrinkling, staining of the teeth, yellowing of the fingernails, and bad breath. Nicotine speeds up the process by which the body uses and eliminates drugs, making medications less effective. In addition, recent research suggests smoking significantly increases the risk for Alzheimer's disease.[129]

## Environmental Tobacco Smoke

Although fewer Americans smoke than in the past, air pollution from smoking in public places continues to be a problem. **Environmental tobacco smoke (ETS)** is divided into two categories: mainstream and sidestream smoke. **Mainstream smoke** refers to smoke drawn through tobacco while inhaling; **sidestream smoke** (commonly called *secondhand smoke*) refers to smoke from the burning end of a cigarette or smoke exhaled by a smoker. People who breathe smoke from someone else's smoking product are said to be *involuntary* or *passive* smokers.

Over a span of 10 years, detectable levels of nicotine exposure in nonsmoking Americans decreased from 87.9 percent to 40.1 percent,[130] due to the growing number of laws that ban smoking in work and public places.

Children are more heavily exposed to ETS than adults. Over 53 percent of U.S. children aged 3 to 11 years—or 22 million children—are exposed.[131] Disparities in ETS also occur among ethnic and racial lines and among income levels. African Americans have been found to have higher levels of exposure to ETS than whites and Latinos. ETS exposure is also higher among low-income persons.[132]

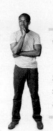

WHICH **PATH** WOULD YOU TAKE **?**
Scan the QR code to see how different smoking choices YOU make today can affect your overall health tomorrow.

## Risks from Environmental Tobacco Smoke

According to the Centers for Disease Control and Prevention (CDC), secondhand smoke has about 2 times more tar and nicotine, 5 times more carbon monoxide, and 50 times more ammonia than mainstream smoke.[133] Every year, ETS is estimated to be responsible for approximately 3,400 lung cancer deaths in nonsmoking adults, 46,000 coronary and heart disease deaths in nonsmoking adults, and higher risk of sudden infant death syndrome.[134]

The Environmental Protection Agency has designated secondhand smoke as a known carcinogen. There are more than 69 cancer-causing agents found in secondhand smoke.[135] There is also strong evidence that secondhand smoke interferes with normal functioning of the heart, blood, and vascular systems, significantly increasing the risk for heart disease and having immediate effects on the cardiovascular system. Studies indicate that nonsmokers exposed to secondhand smoke were 20 to 30 percent more likely to have coronary heart disease than nonsmokers not exposed to smoke.[136]

## LO 8 | QUITTING

Describe methods and benefits of smoking cessation.

Approximately 70 percent of U.S. adult smokers want to quit smoking, and up to 44 percent make a serious attempt to quit each year.[137] However, only 4 to 7 percent succeed. To successfully quit, smokers must break both the physical addiction to nicotine and the psychological habit of lighting up. Quitting is often a lengthy process involving several unsuccessful attempts before success is finally achieved; even successful quitters suffer occasional slips. Smokers unable to quit can expect to lose at least one decade of life compared to those who do not smoke.

## Benefits of Quitting

Many body tissues damaged by smoking can repair themselves. As soon as a smoker stops, the

**environmental tobacco smoke (ETS)** Smoke from tobacco products, including secondhand and mainstream smoke.

**mainstream smoke** Smoke that is drawn through tobacco while inhaling.

**sidestream smoke** Smoke from the burning end of a cigarette, pipe, or cigar or exhaled by nonsmokers; commonly called *secondhand smoke*.

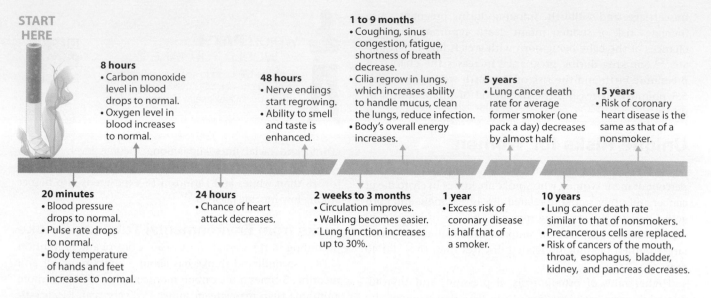

**START HERE**

**8 hours**
- Carbon monoxide level in blood drops to normal.
- Oxygen level in blood increases to normal.

**48 hours**
- Nerve endings start regrowing.
- Ability to smell and taste is enhanced.

**1 to 9 months**
- Coughing, sinus congestion, fatigue, shortness of breath decrease.
- Cilia regrow in lungs, which increases ability to handle mucus, clean the lungs, reduce infection.
- Body's overall energy increases.

**5 years**
- Lung cancer death rate for average former smoker (one pack a day) decreases by almost half.

**15 years**
- Risk of coronary heart disease is the same as that of a nonsmoker.

**20 minutes**
- Blood pressure drops to normal.
- Pulse rate drops to normal.
- Body temperature of hands and feet increases to normal.

**24 hours**
- Chance of heart attack decreases.

**2 weeks to 3 months**
- Circulation improves.
- Walking becomes easier.
- Lung function increases up to 30%.

**1 year**
- Excess risk of coronary disease is half that of a smoker.

**10 years**
- Lung cancer death rate similar to that of nonsmokers.
- Precancerous cells are replaced.
- Risk of cancers of the mouth, throat, esophagus, bladder, kidney, and pancreas decreases.

**FIGURE 8.13** When Smokers Quit Within 20 minutes of smoking that last cigarette, the body begins a series of changes that continues for years. However, by smoking just one cigarette a day, the smoker loses all these benefits, according to the American Cancer Society.

body begins the repair process (**FIGURE 8.13**). Within 8 hours, carbon monoxide and oxygen levels return to normal, and "smoker's breath" disappears. Circulation and the senses of taste and smell improve within weeks. Often, within a month of quitting, the mucus that clogs airways is broken up and eliminated. Circulation and the senses of taste and smell improve within weeks. Many ex-smokers say that they have more energy, sleep better, and feel more alert.

> **nicotine withdrawal** Symptoms, including nausea, headaches, irritability, and intense tobacco cravings, suffered by nicotine-addicted individuals who stop using tobacco.

The risk of dying from a heart attack falls by half after only 1 year without smoking and declines steadily thereafter. At the end of 10 smoke-free years, the ex-smoker can expect to live out his or her normal life span, and after about 15 years without smoking, the ex-smoker's risk of coronary heart disease is similar to that of people who have never smoked.[138]

Another significant benefit of quitting smoking is saving money. A single pack of cigarettes ranges from $5.00 (including tax) to as much as $11.00 to $14.50 in the most expensive states; a pack-a-day smoker in an area where cigarettes cost $8.00 per pack spends $56.00 per week, or $2,912 per year.[139]

## How Can You Quit?

Smokers wishing to quit have several options. Most who succeed quit "cold turkey"—they decide simply not to smoke again. Others focus on gradual reduction in smoking levels, which can reduce risks over time. Some rely on short-term programs based on behavior modification and a system of self-rewards. Still others turn to treatment centers, community outreach programs, or a telephone helpline. Finally, some people work privately with their physicians to reach their goal. Programs that combine several approaches have shown the most promise.

## Breaking the Nicotine Addiction

Nicotine addiction may be one of the toughest addictions to overcome. Symptoms of **nicotine withdrawal** include irritability, restlessness, nausea, vomiting, and intense cravings for tobacco (see **TABLE 8.2**). The evidence is strong that consistent pharmacological treatments can help a smoker quit: An estimated 25 to 33 percent of people who have used nicotine replacement therapy or smoking-cessation medications continue to abstain from cigarettes for over 6 months.[140] The **Skills for Behavior Change** box presents one of the American Cancer Society's approaches for quitting smoking.

**Nicotine Replacement Products** Nontobacco products that replace depleted levels of nicotine in the bloodstream have helped some people stop using tobacco. The two most common are nicotine chewing gum and the nicotine patch, both available over the counter. The FDA has also approved a nicotine nasal spray, a nicotine inhaler, and nicotine lozenges.

Nicotine gum delivers about as much nicotine as a cigarette does. Users experience no withdrawal symptoms and fewer cravings for nicotine as the dosage is reduced until they are completely weaned—users chew up to 20 pieces of gum a day for 1 to 3 months. Nicotine-containing lozenges are available in two strengths, and a 12-week program of use is recommended to allow users to taper off the drug.

The nicotine patch is generally used in conjunction with a comprehensive smoking-behavior cessation program. A small, thin patch delivers a continuous flow of nicotine through the skin, helping to relieve cravings. Patches can be bought with or without a prescription and are available in different dosages. The FDA recommends using the patch for a total of 3 to 5

# TABLE 8.2 | Coping Strategies for Common Smoking Withdrawal Problems

| Withdrawal Challenge | Estimated Length of Symptoms | Coping Strategies* |
|---|---|---|
| Anger, frustration, and irritability | Peaks in first week after quitting, but can last 2–4 weeks. | Avoid caffeine, which can amp up an already agitated mood. Get a massage; try deep breathing or exercise. |
| Anxiety | Builds over the first 3 days, and may last up to 2 weeks. | Same strategies as above. Also remind yourself that the symptoms usually pass by themselves over time. |
| Mild depression | One month or less. | Be with supportive friends, increase physical activity, make a list of things that are upsetting you, and write down possible solutions. If depression lasts longer than a month, seek medical advice. |
| Weight gain | Usually begins in the early weeks and continues through the first year after quitting. | Studies show nicotine replacement products such as gum and lozenges can help counter weight gain. You may also ask your doctor about the drug bupropion (brand name Zyban), which has also been shown to counter weight gain. |

*Asking your doctor for nicotine-replacement products or other medications is a valid coping strategy for any of the withdrawal challenges listed here.

**Source:** Adapted from National Cancer Institute, "Handling Withdrawal Symptoms When You Decide to Quit," National Cancer Institute Fact Sheet, 2010, www.cancer.gov

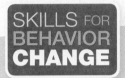

## SKILLS FOR BEHAVIOR CHANGE

### TIPS FOR QUITTING SMOKING

Ready to quit tobacco? These strategies can help:

▶ Ask smokers who live with you to keep cigarettes out of sight and not offer you any.

▶ Use the four Ds: deep breaths, drink water, do something else, and delay (tell yourself you'll smoke in 10 minutes when the urge hits).

▶ Keep "mouth toys" handy: Hard candy, chewing gum, toothpicks, or carrot or celery sticks can help.

▶ Ask your doctor about nicotine gum, patches, nasal sprays, inhalers, or lozenges.

▶ Make an appointment with your dental hygienist to have your teeth cleaned.

▶ Examine those associations that trigger your urge to smoke.

▶ Spend your time in places that don't allow smoking.

▶ Take up a new sport, exercise program, hobby, or organizational commitment. This will help shake up your routine and distract you from smoking.

months. During this time, the dose of nicotine is gradually reduced until the smoker is fully weaned from the drug. The patch costs less than a pack of cigarettes—about $4 per patch.

Each patch typically lasts 16 hours—and some insurance plans will pay for it.[141]

The nasal spray, which requires a prescription, is much more powerful and delivers nicotine to the bloodstream faster than gum, lozenges, or the patch. Patients are warned to be careful not to overdose; as little as 40 mg nicotine taken at once could be lethal. The FDA has advised that it should be used for no more than 3 months and never for more than 6 months, so that smokers don't become dependent. The FDA also advises that no one who experiences nasal or sinus problems, allergies, or asthma should use it.

The nicotine inhaler, which also requires a prescription, consists of a mouthpiece and cartridge. By puffing on the mouthpiece, the smoker inhales air saturated with nicotine, which is absorbed through the lining of the mouth, entering the body much more slowly than does the nicotine in cigarettes. Using the inhaler mimics the hand-to-mouth actions used in smoking and causes the back of the throat to feel as it would when inhaling tobacco smoke.

## Smoking Cessation Medications
Bupropion (brand name Zyban), an antidepressant, is FDA approved as a smoking-cessation aid. Varinicline (brand name Chantix) reduces nicotine cravings and the urge to smoke, and blocks the effects of nicotine at nicotine receptor sites in the brain. Both drugs may cause changes in behavior such as agitation, depression, hostility, and suicidal thoughts or actions. People taking one of these drugs who experience any unusual changes in mood are advised to stop taking the drug immediately and contact their health care professional.[142]

### Alcohol and Tobacco: Are Your Habits Placing You at Risk?

## 1 What's Your Risk of Alcohol Abuse?

Many college students engage in potentially dangerous drinking behaviors. Do you have a problem with alcohol use? Take the following quiz to see.

**1.** How often do you have a drink containing alcohol?
- ⓪ Never
- ① Monthly or less
- ② 2 to 4 times a month
- ③ 2 to 3 times a week
- ④ 4 or more times a week

**2.** How many alcoholic drinks do you have on a typical day when you are drinking?
- ⓪ 1 or 2
- ① 3 or 4
- ② 5 or 6
- ③ 7 to 9
- ④ 10 or more

**3.** How often do you have six drinks or more on one occasion?
- ⓪ Never
- ① Less than monthly
- ② Monthly
- ③ Weekly
- ③ Daily or almost daily

**4.** How often during the past year have you been unable to stop drinking once you had started?
- ⓪ Never
- ① Less than monthly
- ② Monthly
- ③ Weekly
- ④ Daily or almost daily

**5.** How often during the past year have you failed to do what was normally expected from you because of drinking?
- ⓪ Never
- ① Less than monthly

- ② Monthly
- ③ Weekly
- ④ Daily or almost daily

**6.** How often during the past year have you needed a first drink in the morning to get yourself going after a heavy drinking session?
- ⓪ Never
- ① Less than monthly
- ② Monthly
- ③ Weekly
- ④ Daily or almost daily

**7.** How often during the past year have you had a feeling of guilt or remorse after drinking?
- ⓪ Never
- ① Less than monthly
- ② Monthly
- ③ Weekly
- ④ Daily or almost daily

**8.** How often during the past year have you been unable to remember what happened the night before because you had been drinking?
- ⓪ Never
- ① Less than monthly
- ② Monthly
- ③ Weekly
- ④ Daily or almost daily

**9.** Have you or someone else been injured as a result of your drinking?
- ⓪ No

- ① Yes, but not in the past year
- ② Yes, during the past year

**10.** Has a relative, friend, or a doctor or other health care professional been concerned about your drinking or suggested you cut down?
- ⓪ No
- ① Yes, but not in the past year
- ② Yes, during the past year

### Interpreting Part 1

**Scores above 8:** Your drinking patterns are putting you at high risk for illness, unsafe sexual situations, or alcohol-related injuries, and may even affect your academic performance.

**Source:** T. Babor et al., "The Alcohol Use Disorders Identification Test: Interview Version," *Audit: The Alcohol Use Disorders Identification Test,* 2nd Edition. Copyright © 2001.

## YOUR PLAN FOR **CHANGE**

This **ASSESS YOURSELF** activity gave you the chance to evaluate your alcohol consumption. If some of your answers surprised you or if you were unsure how to answer some of the questions, consider taking steps to change your behavior.

**TODAY,** YOU CAN:

☐ Start a journal of your drinking habits to track how much alcohol you consume and what you spend on it.

☐ If you have a family history of alcohol abuse or addiction, consider whether your current use is healthy or is likely to create problems for you in the future.

**WITHIN THE NEXT TWO WEEKS,** YOU CAN:

☐ Make your first drink at a party something nonalcoholic.

☐ Intersperse alcoholic drinks with nonalcoholic beverages to help you pace yourself.

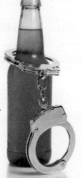

**BY THE END OF THE SEMESTER,** YOU CAN:

☐ Commit yourself to limiting your alcohol intake at every social function.

☐ Cultivate friendships and explore activities that do not center on alcohol. If your friends drink heavily, you may need to step back from the group for a while or make an effort to meet new people who do not make drinking a major focus of their social activity.

## 2 Why Do You Smoke?

Identifying why you smoke can help you develop a plan to quit. Answer the following questions and evaluate your reasons for smoking.

1. I smoke to keep from slowing down.

   ❏ Often ❏ Sometimes ❏ Never

2. I feel more comfortable with a cigarette in my hand.

   ❏ Often ❏ Sometimes ❏ Never

3. Smoking is pleasant and enjoyable.

   ❏ Often ❏ Sometimes ❏ Never

4. I light up a cigarette when something makes me angry.

   ❏ Often ❏ Sometimes ❏ Never

5. When I run out of cigarettes, it's almost unbearable until I get more.

   ❏ Often ❏ Sometimes ❏ Never

6. I smoke cigarettes automatically without even being aware of it.

   ❏ Often ❏ Sometimes ❏ Never

7. I reach for a cigarette when I need a lift.

   ❏ Often ❏ Sometimes ❏ Never

8. Smoking relaxes me in a stressful situation.

   ❏ Often ❏ Sometimes ❏ Never

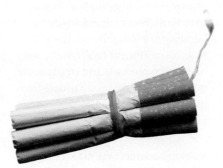

### Interpreting Part 2

Use your answers to identify some of the key reasons why you smoke, then use the tips presented in this chapter to develop a plan for quitting.

**Source:** Abridged and adapted from National Institutes of Health, *Why Do You Smoke?*, NIH Pub. No. 93-1822 (Washington, DC: U.S. Department of Health and Human Services, 1990).

## YOUR PLAN FOR CHANGE

This **ASSESS YOURSELF** activity gave you the chance to evaluate your current smoking habits. Regardless of your current level of nicotine addiction, if you smoke at all, now is the time to take steps toward kicking the habit.

**TODAY,** YOU CAN:

☐ Develop a plan to kick the tobacco habit. The first step in quitting smoking is to identify why you want to quit. Write your reasons down and carry a copy of it with you. Every time you are tempted to smoke, go over your reasons for stopping.

☐ Think about the times and places you usually smoke. What could you do instead of smoking at those times? Make a list of positive tobacco alternatives.

**WITHIN THE NEXT TWO WEEKS,** YOU CAN:

☐ Pick a day to stop smoking, and tell a family member or friend to gain support and accountability.

☐ Throw away all your cigarettes, lighters, and ashtrays.

**BY THE END OF THE SEMESTER,** YOU CAN:

☐ Focus on the positives. Now that you have stopped smoking, your mind and body will begin to feel better. Make a list of the good things about not smoking. Carry a copy with you, and look at it whenever you have the urge to smoke.

☐ Reward yourself for stopping. Go to a movie, go out to dinner, or buy yourself a gift.

☐ If you are having difficulty quitting, consult with your campus health center or your doctor to discuss medications or other therapies that may help you quit.

## CHAPTER **REVIEW**

 To hear an MP3 Tutor Session, scan here or visit the Study Area in **MasteringHealth**.

### LO **1** | Alcohol: An Overview

- Alcohol is a central nervous system (CNS) depressant used by about half of all Americans. Alcohol's effect on the body is measured by the blood alcohol concentration (BAC). The higher the BAC, the greater the drowsiness and impaired judgment and motor function.

### LO **2** | Alcohol and Your Health

- Excessive alcohol consumption can cause long-term damage to the nervous system and cardiovascular system, liver disease, and increased risk for cancer. Alcohol-impaired drivers are responsible for about 1 in 3 car crash deaths. College students have high rates of alcohol-related crashes. Drinking during pregnancy can cause fetal alcohol spectrum disorders (FASD).

### LO **3** | Alcohol Use in College

- Large numbers of college students report drinking in the past 30 days. Negative consequences associated with alcohol use among college students include academic problems, traffic accidents, unplanned sex, hangovers, alcohol poisoning, injury to self or others, and dropping out of school.

### LO **4** | Abuse and Dependence

- Alcohol use becomes alcoholism when it interferes with school, work, or social and family relationships or entails violations of the law. Causes of alcoholism include biological, family, social, and cultural factors. Treatment options include detoxification at private medical facilities, therapy (family, individual, or group), and self-help programs. Most recovering alcoholics relapse (over half within 3 months) because alcoholism is a behavioral addiction as well as a chemical addiction.

### LO **5** | Tobacco Use in the United States

- Tobacco use involves many social and political issues, including advertising targeted at youth and women, the fastest-growing populations of smokers. Smoking costs the United States between $289 and $333 billion per year.
- College students are heavily targeted by tobacco marketing and advertising campaigns. College students smoke to reduce stress, to fit in socially, and because they are addicted. The FDA requires prominent health warnings on tobacco products and enacts other policies to prevent young people from using tobacco products.

### LO **6** | Effects of Tobacco

- Smoking delivers over 7,000 chemicals to the lungs of smokers. Tobacco comes in smoking and smokeless forms; both contain nicotine, an addictive psychoactive substance.

### LO **7** | Health Hazards of Tobacco Products

- Health hazards of smoking include markedly higher rates of cancer, heart and circulatory disorders, respiratory diseases, sexual dysfunction, fertility problems, low birth weight babies, and gum diseases. Smokeless tobacco increases risks for oral cancer and other oral problems. Environmental tobacco smoke puts nonsmokers at greater risk for cancer and heart disease.

### LO **8** | Quitting

- To quit, smokers must kick a chemical addiction and a behavioral habit. Nicotine-replacement products or drugs such as Zyban and Chantix can help wean smokers off nicotine. Therapy methods can also help.

## **THINK** ABOUT IT!

### LO **1** | Alcohol: An Overview

1. Would a person be more intoxicated after having four gin and tonics instead of four beers? Why or why not?

### LO **2** | Alcohol and Your Health

2. At what point in your life should you start worrying about the long-term effects of alcohol abuse?

### LO **3** | Alcohol Use in College

3. When it comes to drinking alcohol, how much is too much? How can you avoid drinking amounts that will affect your judgment? If you see a friend having too many drinks at a party, what actions could you take?

4. What are some of the most common negative consequences college students experience as a result of drinking? What negative impacts do students experience as a result of other students' excessive drinking?

### LO **4** | Abuse and Dependence

5. Describe the difference between a problem drinker and an alcoholic. What factors can cause someone to become an alcoholic?

### LO **5** | Tobacco Use in the United States

6. What tactics do tobacco companies use to target different groups of people?

7. What are some of the main reasons college students choose to use tobacco?

### LO **6** | Effects of Tobacco

8. Discuss the various ways that tobacco is used. Is any method less addictive or less hazardous to health than another?

### LO **7** | Health Hazards of Tobacco Products

9. Discuss health hazards associated with tobacco. Who should be responsible for the medical expenses of smokers? Insurance companies? Smokers themselves?

### LO **8** | Quitting

10. Describe the various methods of tobacco cessation. Which would be most effective for you? Why?

# POP QUIZ

## LO 1 | Alcohol: An Overview

1. If a man and a woman drink the same amount of alcohol, the woman's blood alcohol concentration (BAC) will be approximately
   a. the same as the man's BAC.
   b. 60% higher than the man's BAC.
   c. 30% higher than the man's BAC.
   d. 30% lower than the man's BAC.

## LO 2 | Alcohol and Your Health

2. Which of the following is *not* a potential long-term effect of alcohol use?
   a. Increased risk of some cancers
   b. Increased risk of liver damage
   c. Increased risk of eye disorders
   d. Increased risk of nervous system damage

## LO 3 | Alcohol Use in College

3. Which of the following is *false*?
   a. College students drink in an effort to deal with stress and boredom.
   b. College students tend to underestimate the amount that their peers drink.
   c. Rape is linked to binge drinking.
   d. Consumption of alcohol is the number one cause of preventable death among undergraduates.

4. When Amanda goes out on the weekends, she usually has four to five beers in a row. This type of high-risk drinking is called
   a. tolerance.
   b. alcoholic addiction.
   c. alcohol overconsumption.
   d. binge drinking.

## LO 4 | Abuse and Dependence

5. The alcohol withdrawal syndrome that results in confusion, delusion, agitated behavior, and hallucination is known as
   a. automatic detoxification.
   b. delirium tremens.
   c. acute withdrawal.
   d. transient hyperirritability.

## LO 5 | Tobacco Use in the United States

6. Which of the following does *not* contribute to college students' vulnerability to tobacco?
   a. Targeting by tobacco marketers
   b. The new, stressful environment of college
   c. Presence of tobacco products on campus
   d. Lack of information about the dangers of smoking

## LO 6 | Effects of Tobacco

7. What does nicotine do to cilia in the lungs?
   a. Instantly destroys them
   b. Thickens them
   c. Paralyzes them
   d. Accumulates on them

8. What effect does carbon monoxide have on a smoker's body?
   a. It accumulates on the alveoli in the lungs, making breathing difficult.
   b. It increases heart rate.
   c. It interferes with the ability of red blood cells in the blood to carry oxygen.
   d. It dulls taste and smell.

## LO 7 | Health Hazards of Tobacco Products

9. A major health risk of chewing tobacco is
   a. lung cancer.
   b. leukoplakia.
   c. heart disease.
   d. emphysema.

## LO 8 | Quitting

10. How quickly will an individual begin to see health benefits after quitting smoking?
    a. Within 8 hours
    b. Within a month
    c. Within a year
    d. Never

*Answers to the Pop Quiz can be found on page A-1. If you answered a question incorrectly, review the section identified by the Learning Outcome. For even more study tools, visit MasteringHealth.*

# ACCESS YOUR HEALTH ON THE INTERNET

The following websites explore further topics and issues related to personal health. Visit MasteringHealth for links to the websites and RSS feeds.

*Alcoholics Anonymous.* This website provides general information about AA and the 12-step program. **www.aa.org**

*American Lung Association.* This site offers a wealth of information regarding smoking trends, environmental smoke, and advice on smoking cessation. **www.lungusa.org**

*ASH (Action on Smoking and Health).* The nation's oldest and largest antismoking organization, ASH fights smoking and protects nonsmokers' rights. **www.ash.org**

*College Drinking: Changing the Culture.* This resource center targets three audiences: the student population as a whole, the college and its surrounding environment, and the individual at risk or alcohol-dependent drinker. **www.collegedrinkingprevention.gov**

*Students against Destructive Decisions.* SADD is an organization of students dedicated to raising awareness about the dangers of underage drinking, drug use, and impaired driving, among other destructive decisions. **www.sadd.org**

*The Tobacco Atlas.* This book and website, produced by the World Lung Foundation and the American Cancer Society, cover a range of topics including the history of tobacco use, prevalence of use, youth smoking, secondhand smoke, quitting, and more. **www.tobaccoatlas.com**

# 9 Nutrition: Eating for a Healthier You

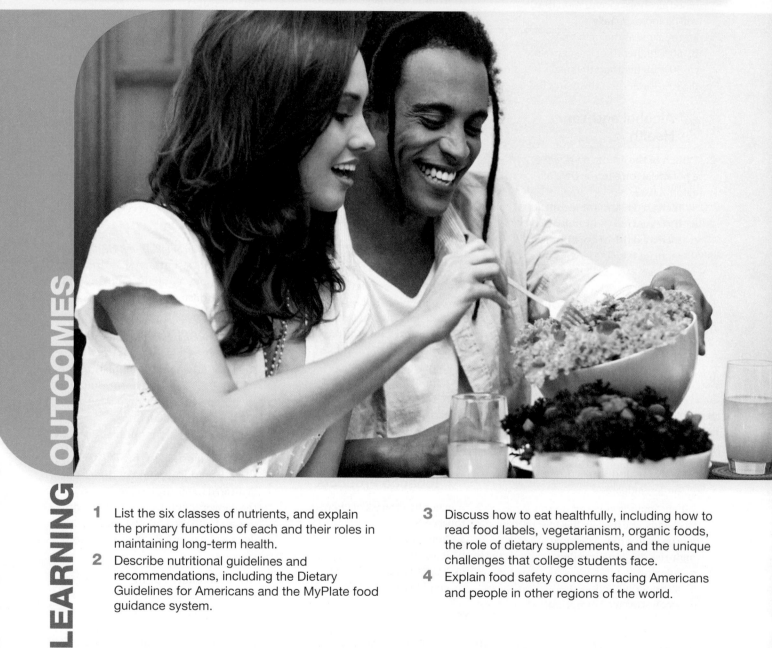

## LEARNING OUTCOMES

**1** List the six classes of nutrients, and explain the primary functions of each and their roles in maintaining long-term health.

**2** Describe nutritional guidelines and recommendations, including the Dietary Guidelines for Americans and the MyPlate food guidance system.

**3** Discuss how to eat healthfully, including how to read food labels, vegetarianism, organic foods, the role of dietary supplements, and the unique challenges that college students face.

**4** Explain food safety concerns facing Americans and people in other regions of the world.

**A**dvice about food comes at us from all directions: from the Internet, popular magazines, television, friends, and neighbors. Even when backed by research, this advice can be contradictory. Some studies indicate that a balanced high-fat diet can be healthful, whereas other studies support consuming a low-fat diet. Choosing what to eat and how much to eat from this media-driven array of food advice can be mind-boggling. For some, this can cause unnecessary anxiety about eating and lead to a lifetime of cycling on and off diets.[1] Why does something that can be a source of pleasure end up being a problem for so many of us? What influences our eating habits, and how can we learn to eat more healthfully?

The answers to these questions aren't as simple as they may seem. When was the last time you ate because you felt truly hungry? True **hunger** occurs when our brains initiate a physiological response that prompts us to seek food for the energy and **nutrients** that our bodies require to maintain proper functioning. Often, people in the United States don't eat in response to hunger—instead, we eat because of **appetite**, a learned psychological desire to consume food. Hunger and appetite are not the only forces influencing our desire to eat. Cultural factors, food advertising, perceived nutritional value, social interaction, emotions, and financial means are other factors.

**Nutrition** is the science that investigates the relationship between physiological function and the essential elements of the foods we eat. With an understanding of nutrition, you will be able to make more informed choices about your diet. Your health depends largely on what you eat, how much you eat, and the amount of exercise that you get throughout your life. The next few chapters focus on fundamental principles of nutrition, weight management, and exercise.

## LO 1 | ESSENTIAL NUTRIENTS FOR HEALTH

List the six classes of nutrients, and explain the primary functions of each and their roles in maintaining long-term health.

Food provides the chemicals we need for activity and body maintenance. Our bodies cannot synthesize certain *essential nutrients* (or cannot synthesize them in adequate amounts); we must obtain them from the foods we eat. Of the six groups of essential nutrients, the four we need in the largest amounts—water, proteins, carbohydrates, and fats—are called *macronutrients*. The other two groups—vitamins and minerals—are needed in smaller amounts, so they are called *micronutrients*.

Before the body can use food, the digestive system must break down larger food particles into smaller, more usable forms. The **digestive process** is the sequence of functions by which the body breaks down foods into molecules small enough to be absorbed, and excretes the wastes.

## Recommended Intakes for Nutrients

In the next sections, we discuss each nutrient group and identify how much of each you need. These recommended amounts are known as the **Dietary Reference Intakes (DRIs)** and are published by the Food and Nutrition Board of the Institute of Medicine. The DRIs establish the amount of each nutrient needed to prevent deficiencies or reduce the risk of chronic disease, as well as identify maximum safe intake levels for healthy people. The DRIs are umbrella guidelines and include the following categories:

- **Recommended Dietary Allowances (RDAs)** are daily nutrient intake levels meeting the nutritional needs of 97 to 98 percent of healthy individuals.
- **Adequate Intakes (AIs)** are daily intake levels assumed to be adequate for most healthy people. AIs are used when there isn't enough research to support establishing an RDA.
- **Tolerable Upper Intake Levels (ULs)** are the highest amounts of a nutrient that an individual can consume daily without risking adverse health effects.
- **Acceptable Macronutrient Distribution Ranges (AMDRs)** are ranges of protein, carbohydrate, and fat intake that provide adequate nutrition, and they are associated with a reduced risk for chronic disease.

Whereas the RDAs, AIs, and ULs are expressed as amounts—usually milligrams (mg) or micrograms (μg)—AMDRs are expressed as percentages. The AMDR for protein, for example, is 10 to 35 percent, meaning that no less than 10 percent and no more than 35 percent of the calories you consume should come from proteins. But that raises a new question: What are calories?

**hunger** The physiological impulse to seek food.

**nutrients** The constituents of food that sustain humans physiologically: water, proteins, carbohydrates, fats, vitamins, and minerals.

**appetite** The learned desire to eat; normally accompanies hunger but is more psychological than physiological.

**nutrition** The science that investigates the relationship between physiological function and the essential elements of foods eaten.

**digestive process** The process by which the body breaks down foods into smaller components and either absorbs or excretes them.

**Dietary Reference Intakes (DRIs)** Set of recommended intakes for each nutrient published by the Institute of Medicine.

**HEAR IT! PODCAST**

Want a study podcast for this chapter? Download **Nutrition: Eating for Optimum Health**, available on **MasteringHealth**™

# Calories

A *kilocalorie* is a unit of measure used to quantify the amount of energy in food. On nutrition labels and in consumer publications, the term is shortened to **calorie**. *Energy* is defined as the capacity to do work. We derive energy from the energy-containing nutrients in the foods we eat. These energy-containing nutrients—proteins, carbohydrates, and fats—provide calories. Vitamins, minerals, and water do not. **TABLE 9.1** shows the caloric needs for various individuals.

# Water: A Crucial Nutrient

Humans can survive for several weeks without food but only for about 1 week without water. **Dehydration**, a state of abnormal depletion of body fluids, can develop within a single day, especially in a hot climate. Too much water can also pose a serious risk to your health. This condition, *hyponatremia,* is characterized by low sodium levels.

The human body consists of 50 to 70 percent water by weight. The water in our system bathes cells; aids in fluid, electrolyte, and acid-base balance; and helps regulate body temperature. Water is the major component of our blood, which carries oxygen, nutrients, and hormones and other substances to body cells and removes metabolic wastes.

Individual needs for water vary drastically according to dietary factors, age, size, overall health, environmental temperature and humidity levels, and exercise. The general recommendations for women are approximately 9 cups of total water from all beverages and foods each day and for men an average of 13 cups.[2] We usually get the fluids we need each day through the water and other beverages we consume, as well as through the food we eat. In fact, fruits and vegetables are 80 to 95 percent water, meats are more than 50 percent water, and even dry bread and cheese are about 35 percent water! Contrary to popular opinion, caffeinated drinks, including coffee, tea, and soda, also count toward total fluid intake. Consumed in moderation, caffeinated beverages have not been found to dehydrate people whose bodies are used to caffeine.[3]

There are situations in which a person needs additional fluids in order to stay properly hydrated. It is important to drink extra fluids when you have a fever or an illness involving vomiting or diarrhea. Anyone with kidney function problems or who tends to develop kidney stones may need more water, as may people with diabetes or cystic fibrosis. The elderly and very young also may have increased water needs. When the weather heats up, or when you exercise, work,

**calorie** A unit of measure that indicates the amount of energy obtained from a particular food.

**dehydration** Abnormal depletion of body fluids; a result of lack of water.

**proteins** Large molecules made up of chains of amino acids; essential constituents of all body cells.

**amino acids** The nitrogen-containing building blocks of protein.

**essential amino acids** The nine basic nitrogen-containing building blocks of human proteins that must be obtained from foods.

## DO IT! NUTRITOOLS

Complete the **Know Your Protein Sources** activity, available on MasteringHealth™

## TABLE 9.1 | Estimated Daily Calorie Needs

| | Calorie Range | | |
|---|---|---|---|
| | Sedentary[a] | | Active[b] |
| **Children** | | | |
| 2–3 years old | 1,000 | → | 1,400 |
| **Females** | | | |
| 4–8 years old | 1,200 | → | 1,800 |
| 9–13 | 1,400 | → | 2,200 |
| 14–18 | 1,800 | → | 2,400 |
| 19–30 | 1,800 | → | 2,400 |
| 31–50 | 1,800 | → | 2,200 |
| 51+ | 1,600 | → | 2,200 |
| **Males** | | | |
| 4–8 years old | 1,200 | → | 2,000 |
| 9–13 | 1,600 | → | 2,600 |
| 14–18 | 2,000 | → | 3,200 |
| 19–30 | 2,400 | → | 3,000 |
| 31–50 | 2,200 | → | 3,000 |
| 51+ | 2,000 | → | 2,800 |

[a] A lifestyle that includes only the light physical activity associated with typical day-to-day life.

[b] A lifestyle that includes physical activity equivalent to walking more than 3 miles per day at 3 to 4 miles per hour, in addition to the light physical activity associated with typical day-to-day life.

**Source:** U.S. Department of Agriculture and U.S. Department of Health and Human Services, *Dietary Guidelines for Americans, 2010*, 7th ed. (Washington, DC: U.S. Government Printing Office).

or engage in other activities in which you sweat profusely, extra water is needed to keep your body's core temperature within a normal range. If you are an athlete and wonder about water consumption, visit the American College of Sports Medicine's website (www.acsm.org) to download its brochure, "Selecting and Effectively Using Hydration for Fitness."[4]

# Proteins

Next to water, **proteins** are the most abundant substances in the human body. Proteins are major components of living cells and are called the "body builders" because of their role in developing and repairing bone, muscle, skin, and blood cells. They are the key elements of antibodies that protect us from disease, enzymes that control chemical activities in the body, and many hormones that regulate body functions. Proteins also supply an alternative source of energy to cells when fats and carbohydrates are not available. Specifically, every gram of protein you eat provides 4 calories. (There are about 28 grams in an ounce by weight.) Adequate protein in the diet is vital to many body functions and ultimately to survival.

Your body breaks down proteins into smaller nitrogen-containing molecules known as **amino acids,** the building blocks of protein. Nine of the 20 different amino acids needed by the body are termed **essential amino acids,** which means the body must obtain them from the diet; the other 11 amino

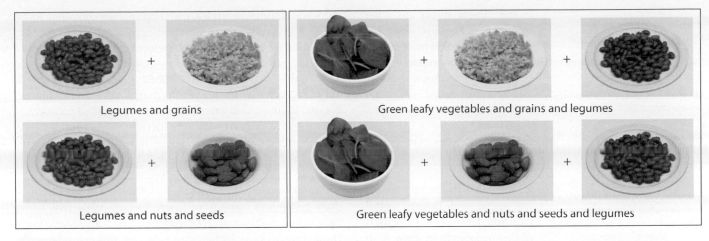

**FIGURE 9.1** **Foods Providing Complementary Amino Acids** Complementary combinations of plant-based foods can provide all essential amino acids. In some cases, you might need to combine three sources of protein to supply all nine; however, the foods do not necessarily have to be eaten in the same meal. Here, two of the limited amino acids in leafy green vegetables are supplied by either grains or nuts and seeds, and the third is found in legumes.

acids are considered nonessential because the body can make them. Dietary protein that supplies all the essential amino acids is called **complete protein**. Typically, protein from animal products is complete.

Nearly all proteins from plant sources are **incomplete proteins** that lack one or more of the essential amino acids. However, it is easy to combine plant foods to produce a complete protein meal (**FIGURE 9.1**). Plant foods rich in incomplete proteins include *legumes* (beans, lentils, peas, peanuts, and soy products); *grains* (e.g., wheat, corn, rice, and oats); and *nuts and seeds*. Certain vegetables, such as leafy green vegetables and broccoli, also contribute valuable plant proteins. Consuming a variety of foods from these categories will provide all the essential amino acids.

Although protein deficiency poses a threat to the global population, few Americans suffer from protein deficiencies. In fact, the average American consumes more than 79 grams of protein daily, much of it from high-fat animal flesh and dairy products.[5] The AMDR for protein is 10 to 35 percent of calories. Adults should consume about 0.8 gram (g) per kilogram (kg) of body weight.[6] To calculate your protein needs, divide your body weight in pounds by 2.2 to get your weight in kilograms, then multiply by 0.8. The result is your recommended protein intake per day. For example, a woman who weighs 130 pounds should consume about 47 grams of protein each day. A 6-ounce steak provides 53 grams of protein—more than she needs!

People who need to eat extra protein include pregnant women and patients fighting a serious infection, recovering from surgery or blood loss, or recovering from burns. In these instances, proteins that are lost to cellular repair and development need to be replaced. Athletes also require more protein to build and repair muscle fibers.[7] In addition, a sedentary person may find it easier to stay in energy balance when consuming a diet with a higher percentage of protein and a lower percentage of carbohydrate. Why? Proteins make a person feel full for a longer period of time because protein takes longer to digest than carbohydrates. Protein also releases certain satiety hormones that contribute to feeling full longer.

# Carbohydrates

**Carbohydrates** supply us with the energy we need to sustain normal daily activity. In comparison to proteins or fats, carbohydrates are broken down more quickly and efficiently, yielding a fuel called glucose. All body cells can burn glucose for fuel; moreover, glucose is the only fuel that red blood cells can use and is the primary fuel for the brain. Carbohydrates are the best fuel for moderate to intense exercise because they can be readily broken down to glucose even when we're breathing hard and our muscle cells are getting less oxygen.

Like proteins, carbohydrates provide 4 calories per gram. The RDA for adults is 130 grams of carbohydrate per day.[8] There are two major types: simple and complex.

**Simple Carbohydrates** **Simple carbohydrates** or *simple sugars* are found naturally in fruits, many vegetables, and dairy. The most common form of simple carbohydrates is *glucose*. Fruits and berries contain *fructose* (commonly called *fruit sugar*). Glucose and fructose are **monosaccharides**. Eventually, the human body converts all types of simple sugars to glucose to provide energy to cells.

**Disaccharides** are combinations of two monosaccharides. Perhaps the best-known example is *sucrose* (granulated table sugar). *Lactose* (milk sugar), found in milk and milk products, and

**complete proteins** Proteins that contain all nine of the essential amino acids.

**incomplete proteins** Proteins that lack one or more of the essential amino acids.

**carbohydrates** Basic nutrients that supply the body with glucose, the energy form most commonly used to sustain normal activity.

**simple carbohydrates** A carbohydrate made up of only one sugar molecule, or of two sugar molecules bonded together; also called simple sugars.

**monosaccharides** A sugar that is not broken down further during digestion, including fructose and glucose.

**disaccharides** Combinations of two monosaccharides such as lactose, maltose, and sucrose.

**DO IT!** NUTRITOOLS
Complete the **Know Your Carbohydrate Sources** activity, available on MasteringHealth™

**complex carbohydrates** A carbohydrate that can be broken down during digestion into monosaccharides or disaccharides; also called a polysaccharide.

**starches** Polysaccharides that are the storage forms of glucose in plants.

**glycogen** The polysaccharide form in which glucose is stored in the liver and, to a lesser extent, in muscles.

**fiber** The indigestible portion of plant foods that helps move food through the digestive system and softens stools by absorbing water.

**whole grains** Grains that are milled in their complete form and thus include the bran, germ, and endosperm, with only the husk removed.

*maltose* (malt sugar) are other examples of common disaccharides. Disaccharides must be broken down into monosaccharides before the body can use them.

Sugar is found in high amounts in a wide range of processed food products. A classic example is the amount of sugar in one can of soda: more than 10 teaspoons per can! Moreover, such diverse items as ketchup, barbecue sauce, and flavored coffee creamers derive 30 to 65 percent of their calories from sugar. Read food labels carefully before purchasing. If *sugar* or one of its aliases (including *high fructose corn syrup* and *cornstarch*) appears near

the top of the ingredients list, then that product contains a lot of sugar and is probably not your best nutritional bet. Also, most labels list the amount of sugar as a percentage of total calories.

## Complex Carbohydrates: Starches and Glycogen
**Complex carbohydrates** are found in grains, cereals, legumes, and other vegetables. Also called *polysaccharides*, they are formed by long chains of monosaccharides. Like disaccharides, they must be broken down into simple sugars before the body can use them. *Starches, glycogen,* and *fiber* are the main types of complex carbohydrates.

**Starches** make up the majority of the complex carbohydrate group and come from flours, breads, pasta, rice, corn, oats, barley, potatoes, and related foods. The body breaks down these complex carbohydrates into glucose, which can be easily absorbed by cells and used as energy or stored in the muscles and the liver as **glycogen**. When the body requires a sudden burst of energy, it breaks down glycogen into glucose.

## Complex Carbohydrates: Fiber
**Fiber,** sometimes referred to as "bulk" or "roughage," is the indigestible portion of plant foods that helps move foods through the digestive system, delays absorption of cholesterol and other nutrients, and softens stools by absorbing water. Dietary fiber is found only in plant foods, such as fruits, vegetables, nuts, and grains.[9]

Fiber is either *soluble* or *insoluble*. Soluble fibers, such as pectins, gums, and mucilages, dissolve in water, form gel-like substances, and can be digested easily by bacteria in the colon. Major food sources of soluble fiber include citrus fruits, berries, oat bran, dried beans, and some vegetables. Insoluble fibers, such as lignins and cellulose, typically do not dissolve in water and cannot be fermented by bacteria in the colon. They are found in most fruits and vegetables and in **whole grains**, such as brown rice, wheat, bran, and whole-grain breads and cereals (see **FIGURE 9.2**). The AMDR for carbohydrates is 45 to

Studies have shown that eating 2.5 servings of whole grains per day can reduce cardiovascular disease risk by as much as 21%. But are people getting the message? One nutrition study showed that only 8% of U.S. adults consume 3 or more servings of whole grains each day, and 42% ate no whole grains at all on a given day.

**Source:** Huang, T., et al. "Consumption of Whole Grains and Cereal Fiber and Total and Cause-specific Mortality: Prospective Analysis of 367,442 Individuals," *BMC Medicine* 13, no 1(2015): 59, doi: 10.1186/s12916-015-0294-7

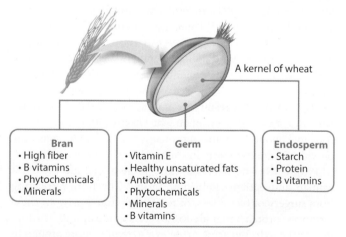

A kernel of wheat

| Bran | Germ | Endosperm |
|---|---|---|
| • High fiber | • Vitamin E | • Starch |
| • B vitamins | • Healthy unsaturated fats | • Protein |
| • Phytochemicals | • Antioxidants | • B vitamins |
| • Minerals | • Phytochemicals | |
| | • Minerals | |
| | • B vitamins | |

**FIGURE 9.2  Anatomy of a Whole Grain** Whole grains are more nutritious than refined grains because they contain the bran, germ, and endosperm of the seed—sources of fiber, vitamins, minerals, and beneficial phytochemicals (chemical compounds that occur naturally in plants).

**Source:** Adapted from Joan Salge Blake, Kathy D. Munoz, and Stella Volpe, *Nutrition: From Science to You*, 1st ed. © 2010, page 138. Printed and electronically reproduced by permission of Pearson Education, Inc., Upper Saddle River, New Jersey.

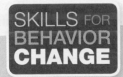

## SKILLS FOR BEHAVIOR CHANGE

### BULK UP YOUR FIBER INTAKE!

▶ Whenever possible, select whole-grain breads, especially those low in fat and sugars. Choose breads with 3 or more grams of fiber per serving. Read labels—just because bread is brown doesn't mean it is better for you.

▶ Eat whole, unpeeled fruits and vegetables rather than drinking their juices. The fiber in the whole fruit tends to slow blood sugar increases and helps you feel full longer.

▶ Substitute whole-grain pastas, bagels, and pizza crust for the refined, white flour versions.

▶ Add wheat crumbs or grains to meat loaf and burgers to increase fiber intake.

▶ Enhance your fiber intake with quinoa, an edible seed that is also high in protein.

▶ Toast grains to bring out their nutty flavor and make foods more appealing.

▶ Sprinkle ground flaxseed on cereals, yogurt, and salads, or add to casseroles, burgers, and baked goods. Flaxseeds have a mild flavor and are also high in beneficial fatty acids.

60 percent of total calories, and health experts recommend that the majority of this intake be fiber-rich carbohydrates.

Fiber protects against obesity, colon and rectal cancers, heart disease, constipation, and possibly even type 2 diabetes, so most experts believe that Americans should double their current consumption of dietary fiber—to 25 grams per day for women and 38 grams per day for men.[10] What's the best way to increase your intake of dietary fiber? Eat fewer refined carbohydrates in favor of more fiber-rich carbohydrates, including whole-grain breads and cereals, fresh fruits, legumes and other vegetables, nuts, and seeds. As with most nutritional advice, however, too much of a good thing can pose problems. A sudden increase in dietary fiber may cause flatulence (intestinal gas), cramping, or bloating. Consume plenty of water or other (sugar-free!) liquids to reduce such side effects. Find out more about the benefits of fiber in the **Skills for Behavior Change** box.

## Fats

**Fats**, perhaps the most misunderstood nutrient, are the most energy dense, providing 9 calories per gram. Fats are a significant source of our body's fuel. Fats also play a vital role in maintaining healthy skin and hair, insulating body organs against shock, maintaining body temperature, and promoting healthy cell function. Fats make foods taste better and carry the fat-soluble vitamins A, D, E, and K to cells. They also make you feel full after eating.

Despite the fact that fats perform all these functions, we are constantly urged to cut back on them, because some fats are less healthy than others and because excessive consumption of fats can lead to weight gain and cardiovascular disease.

**Triglycerides** make up about 95 percent of total body fat and are the most common form of fat in foods. When we consume too many calories from any source, the liver converts the excess into triglycerides, which are stored in fat cells throughout our bodies. The remaining 5 percent of body fat is composed of substances such as **cholesterol.** The ratio of total cholesterol to a group of compounds called **high-density lipoproteins (HDLs)** is important in determining risk for heart disease. Lipoproteins facilitate the transport of cholesterol in the blood. High-density lipoproteins are capable of transporting more cholesterol than are **low-density lipoproteins (LDLs).** Whereas LDLs transport cholesterol to the body's cells, HDLs transport circulating cholesterol to the liver for metabolism and elimination from the body. Past research has indicated that people with a high percentage of HDLs appear to be at lower risk for developing cholesterol-clogged arteries. However, new research has raised questions about the role of HDL and LDL in cardiovascular health. (See Chapter 12 for information about recent research on cholesterol, inflammation, and other risks for cardiovascular disease.)

**fats** Basic nutrients composed of carbon and hydrogen atoms; needed for the proper functioning of cells, insulation of body organs against shock, maintenance of body temperature, and healthy skin and hair.

**triglycerides** The most common form of fat in our food supply and in the body; made up of glycerol and three fatty acid chains.

**cholesterol** A substance that, like fats, is not soluble in water. It is found in animal-based foods and is synthesized by the body. Although essential to functioning, cholesterol circulating in the blood can accumulate on the inner walls of blood vessels.

**high-density lipoproteins (HDLs)** Compounds that facilitate the transport of cholesterol in the blood to the liver for metabolism and elimination from the body.

**low-density lipoproteins (LDLs)** Compounds that facilitate the transport cholesterol in the blood to the body's cells.

**saturated fats** Fats that are unable to hold any more hydrogen in their chemical structure; derived mostly from animal sources; solid at room temperature.

**unsaturated fats** Fats that have room for more hydrogen in their chemical structure; derived mostly from plants; liquid at room temperature.

## WHY SHOULD I CARE?

Cholesterol can accumulate on the inner walls of arteries and narrow the channels through which blood flows. This buildup, called plaque, is a major cause of atherosclerosis, a component of cardiovascular disease.

**Types of Dietary Fats** Triglycerides contain *fatty acid* chains of oxygen, carbon, and hydrogen atoms. Fatty acid chains that cannot hold any more hydrogen in their chemical structure are called **saturated fats.** They generally come from animal sources, such as meat, dairy, and poultry products, and are solid at room temperature. **Unsaturated fats** have room for additional hydrogen atoms in their chemical structure and are liquid at room temperature. They generally come from plants and include most vegetable oils.

The terms *monounsaturated fatty acids* (*MUFAs*) and *polyunsaturated fatty acids* (*PUFAs*) refer to the relative number of hydrogen atoms that

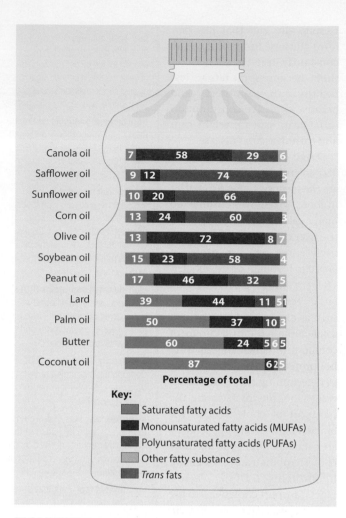

| Oil | Saturated | Monounsaturated | Polyunsaturated | Other | Trans |
|---|---|---|---|---|---|
| Canola oil | 7 | 58 | 29 | 6 | |
| Safflower oil | 9 | 12 | 74 | 5 | |
| Sunflower oil | 10 | 20 | 66 | 4 | |
| Corn oil | 13 | 24 | 60 | 3 | |
| Olive oil | 13 | 72 | 8 | 7 | |
| Soybean oil | 15 | 23 | 58 | 4 | |
| Peanut oil | 17 | 46 | 32 | 5 | |
| Lard | 39 | 44 | 11 | 5 | 1 |
| Palm oil | 50 | 37 | 10 | 3 | |
| Butter | 60 | 24 | 5 | 6 | 5 |
| Coconut oil | 87 | 6 | 2 | 5 | |

**Percentage of total**

**Key:**
- Saturated fatty acids
- Monounsaturated fatty acids (MUFAs)
- Polyunsaturated fatty acids (PUFAs)
- Other fatty substances
- *Trans* fats

**FIGURE 9.3** Percentages of Saturated, Polyunsaturated, Monounsaturated, and *Trans* Fats in Common Vegetable Oils

are missing in a fatty acid chain. Peanut, canola, and olive oils are high in monounsaturated fats, which appear to lower LDL levels and increase HDL levels. Corn, sunflower, and safflower oils are high in polyunsaturated fats. For a breakdown of the types of fats in common vegetable oils, see **FIGURE 9.3**.

Two specific types of polyunsaturated fatty acids essential to a healthful diet are *omega-3 fatty acids* (found in many types of fatty fish; dark green, leafy vegetables; walnuts; and flaxseeds) and *omega-6 fatty acids* (found in corn, soybean, peanut, sunflower, and cottonseed oils). Both are classified as *essential fatty acids*—that is, those we must receive from our diets—because the body cannot synthesize them yet requires them for functioning. The most important fats within these groups are *linoleic acid*, an omega-6 fatty acid, and *alpha-linolenic acid,* an omega-3 fatty acid. The body needs these to make hormone-like compounds that control immune function, pain perception, and inflammation, to name a few key benefits. You may also have heard of EPA (eicosapentaenoic) and DHA (docosahexaenoic acid). These are derivatives of alpha-linolenic acid that are found abundantly in oily fish such as salmon and tuna and are associated with a reduced risk for heart disease.[11]

**trans fats (*trans* fatty acids)**
Fatty acids that are produced when polyunsaturated oils are hydrogenated to make them more solid.

The AMDR for fats is 20 to 35 percent of calories, with 5 to 10 percent coming from essential fatty acids. Within this range, we should minimize our intake of saturated fats.

## Avoiding *Trans* Fatty Acids
For decades, Americans shunned butter, cream, and other foods high in saturated fats. What they didn't know is that some processed foods low in animal fats, such as margarine, could be just as harmful. These processed foods contain **trans fatty acids**. Research shows that just a 2 percent caloric intake of these fats is associated with a 23 percent increased risk for heart disease and a 47 percent increased chance of sudden cardiac death.[12]

Although a small amount of *trans* fatty acids do occur in some animal products, the great majority are in processed foods made with partially hydrogenated oils (PHOs).[13] PHOs are produced when food manufacturers add hydrogen to a plant oil, solidifying it, helping it resist rancidity, and giving the food in which it is used a longer shelf life. The hydrogenation process straightens out the fatty acid chain so that it is more like a saturated fatty acid, and it has similar harmful effects, lowering HDLs and raising LDLs. *Trans* fats have been used in margarines, many commercial baked goods, and restaurant deep-fried foods.

In 2013, the U.S. Food and Drug Administration (FDA) issued a preliminary determination that PHOs are no longer recognized as safe for consumption. If it is finalized, foods

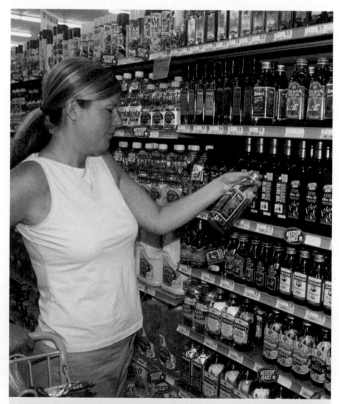

All fats are not the same, and your body needs some fat to function. Try to reduce saturated fats, which are in meat, full-fat dairy, and poultry products, and avoid *trans* fats, which typically come in stick margarines, commercially baked goods, and deep-fried foods. Replace these with unsaturated fats, such as those in plant oils, fatty fish, and nuts and seeds.

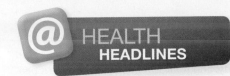

## COCONUT OIL
*Friend or Foe?*

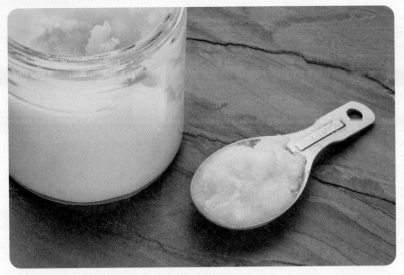

If you're a label reader, you've probably noticed coconut oil on the ingredients list of milk, spreads, and yogurt, or even seen jars filled with a solid milky-white fat on the grocery store shelves. Once thought of as an unhealthy, saturated fat, coconut oil is making a comeback, and is being touted as a healthy alternative to other oils.

The difference between coconut oil and other more commonly used oils is that 87 percent of the fatty acids in coconut oil are mostly saturated. Olive oil, in comparison, is 15 percent saturated. Coconut oil also doesn't contain any polyunsaturated essential fatty acids, but is rich in vitamin E and a variety of phytochemicals. Does coconut oil provide unique health benefits beyond those nutrients?

Some have touted coconut oil may reduce the risk of heart disease, improve weight loss, cure Alzheimer's disease, or protect against infections. The original study that started this craze was observing Polynesian people who have little heart disease but ingest mostly fat from coconuts. The researchers did not explore whether consuming coconut oil reduced the risk of heart disease. There is also no scientific evidence that switching to coconut oil from polyunsaturated oils improves weight loss, cures Alzheimer's disease, or protects against infections.

Health professionals are divided over whether to recommend replacing heart-healthy polyunsaturated vegetable oils with coconut oil. There is a larger body of research in humans that monounsaturated and polyunsaturated fatty acids lower blood cholesterol levels and reduce the risk of heart disease, but little evidence that coconut oil is beneficial for heart health, weight loss, or Alzheimer's. At this point, most health professionals advise against adding coconut oil to your diet.

**Sources:** Tropical Traditions, "What is Virgin Coconut Oil?," Accessed April 2015, www.tropical-traditions.com/what_is_virgin_coconut_oil.htm; F. Hamam, "Specialty Lipids in Health and Disease," *Food and Nutrition Sciences* 4 (2013): 63–70; American Heart Association, "Fats and Oils: AHA Recommendations," Accessed April 2015, Available at www.heart.org.

---

containing PHOs will no longer be sold legally in the United States.[14] In the meantime, *trans* fats are being removed from most foods, and if they are present, they must be clearly indicated on food packaging. If you see the words *partially hydrogenated oils, fractionated oils, shortening, lard,* or *hydrogenation* on a food label, then *trans* fats are present.

### New Fat Advice: Is More Fat Ever Better?
Some researchers worry that we have gone too far in our anti-fat frenzy. In fact, some studies have shown that balanced high-fat diets produce significant improvements in weight loss, blood fat, and blood glucose measures.[15] Balance is the key. No more than 7 to 10 percent of your total calories should come from saturated fat, and no more than 35 percent should come from all forms of fat.[16] Follow these guidelines to add more healthy fats to your diet:

- Eat fatty fish (herring, mackerel, salmon, sardines, or tuna) at least twice weekly.
- Use olive, peanut, soy, and canola oils instead of butter or lard. See **Health Headlines** for more information on coconut oil.

- Add healthy amounts of green leafy vegetables, walnuts, walnut oil, and ground flaxseed to your diet.

Follow these guidelines to reduce your overall intake of less-healthy fats:

- Read the Nutrition Facts on food labels to find out how much fat is in your food.
- Chill meat-based soups and stews, scrape off any fat that hardens on top, and then reheat to serve.
- Fill up on fruits and vegetables.
- Hold the creams and sauces.
- Avoid all products with *trans* fatty acids. For healthy toppings on your bread, try vegetable spreads, bean spreads, nut butters, sugar-free jams, fat-free cheese, etc.
- Choose lean meats, fish, or skinless poultry. Broil or bake whenever possible. Drain off fat after cooking.

**DO IT! NUTRITOOLS**
Complete the **Know Your Fat Sources** activity, available on **MasteringHealth**™

- Choose fewer cold cuts, bacon, sausages, hot dogs, and organ meats.
- Select nonfat and low-fat dairy products.

# Vitamins

**Vitamins** are organic compounds that promote growth and are essential to life and health. Every minute of every day, vitamins help maintain nerves and skin, produce blood cells, build bones and teeth, heal wounds, and convert food energy to body energy—and they do all this without adding any calories to your diet.

Vitamins are classified as either *fat soluble,* which means they are absorbed through the intestinal tract with the help of fats, or *water soluble,* which means they are dissolved easily in water. Vitamins A, D, E, and K are fat soluble; B-complex vitamins and vitamin C are water soluble. Fat-soluble vitamins tend to be stored in the body, and toxic levels can accumulate if people regularly consume more than the UL. Excesses of water-soluble vitamins generally are excreted in the urine and rarely cause toxicity problems. See **TABLE 9.2** for functions, recommended intake amounts, and food sources of specific vitamins.

**Vitamin D** Vitamin D, the sunshine vitamin, is formed from a compound in the skin when exposed to the sun's ultraviolet rays. In most people, an adequate amount of vitamin D can be synthesized with 5 to 30 minutes of sun on the face, neck, hands, arms, and legs twice a week, without sunscreen.[17]

## TABLE 9.2 | A Guide to Vitamins

| Vitamin Name | Primary Functions | Recommended Intake | Reliable Food Sources |
|---|---|---|---|
| Thiamin | Carbohydrate and protein metabolism | Men: 1.2 mg/day<br>Women: 1.1 mg/day | Pork, fortified cereals, enriched rice and pasta, peas, tuna, legumes |
| Riboflavin | Carbohydrate and fat metabolism | Men: 1.3 mg/day<br>Women: 1.1 mg/day | Beef liver, shrimp, dairy foods, fortified cereals, enriched breads and grains |
| Niacin | Carbohydrate and fat metabolism | Men: 16 mg/day<br>Women: 14 mg/day | Meat/fish/poultry, fortified cereals, enriched breads and grains, canned tomato products |
| Vitamin $B_6$ | Carbohydrate and amino acid metabolism | Men and women aged 19–50: 1.3 mg/day | Garbanzo beans, meat/fish/poultry, fortified cereals, white potatoes |
| Folate | Amino acid metabolism and DNA synthesis | Men: 400 µg/day<br>Women: 400 µg/day | Fortified cereals, enriched breads and grains, spinach, legumes, spinach, liver |
| Vitamin $B_{12}$ | Formation of blood cells and nervous system | Men: 2.4 µg/day<br>Women: 2.4 µg/day | Shellfish, all cuts of meat/fish/poultry, dairy foods, fortified cereals |
| Pantothenic acid | Fat metabolism | Men: 5 mg/day<br>Women: 5 mg/day | Meat/fish/poultry, shiitake mushrooms, fortified cereals, egg yolks |
| Biotin | Carbohydrate, fat, and protein metabolism | Men: 30 µg/day<br>Women: 30 µg/day | Nuts, egg yolks |
| Vitamin C | Collagen synthesis; iron absorption, and promotes healing | Men: 90 mg/day<br>Women: 75 mg/day<br>Smokers: 35 mg more per day than RDA | Sweet peppers, citrus fruits and juices, broccoli, strawberries, kiwi |
| Vitamin A | Immune function, maintains epithelial cells, healthy bones and vision | Men: 900 µg<br>Women: 700 µg | Beef and chicken liver, egg yolks, milk<br>Carotenoids found in spinach, carrots, mango, apricots, cantaloupe, pumpkin, yams |
| Vitamin D | Promotes calcium absorption and healthy bones | Adult aged 19–70: 15 µg/day (600 IU/day) | Canned salmon and mackerel, milk, fortified cereals |
| Vitamin E | Protects cell membranes, and acts as a powerful antioxidant | Men: 15 mg/day<br>Women: 15 mg/day | Sunflower seeds, almonds, vegetable oils, fortified cereals |
| Vitamin K | Blood coagulation and bone metabolism | Men: 120 µg/day<br>Women: 90 µg/day | Kale, spinach, turnip greens, Brussels sprouts |

**Note:** RDA: Recommended Dietary Allowance; AI: Adequate Intakes; UL: Tolerable Upper Level Intakes. Values are for all adults aged 19 and older, except as noted. Values increase among women who are pregnant or lactating.

**Source:** Data from J. Thompson and M. Manore, Nutrition: An Applied Approach, 2nd ed., © 2009; The National Academies, "Dietary Reference Intakes for Calcium and Vitamin D," 2011, www.iom.edu.

However, the sun is not high enough in the sky during late fall to early spring in northern climates to allow for vitamin D synthesis. For people who cannot rely on the sun to meet their daily vitamin D needs, consuming vitamin D–fortified milk, yogurt, soy milk, cereals, and fatty fish, such as salmon, can also supply this vitamin.

Vitamin D is essential for the body's regulation of calcium, the primary mineral component of bone. It also assists in the process of calcification by which bone minerals are crystallized. For these reasons, a deficiency of vitamin D can promote loss of bone density and strength, a condition called *osteoporosis*. Two other bone disorders, *rickets* in children, and its adult version, *osteomalacia,* both of which cause softening and distortion of the bones, can also be prevented with adequate intake of vitamin D.[18] Vitamin D also helps fight infections, lowers blood pressure, reduces the risk of developing diabetes mellitus, and may reduce the growth of cancer cells. Breast and prostate cancer, heart disease, and stroke have also been connected to inadequate vitamin D.

More is not always better, however.[19] Too much vitamin D, generally from excessive intake of vitamin D supplements, can reduce appetite and cause nausea, vomiting, and constipation. Excess vitamin D can also affect the nervous system, cause depression, and deposit calcium in the soft tissues of the kidneys, lungs, blood vessels, and heart.

**Folate** One of the B vitamins, folate is needed for the production of compounds necessary for DNA synthesis in body cells. It is particularly important for proper cell division during embryonic development; folate deficiencies during the first few weeks of pregnancy, typically before a woman even realizes she is pregnant, can prompt a neural tube defect such as spina bifida, in which the primitive tube that eventually forms the brain and spinal cord fails to close properly. The FDA requires that all bread, cereal, rice, and pasta products sold in the United States be fortified with folic acid, the synthetic form of folate, to reduce the incidence of neural tube defects.

> **vitamins** Essential organic compounds that promote metabolism, growth, and reproduction and help maintain life and health.
>
> **minerals** Inorganic, indestructible elements that aid physiological processes.

# Minerals

**Minerals** are inorganic, indestructible elements that aid physiological processes within the body. Without minerals, vitamins could not be absorbed. Minerals are readily excreted and, with a few exceptions, are usually not toxic. *Major minerals* are the minerals that the body needs in fairly large amounts: sodium, calcium, phosphorus, magnesium, potassium, sulfur, and chloride. *Trace minerals* include iron, zinc, manganese, copper, fluoride, selenium, chromium, and iodine. Only very small amounts of trace minerals are needed, and serious problems may result if excesses or deficiencies occur (see **TABLE 9.3**).

**Sodium** Sodium is necessary for the regulation of blood volume and blood pressure, fluid balance, transmission of nerve impulses, heart activity, and certain metabolic functions. It enhances flavors, acts as a preservative, and tenderizes meats, so it's often present in high quantities in the foods

## TABLE 9.3 | A Guide to Minerals

| Mineral Name | Primary Functions | Recommended Intake | Reliable Food Sources |
|---|---|---|---|
| Sodium | Fluid and acid-base balance; nerve impulses and muscle contraction | Adults: 1.5 g/day (1,500 mg/day) | Table salt, pickles, most canned soups, snack foods, lunch meats, tomato products |
| Potassium | Fluid balance; nerve impulses and muscle contraction | Adults: 4.7 g/day (4,700 mg/day) | Most fresh fruits and vegetables: potato, banana, tomato juice, orange juice, melon |
| Phosphorus | ATP, fluid balance and bone formation | Adults: 700 mg/day | Milk/cheese/yogurt, soy milk and tofu, legumes nuts, poultry |
| Selenium | Regulates thyroid hormones and reduces oxidative stress | Adults: 55 µg/day | Seafood, milk, whole grains, and eggs |
| Calcium | Part of bone; muscle contraction, acid base balance, and nerve transmission | Adults 1,000 mg/day | Milk/yogurt/cheese, sardines, collard greens and spinach, calcium-fortified juices |
| Magnesium | Part of bone; muscle contraction | Men: 400 mg/day<br>Women: 310 mg/day | Spinach, kale, collard greens, whole grains, seeds, nuts, legumes |
| Iodine | Synthesis of thyroid hormones | Adults: 150 µg/day | Iodized salt, saltwater seafood |
| Iron | Part of hemoglobin and myoglobin | Men: 8 mg/day<br>Women 18 mg/day | Meat/fish/poultry, fortified cereals, legumes |
| Zinc | Immune system function; growth and sexual maturation | Men: 11 mg/day<br>Women: 8 mg/day | Meat/fish/poultry, fortified cereals, legumes |

**Note:** Values are for all adults aged 19 and older.

**Source:** Data from J. Thompson and M. Manore, Nutrition: An Applied Approach, 2nd ed., © 2009; The National Academies, "Dietary Reference Intakes for Calcium and Vitamin D," 2011, www.iom.edu.

we eat. A common misconception is that table salt and sodium are the same thing: Table salt is a compound containing both sodium and chloride. It accounts for only 15 percent of our sodium intake. The majority of sodium in our diet comes from processed foods that are infused with sodium to enhance flavor and for preservation. Pickles, fast foods, salty snacks, processed cheeses, canned and dehydrated soups, frozen dinners, many breads and bakery products, and smoked meats and sausages often contain several hundred milligrams of sodium per serving.

> Even if you never use table salt, you still may be getting excess sodium in your diet.

The AI for sodium is just 1,500 milligrams, which is about 0.65 of a teaspoon.[20] The latest National Health and Nutrition Examination Survey (NHANES) estimated that the average American over 2 years of age consumes 3,463 milligrams of sodium per day, or about 1.5 teaspoons.[21]

Both the Institute of Medicine and the American Heart Association recommend consuming no more than the AI for sodium.[22] Why is high sodium intake a concern? Salt-sensitive individuals respond to a high-sodium diet with an increase in blood pressure (hypertension), which contributes to heart disease and strokes. Although the cause of the majority of cases of hypertension is unknown, lowering sodium intake reduces the risk.

**Calcium** Calcium plays a vital role in building strong bones and teeth, muscle contraction, blood clotting, nerve impulse transmission, heartbeat regulation, and fluid balance within cells. The issue of calcium consumption has gained national attention with the rising incidence of osteoporosis among older adults. Most Americans do not consume the recommended 1,000 to 1,200 milligrams of calcium per day.[23]

Milk is one of the richest sources of dietary calcium. Calcium-fortified orange juice and soymilk are good alternatives if you do not drink dairy milk. Many green leafy vegetables are good sources of calcium, but some contain oxalic acid, which makes their calcium harder to absorb. Spinach, chard, and beet greens are not particularly good sources of calcium, whereas broccoli, cauliflower, and many peas and beans offer good supplies.

It is generally best to take calcium throughout the day, consuming it with foods containing protein, vitamin D, and vitamin C for optimal absorption. Many dairy products are both excellent sources of calcium and fortified with vitamin D, which is known to improve calcium absorption.

Do you consume carbonated soft drinks? Be aware that the added phosphoric acid (phosphate) in these drinks can cause you to excrete extra calcium, which may result in calcium loss from your bones. One study of 2,500 men and women found that in women who consumed at least three cans of cola per week, even diet cola, bone density of the hip was 4 to 5 percent lower than in women who drank fewer than one cola per month. Colas

**anemia** Condition that results from the body's inability to produce adequate hemoglobin.

did not seem to have the same effect on men.[24] There may also be a "milk displacement" effect, meaning that people who drank soda were not drinking milk, thereby decreasing their calcium intake.

**Iron** Worldwide, iron deficiency is the most common nutrient deficiency, affecting more than 2 billion people, nearly 30 percent of the world's population.[25] In the United States, iron deficiency is less prevalent, but it is still the most common micronutrient deficiency.[26] Women aged 19 to 50 need about 18 milligrams of iron per day, and men aged 19 to 50 need about 8 milligrams.

Iron deficiency can lead to *iron-deficiency anemia*. **Anemia** results from the body's inability to produce adequate amounts of hemoglobin (the oxygen-carrying component of the blood). Anemia can also result from blood loss, cancer, ulcers, and other conditions. When iron-deficiency anemia occurs, body cells receive less oxygen. As a result, the iron-deficient person feels tired. Iron is also important for energy metabolism, DNA synthesis, and other body functions.

Iron overload or iron toxicity due to ingesting too many iron-containing supplements is the leading cause of accidental poisoning in small children in the United States. Symptoms of toxicity include nausea, vomiting, diarrhea, rapid heartbeat, weak pulse, dizziness, shock, and confusion. Excess iron intake

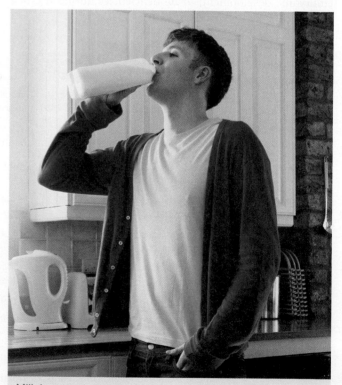

Milk is a great source of calcium and other nutrients. If you don't like milk or can't drink it, make sure to get enough calcium—at least 1,000 milligrams a day—through other sources.

## Beneficial Non-Nutrient Components of Foods

Increasingly, nutrition research is focusing on components of foods that interact with nutrients to promote human health rather than solely as sources of macro- and micronutrients.[28] Foods that may confer health benefits beyond the nutrients they contribute to the diet—whole foods, fortified foods, enriched foods, or enhanced foods—are called **functional foods.** When functional foods are included as part of a varied diet, they have the potential to positively impact health.[29]

Some of the most popular functional foods today are those containing **antioxidants.** These substances appear to protect against oxidative stress, a complex process in which *free radicals* (atoms with unpaired electrons) destabilize other atoms and molecules, prompting a chain reaction that can damage cells, cell proteins, or genetic material in the cells. Free radical formation is a natural process that cannot be avoided, but antioxidants combat it by donating their electrons to stabilize free radicals, activating enzymes that convert free radicals to less-damaging substances, or reducing or repairing the damage they cause.

Among the more commonly cited antioxidants are vitamins C and E, as well as the minerals copper, iron, manganese, selenium, and zinc. Other potent antioxidants are **phytochemicals,** compounds that occur naturally in plants and are thought to protect them against ultraviolet radiation, pests, and other threats. Common examples include the *carotenoids,* pigments found in red, orange, and dark green fruits and vegetables. Beta-carotene, the most researched carotenoid, is a precursor of vitamin A, meaning that vitamin A can be produced in the body from beta-carotene. Both vitamin A and beta-carotene have antioxidant properties. Phenolic phytochemicals, which include a group known as flavonoids, are found in an array of fruits and vegetables as well as soy products, tea, and chocolate. Like carotenoids, they are thought to have antioxidant properties that may prevent cardiovascular disease.[30]

To date, many such claims about the health benefits of antioxidant nutrients and phytochemicals have not been fully investigated. However, studies do show that individuals deficient in antioxidant vitamins and minerals have an increased risk for age-related diseases, and that antioxidants consumed in whole foods, mostly fruits and vegetables, may reduce these individuals' risks.[31] In contrast, antioxidants consumed as supplements do not confer such a benefit, and may be harmful. For example, researchers have long theorized that because many cancers

result from DNA damage, and because vitamin E appears to protect against such damage, vitamin E would also reduce cancer risk. Surprisingly, the great majority of studies have demonstrated no effect or, in some cases, a negative effect.[32]

Foods rich in nutrients and phytochemicals are increasingly being referred to as "superfoods." Do they live up to their name? See the **Health Headlines** box on page 274.

> **functional foods** Foods believed to have specific health benefits beyond their basic nutrients.
>
> **antioxidants** Substances believed to protect against oxidative stress and resultant tissue damage.
>
> **phytochemicals** Naturally occurring non-nutrient plant chemicals believed to have beneficial health effects.

## LO 2 | NUTRITIONAL GUIDELINES

Describe nutritional guidelines and recommendations, including the Dietary Guidelines for Americans and the MyPlate food guidance system.

Today, Americans consume more calories than ever before. From 1970 to 2010, average calorie consumption increased from 2,169 to 2,614 calories per day (see **FIGURE 9.4**).[33] In general, it isn't the actual amount of food, but rather the number of calories in the foods we choose to eat, that has increased. When these trends are combined with our increasingly sedentary lifestyle, it is not surprising that we have seen a dramatic rise in obesity.[34]

The Center for Nutrition Policy and Promotion at the U.S. Department of Agriculture (USDA) publishes two dietary tools created for consumers to make healthy eating easy: the *2010 Dietary Guidelines for Americans* and the MyPlate food guidance system.

## Dietary Guidelines for Americans, 2010

The Dietary Guidelines for Americans are a set of recommendations for healthy eating created by the U.S. Department of Health and Human Services and the USDA. These guidelines are revised every 5 years. New recommendations are currently being reviewed, and final approval is likely in the fall of 2015. The information in *2010 Dietary Guidelines for Americans* was designed to help bridge the gap between the standard American diet and the key recommendations that aim to combat the growing obesity epidemic by balancing calories with adequate physical activity.[35]

Blueberries are a great source of antioxidants.

**Balancing Calories to Manage Weight** The recommendations in *Dietary Guidelines for Americans* were developed to prevent overnutrition, especially when it comes to kilocalories. People who are successful at maintaining a

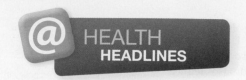
# HEALTH CLAIMS OF SUPERFOODS

Functional foods contain both nutrients and other active compounds that may improve overall health, reduce the risk for certain diseases, or delay aging. If the term "functional foods" strikes you as a bit stodgy, you're not alone. In food advertisements, fitness and food magazines, and even among health care organizations, these foods are increasingly being referred to as "superfoods." For instance, Harvard Medical School recently published a list of 12 superfoods, including broccoli, beans, salmon, oatmeal, Greek yogurt, and dark chocolate. Do superfoods live up to their new name? Let's look at a few.

Salmon is a rich source of the omega-3 fatty acids EPA and DHA, which combat inflammation, improve HDL/LDL blood profiles, and reduce the risk for cardiovascular disease. DHA may also promote a healthy nervous system, reducing the risk for age-related dementia.

Yogurt makes it onto most superfood lists because it contains living, beneficial bacteria called probiotics. You will see their genus name, for example, *Lactobacillus* or *Bifidobacterium*, in the

**Yogurt and kefir (a fermented milk drink) are dairy products containing beneficial bacteria called *probiotics*.**

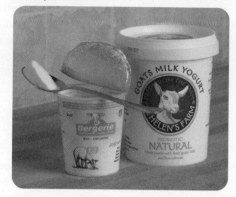

list of ingredients on the product's label. Probiotics colonize the large intestine, where they help complete digestion, produce certain vitamins, and may reduce the risk of diarrhea and other bowel disorders, boost immunity, and help regulate body weight.

Cocoa is particularly rich in a class of chemicals called flavonols that have been shown in many studies to reduce the risk for cardiovascular disease, diabetes, and even arthritis. Dark chocolate has

a higher level of flavonols than milk chocolate.

Given such claims, it's easy to get carried away by the idea that superfoods, like superheros, have superpowers. But eating a square of dark chocolate won't rescue you from the ill effects of a fast-food burger and fries. What matters is your whole diet. Focus on including superfoods as components of a varied diet rich in fresh fruits, legumes and other vegetables, whole grains, lean sources of protein, and nuts and seeds. These are the "everyday heroes" of a super-healthful diet.

**Sources:** Academy of Nutrition and Dietetics, "Position of the Academy of Nutrition and Dietetics: Functional Foods," *Journal of the Academy of Nutrition and Dietetics* 113 (2013): 1096–1103; D. Swanson, R. Block, and S .A. Mousa, "Omega-3 Fatty Acids EPA and DHA: Health Benefits Throughout Life," *Advances in Nutrition* 3, no. 1 (2012): 1–7; R. Krajmalnik-Brown et al., "Effects of Gut Microbes on Nutrient Absorption and Energy Regulation," *Nutrition in Clinical Practice* 27, no. 2 (2012): 201–14; L. Hooper et al., "Effects of Chocolate, Cocoa, and Flavan-3-ols on Cardiovascular Health: A Systematic Review and Meta-Analysis of Randomized Trials," *American Journal of Clinical Nutrition* 95, no. 3 (2012): 740–53, doi: 10.3945/ajcn.111.023457

healthy body weight do so by controlling their intake of kilocalories and being more active. To decrease the number of kilocalories you eat, avoid oversized portions, switch from whole milk to fat-free or 1 percent milk, fill your plate with vegetables and fruit, and increase your physical activity at each stage of life. Remember to enjoy your food, but eat less of it.

## Foods and Food Components to Reduce

The recommendations set forth in *Dietary Guidelines for Americans* promote eating more nutrient dense foods and beverages. A healthy eating pattern limits your intake of saturated fats to 10 percent of total kilocalories by eating less meat and butter and switching from whole-milk products to low-fat or nonfat dairy.[36] Reduce your cholesterol intake to 300 milligrams or less by consuming fewer animal products; reduce foods high in sodium, including processed and canned foods, to 2,300 milligrams, or as low as 1,500 milligrams, if you have high blood pressure.[37] Limit your intake of refined grains, *trans* fats, and added sugars. If you drink alcohol, drink in moderation; limit to one drink per day for women and two drinks per day for men.

## Foods and Nutrients to Increase

A healthy diet emphasizes a variety of protein foods including seafood, lean meat and poultry, eggs, beans, peas, soy products, and unsalted nuts and seeds. Protein foods that are higher in solid fats, such as red meat, should be replaced with protein foods that are lower in solid fats. A healthy diet is rich in plant-based foods, including leafy green, red, and orange vegetables, and whole grains.

## Building Healthy Eating Patterns

A healthy eating pattern takes time to establish. Set a goal that you can achieve over time. Begin by accounting for all foods and beverages you eat each day; assess how they meet your nutrient goals over time with a healthy balance of kilocalories to maintain your weight. Don't just cut high-sugar, high-fat, and processed foods; focus on adding healthy foods such as fruits, vegetables, and whole grains to your eating patterns. Pack healthy lunches and snacks to take with you to avoid fast foods. Control portions by measuring out your snacks rather than eating from the package. Don't skip meals,

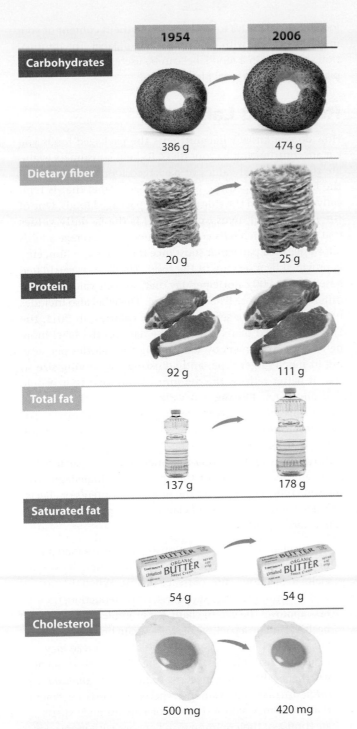

| | 1954 | 2006 |
|---|---|---|
| **Carbohydrates** | 386 g | 474 g |
| **Dietary fiber** | 20 g | 25 g |
| **Protein** | 92 g | 111 g |
| **Total fat** | 137 g | 178 g |
| **Saturated fat** | 54 g | 54 g |
| **Cholesterol** | 500 mg | 420 mg |

**FIGURE 9.4** Trends in Per Capita Nutrient Consumption
Since 1954, Americans' daily caloric intake has increased by about 25%, as has daily consumption of carbohydrates, fiber, and protein. Daily total fat intake has increased by 30%.

**Source:** Data are from USDA/Center for Nutrition Policy and Promotion, Nutrient Availability, updated February 2014, www.ers.usda.gov/data-products/food-availability-(per-capita)-data-system/.aspx#26715.

especially breakfast. Reduce the risk of foodborne illnesses by following good food safety practices. And finally, make eating fun and enjoyable!

# MyPlate Food Guidance System

To help consumers understand and implement the Dietary Guidelines, the USDA has developed an easy-to-follow graphic and guidance system called MyPlate, which can be found at www.choosemyplate.gov and is illustrated in **FIGURE 9.5**. The MyPlate food guidance system takes into consideration the dietary and caloric needs for a wide variety of individuals, such as pregnant or breast-feeding women, those trying to lose weight, and adults with different activity levels. The interactive website can create personalized dietary and exercise recommendations based on the individual information you enter.

**Eat Nutrient-Dense Foods** Although eating the proper number of servings from MyPlate is important, it is also important to recognize that there are large caloric, fat, and energy differences among foods within a given food group. For example, salmon and hot dogs provide vastly different nutrient levels per calorie. Salmon is rich in essential fatty acids and is considered nutrient dense—dense in nutrients compared to kilocalories. Hot dogs, which are not nutrient dense, are loaded with kilocalories, saturated fats, cholesterol, and sodium—all substances we should limit. It is important to eat foods that have a high nutritional value for their caloric content.

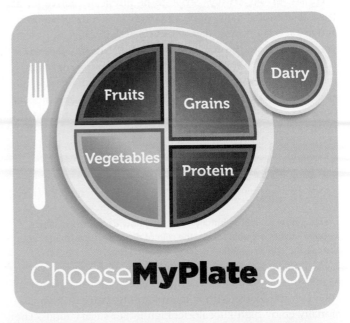

**FIGURE 9.5** The MyPlate System The USDA MyPlate food guidance system takes a new approach to dietary and exercise recommendations. Each colored section of the plate represents a food group, and an interactive tool at www .choosemyplate.gov helps you analyze and track your foods and physical activity, and provides helpful tips to personalize your plan.

**Source:** U.S. Department of Agriculture, 2010, www.choosemyplate.gov.

## Reduce Empty Calorie Foods

Avoid *empty calories*, that is, high-calorie foods and drinks with little nutritional value. MyPlate recommends we limit our intake of sugary drinks as well as the following sugar- and fat-laden items:[38]

- **Cakes, cookies, pastries, and donuts.** One slice of chocolate cake contains 77 percent empty calories.
- **Cheese.** Switching from whole milk mozzarella cheese to nonfat mozzarella cheese saves you 76 empty calories per ounce.
- **Pizza.** One slice of pepperoni pizza adds 139 empty calories to your meal.
- **Ice cream.** More than 75 percent of the 275 calories in ice cream are empty calories.
- **Sausages, hot dogs, bacon, and ribs.** Adding a sausage link to your breakfast adds 96 empty calories.
- **Wine, beer, and all alcoholic beverages.** A whopping 155 empty calories are consumed with each 12 fluid ounces of beer.
- **Refined grains, including crackers, cookies, and white rice.** Switching to whole wheat versions can save you 25 fat-laden empty calories per serving.

**Physical Activity** Strive to be physically active for at least 30 minutes daily, preferably with moderate to vigorous activity levels on most days. Physical activity does not mean you have to go to the gym, jog 3 miles a day, or hire a personal trainer. Any activity that gets your heart pumping counts, including gardening and other yard work, playing basketball, and dancing. MyPlate personalized plans offer recommendations for weekly physical activity. (For more on physical fitness, see Chapter 11.)

## LO 3 | HOW CAN I EAT MORE HEALTHFULLY?

Discuss how to eat healthfully, including how to read food labels, vegetarianism, organic foods, the role of dietary supplements, and the unique challenges that college students face.

Many Americans believe eating healthfully means giving up their favorite foods. With a little planning, you can still occasionally enjoy high-kilocalorie, high-fat, or sugary foods. The key to following a healthy eating pattern is to achieve balance between food groups, choose a variety of foods each day, and moderate the amounts of food you eat. A healthful eating plan also includes foods that are nutrient dense and low in energy density or kilocalories.

Whether you follow a vegetarian diet, eat only organic foods, take dietary supplements, or choose to eat locally grown foods, there are ways to improve the nutrient content of your meals. Let's begin with how to read a food label. The information contained in a food label can be useful when it comes to planning a healthy meal plan.

## Read Food Labels

How do you know what nutrients the packaged foods you eat are contributing to your diet? To help consumers evaluate the nutritional values of packaged foods, the FDA and the USDA developed the Nutrition Facts label that is typically displayed on the side or back of packaged foods. One of the most helpful items on the label is the **% daily values (%DVs)** list, which tells you how much of an average adult's allowance for a particular substance (fat, fiber, calcium, etc.) is provided by a serving of the food. The %DV is calculated based on a 2,000 calorie per day diet, so your values may be different from those listed on a label. The label also includes information on the serving size and calories. In 2014, the FDA announced plans to make the data on the label more helpful for consumers by identifying the calories per serving in much larger type, and adjusting the serving size so that it better reflects the amount of the food that people typically eat.[39] **FIGURE 9.6** walks you through a typical Nutrition Facts label and the proposed label changes. For the latest information on the new label, go to www.FDA.gov and search "Nutrition Facts label."

Food labels contain other information as well, such as the name and manufacturer of the product, an ingredients list, and sometimes claims about the product's contents or effects. The FDA allows three types of claims on the packages of foods and dietary supplements:[40]

- Health claims describe a relationship between a food product and health promotion or disease prevention. It cannot claim to diagnose, cure, or treat a disease. When the current scientific evidence supports the risk reduction, the FDA approves the health claim. For example, an approved health claim on a package of whole-grain bread may state, "In a low-fat diet, whole-grain foods like this bread may reduce the risk of heart disease." The FDA can also evaluate whether health claims meet the standard for *significant scientific agreement* (SSA) among experts. If there is agreement that a food may reduce your risk of a disease and experts are confident their opinion won't change with more scientific study, the health claim is approved.
- Nutrient content claims indicate a specific nutrient is present at a certain level. For example, a product label might

**% daily values (%DVs)** Percentages listed as "% DV" on food and supplement labels; identify how much of each listed nutrient or other substance a serving of food contributes to a 2,000 calorie/day diet.

# 50%

OF ADULTS DRINK AT LEAST ONE **SUGARY** DRINK A DAY.

## Sample Label for Macaroni and Cheese

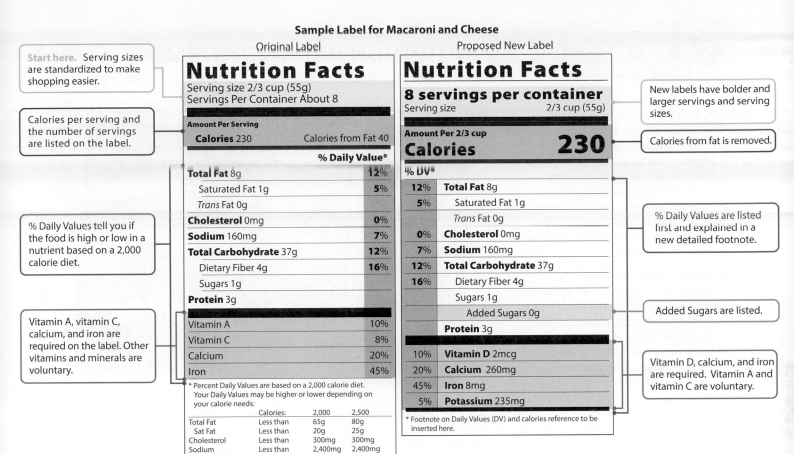

Original Label

**Start here.** Serving sizes are standardized to make shopping easier.

Calories per serving and the number of servings are listed on the label.

% Daily Values tell you if the food is high or low in a nutrient based on a 2,000 calorie diet.

Vitamin A, vitamin C, calcium, and iron are required on the label. Other vitamins and minerals are voluntary.

### Nutrition Facts
Serving size 2/3 cup (55g)
Servings Per Container About 8

**Amount Per Serving**

**Calories** 230          Calories from Fat 40

                                    **% Daily Value***

| | % |
|---|---|
| **Total Fat** 8g | **12**% |
| Saturated Fat 1g | **5**% |
| *Trans* Fat 0g | |
| **Cholesterol** 0mg | **0**% |
| **Sodium** 160mg | **7**% |
| **Total Carbohydrate** 37g | **12**% |
| Dietary Fiber 4g | **16**% |
| Sugars 1g | |
| **Protein** 3g | |
| Vitamin A | 10% |
| Vitamin C | 8% |
| Calcium | 20% |
| Iron | 45% |

\* Percent Daily Values are based on a 2,000 calorie diet. Your Daily Values may be higher or lower depending on your calorie needs:

| | | Calories: | 2,000 | 2,500 |
|---|---|---|---|---|
| Total Fat | Less than | | 65g | 80g |
| Sat Fat | Less than | | 20g | 25g |
| Cholesterol | Less than | | 300mg | 300mg |
| Sodium | Less than | | 2,400mg | 2,400mg |
| Total Carbohydrate | | | 300g | 375g |
| Dietary Fiber | | | 25g | 30g |

Proposed New Label

### Nutrition Facts
**8 servings per container**
Serving size                    2/3 cup (55g)

**Amount Per 2/3 cup**
**Calories**                    **230**

**% DV***

| | |
|---|---|
| 12% | **Total Fat** 8g |
| 5% | Saturated Fat 1g |
| | *Trans* Fat 0g |
| 0% | **Cholesterol** 0mg |
| 7% | **Sodium** 160mg |
| 12% | **Total Carbohydrate** 37g |
| 16% | Dietary Fiber 4g |
| | Sugars 1g |
| | Added Sugars 0g |
| | **Protein** 3g |
| 10% | **Vitamin D** 2mcg |
| 20% | **Calcium** 260mg |
| 45% | **Iron** 8mg |
| 5% | **Potassium** 235mg |

\* Footnote on Daily Values (DV) and calories reference to be inserted here.

New labels have bolder and larger servings and serving sizes.

Calories from fat is removed.

% Daily Values are listed first and explained in a new detailed footnote.

Added Sugars are listed.

Vitamin D, calcium, and iron are required. Vitamin A and vitamin C are voluntary.

**FIGURE 9.6** Reading a Food Label

**Sources:** U.S. Food and Drug Administration, "How to Understand and Use the Nutrition Facts Panel," April 2015, www.fda.gov/Food/IngredientsPackagingLabeling/LabelingNutrition/ucm274593.htm; U.S. Food and Drug Administration, "Proposed Changes to the Nutrition Facts Label," August 2014, www.fda.gov/Food/GuidanceRegulation/GuidanceDocumentsRegulatoryInformation/LabelingNutrition/ucm385663.htm

▶ **VIDEO TUTOR**
Understanding Food Labels

---

say "High in fiber" or "Low in fat" or "This product contains 100 calories per serving." Nutrient content claims can use the following words: *more, less, fewer, good source of, free, light, lean, extra lean, high, low, reduced.*

■ Structure and function claims describe the effect that a component in the food product has on the body. For example, the label of a carton of milk is allowed to state, "Calcium builds strong bones."

In addition to food labels, shoppers are increasingly being guided in their food choices by nutritional rating systems. What are these systems, and can they help you make smarter choices? See the **Student Health Today** box on the next page for answers.

**SEE IT! VIDEOS**

Learn how the new FDA mandate with affect packaging labels. Watch **Changes Coming to Nutrition Labels,** available on MasteringHealth™

**Front of Package Labeling** The FDA has proposed new guidelines for the nutrition labeling on the front of packages to help consumers choose healthy foods. Currently, the

labeling on the front of packages is unregulated and may cause confusion for consumers.

The *Facts Up Front* initiative is a voluntary labeling system that can be used by manufacturers to provide quick, accurate information for the consumer. The most important information from the Nutrition Facts panel is placed on the front of the package. As shown in **FIGURE 9.7**, Facts Up Front illustrates the kilocalories, saturated fat, sodium, and added sugars per serving. If a serving of the food contains more than 10 percent of a vitamin or mineral, the manufacturer can also include

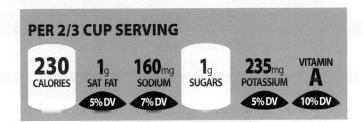

**FIGURE 9.7 Facts Up Front** Information is placed on the front of the package for a quick and accurate picture of the nutritional content of a serving of the food.

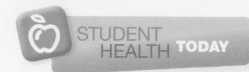
# NUTRITION RATING SYSTEMS

Next time you're at the grocery store, take a close look at the tags on the store shelves. Do you see anything different—stars, perhaps, or numbers inside blue hexagons? If so, you're looking at one of several new nutrition rating systems. Nutrition scientists and physicians designed these systems to help consumers quickly locate healthful foods. Four of the most popular systems in American markets are as follows:

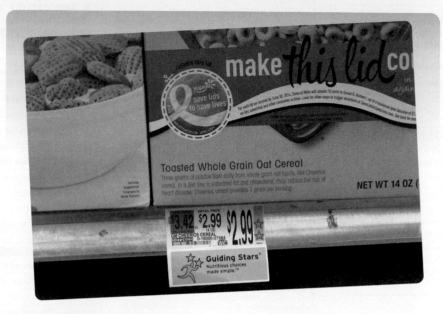

- **Guiding Stars.** This system rates the nutritional quality of foods using information from the Nutrition Facts label and the food's ingredients list. Foods are rated with from zero to three stars, with three indicating the highest nutritional quality. A fresh tomato, for example, gets three stars. When the program was implemented, all foods sold by the participating retailers were evaluated, and less than one fourth earned even a single star. What the system lacks in subtlety it makes up for in simplicity—even consumers who haven't been introduced to it can almost instantly understand the basic message behind it: The product with the most stars "wins."

- **NuVal.** The NuVal System uses a scale of 1 to 100. The higher the number, the higher the nutritional quality. In rating each food, the system considers more than 30 dietary components—not just nutrients, but fiber, antioxidants, and other food components known to affect health. In this system, a tomato gets a top score of 100 points. The 100-point rating scale allows consumers to make more subtle distinctions between very similar foods; for example, two brands of whole-grain bread get scores of 48 versus 29. Although the consumer doesn't need to stop and research the food, the ranking suggests real differences, and in fact, the bread with the higher score is lower in calories and sodium, higher in calcium, and has twice the dietary fiber per slice.

- **American Heart Association Heart Check.** The AHA Heart Check is based on foods that contain sufficient nutrients to promote heart health. To receive a Heart Check rating, the food must meet specific nutrient requirements in six different food categories based on total fat, saturated and *trans* fat, cholesterol, and sodium. For example, to receive a Heart Check rating, a serving of food must not contain more than 20 milligrams of cholesterol. Products that contain partially hydrogenated oils are ineligible to receive a Heart Check rating. Each serving must also contain 10 percent or more of the Daily Value of at least one of these nutrients: dietary fiber, vitamin A, vitamin C, iron, protein, or calcium.

- **Aggregate Nutrient Density Index (ANDI).** This index ranks foods based on the number of micronutrients per calorie and takes into account as many known beneficial phytochemicals as possible. It does not, however, consider macronutrient density, such as the amount of high-quality protein or essential fatty acids in the food. A top score is 1,000. How does this system rate our tomato? It gets just 164 points! In contrast, kale gets a top score of 1,000. Again, the difference is in the calorie/micronutrient ratio: A medium-sized tomato and two thirds of a cup of kale have about the same number of calories, yet the kale has about 7 times as much vitamin A and 3.5 times as much vitamin C.

Do these ranking systems prompt shoppers to choose more healthful foods? Research suggests they just might. An evaluation in the *American Journal of Clinical Nutrition* found that the systems reduce the time and effort consumers spend in making food choices, as compared with more detailed labels and have the potential to help them choose more healthful foods. That's important because, as an evaluation of the NuVal system from the Harvard School of Public Health found, people who eat food with higher scores have a lower risk of cardiovascular disease and diabetes, and may even enjoy a longer life.

**Sources:** S. A. Gerrior, "Nutrient Profiling Systems: Are Science and the Consumer Connected?," *American Journal of Clinical Nutrition* 91, no. 4 (2010): 1116S–17S; L. M. Fischer et al., "Development and Implementation of the Guiding Stars Nutrition Guidance Program," *American Journal of Health Promotion* 26, no. 2 (2011): e55–63, doi: 10.4278/ajhp.100709-QUAL-238; S. E. Chiuve, L. Sampson, and W. C. Willett, "The Association between a Nutritional Quality Index and Risk of Chronic Disease," *American Journal of Preventive Medicine* 40, no. 5 (2011): 505–13, doi: 10.1016/j.amepre.2010.11.022. A. H. Lichtenstein et al., "Food-intake Patterns Assessed by Using Front-of-Pack Labeling Program Criteria Associated with Better Diet Quality and Lower Cardiometabolic Risk," *American Journal of Clinical Nutrition* 99 (2013): 454–62, doi:10.3945/ajcn.113.071407

that information on the front of the package.

## Understand Serving Sizes

MyPlate presents personalized dietary recommendations based on servings of particular nutrients. But how much is one serving? Is it different from a portion? Although these two terms are often used interchangeably, they actually mean very different things. A *serving* is the recommended amount you should consume, whereas a *portion* is the amount you choose to eat at any one time. The saying "your eyes are bigger than your stomach" is rooted in truth—most of us select portions that are much bigger than recommended servings. See **FIGURE 9.8** for a handy pocket guide with tips on recognizing serving sizes.

Unfortunately, we don't always get a clear picture from food producers and advertisers about what a serving really is. Consider a bottle of chocolate milk: The food label may list one serving size as 8 fluid ounces and 150 calories. However, note the size of the entire bottle. If it holds 16 ounces, drinking the whole thing serves up 300 calories.

## Vegetarianism: A Healthy Diet?

The word **vegetarian** means different things to different people. Strict vegetarians, or *vegans*, avoid all foods of animal origin, including dairy products and eggs. Their diet is based on vegetables, grains, fruits, nuts, seeds, and legumes. Far more common are *lacto-vegetarians*, who eat dairy products but avoid flesh foods and eggs. *Ovo-vegetarians* add eggs to a vegan diet, and *lacto-ovo-vegetarians* eat both dairy products and eggs. *Pesco-vegetarians* eat fish, dairy products, and eggs, and *semi-vegetarians* eat chicken, fish, dairy products, and eggs. Some people in the semivegetarian category prefer to call themselves "non–red meat eaters."

According to a poll conducted by the Vegetarian Resource Group, more than 4 percent of U.S. adults, approximately 9 million people, are vegetarians.[41] Other surveys have shown that 5 percent of Americans consider themselves to be "vegetarian" and 2 percent stated they are vegans.[42]

Common reasons for pursuing a vegetarian lifestyle include concern for animal welfare, the environmental costs of meat production, food safety, personal health, weight loss, and weight maintenance. Generally, people who follow a balanced vegetarian diet weigh less and have better cholesterol levels, fewer problems with irregular bowel movements (constipation and diarrhea), and a lower risk of heart disease than do nonvegetarians. A recent analysis of 29 studies involving a total of more than 20,000 participants found that people who follow a vegetarian diet have an average blood pressure several points lower than that of

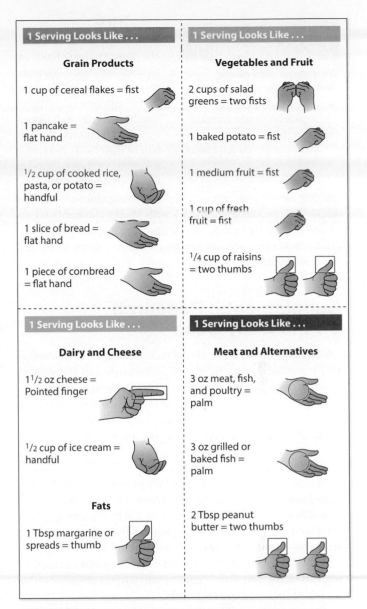

**FIGURE 9.8 Serving Size Card** One of the challenges of following a healthy diet is judging how big a portion size should be and how many servings you are really eating. The comparisons on this card can help you recall what a standard food serving looks like. For easy reference, photocopy or cut out this card, fold on the dotted lines, and keep it in your wallet. You can even laminate it for long-term use.

**Sources:** National Heart, Lung and Blood Institute, "Serving Size Card," Accessed April 2015, http://hp2010.nhlbihin.net/portion/servingcard7.pdf; National Dairy Council, "Serving Size Comparison Chart," Accessed April 2015, www.healthyeating.org /Portals/0/Documents/Schools/ Parent%20Ed/Portion_Sizes_Serving_Chart.pdf

nonvegetarians.[43] Some studies suggest that vegetarianism may also reduce the risk of some cancers, particularly colon cancer.[44]

With proper meal planning, vegetarianism provides a healthful alternative to a meat-based diet. Eating a variety of healthful foods throughout the day helps to ensure proper nutrient intake. Vegan diets are of greater concern than diets that include dairy products and eggs. Vegans may be deficient in vitamins B$_2$ (riboflavin),

> **vegetarian** A person who follows a diet that excludes some or all animal products.

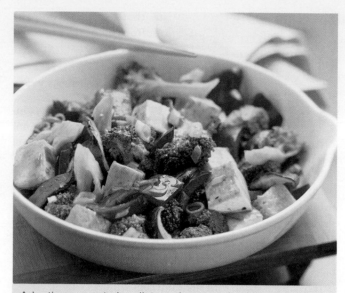

## WHAT DO YOU THINK?

**Why are so many people becoming vegetarians?**

- How easy is it to be a vegetarian on your campus?
- What concerns about vegetarianism do you have, if any?

$B_{12}$, and D, as well as calcium, iron, zinc, and other minerals; however, many foods are fortified with these nutrients, or vegans can obtain them from supplements. Vegans also have to pay more attention to the amino acid content of their foods, but eating a variety of types of plant foods throughout the day will provide adequate amounts of protein. Pregnant women, older adults, sick people, and families with young children who are vegans need to take special care to ensure that their diets are adequate. In all cases, seek advice from a health care professional if you have questions.

Adopting a vegetarian diet can be a very healthy way to eat. Take care to prepare your food healthfully by avoiding added sugars and excessive sodium. Make sure you get complementary essential amino acids throughout the day. Meals like this tofu and vegetable stir-fry can be further enhanced by adding a whole grain, such as brown rice.

## Supplements: Research on the Daily Dose

**Dietary supplements** are products containing one or more dietary ingredients taken by mouth and intended to supplement existing diets. Ingredients range from vitamins, minerals, and herbs to enzymes, amino acids, fatty acids, and organ tissues. They can come in tablet, capsule, liquid, powder, and other forms. Because consumers see dietary supplements as an easy fix to improve their less than healthy diets, sales have skyrocketed.

It is important to note that dietary supplements are not regulated like foods or drugs. The FDA does not evaluate the safety and efficacy of supplements prior to their marketing, and it can take action to remove a supplement from the market only after the product has been proved harmful. Currently, the United States has no formal guidelines for supplement marketing and safety, and supplement manufacturers are responsible for self-monitoring their activities.

Do you really need to take dietary supplements? The Office of Dietary Supplements, part of the National Institutes of Health, states that some supplements may help ensure that you get adequate amounts of essential nutrients if you don't consume a variety of foods, as recommended in the *Dietary Guidelines for Americans*. However, dietary supplements are not intended to prevent or treat disease, and recently the U.S. Preventive Services Task Force concluded that there is insufficient evidence to recommend that healthy people take multivitamin/mineral supplements to prevent cardiovascular disease or cancer.[45] Those who may benefit from using multivitamin/mineral supplements include pregnant and breast-feeding women, older adults, vegans, people on a very low-calorie weight-loss diets, alcohol-dependent individuals, and patients with malabsorption problems or other significant health problems.

**dietary supplements** Products taken by mouth and containing dietary ingredients such as vitamins and minerals that are intended to supplement existing diets.

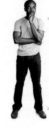

The wisdom of taking other types of supplements, as opposed to consuming nutrients in whole foods, is also unproven. For example, the benefit of fish consumption in reducing the risk for cardiovascular disease is well-established, but studies have shown conflicting results about fish-oil supplements.[46]

Taking high-dose supplements of the fat-soluble vitamins A, D, and E can be harmful or even fatal. Too much vitamin A, for example, can damage the liver, and excessive vitamin E

### WHICH PATH WOULD YOU TAKE?

Scan the QR code to see how different dietary choices YOU make today can affect your overall health tomorrow.

increases the risk for a stroke.[47] The Academy of Nutrition and Dietetics recommends that, though some people benefit from taking supplements, a healthy diet is the best way to give your body what it needs.[48] Be aware that supplements can interact with certain medications, including aspirin, diuretics, and steroids, which may result in potential problems.

If you do decide to take a multivitamin, choose brands that contain the US Pharmacopeia or Consumer Lab seal. This ensures that the supplement has been reviewed, is free of toxic ingredients, and contains the ingredients stated on the label. Store your supplements in a dark, dry place (not the bathroom or other damp spots), make sure they are out of reach of small children, and check the expiration date.

## Eating Well in College

Many college students find it hard to fit a well-balanced meal into the day, but breakfast and lunch are important if you are to keep energy levels up and get the most out of your classes. Eating a complete breakfast that includes fiber-rich carbohydrates, protein, and healthy unsaturated fat (such as a banana, peanut butter and whole-grain bread sandwich or a bowl of oatmeal topped with dried fruit and nuts) is key. If you are short on time, bring a container of yogurt and a handful of almonds to your morning class.

If your campus is like many others, your lunchtime options include a variety of fast-food restaurants. Generally speaking, you can eat more healthfully and for less money if you bring food from home or eat at your campus dining hall. If you must eat fast food, follow the tips below to get more nutritional bang for your buck:

- Ask for nutritional analyses of menu items. Most fast-food chains now have them.
- Order salads, but be careful about what you add to them. Taco salads and Cobb salads are often high in fat, calories, and sodium. Ask for low-fat dressing on the side, and use it sparingly. Stay away from high-fat add-ons, such as bacon bits, croutons, and crispy noodles.
- If you crave french fries, try baked "fries," which may be lower in fat.
- Avoid giant sizes, and refrain from ordering extra sauce, bacon, cheese, and other toppings that add calories, sodium, and fat.
- Limit sodas and other beverages that are high in added sugars.
- At least once per week, swap a vegetable-based meat substitute into your fast-food choices. Most places now offer veggie burgers and similar products, which provide excellent sources of protein and often have less fat and fewer calories.

In the dining hall, try these ideas:

- Choose lean meats, grilled chicken, fish, or vegetable dishes. Avoid fried chicken, fatty cuts of red meat, or meat dishes smothered in creamy or oily sauce.
- Hit the salad bar and load up on leafy greens, beans, tuna, or tofu. Choose items such as avocado or nuts for "good" fat. Go easy on the dressing, or substitute vinaigrette or low-fat dressings.

**COLLEGE MALES SPEND AN AVERAGE OF**

# $99.17

**AND COLLEGE FEMALES SPEND AN AVERAGE OF $52.11 ON FAST FOOD IN A MONTH.**

- When choosing items from a made-to-order food station, ask the preparer to hold the butter or oil, mayonnaise, sour cream, or cheese- or cream-based sauces.
- Avoid going back for seconds and consuming large portions.
- If there is something you'd like but don't see in your dining hall, speak to your food service manager and provide suggestions.
- Pass on high-calorie, low-nutrient foods such as sugary cereals, ice cream, and other sweet treats. Choose fruit or low-fat yogurt to satisfy your sweet tooth.

Between classes, avoid vending machines. Reach into your backpack for an apple, banana, some dried fruit and nuts, a single serving of unsweetened applesauce, or whole-grain crackers spread with peanut butter. Energy bars can be a nutritious option if you choose right. Check the Nutrition Facts label for bars that are below 200 calories and provide at least 3 grams of dietary fiber. Cereal bars usually provide less protein than energy bars; however, they also tend to be much lower in calories and sugar, and high in fiber.

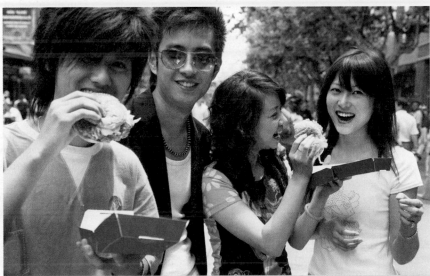

Meals like this one may be convenient, but they are high in saturated fat, sodium, refined carbohydrates, and calories. Even when you are short on time and money, it is possible—and worthwhile—to make healthier choices. If you are ordering fast food, opt for foods prepared by baking, roasting, or steaming; ask for the leanest meat option; and request that sauces, dressings, and gravies be served on the side.

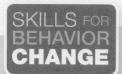
Maintaining a nutritious diet within the confines of student life can be challenging. However, if you take the time to plan healthy meals, you will find that you are eating better, enjoying it more, and actually saving money. The **Money & Health** box examines ways to include fruits and vegetables in your diet without breaking the bank.

## LO 4 | FOOD SAFETY: A GROWING CONCERN

Explain food safety concerns facing Americans and people in other regions of the world.

Eating unhealthy food is one thing. Eating food that has been contaminated with a pathogen, toxin, or other harmful substance is quite another. As outbreaks of foodborne illness (commonly called food poisoning) make the news, the food industry has come under fire. The Food Safety Modernization Act, passed into law in 2011, included new requirements for

**organic** Grown without use of toxic and persistent pesticides, chemicals, or hormones.

food processors to take actions to prevent contamination of foods. The act gave the FDA greater authority to inspect food-manufacturing facilities and to recall contaminated foods.[49]

## Choosing Organic or Locally Grown Foods

Concerns about the health effects of chemicals used to grow and produce food have led many people to turn to foods that are **organic**—foods and beverages developed, grown, or raised without the use of toxic and persistent pesticides or fertilizers, antibiotics, or hormones. Any food sold in the United States as organic has to meet criteria set by the USDA under the National Organic Rule and can carry a USDA seal verifying products as "certified organic." Under this rule, a product that is certified may carry one of the following terms: "100 percent Organic" (100% compliance with organic criteria), "Organic" (must contain at least 95% organic materials), "Made with Organic Ingredients" (must contain at least 70% organic ingredients), or "Some Organic Ingredients" (contains less than 70% organic ingredients—usually listed individually). To be labeled with any of the above terms, the foods also must be produced without genetic modification or germ-killing radiation. However, reliable monitoring systems to ensure credibility are still under development. See the **Skills for Behavior Change** box for a breakdown of natural versus organic foods.

The market for organic foods has been increasing faster than food sales in general for many years. Whereas only a small subset of the population once bought organic, 81 percent of all U.S. families are now buying organic foods at least occasionally.[50] In 2012, annual organic food sales were estimated to be $31 billion and are expected to rise to $35 billion in 2014.[51]

Is organic food really more nutritious? That depends on what aspect of the food is being studied and how the research is conducted. Two recent review studies, both of which examined decades of research into the nutrient quality of organic versus traditionally grown foods, reached opposite conclusions: One found organic foods more nutritious, and the other did not.[52] However, we do know that pesticide residues remain on conventionally grown produce. The U.S. Environmental Protection Agency warns that food pesticides can lead to health problems like cancer, nerve damage, and birth defects.[53] In 2013, the USDA reported that 3.7 percent of food samples harvested in 2011 had pesticide residues that exceeded the established tolerance level or had residues of pesticides for which no

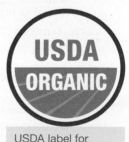

USDA label for organic foods.

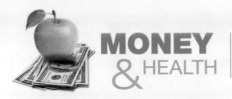

# MONEY & HEALTH | ARE FRUITS AND VEGGIES BEYOND YOUR BUDGET?

Many people on a tight budget, including college students, think that fruits and vegetables are beyond their budget. Maybe a carton of orange juice and a package of carrots are affordable, but five to nine servings a day? No way.

If that sounds like you, it's time for some facts. In 2011, the U.S. Department of Agriculture published data showing that the average American family spends more money on food than is necessary to consume a nutritious diet—one that includes the recommended servings of fruits and vegetables. The report concluded that, contrary to popular opinion, people on a tight budget can eat healthfully, including plenty of fruits and vegetables, and spend less on food.

So how do you do it? Here are some tips:

■ Focus on five fresh favorites. Throughout the United States, five of the least expensive, perennially available fresh vegetables are carrots, eggplant, lettuce, potatoes, and summer squash. Five fresh fruit options are apples, bananas, pears, pineapple, and watermelon.

■ Buy small amounts frequently. Most items of fresh produce keep only a few days, so buy amounts that you know you'll be able to eat or freeze.

■ Celebrate the season. From apples to zucchini, when fruits and veggies are in season, they cost less. If you can freeze them, stock up. If not, enjoy them fresh while you can.

■ Do it yourself. Avoid prewashed, precut fruits and vegetables, including salad greens. They cost more and often spoil faster. Also choose frozen 100 percent juice concentrate and add the water yourself.

■ Buy canned or frozen on sale, in bulk. Canned and frozen produce, especially when it's on sale, may be much less expensive than fresh. Most frozen items are just as nutritious as fresh, and can be even more so, depending on how long ago the fresh food was harvested. For canned items, choose fruits without added sugars and vegetables without added salt or sauces. Bear

in mind that beans are legumes and count as a vegetable choice. Low-sodium canned beans are one of the most affordable, convenient, and nutritious foods you can buy. If you can't find low-sodium beans, just rinse them before heating.

■ Fix and freeze. Make large batches of homemade soup, vegetable stews, and pasta sauce and store them in single-serving containers in your freezer.

■ Grow your own. All it takes is one sunny window, a pot, soil, and a packet of seeds. Lettuce, spinach, and fresh herbs are particularly easy to grow indoors in small spaces.

**Sources:** U.S. Department of Agriculture, *Eating Healthy on a Budget: The Consumer Economics Perspective*, September 2011, www .choosemyplate.gov/food-groups/downloads/ ConsumerEconomicsPerspective.pdf; U.S. Department of Agriculture, Center for Nutrition Policy and Promotion, *Smart Shopping for Veggies and Fruits,* September 2011, www .choosemyplate.gov/food-groups/downloads/ TenTips/DGTipsheet9SmartShopping.pdf; U.S. Centers for Disease Control and Prevention, *Fruits & Veggies: More Matters, 30 Ways in 30 Days to Stretch Your Fruit & Vegetable Budget,* September 2011, www.fruitsandveggiesmatter. gov/downloads/Stretch_FV_Budget.pdf

---

tolerance level has been established.[54] Both agencies advise consumers to wash fruits and vegetables before cooking or consuming them.

The word **locavore** has been coined to describe people who eat mostly food grown or produced locally, usually within close proximity to their homes. Farmers' markets or homegrown foods or those grown by independent farmers are thought to be fresher and to require far fewer resources to get them to market and keep them fresh for longer periods of time. Locavores believe that locally grown food is preferable to foods produced by large corporations or supermarket-based organic foods, as they make a smaller impact on the environment. The locavore movement is less concerned about foods that are grown organically as they are about buying locally grown foods.

## Foodborne Illnesses

Are you concerned that the chicken you are buying doesn't look pleasingly pink or your "fresh" fish smells a little *too* fishy? You may have good reason to be worried. Scientists estimate that

foodborne illnesses sicken 1 in 6 Americans (over 48 million people) and cause some 128,000 hospitalizations and 3,000 deaths in the United States annually.[55] Although the incidence of infection with certain microbes has declined, current data from the U.S. Centers for Disease Control and Prevention (CDC) show a lack of recent progress in reducing foodborne infections and highlight the need for improved prevention.[56]

**locavore** A person who primarily eats food grown or produced locally.

Several common types of bacteria and viruses, including the bacteria salmonella, listeria, and campylobacter and the virus norovirus, cause most foodborne infections and illnesses. Foodborne illnesses can also be caused by a toxin in food that was originally produced by a bacterium or other microbe in the food. These toxins can produce illness even if the microbes that produced them are no longer there. For example, the illness listeriosis is caused by the

**SEE IT! VIDEOS**
Is organic produce better for you?
Watch **Organic Produce,** available on **MasteringHealth**™

## SEE IT! VIDEOS

What can the FDA do to make food safe? Watch **FDA Proposes New Food Safety Rules**, available on MasteringHealth™

bacterium *Listeria monocytogenes*, which seriously affects approximately 1,600 individuals in the United States annually, with pregnant women being 10 times more likely than others to become infected.[57] This bacterium is found in the intestinal tracts of humans and animals, milk, soil, and leafy vegetables and can grow slowly at refrigerator temperatures.[58] Potential food sources include ready-to-eat foods such as hot dogs, luncheon meats, cold cuts, fermented or dry sausage, other deli-style meat and poultry, soft cheeses, and unpasteurized milk.[59] Illness from listeria causes fever, chills, headache, abdominal pain and diarrhea; it may later develop into more serious illness in high-risk individuals such as pregnant women.[60]

Signs of foodborne illnesses vary tremendously and usually include one or several symptoms: diarrhea, nausea, cramping, and vomiting. Depending on the amount and virulence of the pathogen, symptoms may appear as early as 30 minutes after eating contaminated food or as long as several days or weeks later. Most of the time, symptoms occur 5 to 8 hours after eating and last only a day or two. For certain populations, such as the very young; older adults; or people with severe illnesses such as cancer, diabetes, kidney disease, or AIDS, foodborne diseases can be fatal.

Several factors contribute to foodborne illnesses. Since fresh foods are not in season much of the year, the United States imports $18 billion in fresh fruits and vegetables from other countries, often from great distances. These countries include Mexico (36% of imports), several Central and South American countries (about 25%), and China (8%).[61] Although we are

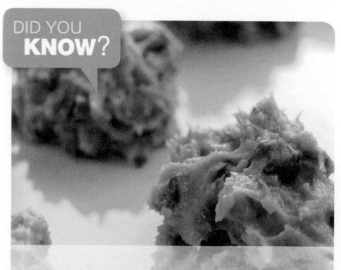

Most college students claim they understand and practice food safety guidelines. For instance, in one survey, 88% said they understood the importance of hand washing in preventing foodborne illness. Yet only 49% of those surveyed actually washed their hands always or most of the time before meals.

**Source:** Data are from B.A. Miko et al., "Personal and Household Hygiene, Environmental Contamination, and Health in Undergraduate Residence Halls in New York City, 2011," *PLoS One* 8, no. 11 (2013): e81460.

CLEAN   SEPARATE   COOK   CHILL

**FIGURE 9.9** The Four Core Practices
This logo reminds consumers how to prevent foodborne illness.

**Source:** Partnership for Food Safety Education, 2919, www.fightbac.org/safe-food-handling

told when we travel to developing and transitioning countries to "boil it, peel it, or don't eat it," we bring these imported foods into our kitchens at home and eat them, often without washing them—or knowing how they were handled or treated during harvest or production.

Food can become contaminated in the field by being watered with tainted water, fertilized with animal manure, or harvested by people who have not washed their hands properly after using the toilet. Food-processing equipment, facilities, or workers may contaminate food, or it can become contaminated if not kept clean and cool during transport or on store shelves. To give you an idea of the implications, studies have shown that the bacterium *Escherichia coli* can survive in cow manure for up to 70 days and can multiply in crops grown with manure unless heat or additives such as salt or preservatives are used to kill the microbes.[62] There are no regulations that prohibit farmers from using animal manure to fertilize crops. In addition, *E. coli* quickly reproduces in summer months as cattle await slaughter in crowded, overheated pens. This increases the chances of meat coming to market already contaminated.

## Avoiding Risks in the Home

Part of the responsibility for preventing foodborne illness lies with consumers—more than 30 percent of all foodborne illnesses result from unsafe handling of food at home. Four basic steps reduce the likelihood of contaminating your food (see **FIGURE 9.9**). Among the most basic precautions are to wash your hands and to wash all produce before eating it. Also, avoid cross-contamination in the kitchen by using separate cutting boards and utensils for meats and produce. Temperature control is also important—refrigerators must be set at 40°F or lower. Cook meats to the recommended temperature to kill contaminants before eating. Keep hot foods hot and cold foods cold to avoid unchecked bacterial growth. Eat leftovers within 3 days, and if you're unsure how long something has been sitting in the fridge, don't take chances. When in doubt, throw it out. See the **Skills for Behavior Change** box for more tips about reducing risk of foodborne illness.

## Food Sensitivities, Allergies, and Intolerances

About 33 percent of people today *think* they have a food allergy; however, it is estimated that only 5 percent of children and 4 percent of adults actually do.[63] Still, the prevalence of

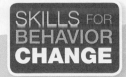
reported food allergies is on the rise. Data suggest the prevalence of peanut allergies among children tripled between 1997 and 2008.[64]

A **food allergy,** or hypersensitivity, is an abnormal response to a component—usually a protein—in food that is triggered by the immune system. Symptoms of an allergic reaction vary in severity and may include a tingling sensation in the mouth; swelling of the lips, tongue, and throat; difficulty breathing; skin hives; vomiting; abdominal cramps; and diarrhea. Approximately 100 to 200 deaths per year occur as a result of more severe reactions called *anaphylaxis* that cause widespread inflammation and cardiovascular problems such as a sudden drop in blood pressure.[65] Anaphylaxis may occur within

Peanuts are among the eight most common food allergens.

seconds to hours after eating the foods to which one is allergic.

The Food Allergen Labeling and Consumer Protection Act (FALCPA) requires food manufacturers to label foods clearly to indicate the presence of (or possible contamination by) any of the eight major food allergens: milk, eggs, peanuts, wheat, soy, tree nuts (walnuts, pecans, cashews, pistachios, etc.), fish, and shellfish. Al- though over 160 foods have been identified as allergy triggers, these eight foods account for 90 percent of all food allergies in the United States.[66]

**Celiac disease** is an autoimmune disorder that causes malabsorption of nutrients from the small intestine in genetically susceptible people. It is thought to affect over 2 million Americans, most of whom are undiagnosed.[67] When a person with celiac disease consumes gluten— a protein found in wheat, rye, and barley—the person's immune system responds with inflammation. This degrades the lining of the small intestine and reduces nutrient absorption. Pain, abdominal cramping, often diarrhea, and other symptoms follow in the short term. Untreated, celiac disease can lead to long-term health problems, such as nutritional deficiencies, tissue wasting, osteoporosis, seizures, liver disease, and cancer of the small intestine. Individuals diagnosed with celiac disease are encouraged to consult a dietitian for help designing a gluten-free diet. For more information on gluten-free diets, read **Health Headlines: Gluten-Free Diets** on the next page.

**Food intolerance** can cause you to have symptoms of digestive upset, but the upset is not the result of an immune system response. Probably the best example of a food intolerance is *lactose intolerance,* a problem that affects about 1 in every 10 American adults.[68] Lactase is an enzyme produced by the small intestine that degrades lactose, the sugar in dairy products. If you don't have enough lactase, you cannot digest lactose, and it remains in the gut to be used by bacteria. Gas is formed, and you experience bloating, abdominal pain, and sometimes diarrhea. The prevalence of primary lactose intolerance varies according to race; Americans of European descent typically have rates of lactose intolerance as low as 2 to 3 percent, whereas 24 percent or more of minority populations are lactose intolerant.[69] Food intolerance also occurs in response to some food additives, such as the flavor enhancer monosodium glutamate (MSG), certain dyes, sulfites, gluten, and other substances. In some cases, the food intolerance may have psychological triggers.

If you suspect that you have a food allergy, celiac disease, or a

**food allergy** Overreaction by the immune system to normally harmless proteins in foods, which are perceived as allergens. In response, the body produces antibodies, triggering allergic symptoms.

**celiac disease** An inherited immune disorder causing malabsorption of nutrients from the small intestine and triggered by the consumption of gluten, a protein found in certain grains.

**food intolerance** Adverse effects that result when people who lack the digestive chemicals needed to break down certain substances eat those substances.

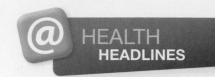
# GLUTEN-FREE DIETS

Gluten-free diets have become a fad. The number of individuals consuming a gluten-free diet is fueling a market of gluten-free products. In a 5-year period ending in 2014, gluten-free products grew by more than 34 percent. There are more people following a gluten-free diet than there are diagnosed with celiac disease, a condition that worsens when gluten is consumed. Is this healthy?

A gluten-free diet is an eating plan that leaves out gluten, a protein found in wheat, barley, rye, and triticale, a cross between wheat and rye. Eating a gluten-free diet improves control of the symptoms and complications for those individuals who have celiac disease, Hashimoto's, or who are gluten sensitive.

Going gluten free for people who do not have gluten sensitivities is not necessarily healthier when it means eliminating many common, nutritious foods. Gluten itself doesn't provide any nutritional benefits, but the foods that contain gluten do. These foods are rich in dietary fiber, vitamins, and minerals. Many gluten-free products are made with refined, unenriched gluten-free grains, such as sorghum and rice flours, which are low in essential nutrients and high in fat and kilocalories—not to mention expensive. For this reason, there are no real benefits to eating a gluten-free

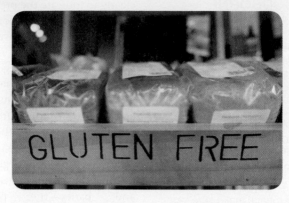

diet unless you are gluten sensitive, or have been diagnosed with an autoimmune disorder such as Hashimoto's or celiac disease. In fact, people who follow a gluten-free diet may have low levels of certain vitamins and nutrients in their diets, including iron, calcium, fiber, and the B vitamins riboflavin, thiamin, folate, and niacin.

Switching to a gluten-free diet may seem daunting at first. It's a good idea to consult a dietitian for advice about how to avoid gluten while still eating a healthy, balanced diet. Many healthy foods are naturally free of gluten, including beans, nuts, seeds, legumes, eggs, meats, fish, poultry, fruits, vegetables, and low-fat dairy foods. When buying foods on a gluten-free diet, fresh, unprocessed foods are the best choice.

Certain grains that are naturally gluten free, such as oats, can be contaminated when gluten-free foods come into contact

with gluten-containing foods during manufacturing. You might inadvertently cross-contaminate foods yourself if you prepare gluten-free foods on the same surfaces as wheat breads or other gluten-containing foods. For instance, toasting gluten-free bread in the same toaster you use to toast wheat bread can result in cross-contamination.

Processed foods may also be labeled as "certified gluten-free." The FDA requires that, to use a gluten-free label, the product must contain less than 20 parts per million of gluten. It's best to read the ingredient list before buying. Even if the label states the product is wheat free, it still may contain gluten.

**Sources:** Packaged Facts, *Gluten-free Foods and Beverages in the US*, 5th ed. (Rockville, MD: Packaged Foods, 2015.) Available from www.packagedfacts.com/Gluten-Free-Foods-8108350/; G. A. Gaesser, and S. S. Angadi, "Gluten-free Diet: Imprudent Dietary Advice for the General Population?," *Journal of the Academy of Nutrition and Dietetics* 112, no. 9 (2012): 1300–1333; S. J. Shepherd and P. R. Gibson, "Nutritional Inadequacies of the Gluten-free Diet in Both Recently-Diagnosed and Long-Term Patients with Celiac Disease," *Journal of Human Nutrition and Dietetics* 26, no. 4 (2013): 349–58, doi: 10.1111/jhn.12018; T. B. Koerner et al., "Gluten Contamination in the Canadian Commercial Oat Supply," *Food Additives and Contaminants Part A, Chemistry, Analysis, Control, Exposure and Risk Assessment*, 28, no. 6 (2013): 705–710, doi: 10.1080/19440049.2011.579626; May Clinic, "Gluten-Free Diet," November 25, 2014, www.mayoclinic.org/healthy-lifestyle/nutrition-and-healthy-eating/in-depth/gluten-free-diet/art-20048530

food intolerance, see your doctor. Because these diseases can have some common symptoms, as well as share symptoms with other gastrointestinal disorders, clinical diagnosis is essential.

## Genetically Modified Food Crops

Genetically modified crop farming is expanding rapidly around the world. Genetic modification involves the insertion or deletion of genes into the DNA of an organism. In the case of **genetically modified (GM) foods**, usually this genetic cutting and pasting is done to enhance production, for example, by making disease- or insect-resistant plants, improving yield, or controlling weeds. In addition, GM foods are sometimes created to improve the color and appearance of foods or

to enhance specific nutrients. For example, in regions where rice is a staple and vitamin A deficiency and iron-deficiency anemia are leading causes of morbidity and mortality, GM technology has been used to create varieties of rice high in vitamin A and iron. Another use under development is the production and delivery of vaccines through GM foods.

The long-term safety of GM foods—for humans and other species—is still in question. The American Association for the Advancement of Science reports that foods containing GM ingredients are no more a risk than are the same foods composed of crops modified over time with conventional plant breeding techniques, and the World Health Organization states that no adverse effects on human health have been shown from consumption of GM foods in countries that have approved their use.[70] The debate surrounding GM foods is not likely to end soon; see the **Points of View** box for more on this debate.

**genetically modified (GM) foods** Foods derived from organisms whose DNA has been altered using genetic engineering techniques.

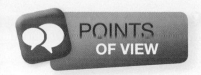

# Genetically Modified Foods
*Boon or Bane?*

Farmers in the United States have widely accepted GM crops. Genetically modified (GM) foods do not occur naturally but have been altered by introducing a gene from a different organism. Soybeans and cotton are the most common GM crops, followed by corn. On supermarket shelves, an estimated 75 percent of processed foods are genetically modified. Even much of the produce you buy in stores has been genetically modified, including tomatoes, corn, potatoes, squash, and soybeans.

State governments, industry, and scientists tout the benefits of genetically modified foods for health, agriculture, and the ecosystem, including feeding the world's population. In contrast, consumer activists, environmental organizations, religious groups, and health advocates warn of unexpected health risks and environmental and socioeconomic consequences. Consumers question whether genetically modified plants are safe to eat. By 2014, two states—Connecticut and Maine—had enacted GMO-labeling laws. However, the legislation doesn't go into effect until nearby states enact similar labeling laws. The FDA continues to evaluate the safety issues of genetically modified foods and future regulations to protect the world's food supply.

Below are some of the main points for and against the development of GM food.

## Arguments for the Development of GM Foods

- People have been manipulating food crops—primarily through selective breeding—since the beginning of agriculture. Genetic modification is fundamentally the same thing, just more precise.
- Modified fruits and vegetables produce higher levels of antioxidants, which reduce the risk of heart disease and cancer, and vitamin A to prevent blindness.
- Genetically modified seeds and products are tested for safety, and there has never been a substantiated claim for a human illness resulting from consumption of a GM food.
- Genetically modified crops have the potential to reduce world hunger: They can be created to grow more quickly than conventional crops, increasing productivity and allowing for faster cycling of crops, which means more food yield. In addition, nutrient-enhanced crops can address malnutrition, and crops engineered to resist spoiling or damage can allow for transportation to areas affected by drought or natural disaster.

## Arguments against the Development of GM Foods

- Genetic modification may cause an allergic reaction. Allergic reactions occur in humans when their immune system recognizes a protein as a foreign invader. Research in vitro studies suggests that some GM foods may cause allergic reactions.
- GM foods have the potential to reduce absorption of essential nutrients. For example, if the gene inserted to make the new GM food increases the phytate content of the food, which reduces the absorption of certain minerals, such as calcium and iron. Modified soy products may also produce less phytoestrogens known to reduce the risk of heart disease and cancer.
- Plants naturally produce low levels of substances that are toxic to humans. While these toxins do not produce problems for humans, there is a concern that adding a new gene to produce a GM plant may cause the new plant to produce toxins at higher levels that could be dangerous if eaten. For instance, GM potatoes produce higher levels of glycoalkaloids.

## WHERE DO YOU STAND?

- Do you think GM foods are more helpful or harmful?
- What are your greatest concerns over GM foods? What do you think are their greatest benefits?
- In what ways could the creators of GM foods address the concerns of those opposed to them?

- What sort of regulation do you think the government should have with regard to the creation, cultivation, and sale of GM foods?
- Currently, there are no GM livestock; however, many livestock are fed GM feed or feed that includes additives and vaccines produced by GM microorganisms. Do you feel any differently about directly consuming GM crops versus eating the flesh, milk, or eggs of an animal that has been fed on GM crops?

**Sources:** U.S. Department of Agriculture, Economic Research Service, "Adoption of Genetically Engineered Crops in the U.S.," July 2013, www.ers.usda.gov/data-products/adoption-of-genetically-engineered-crops-in-the-us.aspx; Center for Food Safety, "About Genetically Engineered Foods," Accessed March 2014, www.centerforfoodsafety.org/issues/311/ge-foods/about-ge-foods; A. Bakshi, "Potential Adverse Health Effects of Genetically Modified Crops," *Journal of Toxicology and Environmental Health, Part B: Critical Reviews* 6, no. 3 (2003): 211–25.

# ASSESS | YOURSELF

## How Healthy Are Your Eating Habits?

**LIVE IT!** ASSESS YOURSELF
An interactive version of this assessment is available online in MasteringHealth™

## 1 Keep Track of Your Food Intake

Keep a food diary for 5 days, writing down everything you eat or drink. Be sure to include the approximate amount or portion size. Add up the number of servings from each of the major food groups on each day and enter them into the chart below.

| Number of Servings: | | | | | | |
|---|---|---|---|---|---|---|
| | Day 1 | Day 2 | Day 3 | Day 4 | Day 5 | Average |
| Fruits | | | | | | |
| Vegetables | | | | | | |
| Grains | | | | | | |
| Protein Foods | | | | | | |
| Dairy | | | | | | |
| Fats and Oils | | | | | | |
| Sweets | | | | | | |

## 2 Evaluate Your Food Intake

Now compare your consumption patterns to the MyPlate recommendations. Look at **TABLE 9.1** (page 264) and **FIGURE 9.5** (page 275) and visit **www.choosemyplate.gov** to evaluate your daily caloric needs and the recommended consumption rates for the different food groups. How does your diet match up?

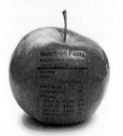

| | Less than the Recommended Amount | About Equal to the Recommended Amount | More than the Recommended Amount |
|---|---|---|---|
| 1. How does your daily fruit consumption compare to the recommendation for you? | ○ | ○ | ○ |
| 2. How does your daily vegetable consumption compare to the recommendation for you? | ○ | ○ | ○ |

| | Less than the Recommended Amount | About Equal to the Recommended Amount | More than the Recommended Amount |
|---|---|---|---|
| 3. How does your daily grain consumption compare to the recommendation for you? | ○ | ○ | ○ |
| 4. How does your daily protein food consumption compare to the recommendation for you? | ○ | ○ | ○ |
| 5. How does your daily dairy food consumption compare to the recommendation for you? | ○ | ○ | ○ |
| 6. How does your daily calorie consumption compare to the recommendation for your age and activity level? | ○ | ○ | ○ |

### Scoring 2

If you found that your food intake is consistent with the MyPlate recommendations, congratulations! If you are falling short in a major food group or are overdoing it in certain categories, consider taking steps to adopt healthier eating habits. Following are some additional assessments to help you figure out where your diet is lacking.

**Source:** J. S. Blake, K. D. Munoz, and S. Volpe, *Nutrition: From Science to You,* 3rd ed., © 2016. Reprinted and electronically reproduced by permission of Pearson Education, Inc., Upper Saddle River, New Jersey.

The **ASSESS YOURSELF** activity gave you the chance to evaluate your current nutritional habits. Once you have considered these results, you can decide whether you need to make changes in your daily eating for long-term health.

**TODAY,** YOU CAN:

☐ Start keeping a more detailed food log. The easy-to-use SuperTracker at www.supertracker.usda.gov can help you keep track of your food intake and analyze what you eat. Take note of the nutritional content of the various foods you eat and write down particulars about the number of calories, grams of saturated fat, grams of sugar, milligrams of sodium, and so on of each food. Try to find specific weak spots: Are you consuming too many calories or too much salt or sugar? Do you eat too little calcium or iron? Use the SuperTracker to plan a healthier food intake to overcome these weak spots.

☐ Take a field trip to the grocery store. Forgo your fast-food dinner and instead spend time in the produce section of the supermarket. Purchase your favorite fruits and vegetables, and try something new to expand your tastes.

**WITHIN THE NEXT TWO WEEKS,** YOU CAN:

☐ Plan at least three meals that you can make at home or in your dorm room, and purchase the ingredients you'll need ahead of time. Something as simple as a chicken sandwich on whole-grain bread will be more nutritious, and probably cheaper, than heading out for a fast-food meal.

☐ Start reading labels. Be aware of the amount of calories, sodium, sugars, and saturated fats in prepared foods; aim to buy and consume those that are lower in all of these and are higher in micronutrients and fiber.

**BY THE END OF THE SEMESTER,** YOU CAN:

☐ Get in the habit of eating a healthy breakfast every morning. Combine whole grains, proteins, and fruit in your breakfast—for example, eat a bowl of cereal with soy milk and bananas or a cup of low-fat yogurt with granola and berries. Eating a healthy breakfast will jump-start your metabolism, prevent drops in blood glucose levels, and keep your brain and body performing at their best through your morning classes.

☐ Commit to one or two healthful changes to your eating patterns for the rest of the semester. You might resolve to eat five servings of fruits and vegetables every day, to switch to low-fat or nonfat dairy products, to stop drinking soft drinks, or to use only olive oil in your cooking. Use your food diary to help you spot places where you can make healthier choices on a daily basis.

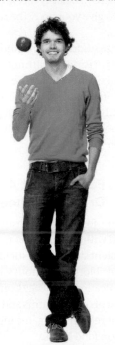

## CHAPTER REVIEW

To hear an MP3 Tutor Session, scan here or visit the Study Area in **MasteringHealth**.

### LO 1 | Essential Nutrients for Health

- Nutrition is the science of the relationship between physiological function and the essential elements of the foods we eat. The Dietary Reference Intakes (DRIs) are recommended nutrient intakes for healthy people.
- The essential nutrients include water, proteins, carbohydrates, fats, vitamins, and minerals. Water makes up 50 to 60 percent of our body weight and is necessary for nearly all life processes. Proteins are major components of our cells and tissues and are key elements of antibodies, enzymes, and hormones. Carbohydrates are our primary sources of energy. Fats provide energy while we are at rest and for long-term activity. They also play important roles in maintaining body temperature, cushioning and protecting organs, and promoting healthy cell function. Vitamins are organic compounds, and minerals are inorganic elements. We need these micronutrients in small amounts to maintain healthy body structure and function.

### LO 2 | Nutritional Guidelines

- A healthful diet is adequate, moderate, balanced, varied, and nutrient dense. The Dietary Guidelines for Americans and the MyPlate plan provide guidelines for healthy eating. These recommendations, developed by the USDA, place emphasis on balancing calories and understanding which foods to increase and which to decrease.
- The Nutrition Facts label on food labels identifies the serving size, number of calories per serving, and amounts of various nutrients, as well as the %DV, which is the percentage of recommended daily values those amounts represent.

### LO 3 | How Can I Eat More Healthfully?

- With a little menu planning, vegetarianism can be a healthful lifestyle choice, providing plenty of nutrients, plus fiber and phytochemicals, typically with less saturated fat and fewer calories.
- Although some people may benefit from taking vitamin and mineral supplements, a healthy diet is the best way to give your body the nutrients it needs.
- College students face unique challenges in eating healthfully. Learning to make better choices, to eat healthfully on a budget, and to eat nutritionally in the dorm are all possible when you use the information in this chapter.

### LO 4 | Food Safety: A Growing Concern

- Organic foods are grown and produced without the use of toxic and persistent synthetic pesticides, fertilizers, antibiotics, hormones, or genetic modification. The USDA offers certification of organic farms and regulates claims regarding organic ingredients used on food labels.
- Foodborne illnesses can be traced to contamination of food at any point from fields to the consumer's kitchen. To keep food safe at home, follow four steps: Clean, separate, cook, and chill.
- Food allergies, celiac disease, food intolerances, GM foods, and other food safety and health concerns are becoming increasingly important to health-wise consumers. Recognizing potential risks and taking steps to prevent problems are part of a sound nutritional plan.

## POP QUIZ

Visit **MasteringHealth** to personalize your study plan with Chapter Review Quizzes and Dynamic Study Modules.

### LO 1 | Essential Nutrients for Health

1. What is the most crucial nutrient for life?
   a. Water
   b. Fiber
   c. Minerals
   d. Starch

2. Which of the following nutrients is critical for the repair and growth of body tissue?
   a. Carbohydrates
   b. Proteins
   c. Vitamins
   d. Fats

3. Which of the following substances helps move food through the digestive tract?
   a. Folate
   b. Fiber
   c. Minerals
   d. Starch

4. What substance provides energy, promotes healthy skin and hair, insulates body organs, helps maintain body temperature, and contributes to healthy cell function?
   a. Fats
   b. Fibers
   c. Proteins
   d. Carbohydrates

5. Which of the following fats is a healthier fat to include in the diet?
   a. *Trans* fat
   b. Saturated fat
   c. Unsaturated fat
   d. Hydrogenated fat

6. Which vitamin maintains bone health?
   a. $B_{12}$
   b. D
   c. $B_6$
   d. Niacin

## LO 2 | Nutritional Guidelines

7. Which of the following foods would be considered a healthy, *nutrient-dense* food?
   a. Nonfat milk
   b. Cheddar cheese
   c. Soft drink
   d. Potato chips

8. The *Dietary Guidelines for Americans 2010* recommend that you
   a. stop smoking and walk daily.
   b. sleep 8 hours a night and jog every other day.
   c. maintain a kilocalorie balance over time and stop smoking.
   d. maintain a kilocalorie balance over time and sustain a healthy body weight.

## LO 3 | How Can I Eat More Healthfully?

9. Carrie eats dairy products and eggs, but she does not eat fish, poultry, or meat. Carrie is considered a(n)
   a. vegan.
   b. lacto-ovo-vegetarian.
   c. ovo-vegetarian.
   d. pesco-vegetarian.

## LO 4 | Food Safety: A Growing Concern

10. Lucas's doctor diagnoses him with celiac disease. Which of the following foods should Lucas cut out of his diet to eat gluten free?
    a. Shellfish
    b. Eggs
    c. Peanuts
    d. Wheat

*Answers to the Pop Quiz can be found on page A-1. If you answered a question incorrectly, review the section tagged by the Learning Outcome. For even more study tools, visit MasteringHealth.*

# THINK ABOUT IT!

## LO 1 | Essential Nutrients for Health

1. Which factors influence a person's dietary patterns and behaviors? What factors have been the greatest influences on your eating behaviors?

2. What are the major types of nutrients that you need to obtain from the foods you eat? What happens if you fail to get enough of some of them? Are there significant differences between men and women in particular areas of nutrition?

## LO 2 | Nutritional Guidelines

3. What are the four main recommendations from the *Dietary Guidelines for Americans 2010*? What can you do to balance your kilocalories to maintain a healthy body weight?

4. What are the major food groups in the MyPlate plan? From which groups do you eat too few servings? What can you do to increase or decrease your intake of selected food groups?

## LO 3 | How Can I Eat More Healthfully?

5. Distinguish among varieties of vegetarianism. Which types are most likely to lead to nutrient deficiencies? What can be done to ensure that even the most strict vegetarian receives enough of the major nutrients?

6. What are the major problems that many college students face when trying to eat the right foods? List five actions that you and your classmates could take immediately to improve your eating.

## LO 4 | Food Safety: A Growing Concern

7. What are the major risks for foodborne illnesses, and what can you do to protect yourself?

8. How does a food intolerance differ from a food allergy?

# ACCESS YOUR HEALTH ON THE INTERNET

The following websites explore further topics and issues related to personal health. Visit MasteringHealth for links to the websites and RSS feeds.

*Academy of Nutrition and Dietetics.* The academy provides information on a full range of dietary topics, including sports nutrition, healthful cooking, and nutritional eating; the site also links to scientific publications and information on scholarships and public meetings. **www.eatright.org**

*U.S. Food and Drug Administration (FDA).* The FDA provides information for consumers and professionals in the areas of food safety, supplements, and medical devices. There are links to other sources of information about nutrition and food. **www.fda.gov**

*Food and Nutrition Information Center.* This site offers a wide variety of information related to food and nutrition. **http://fnic.nal.usda.gov**

*National Institutes of Health: Office of Dietary Supplements.* This is the site of the International Bibliographic Database of Information on Dietary Supplements (IBDIDS), updated quarterly. **http://dietary-supplements.info.nih.gov**

*U.S. Department of Agriculture, USDA: Choose MyPlate.* The USDA offers a personalized nutrition and physical activity plan based on the MyPlate program, sample menus and recipes, and a full discussion of the *Dietary Guidelines for Americans.* **www.choosemyplate.gov**

*U.S. Department of Health and Human Services: Food Safety.* This is the official gateway site to food safety information provided by the federal government, including recalls and alerts, news, and tips for reporting problems. **www.foodsafety.gov**

# 10 Reaching and Maintaining a Healthy Weight

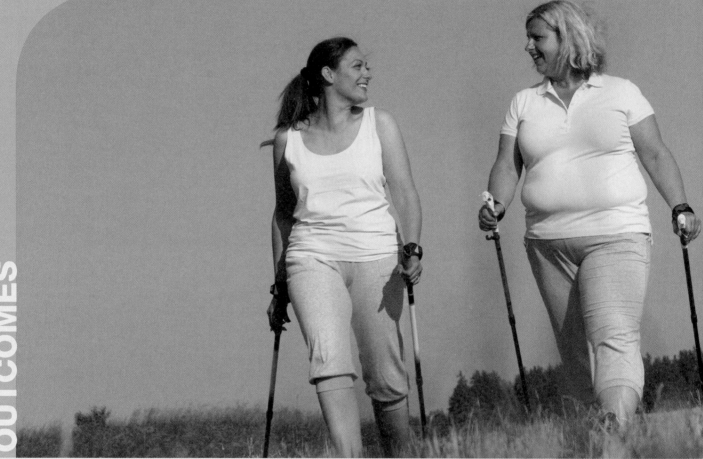

## LEARNING OUTCOMES

**1** Describe the current epidemic of overweight/obesity in the United States and globally, and demonstrate understanding of health risks associated with excess weight.

**2** Describe factors that put people at risk for problems with obesity, distinguishing between controllable and uncontrollable factors.

**3** Discuss reliable options for determining a healthy weight and body fat percentage.

**4** Explain the effectiveness and potential pros/cons of various weight control strategies, including exercise, diet, lifestyle modification, supplements/diet drugs, surgery, and other options.

The United States currently has the dubious distinction of being among the fattest developed nations on Earth. Young and old, rich and poor, rural and urban, educated and uneducated, Americans share one thing in common—they are fatter than virtually all previous generations.[1] The word **obesogenic** refers to environmental conditions that promote obesity, such as the availability and marketing of unhealthy foods, social and cultural norms that lead to high calorie consumption and lack of physical activity—an apt descriptor of our society.

## LO 1 | OVERWEIGHT AND OBESITY: A GROWING CHALLENGE

Describe the current epidemic of overweight/obesity in the United States and globally, and demonstrate understanding of health risks associated with excess weight.

Today **obesity** is often categorized by class, reflecting both severity and increasing risks based on percent body fat. *Obesity* refers to a body weight that is more than 20 percent above recommended levels for health or a **body mass index (BMI)** over 30. *Class 1 obesity* refers to those with a BMI ≥30 but less than 35. *Class 2 obesity* includes those with a BMI of ≥35, but less than 40, and *Class 3 obesity* includes those with a BMI ≥40, often referred to as *morbidly obese*.[2] Less extreme, but still damaging, is *overweight*, which is body weight more than 10 percent above healthy levels or a BMI between 25 and 29.

## Overweight and Obesity in the United States

**FIGURE 10.1** illustrates just how high levels of obesity have risen in the United States, as a percentage of the population, since the 1960s. Indeed, the prevalence of obesity has steadily increased in recent decades, with disproportionate risks among some populations.[3] Children aged 2 to 5 have shown slight decreases overall in prevalence in recent years. Children and adolescents living in low-income, low-education, and higher-unemployment homes are at significantly greater risk of developing obesity, while those from higher income homes with more educated parents have decreasing risk.[4] More than 69 percent of U.S. adults overall (over 178 million people) are overweight or obese.[5] Rates of obesity are 34 percent among men and 36 percent for women, and rates of extreme obesity are on the rise.[6]

Research points to higher obesity rates and risks among some ethnic groups in the United States. Hispanic men (80 percent) and non-Hispanic white men (73 percent) are more likely to be overweight/obese than are non-Hispanic black men

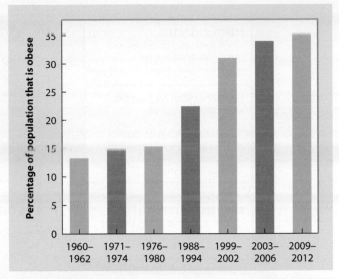

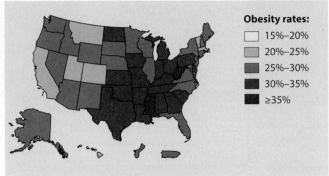

**FIGURE 10.1** Obesity in the United States

**Sources:** Centers for Disease Control and Prevention, "Health, United States, 2013, Table 69. Healthy weight, overweight, and obesity among adults aged 20 and over, by selected characteristics: United States, selected years 1960–1962 through 2009–2012," 2013, www.cdc.gov/nchs/data/hus/2013/069 .pdf; Centers for Disease Control and Prevention, "Obesity Prevalence Maps 2013," www.cdc.gov/obesity/data/prevalence-maps.html

(69 percent). Non-Hispanic black women (82 percent) and Hispanic women (76 percent) are more likely to be overweight or obese than are non-Hispanic white women (61 percent).[7] In sharp contrast, between 51 and 68 percent of Asian populations are at a healthy weight.[8]

## An Obesogenic World

The United States is not alone in the obesity epidemic. In fact, obesity has more than doubled globally since 1980, with over 1.9 billion overweight and 600 million obese adults.[9] While obesity was once predominantly a problem in high-income countries, today increasing numbers of low- and middle-income countries have overweight/obesity

**obesogenic** refers to environmental conditions that promote obesity, such as the availability of unhealthy foods, social and cultural norms that lead to high calorie consumption and lack of physical activity.

**obesity** Having a body weight more than 20 percent above healthy recommended levels; in an adult, a BMI of 30 or more.

**body mass index (BMI)** A number calculated from a person's weight and height that is used to assess risk for possible present or future health problems.

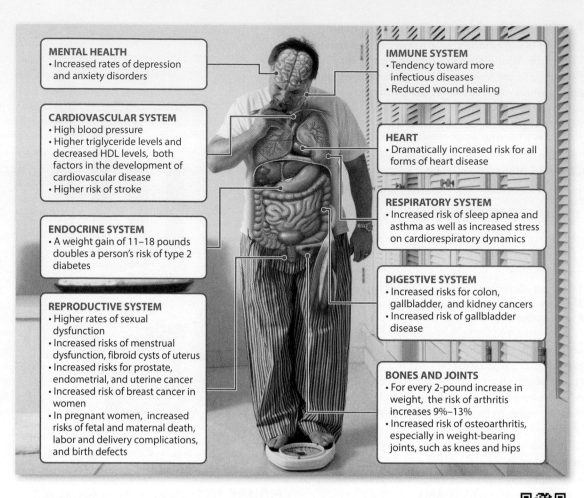

**FIGURE 10.2** Potential Negative Health Effects of Overweight and Obesity

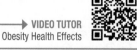

**VIDEO TUTOR**
Obesity Health Effects

**globesity** Global rates of obesity

problems.[10] The global epidemic of high rates of overweight and obesity in multiple regions of the world has come to be known as **globesity**.

## Health Risks of Excess Weight

Although smoking is still the leading cause of preventable death in the United States, obesity is rapidly gaining ground. Cardiovascular disease (CVD), stroke, cancer, hypertension, diabetes, depression, digestive problems, gallstones, sleep apnea, osteoarthritis, certain cancers, and other ailments lead the list of life-threatening, weight-related problems. **FIGURE 10.2** summarizes these and other potential health consequences of obesity.

Consider the following facts about specific risks for obese individuals compared to their nonobese counterparts:[11]

- They have a 104 percent increase in risk of heart failure.
- BMI greater than 30 reduces their life expectancy by 2 to 4 years.
- BMI greater than 40 costs 8 to 10 years of life expectancy—similar to a long-term smoker.

- Obese adolescents have a 16-times increased risk of becoming severely obese adults, and at current prevalence rates, will result in 1.5 million life years lost.[12]

Diabetes, strongly associated with overweight and obesity, is another major concern. Over 29 million Americans have diabetes, and another 86 million adults have pre-diabetes.[13] **Focus On: Minimizing Your Risk for Diabetes** discusses the devastating effects of obesity on diabetes-related risks and the benefits of prevention. (See the **Money & Health** box for information on the costs of obesity.)

CVD and chronic, killer diseases are not the only risks associated with overweight and obesity. The costs of social isolation, bullying in school, stigmatization, discrimination, and diminished quality of life can also be devastating. Obese individuals suffer more major disability and difficulty with activities of daily living (ADLs) than do their nonobese counterparts. They are also more likely to experience falls and injury, with the exception of morbidly obese individuals—who may fall less—perhaps because they are less active, and seem to be less prone to injury when they fall.[14]

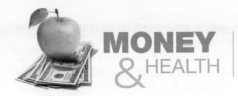

# MONEY & HEALTH | "LIVING LARGE" CAN BE INCREASINGLY COSTLY

*"The startling economic costs of obesity, often borne by the nonobese, could become the epidemic's second-hand smoke."*

—Sharon Begley, "As America's Waistline Expands, Costs Soar," Reuters, April 30, 2012.

A large body of literature points to evidence that as BMI increases, healthcare consumption and associated costs also increase. Consider the following:

- Obesity is believed to be one of the three largest human-generated social burdens in the world.
- More than 2.1 billion people, almost 30 percent of the world's population, are overweight or obese—more than 2.5 times the number of people who are undernourished.
- Obesity is responsible for nearly 5 percent of all the deaths each year globally. Its economic impact hits international gross domestic product hard, costing nearly $2.0 trillion—right up there with smoking ($2.1 trillion), armed violence ($2.1 trillion), war and terrorism ($2.1 trillion), and alcoholism ($1.4 trillion).
- Obese populations have a 36 percent higher annual health care cost than healthy-weight populations. Lifetime medical costs for major diseases increase by over 50 percent for obese individuals—twice that amount for severely obese.
- More than double previous estimates, almost 21 percent of U.S. health care costs can be attributed to obesity. By some estimates, morbidly obese individuals may cost between $6,500 and $15,000 dollars more per year

in additional health care costs when factors such as longer hospital stays, recovery, and increased medications are included.

- Obese populations incur 37 percent higher prescription drug costs than healthy-weight populations
- Obese individuals miss nearly 2 days of work more than their healthy weight counterparts, accounting for between 6.5 to 12.6 percent of total absenteeism costs each year.
- Obese individuals are more likely to suffer from "presenteeism" where they are less likely to be productive and have less stamina than their healthy-weight counterparts.
- Obesity may mean increased transportation costs for more fuel consumption and larger vehicles/seats, bigger ambulances, and other issues.
- A recent study of 150,000 Swedish brothers indicated that *being obese is as costly as not having an undergraduate degree*; an "obesity penalty" is equivalent to earning over 16 percent less than their normal weight counterparts.

Many insurance companies are charging more for people who are overweight and refuse to participate in available "wellness" programs. In fact, the U.S. Patient Protection and Affordable Care Act has a provision that allows employers to charge obese workers significantly higher premiums (between 30 and 50 percent more in some cases!) for their health insurance if they don't make a good faith effort to reduce their health risks and must provide support for services to help them lose weight. Some workplaces offer counseling and

free gym memberships for those struggling with their weight. Are these fair? Many argue that such penalties unfairly reflect a form of obesity stigma and size discrimination, whereas others argue that those within a normal weight range shouldn't have to subsidize excess costs. Still others argue that this is a slippery slope on the way to paying more for factors like eating high-fat foods and having high cholesterol, having too many beers in a week, or even unintended pregnancy.

Currently, there is much debate about these extra costs, even as many insurers and businesses implement policies and programs to motivate employees and members of insurance groups to take action, "or else."

**Sources:** A. Dee et al., "The Direct and Indirect Costs of Both Overweight and Obesity: A systematic Review," *BMC Research Notes* 7, no. 1 (2014): 242, doi: 10.1186/1756-0500-7-242; R. Hammond and R. Levine, "The Economic Impact of Obesity in the United States," *Diabetes, Metabolic Syndrome and Obesity: Targets and Therapy* 3 (2010): 285–95; T. Andreyeva et al., "State-Level Estimates of Obesity-Attributable Costs of Absenteeism," *Journal of Occupational and Environmental Medicine* 56, no. 11 (2014): 1120–27; P. Lunderg et al., "Body Size, Skills and Income: Evidence from 150,000 Teenage Siblings," *Demography* 51, no. 5 (2014): 1573–96; C. Roberts, et al., "Patchy Progress on Obesity Prevention: Emerging Examples, Entrenched Barriers and New Thinking," *The Lancet* (2015), dx.doi.org/10.1016/S0140-6736(14)61744-x. (Epub ahead of print.); McKinsey & Company, "How the World Could Better Fight Obesity," November 2014, www.mckinsey.com/insights/economic_studies/how_the_world_could_better_fight_obesity; J. Cawley and C. Meyerhoefer, "The Medical Care Costs of Obesity: An Instrumental Variables Approach," *Journal of Health Economics* 31, no. 1 (2012): 219, doi: 10.1016/j.jhealeco.2011.10.003; E. A. Finkelstein et al., "The Costs of Obesity in the Workplace," *Journal of Occupational and Environmental Medicine* 52, no. 10 (2012): 971–76.

## LO 2 | FACTORS CONTRIBUTING TO OVERWEIGHT AND OBESITY

**Describe factors that put people at risk for problems with obesity, distinguishing between controllable and uncontrollable factors.**

The reasons for our soaring rates of overweight and obesity are complex, and not all of them are within easy individual

control. Although diet and exercise are two major contributors, other factors, including genetics and physiology, are also important. Newer thinking regarding reducing obesity risk involves a more ecological approach that seeks to change obesogenic environmental and contextual factors. Learned behaviors in the home; influences at school and in social environments; media influences; and the environments where we live, work, and play are important to our weight profiles.[15]

# Genetic and Physiological Factors

Are some people born to be fat? Genes, hormones, and other aspects of your physiology seem to influence whether you become obese or thin.

**Genes: A Variety of Theories** In spite of decades of research, the exact role of genes in one's predisposition toward obesity remains in question. Countless observational studies back up the theory that fat parents tend to have fat children. Whether that is due to learned eating and exercise behaviors, environmental cues, genes, or a combination is unclear. Early support for a genetic basis for obesity came from twin research. Researchers found that adopted individuals tend to be similar in weight to their biological parents and that identical twins are twice as likely to weigh the same as are fraternal twins, even if they are raised separately.[16] Subsequent research supported this theory, exploring the fact that obesity involves complex gene-gene and gene-environmental interactions: One gene in particular, the *FTO* gene, may be among the most important.[17] Much of this work has centered on the role of genes such as FTO on regulation the hormone ghrelin—a key factor in eating behavior.[18] Specifically, people with certain genetic variations may tend to graze for food more often, eat more meals, and consume more calories every day, as well as display patterns of seeking out high-fat food groups. Also, different genes may influence weight gain at certain periods of life, particularly during adolescence and young adulthood.[19] Rather than acting individually, the effects of the genes may be in clusters, influencing the regulation of food intake through action in the central nervous system, as well as influencing fat cell synthesis and functioning.

So, if your genes play a key role in obesity tendencies, are you doomed to a lifelong battle with your weight? Probably not. A healthy lifestyle may be able to override "obesity" genes. Results of a major European study found that the effects of the *FTO* gene on obesity is over 30 percent less among physically active adults. Those who seemed to be beating their obesity tendencies exercised at least 90 minutes a day compared to those who exercised 30 minutes.[20]

One potential genetic basis for obesity was identified as a result of observational studies of certain Native American and African tribes. Labeled the *thrifty gene theory*, researchers noted higher body fat and obesity levels in some of these tribes than in the general population.[21] Because their ancestors struggled through centuries of famine, members of the tribes appear to have survived by adapting metabolically to periods of famine with slowed metabolism. Over time, ancestors may have passed on a genetic, hormonal, or metabolic predisposition toward fat storage that makes losing fat more difficult. Critics of this theory believe that there are many other factors that influence obesity development, most of which focus on *obesogenic* behaviors and environments.

**Metabolic Rates** Several aspects of your metabolism also help determine whether you gain, maintain, or lose weight. Each of us has an innate energy-burning capacity called **basal metabolic rate (BMR)**—the minimum rate at which the body uses energy to maintain basic vital functions. A BMR for the average, healthy adult is usually between 1,200 and 1,800 calories per day. Technically, to measure BMR, a person would be awake, but all major stimuli (including stressors to the sympathetic nervous system and digestion) would be at rest. Usually, the best time to measure BMR is after 8 hours of sleep and after a 12-hour fast.

A more practical way of assessing your energy expenditure levels is the **resting metabolic rate (RMR)**. Slightly higher than the BMR, the RMR includes the BMR plus any additional energy expended through daily sedentary activities such as food digestion, sitting, studying, or standing. The **exercise metabolic rate (EMR)** accounts for the remaining percentage of all daily calorie expenditures and refers to the energy expenditure that occurs during physical activity. For most of us, these calories come from light daily activities, such as walking, climbing stairs, and mowing the lawn.

Your BMR and RMR fluctuate through life, and are highest during infancy, puberty, and pregnancy. Generally, the younger you are, the higher your BMR, partly because cells undergo rapid subdivision during periods of growth, consuming lots of energy. After age 30, a person's BMR slows down 1 to

---

**basal metabolic rate (BMR)**
The rate of energy expenditure by a body at complete rest in a neutral environment.

**resting metabolic rate (RMR)**
The energy expenditure of the body under BMR conditions plus other daily sedentary activities.

**exercise metabolic rate (EMR)**
The energy expenditure that occurs during exercise.

---

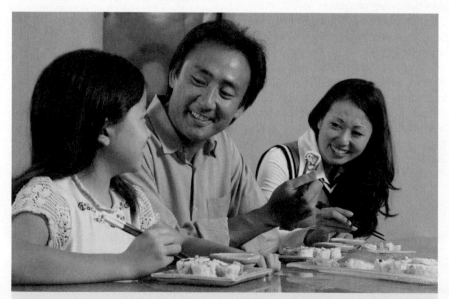

Many factors help determine weight and body type, including heredity and genetic makeup, environment, and learned eating patterns, which are often connected to family habits.

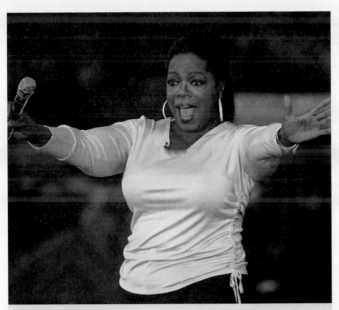

Oprah Winfrey has been candid about her struggles with yo-yo dieting. Such a pattern disrupts the body's metabolism and makes future weight loss more difficult and permanent changes even harder to maintain.

2 percent a year; older people commonly find an extra helping of ice cream harder to burn off. Slower BMR, coupled with less activity, age-related muscle loss, and shifting priorities from fitness to family and career obligations contribute to the weight gain of many middle-aged people.

Anyone who has ever lost weight only to reach a point at which, try as they might, they can't lose another ounce, may be a victim of **adaptive thermogenesis,** whereby the body slows metabolic activity and energy expenditure as a form of defensive protection against possible starvation. With increased weight loss may come increased hunger sensations, slowed energy expenditure, and a tendency to regain weight or make further weight loss more difficult.[22]

**Yo-yo diets** refer to when people cycle between periods of weight loss and gain. Typically, after weight loss, BMR is lower due to the fact that they body has less muscle mass and weight and requires less energy for basic functioning. When dieters resume eating after their weight loss, due to the related BMR decrease, calories burn more slowly, and they regain weight. Repeated cycles of dieting and regaining weight may actually increase the likelihood of getting heavier over time. Increased age and overall loss of muscle mass through inactivity also tend to result in lowered BMR.

On the other side of the BMR equation is **set point theory,** which suggests that our bodies fight to maintain weight around a narrow range or set point. If we go on a drastic starvation diet or fast, BMR slows to conserve energy. Set point theory, which suggests that our own bodies may sabotage our weight loss efforts by holding on to calories, explaining why people tend to stay near a certain weight threshold and why moving to a different level of weight loss is difficult. The good news is that set points can be changed; however, these changes may take time to be permanent.

## Hormonal Influences

Obese people may be more likely than thin people to satisfy their appetite and eat for reasons other than nutrition.[23] In some instances, the problem with overconsumption may be related more to **satiety** than it is to appetite or hunger. People generally feel satiated, or full, when they have satisfied their nutritional needs and their stomach signals "no more."

One hormone, produced in the stomach, that researchers suspect may influence satiety and play a role in keeping weight off is *ghrelin,* sometimes referred to as "the hunger hormone." Initial interest in ghrelin was the result of an early study that focused on a small group of obese people who had lost weight over a 6-month period.[24] The researchers noted that ghrelin levels rose before every meal and fell drastically shortly afterward, suggesting that the hormone plays a role in appetite stimulation. Since then, ghrelin has been shown to be an important growth hormone that plays a key role in the regulation of appetite and food intake control, gastrointestinal motility, gastric acid secretion, endocrine and exocrine pancreatic secretions, glucose and lipid metabolism, and cardiovascular and immunological processes.[25]

Another hormone that has gained increased attention and research is *leptin,* an appetite regulator produced by fat cells in mammals. As fat tissue increases, levels of leptin in the blood increase, and when levels of leptin in the blood rise, appetite drops. Scientists believe leptin serves as a form of "adipostat" that signals you are getting full, slows food intake, and promotes energy expenditure.[26] For unknown reasons, obese people seem to have faulty leptin receptors, although it may be that environmental cues are stronger than biological signals in some individuals.

**adaptive thermogenesis** Theoretical mechanism by which the brain regulates metabolic activity according to caloric intake.

**yo-yo diets** Cycles in which people diet and regain weight.

**set point theory** Theory that a form of internal thermostat controls our weight and fights to maintain this weight around a narrowly set range.

**satiety** The feeling of fullness or satisfaction at the end of a meal.

**hyperplastic obesity** A condition characterized by an excessive number of fat cells.

**hypertrophy** The act of swelling or increasing in size, as with cells.

## Fat Cells and Predisposition to Fatness

Some obese people may have excessive numbers of fat cells. Where an average-weight adult has approximately 25 to 35 billion fat cells and a moderately obese adult 60 to 100 billion, an extremely obese adult has as many as 200 billion.[27] This condition, **hyperplastic obesity,** usually appears in early childhood and perhaps, due to the mother's dietary habits, even prior to birth. The most critical periods for the development of hyperplasia are the last 2 to 3 months of fetal development, the first year of life, and the period between ages 9 and 13. Central to this theory is the belief that the number of fat cells in a body does not increase appreciably during adulthood. However, the ability of each of these cells to swell (**hypertrophy**) and shrink does carry over into adulthood. People with large numbers of fat cells may be able to lose weight by decreasing the size of each cell in adulthood, but with the next calorie binge, cells swell and sabotage

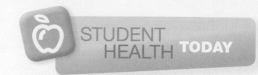
# BEWARE OF PORTION INFLATION AT RESTAURANTS

From burgers and fries to meat-and-potato or pasta meals, today's popular restaurant foods dwarf their earlier counterparts. For example, a 25-ounce prime rib dinner served at one local steak chain contains nearly 3,000 calories and 150 grams of fat. That's 1.5 times the calories and two to three times the fat that most adults need in a whole day!

Many researchers believe that the main reason Americans are gaining weight is that people no longer recognize a normal serving size. The National Heart, Lung, and Blood Institute has developed a pair of "Portion Distortion" quizzes that show how today's portions compare with those of 20 years ago. Test your knowledge of portion size online at www.nhlbi.nih.gov/health/educational/wecan/eat-right/portion-distortion.htm.

To make sure you're not overeating when you dine out, follow these strategies:

- Order the smallest size available. Focus on taste and quality, rather than quantity. When you eat huge amounts at the all-you-can-eat buffet, focus on how you feel. Get used to eating less,

**Today's bloated portions.**

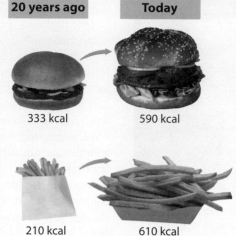

| 20 years ago | Today |
|---|---|
| 333 kcal | 590 kcal |
| 210 kcal | 610 kcal |

eating slowly, and enjoying what you eat.
- Take your time, and let your fullness indicator have a chance to kick in while there is still time to quit. Chew more, talk more, set your fork down more often between bites.

- Order condiments and dressings on the side and don't use the entire container! Lightly dip your food in dressings or gravies rather than pouring on extra calories.
- Order a healthy, protein-rich appetizer as your main meal, and a small salad or vegetable. Happy hour menus often offer great smaller choices.
- Split an entrée with a friend, and order a side salad for each of you. Alternately, put half of your meal in a takeout box immediately, and finish the rest at the restaurant.
- Avoid buffets and all-you-can-eat establishments. If you go to them, use small plates and fill them with salads, vegetables and other high-protein, low-calorie, low-fat options. Pay careful attention to newly required menu labeling for fast-food restaurants. These can be helpful in making sure you choose the best alternative for healthy dining.

**Source:** Data are from National Heart, Lung, and Blood Institute, "Portion Distortion," Accessed April 1, 2015, www.nhlbi.nih.gov/health/educational/wecan/eat-right/portion-distortion.htm

weight-loss efforts. Weight gain may be tied to both the number of fat cells in the body and the capacity of individual cells to enlarge.

## Environmental Factors

Environmental factors have come to play a large role in weight maintenance. Automobiles, remote controls, desk jobs, and sedentary habits contribute to decreased physical activity and energy expenditure. Coupled with our culture of eating more, it's a recipe for weight gain.

U.S. ADULTS GET

# 11.3%

OF TOTAL DAILY **CALORIES** FROM FAST FOODS—DOWN FROM 12.8% IN 2007–2008.

**Greater Access to High-Calorie Foods** More foods that are high in calories and low in nutrients exist today compared to the past. There are many environmental factors that can prompt us to consume them:

- Because of constant advertising, we are bombarded with messages to eat, eat, eat, and taste often trumps nutrition.
- Super-sized portions are now the norm (see the **Student Health Today** box), leading to increased calorie and fat intake.
- Widespread availability of high-calorie coffee and sugary drinks lure people in for a form of break/reward between meals, which really add up in calories over time.
- Families have increased reliance on restaurant and store-bought convenience foods, which tend to be higher in calories than food made from scratch.
- Bottle-feeding infants may increase energy intake relative to breast-feeding.
- Misleading food labels confuse consumers about serving sizes.

Although we still consume about 500 calories per day more today than we did in 1970, daily consumption of some foods

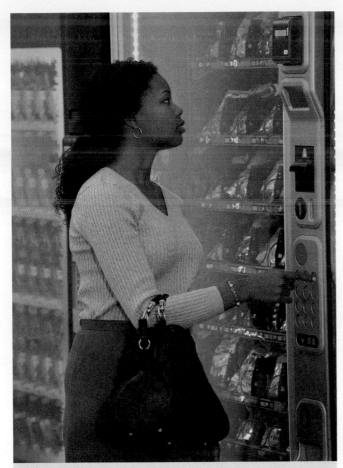

The easy availability of high-calorie foods, such as those found in most vending machines, is one of the environmental factors contributing to the obesity problem in the United States today.

The above differences in statistics are, in part, a reflection of the fact that data are largely based on self-reporting, and people over-estimate their daily exercise level and intensity. Complicating the problem further is a hodgepodge of terminology for determining activity levels and more than one fitness measure, so defining yourself as "active" can mean very different things for different people.

## WHAT DO YOU THINK?

Can you think of factors in your particular environment that might contribute to your own risks for obesity or risks to your family and friends?

- What are they and how do they increase the risks?
- What actions could you take to combat them?

## Psychosocial and Socioeconomic Factors

The relationship of weight problems to emotional insecurities, needs, and wants remains difficult to assess. What we do know is eating tends to be a focal point of people's lives and is in part a social ritual associated with companionship, celebration, and enjoyment. *Comfort food* is also used to help you feel good when other things in life are not going well. Our friends and loved ones are often key influences in our eating behaviors. In fact, according to recent research, young adults who are overweight and obese tend to befriend and date overweight and obese people in much the same way that smokers or exercisers tend to hang out with other smokers or exercisers. People may gain or lose weight based on support for loss or social undermining of weight loss attempts ("Let's go out for ice cream!").[31]

Socioeconomic status can have a significant effect on risk for obesity. When times are tough, people tend to eat more inexpensive, high-calorie processed foods. People living in poverty may have less access to fresh, nutrient-dense foods and have less time to cook nutritious meals due to shiftwork, longer commutes, or multiple jobs.[32] Counselors, fitness center memberships, and other supports for weight loss are often too expensive or unavailable. Additionally, unsafe neighborhoods and poor infrastructure, such as lack of sidewalks or parks, can make it difficult for less-affluent people to exercise.[33]

appears to be declining in the last decade. For example, annual consumption of sugars, including *high fructose corn syrup* was 119 pounds per person in 1970, increasing to 151 pounds per person in 1999. Today's consumption has decreased to 139 pounds per person.[28] If we are consuming less, why aren't we seeing major changes in obesity rates? One possibility is that we are exercising less than ever, thereby offsetting potential weight loss.[29]

**Lack of Physical Activity** Although heredity, metabolism, and environment all have an impact on weight management, the way we live our lives is also responsible. In general, Americans are eating more and moving less than ever before—becoming overfat as a result.

According to data from the 2014 *National Health Interview Survey*, 50 percent of adults 18 and over in the United States met the guidelines for aerobic activity through involvement in leisure time activity. However, a recent Behavioral Risk Factor Surveillance System (*BRFSS*) survey reported that only 21% percent of adults engaged in enough aerobic and muscle strengthening exercise to meet the guidelines.[30]

## LO 3 | ASSESSING BODY WEIGHT AND BODY COMPOSITION

Discuss reliable options for determining a healthy weight and body fat percentage.

Everyone has his or her own ideal weight, based on individual variables such as body structure, height, and fat distribution. Traditionally, experts used measurement techniques such as height-weight charts to determine whether an individual was an ideal weight, overweight, or obese. These charts can be misleading because they don't take body composition—a person's

**underweight** Having a body weight more than 10 percent below healthy recommended levels; in an adult, having a BMI below 18.5.

**healthy weight** Those with BMIs of 18.5 to 24.9, the range of lowest statistical health risk

**overweight** Having a body weight more than 10 percent above healthy recommended levels; in an adult, having a BMI of 25 to 29.9.

**morbidly obese** Having a body weight 100 percent or more above healthy recommended levels; in an adult, having a BMI of 40 or more.

**super obese** Having a body weight higher than morbid obesity; in an adult, having a BMI of 50 or more.

ratio of fat to lean muscle—or fat distribution into account. More accurate measures of evaluating healthy weight and disease risk focus on a person's percentage of body fat and how that fat is distributed in his or her body.

It's important to remember that body fat isn't all bad. In fact, some fat is essential for healthy body functioning. Fat regulates body temperature, cushions and insulates organs and tissues, and is the body's main source of stored energy. Body fat is composed of two types: essential fat and storage fat. *Essential fat* is the fat necessary for maintenance of life and reproductive functions. *Storage fat,* the nonessential fat that many of us try to shed, makes up the remainder of our fat reserves. Being **underweight,** or having extremely low body fat, can cause a host of problems, including hair loss, visual disturbances, skin problems, a tendency to fracture bones easily, digestive system disturbances, heart irregularities, gastrointestinal problems, difficulties in maintaining body temperature, and loss of menstrual period in women.

# Body Mass Index (BMI)

As mentioned in earlier discussion, BMI is a description of body weight relative to height—numbers that are highly correlated with your total body fat. Find your BMI in inches and pounds in **FIGURE 10.3**, or calculate your BMI now by dividing your weight in kilograms by height in meters squared. The mathematical formula is

$$BMI = weight\ (kg)/height\ squared\ (m^2)$$

A BMI calculator is also available from the National Heart, Lung, and Blood Institute at www.nhlbi.nih.gov/guidelines/obesity/BMI/bmicalc.htm.

Desirable BMI levels may vary with age and by sex; however, most BMI tables for adults do not account for such variables. **Healthy weight** is defined as having a BMI of 18.5 to 24.9, the range of lowest statistical health risk.[34] A BMI of 25 to 29.9 indicates **overweight** and potentially significant health risks. A BMI of 30 to 39.9 is classified as **obese.** A BMI of 40 to 49.9 is **morbidly obese,** and a new category of BMI of 50 or higher—one increasing in numbers—has been labeled as **super obese.**[35] In 2011–2012, over 6 percent of American adults were morbidly obese, with a BMI over 40.[36]

**Limitations of BMI** Like other assessments of fatness, the BMI has its limitations. Water, muscle, and bone mass are not included in BMI calculations, and BMI levels don't account for the fact that muscle weighs more than fat. BMI levels can be inaccurate for people who are under 5 feet tall, are highly muscled, or who are older and have little muscle mass. Although a combination of measures might be most reliable in assessing fat levels, BMI continues to be a quick, inexpensive, and useful tool for developing basic health recommendations.[37]

**Youth and BMI** Today, over 30 percent of youth in America are obese, three times higher than rates in the 1980s.[38] Although the labels *obese* and *morbidly obese* have been used for years for adults, there is growing concern that such labels increase bias and *obesity stigma* against youth.[39] BMI ranges above a normal weight for children and teens are often labeled differently, as

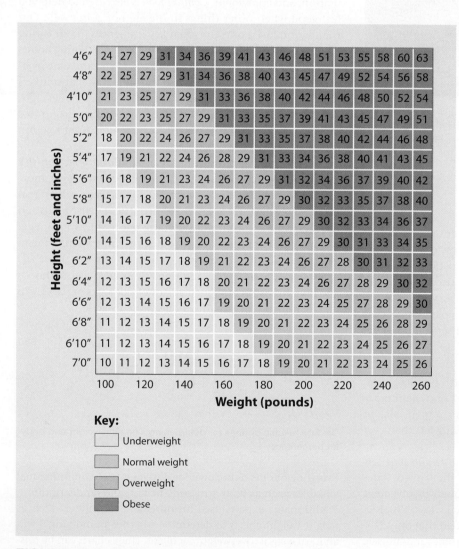

| Height (feet and inches) | 100 | 120 | 140 | 160 | 180 | 200 | 220 | 240 | 260 |
|---|---|---|---|---|---|---|---|---|---|
| 4'6" | 24 27 | 29 31 | 34 36 | 39 41 | 43 46 | 48 51 | 53 55 | 58 60 | 63 |
| 4'8" | 22 25 | 27 29 | 31 34 | 36 38 | 40 43 | 45 47 | 49 52 | 54 56 | 58 |
| 4'10" | 21 23 | 25 27 | 29 31 | 33 36 | 38 40 | 42 44 | 46 48 | 50 52 | 54 |
| 5'0" | 20 22 | 23 25 | 27 29 | 31 33 | 35 37 | 39 41 | 43 45 | 47 49 | 51 |
| 5'2" | 18 20 | 22 24 | 26 27 | 29 31 | 33 35 | 37 38 | 40 42 | 44 46 | 48 |
| 5'4" | 17 19 | 21 22 | 24 26 | 28 29 | 31 33 | 34 36 | 38 40 | 41 43 | 45 |
| 5'6" | 16 18 | 19 21 | 23 24 | 26 27 | 29 31 | 32 34 | 36 37 | 39 40 | 42 |
| 5'8" | 15 17 | 18 20 | 21 23 | 24 26 | 27 29 | 30 32 | 33 35 | 37 38 | 40 |
| 5'10" | 14 16 | 17 19 | 20 22 | 23 24 | 26 27 | 29 30 | 32 33 | 34 36 | 37 |
| 6'0" | 14 15 | 16 18 | 19 20 | 22 23 | 24 26 | 27 29 | 30 31 | 33 34 | 35 |
| 6'2" | 13 14 | 15 17 | 18 19 | 21 22 | 23 24 | 26 27 | 28 30 | 31 32 | 33 |
| 6'4" | 12 13 | 15 16 | 17 18 | 20 21 | 22 23 | 24 26 | 27 28 | 29 30 | 32 |
| 6'6" | 12 13 | 14 15 | 16 17 | 19 20 | 21 22 | 23 24 | 25 27 | 28 29 | 30 |
| 6'8" | 11 12 | 13 14 | 15 17 | 18 19 | 20 21 | 22 23 | 24 25 | 26 28 | 29 |
| 6'10" | 11 12 | 13 14 | 15 16 | 17 18 | 19 20 | 21 22 | 23 24 | 25 26 | 27 |
| 7'0" | 10 11 | 12 13 | 14 15 | 16 17 | 18 19 | 20 21 | 22 23 | 24 25 | 26 |

**Weight (pounds)**

**Key:**
- Underweight
- Normal weight
- Overweight
- Obese

**FIGURE 10.3** Body Mass Index (BMI)

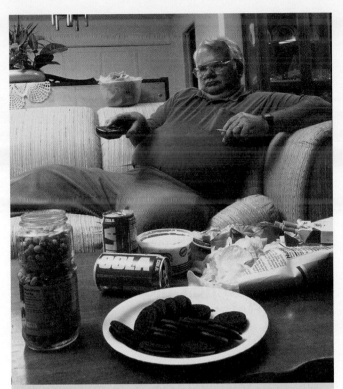

Abdominal obesity puts individuals at increased risk of CVD, stroke, and diabetes, particularly among men.

"at risk of overweight" and "overweight," to avoid the sense of shame such words may cause. In addition, BMI ranges for children and teens take into account normal differences in body fat between boys and girls and the differences in body fat that occur at various ages. Specific guidelines for calculating youth BMI are available at the Centers for Disease Control and Prevention website, www.cdc.gov.

## Waist Circumference and Ratio Measurements

Knowing where your fat is carried may be more important than knowing how much you carry. Men and postmenopausal women tend to store fat in the upper regions of the body, particularly in the abdominal area. Premenopausal women usually store fat in the lower regions of their bodies, particularly the hips, buttocks, and thighs. Waist circumference measurements, including *waist circumference* only, the *waist circumference-to-hip ratio*, and the *waist circumference-to-height ratio*, have all been used to measure abdominal fat as an indicator of obesity and health risk. Where you carry the weight may be of particular importance in determining whether you develop diabetes, cardiovascular disease, hypertension, or stroke.[40]

A waistline greater than 40 inches (102 centimeters) in men and 35 inches (88 centimeters) in women may be particularly indicative of greater health risk.[41] If a person is less than 5 feet tall or has a BMI of 35 or above, waist circumference standards used for the general population might not apply.

The waist circumference-to-hip ratio measures regional fat distribution. A waist-to-hip ratio greater than 1 in men and 0.8 in women indicates increased health risks.[42] Newer research has pointed to waist-to-hip ratio being more effective than waist circumference alone or BMI use when measuring body fat in children and adolescents.[43] A waist circumference-to-height ratio is a simple screening tool that says that your waist should be approximately one half of your height; if you were 70 inches tall, your waist shouldn't be more than 35 inches.

## Measures of Body Fat

There are numerous ways to assess whether your body fat levels are too high. One low-tech way is simply to look in the mirror or consider how your clothes fit now compared with how they fit last year. For those who wish to take a more precise measurement of their percentage of body fat, more accurate techniques are available, several of which are described and depicted in **FIGURE 10.4**. These methods usually involve the help of a skilled professional and typically must be done in a lab or clinical setting. Before undergoing any procedure, make sure you understand the expense, potential for accuracy, risks, and training of the tester. Also, consider why you are seeking this assessment and what you plan to do with the results.

Although opinion varies somewhat, most experts agree that men's bodies should contain between 8 and 20 percent total body fat, and women should be within the range of 20 to 30 percent (see **TABLE 10.1**). Generally, men who exceed 22

TABLE **10.1** | Body Fat Percentage Norms for Men and Women*

| Age (Men) | Very Lean | Excellent | Good | Fair | Poor | Very Poor |
|---|---|---|---|---|---|---|
| 20–29 | <7% | 7%–10% | 11%–15% | 16%–19% | 20%–23% | >23% |
| 30–39 | <11% | 11%–14% | 15%–18% | 19%–21% | 22%–25% | >25% |
| 40–49 | <14% | 14%–17% | 18%–20% | 21%–23% | 24%–27% | >27% |
| 50–59 | <15% | 15%–19% | 20%–22% | 23%–24% | 25%–28% | >28% |
| 60–69 | <16% | 16%–20% | 21%–22% | 23%–25% | 26%–28% | >28% |
| 70–79 | <16% | 16%–20% | 21%–23% | 24%–25% | 26%–28% | >28% |
| Age (Women) | Very Lean | Excellent | Good | Fair | Poor | Very Poor |
| 20–29 | <14% | 14%–16% | 17%–19% | 20%–23% | 24%–27% | >27% |
| 30–39 | <15% | 15%–17% | 18%–21% | 22%–25% | 26%–29% | >29% |
| 40–49 | <17% | 17%–20% | 21%–24% | 25%–28% | 29%–32% | >32% |
| 50–59 | <18% | 18%–22% | 23%–27% | 28%–30% | 31%–34% | >34% |
| 60–69 | <18% | 18%–23% | 24%–28% | 29%–31% | 32%–35% | >35% |
| 70–79 | <18% | 18%–24% | 25%–29% | 30%–32% | 33%–36% | >36% |

*Assumes nonathletes. For athletes, recommended body fat is 5 to 15 percent for men and 12 to 22 percent for women. Please note that there are no agreed-upon national standards for recommended body fat percentage.

**Source:** Based on data from The Cooper Institute, Dallas, Texas, www.cooperinstitute.org

**Underwater (hydrostatic) weighing:**
Measures the amount of water a person displaces when completely submerged. Fat tissue is less dense than muscle or bone, so body fat can be computed within a 2%–3% margin of error by comparing weight underwater and out of water.

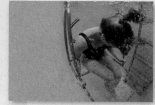

**Skinfolds:**
Involves "pinching" a person's fold of skin (with its underlying layer of fat) at various locations of the body. The fold is measured using a specially designed caliper. When performed by a skilled technician, it can estimate body fat with an error of 3%–4%.

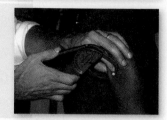

**Bioelectrical impedance analysis (BIA):**
Involves sending a very low level of electrical current through a person's body. As lean body mass is made up of mostly water, the rate at which the electricity is conducted gives an indication of a person's lean body mass and body fat. Under the best circumstances, BIA can estimate body fat with an error of 3%–4%.

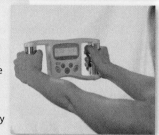

**Dual-energy X-ray absorptiometry (DXA):**
The technology is based on using very-low-level X ray to differentiate between bone tissue, soft (or lean) tissue, and fat (or adipose) tissue. The margin of error for predicting body fat is 2%–4%.

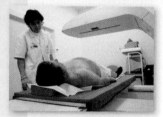

**Bod Pod:**
Uses air displacement to measure body composition. This machine is a large, egg-shaped chamber made from fiberglass. The person being measured sits in the machine wearing a swimsuit. The door is closed and the machine measures how much air is displaced. That value is used to calculate body fat, with a 2%–3% margin of error.

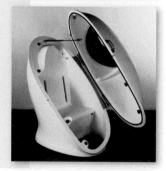

**FIGURE 10.4** Overview of Various Body Composition Assessment Methods

**Source:** Adapted from J. Thompson and M. Manore, *Nutrition: An Applied Approach My Plate Edition*, 3rd edition, © 2012. Printed and electronically reproduced by permission of Pearson Education, Inc., Upper Saddle River, New Jersey.

percent body fat and women who exceed 35 percent are considered overweight, but these ranges vary with age and stages of life. In addition, there are percentages of body fat below which a person is considered underweight, and health is compromised. In men, this lower limit is approximately 3 to 7 percent of total body weight and in women it is approximately 8 to 15 percent.

Explain the effectiveness and potential pros/cons of various weight control strategies, including exercise, diet, lifestyle modification, supplements/diet drugs, surgery, and other options.

At some point in our lives, almost all of us will decide to lose weight. Many will have mixed success. Failure is often related to thinking about losing weight in terms of short-term "dieting" rather than adjusting long-term behaviors. Drugs and intensive counseling can contribute to positive weight loss, but even then, many people regain weight after treatment. Maintaining a healthful body takes constant attention and nurturing. The **Student Health Today** box looks at characteristics of successful weight losers.

## Understanding Calories and Energy Balance

A *calorie* is a unit of measure that indicates the amount of energy gained from food or expended through activity. Each time you consume 3,500 calories more than your body needs to maintain weight, you gain a pound of storage fat. Conversely, each time your body expends an extra 3,500 calories, you lose a pound of fat. If you consume 140 calories (the amount in one can of regular soda) more than you need every single day and make no other changes in diet or activity, you would gain 1 pound in 25 days (3,500 calories ÷ 140 calories per day = 25 days). Conversely, if you walk for 30 minutes each day at a pace of 15 minutes per mile (172 calories burned) in addition to your regular activities, you would lose 1 pound in 20 days (3,500 calories ÷ 172 calories per day = 20.3 days). **FIGURE 10.5** illustrates the concept of energy balance.

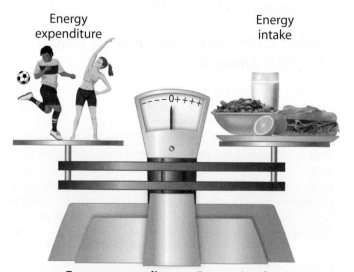

Energy expenditure = Energy intake

**FIGURE 10.5** The Concept of Energy Balance If you consume more calories than you burn, you gain weight. If you burn more than you consume, you lose weight. If both are equal, your weight will not change.

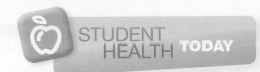

# WHO WINS IN LOSING?
## Characteristics of Successful Losers

Millions of Americans start their New Year with the most popular resolution: to lose weight and keep it off. Even so, the majority who lose some weight ultimately regain it. But what about those few losers who manage to keep it off?

In general, the literature indicates success rates between 2 and 15 percent, using a variety of weight and BMI parameters, as well as timelines for defining success. From there, success measures look at short-term initial success, 6-month success, and 1-year success, with few studies looking at success rates past 24 months. Based on these studies, characteristics of those likely to be successful include the following:

- High self-esteem, self-efficacy, and realistic body image.
- A strong locus of control—being motivated by internal rather than external factors.
- Having awareness of their current risks and reasonable knowledge of healthy nutrition.
- Having supportive friends and family.
- Utilizing community resources.
- Journaling and tracking calories, nutrients, and/or portion sizes; they also regularly monitor weight.
- Ultimately aiming to follow a healthy, realistic eating and exercise pattern.
- Incorporating some type of incentive into their program
- Praising small successes and avoiding becoming discouraged by setbacks.

A recent meta-analysis of some of the most comprehensive research studies to

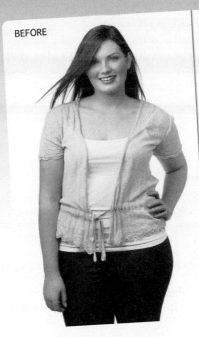

BEFORE      AFTER

date indicated that behavioral interventions that focus on diet and exercise show small but significant weight loss and that long-term maintenance is aided by selected pharmaceutical aids. Those who focus on the above are most likely to win at the losing game.

**Sources:** J. Kassier and M. Angell, "Losing Weight—An Ill-Fated New Year's Resolution," *New England Journal of Medicine* 338, no. 1 (1998): 52–54; S. Dombrowski et al. "Long Term Maintenance of Weight Loss with Non-surgical Interventions in Obese Adults: Systematic Review and Meta-analyses of Randomized Controlled Trials," *British Medical Journal* 348 (2014): g2646; Look AHEAD Research Group, "Eight Year Weight Losses with an Intensive Lifestyle Intervention: The Look Ahead Study," *Obesity* 22, no 1 (2014): 5–13; M. Butryn et al., "Consistent Self-Monitoring of Weight: A Key Component of Successful Weight Loss Maintenance," *Obesity* 15, no. 12 (2007): 3091–3096; T. Wadden et al., "One Year Weight Losses in the Look Ahead Study: Factors Associated with Success," *Obesity* 17, no. 4 (2009): 713–22; J. Moreno and C. Johnston, "Success Habits of Weight Losers," *American Journal of Lifestyle Medicine* 6, no. 2 (2012): 113–15; Centers for Disease Control and Prevention, "Keeping It Off," September 2011, www.cdc.gov/healthyweight/losing_weight/keepingitoff.html; S. Ramage et al., "Healthy Strategies for Successful Weight Loss and Weight Maintenance: A Systematic Review," *Applied Physiology, Nutrition, and Metabolism* 39, no. 1 (2013): 1–20; S. Simpson et al., "What Is the Most Effective Way to Maintain Weight Loss in Adults?," *British Medical Journal,* 343 (2011):d8042.

# Diet and Eating Behaviors

Successful weight loss requires shifting energy balance. The first part of the equation is to reduce calorie intake through modifying eating habits and daily diet.

**Improving Your Eating Habits** Before you can change an unhealthy eating habit, you must first determine what causes or triggers it. Keeping a detailed daily log of eating triggers—when, what, where, and how much you eat—for at least a week can give clues about what causes you to want unneeded food. Typically, dietary triggers center on patterns and problems in everyday living rather than real hunger pangs. For example, your daily commute might take you past your favorite fast food restaurant. Or maybe there are numerous vending machines on campus. Many people eat compulsively when stressed; however, for other people, the same circumstances diminish their appetite, causing them to lose weight. See the

Skills for Behavior Change box for tips on healthy snacking, and see **FIGURE 10.6** for ways to adjust your eating triggers.

## Choosing a Diet Plan

Once you have determined your triggers, begin to devise a plan for improved eating by doing the following:

- Seeking assistance from reputable sources such as MyPlate (www.choosemyplate.gov), a registered dietitian (RD), some physicians, health educators, or exercise physiologists with nutritional training.
- Being wary of nutritionists or nutritional life coaches, since there is no formal credential for those titles.
- Avoiding weight-loss programs that promise quick, "miracle" results or that are run by "trainees," often people with short courses on nutrition and exercise that are designed to sell products or services.
- Assessing the nutrient value of any prescribed diet, verifying dietary guidelines are consistent with reliable nutrition research, and analyzing the suitability of the diet to your tastes, budget, and lifestyle.

Any diet that requires radical behavior changes or sets up artificial dietary programs through prepackaged products is likely to fail. The most successful plans allow you to make food choices in real-world settings and do not ask you to

| If your trigger is . . . | then ➤ try this strategy . . . |
|---|---|
| A stressful situation | Acknowledge and address feelings of anxiety or stress, and develop stress management techniques to practice daily. |
| Feeling angry or upset | Analyze your emotions and look for a noneating activity to deal with them, such as taking a quick walk or calling a friend. |
| A certain time of day | Change your eating schedule to avoid skipping or delaying meals and overeating later; make a plan of what you'll eat ahead of time to avoid impulse or emotional eating. |
| Pressure from friends and family | Have a response ready to help you refuse food you do not want, or look for healthy alternatives you can eat instead when in social settings. |
| Being in an environment where food is available | Avoid the environment that causes you to want to eat: Sit far away from the food at meetings, take a different route to class to avoid passing the vending machines, shop from a list and only when you aren't hungry, arrange nonfood outings with your friends. |
| Feeling bored and tired | Identify the times when you feel low energy and fill them with activities other than eating, such as exercise breaks; cultivate a new interest or hobby that keeps your mind and hands busy. |
| The sight and smell of food | Stop buying high-calorie foods that tempt you to snack, or store them in an inconvenient place, out of sight; avoid walking past or sitting or standing near the table of tempting treats at a meeting, party, or other gathering. |
| Eating mindlessly or inattentively | Turn off all distractions, including phones, computers, television, and radio, and eat more slowly, savoring your food and putting your fork down between bites so you can become aware of when your hunger is satisfied. |
| Spending time alone in the car | Get a book on tape to listen to, or tape your class notes and use the time for studying. Keep your mind off food. Don't bring money into the gas station where snacks are tempting. |
| Alcohol use | Drink plenty of water and stay hydrated. Seek out healthy snack choices. After a night out, brush your teeth immediately upon getting home and stay out of the kitchen. |
| Feeling deprived | Allow yourself to eat "indulgences" in moderation, so you won't crave them; focus on balancing your calorie input to calorie output. |
| Eating out of habit | Establish a new routine to circumvent the old, such as taking a new route to class so you don't feel compelled to stop at your favorite fast-food restaurant on the way. |
| Watching television | Look for something else to occupy your hands and body while your mind is engaged with the screen: Ride an exercise bike, do stretching exercises, doodle on a pad of paper, or learn to knit. |

**FIGURE 10.6** Avoid Trigger-Happy Eating

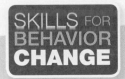
## TIPS FOR SENSIBLE SNACKING

▶ **Keep healthy munchies around.** Buy 100 percent whole wheat breads, and if you need something to spice that up, use low-fat or soy cheese, low-fat cream cheese, peanut butter, hummus, or other high-protein healthy favorites. Some baked or popped crackers are low in fat and calories and high in fiber.

▶ **Keep "crunchies" on hand.** Apples, pears, green or red pepper sticks, popcorn, snap peas, and celery all are good choices. Wash the fruits and vegetables and cut them up to carry with you; eat them when a snack attack comes on.

▶ **Choose natural beverages.** Drink plain water, 100 percent juice in small quantities, or other low-sugar choices to satisfy your thirst. Hot tea, coffee (black), or soup broths are also good choices.

▶ **Eat nuts instead of candy.** Although relatively high in calories, nuts are also loaded with healthy fats and are healthy when consumed in moderation.

▶ **If you must have a piece of chocolate, keep it small and dark.** Dark chocolate has more antioxidants.

▶ **Avoid high-calorie energy bars.** Eat these only if you are exercising hard and don't have an opportunity to eat a regular meal. Select ones with a good mixture of fiber and protein and that are low in fat, sugar, and calories.

sacrifice everything you enjoy. See **TABLE 10.2** for an analysis of some popular diets marketed today. For information on other plans, check out the regularly updated list of reviews on the website of the Academy of Nutrition and Dietetics (formerly the American Dietetic Association) at www.eatright.org.

# Including Exercise

Any increase in the intensity, frequency, and duration of daily exercise can lead to an increase in muscle mass, which can have a significant impact on total calorie expenditure because lean (muscle) tissue is more metabolically active than fat tissue. Exact estimates vary, but experts currently think that 2 to 50 more calories per day are burned per pound of muscle than each pound of fat tissue. Thus, the base level of calories needed to maintain a healthy weight varies greatly from person to person.

The number of calories spent through physical activity depends on three factors:

1. The number and proportion of muscles used
2. The amount of weight moved
3. The length of time the activity takes

An activity involving both the arms and legs burns more calories than one involving only the legs. An activity performed by a heavy person burns more calories than the same activity performed by a lighter person. And, an activity performed for 40 minutes requires twice as much energy as the same activity performed for only 20 minutes.

## TABLE 10.2 | Analyzing Popular Diet Programs

| Diet Name | Basic Principles | Good for Diabetes and Heart Health? | Weight Loss Effectiveness | Pros, Cons, and Other Things to Consider |
|---|---|---|---|---|
| **DASH (Dietary Approaches to Stop Hypertension)** | A balanced plan developed to fight high blood pressure. Eat fruits, veggies, whole grains, lean protein, and low-fat dairy. Avoid sweets, fats, red meat, and sodium. | Yes | Not specifically designed for weight loss. | A balanced, safe and healthy diet, rated the no. 1 best diet overall by 2015 *U.S. News & World Report*. Although not designed for weight reduction per se, it is regarded as very effective in improving cholesterol levels and other biomarkers long term. |
| **TLC (Therapeutic Lifestyle Change)** | Developed by NIH. Focus on CVD risk reduction with fruits and veggies, lean protein, low fat, etc. Balanced and effective. | Yes | Weight loss likely; cholesterol key. | Safe, balanced, and healthy diet rated no. 2 diet by 2015 *U.S. News & World Report*. Particularly good for heart health. |
| **Mediterranean** | A plan that emphasizes fruits, vegetables, fish, whole grains, beans, nuts, legumes, olive oil, and herbs and spices. Poultry, eggs, cheese, yogurt, and red wine can be enjoyed in moderation, whereas sweets and red meat are saved for special occasions. | Yes | Effective | Widely considered to be one of the more healthy, safe, and balanced diets. Weight loss may not be as dramatic but long-term health benefits have been demonstrated. Tied for third best diet overall—with the Mayo Clinic and Weight Watchers—by 2015 *U.S. News & World Report*. Relatively easy to follow. |
| **Weight Watchers** | The program assigns every food a point value based on its nutritional values and how hard your body has to work to burn it off. Total points allowed depend on activity level and personal weight goals. In-person group meetings or online membership are options. | Yes (depending on individual choices) | Effective | Experts consider Weight Watchers effective and easy to follow for both short- and long-term weight loss. Other pluses include an emphasis on group support and room for occasional indulgences. But while not as expensive as some plans, there are membership fees. Tied for third best diet overall in 2015 *U.S. News & World Report*. |

*continued*

TABLE **10.2** | Analyzing Popular Diet Programs (*continued*)

| Diet Name | Basic Principles | Good for Diabetes and Heart Health? | Weight Loss Effectiveness | Pros, Cons, and Other Things to Consider |
|---|---|---|---|---|
| **Jenny Craig** | Prepackaged meals do the work of restricting calorie intake. Members get personalized meal and exercise plans, plus weekly counseling sessions. | Yes | Effective short term, long-term results dependent on adopting healthful eating later. | Support and premade meals make weight loss easier; however, it may be difficult to maintain for the long run. Cons include cost, which will run hundreds of dollars per month for food alone, plus membership fees. Lactose- and gluten-intolerant individuals cannot join due to available foods. |
| **Biggest Loser** | Four servings a day of fruits and vegetables, three of protein foods, two of whole grains, and no more than 200 calories of "extras" like desserts. Exercise, food journals, portion control, and calculating personal calorie allowances are all stressed. | Yes | Effective | This diet is effective at weight loss. Ranked no. 1 by *U.S. News and World Report*, 2015 for those with pre-diabetes or diabetes. Helps reduce blood glucose levels and reduces other biomarkers such as cholesterol, triglycerides, etc. |
| **Nutrisystem** | Low-calorie, prepackaged meals are ordered online and delivered to your home. | Not for heart health per se, but may help reduce diabetes risks. | Effective short-term, long-term results dependent on adopting healthful eating later. | Nutrisystem is quite safe, easier to follow than many other diets, and has few nutritional deficiencies if followed as directed, according to experts. It is also expensive (similar to Jenny Craig) due to the cost of ordering food and may not help you learn to eat healthfully after diet is done. |
| **Medifast** | Dieters eat six meals a day, five of them 100-calorie Medifast products. After goal weight loss, people wean from Medifast food and gradually add back in starchy veggies, whole grains, fruit, and low-fat dairy products. | Likely yes | Effective in short term; long-term results unproven. | Medifast scored above average in short-term weight loss but gets lower marks for keeping weight off. Because of the extremely low calorie intakes on the program, it is hard to stay on the program for long; doesn't teach healthy eating as part of plan. |
| **Low Carb Diets (Atkins, South Beach, and other variations)** | Carbs—sugars and "simple starches" like potatoes, white bread, and rice—are avoided, and some minimize all carb-based foods. Emphasis on proteins and fat from meat and eggs are embraced. | Not likely with so much fat eaten. | Effective in short term, mixed long-term results. | Low carb diets in most forms are often extremely effective at short-term weight loss, but many experts worry that fat intake is up to three times higher than standard daily recommendations and some even omit fruits, vegetables, and healthy grains. |
| **Paleo** | Based on the theory that digestive systems have not evolved to deal with many modern foods such as diary, legumes, grains and sugar, this plan emphasizes meats, fish, poultry, fruits, and vegetables. | Unknown (too few studies) | Unknown (too few studies) | Gets low marks by health and nutrition experts due to avoidance of grains, legumes, and dairy and higher fat than the government recommends. Missing essential nutrients, costly to maintain. It can be hard to follow long term and has had only a few very small studies done to document effectiveness. |
| **Fast Diet (also known as the 5:2 diet or Intermittent Fasting Diet)** | Based on the theory that by drastically reducing calories on two days (500 cal/day) each week and eating normally the other five, you will lose weight. | Not likely as it doesn't follow guidelines for carbohydrates. Should talk with registered dietician or health care provider. | Effective, but weight loss is relatively slow unless calorie intake is monitored on non-fast days and exercise is part of regimen. | Exceeds dietary guidelines for fat and protein and falls short on carbohydrate recommendation. Does encourage fruits and veggies, but feast and famine regimen is hard to sustain. |

**Source:** Opinions on diet pros and cons are based on *U.S. News & World Report*, "Best Diet Rankings," 2015, http://health.usnews.com/best-diet/best-over-all-diets?int=9c2508; dietary reviews are available online from registered dieticians at the Academy of Nutrition and Dietetics, 2015, http://www.eatrightpro.org/resources/media/trends-and-reviews.

# Keeping Weight Control in Perspective

Weight loss is a struggle for many people, and many factors influence success or failure. To reach and maintain a healthy weight, develop a program of exercise and healthy eating behaviors that you can maintain. Remember, you didn't gain your weight in a week or two, and it is both unrealistic and potentially dangerous to take drastic weight loss measures. Instead, try to lose a healthy 1 to 2 pounds during the first week, and stay with this slow and easy regimen. Adding exercise and cutting back on calories to expend about 500 calories more than you consume each day will help you lose weight at a rate of 1 pound per week. You may find tracking your intake and activity easier with one of the apps described in the **Tech & Health** box on the next page. See the **Skills for Behavior Change** box for strategies to help your weight management program succeed.

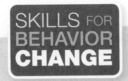

## WHY SHOULD I CARE?

It may be easy to grab a fast-food meal, but unless you are very physically active, your body will likely store that "super-sized" meal as fat, which is anything but easy to lose. Eating 500 extra calories a day—less than the average hamburger—can lead to a pound of weight gain in just a week's time. A 150-pound person would need to walk for about 90 minutes at 4 mph to burn that off. if you walk slower, it would take even longer.

One particularly dangerous potential complication of VLCDs is *ketoacidosis*, a condition that occurs when your cells don't have enough of the glucose they need for energy. When this happens, the body begins to burn fat for energy, producing *ketones*—acidic chemicals that can cause major risks to health. As ketones increase initially, you may not feel hungry or thirsty and weight loss may occur. As levels increase, you may begin to develop *ketosis*, which can progress to *ketoacidosis* or acidic blood levels. Early symptoms may include excessive thirst, excessive urination, and high blood sugar, progressing to extreme fatigue, nausea, vomiting, abdominal pain, "fruity breath," fainting, possible coma, and death. Extreme diets that allow very few carbohydrates and/or calories are often the culprits. People with untreated type 1 diabetes and individuals with anorexia or bulimia are also at high risk.

> **very-low-calorie diets (VLCDs)** Diets with a daily calorie value of 400 to 700 calories.

## Considering Drastic Weight-Loss Measures?

When nothing seems to work, people become frustrated and pursue high-risk, unproven methods of weight loss or seek medical interventions. Dramatic weight loss may be recommended in cases of extreme health risk. Even in such situations, drastic dietary, pharmacological, or surgical measures should be considered carefully and discussed with several knowledgeable, licensed health professionals working in accredited facilities.

**Very-Low-Calorie Diets** In severe cases of obesity that are not responsive to traditional dietary strategies, medically supervised, powdered formulas with daily values of 400 to 700 calories plus vitamin and mineral supplements may be given to patients. Many of these diets emphasize high protein and very low carbohydrates. Such **very-low-calorie diets (VLCDs)** should never be undertaken without strict medical supervision. They do not teach healthy eating, and persons who manage to lose weight on VLCDs may experience significant weight regain. Problems associated with any form of severe caloric restriction include blood sugar imbalance, cold intolerance, constipation, decreased BMR, dehydration, diarrhea, emotional problems, fatigue, headaches, heart irregularities, kidney infections and failure, loss of lean body tissue, weakness, and the potential for coma and death.

## SEE IT! VIDEOS

Do you snack like crazy when you're watching an exciting movie? Watch **Fast Paced Movies, Television Shows May Lead to More Snacking** in the Study Area of MasteringHealth™

## SKILLS FOR BEHAVIOR CHANGE

### KEYS TO SUCCESSFUL WEIGHT MANAGEMENT

**Make a Plan**
▶ Establish short- and long-term plans. What are the diet and exercise changes you can make this week? Once you do 1 week, plot a course for 2 weeks, and so on.
▶ Look for balance. Remember it's calories taken in and burned over time that make the difference.

**Change Your Habits**
▶ Be adventurous. Expand your usual foods to enjoy a wider variety.
▶ Eat small portions, less often and savor the flavor.
▶ Notice whether you are hungry before starting a meal. Eat slowly, noting when you start to feel full, and *stop* before you are full.
▶ Eat breakfast, especially low-fat foods with whole grains and protein. This will prevent you from being too hungry and overeating at lunch.
▶ Keep healthful snacks on hand for when you get hungry.

**Incorporate Exercise**
▶ Be active and slowly increase your time, speed, distance, or resistance levels.
▶ Vary your physical activity. Find activities that you really love and try things you haven't tried before.
▶ Find an exercise partner to help you stay motivated.

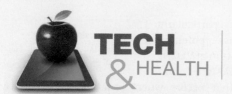

# TECH & HEALTH

## TRACKING YOUR DIET OR WEIGHT LOSS? *There's an App for That*

Studies consistently report that people who keep detailed food and exercise journals lose more weight and keep it off longer than those who do not. Want to track what you ate today in terms of total calories and amount of nutrients? There's an app for that. Want to track your walking, running, swimming, lifting, and sleeping activities? There are apps for that, too.

The best programs combine food and physical activity logs, so if you splurge on dessert, you can figure out how many miles you'll need to jog to burn it off. These apps often feature calculators for determining daily calorie intake goals as well as barcode scanners that allow you to quickly add packaged foods to your log. Here are just a few:

- **Lose It!** by FitNow. (Basic Plan Free: Android, iPhone and iPad, Nook tablet, PCs. $39.95 for year subscription to Premium plan), www.loseit.com
- Simple to use, comprehensive database of foods, phone scanning of bar codes, and activities designed to help you log meals and track exercise. Premium model connects to scale for weight-loss monitoring and tracks key health indicators.
- **Restaurant Weight Watcher.** (Modest cost; Android only), http://ellisapps .com Lists nutrition information for the menus of over 200 restaurants and continues to add new ones.

- **MyFitnessPal Calorie Counter & Diet Tracker** (Free: iPhone, Android, Blackberry, PCs) www.myfitnesspal.com A combination of diet and fitness goals as well as a nutritional analysis of what you are eating and your exercise levels. Can scan bar codes on food to help you monitor what you are buying and make healthy choice.
- **Diet Point • Weight Loss** (Free: Android and iPhone) www.dietpointed.com/ Weight loss assistant that offers 55 unique diet plans, from low-carb to vegan to paleo, including grocery lists, instructions, and reminders. Includes BMI and BMR calculator that tracks energy expenditure as well as exercise tracking.

## Weight Loss Supplements and Over the Counter Drugs

Thousands of over-the-counter supplements and drugs that claim to make weight loss fast and easy are available for purchase. It's important to note that U.S. Food and Drug Administration (FDA) approval is not required for over-the-counter "diet aids" or supplements. The lack of regular and continuous monitoring of supplements in the United States leaves consumers vulnerable to fraud and potentially toxic "remedies." Most dietary supplements contain stimulants, such as caffeine, or diuretics, and their effectiveness in promoting weight loss has been largely untested and unproved by any scientific studies. In many cases, the only thing that users lose is money. Virtually all persons who used supplements and diet pills in review studies regained their weight once they stopped taking them.[44]

Supplements containing *Hoodia gordonii,* an African, cactus-like plant, have become popular in recent years, and there are many off-market brands produced, including some that contain more unproven ingredients such as bitter orange and other stimulants. Even so, no convincing evidence has been shown for or against *Hoodia gordonii*; to date, it is not FDA approved and has not been tested in clinical trials.[45]

Products containing *ephedra* can cause rapid heart rate, tremors, seizures, insomnia, headaches, and raised blood pressure, all without significant effects on long-term weight control. *St. John's wort* and other alternative medicines reported to enhance serotonin, suppress appetite, and reduce the side effects of depression have not been shown to be effective in weight loss, either.

Historically, FDA-approved diet pills have been available only by prescription and are closely monitored. These lines were blurred in 2007 when the FDA approved the first over-the-counter weight loss pill—a half-strength version of the prescription drug *orlistat* (brand name *Xenical*), marketed as Alli. This drug inhibits the action of lipase, an enzyme that helps the body to digest fats, causing about 30 percent of fats consumed to pass through the digestive system undigested, leading to reduced overall caloric intake. Known side effects of orlistat include gas with watery fecal discharge; oily stools and spotting; frequent, often unexpected, bowel movements; and possible deficiencies of fat-soluble vitamins.

## Prescription Weight Loss Drugs

In 2012, the FDA approved the first new weight loss drugs in nearly 13 years. These new drugs, *Belviq* and *Qsymia,* were met with much controversy and carry several warnings and restrictions. Qsymia is an appetite suppressant and antiseizure drug that reduces the desire for food. Belviq affects serotonin levels, helping patients feel full. Newer drugs, such as

# 39.5%

OF ADULTS AGED 40–59 ARE **OBESE**, FOLLOWED BY 30.3% OBESITY IN THE 20–39 AGE GROUP, AND 35.4% OBESITY IN THE 60+ AGE GROUP.

*Contrave* combine antidepressants with other approved drugs and carry warnings specific to both. Other weight loss drugs that have been on the market for some time, such as *Meridia*, continue to be marketed. Before taking any weight loss supplements and herbal remedies or prescription drugs, you should always discuss risks, benefits, and options with your doctor and carefully read FDA warnings.

When used as part of a long-term, comprehensive weight-loss program, weight-loss drugs can potentially help those who are severely obese lose up to 10 percent of their weight and maintain the loss. The challenge is to develop an effective drug that can be used over time without adverse effects or abuse, and no such drug currently exists. A classic example of supposedly safe drugs that were later found to have dangerous side effects are Pondimin and Redux, known as *fen-phen* (from their chemical names fenfluramine and phentermine), two of the most widely prescribed diet drugs in U.S. history.[46] When they were found to damage heart valves and contribute to pulmonary hypertension, a massive recall and lawsuit ensued.

### Surgery

When all else fails, particularly for people who are severely overweight and have weight-related diseases, a person may be a candidate for weight-loss surgery. Generally,

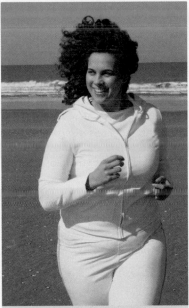

Participating in daily physical activity is key to managing your weight, as well as overall fitness and health.

these surgeries fall into one of two major categories: *restrictive surgeries,* such as gastric banding or lap banding, that limit food intake, and *malabsorption surgeries,* such as gastric bypass, which decrease the absorption of food into the body.

To select the best option, a physician will consider that operation's benefits and risks, the patient's age, BMI, eating behaviors, obesity-related health conditions, mental history, dietary history, and previous operations. Like drugs prescribed for weight loss, surgery for obesity also carries risks for consumers.[47] Some health advocates have proposed that obesity be classified as a disability (see the **Points of View** box on the next page), which could potentially affect a physician's decision on recommending surgery.

In gastric banding and other restrictive surgeries, the surgeon uses an inflatable band to partition off part of the stomach. The band is wrapped around that part of the stomach and is pulled tight, like a belt, leaving only a small opening between the two parts of the stomach. The upper part of the stomach is smaller, so the person feels full more quickly, and food digestion slows so that the person also feels full longer. Although the bands are designed to stay in place, they can be removed surgically. They can also be inflated to different levels to adjust the amount of restriction.

*Sleeve gastrectomy* is another form of restrictive weight loss that is often done laparoscopically. In this surgery, about 75 percent of the stomach is removed, leaving only a tube (about the size of a banana) or sleeve that is connected directly to the intestines. Usually, this procedure is done on extremely obese or ill patients who need an interim, less invasive procedure before more invasive gastric bypass. However, this procedure isn't reversible and potential risks may be higher.

*Gastric bypass* is one of the most common types of weight loss surgery and it combines restrictive and malabsorption elements. It can be done laparoscopically or via full open surgery. In this surgery, a major section (as much as 70%) of the stomach is sutured off, restricting the amount of food you can eat and absorb. The remaining pouch is hooked up directly to the small intestine. Results are fast and dramatic, with health issues related to obesity, such as diabetes, high blood pressure, arthritis, sleep apnea, and other problems diminishing or being reduced drastically in a short time.

While weight loss tends to be maintained and health problems decline, there are many risks, including nutritional deficiencies, blood clots in the legs, a leak in a staple line in the stomach, pneumonia, infection, and although rare, even death.

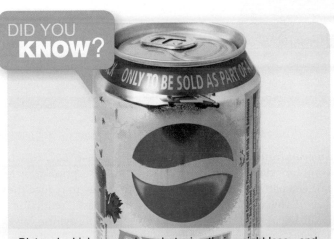

**DID YOU KNOW?**

Diet soda drinkers may be sabotaging their weight loss—and increasing risks for a variety of health problems! In fact, diet soda drinkers may consume more calories than sugared soda drinkers. Why? Artificial sweeteners may change perceptions of fullness and increase appetite. Others suggest a form of "cognitive distortion" whereby we justify a few more snacks or dessert because our drinks have fewer calories.

**Sources:** S. N. Bleich, J. A. Wolfson, and S. Vine, "Diet-Beverage Consumption and Caloric Intake among US Adults, Overall and by Body Weight," *American Journal of Public Health* 104, no. 3 (2014): e72–e78

**SEE IT!** VIDEOS

How can you control your urge to go overboard with meal portions? Watch **Experiment Shows Portion Control Is the Key to Healthy Eating** on **MasteringHealth**™

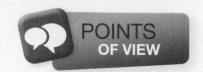

# Obesity
## *Is It a Disability?*

A person 150 to 200 pounds overweight can have difficulty walking, running, standing, and doing other daily tasks. Some believe obesity should be considered a disability legally entitling individuals to certain health benefits and accommodations. Others believe that labeling obesity a disability would add to its stigma and create more problems than it solves.

The federal Americans with Disabilities Act (ADA) defines *disability* as "a physical or mental impairment that substantially limits one or more of the major life activities of [an] individual." Currently, people must have BMIs over 40, or be at least 100 pounds overweight with an underlying disorder before the ADA classifies them as disabled. These strict criteria mean the ADA currently receives few valid claims relating to obesity.

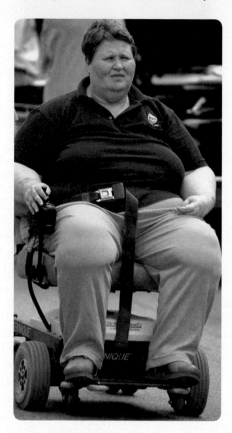

### Arguments Favoring Disability Status for Obese People

- Labeling obesity as a disability would provide obese individuals with increased options for health insurance.
- Labeling would protect individuals against weight-based discrimination.
- Labeling would help persons with chronic diseases that require use of walkers, wheelchairs, and other special accommodations at work or home to receive them.

### Arguments Opposing Disability Status for Obese People

- Some doctors worry that defining obesity as a disability would make them vulnerable to lawsuits from obese patients who don't want to discuss their weight. Such a threat would prevent doctors from discussing obesity with their overweight patients and recommending specific actions.
- Issues of unfair insurance or job practices could be handled with antidiscrimination laws, not disability status.
- Not all obese people are disabled by their weight, so labeling them all as such would be discriminatory.

### WHERE DO YOU STAND?

- What consequences might result from classifying overweight or obese individuals as disabled?
- Do you think labeling obesity as a disability would alter the way our society perceives and behaves toward overweight and obese individuals? If so, how?

---

Another risk is rapid gastric emptying, commonly referred to as "dumping," in which undigested foods rush through the small intestine, causing cramping and problems with uncontrollable diarrhea.[48] Because the stomach pouch that remains after surgery is only the size of a lime, the person can drink only a few tablespoons of liquid and consume only a very small amount of food at a time. For this reason, other possible side effects include nausea, vitamin and mineral deficiencies, and dehydration. Additional risks include the potential for excess bleeding, ulcers, hernia, and the typical risks from anesthesia.

A technique gaining in popularity because it's even more effective than gastric bypass for rapid weight loss, is the *biliopancreatic diversion* or *duodenal switch procedure,* which combines elements of restrictive and malabsorption surgeries. The patient receives a partial gastrectomy to reduce the size of the stomach (less than gastric bypass's reduction) while bypassing less of the small intestine. The pyloric valve remains intact, which helps prevent dumping syndrome, ulcers, blockages, and other problems that can occur with other techniques. This surgery is one of the most difficult and highest risk surgeries for patients, with the risk of death and other complications higher than those of other options.[49]

Considerable research has demonstrated exciting, unexpected results from gastric surgeries: Even prior to weight

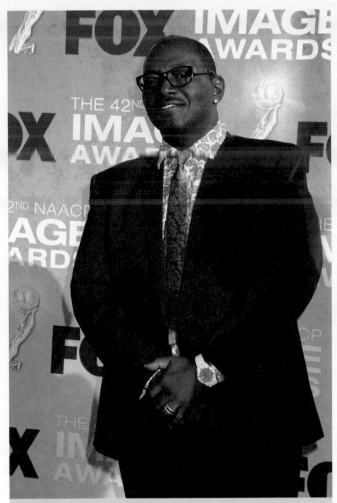

Former *American Idol* judge and record producer Randy Jackson and NBC weatherman Al Roker each have undergone gastric bypass surgery to shed well over 100 pounds and reduce the risks of serious chronic diseases such as type 2 diabetes.

loss, patients have shown complete remission of type 2 diabetes in the majority of cases, with drastic reductions in blood glucose levels in others.[50] While extremely promising, newer research indicates that about one third of those who have gastric surgery with remission of diabetic symptoms will relapse and begin to show diabetic symptoms within 5 years after surgery. For those at high risk from these diseases, the choice of undergoing a high-risk surgery may ultimately be similar to the risk of maintaining their current weight.

Unlike surgeries that help make weight loss easier, *liposuction* is a surgical procedure in which fat cells are actually removed from specific areas of the body. Generally, liposuction is considered cosmetic surgery rather than true weight-loss surgery, even though people who have it lose weight and contour their bodies. Liposuction is not risk-free. If you are considering this procedure, check the credentials of the surgeon, the certification of the facility, and the proximity to emergency care if problems arise.

## Trying to Gain Weight

For some people, trying to gain weight is a challenge. If you have trouble, the first priority is to determine why you cannot gain weight. Perhaps you're an athlete and you burn more calories than you eat. Perhaps you're stressed out and skip meals to increase study time. Among older adults, senses of taste and smell may decline, making food less pleasurable to eat. Visual problems and other disabilities may make meals more difficult to prepare, and dental problems may make eating more difficult. People who engage in extreme energy-burning sports and exercise routines may be at risk for caloric and nutritional deficiencies, which can lead not only to weight loss, but also to immune system problems and organ dysfunction; weakness, which leads to falls and fractures; slower recovery from diseases; and a host of other problems. Underweight individuals need to examine diet and exercise behaviors and take steps achieve and maintain a healthy weight.

## WHAT DO YOU THINK?

If you wanted to lose weight, what strategies would you most likely choose?

- Which strategies, if any, have worked for you before?
- What factors might serve to help or hinder your weight loss efforts?

**SEE IT! VIDEOS**

Could a diet high in protein and fats lead to weight loss? Watch **Low-Carb Diet Trumps Low Fat in Weight-Loss Study** in the Study Area of **MasteringHealth**™

If you are overweight or obese, complete each of the following questions by circling the response(s) that best represents your situation or attitudes, then total your points for each section.

## Section 1 Family, Weight, and Diet History

1. How many people in your immediate family (parents or siblings) are overweight or obese?

   a. No one is overweight or obese (0 points)

   b. One person (1 point)

   c. Two people (2 points)

   d. Three or more people (3 points)

2. During which periods of your life were you overweight or obese? (Circle all that apply.)

   a. Birth through age 5 (1 point)

   b. Ages 6 to 11 (1 point)

   c. Ages 12 to 13 (1 point))

   d. Ages 14 to 18 (2 points)

   e. Ages 19 to present (2 points)

3. How many times in the last year have you made a major effort to lose weight but had little or no success?

   a. None. (0 points)

   b. I've thought about it, but never tried. (1 point)

   c. I have tried 2 to 3 times. (1 point)

   d. I have tried at least once a month. (2 points)

   e. I have too many times to count. (3 points)

   Total points: _____

### Scoring

A score higher than 4 suggests you may have several challenges ahead as you begin a weight loss program. Your weight is often a product of learned patterns of eating and exercise. If you've tried repeatedly to lose and have not been successful, you may have to reframe your thinking and try something new.

## Section 2 Readiness to Change

1. What is/are your main reason(s) for wanting to lose weight? (Circle all that apply.)

   a. I want to please someone I know or attract a new person. (0 points)

   b. I want to look great and/or fit into smaller size clothes for an upcoming event (wedding, vacation, date, etc.). (1 point)

   c. Someone I know has had major health problems because of being overweight/obese. (1 point)

   d. I want to improve my health and/or have more energy. (2 points)

   e. I was diagnosed with a weight-related health problem. (2 points)

2. What do you think about your weight and body shape? (Circle all that apply.)

   a. I'm fine with being overweight, and if others don't like it, tough! (0 points)

   b. My weight hurts my energy levels and my performance. (1 points)

   c. I feel good about myself, but think I will be happier if I lose weight. (1 points)

   d. I'm self-conscious about my weight and uncomfortable in my skin. (1 point)

   e. I'm really worried I will have a major health problem if I don't change my behaviors now. (2 points)

3. Which of the following statements describes you? (Circle all that apply.)

   a. I think about food several times a day, even when I'm not hungry. (0 point)

   b. There are some foods or snacks that I can't stay away from, and I eat them even when I'm not hungry. (0 point)

   c. I tend to eat more meat and fatty foods and seldom get enough fruits and veggies. (0 points)

   d. I've thought about the weaknesses in my diet and have some ideas about what I need to do. (1 point)

   e. I haven't really tried to eat a "balanced" diet, but I know that I need to start now. (1 point)

4. When you binge or eat things you shouldn't, what are you likely to do? (Circle all that apply.)

   a. Not care and go off of my diet. (0 points)

   b. Feel guilty for a while, but then do it again the next time I am out. (0 points)

   c. Fast for the next day or two to help balance the high consumption day. (0 points)

   d. Plan ahead for next time and have options in mind so that I do not continue to overeat. (1 point)

   e. Acknowledge that I have made a slip and get back on my program the next day. (1 point)

5. On a typical day, what are your eating patterns? (Circle all that apply.)

   a. I skip breakfast and save my calories for lunch and dinner. (0 point)

   b. I never really sit down for a meal. I am a "grazer" and eat whatever I find that is readily available. (0 point)

   c. I try to eat at least five servings of fruits and veggies and restrict saturated fats in my diet. (1 points)

   d. I eat several small meals, trying to be balanced in my portions and getting foods from different food groups. (1 points)

6. How would you describe your current support system for helping you lose weight? (Circle all that apply.)

   a. I believe I can do this best by doing it on my own. (0 points)

   b. I am not aware of any sources that can help me. (0 points)

   c. I have two to three friends or family members I can count on to help me. (1 point)

   d. There are counselors on campus with whom I can meet to plan a successful approach to weight loss. (1 point)

   e. I have the resources to join Weight Watchers or other community or online weight loss programs. (1 point)

7. How committed are you to exercising? (Circle all that apply.)

   a. Exercise is uncomfortable, embarrassing, and/or I don't enjoy it. (0 points)

   b. I don't have time to exercise. (0 points)

   c. I'd like to exercise, but I'm not sure how to get started. (1 point)

   d. I've visited my campus recreation center or local gym to explore my options. (2 points)

   e. There are specific sports or physical activities I do already, and I can plan to do more of them. (2 points)

8. What statement best describes your motivation to start a weight loss/lifestyle change program?

   a. I don't want to start losing weight. (0 points)

   b. I am thinking about it sometime in the distant future. (0 points)

   c. I am considering starting within the next few weeks; I just need to make a plan. (1 point)

   d. I'd like to start in the next few weeks, and I'm working on a plan. (2 points)

   e. I already have a plan in place, and I'm ready to begin tomorrow. (3 points)

Total points: _____

## Scoring

A score higher than 8 indicates that you may be ready to change; the higher your score above 8, the more successful you may be. Take a close look at areas that you could work on. Your behaviors, resources, readiness to change, and overall plan for change may give you the extra edge necessary to be successful.

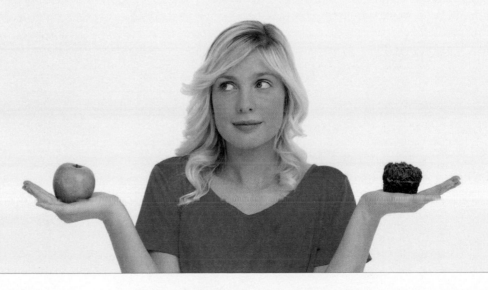

# YOUR PLAN FOR CHANGE

The **ASSESS YOURSELF** identifies six areas of importance in determining your readiness for weight loss. If you wish to lose weight to improve your health, understanding your attitudes about food and exercise will help you succeed.

**TODAY,** YOU CAN:

☐ Set SMART goals for weight loss and give them a reality check: Are they **s**pecific, **m**easurable, **a**chievable, **r**elevant, and **t**ime oriented? For example, rather than aiming to lose 15 pounds this month (which probably wouldn't be healthy or achievable), set a comfortable goal to lose 1 pound per week by diet and exercise changes.

☐ Keep a food log to identify the triggers that influence your eating habits. Think about what you can do to eliminate or reduce the influence of your two most common food triggers.

**WITHIN THE NEXT TWO WEEKS,** YOU CAN:

☐ Get in the habit of incorporating more fruits, vegetables, and whole grains in your diet and eating less fat. The next time you make dinner, look at the proportions on your plate. If vegetables and whole grains do not take up most of the space, substitute 1 cup of the meat, non-whole grains, or cheese in your meal with 1 cup of legumes, salad greens, or a favorite vegetable.

☐ Ramp up your exercise in small increments. Visit your campus recreation center or a local gym, and familiarize yourself with the equipment and facilities that are available. Try a new machine or sports activity, and experiment until you find something you really like.

**BY THE END OF THE SEMESTER,** YOU CAN:

☐ Get in the habit of grocery shopping every week and buying healthy, nutritious foods while avoiding high-fat, high-sugar, or overly processed foods. As you make healthy foods more available and unhealthy foods less available, you'll find it easier to eat better.

☐ Chart your progress and reward yourself as you meet your goals. Do something fun like see a movie, or buy that new pair of skinny jeans you've been wanting for (which will likely fit better than before!).

# STUDY PLAN

Customize your study plan—and master your health!—in the Study Area of MasteringHealth™

## CHAPTER REVIEW

 To hear an MP3 Tutor Session, scan here or visit the Study Area in MasteringHealth.

**LO 1 | Overweight and Obesity: A Growing Challenge**

- Overweight, obesity, and weight-related health problems have reached epidemic levels. *Globesity,* or global rates of obesity, threatens the health of many countries. Societal costs from obesity include increased health care costs and lowered worker productivity. Individual health risks from overweight and obesity include increased chance of developing cardiovascular diseases, arthritis, stroke, diabetes, gastrointestinal problems, low back pain, and a number of other diseases. Overweight individuals are also at risk of struggling with depression, low self-esteem, and high levels of stress.

**LO 2 | Factors Contributing to Overweight and Obesity**

- It is important to consider environmental, cultural, and socioeconomic factors when working to prevent obesity. In addition to genetics, metabolism, hormonal influences, excess fat cells, and physical risks, key environmental influences, such as poverty, socioeconomic status, education level, and lack of access to nutritious food, and lifestyle factors, including sedentary lifestyle and high calorie consumption, all make weight loss challenging.

**LO 3 | Assessing Body Weight and Body Composition**

- Percentage of body fat is a fairly reliable indicator for levels of overweight and obesity. There are many different methods of assessing body fat. Body mass index (BMI) is one of the most commonly accepted measures of weight based on height. *Overweight* is most commonly defined as a BMI of 25 to 29.9 and *obesity* as a BMI of 30 or greater. Waist circumference, or the amount of fat in the belly region, is believed to be related to the risk for several chronic diseases, particularly type 2 diabetes.

**LO 4 | Managing Your Weight**

- Increased physical activity, a balanced, healthy diet that controls caloric intake, and other strategies are recommended for controlling your weight. When these options fail and risks increase, doctor-recommended prescription medications, weight loss surgery, and other strategies are used to maintain or lose weight. However, sensible eating behavior and aerobic exercise and exercise that builds muscle mass offer the best options for weight loss and maintenance.

## POP QUIZ

Visit **MasteringHealth** to personalize your study plan with Chapter Review Quizzes and Dynamic Study Modules.

**LO 1 | Overweight and Obesity: A Growing Challenge.**

1. All of the following statements are true *except* which?
   a. Hispanic and non-Hispanic white men are more likely to be overweight/obese than non-Hispanic Black or Asian men.
   b. Children and adolescents living in higher income homes where parents are more educated have a greatly increased risk of obesity over those living in low income homes where parents are less educated and/or unemployed.
   c. Non-Hispanic black and Hispanic women are more likely to be overweight or obese than non-Hispanic white women.
   d. The United States has the distinction of being one of the fattest developed nations on earth.

**LO 2 | Factors Contributing to Overweight and Obesity**

2. The rate at which your body consumes food energy to sustain basic functions is your
   a. basal metabolic rate.
   b. resting metabolic rate.
   c. body mass index.
   d. set point.

3. All of the following statements are true *except* which?
   a. A slowing basal metabolic rate may contribute to weight gain after age 30.
   b. Hormones are increasingly implicated in hunger impulses and eating behavior.
   c. The more muscles you have, the fewer calories you will burn.
   d. Yo-yo dieting can make weight loss more difficult.

**LO 3 | Assessing Body Weight and Body Composition**

4. The proportion of your total weight that is made up of fat is called
   a. body composition.
   b. lean mass.
   c. percentage of body fat.
   d. BMI.

5. All of the following statements about BMI are true *except* which?
   a. BMI is based on height and weight measurements.
   b. BMI is accurate for everyone, including athletes with high amounts of muscle mass.
   c. Very low and very high BMI scores are associated with greater risk of mortality.
   d. BMI stands for "body mass index."

6. Which of the following body circumferences is most strongly associated with risk of heart disease and diabetes?
   a. Hip circumference
   b. Chest circumference
   c. Waist circumference
   d. Thigh circumference

7. One pound of additional body fat is created through consuming how many extra calories?
   a. 1,500 calories
   b. 3,500 calories
   c. 5,000 calories
   d. 7,000 calories

8. To lose weight, you must establish a(n)
   a. negative caloric balance.
   b. isocaloric balance.
   c. positive caloric balance.
   d. set point.

9. Successful weight maintainers are most likely to do which of the following?
   a. Eat two large meals a day before 1 P.M.
   b. Skip meals
   c. Drink diet sodas
   d. Eat high-volume but low-calorie density foods

10. Successful, healthy weight loss is characterized by
    a. a lifelong pattern of healthful eating and exercise.
    b. cutting out all fats and carbohydrates and eating a lean, mean, high-protein diet.
    c. never eating foods that are considered bad for you and rigidly adhering to a plan.
    d. a pattern of repeatedly losing and regaining weight.

*Answers to the Pop Quiz can be found on page A-1. If you answered a question incorrectly, review the section tagged by the Learning Outcome. For even more study tools, visit MasteringHealth.*

# THINK ABOUT IT!

### LO **1** | Overweight and Obesity: A Growing Challenge

1. Why do you think that obesity rates are rising in both developed and less-developed regions of the world? What strategies can we take collectively and individually to reduce risks of obesity nationally? Internationally?

### LO **2** | Factors Contributing to Overweight and Obesity

2. List the risk factors for your being overweight or obese right now. Which seem most likely to determine whether you will be obese in middle age?

### LO **3** | Assessing Body Weight and Body Composition

3. Which measurement would you choose to assess your fat levels? Why?

### LO **4** | Managing Your Weight

4. Are you satisfied with your body weight? If so, what do you do to maintain a healthy weight? If not, what are some lifestyle changes you could make to improve your weight and overall health?

# ACCESS YOUR HEALTH ON THE INTERNET

Visit **MasteringHealth** for links to the websites and RSS feeds. The following websites explore further topics and issues related to personal health. For links to these websites, visit MasteringHealth.

*Academy of Nutrition and Dietetics.* This site includes recommended dietary guidelines and other current information about weight control. **www.eatright.org**

*Weight Control Information Network.* This is an excellent resource for diet and weight control information. **http://win.niddk.nih.gov/index.htm**

*The Rudd Center for Food Policy and Obesity.* This website provides excellent information on the latest in obesity research, public policy, and ways we can stop the obesity epidemic at the community level. **www.uconnruddcenter.org/**

*The Obesity Society.* Key site for information/education about our national obesity epidemic, including statistics, research, consumer issues, and fact sheets. **www.obesity.org**

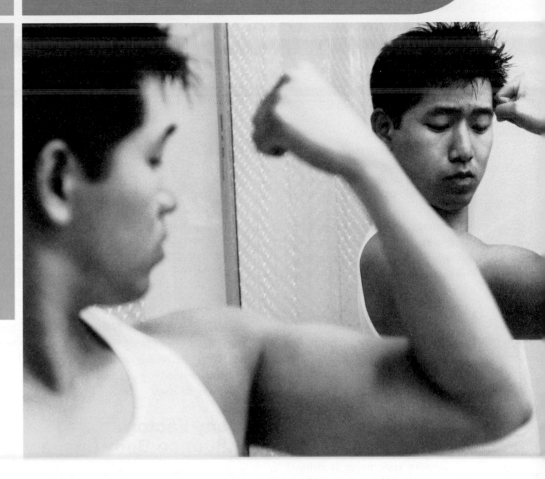

# FOCUS ON

# Enhancing Your Body Image

Dissatisfaction with one's appearance and shape is an all-too-common feeling in today's society that can foster unhealthy attitudes and thought patterns, as well as disordered eating and exercising behaviors.

## LEARNING OUTCOMES

1 Define body image, list the factors that influence it, and identify the difference between being dissatisfied with your appearance and body image disorders.

2 Describe the signs and symptoms of disordered eating, as well as the physical effects and treatment options for anorexia nervosa, bulimia nervosa, orthorexia nervosa, and binge-eating disorder.

3 List the criteria, symptoms, and treatment for exercise disorders such as muscle dysmorphia and female athlete triad.

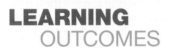

hen you look in the mirror, do you like what you see? If you feel disappointed, frustrated, or even angry, you're not alone. Preoccupation with appearance and a distorted image of how we look is a major problem for a wide range of people. In a UK study, 93 percent of the women reported negative thoughts about their appearance during the past week and wanted to lose weight, even though the majority were in the underweight or normal weight ranges.[1] Concerns about weight seem to be central to many people's body dissatisfaction. As body mass increases, dissatisfaction increases, particularly during transitional periods in life. Females, in particular, seem to experience peak levels of body dissatisfaction when transitioning from high school to young adulthood.[2] Sadly, dissatisfaction with your body can result in behaviors that disrupt your relationships, affect your mental health, and lead to life-threatening illness. Developing and maintaining a healthy body image can enhance your interactions with others, reduce stress, give you an increased sense of personal empowerment, and bring confidence and joy to your life.

# 80%

OF ADULT AMERICAN WOMEN REPORT DISSATISFACTION WITH THEIR **APPEARANCE**.

## LO 1 | **WHAT** IS BODY IMAGE?

Define body image, list the factors that influence it, and identify the difference between being dissatisfied with your appearance and body image disorders.

**Body image** refers to what you believe or emotionally feel about your body's shape, weight, and general appearance. More than what you see in the mirror, it includes the following:

- How you see yourself in your mind
- What you believe about your own appearance (including memories, assumptions, and generalizations)
- How you feel about your body, including your height, shape, and weight
- How you sense and control your body as you move

A *negative body image* is defined as either a distorted perception of your shape or feelings of discomfort, shame, or anxiety about your body. It may involve being certain that only people other than you are attractive and that your body is a sign of personal failure. In contrast, a *positive body image* is a true perception of your appearance: You see yourself as you really are. You understand that everyone is different, and you celebrate your uniqueness—including your perceived "flaws," which you know have nothing to do with your value as a person.

Is your body image negative or positive—or somewhere in between? Researchers have developed a body image continuum that may help you

---

**body image** How you see yourself in your mind, what you believe about your appearance, and how you feel about your body.

Although the exact nature of the "in" look may change from generation to generation, unrealistic images of both male and female celebrities are nothing new. In the 1960s, images of brawny film stars such as Clint Eastwood dominated the media. The physique of today's male celebrities is even more muscular and still very difficult for most to achieve themselves.

decide (see **FIGURE 1**). Notice that the continuum identifies behaviors associated with particular states, from total dissociation with one's body to body not being an issue.

## Many Factors Influence Body Image

You're not born with a body image, but you do begin to develop one at an early age. Let's look more closely at the factors that probably played a role in the development of your body image.

### The Media and Popular Culture

Media images tend to set the standard for what we find attractive, leading some people to go to dangerous extremes to have the biggest biceps or fit into size zero jeans. Changing our bodies or body parts to better achieve what current society feels is beautiful has long been part of American culture. During the early twentieth century, while men idolized the strong, hearty outdoorsman President Teddy Roosevelt, women pulled their corsets ever tighter to achieve unrealistically tiny waists. In the 1920s and 1930s, men emulated the burly cops and robbers in

gangster films, while women dieted and bound their breasts to achieve the boyish "flapper" look. By the 1960s, tough guys were the male ideal, whereas rail-thin supermodels embodied the nation's standard of female beauty. Today's societal obsession around appearance—even when many images are airbrushed or Photoshopped—isn't much different.

Social media popularity has also increased concerns regarding negative body images.[3] Many social media sites actively warn against posts promoting or glorifying self-harm, but even messages promoting unhealthy body images can still be hard to avoid. Such messages are often disguised as a type of encouragement—images of unrealistically thin bodies are coupled with catch phrases telling young people to get "thin" or avoid being "fat."[4] See **Student Health Today** on page 320 for more on "thinspiration."

Today, more than 69 percent of American adults 20 years and older are overweight or obese; thus, a significant disconnect exists between the media's idealized images of male and female bodies and the typical American body.[5] We are bombarded with unrealistic images of "beauty." In fact, one study conducted with college women of

| Body hate/<br>disassociation | Distorted body<br>image | Body preoccupied/<br>obsessed | Body acceptance | Body ownership |
|---|---|---|---|---|
| I often feel separated and distant from my body—as if it belonged to someone else.<br><br>I hate my body, and I often isolate myself from others.<br><br>I don't see anything positive or even neutral about my body shape and size.<br><br>I don't believe others when they tell me I look okay.<br><br>I hate the way I look in the mirror. | I spend a significant amount of time exercising and dieting to change my body.<br><br>My body shape and size keeps me from dating or finding someone who will treat me the way I want to be treated.<br><br>I have considered changing (or have changed) my body shape and size through surgical means.<br><br>I wish I could change the way I look in the mirror. | I weigh and measure myself a lot.<br><br>I spend a significant amount of time viewing myself in the mirror.<br><br>I compare my body to others.<br><br>I have days when I feel fat.<br><br>I accept society's ideal body shape and size as the best body shape and size.<br><br>I'd be more attractive if I were thinner, more muscular, etc. | I pay attention to my body and my appearance because it is important to me, but it only occupies a small part of my day.<br><br>I would like to change some things about my body, but I spend most of my time highlighting my positive features.<br><br>My self-esteem is based on my personality traits, achievements, and relationships—not just my body image. | I feel fine about my body.<br><br>I don't worry about changing my body shape or weight.<br><br>I never weigh or measure myself.<br><br>My feelings about my body are not influenced by society's concept of an ideal body shape.<br><br>I know that the significant others in my life will always love me for who I am, not for how I look. |

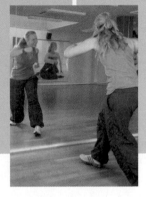

VIDEO TUTOR
Body Image Continuum

**FIGURE 1 Body Image Continuum** This continuum shows a range of attitudes and behaviors toward body image. Functioning at either extreme—not caring at all or being obsessed—leads to problems. When you are functioning in the "body acceptance" area, you are taking care of your body and emotions.

**Source:** Adapted from Smiley/King/Avery, "Eating Issues and Body Image Continuum," Campus Health Service 1996. Copyright © 1997 Arizona Board of Regents for University of Arizona.

multiple ethnicities found that female body dissatisfaction was attributed to perceptions of celebrity role models and Western culture's thin idealization.[6]

## Family, Community, and Cultural Groups

The people with whom we most often interact—our family members, friends, and others—strongly influence the way we see ourselves. Parents are especially influential in body image development. For instance, it's common and natural for fathers of adolescent girls to experience feelings of discomfort related to their daughters' changing bodies. If they are able to navigate these feelings successfully and validate the acceptability of their daughters' appearance throughout puberty, they'll help their daughters maintain a positive body image. In contrast, even subtle judgments about their daughters' changing bodies may prompt girls to question how males view their bodies in general. In addition, mothers who model body acceptance or body ownership may be more likely to foster a positive body image in their daughters, whereas mothers who are frustrated with or ashamed of their own bodies may foster negative attitudes.

Interactions with siblings and other relatives, peers, teachers, coworkers, and other community members can also influence body image development. For instance, peer harassment (teasing and bullying) is widely acknowledged to contribute to a negative body image. Associations within one's cultural group are also a factor. For example, studies have found that European American females experience the highest rates of body dissatisfaction, and as a minority group becomes more acculturated into the mainstream and exposed to media, the body dissatisfaction levels of women in that group increase.[7]

## Physiological and Psychological Factors

Recent neurological research suggests that people who have been diagnosed with a body image disorder show differences in the brain's ability to regulate mood-linked

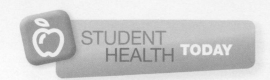

# THINSPIRATION AND THE ONLINE WORLD OF ANOREXIA

The pro-anorexia movement has a host of websites, chat rooms, blogs, and discussion boards mostly created and hosted by girls and women struggling with eating disorders. With dangerous and incorrect information about restrictive eating, metabolism, binging, and laxative abuse, many include "thinspiration"—pictures and quotes intended to inspire visitors to thinness—as well as tips and tricks to hide and maintain disordered eating.

Despite the support and understanding that participating women get from each other, they also encourage each other to remain sick. Ambivalent messages about thinness and weight loss coincide with how many visitors feel about their own eating disorder. Many sites claim it is not their intention to recruit new "members"; on the same site, though, you may find tips on "how to become anorexic."

Recently, France voted to punish anyone encouraging people to become dangerously thin with a year in prison and a fine of roughly $11,000. While French authorities have focused on fashion websites, which encourage women to keep their weight as low as possible, pro-anorexia sites are clear violators. Brazil, Italy, and Spain have all taken action against skinny models in fashion shows.

**Sources:** K. Davis, "Ana & Mia: The Online World of Anorexia and Bulimia," *OHPE Bulletin* 244, no. 1 (2002), www.ohpe.ca/node/160; National Eating Disorder Information Centre, www.nedic.ca; MPA Website, Accessed May 2015, www.myproana.com/index.php/blogs/; P. Allen and I. Sparks, " France Cracks Down on 'Pro-Anorexia" Websites that Encourage Young Women to Keep Their Weight as Low as Possible," *The Daily Mail*, April 2, 2015, www.dailymail.co.uk/news/article-3023026/France-cracks-pro-anorexia-websites-encourage-young-women-weight-low-possible.html

---

chemicals called *neurotransmitters*.[8] Poor regulation of neurotransmitters is also involved in depression, anxiety disorders, and obsessive-compulsive disorder. One study linked distortions in body image, particularly the face, to a malfunction in the brain's visual processing region that was revealed by magnetic resonance imaging (MRI) scanning.[9]

## Building a Positive Body Image

To develop a more positive body image, start by challenging some commonly held myths and attitudes in contemporary society.[10]

**Myth 1: How you look is more important than who you are.** Do you think your weight is important in defining who you are? How much does it matter to you to have thin and attractive friends? How important do you think being thin is for attracting your ideal partner?

**Myth 2: Anyone can be slender and attractive if they work at it.** When you see someone who is extremely thin, what assumptions do you make about that person? When you see someone who is overweight or obese, what assumptions do you make? Have you ever berated yourself for not having the "willpower" to change some aspect of your body?

**Myth 3: Extreme dieting is an effective weight-loss strategy.** Do you believe in trying fad diets or "quick-weight-loss" products? How far would you be willing to go to attain the "perfect" body?

**Myth 4: Appearance is more important than health.** How do you evaluate whether a person is healthy? Is your desire to change some aspect of your body motivated by health reasons or by concerns about appearance?

For ways to bust these toxic myths and attitudes and to build a more positive body image, check out the **Skills for Behavior Change** box.

## Body Image Disorders

Although most Americans are dissatisfied with some aspect of their appearance, very few have a true body image

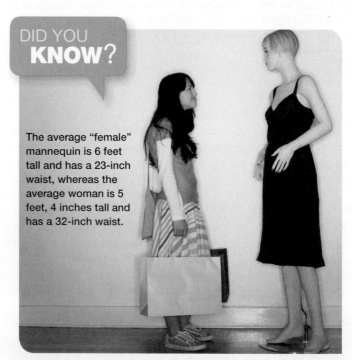

**DID YOU KNOW?**

The average "female" mannequin is 6 feet tall and has a 23-inch waist, whereas the average woman is 5 feet, 4 inches tall and has a 32-inch waist.

**Sources:** R. Duyff, *American Dietetic Association Complete Food and Nutrition Guide*, 4th ed. (Hoboken, NJ: John Wiley & Sons, Inc., 2012), 50; C. Fryar, Q. Gu, and C. Ogden, "Anthropometric Reference Data for Children and Adults: United States, 2007–2010," National Center for Health Statistics, *Vital and Health Statistics*, Series 11, no. 252 (2012), www.cdc.gov/nchs/data/series/sr_11/sr11_252.pdf

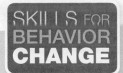
## TEN STEPS TO A POSITIVE BODY IMAGE

One way to turn negative thoughts positive is to think about how to look more healthfully and happily at yourself and your body. The more you try, the better you will feel about who you are and the body you naturally have.

▶ **Step 1.** Appreciate all of the amazing things your body does for you—running, dancing, breathing, laughing, dreaming.

▶ **Step 2.** Make a list of things you like about yourself—things that aren't related to how much you weigh or how you look. Add to it as you notice things.

▶ **Step 3.** Remind yourself that true beauty is not skin deep. When you feel good about yourself and who you are, you carry yourself with a sense of confidence, self-acceptance, and openness that makes you beautiful.

▶ **Step 4.** Look at yourself as a whole person. When you see yourself in a mirror or in your mind, choose not to focus on specific body parts.

▶ **Step 5.** Surround yourself with positive people. It is easier to feel good about yourself when you are around those who are supportive and who recognize the importance of liking yourself as you naturally are.

▶ **Step 6.** Shut down those voices in your head that tell you your body is not "right" or that you are a "bad" person.

▶ **Step 7.** Wear comfortable clothes that make you feel good about your body. Work with your body, not against it.

▶ **Step 8.** Become a critical viewer of social and media messages. Pay attention to images, slogans, and attitudes that make you feel bad about your appearance.

▶ **Step 9.** Show appreciation for your body. Take a bubble bath, make time for a nap, or find a peaceful place outside to relax.

▶ **Step 10.** Use the time and energy you might have spent worrying about food, calories, and your weight to do something to help others. Reaching out to other people can help you feel better about yourself and make a positive change in our world.

**Source:** "10 Steps to Positive Body Image," from National Eating Disorders Association website, April 22, 2013. Copyright © 2013 National Eating Disorders Association. Reprinted with permission. For more information visit **www.NationalEatingDisorders.org** or call NEDA's helpline 1-800-931-2237.

**body dysmorphic disorder (BDD)** Psychological disorder characterized by an obsession with one's appearance and a distorted view of one's body or with a minor or imagined flaw in appearance.

**social physique anxiety (SPA)** A desire to look good that has a destructive effect on a person's ability to function well in social interactions and relationships.

estimated that 10 percent of people seeking dermatology or cosmetic treatments have BDD.[13] Not only do such actions fail to address the underlying problem, but also they are actually considered diagnostic signs of BDD. Psychiatric treatment, including psychotherapy and/or antidepressant medications, can help.

## Social Physique Anxiety

An emerging problem for both young men and women is **social physique anxiety (SPA).** The desire to "look good" becomes so strong it has a destructive and sometimes disabling effect on the person's ability to

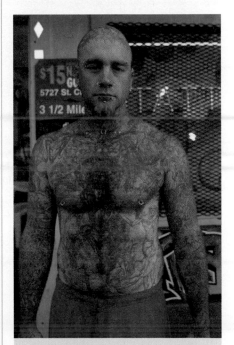

It's not always easy to spot people who are highly dissatisfied with their bodies. People who cover their bodies with tattoos may have a strong sense of self-esteem. On the other hand, extreme tattooing can be an outward sign of a severe body image disturbance known as body dysmorphic disorder.

disorder. However, several diagnosable body image disorders affect a small percentage of the population. Two of the most common are body dysmorphic disorder and social physique anxiety.

## Body Dysmorphic Disorder

Approximately 1 percent of people in the United States suffer from **body dysmorphic disorder (BDD).**[11] Persons with BDD are obsessively concerned with their appearance and have a distorted view of their own body shape, size, weight, perceived lack of muscles, facial blemishes, size of body parts, etc. Although the cause of the disorder isn't known, an anxiety disorder or obsessive-compulsive disorder is often present as well. Contributing factors may include genetic susceptibility, childhood teasing, physical or sexual abuse, low self-esteem, and rigid sociocultural expectations of beauty.[12]

People with BDD may try to fix their perceived flaws through abuse of steroids, excessive bodybuilding, cosmetic surgeries, extreme tattooing, or other appearance-altering behaviors. It is

| Eating disordered | Disruptive eating patterns | Food preoccupied/ obsessed | Concerned in a healthy way | Food is not an issue |
|---|---|---|---|---|
| I worry about what I will eat or when I will exercise all the time. | My food and exercise concerns are starting to interfere with my school and social life. | I think about food a lot. | I pay attention to what I eat in order to maintain a healthy body. | I am not concerned about what or how much I eat. |
| I follow a very rigid eating plan and know precisely how many calories, fat grams, or carbohydrates I eat every day. | I use food to comfort myself. | I'm obsessed with reading books and magazines about dieting, fitness, and weight control. | Food and exercise are important parts of my life, but they only occupy a small part of my time. | I feel no guilt or shame no matter what I eat or how much I eat. |
| I feel incredible guilt, shame, and anxiety when I break my diet. | I have tried diet pills, laxatives, vomiting, or extra time exercising in order to lose or maintain my weight. | I sometimes miss school, work, and social events because of my diet or exercise schedule. | I enjoy eating, and I balance my pleasure with my concern for a healthy body. | Exercise is not really important to me. I choose foods based on cost, taste, and convenience, with little regard to health. |
| I regularly stuff myself and then exercise, vomit, or use laxatives to get rid of the food. | I have fasted or avoided eating for long periods of time in order to lose or maintain my weight. | I divide food into "good" and "bad" categories. | I usually eat three balanced meals daily, plus snacks, to fuel my body with adequate energy. | My eating is very sporadic and irregular. |
| My friends and family tell me I am too thin, but I feel fat. | If I cannot exercise to burn off calories, I panic. | I feel guilty when I eat "bad" foods or when I eat more than what I feel I should be eating. | I am moderate and flexible in my goals for eating well and being physically active. | I don't worry about meals; I just eat whatever I can, whenever I can. |
| I am out of control when I eat. | I feel strong when I can restrict how much I eat. | I am afraid of getting fat. | Sometimes I eat more (or less) than I really need, but most of the time I listen to my body. | I enjoy stuffing myself with lots of tasty food at restaurants, holiday meals, and social events. |
| I am afraid to eat in front of others. | I feel out of control when I eat more than I wanted to. | I wish I could change how much I want to eat and what I am hungry for. | | |
| I prefer to eat alone. | | | | |

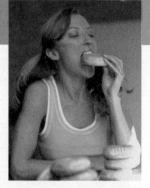
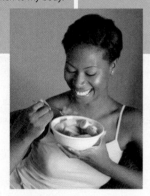

**FIGURE 2** Eating Issues Continuum This continuum shows progression from eating disorders to normal eating. Being concerned in a healthy way is the goal, rather than functioning at either extreme.

**Source:** Adapted from Smiley/King/Avery, "Eating Issues and Body Image Continuum," Campus Health Service 1996. Copyright © 1997 Arizona Board of Regents for University of Arizona.

function effectively in relationships and interactions with others. People suffering from SPA spend a disproportionate amount of time fixating on their bodies, working out, and performing tasks that are ego centered and self-directed, rather than focusing on interpersonal relationships and general tasks.[14] Experts speculate that this anxiety may contribute to disordered eating.

**disordered eating** A pattern of atypical eating behaviors that is used to achieve or maintain a lower body weight.

## LO 2 | DISORDERED EATING AND EATING DISORDERS

Describe the signs and symptoms of disordered eating, as well as the physical effects and treatment options for anorexia nervosa, bulimia nervosa, orthorexia nervosa, and binge-eating disorder.

- - - - - - - - - - - - - - - - - - - - - - - - - -

People with a negative body image can fixate on a wide range of self-perceived "flaws." The so-called flaw that distresses the majority of people with negative body image is feeling overweight.

Some people channel weight-related anxiety into self-defeating thoughts and harmful behaviors. The far left of the eating issues continuum (**FIGURE 2**) identifies a pattern of thoughts and behaviors associated with **disordered eating**, including chronic dieting, rigid eating patterns, abusing diet pills and laxatives, self-induced vomiting, and many others.

Few people who exhibit disordered eating patterns progress to a clinical **eating disorder.** The eating disorders defined by the American Psychiatric Association (APA) in the *Diagnostic and*

*Statistical Manual of Mental Disorders, Fifth Edition (DSM-5)* are *anorexia nervosa, bulimia nervosa, binge-eating disorder,* and a cluster of less-distinct conditions collectively referred to as other specified feeding or eating disorder (OSFED).[15]

Twenty million women and 10 million men in the United States will suffer from some sort of eating disorder over their lifetimes.[16] Although anorexia nervosa and bulimia nervosa used to affect people primarily in their teens and twenties, increasing numbers of children as young as 7 have been diagnosed, as have women as old as 80.[17] In 2014, 2.1 percent of college students self-reported as having anorexia or bulimia.[18] Disordered eating and eating disorders are also common among ballet dancers and athletes, particularly athletes in sports with an aesthetic component (e.g., figure skating or gymnastics) or tied to a weight class (e.g., tae kwon do, judo, or wrestling).[19]

Eating disorders are on the rise among men, who make up nearly 25 percent of all anorexia and bulimia patients.[20] Many men suffering from eating disorders fail to seek treatment because these illnesses are traditionally thought of as a woman's problem.

What factors put individuals at risk? Many people with eating disorders feel disenfranchised in other aspects of their lives and try to gain a sense of control through food. Many are clinically depressed, suffer from obsessive-compulsive disorder, or have other psychiatric problems. In addition, individuals with low self-esteem, negative body image, and a high tendency for perfectionism are at risk.[21]

## Anorexia Nervosa

**Anorexia nervosa** is a persistent, chronic eating disorder characterized by deliberate food restriction and severe, life-threatening weight loss. It has the highest

**SEE IT!** VIDEOS

How do you treat the most common but least well known eating disorder?

Watch **EDNOS: Most Dangerous, Unheard of Eating Disorder** on **MasteringHealth**™

death rate (20%) of any psychological illness.[22] It involves self-starvation motivated by an intense fear of gaining weight and an extremely distorted body image. Initially, most people with anorexia nervosa lose weight by reducing total food intake, particularly of high-calorie foods. Eventually, they progress to restricting their intake of almost all foods. The little they do eat, they may purge through vomiting or using laxatives. Although they lose weight, people with anorexia nervosa never feel thin enough. An estimated 0.3 percent of females suffer from anorexia nervosa in their lifetime.[23]

**FIGURE 3** illustrates physical symptoms and negative health consequences associated with anorexia nervosa.

Causes of anorexia nervosa are complex and variable. Many people with anorexia have other coexisting psychiatric problems, including low self-esteem, depression, an anxiety disorder such as obsessive-compulsive disorder, and substance abuse. Some people have a history of being physically or sexually abused, and others have troubled interpersonal relationships. Cultural norms that value appearance and glorify thinness as beauty are factors, as are weight-based shame, peer comparisons, and weight bias.[24] Physical factors are thought to include an imbalance of neurotransmitters and genetic susceptibility.[25]

## Bulimia Nervosa

Individuals with **bulimia nervosa** often binge on huge amounts of

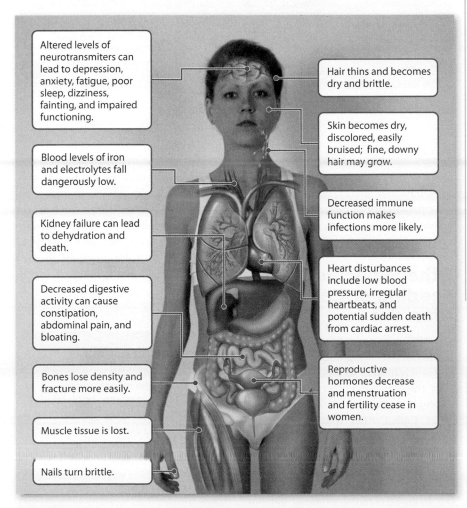

Altered levels of neurotransmiters can lead to depression, anxiety, fatigue, poor sleep, dizziness, fainting, and impaired functioning.

Blood levels of iron and electrolytes fall dangerously low.

Kidney failure can lead to dehydration and death.

Decreased digestive activity can cause constipation, abdominal pain, and bloating.

Bones lose density and fracture more easily.

Muscle tissue is lost.

Nails turn brittle.

Hair thins and becomes dry and brittle.

Skin becomes dry, discolored, easily bruised; fine, downy hair may grow.

Decreased immune function makes infections more likely.

Heart disturbances include low blood pressure, irregular heartbeats, and potential sudden death from cardiac arrest.

Reproductive hormones decrease and menstruation and fertility cease in women.

**FIGURE 3** What Anorexia Nervosa Can Do to the Body

**eating disorder** A psychiatric disorder characterized by severe disturbances in body image and eating behaviors.

**anorexia nervosa** Eating disorder characterized by deliberate food restriction, self-starvation, or extreme exercising to achieve weight loss, and an extremely distorted body image.

**bulimia nervosa** Eating disorder characterized by binge eating followed by inappropriate purging measures or compensatory behavior, such as vomiting or excessive exercise, to prevent weight gain.

food—often with a feeling of being out of control—and then engage in some kind of purging or compensatory behavior, such as vomiting, taking laxatives, or exercising excessively, to lose the calories they have just consumed. People with bulimia are obsessed with their bodies, weight gain, and appearance, but unlike those with anorexia, their problem is often hidden from the public eye because their weight may fall within a normal range or they may be overweight. Up to 3 percent of adolescents and young women are bulimic; rates among men are about 10 percent of the rate among women.[26]

**FIGURE 4** illustrates the physical symptoms and negative health consequences associated with bulimia nervosa.

A combination of genetic and environmental factors is thought to cause bulimia nervosa.[27] A family history of obesity, an underlying anxiety disorder, and an imbalance in neurotransmitters are all possible contributing factors. In support of the role of neurotransmitters, a study showed that brain circuitry involved in regulating impulsive behavior seems to be less active in women with bulimia than in healthy women.[28] However, it is unknown whether such differences exist before bulimia develops or arise as a consequence of the disorder.

## Binge-Eating Disorder

Individuals with **binge-eating disorder** gorge themselves, but do not take excessive measures to lose the weight gained. Thus, they are often clinically obese. Binge-eating episodes are typically characterized by eating large amounts of food rapidly, even when not feeling

---

binge-eating disorder A type of eating disorder characterized by gorging on food once a week or more, but not typically followed by a purge.

other specified feeding or eating disorder (OSFED) Eating disorders that are a true psychiatric illness but that do not fit the strict diagnostic criteria for anorexia nervosa, bulimia nervosa, or binge-eating disorder.

orthorexia nervosa An eating disorder characterized by fixation on food quality and purity.

---

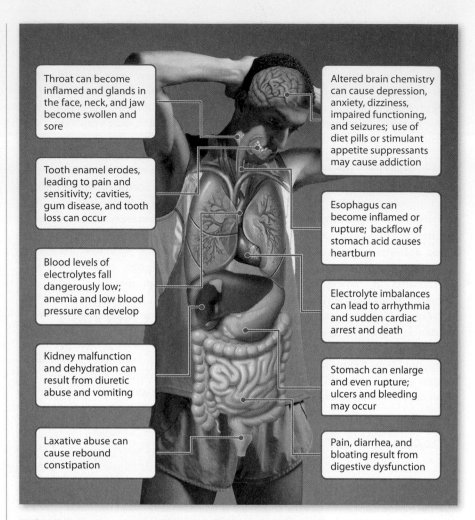

Throat can become inflamed and glands in the face, neck, and jaw become swollen and sore

Tooth enamel erodes, leading to pain and sensitivity; cavities, gum disease, and tooth loss can occur

Blood levels of electrolytes fall dangerously low; anemia and low blood pressure can develop

Kidney malfunction and dehydration can result from diuretic abuse and vomiting

Laxative abuse can cause rebound constipation

Altered brain chemistry can cause depression, anxiety, dizziness, impaired functioning, and seizures; use of diet pills or stimulant appetite suppressants may cause addiction

Esophagus can become inflamed or rupture; backflow of stomach acid causes heartburn

Electrolyte imbalances can lead to arrhythmia and sudden cardiac arrest and death

Stomach can enlarge and even rupture; ulcers and bleeding may occur

Pain, diarrhea, and bloating result from digestive dysfunction

**FIGURE 4** What Bulimia Nervosa Can Do to the Body

hungry, and feeling guilty or depressed after overeating.[29]

A national survey reported a lifetime prevalence of binge-eating disorder in the study participants of 1.4 percent.[30]

## Other Specified Feeding or Eating Disorder

The APA recognizes that some patterns of disordered eating qualify as a legitimate psychiatric illness but don't fit into the strict diagnostic criteria for anorexia, bulimia, or binge-eating disorder. Called **other specified feeding or eating disorders (OSFED),** this group of disorders includes five specific subtypes: *night eating syndrome, purging disorder, binge-eating disorder of low frequency/limited duration, bulimia*

*nervosa of low frequency/duration, and atypical anorexia nervosa.* Atypical anorexia nervosa is defined in this category as displaying anorexic features without low weight.[31] All of these subtypes can cause remarkable distress or impairment but don't exhibit the full criteria of another feeding or eating disorder.

### WHAT DO YOU THINK?

Is attention to the national obesity epidemic likely to worsen problems with eating disorders? Why or why not?

■ What do you think can be done to increase awareness of eating disorders in the United States?

■ Can you think of ways to prevent eating disorders?

## Orthorexia Nervosa

Literally meaning "fixation on righteous eating," **orthorexia nervosa** is an unhealthy obsession with what would otherwise be healthy eating. What typically begins as a simple attempt to eat more healthfully can become a fixation with food quality and purity. Those with orthorexia nervosa become consumed with what and how much to eat and how to deal with eating mistakes. Eventually, food choices become so restrictive that health suffers.

## Treatment for Eating Disorders

Because eating disorders are caused by a combination of factors, there are no simple solutions. Without treatment, approximately 20 percent of people with a serious eating disorder will die as a result; with treatment, long-term full recovery rates range from 44 to 76 percent for anorexia nervosa and from 50 to 70 percent for bulimia nervosa.[32]

Treatment often focuses first on reducing the threat to life. Once the patient is stabilized, long-term therapy focuses on the psychological, social, environmental, and physiological factors that have led to the problem. Through therapy, the patient works on adopting new eating behaviors, building self-confidence, and finding healthy ways to deal with life's problems. Support groups can help the family and the individual learn positive actions and interactions. Treatment of an underlying anxiety disorder or depression may also be a focus.

## Helping Someone with Disordered Eating

Although every situation is different, there are several things you can do if you suspect someone you know is struggling with disordered eating:[33]

- **Learn** as much as you can about disordered eating.
- **Know the facts** about weight, nutrition, and exercise. Accurate

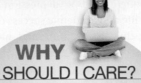

### WHY SHOULD I CARE?

Although exercising is generally beneficial to your health, doing it compulsively can lead to broken bones, joint injuries, and even depression—all of which can put you out of commission for the other things you enjoy. Remember that moderation is essential and taking rest days is important to your health.

information can help you reason against excuses used to maintain a disordered eating pattern.

- **Be honest** and talk openly about your concerns.
- **Be caring, but be firm** because caring about your friend does not mean allowing him or her to manipulate you. Your friend must be responsible for his or her actions and the

consequences of those actions. Avoid making statements that you cannot or will not uphold.

- **Compliment** your friend's personality, successes, and accomplishments.
- **Be a good role model** for healthy eating, exercise, and self-acceptance.
- **Tell someone**, and don't wait until your friend's life is in danger. Addressing disordered eating patterns in their beginning stages offers your friend the best chance for working through these issues and becoming healthy again.

There are many resources for people who are considering seeking help or finding out if they are at risk for developing an eating disorder. The National Eating Disorders Association has a general online screening tool allowing individuals to assess their own patterns to determine if they should seek professional help (www.nationaleatingdisorders.org/online-eating-disorder-screening). They also have additional information and a helpline (1-800-931-2237) for guidance, treatment referrals, and support.[34]

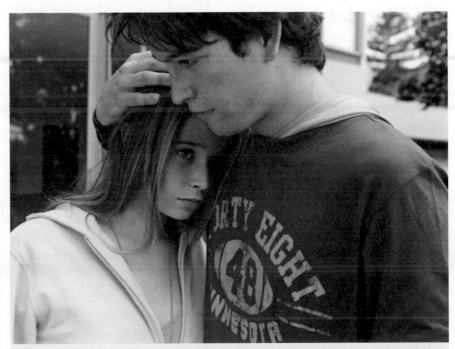

When talking to a friend about an eating disorder or disordered eating patterns, avoid casting blame, preaching, or offering unsolicited advice. Instead, be a good listener, let the person know that you care, and offer your support.

## LO 3 | EXERCISE DISORDERS

List the criteria, symptoms, and treatment for exercise disorders such as muscle dysmorphia and female athlete triad.

Although exercise is generally beneficial, in excess it can be a problem. In addition to being a common compensatory behavior used by people with anorexia or bulimia, exercise can become a compulsion or contribute to more complex disorders such as muscle dysmorphia or the female athlete triad.

## Compulsive Exercise

In a recent study, researchers showed that participants used excessive exercise or **compulsive exercise** as a way to regulate their emotions.[35] Also called *anorexia athletica,* compulsive exercise is characterized not by a *desire* to exercise but a *compulsion;* that is, the person struggles with guilt and anxiety if he or she doesn't work out. Compulsive exercisers, like people with eating disorders, often define their self-worth externally. They overexercise in order to feel more in control of their lives. Disordered eating or an eating disorder is often part of the picture.

Compulsive exercise can contribute to a variety of injuries. It can also put significant stress on the heart, especially if combined with disordered eating. Psychologically, people who engage in compulsive exercise are often plagued by anxiety and/or depression. Their social life and academic success can suffer as they fixate more and more on exercise.

## Muscle Dysmorphia

**Muscle dysmorphia** is a form of body image disturbance and exercise disorder in which a person (usually male) believes his body is insufficiently lean or muscular.[36] Men who have muscle dysmorphia believe, despite looking normal or even unusually brawny, that they look "puny." Because of their adherence to a meticulous diet and time-consuming workout schedule, and their shame over their perceived appearance flaws, important social or occupational activities may fall by the wayside. Other behaviors characteristic of muscle dysmorphia include comparing oneself unfavorably to others, checking one's appearance in the mirror, and camouflaging one's appearance. Men with muscle dysmorphia also are likely to abuse anabolic steroids and dietary supplements.[37]

## The Female Athlete Triad

In an effort to be the best, some women may put themselves at risk for developing a syndrome called the **female athlete triad.** *Triad* means "three," and the three interrelated problems are low energy (food) intake, typically prompted by disordered eating behaviors; menstrual dysfunction such as amenorrhea; and poor bone density (**FIGURE 5**).[38]

How does the female athlete triad develop, and what makes it so dangerous? First, a chronic pattern of low energy intake and intensive exercise alters normal body functions. For example, when an athlete restricts her

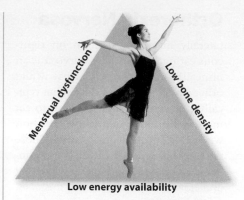

**FIGURE 5** The Female Athlete Triad

eating, she can deplete her body stores of nutrients essential to health. At the same time, her body begins to burn its stores of fat tissue for energy. Adequate body fat is essential to maintaining healthy levels of the female reproductive hormone *estrogen;* when an athlete isn't getting enough food, estrogen levels decline. This can manifest as amenorrhea: The body is using all calories to keep the athlete alive, and nonessential body functions such as menstruation cease. In addition, fat-soluble vitamins, calcium, and estrogen are all essential for dense, healthy bones, so their depletion weakens the athlete's bones, leaving her at high risk for fracture.

The female athlete triad is particularly prevalent in women who participate in highly competitive individual sports or activities that emphasize leanness and require body-contouring clothing. Gymnasts, figure skaters, cross-country runners, and ballet dancers are among those at highest risk for the female athlete triad.

**SEE IT! VIDEOS**

Can you go too far with extreme exercise? Watch **Young Boys Exercising to Extremes,** available on MasteringHealth™

---

**compulsive exercise** Disorder characterized by a compulsion to engage in excessive amounts of exercise and feelings of guilt and anxiety if the level of exercise is perceived as inadequate.

**muscle dysmorphia** Body image disorder in which men believe that their bodies are insufficiently lean or muscular.

**female athlete triad** A syndrome of three interrelated health problems seen in some female athletes: disordered eating, amenorrhea, and poor bone density.

## Are Your Efforts to Be Thin Sensible—Or Are You Spinning Out of Control?

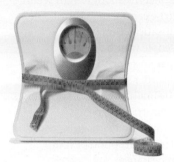

Just because you weigh yourself, count calories, or work out every day doesn't necessarily mean you have any of the health concerns discussed in this chapter. On the other hand, efforts to lose a few pounds can spiral out of control. To assess whether your efforts to be thin are harmful to you, take the following quiz from the National Eating Disorders Association (NEDA).

| | | | |
|---|---|---|---|
| 1. | I constantly calculate numbers of fat grams and calories. | T | F |
| 2. | I weigh myself often and find myself obsessed with the number on the scale. | T | F |
| 3. | I exercise to burn calories and not for health or enjoyment. | T | F |
| 4. | I sometimes feel out of control while eating. | T | F |
| 5. | I often go on extreme diets. | T | F |
| 6. | I engage in rituals to get me through mealtimes and/or secretively binge. | T | F |
| 7. | Weight loss, dieting, and controlling my food intake have become my major concerns. | T | F |
| 8. | I feel ashamed, disgusted, or guilty after eating. | T | F |
| 9. | I constantly worry about the weight, shape, and/or size of my body. | T | F |
| 10. | I feel my identity and value are based on how I look or how much I weigh. | T | F |

If any of these statements is true for you, you could be dealing with disordered eating. If so, talk about it! Tell a friend, parent, teacher, coach, youth group leader, doctor, counselor, or nutritionist what you're going through. Check out the NEDA's Sharing with EEEase handout at www.nationaleatingdisorders.org/sharing-eeease for help planning what to say the first time you talk to someone about your eating and exercise habits.

**Source:** Adapted from "NEDA Screening for Eating Disorders" by the National Eating Disorders Association (NEDA) and Screening for Mental Health, Inc. (SMH), from NEDA website. Copyright © 2013 NEDA and SMH. Reprinted with permission.

## YOUR PLAN FOR **CHANGE**

The **ASSESS YOURSELF** activity gives you a chance to evaluate your feelings about your body. Below are some steps you can take to improve your body image.

**TODAY,** YOU CAN:

☐ Talk back to the media. Write letters to advertisers and magazines that depict unhealthy and unrealistic body types. Boycott their products or start a blog commenting on harmful body image messages in the media.

☐ Just for today, eat the recommended number of servings from every food group at every meal. And don't count calories!

**WITHIN THE NEXT TWO WEEKS,** YOU CAN:

☐ Find a photograph of a person you admire for his or her contributions to humanity. Put it up next to your mirror to remind yourself that true beauty comes from within and benefits others.

☐ Start a journal. Each day, record one thing you are grateful for that has nothing to do with your appearance. At the end of each day, record one small thing you did to make someone's world a little brighter.

**BY THE END OF THE SEMESTER,** YOU CAN:

☐ Establish a group of friends who support you for who you are, not what you look like and who get the same support from you. Form a group on a favorite social-networking site, and keep in touch, especially when you feel troubled by self-defeating thoughts or have the urge to engage in unhealthy behaviors.

☐ Borrow from the library or purchase one of the many books on body image now available, and read it!

## CHAPTER REVIEW

 To head an MP3 Tutor Session, scan here or visit the Study Area in **MasteringHealth.**

### LO 1 | What Is Body Image?

■ Body image refers to what you believe or emotionally feel about your body's shape, weight, and general appearance.

### LO 2 | Disordered Eating and Eating Disorders

■ Millions of Americans will struggle with an eating disorder at some point in their lives. Media, family, community, cultural groups, and psychological and physiological factors all influence body image.

■ Anorexia nervosa is a persistent, chronic eating disorder characterized by deliberate food restriction and severe, life-threatening weight loss.

■ Individuals with bulimia nervosa rapidly consume large amounts of food and purge either with vomiting or laxative abuse or by using non-purging techniques such as excessive exercise and/or fasting.

■ Individuals with binge-eating disorder gorge themselves but do not take excessive measures to lose weight.

■ Orthorexia nervosa is an unhealthy obsession with a rigid diet focused on food quality and purity.

■ Eating disorders are caused by a combination of many factors, and there are no simple solutions. Without treatment, approximately 20 percent of people with a serious eating disorder will die from it. Long-term treatment focuses on the psychological, social, environmental, and physiological factors that have led to the problem.

### LO 3 | Exercise Disorders

■ Compulsive exercise is used as a way to regulate emotions. Also called *anorexia athletica,* compulsive exercise is characterized by a compulsion to exercise, resulting in guilt and anxiety if the person doesn't work out.

■ Muscle dysmorphia, typically found in men, is characterized by a distorted belief that their body is insufficiently muscular or lean. As a result, they spend an inordinate amount of time working out.

■ The female triad syndrome occurs when female athletes restrict their food intake and train intensively, altering their normal body functions. Three interrelated problems occur: low energy intake; menstrual dysfunction, and poor bone density.

■ Treatment requires a multidisciplinary approach involving the coach, psychologist, and family members.

## POP QUIZ

Visit **MasteringHealth** to personalize your study plan with Chapter Review Quizzes and Dynamic Study Modules.

### LO 1 | What Is Body Image?

1. All of the statements about body image are true *except* which?
   a. The obsession with having big biceps or being able to wear size zero skinny jeans began in the late 1990s.
   b. Concerns about weight seems to be central to many people's dissatisfaction with their body.
   c. People who have been diagnosed with a body image disorder show differences in the brain's ability to regulate neurotransmitters.
   d. Positive body image is possessing a true perception of your appearance.

### LO 2 | Disordered Eating and Eating Disorders

2. Orthorexia nervosa is
   a. an excessive focus on eating foods high in calcium and vitamin D.
   b. characterized by a fixation on the quality and purity of food.
   c. an obsession with bone health.
   d. a condition that results from binging and purging.

### LO 3 | Exercise Disorders

3. Muscle dysmorphia
   a. is a muscular disease that results from an autoimmune disorder.
   b. occurs only in women.
   c. results in menstrual dysfunction.
   d. occurs most often in men.

*Answers to the Pop Quiz questions can be found on page A-1. If you answered a question incorrectly, review the section identified by the Learning Outcome. For even more study tools, visit MasteringHealth.*

# 11 Improving Your Personal Fitness

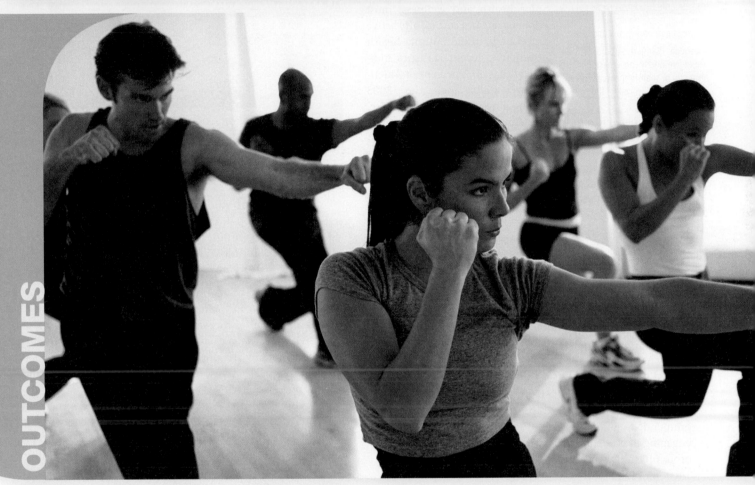

**M**ost Americans are aware of the wide range of physical, social, and mental health benefits of physical activity and know that they should be more physically active. The physiological changes in the body that result from regular physical activity reduce the likelihood of coronary artery disease, high blood pressure, type 2 diabetes, obesity, and other chronic diseases. Furthermore, engaging in physical activity regularly helps to control stress, increases self-esteem, and contributes to that "feel-good" feeling.

**physical activity** Refers to all body movements produced by skeletal muscles, resulting in substantial increases in energy expenditure.

**exercise** Planned, structured, and repetitive bodily movement done to improve or maintain one or more components of physical fitness.

Despite knowledge of the importance of physical activity for health and wellness, most people are not sufficiently active to obtain these optimal health benefits. Recent statistics indicate that 50.2 percent of American adults met the 2008 guidelines for aerobic exercise, and 29.6 percent met the guidelines for strengthening exercise.[1] However, only 20.2 percent reported meeting the guidelines for both aerobic and strengthening exercise, and 26.3 percent reported no leisure activities.[2] These statistics are based on activity reported during one's "down" time in the previous month.[3] The growing percentage of Americans who live physically inactive lives has been linked to the current high incidences of obesity, type 2 diabetes, and other chronic and mental health diseases.[4]

In general, college students are more physically active than older adults, but a recent survey indicated that 51.0 percent of college women and 47.0 percent of college men do not meet recommended guidelines for engaging in moderate or vigorous physical activities.[5]

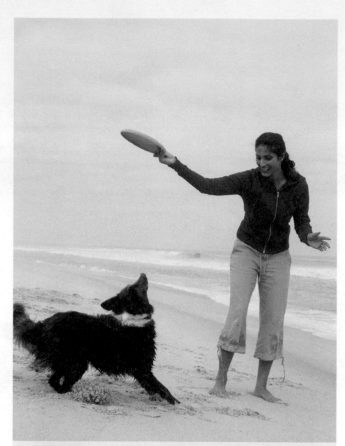

Activities such as walking and playing with your dog count toward your recommended daily physical activity.

## WHAT DO YOU THINK?

Why do you think most college students aren't more physically active?

- Why do you think women are less likely than men to obtain sufficient levels of physical activity?

- Do you think your college or university years are a good time to become more physically active? Why or why not?

## LO 1 | PHYSICAL ACTIVITY FOR HEALTH

Describe the health benefits of being physically active.

- - - - - - - - - - - - - - - - - - - - - - - - - - - - - - - - -

**Physical activity** refers to all body movements produced by skeletal muscles that result in substantial increases in energy expenditure. Physical activities can vary by intensity: light, moderate, or vigorous. For example, walking on a flat surface at a casual pace requires little effort (light), whereas

walking uphill is more intense and harder to do (moderate). Jogging and running are examples of vigorous intensity physical activities. There are three general categories of physical activity defined by the purpose for which they are done: leisure-time physical activity, occupational physical activity, and lifestyle physical activity.

**Exercise** is defined as planned, repetitive, and structured bodily movement undertaken to maintain or better any number of physical fitness components—for example, cardiorespiratory fitness, muscular strength or endurance, or flexibility. Although all exercise is physical activity, not all physical activity would be considered exercise. For example, walking from your car to class is physical activity, whereas going for a brisk 30-minute walk to maintain a healthy body weight is considered exercise.

# 150 MINUTES

OF MODERATE PHYSICAL ACTIVITY A WEEK—ALONG WITH STRENGTH EXERCISES TWO DAYS A WEEK—PROVIDES SUBSTANTIAL **HEALTH BENEFITS**. MORE IS EVEN BETTER!

Adding more physical activity to your day, like walking or cycling to school, can benefit your health. In fact, it is estimated that if the number of adults meeting the 2008 Physical Activity Guidelines (see **TABLE 11.1**) increased by 25 percent, there would be 1.3 million fewer deaths per year and the life expectancy would increase. In the United Stated, it is estimated that physical inactivity is responsible for 6.7 percent of the cases of coronary heart disease, 8.3 percent cases of type 2 diabetes, 12.4 percent cases of breast cancer, and 12.0 percent cases of colon cancer. Furthermore, physical inactivity accounts for approximately 10.8 percent of deaths in the United States.[6]

Regular participation in physical activity improves more than 50 different physiological, metabolic, and psychological aspects of human life. **FIGURE 11.1** summarizes some of these major health-related benefits.

## Reduced Risk of Cardiovascular Diseases

Aerobic exercise is good for the heart and lungs and reduces the risk for heart-related diseases. It improves blood flow and eases

## WHY SHOULD I CARE?

Being physically active reduces your risk for many chronic diseases. That may not seem like an immediate concern, but there are a lot more immediate benefits: Becoming physically fit can help improve your physical appearance and sense of self-esteem, boost your resistance to diseases like colds and flus, reduce your stress level, improve your sleep, and help you concentrate. All that, and it's fun, too!

the performance of everyday tasks. Regular exercise makes the cardiovascular and respiratory systems more efficient by strengthening the heart muscle, enabling more blood to be pumped with each stroke, and increasing the number of *capillaries* (small blood vessels that allow gas exchange between blood and surrounding tissues) in trained skeletal muscles, which supply more blood to working muscles. Exercise also improves the respiratory system by increasing the amount of oxygen that is inhaled with each breath and distributed to body tissues.[7]

Regular physical activity can reduce hypertension, or chronic high blood pressure, a cardiovascular disease itself, and a significant risk factor for other coronary heart diseases and stroke (see Chapter 12).[8] Regular aerobic exercise also improves the blood lipid profile. It typically increases high-density lipoproteins (HDLs, or "good" cholesterol), which are associated with lower risk for coronary artery disease because of their role in removing plaque built up in the arteries.[9] Triglycerides (a blood fat) typically decrease with aerobic exercise. Low-density lipoproteins (LDLs, or "bad" cholesterol) and total cholesterol are often improved with exercise due to weight loss and the improvements in HDL and triglycerides.

## TABLE 11.1 | 2008 Physical Activity Guidelines for Americans

| | Key Guidelines for Health* | For Additional Fitness or Weight Loss Benefits* | Additional Exercises |
|---|---|---|---|
| **Adults** | 150 min/week moderate-intensity physical activity<br><br>OR<br><br>75 min/week of vigorous-intensity physical activity<br><br>OR<br><br>Equivalent combination of moderate- and vigorous-intensity physical activity (e.g., 100 min moderate intensity + 25 min vigorous intensity) | 300 min/week moderate-intensity physical activity<br><br>OR<br><br>150 min/week of vigorous-intensity physical activity<br><br>OR<br><br>Equivalent combination of moderate- and vigorous-intensity physical activity (e.g., 200 min moderate intensity + 50 min vigorous intensity)<br><br>OR<br><br>More than the previously described amounts | Muscle-strengthening activities for all the major muscle groups at least 2 days/week |
| **Older Adults** | If unable to follow above guidelines, then as much physical activity as their condition allows | If unable to follow above guidelines, then as much physical activity as their condition allows | In addition to muscle-strengthening activities, those with limited mobility should add exercises to improve balance and reduce risk of falling. |
| **Children and Youth** | 60 min or more of moderate- or vigorous-intensity physical activity daily; should include at least 3 days/week or vigorous activity | At least 60 min of moderate- or vigorous-intensity physical activity on every day of the week | Include muscle-strengthening activities at least 3 days/week. Include bone-strengthening activities at least 3 days/week. |

*Avoid inactivity (some activity is better than none), accumulate physical activity in sessions of 10 minutes or more at one time, and spread activity throughout the week.
**Source:** Office of Disease Prevention and Health Promotion, U.S. Department of Health and Human Services, *2008 Physical Activity Guidelines for Americans: Be Active, Healthy, and Happy!* (Washington, DC: U.S. Department of Health and Human Services, 2008), ODPHP Publication no. U0036, www.health.gov

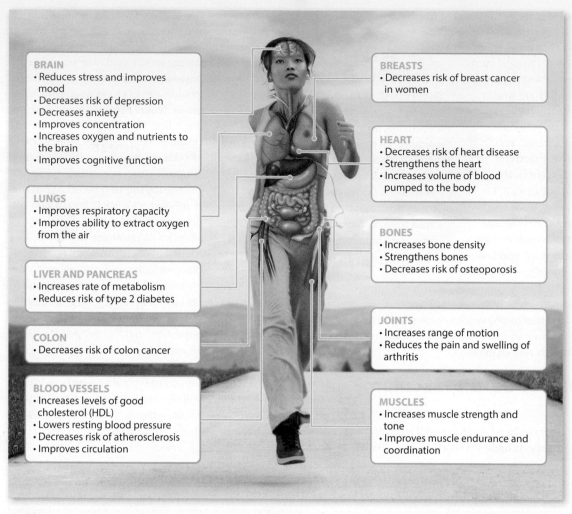

**BRAIN**
- Reduces stress and improves mood
- Decreases risk of depression
- Decreases anxiety
- Improves concentration
- Increases oxygen and nutrients to the brain
- Improves cognitive function

**LUNGS**
- Improves respiratory capacity
- Improves ability to extract oxygen from the air

**LIVER AND PANCREAS**
- Increases rate of metabolism
- Reduces risk of type 2 diabetes

**COLON**
- Decreases risk of colon cancer

**BLOOD VESSELS**
- Increases levels of good cholesterol (HDL)
- Lowers resting blood pressure
- Decreases risk of atherosclerosis
- Improves circulation

**BREASTS**
- Decreases risk of breast cancer in women

**HEART**
- Decreases risk of heart disease
- Strengthens the heart
- Increases volume of blood pumped to the body

**BONES**
- Increases bone density
- Strengthens bones
- Decreases risk of osteoporosis

**JOINTS**
- Increases range of motion
- Reduces the pain and swelling of arthritis

**MUSCLES**
- Increases muscle strength and tone
- Improves muscle endurance and coordination

**FIGURE 11.1** Some Health Benefits of Regular Exercise

▶ **VIDEO TUTOR**
Health Benefits of Regular Exercise

# Reduced Risk of Metabolic Syndrome and Type 2 Diabetes

Regular physical activity reduces the risk of metabolic syndrome, a combination of heart disease and diabetes risk factors that produces a synergistic increase in risk.[10] Specifically, metabolic syndrome includes high blood pressure, abdominal obesity, low levels of HDLs, high levels of triglycerides, and impaired glucose tolerance.[11] Regular participation in moderate-intensity physical activities reduces risk for each factor individually and collectively.[12]

Research indicates that a healthy dietary intake combined with sufficient physical activity could prevent many of the current cases of type 2 diabetes.[13] In a major national clinical trial, researchers found that exercising 150 minutes per week and eating fewer calories and less fat could prevent or delay the onset of type 2 diabetes.[14] (For more on diabetes prevention and management, see **Focus On: Minimizing Your Risk for Diabetes** on page 386.)

# Reduced Cancer Risk

After decades of research, most cancer epidemiologists believe that 25 percent to 37 percent of cancers can be avoided by healthier lifestyle and environmental choices.[15] In fact, a report released by the World Cancer Research Fund, in conjunction with the American Institute for Cancer Research, stated that one third of cancers could be prevented by being physically active and eating well.[16] Regular physical activity appears to lower the risk for some specific cancers, particularly colon, rectal, and breast cancer.[17] Research on exercise and breast cancer survivors has shown that physical activity helps patients more effectively deal with treatment for the disease and improves survival rates.[18]

# Improved Bone Mass and Reduced Risk of Osteoporosis

A common affliction for older people is *osteoporosis,* a disease characterized by low bone mass and deterioration of bone tissue, which increases fracture risk. Regular weight-bearing and strength-building physical activities are recommended to maintain bone health and prevent osteoporotic fractures. Although men and women are both negatively affected by osteoporosis, it is more common in women. Bone mass levels are significantly higher among active individuals than among sedentary persons.[19] However, it appears that the full bone-related benefits of physical activity can only be achieved with sufficient hormone levels (estrogen in women, testosterone in men) and adequate calcium, vitamin D, and total caloric intakes.[20]

## Improved Weight Management

For many people, the desire to lose weight or maintain a healthy weight is the main reason for physical activity. On the most basic level, physical activity requires your body to generate energy through calorie expenditure; if calories expended exceed calories consumed over a span of time, the net result will be weight loss. Some activities are more intense or vigorous than others and result in more calories used. **FIGURE 11.2** shows the caloric cost of various activities when done for 30 minutes.

In addition to the calories expended during activity, physical activity has a direct positive effect on metabolic rate, keeping it elevated for several hours following vigorous physical activities. This increase in metabolic rate can lead to body composition changes that favor weight management. After weight loss, increased physical activity also improves your chances of maintaining the weight loss. If you are currently at a healthy body weight, regular physical activity can prevent significant weight gain.[21]

> If you want to lose weight, you need to move more and often!

## Improved Immunity

Research shows that regular moderate-intensity physical activity reduces individual susceptibility to disease.[22] Just how regular physical activity positively influences immunity is not well understood. We know that moderate-intensity physical activity temporarily increases the number of white blood cells, which are responsible for fighting infection.[23] Often, the relationship of physical activity to immunity, or more specifically to disease susceptibility, is described as a J-shaped curve. Susceptibility to disease decreases with moderate activity, but then increases as you move to extreme levels of physical activity or exercise or if you continue to exercise without adequate recovery time and/or dietary intake.[24] Athletes engaging in marathon-type events or very intense physical training programs have been shown to be at greater risk for upper respiratory tract infections in the first 8 hours after an intense exercise session.[25]

## Improved Mental Health and Stress Management

Most people who engage in regular physical activity are likely to notice the psychological benefits, such as feeling better about oneself and an overall sense of well-being. Although these mental health benefits are difficult to quantify, they are frequently mentioned as reasons for continuing to be physically active. Learning new skills, developing increased ability and capacity in recreational activities, and sticking with a physical activity plan also improve self-esteem. In addition, regular physical activity can improve a person's physical appearance, further increasing self-esteem.

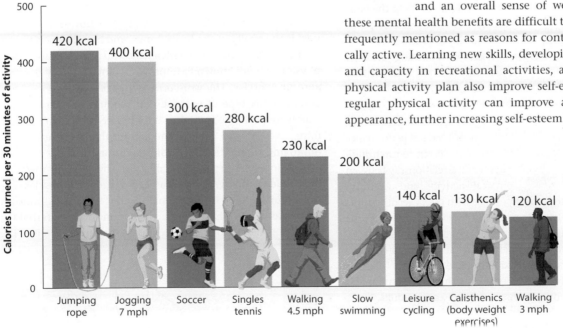

**FIGURE 11.2** **Calories Burned by Different Activities** The harder your physical activity, the more energy you expend. Estimated calories burned for various moderate and vigorous activities are listed for 30 minutes of activity. Note that the number of calories burned depends on body weight (generally, the higher your body weight, the greater the number of calories you'll burn).

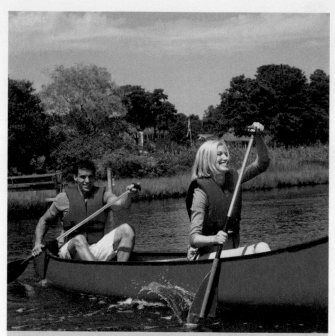

Although physical activity actually stimulates the stress response, a physically fit body adapts efficiently to the eustress of it, and as a result is better able to tolerate and effectively manage stress of all kinds.

particularly among those who have several risk factors and who use physical activity as a means of risk reduction.[31] Results from a study of nearly a million subjects showed that the largest benefits from physical activity occur in sedentary individuals who add a little physical activity to their lives, with additional benefits as physical activity levels increase.[32] Additionally, data from a national sample show that a sedentary lifestyle as associated with a reduced ability to perform activities of daily living.[33] The more sedentary time adults report, the greater reduction in the ability to perform activities of daily living. It is not just structured exercise that is important, but moving as much as possible and sitting as little as possible.

## LO 2 | PHYSICAL ACTIVITY FOR FITNESS AND PERFORMANCE

Distinguish between the physical activity required for health, physical fitness, and performance.

**Physical fitness** refers to a set of attributes that are either health or skill related.

## Health-Related Components of Physical Fitness

The health-related attributes—cardiorespiratory fitness, muscular strength and endurance, flexibility, and body composition—allow you to perform moderate- to vigorous-intensity physical activities on a regular basis without getting too tired and with energy left over to handle physical or mental emergencies. **FIGURE 11.3** identifies the major health-related components of physical fitness.

**Cardiorespiratory Fitness** **Cardiorespiratory fitness** is the ability of the heart, lungs, and blood vessels to supply the body with oxygen efficiently. The primary category of physical activity known to improve cardiorespiratory fitness is **aerobic exercise**. The word *aerobic* means "with oxygen" and describes any type of exercise that requires oxygen to make energy for prolonged activity. Aerobic activities, such as swimming, cycling, and jogging, are among the best exercises for improving or maintaining cardiorespiratory fitness.

Cardiorespiratory fitness is measured by determining **aerobic capacity (power)**, the volume of oxygen the muscles consume during exercise. Maximal aerobic power (commonly written as $VO_{2max}$) is defined as the volume of oxygen that the muscles consume per minute during maximal exercise. The

**physical fitness** A balance of health-related attributes that allows you to perform moderate to vigorous physical activities on a regular basis and complete daily physical tasks without undue fatigue.

**cardiorespiratory fitness** The ability of the heart, lungs, and blood vessels to supply oxygen to skeletal muscles during sustained physical activity.

**aerobic exercise** Prolonged exercise that requires oxygen to make energy for activity.

**aerobic capacity (power)** The functional status of the cardiorespiratory system; refers specifically to the volume of oxygen the muscles consume during exercise.

Regular aerobic physical activity can provide a break from stressors. It can improve the way the body handles stress by its effect on neurotransmitters associated with mood enhancement. Physical activity might also help the body recover from the stress response more quickly as fitness increases.[26]

There is increasing evidence that regular physical activity improves cognitive function across the lifespan. Research has associated regular activity with academic and standardized test performance in school.[27] Recent research indicates that the relationship between physical activity and executive cognitive function is reciprocal.[28] Those with poor executive function experienced greater reductions in physical activity over time compared to those with higher function. Promoting physical activity as we age is important to prevent the decline in cognitive function, which in turn can help maintain regular activity.[29] Regular aerobic activity has also been associated with the prevention and improvement of dementia and Alzheimer's disease in adults.[30]

## Longer Life Span

Experts have long debated the relationship between physical activity and longevity. Several studies indicate significant decreases in long-term health risk and increases in years lived,

ONLY 20.2%

OF AMERICAN ADULTS MEET GUIDELINES FOR BOTH CARDIORESPIRATORY AND MUSCULAR **FITNESS**.

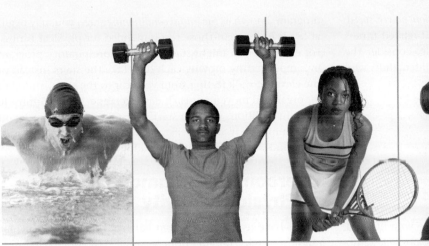

| Cardiorespiratory fitness | Muscular strength | Muscular endurance | Flexibility | Body composition |
|---|---|---|---|---|
| Ability to sustain aerobic whole-body activity for a prolonged period of time | Maximum force able to be exerted by single contraction of a muscle or muscle group | Ability to perform muscle contractions repeatedly without fatiguing | Ability to move joints freely through their full range of motion | The relative proportions of fat mass and fat-free mass in the body |

**FIGURE 11.3** Health-Related Components of Physical Fitness

most common measure of maximal aerobic capacity is a walk or run test on a treadmill. For greatest accuracy, this is done in a lab with specialized equipment and technicians to measure the precise amount of oxygen entering and exiting the body during the exercise session. To get a more general sense of cardiorespiratory fitness, submaximal tests performed in the classroom or field can predict maximal aerobic capacity.

**Muscular Strength** Muscular strength refers to the amount of force a muscle or group of muscles can generate in one contraction. The most common way to assess the strength of a particular muscle or muscle group is to measure the maximum amount of weight you can move one time (and no more) or your one repetition maximum (1 RM).

**Muscular Endurance** Muscular endurance is the ability of a muscle or group of muscles to exert force repeatedly without fatigue or the ability to sustain a muscular contraction. The more repetitions you can perform successfully (e.g., push-ups) or the longer you can hold a certain position (e.g., flexed arm hang), the greater your muscular endurance.

**Flexibility** Flexibility refers to the range of motion, or the amount of movement possible, at a particular joint or series of joints: the greater the range of motion, the greater the flexibility. Various tests measure the flexibility of the body's joints, including range-of-motion tests for specific joints.

**Body Composition** Body composition is the fifth and final health-related component of physical fitness. Body composition describes the relative proportions and distribution of fat and fat-free (muscle, bone, water, organs) tissues in the body. (For more details on body composition, including its measurement, see Chapter 10.)

## Skill-Related Components of Physical Fitness

In addition to the five health-related components of physical fitness, physical fitness for athletes involves attributes that improve their ability to perform athletic tasks. These attributes, called the *skill-related components* of physical fitness, also help recreational athletes and general exercisers increase fitness levels and their ability to perform daily tasks. The skill-related components of physical fitness (also

**muscular strength** The amount of force that a muscle is capable of exerting in one contraction.

**muscular endurance** A muscle's ability to exert force repeatedly without fatiguing or the ability to sustain a muscular contraction for a length of time.

**flexibility** The range of motion, or the amount of movement possible, at a particular joint or series of joints.

**body composition** The relative proportions of fat and fat-free (muscle, bone, water, organs) tissues in the body.

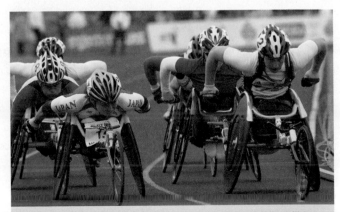

It is important for all people, including those with disabilities, to develop optimal levels of physical fitness and participate in physical activities they enjoy—including competitive sports.

called sport skills) are *agility, balance, coordination, power, speed,* and *reaction time*. Note that some of the skill-related fitness components can impact health. For example, consider the importance of balance and coordination for older adults who are at increased risk for falls.

## LO 3 | COMMITTING TO PHYSICAL FITNESS

Identify lifestyle obstacles to physical activity, describe ways to surmount them, and make a commitment to getting physically fit.

To succeed at incorporating physical fitness into your life, you need to design a fitness program that takes obstacles into account and that is founded on the activities you enjoy most.

### What If I Have Been Inactive for a While?

If you have been physically inactive for the past few months or longer, first make sure that your physician clears you for exercise. Consider consulting a personal trainer or fitness instructor to help you get started. In this phase of a fitness program, known as *the initial conditioning stage,* you may begin at levels lower than those recommended for physical fitness. For example, you might start your cardiorespiratory program by simply getting moving each day. Take the stairs instead of the elevator, walk farther from your car to the store, and plan for organized movement each day, such as a 10- to 15-minute walk. In addition, you can start your muscle fitness program with simple body weight exercises, emphasizing proper technique and body alignment before adding any resistance.

## Overcoming Common Obstacles to Physical Activity

People have real and perceived barriers that prevent regular physical activity, ranging from personal ("I do not have time") to environmental ("I do not have a safe place to be active"). Some people may be reluctant to exercise if they are overweight, feel embarrassed to work out with their more "fit" friends, or feel they lack the knowledge and skills required.

Think about your obstacles to physical activity and write them down. Consider anything that gets in your way of exercising, however minor. Once you honestly evaluate why you are not as physically active as you want to be, review TABLE 11.2 for suggestions on overcoming your hurdles.

## TABLE 11.2 | Overcoming Obstacles to Physical Activity

| Obstacle | Possible Solution |
|---|---|
| Lack of time | ■ Look at your schedule. Where can you find 30-minute time slots? Perhaps you need to focus on shorter times (10 minutes or more) throughout the day.<br>■ Multitask. Read while riding an exercise bike or listen to lectures or podcasts while walking.<br>■ Be physically active during your lunch and study breaks as well as between classes. Skip rope or throw a Frisbee with a friend.<br>■ Select activities that require less time, such as brisk walking or jogging.<br>■ Ride your bike to class, or park (or get off the bus) farther from your destination. |
| Social influence | ■ Invite family and friends to be active with you.<br>■ Join an exercise class to meet new people.<br>■ Explain the importance of exercise and your commitment to physical activity to people who may not support your efforts.<br>■ Find a role model to support your efforts.<br>■ Plan for physically active dates—go for a walk, dancing, or bowling. |
| Lack of motivation, willpower, or energy | ■ Schedule your workout time just as you would any other important commitment.<br>■ Enlist the help of an exercise partner to make you accountable for working out.<br>■ Give yourself an incentive.<br>■ Schedule your workouts when you feel most energetic.<br>■ Remind yourself that exercise gives you more energy.<br>■ Get things ready; for example, if you choose to walk in the morning, set out your clothes and shoes the night before. |
| Lack of resources | ■ Select an activity that requires minimal equipment, such as walking, jogging, jumping rope, or calisthenics.<br>■ Identify inexpensive resources on campus or in the community.<br>■ Use active forms of transportation.<br>■ Take advantage of no-cost opportunities, such as playing catch in the park or green space on campus. |

**Source:** Adapted from National Center for Chronic Disease Prevention and Health Promotion, "How Can I Overcome Barriers to Physical Activity?," Updated May 2011, www.cdc.gov

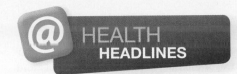
# TRANSPORT YOURSELF!

Before we became a car culture, much of our transportation was human powered. Historically, bicycling and walking were important means of transportation and recreation in the United States. Since World War II, however, the development of automobile-oriented communities has led to a steady decline of bicycling and walking. Currently, less than 12 percent of trips are made by foot or bike, but the number varies according to region of the country and size of the city.

Many people are now embracing a movement toward more active transportation. *Active transportation* means using your own power to get from place to place—whether walking, riding a bike, skateboarding, or roller skating. You can cycle to work or to do errands even if you do not own a bike. Check to see whether your city has a bike share program at http://bikeshare.com. Here are just a few of the many reasons to make active transportation a bigger part of your life:

- **You will be adding more exercise into your daily routine.** People who use active forms of transportation to complete errands are more likely to meet physical activity guidelines.
- **Walking or biking can save you money.** It is significantly less expensive to own a bike than a car when

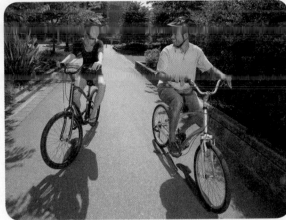

Hop on that bike and join the green revolution! Active transportation is an excellent want to add physical activity to your day, especially on nonexercise days.

you consider gas and maintenance. It is estimated that it is costs 30 times more to maintain a care than a bike! Additionally, those who cycle to work are eligible for up to $20 per month in a tax-free reimbursement!

- **Walking or biking may save you time!** Short commutes of three to five files are usually as fast or faster via bicycle rather than via car.
- **You will enjoy being outdoors.** Research is emerging on the physical and mental health benefits of nature and being outdoors. So much of what we do is inside, with recirculated air and artificial lighting, that our bodies are deficient in fresh air and sunlight.

- **You will make a significant contribution to reducing air pollution.** Choosing to walk or bike instead of driving only 2 days a week can reduce greenhouse gas emissions by an average of 4,000 pounds a year.
- **You will help reduce traffic.** More active commuters means fewer cars on the roads and less traffic congestion.
- **You will contribute to global environmental health.** Reducing vehicle trips will help reduce overall greenhouse gas emissions and the need to source more fossil fuel. Swapping waking or cycling for the car when taking short trips is estimated to save over 10 billion gallons of fuel per year.

**Sources:** Rails-to-Trails Conservancy, "Investing in Trails: Cost-Effective Improvements—for Everyone," 2013, www.railstotrails.org /resourcehandler.ashx?id=3629; M. Woodruff, "13 Reasons You Should Start Biking to Work," *Business Insider,* October 2012, www .businessinsider.com/13-reasons-you-should -bike-to-work-2012-10#ixzz3fFS2Ovre; U.S. Environmental Protection Agency, "Climate Change: What You Can Do: On the Road," Updated April 2014, www.epa.gov/climatechange /wycd/road.html; B. McKenzie, "Modes Less Traveled—Bicycling and Walking to Work in the United States: 2008–2012," U.S. Department of Commerce, May 2014, www.census .gov/prod/2014pubs/acs-25.pdf

## Incorporating Physical Activity in Your Life

When designing your fitness program, there are several factors to consider. First, choose activities that are appropriate for you, convenient, and that you genuinely enjoy. For example, choose jogging because you like to run and there are beautiful trails nearby versus swimming when you do not really like the water and the pool is difficult to get to. Likewise, choose activities that are suitable for your current fitness level. If you are overweight or have not exercised in months, start slowly, plan fun activities, and progress to more challenging physical activities as your physical fitness improves. You may choose to simply walk more in an attempt to achieve the recommended goal

of 10,000 steps per day; keep track with a pedometer. Try to make physical activity a part of your routine by incorporating it into something you already have to do—such as getting to class or work. See the **Health Headlines** box for more on using your transportation for fitness.

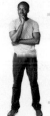

WHICH **PATH** WOULD YOU TAKE **?**

Scan the QR code to see how different physical fitness choices YOU make today can affect your overall health tomorrow.

## Set SMART Goals

To set successful goals, try using the *SMART* system. SMART goals are specific, measurable, action-oriented, realistic, and time-oriented.

A vague goal would be "Improve fitness by exercising more." A SMART goal would be as follows:

- *Specific*—"I'll participate in a resistance-training program that targets all of the major muscle groups 3–5 days per week."
- *Measurable*—"I'll improve my fitness classification from average to good."
- *Action-oriented*—"I'll meet with a personal trainer to learn how to safely do resistance exercises and to plan a workout for the gym and home."
- *Realistic*—"I'll increase the weight I can lift by 20 percent."
- *Time-oriented*—"I'll try my new weight program for 8 weeks, then reassess."

## Use the FITT Principle

To improve your health-related physical fitness (or performance-related physical fitness), use the **FITT** (Frequency, Intensity, Time, and Type)[34] principle to define your exercise program. The FITT prescription (**FIGURE 11.4**) uses the following criteria:

- **Frequency** refers to the number of times per week you need to engage in particular exercises to achieve the desired level of physical fitness in a particular component.
- **Intensity** refers to how hard your workout must be to achieve the desired level of physical fitness.
- **Time,** or the *duration,* refers to how many minutes or repetitions of an exercise are required at a specified intensity during any one session to attain the desired level of physical fitness for each component.
- **Type** refers to what kind of exercises should be performed to improve the specific component of physical fitness.

## The FITT Principle for Cardiorespiratory Fitness

The most effective aerobic exercises for building cardiorespiratory fitness are total body activities involving the large muscle groups of your body. The FITT prescription for cardiorespiratory fitness includes 3 to 5 days per week of vigorous, rhythmic, continuous activity at 64 to 96 percent of your estimated maximal heart rate for 20 to 60 minutes.[35]

**Frequency** The frequency of your program is related to your intensity. If you choose to do moderate-intensity exercises, you should aim for a frequency of at least 5 days (frequency drops to at least 3 days per week with vigorous-intensity activities). Newcomers to exercise can still improve by doing less-intense exercise (light to moderate level), but doing it more days during a week. In this case, follow the recommendations from the Centers for Disease Control and Prevention (CDC) for moderate physical activity (refer to Table 11.1 on page 331).

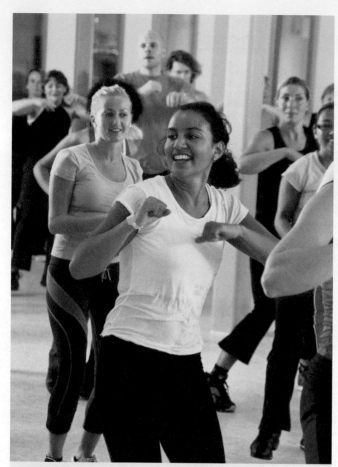

One great way to motivate yourself is to sign up for an exercise class. The structure, schedule, social interaction, and challenge of learning a new skill can be the motivation you need to get moving!

## LO 4 | CREATING YOUR OWN FITNESS PROGRAM

Understand and be able to use the FITT (frequency, intensity, time, and type) principles for the health-related components of physical fitness.

**FITT** Acronym for frequency, intensity, time, and type; the terms that describe the essential components of a program or plan to improve a health-related component of physical fitness.

**frequency** As part of the FITT prescription, refers to how many days per week a person should exercise.

**intensity** As part of the FITT prescription, refers to how hard or how much effort is needed when a person exercises.

**time** As part of the FITT prescription, refers to the duration of an exercise session.

**type** As part of the FITT prescription, refers to what kind of exercises a person needs to do.

The first step in creating a personal physical fitness program is identifying your goals. Do you want to be better at sports or feel better about your body? Is your goal to manage stress or reduce your risk of chronic diseases? Perhaps your most vital goal will be to establish a realistic schedule of diverse physical activities that you can maintain and enjoy throughout your life. Your physical fitness goals and objectives should be both achievable for you and in line with what you truly want.

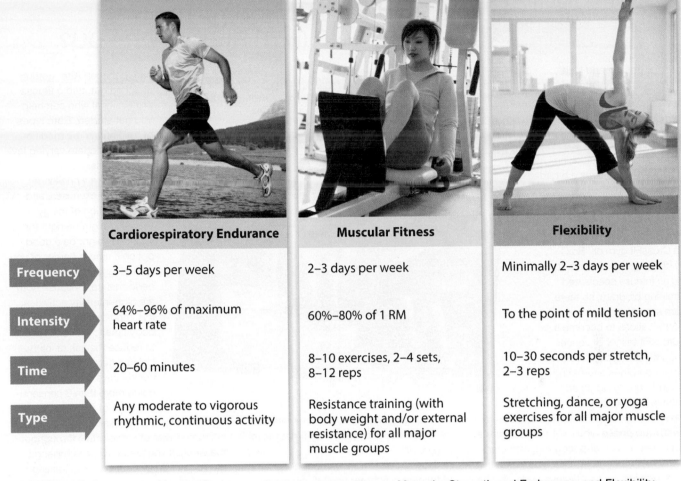

| | Cardiorespiratory Endurance | Muscular Fitness | Flexibility |
|---|---|---|---|
| **Frequency** | 3–5 days per week | 2–3 days per week | Minimally 2–3 days per week |
| **Intensity** | 64%–96% of maximum heart rate | 60%–80% of 1 RM | To the point of mild tension |
| **Time** | 20–60 minutes | 8–10 exercises, 2–4 sets, 8–12 reps | 10–30 seconds per stretch, 2–3 reps |
| **Type** | Any moderate to vigorous rhythmic, continuous activity | Resistance training (with body weight and/or external resistance) for all major muscle groups | Stretching, dance, or yoga exercises for all major muscle groups |

**FIGURE 11.4** The FITT Principle Applied to Cardiorespiratory Fitness, Muscular Strength and Endurance, and Flexibility

**Intensity** The most common methods used to determine the intensity of cardiorespiratory endurance exercises are target heart rate, rating of perceived exertion, and the talk test. The exercise intensity required to improve cardiorespiratory endurance is a heart rate between 64 and 96 percent of your maximum heart rate (moderate to vigorous intensity). Before calculating your **target heart rate**, you must first estimate your maximal heart rate with the formula [207 – 0.7(age)]. The example below is based on a 20-year-old. Substitute your age to determine your own maximal heart rate, then multiply by 0.64 and 0.94 to determine the lower and upper limits of your target range.

1. 207 – 0.7(20) = maximal heart rate for a 20-year old
2. 207 – 14 = 193 (maximal heart rate)
3. 193(0.64) = 123.52 (lower target limit)
4. 193.5(0.94) = 185.28 (upper target limit)
5. Target range = 124–186 beats per minute

To determine how close you are to your target heart rate, take your pulse. Lightly place your index and middle fingers (not your thumb) over the carotid artery in your neck or on the radial artery on the inside of your wrist (**FIGURE 11.5**). Count your pulse while exercising, if possible, or start counting your pulse immediately after you stop exercising, as your heart rate decreases rapidly when you stop. Using a watch or a clock, take your pulse for 10 seconds (the first pulse is "0" if you are starting a stopwatch, but 1 if you are using a watch that is already running) and multiply this number by 6 to get the number of beats per minute.

**target heart rate** The heart rate range of aerobic exercise that leads to improved cardiorespiratory fitness (i.e., 64% to 96% of maximal heart rate).

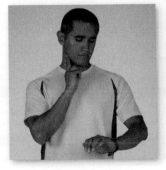

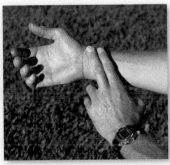

ⓐ Carotid pulse   ⓑ Radial pulse

**FIGURE 11.5** Taking a Pulse Palpation of the carotid (neck) or radial (wrist) artery is a simple way of determining heart rate.

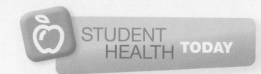
# IS HIGH INTENSITY INTERVAL TRAINING (HIIT) RIGHT FOR YOU?

CrossFit and high-intensity interval training (HIIT) are two methods of training that are increasing in popularity. CrossFit is a strength and conditioning program that utilizes a broad range of high-intensity functional movements and activities. CrossFit is typically performed in a CrossFit gym or "Box" within a group or class. It is an intense specialized training program, so there are special requirements and certifications to become a CrossFit trainer or coach.

HIIT is a type of training that combines alternating high-intensity bouts and active rest bouts within your exercise session. For example, after the warm-up phase, you might do 2 minutes of a near-maximal-paced run, and then jog for 2 minutes to rest. This type of training can provide a very efficient workout. The volume of exercise is generally less than a continuous bout at a constant pace, but similar fitness gains can be seen with the lower volume of exercise as with the

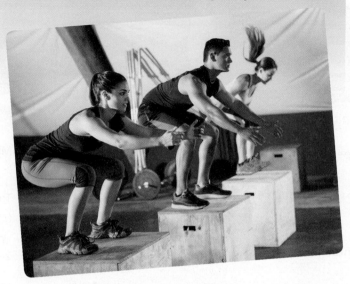

CrossFit and high-intensity interval training (HIIT) are two methods of training that are increasing in popularity. If you're healthy enough—and up for the challenge—they might be right for you.

tradition exercise bout. The intervals can be varied depending on your fitness level and goals.

How do you know whether either type of training is right for you? If you are a beginner, have risk factors for cardiovascular disease or musculoskeletal disorders, are obese, or have been sedentary, make sure you get clearance from your health

care provider. After getting checked out, find a fitness professional who can help you get started. Both types of training can be modified to accommodate varying levels of fitness.

If you like a challenge, a variety of exercises, and the motivation of the gym, CrossFit might be right for you. HIIT might be a good option if time is barrier or you are trying to improve your performance. Because both are high-intensity activities, it is important to allow your body time to rest and recover to reduce the risk of injury. Using different activities on consecutive days and not doing more than 3 consecutive days of exercise are recommendations for CrossFit. HIIT should be alternated with other activities throughout the week. If you are up for the challenge, give one of these nontraditional training programs a try.

**Sources:** CrossFit, /www.crossfit.com/; L. Kravitz, "High-Intensity Interval Training," ACSM, www.acsm.org/docs/brochures/high-intensity-interval-training.pdf

---

Another way to determine the intensity of cardiorespiratory exercise intensity is to use Borg's rating of perceived exertion (RPE) scale. **Perceived exertion** refers to how hard you feel you are working, which you might base on your heart rate,

**perceived exertion** The subjective perception of effort during exercise that can be used to monitor exercise intensity

breathing rate, sweating, and level of fatigue. This scale uses a rating from 6 (no exertion at all) to 20 (maximal exertion). An RPE of 12 to 16 is generally recommended for training the cardiorespiratory system.

The easiest method of measuring cardiorespiratory exercise intensity is the "talk test." A "moderate" level of exercise (heart rate at 64 to 76 percent of maximum) is a conversational level of exercise. At this level you are able to talk with a partner while exercising. If you can talk, but only in short fragments and not sentences, you may be at a "vigorous" level of exercise (heart rate at 76 to 96 percent of maximum). If you are breathing so hard that speaking at all is difficult, the intensity of your exercise may be too high. Conversely, if you are able to sing or

laugh heartily while exercising, the intensity of your exercise is light and may be insufficient for maintaining or improving cardiorespiratory fitness.

**Time** For cardiorespiratory fitness benefits, the American College of Sports Medicine (ACSM) recommends that vigorous activities be performed for at least 20 minutes at a time, and moderate activities for at least 30 minutes.[36] See also the **Student Health Today** box for information on a few exercise programs that can really give you a lot of bang for your buck. Free time for exercise can vary from day to day, so you can also set a time goal for the entire week as long as you keep your sessions to at least 10 minutes (150 minutes per week for moderate intensity, and 75 minutes per week for vigorous intensity).

**Type** Any sort of rhythmic, continuous, and physical activity that can be done for 20 or more minutes will improve cardiorespiratory fitness. Examples include walking briskly, cycling, jogging, fitness classes, and swimming.

# The FITT Principle for Muscular Strength and Endurance

The FITT prescription for muscular strength and endurance includes 2 to 3 days per week of exercises that train the major muscle groups, using enough sets, repetitions, and resistance to maintain or improve muscular strength and endurance.[37]

**Frequency** For frequency, training the major muscle groups 2 to 3 days a week is recommended. It is believed that overloading the muscles, a normal part of resistance training described below, causes microscopic tears in muscle fibers, and the rebuilding process that increases the muscle's size and capacity takes about 24 to 48 hours. Thus, resistance training exercise programs should include at least 1 day of rest between workouts before the same muscles are overloaded again. But don't wait too long between workouts: One of the important principles of strength training is the idea of *reversibility*. Reversibility means that if you stop exercising, the body responds by deconditioning. Within 2 weeks, muscles begin to revert to their untrained state.[38] The saying "use it or lose it" applies!

**Intensity** To determine the intensity of exercise needed to improve muscular strength and endurance, you need to know the maximum amount of weight you can lift (or move) in one contraction. This value is called your **one repetition maximum (1 RM)**. Once your 1 RM is determined, it is used as the basis for intensity recommendations for improving muscular strength and endurance. Muscular strength is improved when resistance loads are greater than 60 percent of your 1 RM, whereas muscular endurance is improved using loads less than 50 percent of your 1 RM.

Everyone begins a resistance-training program at an initial level of strength. To become stronger, you must *overload* your muscles, that is, regularly create a degree of tension in your muscles that is greater than what they are accustomed to.

Overloading them forces your muscles to adapt by getting larger, stronger, and capable of producing more tension. If you "underload" your muscles, you will not increase strength. If you create too great an overload, you may experience muscle injury, muscle fatigue, and potentially a loss in strength.

> **one repetition maximum (1 RM)** The amount of weight or resistance that can be lifted or moved only once.

**Time** The time recommended for muscular strength and endurance exercises is measured, not in minutes of exercise, but rather in repetitions and sets.

- **Repetitions and sets.** To increase muscular strength, you need higher intensity and fewer repetitions and sets: Use a resistance of at least 60 percent of your 1 RM, performing 8 to 12 repetitions per set, with two to four sets performed overall. If improving muscular endurance is your goal, use less resistance and more repetitions: Perform one to two sets of 15 to 25 repetitions using a resistance that is less than 50 percent of your 1 RM.
- **Rest periods.** Resting between exercises is crucial to reduce fatigue and help with performance and safety in subsequent sets. A rest period of 2 to 3 minutes is recommended when using the guidelines for general health benefits. However, the rest period when working to develop strength or endurance will vary. Note that the rest period refers specifically to the muscle group being exercised. For example, you can alternate a set of push-ups with curl-ups, as the muscle groups worked in one set can rest while you are working the other muscle groups.

**Type** To improve muscular strength or endurance, it is recommended that resistance training use either the body's weight or devices that provide a fixed or variable resistance (see **TABLE 11.3**). When selecting strength-training exercises,

## TABLE 11.3 | Methods of Providing Muscular Resistance

| Body Weight Resistance (Calisthenics) | Fixed Resistance | Variable Resistance |
|---|---|---|
| | | |
| ■ Uses your own body weight to develop muscular strength and endurance | ■ Provides a constant resistance throughout the full range of movement | ■ Resistance altered so that the muscle's effort is consistent throughout the full range of motion |
| ■ Improves overall muscular fitness and, in particular, core body strength and overall muscle tone | ■ Requires balance and coordination; promotes development of core body strength | ■ Provides more controlled motion and isolates certain muscle groups |
| **Examples:** Push-ups, pull-ups, curl-ups, dips, leg raises, chair sits, etc. | **Examples:** Free weights, such as barbells, dumbbells, medicine balls, and kettlebells | **Examples:** Weight machines in gyms and homes |

## Foods for Exercise and Recovery

To make the most of your workouts, follow the recommendations from the MyPlate plan and make sure that you eat sufficient carbohydrates, the body's main source of fuel. Your body stores carbohydrates as glycogen primarily in the muscles and liver and then uses this stored glycogen for energy when you are physically active. Fats are also an important source of energy, packing more than double the energy per gram compared to carbohydrates. Protein plays a role in muscle repair and growth, but is not normally a source of energy.

When you eat is almost as important as what you eat. Eating a large meal before exercising can cause upset stomach, cramping, and diarrhea, because your muscles have to compete with your digestive system for energy. After a large meal, wait 3 to 4 hours before you begin exercising. Smaller meals (snacks) can be eaten about an hour before activity. Not eating at all before a workout can cause low blood sugar levels that in turn cause weakness and slower reaction times.

**hyponatremia or water intoxication** Overconsumption of water, which leads to a dilution of sodium concentration in the blood, with potentially fatal results.

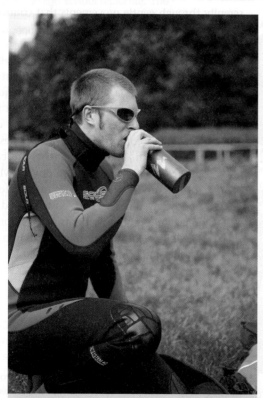

The American College of Sports Medicine and the National Athletic Trainers' Association recommend consuming 14 to 22 ounces of fluid several hours prior to exercise and about 6 to 12 ounces per 15 to 20 minutes during—assuming you are sweating.

After your workout, help your muscles recover by eating a snack or meal that contains plenty of carbohydrates and a little protein, too. Today, there is a burgeoning market for dietary supplements that claim to deliver the nutrients needed for muscle recovery, as well as additional "performance-enhancing" ingredients; one thing to keep in mind, especially if you consider these products, is that there are few standards and virtually no Food and Drug Administration (FDA) approval needed for many to grace store shelves. (See Chapter 9 on nutrition for more on supplements).

## Fluids for Exercise and Recovery

In addition to eating well, staying hydrated is also crucial. How much fluid do you need? Keep in mind that the goal of fluid replacement is to prevent excessive dehydration (greater than 2% loss of body weight). The ACSM and the National Athletic Trainers Association recommend consuming 5 to 7 milliliters per kilogram of body weight (approximately 0.7 to 1.07 ounces per 10 pounds body weight) 4 hours prior to exercise.[49] Drinking fluids during exercise is also important, but it is difficult to provide guidelines for how much or when because intake should be based on time, intensity, and type of activity performed. A good way to monitor how much fluid you need to replace is to weigh yourself before and after your workout. The difference in weight is how much you should drink. So, for example, if you lost 2 pounds during a training session, you should drink 32 ounces of fluid.[50]

For exercise sessions lasting less than 1 hour, plain water is sufficient for rehydration. If your exercise session exceeds 1 hour—and you sweat profusely—consider a sports drink containing electrolytes. The electrolytes in these products are minerals and ions such as sodium and potassium that are needed for proper functioning of your nervous and muscular systems. Replacing electrolytes is particularly important for endurance athletes. In endurance events lasting more than 4 hours, an athlete's overconsumption of plain water can dilute the sodium concentration in the blood with potentially fatal results, an effect called **hyponatremia** or **water intoxication**.

Although water is the best choice in most cases, there are situations in which you might need to choose something different. Some people are likely to consume more when their drink is flavored, a point that may be significant in ensuring proper hydration. Recently, research has considered low-fat chocolate milk as a recovery drink.[51] Chocolate milk is a liquid that not only hydrates, but also is a source of sodium, potassium, carbohydrates, and protein. Consuming carbohydrates and protein immediately after exercise will help replenish muscle and liver glycogen stores and stimulate muscle protein synthesis for better recovery from exercise. The protein in milk, whey protein, is ideal because it contains all of the essential amino acids and is rapidly absorbed by the body. Low-fat chocolate milk is a good choice to hydrate and recover after exercise.

## LO 7 | PREVENTING AND TREATING FITNESS-RELATED INJURIES

Explain how to prevent and treat common exercise injuries.

Two basic types of injuries stem from fitness-related activities: traumatic injuries and overuse injuries. **Traumatic injuries** occur suddenly and usually by accident. Typical traumatic injuries are broken bones, torn ligaments and muscles, contusions, and lacerations. If a traumatic injury causes a noticeable loss of function and immediate pain or pain that does not go away after 30 minutes, consult a physician.

**Overuse injuries** result from the cumulative effects of day-after-day stresses. These injuries occur most often in repetitive activities such as swimming, running, bicycling, and step aerobics. The forces that occur normally during physical activity are not enough to cause a ligament sprain or muscle strain as in a traumatic injury, but when these forces are applied daily for weeks or months, they can result in an overuse injury. Factors such as overweight or obesity, running mechanics, and poor choice of shoe can also contribute to overuse injury.

The three most common overuse injuries are *runner's knee, shin splints,* and *plantar fasciitis.* Runner's knee is a general term describing a series of problems involving the muscles, tendons, and ligaments around the knee. *Shin splints* is a general term used for any pain that occurs below the knee and above the ankle in the shin. Plantar fasciitis is an inflammation of the plantar fascia, a broad band of dense, inelastic tissue in the foot. Rest, variation of routine, and stretching are the first lines of treatment for any of these overuse injuries. If pain continues, visit a physician. Orthotics, physical therapy, or steroid shots are possible treatment options.

### WHAT DO YOU THINK?

How do your physical activities put you at risk of injury?

- What changes can you make to your approach to training, your training program, equipment, or footwear to reduce these risks?

## Preventing Injuries

To reduce your risk of overuse or traumatic injuries, use common sense and the proper gear and equipment. Vary your physical activities throughout the week, setting appropriate and realistic short- and long-term goals. Listen to your body when working out. Warning signs include muscle stiffness and soreness, bone and joint pains, and whole-body fatigue that simply does not go away.

**Appropriate Footwear** Proper footwear, replaced in a timely manner, can decrease the likelihood of foot, knee, hip, or back injuries. Biomechanics research has revealed that running is a collision sport—with each stride, the runner's foot collides with the ground with a force three to five times the runner's body weight.[52] Consider the impact for a beginner runner who might have poor mechanics or an overweight individual who participates in weight-bearing activities. The force not absorbed by the running shoe is transmitted upward into the foot, leg, thigh, and back. Our bodies can absorb forces such as these but may be injured by the cumulative effect of repetitive impacts (such as running 40 miles per week). Thus, the shoes' ability to absorb shock is critical—not just for those who run, but for anyone engaged in weight-bearing activities.

> **traumatic injuries** Injuries that are accidental and occur suddenly.
>
> **overuse injuries** Injuries that result from the cumulative effects of day-after-day stresses placed on tendons, muscles, and joints.

In addition to absorbing shock, an athletic shoe should provide a good fit for maximal comfort and performance—see **FIGURE 11.7**. To get the best fit, shop at a sports or fitness specialty store where there is a large selection and the salespeople are trained in properly fitting athletic shoes. Try on shoes later in the day when your feet are largest, and check to make sure there is a little extra room in the toe and that the width is appropriate. Because different activities place different stresses on your feet and joints, you should choose shoes specifically designed for your sport or activity. Shoes of any type should be replaced once they lose their cushioning. A common rule of thumb is that running shoes ought to be replaced after 300 to 500 miles of use, which is typically between 3 and 9 months, depending on your activity level.

**Appropriate Protective Equipment** It is essential to use well-fitted, appropriate protective equipment for your physical activities. For example, using the correct racquet with the proper tension helps prevent the general inflammatory condition known as tennis elbow. As another example, eye injuries can occur in virtually all physical activities, although some activities (such as baseball, basketball, and racquet sports) are more risky than others.[53] As many as 90 percent of eye injuries could be prevented by wearing appropriate eye protection, such as goggles with polycarbonate lenses.[54]

Wearing a helmet while bicycle riding is an important safety precaution. An estimated 66 to 88 percent of head injuries among cyclists can be prevented by wearing a helmet.[55] In a

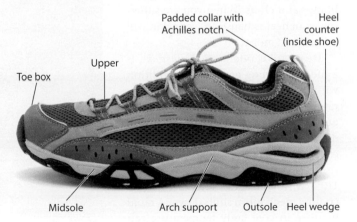

**FIGURE 11.7** Anatomy of a Running Shoe  A good running shoe should fit comfortably; allow room for your toes to move; have a firm, but flexible midsole; and have a firm grip on your heel to prevent slipping.

**heat cramps** Involuntary and forcible muscle contractions that occur during or following exercise in hot and/or humid weather.

**heat exhaustion** A heat stress illness caused by significant dehydration resulting from exercise in hot and/or humid conditions.

**heatstroke** A deadly heat stress illness resulting from dehydration and overexertion in hot and/or humid conditions.

**hypothermia** Potentially fatal condition caused by abnormally low body core temperature.

recent study of college students, 45.8 percent of students who rode a bike in the past 12 months reported never wearing a helmet, and 24.69 percent said they wore one only sometimes or rarely.[56] The direct medical costs from cyclists' failure to wear helmets is an estimated $81 million a year.[57] Cyclists aren't the only ones who should be wearing helmets. People who skateboard, ski, in-line skate, snowboard, play contact sports, or use kickscooters should also wear helmets. Look for helmets that meet the standards established by the American National Standards Institute or the Snell Memorial Foundation.

## Exercising in the Heat

Exercising in hot or humid weather increases your risk of a heat-related illness. In these conditions, your body's rate of heat production can exceed its ability to cool itself. The three different heat stress illnesses, progressive in their level of severity, are heat cramps, heat exhaustion, and heatstroke.

**Heat cramps** (heat-related involuntary and forcible muscle contractions that cannot be relaxed), the least serious problem, can usually be prevented by adequate fluid replacement and a dietary intake that includes the electrolytes lost during sweating.

**Heat exhaustion** is actually a mild form of shock, in which the blood pools in the arms and legs away from the brain and major organs of the body. It is caused by excessive water loss because of intense or prolonged exercise or work in a hot and/or humid environment. Symptoms of heat exhaustion include nausea, headache, fatigue, dizziness and faintness, and, paradoxically, goose bumps and chills. When you are suffering from heat exhaustion, your skin will be cool and moist.

**Heatstroke,** often called *sunstroke,* is a life-threatening emergency condition with a high morbidity and mortality rate.[58] Heatstroke occurs during vigorous exercise when the body's heat production significantly exceeds its cooling capacities. Core body temperature can rise from normal (98.6°F) to 105°F to 110°F within minutes after the body's cooling mechanism shuts down. A rapid increase in core body temperature can cause brain damage, permanent disability, and death. Common signs of heatstroke are dry, hot, and usually red skin;

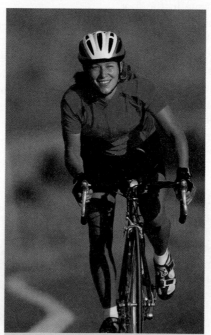

Reducing risk for exercise injuries requires common sense and preventative measures, including wearing protective gear (helmets, knee pads, elbow pads, eyewear).

very high body temperature; and rapid heart rate. If you experience any of the symptoms mentioned here, stop exercising immediately. Move to the shade or a cool spot to rest and drink plenty of cool fluids for heat cramps and exhaustion. If heatstroke is suspected, seek medical attention immediately.

You can prevent heat stress by following certain precautions. First, acclimatize yourself to hot or humid climates. The process of heat acclimatization, which increases your body's cooling efficiency, requires about 10 to 14 days of gradually increased physical activity in the hot environment. Second, reduce your risk of dehydration by replacing fluids before, during, and after exercise. Third, wear clothing appropriate for the activity and the environment—for example, light-colored nylon shorts and a mesh tank top. Finally, use common sense. For example, on a day when the temperature is 85°F and the humidity is around 80 percent, postpone lunchtime physical activity until the evening when it is cooler or exercise indoors where the conditions are controlled.

## Exercising in the Cold

When you exercise in cool weather, especially in windy and damp conditions, your body's rate of heat loss is frequently greater than its rate of heat production. These conditions may lead to **hypothermia**—a condition in which the body's core temperature drops below 95°F.[59] Temperatures need not be frigid for hypothermia to occur; it can also result from prolonged, vigorous exercise in 40°F to 50°F temperatures, particularly if there is rain, snow, or a strong wind.

As body core temperature drops from the normal 98.6°F to about 93.2°F, shivering begins. Shivering—the involuntary contraction of nearly every muscle in the body—increases body temperature by using the heat given off by muscle activity. You may also experience cold hands and feet, poor judgment, apathy, and amnesia. Shivering ceases in most hypothermia victims as body core temperatures drop to between 87°F and 90°F, a sign that the body has lost its ability to generate heat. Death usually occurs at body core temperatures between 75°F and 80°F.[60]

To prevent hypothermia, analyze weather conditions before engaging in outdoor physical activity. Remember that wind and humidity are as significant as temperature. Have a friend join you for safety when exercising outdoors in cold weather, and wear layers of appropriate clothing to prevent excessive heat loss and frostbite (polypropylene or woolen undergarments, a windproof outer garment, and a wool hat and gloves). Keep your head, hands, and feet warm. Finally, do not allow yourself to become dehydrated.[61]

# Treating Injuries

First-aid treatment for virtually all fitness training–related injuries involves **RICE**: **r**est, **i**ce, **c**ompression, and **e**levation.

- *Rest*—is required to avoid further irritation of the injured body part.
- *Ice*—is applied to relieve pain and constrict the blood vessels to reduce internal or external bleeding. To prevent frostbite, wrap the ice or cold pack in a layer of wet toweling or elastic bandage before applying it to your skin. A new injury should be iced for approximately 20 minutes every hour for the first 24 to 72 hours.
- *Compression*—of the injured body part can be accomplished with a 4- or 6-inch-wide elastic bandage; this applies indirect pressure to damaged blood vessels to help stop bleeding. Be careful, though, that the compression wrap does not interfere with normal blood flow. Throbbing or pain indicates that the compression wrap should be loosened.
- *Elevation*—of an injured extremity above the level of your heart also helps control internal or external bleeding by making the blood flow upward to reach the injured area.

Applying ice to an injury such as a sprain can help relieve pain and reduce swelling, but never apply the ice directly to the skin, as that could lead to frostbite.

**RICE** Acronym for the standard first-aid treatment for virtually all traumatic and overuse injuries: rest, ice, compression, and elevation.

## 1 Evaluating Your Cardiorespiratory Endurance (The 1.5-Mile Run Test)

This test assesses your cardiorespiratory endurance level.

### Procedure

Find a local track, typically .25 mile per lap, to perform your test. Run 1.5 miles; use a stopwatch to measure how long it takes to reach that distance. If you become extremely fatigued during the test, slow your pace or walk—do not overstress yourself! If you feel faint or nauseated or experience any unusual pains in your upper body, stop and notify your instructor. Use the chart below to estimate your cardiorespiratory fitness level based on your age and sex. Note that women have lower standards for each fitness category because they have higher levels of essential fat than men do.

### Fitness Categories for 1.5-Mile Run Test

| Men, years | Excellent | Good | Fair | Poor |
|---|---|---|---|---|
| 20–29 | < 10:10 | 10:10–11:29 | 11:30–12:38 | > 12:38 |
| 30–39 | < 10:47 | 10:47–11:54 | 11:55–12:58 | > 12:58 |
| 40–49 | < 11:16 | 11:16–12:24 | 12:25–13:50 | > 13:50 |
| 50–59 | < 12:09 | 12:09–13:35 | 13:36–15:06 | > 15:06 |
| 60–69 | < 13:24 | 13:24–15:04 | 15:05–16:46 | > 16:46 |

| Women, years | Excellent | Good | Fair | Poor |
|---|---|---|---|---|
| 20–29 | < 11:59 | 11:59–13:24 | 13:25–14:50 | > 14:50 |
| 30–39 | < 12:25 | 12:25–14:08 | 14:09–15:43 | > 15:43 |
| 40–49 | < 13:24 | 13:24–14:53 | 14:54–16:31 | > 16:31 |
| 50–59 | < 14:35 | 14:35–16:35 | 16:36–18:18 | > 18:18 |
| 60–69 | < 16:34 | 16:34–18:27 | 18:28–20:16 | > 20:16 |

**Source:** The Cooper Institute, *Physical Fitness Assessments and Norms for Adults and Law Enforcement,* Dallas, Texas. Copyright © 2007 by The Cooper Institute. Reprinted with permission.

## 2 Evaluating Your Muscular Strength and Endurance (Partial Curl-Up Test)

Your abdominal muscles are important for core stability and back support; this test will assess their muscular endurance.

### Procedure

Lie on a mat with your arms by your sides, palms flat on the mat, elbows straight, and fingers extended. Bend your knees at a 90-degree angle. Your instructor or partner will mark your starting finger position with a piece of masking tape aligned with the tip of each middle finger. He or she will also mark with tape your ending position, 10 cm (4 inches) away from the first piece of tape—one ending position tape for each hand.

Set a metronome to 50 beats per minute and curl up at this slow, controlled pace: one curl-up every two beats (25 curl-ups per minute). Curl your head and upper back upward, lifting your shoulder blades off the mat (your trunk should make a 30-degree angle with the mat) and reaching your arms forward along the mat to touch the ending tape. Then curl back down so that your upper back and shoulders touch the floor. During the entire curl-up, your fingers, feet, and buttocks should stay on the mat. Your partner will count the number of correct repetitions you complete. Perform as many curl-ups as you can in 1 minute without pausing, to a maximum of 25.

### Healthy Musculoskeletal Fitness: Norms and Health Benefit Zones: Curl-Ups

| Men, years | Excellent | Good | Fair | Needs Improvement | Women, years | Excellent | Good | Fair | Needs Improvement |
|---|---|---|---|---|---|---|---|---|---|
| 20–29 | 25 | 21–24 | 11–20 | ≤ 10 | 20–29 | 25 | 18–24 | 5–17 | ≤ 4 |
| 30–39 | 25 | 18–24 | 11–17 | ≤ 10 | 30–39 | 25 | 19–24 | 6–18 | ≤ 5 |
| 40–49 | 25 | 18–24 | 6–17 | ≤ 5 | 40–49 | 25 | 19–24 | 4–18 | ≤ 3 |
| 50–59 | 25 | 17–24 | 8–16 | ≤ 7 | 50–59 | 25 | 19–24 | 6–18 | ≤ 5 |
| 60–69 | 25 | 16–24 | 6–15 | ≤ 5 | 60–69 | 25 | 17–24 | 3–16 | ≤ 2 |

**Source:** From *Canadian Physical Activity, Fitness & Lifestyle Approach: CSEP-Health & Fitness Program's Appraisal and Counselling Strategy,* 3rd edition, © 2003. Reprinted with permission from the Canadian Society for Exercise Physiology

# 3 Evaluating Your Flexibility (The Sit-and-Reach Test)

This test measures the general flexibility of your lower back, hips, and hamstring muscles.

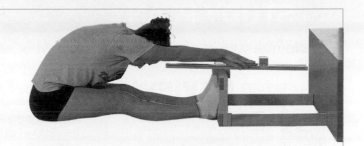

## Procedure

Warm up with some light activity that involves the total body, range-of-motion exercises, and stretches for the lower back and hamstrings. For the test, start by sitting upright, straight-legged on a mat with your shoes removed and soles of the feet flat against a flexometer (sit-and-reach box) at the 10.25-in mark. Inner edges of the soles are placed within 0.75 in of the measuring scale.

Have a partner on hand to record your measurements. Stretch your arms out in front of you and, keeping the hands parallel to each other, slowly reach forward with both hands as far as possible, holding the position for approximately

2 seconds. Your fingertips should be in contact with the measuring portion of the sit-and-reach box. To facilitate a longer reach, exhale and drop your head between your arms while reaching forward. Keep your knees extended the whole time and breathe normally.

Your score is the most distant point (in inches) reached with the fingertips; have your partner make note of this number for you. Perform the test twice, record your best score, and compare it with the norms presented in the following tables.

## Healthy Musculoskeletal Fitness: Norms and Health Benefit Zones: Sit-and-Reach Test*

| Men, years | Excellent (in) | Very Good (in) | Good (in) | Fair (in) | Needs Improvement (in) | Women, years | Excellent (in) | Very Good (in) | Good (in) | Fair (in) | Needs Improvement (in) |
|---|---|---|---|---|---|---|---|---|---|---|---|
| 20–29 | ≥ 15.5 | 13.5–15.5 | 12–13 | 10–11.5 | ≤ 10 | 20–29 | ≥ 16 | 14.5–15.5 | 13–14 | 11–12.5 | ≤ 10.5 |
| 30–39 | ≥ 15 | 13–14.5 | 11–12.5 | 9–10.5 | ≤ 9 | 30–39 | ≥ 16 | 14–15.5 | 12.5–13.5 | 10.5–12 | ≤ 10 |
| 40–49 | ≥ 13.5 | 11.5–13.5 | 9.5–11 | 7–9 | ≤ 6.5 | 40–49 | ≥ 15 | 13.5–14.5 | 12–13 | 10–11.5 | ≤ 9.5 |
| 50–59 | ≥ 13.5 | 11–13.5 | 9.5–10.5 | 6–9 | ≤ 6 | 50–59 | ≥ 15.5 | 13–15 | 12–12.5 | 10–11.5 | ≤ 9.5 |
| 60–69 | ≥ 13 | 10–12.5 | 8–9.5 | 6–7.5 | ≤ 5.5 | 60–69 | ≥ 13.5 | 12–13.5 | 10.5–12 | 9–10 | ≤ 8.5 |

*Note: These norms are based on a sit-and-reach box in which the zero point is set at 10.25 in. When using a box in which the zero point is set at 9 in, subtract 1.2 in from each value in this table.
Source: From *Canadian Physical Activity, Fitness & Lifestyle Approach: CSEP-Health & Fitness Program's Appraisal and Counselling Strategy*, 3rd edition, © 2003. Reprinted with permission from the Canadian Society for Exercise Physiology.

## YOUR PLAN FOR CHANGE

The **ASSESS YOURSELF** activity helped you determine your current level of physical fitness. Based on your results, you may decide that you should take steps to improve one or more components of your physical fitness.

### TODAY, YOU CAN:

☐ Visit your campus fitness facility (or its website) and familiarize yourself with the equipment and resources. Find out what classes it offers, and take home (or print out) a copy of the schedule.

☐ Walk between your classes; make an extra effort to take the long way to get from building to building. Use the stairs instead of the elevator or escalator.

☐ Take an activity break. Spend 5 to 10 minutes between homework projects or just before bed doing some type of activity, such as abdominal crunches, push-ups, or yoga poses.

### WITHIN THE NEXT TWO WEEKS, YOU CAN:

☐ Shop for comfortable workout clothes and appropriate athletic footwear.

☐ Look into group activities on your campus or in your community that you might enjoy.

☐ Ask a friend to join you in your workout once a week. Agree on a date and time in advance so you both will be committed to following through.

☐ Plan for a physically active outing with a friend or date; perhaps you can go dancing, bowling, or shoot hoops. Use active transportation (i.e., walk or cycle) to get to a movie or go out for dinner.

### BY THE END OF THE SEMESTER, YOU CAN:

☐ Establish a regular routine of engaging in physical activity or exercise at least three times a week. Mark your exercise times on your calendar and keep a log to track your progress.

☐ Take your workouts to the next level. If you have been working out at home, try going to a gym or participating in an exercise class. If you are walking, try walking up hills, intermittent jogging, or sign up for a fitness event such as a charity 5K.

## CHAPTER REVIEW

To hear an MP3 Tutor Session, scan here or visit the Study Area in **MasteringHealth**.

### LO 1 | Physical Activity for Health

- Benefits of regular physical activity include reduced risk of cardiovascular diseases, metabolic syndrome and type 2 diabetes, and cancer, as well as improved blood lipoproteins, bone mass, weight control, immunity to disease, mental health, stress management, and life span.

### LO 2 | Physical Activity for Fitness and Performance

- Physical fitness involves achieving minimal levels in the health-related components of fitness: cardiorespiratory, muscular strength, muscular endurance, flexibility, and body composition. Skill-related components of fitness, such as agility, balance, reaction time, speed, coordination, and power, are essential for elite and recreational athletes to increase their performance in and enjoyment of sport.

### LO 3 | Committing to Physical Fitness

- Commit to your new lifestyle of physical activity and increased fitness levels by incorporating fitness activities into your life. If you are new to exercise, start slowly, keep your fitness program simple, and consider consulting your physician and/or a fitness instructor for recommendations. Overcome your barriers or obstacles to exercise by identifying them and then planning specific strategies to address them. Choose activities that are fun and convenient to increase your likelihood of sticking with them.

### LO 4 | Creating Your Own Fitness Program

- The FITT principle can be used to develop a progressive program of physical fitness. For general health

benefits, every adult should participate in moderate-intensity activities for 30 minutes at least 5 days a week. To improve cardiorespiratory fitness, you should engage in vigorous, continuous, and rhythmic activities 3 to 5 days per week at an exercise intensity of 64 to 96 percent of your maximum heart rate for 20 to 30 minutes.

- Three key principles for developing muscular strength and endurance are overload, specificity of training, and reversibility. Muscular strength is improved by engaging in resistance-training exercises two to three times per week, using an intensity of greater than 60 percent of 1 RM, and completing two to four sets of 8 to 12 repetitions. Muscular endurance is improved by engaging in resistance-training exercises two to three times per week, using an intensity of less than 50 percent of 1 RM, and completing one to two sets of 15 to 25 repetitions.

- Flexibility is improved by engaging in two to four repetitions of static stretching exercises at least 2 to 3 days a week, where each stretch is held for 10 to 30 seconds.

### LO 5 | Implementing Your Fitness Program

- Planning to improve your physical fitness involves setting goals and designing a program to achieve these goals. A comprehensive workout should include a warm-up with some light stretching, strength-development exercises, aerobic activities, and a cool-down period with a heavier emphasis on stretching exercises. Core strength training is important for mobility, stability, and preventing back injury. The popular exercise forms of yoga, tai chi, and Pilates all develop core strength as well as flexibility, strength, and endurance.

### LO 6 | Taking in Proper Nutrition for Exercise

- Fueling properly for exercise involves eating a balance of healthy foods 3 to 4 hours before exercise. In exercise sessions lasting an hour or more, performance can benefit from some

additional calories ingested during the exercise session. Hydrating properly for exercise is important for performance and injury prevention. Chocolate milk is a good source of carbohydrates and protein for postexercise recovery.

### LO 7 | Preventing and Treating Common Exercise Injuries

- Physical activity–related injuries are generally caused by overuse or trauma. The most common overuse injuries are plantar fasciitis, shin splints, and runner's knee. Proper footwear and protective equipment help to prevent injuries. Exercising in the heat or cold requires taking special precautions. Minor exercise injuries should be treated with RICE (rest, ice, compression, and elevation).

## POP QUIZ

Visit **MasteringHealth** to personalize your study plan with Chapter Review Quizzes and Dynamic Study Modules.

### LO 1 | Physical Activity for Health

1. What is physical fitness?
   a. The ability to respond to routine physical demands
   b. Having enough physical reserves to cope with a sudden challenge
   c. A balance of cardiorespiratory, muscle, and flexibility fitness
   d. All of the above

2. Which of the following is not a health benefit associated with regular exercise?
   a. Reduced risk for some cancers
   b. Reduced risk for cardiovascular diseases
   c. Elimination of chronic diseases
   d. Improved mental health

### LO 2 | Physical Activity for Fitness and Performance

3. The maximum volume of oxygen consumed by the muscles during exercise defines

a. target heart rate.

b. muscular strength.

c. aerobic capacity.

d. muscular endurance.

4. Flexibility is the range of motion around

   a. specific bones.

   b. a joint or series of joints.

   c. the tendons.

   d. the muscles.

## LO 3 | Committing to Physical Fitness

5. Miguel is thinking about becoming more active. Which of the following is *not* a good piece of advice to offer him?

   a. Incorporate physical activity into your daily life.

   b. Make multiple changes to diet and exercise routines simultaneously.

   c. Identify obstacles to being active.

   d. Set SMART goals.

## LO 4 | Creating Your Own Fitness Program

6. Janice has been lifting 95 pounds while doing three sets of six leg curls. To become stronger, she began lifting 105 pounds while doing leg curls. What principle of strength development does this represent?

   a. Reversibility

   b. Overload

   c. Flexibility

   d. Specificity of training

7. The "talk test" measures

   a. exercise intensity.

   b. exercise time.

   c. exercise frequency.

   d. exercise type.

## LO 5 | Implementing Your Fitness Program

8. At the start of an exercise session, you should always

   a. stretch before doing any activity.

   b. do 50 crunches to activate your core muscles.

   c. warm up with light cardiorespiratory activities.

   d. eat a meal to ensure that you are fueled for the activity.

## LO 6 | Taking in Proper Nutrition for Exercise

9. Chocolate milk is good for

   a. preworkout energy boost.

   b. postworkout recovery.

   c. slimming down.

   d. staying hydrated during exercise.

## LO 7 | Preventing and Treating Common Exercise Injuries

10. Overuse injuries can be prevented by

   a. monitoring the quantity and quality of your workouts.

   b. engaging in only one type of aerobic training.

   c. working out daily.

   d. working out with a friend.

*Answers to the Pop Quiz can be found on page A-1. If you answered a question incorrectly, review the section identified by the Learning Outcome. For even more study tools, visit MasteringHealth.*

# THINK ABOUT IT!

## LO 1 | Physical Activity for Health

1. How do you define *physical fitness*? Identify at least four physiological and psychological benefits of physical activity. How would you promote these benefits to nonexercisers?

## LO 2 | Physical Activity for Fitness and Performance

2. How are muscle strength and muscle endurance different? What are some ways you might work to increase muscle strength and muscle endurance?

## LO 3 | Committing to Physical Fitness

3. What do you do to motivate yourself to engage in physical activity on a regular basis? What and who helps you to be physically active?

## LO 4 | Creating Your Own Fitness Program

4. Describe the FITT prescription for cardiorespiratory fitness, muscular

strength and endurance, and flexibility training.

## LO 5 | Implementing Your Fitness Program

5. Why is core strength important? What are some ways to increase your core strength every day?

## LO 6 | Taking in Proper Nutrition for Exercise

6. Why is when you eat as important as what you eat? How might your exercise preparation and routine differ in hot and cold climates?

## LO 7 | Preventing and Treating Common Exercise Injuries

7. What precautions do you need to take when exercising outdoors in the heat and in the cold?

# ACCESS YOUR HEALTH ON THE INTERNET

Visit **MasteringHealth** for links to the websites and RSS feeds.

The following websites explore further topics and issues related to personal health. For links to the websites below, visit the Study Area in MasteringHealth.

*American College of Sports Medicine.* This site is the link to the American College of Sports Medicine and all its resources. **www.acsm.org**

*American Council on Exercise.* Information is found here on exercise and disease prevention. **www.acefitness.org**

*Centers for Disease Control and Prevention, National Center for Chronic Disease Prevention and Health Promotion, Division of Nutrition, Physical Activity, and Obesity.* This site is a great resource for current information on exercise and health. **www.cdc.gov/nccdphp/dnpao**

*National Strength and Conditioning Association.* This site is a resource for personal trainers and others interested in conditioning and fitness. **www.nsca-lift.org**

# 12 Reducing Your Risk of Cardiovascular Disease and Cancer

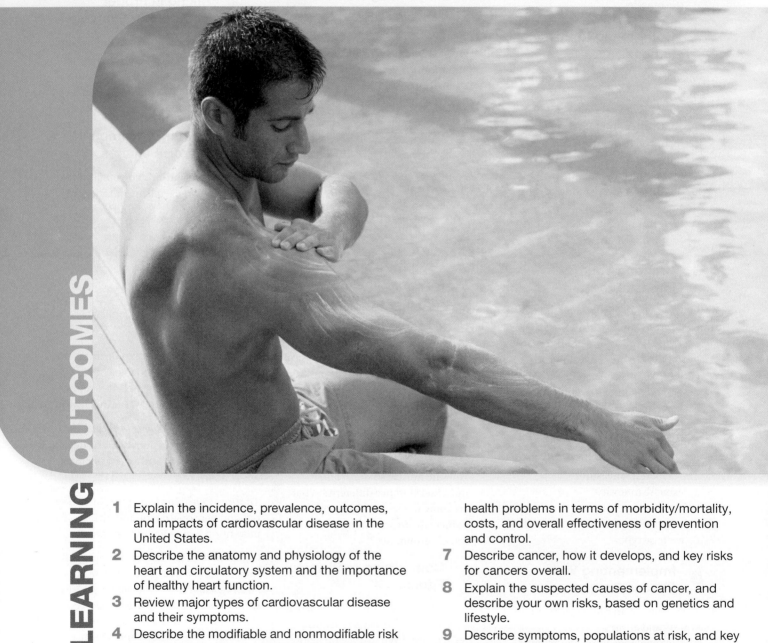

When we think of the major disease killers, images of older individuals dying after a long battle with *cancer* or succumbing to a fast and painful death from *cardiovascular disease* (CVD) like heart attack or stroke often come to mind. In reality, more often than not, cancer and CVD are long-term illnesses that exact a huge toll on individuals young and old, their loved ones, and society. In fact, these two categories of disease are among the greatest contributors to the **global burden of disease (GBD)**, a method of quantifying the burden of premature morbidity, disability, and death for a given disease or disease group.[1] GBD is measured in **disability adjusted years (DALYs)** or years lived in ill health or disability.[2] Today, people in many higher income regions of the world often live longer with diseases such as cancer and CVD due to earlier diagnosis, better treatments, and improved medicines, all of which increase disease costs. Diabetes, another major cause of global disease is discussed in **Focus On: Minimizing Your Risk for Diabetes** beginning on page 386.)

Even though death rates have declined and people may live longer, CVD continues to be the leading cause of death in the world, killing more than 17 million each year. If current trends continue, numbers are projected to grow to nearly 24 million by 2030.[3]

Like CVD, cancer is no slouch when it comes to exacting a heavy global burden. In 2012, over 14 million new cases of cancer were diagnosed and slightly over 8.2 million people died from cancer-related causes.[4] These rates are projected to soar to 21.7 million new cases and 13 million deaths by 2030.[5] Cancers of the lungs, stomach, liver, colon, and female breasts account for the largest percentage of cancer death.[6] Those living in poverty are hit hardest and have the worst prognosis once cancer or CVD are diagnosed, as resources necessary for early and comprehensive diagnosis and treatment are often lacking.[7]

Both CVD and cancer are **chronic diseases**, meaning they are prolonged, do not resolve spontaneously, and are rarely cured completely. As such, they are responsible for significant rates of disability, lost productivity, pain, and suffering, not to mention soaring health care costs. Cardiovascular diseases in particular are closely related to lifestyle factors such as obesity, sedentary behavior, poor nutrition, stress, lack of sleep, tobacco use, and excessive alcohol use. The good news is that in many cases, these lifestyle factors can be changed or modified to decrease disease risks for both CVD and cancer.

## LO 1 | CARDIOVASCULAR DISEASE IN THE UNITED STATES

Explain the incidence, prevalence, outcomes, and impacts of cardiovascular disease in the United States.

Early in 2015, the American Heart Association (AHA) reported that death rates from **cardiovascular disease (CVD)**—diseases associated with the heart and blood vessels, such as high blood pressure, coronary heart disease (CHD), heart failure, stroke, and congenital cardiovascular defects—had declined by nearly 33 percent in the last decade.[8] Sounds great, doesn't it? In spite of the promising decline, nearly 86 million Americans, more than 1 out of every 3 adults, suffer from one or more types of CVD.[9]

Much of the improvement in death rates is due to better diagnosis, early intervention and treatment, and a multi-billion-dollar market in drugs designed to keep the heart and circulatory system ticking along. We've also improved our understanding about diet, activity, and other behaviors that impact risk of CVD. Yet, CVD continues to be a threat (**FIGURE 12.1**).[10] Nearly *one third* of all deaths in the United States have CVD as an underlying cause—more than cancer, chronic lower respiratory diseases, and accidental deaths combined.[11] Some populations are disproportionately affected; 48 percent of African American women and 46 percent of African American men have a variety of cardiovascular disease.[12]

HEAR IT! PODCASTS

Want a study podcast for this chapter? Download **Cardiovascular Disease: Reducing Your Risk** and **Cancer: Reducing Your Risk,** available on

MasteringHealth™

**global burden of disease (GBD)** A method of quantifying the burden of premature morbidity, disability, and death for a given disease or disease groups.

**disability adjusted life years (DALYs)** A measure of overall disease burden expressed as the number of years lost due to ill-health.

**chronic disease** An illness that is prolonged, does not resolve spontaneously, and is rarely cured.

**cardiovascular disease (CVD)** Disease of the heart and blood vessels.

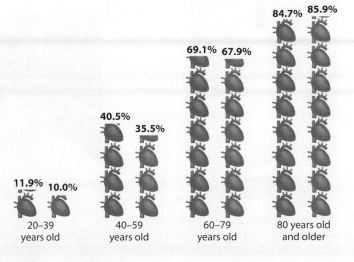

 Men with CVD; each heart = 10% of the population

Women with CVD; each heart = 10% of the population

**FIGURE 12.1** Prevalence of Cardiovascular Diseases (CVDs) in Adults Aged 20 and Older by Age and Sex

**Source:** Data from D. Mozaffarian, et al. "Heart Disease and Stroke Statistics, 2015 Update," *Circulation* 131 (2015): e29–2322).

# 2,150

IS THE NUMBER OF AMERICANS WHO DIE EVERY DAY OF **CVD**. MILLIONS MORE ARE DISABLED OR TAKING MEDICATIONS TO KEEP THEIR CVD UNDER CONTROL.

Although these statistics are grim, the reality is that CVD has been the leading killer of both men and women in the United States every year since 1918, when a pandemic flu killed more people.[13] Recognizing that selected risk factors are key to changing the future course of CVD, the American Heart Association is aiming to improve Americans' cardiovascular health by 20 percent and to reduce death from CVDs and stroke by 20 percent—all by the year 2020.[14] As part of this strategy, the AHA is focusing on **ideal cardiovascular health (ICH)** rather than mortality rates and the disease process. ICH is defined as the absence of clinical indicators of CVD and the simultaneous presence of the following seven behavioral and health factor metrics.[15]

**Behaviors:**
1. Not smoking
2. Recommended physical activity
3. A healthy diet pattern
4. A healthy weight

**Health Factors:**
5. Having optimal total cholesterol without medication
6. Having optimal blood pressure without medication
7. Having optimal fasting blood glucose without medication

How are we doing with respect to these ideal healthy heart measures today? Not so hot. Only 18 percent of U.S. adults meet five or more metrics with ideal levels, whereas 50 percent of children meet five or more metrics.[16] Clearly, we have a long way to go.

The best defense against CVD is to reduce your risks and prevent it from developing in the first place. Considerable research points to the fact that the sooner you start, the better![17]

**ideal cardiovascular health (ICH)** The absence of clinical indicators of CVD and the presence of certain behavioral and health factor metrics.

**cardiovascular system** Organ system, consisting of the heart and blood vessels, that transports nutrients, oxygen, hormones, metabolic wastes, and enzymes throughout the body.

**atria (singular: atrium)** The heart's two upper chambers, which receive blood.

**ventricles** The heart's two lower chambers, which pump blood through the blood vessels.

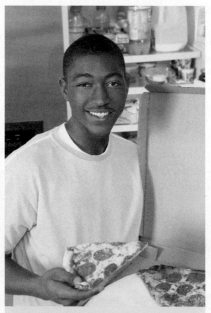

About 25 percent of your blood cholesterol level comes from foods you eat, and this is where you can make real improvements.

## LO 2 | UNDERSTANDING THE CARDIOVASCULAR SYSTEM

Describe the anatomy and physiology of the heart and circulatory system and the importance of healthy heart function.

The **cardiovascular system** is the network of organs and vessels through which blood flows as it carries oxygen and nutrients to all parts of the body. It includes the *heart, arteries, arterioles* (small arteries), *veins, venules* (small veins), and *capillaries* (minute blood vessels). Understanding how your cardiovascular system works and the factors that can impair its functioning will help you understand your risk and how to reduce it.

## The Heart: A Mighty Machine

The heart is a muscular, four-chambered pump, roughly the size of your fist. It is a highly efficient, extremely flexible organ that contracts 100,000 times each day and pumps the equivalent of 2,000 gallons of blood through the body. In a 70-year lifetime, an average human heart beats 2.5 billion times.

Under normal circumstances, the human body contains approximately 6 quarts of blood, which transports nutrients, oxygen, waste products, hormones, and enzymes throughout the body. Blood also aids in regulating body temperature, cellular water levels, and acidity levels of body components, and it helps defend the body against toxins and harmful microorganisms. An adequate blood supply is essential to health and well-being.

The heart has four chambers that work together to circulate blood constantly throughout the body. The two upper chambers of the heart, called **atria,** are large collecting chambers that receive blood from the rest of the body. The two lower chambers, known as **ventricles,** pump the blood out again. Small valves regulate the steady, rhythmic flow of blood between chambers and prevent leakage or backflow between them.

**Heart Function** Heart activity depends on a complex interaction of biochemical, physical, and neurological signals. Here are the four basic steps involved in heart function (see **FIGURE 12.2**):

1. Deoxygenated blood enters the right atrium after having been circulated through the body.
2. From the right atrium, blood moves to the right ventricle and is pumped through the pulmonary artery to the lungs, where it receives oxygen.

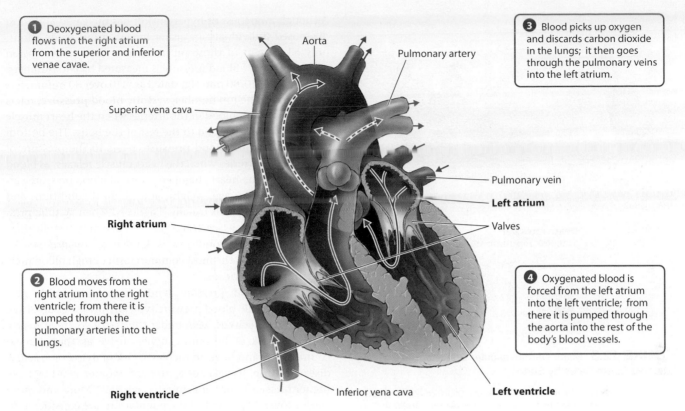

① Deoxygenated blood flows into the right atrium from the superior and inferior venae cavae.

③ Blood picks up oxygen and discards carbon dioxide in the lungs; it then goes through the pulmonary veins into the left atrium.

Aorta

Pulmonary artery

Superior vena cava

Pulmonary vein

**Left atrium**

**Right atrium**

Valves

② Blood moves from the right atrium into the right ventricle; from there it is pumped through the pulmonary arteries into the lungs.

④ Oxygenated blood is forced from the left atrium into the left ventricle; from there it is pumped through the aorta into the rest of the body's blood vessels.

**Right ventricle**

Inferior vena cava

**Left ventricle**

**FIGURE 12.2** Blood Flow within the Heart

3. Oxygenated blood from the lungs then returns to the left atrium of the heart.

4. Blood from the left atrium moves into the left ventricle. The left ventricle pumps blood through the aorta to all body parts.

Various blood vessels perform different parts of this process. **Arteries** carry blood away from the heart; all arteries carry oxygenated blood, *except* for pulmonary arteries, which carry deoxygenated blood to the lungs, where the blood picks up oxygen and gives off carbon dioxide. As the arteries branch off from the heart, they branch into smaller blood vessels called **arterioles,** and then into even smaller blood vessels known as **capillaries.** Capillaries have thin walls that permit the exchange of oxygen, carbon dioxide, nutrients, and waste products with body cells. Carbon dioxide and other waste products are transported to the lungs and kidneys through **veins** and **venules** (small veins).

For the heart to function properly, the four chambers must beat in an organized manner. Your heartbeat is governed by an electrical impulse that directs the heart muscle to move when the impulse travels across it, resulting in a sequential contraction of the four chambers. This signal starts in a small bundle of highly specialized cells, the **sinoatrial node (SA node),** located in the right atrium. The SA node serves as a natural pacemaker for the heart. People with a damaged SA node must often have a mechanical pacemaker implanted to ensure the smooth passage of blood

through the heartbeat's sequential phases.

At rest, the average adult heart beats 70 to 80 times per minute; a well-conditioned heart may beat only 50 to 60 times per minute to achieve the same results. If your resting heart rate is routinely in the high 80s or 90s, it may indicate that you are out of shape or suffering from some underlying illness. When overly stressed, a heart may beat more than 200 times per minute. A healthy heart functions more efficiently and is less likely to suffer damage from overwork.

**arteries** Vessels that carry blood away from the heart to other regions of the body.

**arterioles** Branches of the arteries.

**capillaries** Minute blood vessels that branch out from the arterioles and venules; their thin walls permit exchange of oxygen, carbon dioxide, nutrients, and waste products among body cells.

**veins** Vessels that carry blood back to the heart from other regions of the body.

**venules** Branches of the veins.

**sinoatrial node (SA node)** Cluster of electric pulse–generating cells that serves as a natural pacemaker for the heart.

## LO **3** | **KEY** CARDIOVASCULAR DISEASES

Review major types of cardiovascular disease and their symptoms.

Although there are several types of CVD and derivatives thereof, the key ones we will consider are hypertension, atherosclerosis, peripheral arterial disease (PAD), coronary heart disease (CHD), angina pectoris, arrhythmia, congestive heart

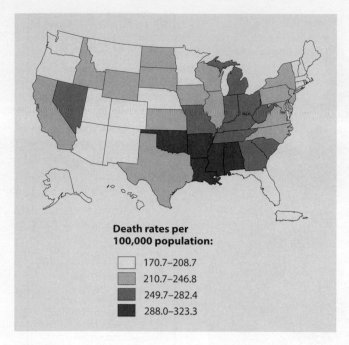

**FIGURE 12.3** Major Cardiovascular Disease Age-Adjusted Death Rates by State

**Death rates per 100,000 population:**
- 170.7–208.7
- 210.7–246.8
- 249.7–282.4
- 288.0–323.3

**Source:** A. S. Go et al., "Heart Disease and Stroke Statistics—2014 Update: A Report from the American Heart Association," *Circulation* 129 (2014): e28–e292.

failure, and stroke. Many forms of CVD are potentially fatal, and **FIGURE 12.3** presents the prevalence CVD-related deaths among adults in the United States.

## Hypertension

Blood pressure measures how hard blood pushes against the walls of vessels as your heart pumps. Sustained high blood pressure is called **hypertension**. Known as the "silent killer," it has few overt symptoms. Untreated hypertension damages blood vessels and increases your chance of angina, heart failure, peripheral artery disease, stroke, and heart attack. Hypertension can also cause kidney damage and contribute to vision loss, erectile dysfunction, and memory problems.[18]

Today, nearly 1 in 3 adults in the United States have high blood pressure; based on current trends, rates may reach 41.4 percent by 2030.[19] There are large disparities in self-reported hypertension by race/ethnicity, age, sex, level of education, and state. At approximately 45 percent, African Americans have the highest rates of high blood pressure in the United States and globally.[20] Rates are also much higher among the elderly, men, and those who don't have a high school education.[21]

**hypertension** Sustained elevated blood pressure.

**systolic blood pressure** The upper number in the fraction that measures blood pressure, indicating pressure on the walls of the arteries when the heart contracts.

**diastolic blood pressure** The lower number in the fraction that measures blood pressure, indicating pressure on the walls of the arteries during the relaxation phase of heart activity.

**prehypertensive** Blood pressure is above normal, but not yet in the hypertensive range.

Although awareness of hypertension has increased and most diagnosed individuals are using hypertension medications, only 53 percent of those on meds have their hypertension under control.[22] Blood pressure is measured by two numbers, for example, 110/80 mm Hg, stated as "110 over 80 millimeters of mercury." The top number, **systolic blood pressure**, refers to the pressure of blood in the arteries when the heart muscle contracts, sending blood to the rest of the body. The bottom number, **diastolic blood pressure**, refers to the pressure of blood on the arteries when the heart muscle relaxes, as blood is reentering the heart chambers. Normal blood pressure varies depending on age, weight, and physical condition, and high blood pressure is usually diagnosed when systolic pressure is 140 or above (see **TABLE 12.1**). When only systolic pressure is high, the condition is known as *isolated systolic hypertension (ISH)*, the most common form of high blood pressure in older Americans.

Systolic blood pressure tends to increase with age, whereas diastolic blood pressure typically increases until age 55 and then declines. Men under the age of 45 are at nearly twice the risk of becoming hypertensive as their female counterparts and have an increased risk of dying of vascular disease within 10 years of a stroke.[23] Women tend to have higher rates of hypertension after age 65.[24] More and more people (over 30 percent of the population) are considered to be **prehypertensive**, meaning that their blood pressure is above normal, but not yet in the hypertensive range. These individuals have a significantly greater risk of becoming hypertensive.[25]

New guidelines for the management/treatment of high blood pressure among those with a history of diabetes, heart disease, or stroke are available. In general, guidelines for treating and managing high blood pressure provide information about maintaining lower blood pressure levels, recommending certain types of meds, as well as optimal times to begin medicating. People 65 and over are usually put on meds when their blood pressure is 150/90 or higher; those under 60 years of age are recommended to take medications at 140/90 or higher,

## TABLE **12.1** | Blood Pressure Classifications

| Classification | Systolic Reading (mm Hg) | | Diastolic Reading (mm Hg) |
|---|---|---|---|
| Normal | Less than 120 | and | Less than 80 |
| Prehypertension | 120–139 | or | 80–89 |
| Hypertension | | | |
| Stage 1 | 140–159 | or | 90–99 |
| Stage 2 | Greater than or equal to 160 | or | Greater than or equal to 100 |
| Hypertensive crisis | Greater than or equal to 180 | or | Greater than or equal to 110 |

**Source:** The American Heart Association, "Understanding Blood Pressure Readings," 2015, http://www.heart.org/HEARTORG/Conditions/HighBloodPressure/HighBloodPressure/Understanding-Blood-Pressure-Readings_UCM_301764_Article.jsp

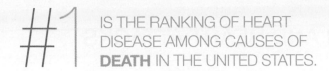 **IS THE RANKING OF HEART DISEASE AMONG CAUSES OF DEATH IN THE UNITED STATES.**

especially if they have kidney disease or diabetes. At current rates, more and more people will begin heart meds at younger and younger ages.[26]

## Atherosclerosis

**Arteriosclerosis,** thickening and hardening of arteries, is a condition that underlies many cardiovascular health problems. **Atherosclerosis** is a type of arteriosclerosis, where fatty substances, cholesterol, cellular waste products, calcium, and fibrin (a clotting material in the blood) accumulate in the inner lining of an artery. *Hyperlipidemia* (abnormally high blood levels of *lipids,* which are non-water-soluble molecules, such as fats and cholesterol) is a key factor in this process, and the resulting buildup is referred to as **plaque.**

As plaque accumulates, it adheres to the inner lining of the blood vessels. Vessel walls become narrow and may eventually block blood flow or rupture. This is similar to putting your thumb over the end of a hose while water is running through it. Pressure builds within arteries just as pressure builds in the hose. If vessels are weakened and pressure persists, the artery may become weak

and eventually burst. Fluctuation in the blood pressure levels within arteries may actually damage their internal walls, making it even more likely that plaque will accumulate.

Atherosclerosis is the most common form of *coronary artery disease (CAD).* It occurs as plaques are deposited in vessel walls and restrict blood flow and oxygen to the body's main coronary arteries on the outer surface of the heart, often eventually resulting in a heart attack (see **FIGURE 12.4**). When circulation is impaired and blood flow to the heart is limited, the heart may become starved for oxygen—a condition commonly referred to as **ischemia.** Sometimes coronary artery disease is referred to as ischemic heart disease.

## Peripheral Artery Disease

When atherosclerosis occurs in the upper or lower extremities, such as in the arms, feet, calves, or legs, and causes narrowing or complete blockage of arteries, it is often called **peripheral artery disease (PAD).** In the United States, over 8.5 million

**arteriosclerosis** A general term for thickening and hardening of the arteries.

**atherosclerosis** Condition characterized by deposits of fatty substances (plaque) on the inner lining of an artery.

**plaque** Buildup of deposits in the arteries.

**ischemia** Reduced oxygen supply to a body part or organ.

**peripheral artery disease (PAD)** Atherosclerosis occurring in the lower extremities, such as in the feet, calves, or legs, or in the arms.

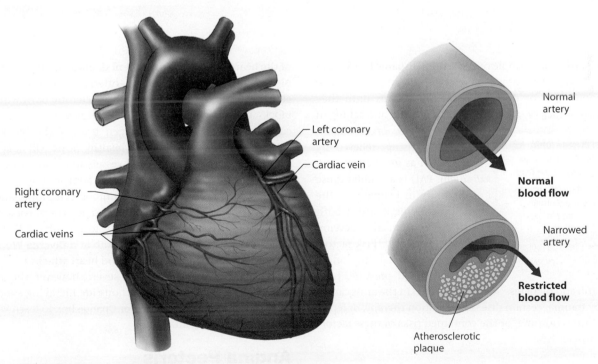

**FIGURE 12.4** **Atherosclerosis and Coronary Heart Disease** The coronary arteries are located on the exterior of the heart and supply blood and oxygen to the heart muscle itself. In atherosclerosis, arteries become clogged by a buildup of plaque. When atherosclerosis occurs in coronary arteries, blood flow to the heart muscle is restricted and a heart attack may occur.

**Sources:** Adapted from Joan Salge Blake, *Nutrition & You,* and Michael D. Johnson, *Human: Biology: Concepts and Current Issues*, 7th ed. Both copyright © 2014 Pearson Education, Inc. Reprinted by permission.

➔ **VIDEO TUTOR** Atherosclerosis and Coronary Artery Disease

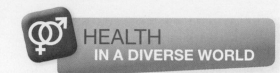
# WOMEN AND HEART ATTACKS

"Having a heart attack" usually brings to mind an older man gasping for breath, clutching his chest, toppling over in the middle of a workout. So, the story of comedian and former talk show host Rosie O'Donnell's heart attack doesn't seem to fit the mold: O'Donnell, 50, didn't immediately know she'd had one. At first, she wondered if she might have strained a muscle. Later she felt hot, clammy, and vomited. Fortunately, she took an aspirin and eventually went to the doctor, despite initially doubting a serious problem. It turned out O'Donnell had an almost complete blockage of a heart artery that required a stent.

Unfortunately, Rosie isn't alone. In fact, heart disease is the number one killer of women, affecting 1 out of every 3 in the United States. Like many chronic diseases, certain populations are disproportionately affected, in part because of late access to diagnosis and treatment—largely the result of being uninsured or underinsured, and lack of nearby information/resources about symptoms and risks. Nearly half of African American women have heart disease.

In addition to the above, women's heart attack symptoms often don't "look" like what people have come to expect. Women who suffer heart attacks under the age of 55 are not only less likely to have classic chest pain or pressure, but they also tend to delay going to the doctor. When they do seek medical attention, they often report atypical symptoms, such as shortness of breath, or pain in the neck, shoulder, arms, and stomach. Many women chalk up heart symptoms to stress, flu, or lack of exercise. Because of treatment delays, women are more likely to have heart damage and to die from a heart attack than are men of the same age.

So how can a woman tell if she is having a heart attack? In addition to the symptoms already mentioned, women may experience chest pressure or pain; radiating pains in the arms, shoulder, neck, jaw, or back; dizziness; abdominal pain; and unexplained feelings of fatigue, anxiety, or weakness—especially during exertion. But the real answer to the question of how to tell if a woman is having a heart attack is this: *Let a doctor* determine that. If you or someone you know has even a few of these symptoms, don't delay. Crush or chew a full strength aspirin and swallow it with water. In addition to being a pain killer, aspirin has blood-thinning properties; taking one can prevent fatal blood clots from forming. Then, have someone drive you to a health care facility for evaluation, or call 9-1-1 to get an ambulance.

**Sources:** J. Cant, W. J. Rogers, R. J. Goldberg, et al., "Association of Age and Sex with Myocardial Infarction Symptom Presentation and In-Hospital Mortality," *Journal of the American Medical Association* 307, no. 8 (2012,): 813–22; National Coalition for Women with Heart Disease, "Women Heart, Are You Having a Heart Attack?," 2014, www.heart.org/HEARTORG/Conditions/HeartAttack/WarningSignsofaHeartAttack/Angina-in-Women-Can-Be-Different-Than-Men. 2015_UCM_448902_Article.jsp

---

people—particularly people over 65, non-Hispanic blacks, and women—have PAD; many receive no treatment because they are asymptomatic or don't recognize symptoms until they have a heart attack or stroke.[27] Others have pain and aching in the legs, calves, or feet upon walking/exercising, relieved by rest (known as *intermittent claudication*). PAD is a leading cause of disability in people over the age of 50. While it strikes both men and women, men develop it more frequently. Risk factors include inflammation, smoking, high blood pressure, high cholesterol, and diabetes.[28] Sometimes PAD in the arms can be caused by trauma, certain diseases, radiation therapy, or repetitive motion syndrome, or the combined risks of these factors and atherosclerosis.

**coronary heart disease (CHD)** A narrowing of the small blood vessels that supply blood to the heart.

**myocardial infarction (MI; heart attack)** A blockage of normal blood supply to an area in the heart.

**angina pectoris** Chest pain occurring as a result of reduced oxygen flow to the heart.

## Coronary Heart Disease

Of all the major cardiovascular diseases, **coronary heart disease (CHD)** is the greatest killer, accounting for nearly 1 in 7 deaths in the United States. Nearly 1 million new and recurrent heart attacks occur in the United States each year.[29] A **myocardial infarction (MI),** or **heart attack,** involves an area of the heart that suffers permanent damage because its normal blood supply has been blocked—often brought on by a blood clot in a coronary artery or an atherosclerotic narrowing that blocks an artery. When blood does not flow readily, there is a corresponding decrease in oxygen flow. If the blockage is extremely minor, an otherwise healthy heart will adapt over time by enlarging existing blood vessels and growing new ones to reroute blood through other areas. Some populations, particularly women, seem to have unique symptoms and fare worse upon having a heart attack than do others. For a variety of reasons, women are more likely to die after a first heart attack than men are.[30] (See the **Health in a Diverse World** box for more information on women and heart attacks.)

When heart blockage is more severe, however, the body is unable to adapt on its own, and outside lifesaving support is critical. See the **Skills for Behavior Change** box to learn what to do in case of a heart attack.

## Angina Pectoris

**Angina pectoris** is a symptom of CHD that occurs when there is not enough oxygen to supply the heart muscle. Nearly 8 million people in the United States suffer from angina symptoms, ranging from indigestion or heartburn-like symptoms to palpitations and crushing chest pain.[31] Although angina pectoris is not a heart attack, it is an indicator of underlying heart

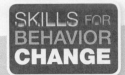
disease. Mild cases may be treated with rest. Drugs such as *nitroglycerin* can dilate veins and provide pain relief. Other medications such as *calcium channel blockers* can relieve cardiac spasms and arrhythmias, lower blood pressure, and slow heart rate. *Beta-blockers* can control potential overactivity of the heart muscle.

## Arrhythmias

Over the course of a lifetime, most people experience some type of **arrhythmia,** an irregularity in heart rhythm that occurs when the electrical impulses in the heart that coordinate heartbeat don't work properly. Often described as a heart "fluttering" or racing, these irregularities send many people to the emergency room, only to find they are fine. A racing heart in the absence of exercise or anxiety may be experiencing *tachycardia,* the medical term for abnormally fast heartbeat. On the other end of the continuum is *bradycardia,* or abnormally slow heartbeat. When a heart goes into **fibrillation,** it beats in a sporadic, quivering pattern, resulting in extreme inefficiency in moving blood through the cardiovascular system. If untreated, fibrillation may be fatal.

Not all arrhythmias are life-threatening. In many instances, excessive caffeine or nicotine consumption can trigger an

episode. However, severe cases may require drug therapy or external electrical stimulus to prevent serious complications. When in doubt, check with your doctor.

## Heart Failure

When the heart muscle is damaged or overworked and lacks the strength to keep blood circulating normally through the body, blood and fluids begin to back up into the lungs and other body tissues, continuing on to the feet, ankles, and legs, along with shortness of breath and tiredness. Known as **heart failure** or **congestive heart failure,** this condition is increasingly common, particularly among those with a history of other heart problems. Nearly 5.7 million adults have heart failure in the United States, with cases estimated to approach 10 million by 2030.[32]

Underlying causes of heart failure may include heart injury from CVD risks, including uncontrolled high blood pressure, rheumatic fever, pneumonia, heart attack, uncontrolled sleep apnea, or other problems. Certain prescription drugs such as NSAIDS and diabetes medications also increase risks, as do chronic drug and alcohol abuse. In some cases, radiation or chemotherapy treatments for cancer cause damage.

Untreated, heart failure can be fatal. However, most cases respond well to treatment that includes *diuretics* ("water pills") to relieve fluid accumulation; drugs, such as *digitalis,* that increase the pumping action of the heart; and drugs called *vasodilators,* which expand blood vessels and decrease resistance, allowing blood to flow more freely and making the heart's work easier.

## Stroke

Like heart muscle, brain cells require a continuous supply of oxygen. A **stroke** (also called a *cerebrovascular accident*) occurs when blood supply to the brain is interrupted. Strokes may be either *ischemic* (caused by plaque formation that narrows blood flow or a clot that obstructs a blood vessel) or *hemorrhagic* (due to a weakening of a blood vessel that causes it to bulge or rupture). An **aneurysm** (a widening or bulge in a blood vessel that may become hemorrhagic) is the most well-known of the hemorrhagic strokes. When any of these events occurs, oxygen deprivation kills brain cells.

Some strokes are mild and cause only temporary dizziness or slight weakness or numbness. More serious interruptions in blood flow may impair speech, swallowing, memory, or motor control in the long term. Other strokes affect parts of the brain that regulate heart and lung function, killing within minutes. According to the American Heart Association, nearly 7 million

**arrhythmia** An irregularity in heartbeat.

**fibrillation** A sporadic, quivering pattern of heartbeat that results in extreme inefficiency in moving blood through the cardiovascular system.

**congestive heart failure (CHF)** An abnormal cardiovascular condition that reflects impaired cardiac pumping and blood flow; pooling blood leads to congestion in body tissues.

**stroke** A condition occurring when the brain is damaged by disrupted blood supply; also called cerebrovascular accident.

**aneurysm** A weakened blood vessel that may bulge under pressure and, in severe cases, burst.

**transient ischemic attacks (TIAs)** Brief interruption of the blood supply to the brain that causes only temporary impairment; often an indicator of impending major stroke.

Americans suffer a stroke every year, and almost 129,000 people die as a result, making it the fourth leading cause of death in the United States.[33] Strokes cause countless levels of disability and suffering; depression is often an issue with patients recovering from strokes.

Even scarier, more young people are having strokes than ever before, possibly due to increased obesity and hypertension.[34] Many strokes are preceded days, weeks, or months earlier by **transient ischemic attacks (TIAs)**, brief interruptions of the blood supply to the brain that cause only temporary impairment. Symptoms of TIAs include dizziness, particularly when first rising in the morning, weakness, temporary paralysis or numbness in the face or other regions, temporary memory loss, blurred vision, nausea, headache, slurred speech, or other unusual physiological reactions. Some people may experience unexpected falls or have blackouts; however, others may have no obvious symptoms. TIAs often indicate an impending major stroke. The earlier a stroke is recognized and treatment started (best results are seen if treatment begins within the first 1–2 hours), the more effective that treatment will be. See the **Skills for Behavior Change** box for tips on recognizing signs and symptoms of a possible stroke.

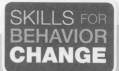

## SKILLS FOR BEHAVIOR CHANGE

### A SIMPLE TEST FOR STROKE

People often ignore, minimize, or misunderstand stroke symptoms. Starting treatment within just a few hours is crucial for the best recovery outcomes. So if you suspect someone is having a stroke, use the tool many emergency teams use to assess what is happening: think FAST.

▶ Facial droop: Ask the person to smile. It is normal for both sides of the face to move equally, and it is abnormal if one side moves less easily.

▶ Arm weakness: Ask the person to raise both arms. It is normal if both arms move equally (or not at all). It is abnormal if one arm drifts or cannot be raised as high as the other.

▶ Speech difficulty: Have the patient restate a sentence such as, You can't teach an old dog new tricks." It is normal if they can say the sentence correctly, and it is abnormal if they use inappropriate words, slur, or cannot speak.

▶ Time to *act* and call 9-1-1. Don't delay if you note 1–3 above. Time is of the essence.

**Source:** Centers for Disease Control, "Stroke Signs and Symptoms," April 2015, www.cdc.gov/stroke/signs_symptoms.htm

One of the greatest U.S. medical successes in recent years has been the decline in stroke fatality rates, which have dropped by one third since the 1980s and continue to fall.[35] Greater awareness of stroke symptoms and faster medical attention, improvements in emergency medicine protocols and medicines, and a greater emphasis on fast rehabilitation and therapy after a stroke have helped many survive. Newer treatments, including *tissue plasminogen activator* or *tPA*, the only FDA-approved treatment for ischemic stroke, dissolves clots and improves blood flow to affected areas, resulting in less damage and better chances of recovery. Various surgical techniques and mechanical devices are being tested that may further improve prognosis for future stroke victims.[36]

## LO 4 | REDUCING YOUR RISKS

Describe the modifiable and nonmodifiable risk factors for cardiovascular disease and methods of prevention.

Recently, the U.S. Burden of Disease Collaborators determined that greatest contributor to CVD was suboptimal diet, followed by tobacco smoking, high body mass index, high blood pressure, high fasting plasma glucose, and physical inactivity.[37] Newer research indicates that for people aged 12 to 39, smoking, high body fat, and high blood glucose increase the chances of dying from CVD-related complications before age 60.[38] As mentioned previously, hypertension doesn't just

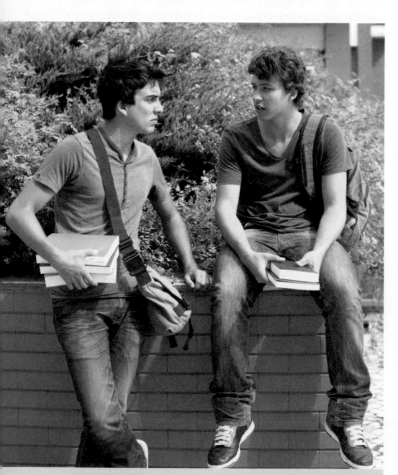

Young men, in particular, are at an elevated risk for stroke.

wreak havoc with your heart and circulatory system; it may eventually lead to cognitive function declines and may increase risk for Alzheimer's disease.[39] **Cardiometabolic risks** are the combined risks that indicate physical and biochemical changes that can lead to both CVD and type 2 diabetes. Some of these risks result from choices and behaviors, and so are modifiable. Others are inherited or intrinsic (such as your age and gender) and cannot be modified.

## Metabolic Syndrome: Quick Risk Profile

A cluster of combined cardiometabolic risks, variably labeled as *syndrome X, insulin resistance syndrome,* and, most recently, **metabolic syndrome** are believed to increase the risk for atherosclerotic heart disease by as much as three times the normal rates. Women are more likely than men to have metabolic syndrome overall. Nearly 23 percent of whites, 19 percent of African Americans, and 34.8 percent of Mexican Americans meet the criteria for metabolic syndrome.[40] Although different professional organizations have slightly different criteria for the syndrome, the National Cholesterol Education Program's Adult Treatment Panel (NCEP/ATP III) is most commonly used. According to these criteria, a person with three or more of the following risks is diagnosed with metabolic syndrome:[41]

- Abdominal obesity (waist measurement of more than 40 inches in men or 35 inches in women).
- Elevated blood fat (triglycerides greater than 150) or on drug treatment for elevated triglycerides
- Low levels of HDL ("good") cholesterol (less than 40 in men and less than 50 in women) or on drug treatment for HDL reduction
- Elevated blood pressure greater than 130/85 or on drug treatment for BP reduction
- Elevated fasting glucose greater than 100 mg/dL (a sign of insulin resistance or glucose intolerance) or on drug treatment for elevated glucose

Metabolic syndrome and other, similar terms have been important for highlighting the relationship between the number of risks a person possesses and that person's likelihood of developing CVD and diabetes. Groups such as the AHA and others are giving increased attention to focusing on multiple risks and emphasizing cardiovascular health in lifestyle interventions.

## Modifiable Risks

It may surprise you that younger adults are not invulnerable to CVD risks. The reality is that from the first moments of your life, you begin to accumulate increasing numbers of risks. Your past and future lifestyle choices may haunt you as you enter your middle and later years of life. Behaviors you choose today and over the coming decades can actively reduce or promote your risk for CVD.[42]

**Avoid Tobacco** Today, approximately 21 percent of U.S. adults age 18 and over are regular smokers in spite of massive efforts aimed at prevention and control (see Chapter 8).[43] Just how great a risk is smoking when it comes to CVD? Consider this:[44]

- Smokers are two to four times more likely to develop CHD than nonsmokers.
- Cigarette smoking doubles a person's stroke risk.
- Smokers are over 10 times more likely to develop peripheral vascular diseases than nonsmokers.

Some believe that nicotine in tobacco forces the heart to work harder to obtain sufficient oxygen. Other chemicals in smoke are thought to damage and inflame the lining of the coronary arteries, allowing cholesterol and plaque to accumulate more easily, increasing blood pressure and forcing the heart to work harder.

The good news is that if you stop smoking, your heart begins to mend itself. After 1 year, a former smoker's risk of heart disease drops by 50 percent. Between 5 to 15 years after quitting, the risk of stroke and CHD becomes similar to that of nonsmokers. Younger, college-age students take note: Studies have shown that those who quit smoking at age 30 reduce their chance of dying prematurely from smoking-related diseases by more than 90 percent.[45]

## Cut Back on Saturated Fat and Cholesterol

Cholesterol is a fatty, waxy substance found in the bloodstream and in body cells. Although we tend to hear only bad things about it, in truth, cholesterol plays an important role in the production of cell membranes and hormones and in other body functions. However, when blood cholesterol levels get

> **cardiometabolic risks** Risk factors that impact both the cardiovascular system and the body's biochemical metabolic processes.
>
> **metabolic syndrome (MetS)** A group of metabolic conditions occurring together that increases a person's risk of heart disease, stroke, and diabetes.

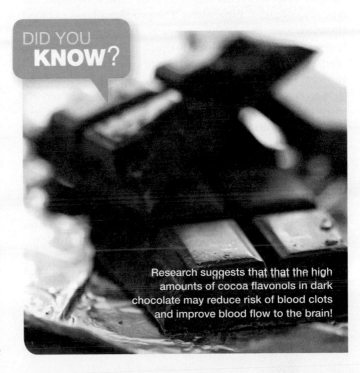

DID YOU **KNOW**?

Research suggests that that the high amounts of cocoa flavonols in dark chocolate may reduce risk of blood clots and improve blood flow to the brain!

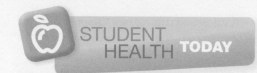
# IS CHOLESTEROL SO BAD?

When blood cholesterol levels get too high, the consensus until recently has been that CVD risk escalates. According to new ACC/AHA report, things might not be quite so black and white. In the report:

- Cholesterol is redeemed as *not being the major culprit* in artery clogging atherosclerosis. Instead, the report suggests we should be limiting saturated and avoiding *trans* fats. That means that eggs and shrimp, which are low in fat and high in protein, are taken off the "eat very little" list.

- Fruits and vegetables get a boost as being beneficial for all potential health outcomes.
- A *healthy diet,* including increases in fruits and vegetables, whole grains, low-fat and non-fat (low-sugar) foods, seafood, legumes, and nuts is emphasized.
- Sugar is a "no no." Intake should be limited to 12 teaspoons per day (less than a can of soda!). Right now, Americans consume over double that amount each day.
- Coffee gets a boost due to its antioxidant benefits.

- Salt consumption recommendations are reduced.

Until we learn more, current recommendations are to consume a balanced, plant-based diet such as the Mediterranean diet.

**Sources:** N.J Stone et al., "ACC/AHA Guidelines on the Treatment of Blood Cholesterol to Reduce Atherosclerotic Cardiovascular Risk in Adult: A Report of the American College of Cardiology/American Heart Association Task force on Practice Guidelines," *Circulation* 129 (2014): S1-S45; N. Stone et al., "Treatment of Blood Cholesterol to Reduce Atherosclerotic Cardiovascular Disease Risk in Adults: Synopsis of the 2013 American College of Cardiology/American Heart Association Cholesterol Guidelines," *Annals of Internal Medicine* 160, no. 5 (2014): 339–43.

---

too high, CVD risk escalates. See **Student Health Today** for info on the gray area around cholesterol.

Seventy-five percent of blood cholesterol is produced by your liver and other cells—mostly out of your control. The other 25 percent comes from the foods you eat. Changing your diet can make real improvements in your overall cholesterol level, even if your total amount is naturally high.

Diets high in saturated fat and *trans* fats are known to raise cholesterol levels, send the body's blood-clotting system into high gear, and make blood more viscous in just a few hours, increasing the risk of heart attack or stroke. Increased blood levels of cholesterol also contribute to atherosclerosis. Total cholesterol level isn't the only level to be concerned about; the type of cholesterol also matters. The two major types of blood cholesterol are *low-density lipoprotein (LDL)* and *high-density lipoprotein (HDL).* Low-density lipoprotein, often referred to as "bad" cholesterol, is believed to build up on artery walls. In contrast, high-density lipoprotein, or "good" cholesterol, appears to remove cholesterol from artery walls, thus serving as a protector. In theory, if LDL levels get too high or HDL levels too low, cholesterol will accumulate inside arteries and lead to cardiovascular problems.

*Triglycerides* have also gained increasing attention as a key factor in CVD risk. When you consume extra calories, the body converts them to triglycerides, which are stored in fat cells. High levels of blood triglycerides are often found in people who have high cholesterol levels, heart problems, diabetes, or who are overweight. As people get older, heavier, or both, their triglyceride and cholesterol levels tend to rise. It is recommended that a baseline cholesterol test (known as a lipid panel or lipid profile) be taken at age 20, with follow-ups every 5 years. This test, which measures triglyceride levels as well as HDL, LDL, and total cholesterol levels, requires that you fast for 12 hours prior to the test, are well hydrated, and avoid coffee and tea prior to testing. Men over the age of 35 and women over the age

of 45 should have their lipid profile checked annually, with more frequent tests for those at high risk. See **TABLE 12.2** for current recommended levels of cholesterol and triglycerides.

## TABLE **12.2** | Recommended Cholesterol Levels for Lower/Moderate Risk Adults

| Total Cholesterol Level (lower numbers are better) | |
|---|---|
| Less than 200 mg/dL | Desirable |
| 200–239 mg/dL | Borderline high |
| 240 mg/dL and above | High |
| **HDL Cholesterol Level (higher numbers are better)** | |
| Less than 40 mg/dL (for men) | Low |
| 60 mg/dL and above | Desirable |
| **LDL Cholesterol Level (lower numbers are better)** | |
| Less than 100 mg/dL | Optimal |
| 100–129 mg/dL | Near or above optimal |
| 130–159 mg/dL | Borderline high |
| 160–189 mg/dL | High |
| 190 mg/dL and above | Very high |
| **Triglyceride Level (lower numbers are better)** | |
| Less than 150 mg/dL | Normal |
| 150–199 mg/dL | Borderline high |
| 200–499 mg/dL | High |
| 500 mg/dL and above | Very high |

**Source:** Adapted from National Heart, Lung, and Blood Institute, National Institutes of Health, *ATP III Guidelines At-A-Glance Quick Desk Reference,* NIH Publication No. 01-3305, Update on Cholesterol Guidelines, 2004, www.nhlbi.nih.gov

In general, LDL (or "bad" cholesterol) is more closely associated with cardiovascular risk than is total cholesterol. Until recently, most authorities agreed that looking only at LDL ignored the positive effects of "good" cholesterol (HDL) and that raising HDL was an important goal. There has been general agreement that the best method of evaluating risk is to examine the ratio of HDL to total cholesterol. If the level of HDL is lower than 35 mg/dL, cardiovascular risk increases dramatically. To reduce risk, the goal has been to manage the ratio of HDL to total cholesterol by lowering LDL levels, raising HDL, or both. New research indicates that trying to raise HDL as a means of preventing negative CVD outcomes may not be as beneficial as once thought.[46]

Drugs that were effective in raising HDL levels had little or no effect on CVD risks or mortality. Regular exercise and a healthy diet low in saturated fat continue to be the best methods for maintaining healthy ratios. See the **Health Headlines** box on page 366 for information about foods and dietary practices that can help maintain healthy cholesterol levels.

About 45 percent of adults aged 20 and over have cholesterol levels at or above 200 mg/dL, and another 16 percent have levels in excess of 240 mg/dL.[47] Over half of all men aged 65 and over and nearly 40 percent of all women aged 65 or older are taking antihyperlipidemia prescription drugs and other medications to reduce blood fats.[48]

**Maintain a Healthy Weight** Researchers are not sure whether high-fat, high-sugar, high-calorie diets are a direct risk for CVD or whether they invite risk by causing obesity, which strains the heart, forcing it to push blood through the many miles of capillaries that supply each pound of fat. A heart that has to continuously move blood through an overabundance of vessels may become damaged. Overweight people are more likely to develop heart disease and stroke even if they have no other risk factors. This is especially true if you're an "apple" (thicker around your upper body and waist) rather than a "pear" (thicker around your hips and thighs).

**Exercise Regularly** Even modest levels of low-intensity physical activity—walking, gardening, housework, dancing—are beneficial if done regularly and over the long term. Exercise can increase HDL, lower triglycerides, and reduce coronary risks in several ways.

**Control Diabetes** Heart disease death rates among adults with diabetes are two to four times higher than the rates for adults without diabetes. At least 65 percent of people with diabetes die of some form of heart disease or stroke.[49] However, through a prescribed regimen of diet, exercise, and medication, they can control much of their increased risk for CVD. (See **Focus On: Minimizing Your Risk for Diabetes** starting on page 386 for more on preventing and controlling diabetes.)

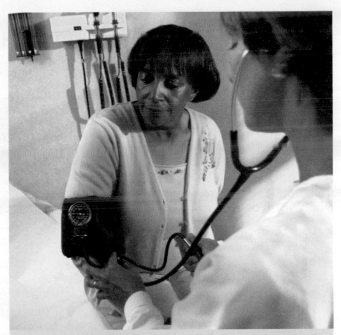

While many behavioral and environmental factors contribute to a person's risk for cardiovascular diseases, research suggests hereditary culprits, too. Find out your family history of CVD and have regular blood pressure and blood cholesterol screenings, as well as avoid lifestyle risks.

**Control Your Blood Pressure** In general, the higher your blood pressure, the greater your risk for CVD. Key factors in increasing blood pressure include obesity, lack of exercise, atherosclerosis, kidney damage from diabetes complications, and other factors.[50] Treatment of hypertension can involve dietary changes (avoiding high sodium and processed foods and cutting calories when appropriate),[51] medication, regular exercise, controlling stress, and getting enough sleep.

**Manage Stress** In recent years, scientists have shown compelling evidence that both acute and chronic stress may trigger acute cardiac events or even sudden cardiac death, as well as increase risks of hypertension, stroke, and elevated cholesterol levels.[52] Financial stressors, pressure to succeed in college and get a great job, pressure to find a partner, and pressure to please significant others can have a tsunamis-like effect on people young and old.[53] See Chapter 3 for more on effects of and coping with stress.

## Nonmodifiable Risks

Unfortunately, not all risk factors for CVD can be prevented or controlled. The most important are the following:

- **Race and ethnicity.** African Americans tend to have the highest overall rates of CVD and hypertension and the lowest rates of physical activity. Mexican Americans have the highest percentage of adults with cholesterol levels exceeding 200 mg/dL and the highest rates of obesity and overweight.[54]

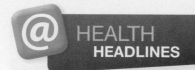

# @ HEALTH HEADLINES

# HEART-HEALTHY SUPER FOODS

The foods you eat play a major role in your CVD risk. While many foods can increase your risk, several have been shown to reduce the chances that cholesterol will be absorbed in the cells, reduce levels of LDL cholesterol, or enhance the protective effects of HDL cholesterol. To protect your heart, include the following in your diet:

- **Dark chocolate.** Dark chocolate contains 70 percent or more of flavonoid-rich cocoa, and much less sugar than milk chocolate. If you must indulge, buy the highest percent cocoa you can find, and savor the 1 to 2 ounces a bit at a time. Moderation is the key.
- **Fish high in omega-3 fatty acids.** Consumption of fish such as salmon, sardines, and herring may help reduce blood pressure and the inflammation that leads to plaque formation; however, new research is showing conflicting results about the benefits of omega-3s.
- **Olive oil.** Using monounsaturated fats in cooking, particularly extra virgin olive oil, helps lower total cholesterol and raise your HDL levels. Canola oil; margarine labeled *trans* fat–free; and cholesterol-lowering margarines such as Benecol, Promise Activ, or Smart Balance are also excellent choices.
- **Whole grains and fiber.** Getting enough fiber each day in the form of 100 percent whole wheat, steel cut oats, oat bran, flaxseed, fruits, and vegetables helps lower LDL or bad cholesterol. Soluble fiber, in particular, seems to keep cholesterol from being absorbed in the intestines.

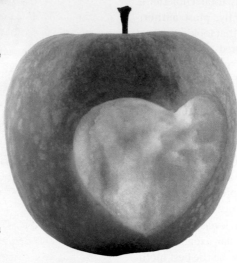

While an "apple a day" may not keep the proverbial doctor away, making sure that fruits and vegetables are part of a balanced diet is key to risk reduction for CVD and other health issues.

- **Plant sterols and stanols.** These essential components of plant membranes are found naturally in vegetables, fruits, and legumes. In addition, many food products, including juices and yogurt, are now fortified with them. These compounds are believed to benefit your heart health by blocking cholesterol absorption in the bloodstream, thus reducing LDL levels.
- **Nuts.** Long maligned for being high in calories, walnuts, almonds, and other nuts are naturally high in omega-3 fatty acids, which are important in lowering cholesterol and good for the blood vessels themselves.
- **Green tea.** Several studies have indicated that green tea may reduce LDL cholesterol. The flavonoids in it act as powerful antioxidants that may protect the cells of the heart and blood vessels;

however, other studies indicate that the FDA should *not* endorse health claims for green tea. Research in support is methodologically weak, and there are safety issues with the wide range of unfiltered tea available on the market.

- **Red wine.** In recent years, many observational studies have indicated that one glass of red wine may be protective and reduce your risk of CHD. Although the research is promising, the American Heart Association is slow to endorse drinking alcohol to reduce CVD risk and instead recommends dietary modification, exercise, and stress reduction, while supporting additional research. While one drink of red wine might be protective, adding additional doses of wine won't help and, in fact, is likely to be harmful.

**Sources:** L. Hooper, C. Kay, A. Abdelhamid et al., "Effects of Chocolate, Cocoa, and Flavan-3-ols on Cardiovascular Health: A Systematic Review and Meta-Analysis of Randomized Trials," *American Journal of Clinical Nutrition* 95, no. 3 (2012): 740–51; American Heart Association, "Alcoholic Beverages and Cardiovascular Disease," 2014, www.heart.org/HEARTORG/GettingHealthy/Nutrition-Center/HealthyEating/Alcohol-and-Heart-Health_UCM_305173_Article.jsp; P. Ronksley, S. Brien, B. Turner et al., "Association of Alcohol Consumption with Selected Cardiovascular Disease Outcomes: A Systematic Review and Meta-Analysis," *British Medical Journal* 342 (2011): 671–81; S. Kalesi, J. Sun, and N. Buys, "Green Tea Catechins and Blood Pressure: A Systematic Review and Meta Analysis of Randomized Controlled Trials," *European Journal of Nutrition,* May 2014, doi: 10.1007/s00394-014-0720-1; M. Murray, C. Walcuk, M. Suh, and P. J. Jones, "Green Tea Catechins and Cardiovascular Risk Factors. Should a Health Claim be Made by U.S. FDA?," *Trends in Food Science and Technology* 41, no. 2 (2015): 188–97; American Heart Association, "Fish and Omega 3 Fatty Acids," May 14, 2014, www.heart.org/HEARTORG/General/Fish-and-Omega-3-Fatty-Acids_UCM_303248_Article.jsp

- **Heredity.** A family history of heart disease increases risk of CVD significantly. The amount of cholesterol you produce, tendencies to form plaque, and other factors seem to have genetic links. The difficulty comes in sorting out genetic influences from the modifiable factors shared by family members, such as environment, stress, dietary habits, and so on. Newer research has focused on studying the interactions between nutrition and genes (*nutrigenetics*) and the role that diet may play in increasing or decreasing risks among certain genetic profiles.[55]

- **Age.** Although cardiovascular disease can affect all ages, over 68 percent of those aged 60 to 79 and 85 percent of those over 80 have one or more CVD issue.[56] Increasing age ups the risk of CVD for all.
- **Gender.** Men are at greater risk for CVD until about age 60, when women begin to catch up, taking the lead at age 80. Otherwise healthy women under age 35 have a fairly low risk, although oral contraceptive use and smoking increase risks. After menopause, or after estrogen levels are otherwise reduced (for example, because of hysterectomy), women's

LDL levels tend to go up, which increases the chance for CVD. Women also have poorer health outcomes and higher death rates than men when they have a heart attack.[57]

## Other Risk Factors Being Studied

Although risk factors for CVD are widely known, most people who die suddenly of a heart attack don't have obvious symptoms before it happens. New tests and emerging risk factors are being studied. Two fairly new CVD risks include high levels of inflammation in the vessels and homocysteine levels.

## Inflammation and C-Reactive Protein

Occurring when tissues are injured by bacteria, trauma, toxins, or heat, among other things, inflammation is increasingly being considered a culprit in atherosclerotic plaque formation. Injured vessel walls are more prone to plaque formation. To date, several factors, including cigarette smoke, high blood pressure, high LDL cholesterol, diabetes mellitus, certain forms of arthritis, gastrointestinal problems, and exposure to toxic substances have all been linked to increased risk of inflammation. However, the greatest risk appears to be from certain infectious disease pathogens, most notably *Chlamydia pneumoniae,* a common cause of respiratory infections; *Helicobacter pylori* (a bacterium that causes ulcers); herpes simplex virus (a virus that most of us have been exposed to); and *Cytomegalovirus* (another herpes virus infecting most Americans before the age of 40). During an inflammatory reaction, **C-reactive proteins** tend to be present at high levels. A recent meta-analysis of over 38 studies with nearly 170,000 subjects has shown a strong association between C-reactive proteins in the blood and increased risks for atherosclerosis and CVD.[58] Blood tests can test these proteins using a highly sensitive assay called *hs-CRP* (high-sensitivity C-reactive protein); if levels are high, action could be taken to reduce inflammation.

The FDA recently approved a new, nonfasting blood test that predicts heart attack in people with no history of heart disease. Known as *PLAC,* the test measures activity of inflammatory enzymes in the blood, which cause plaque to form. More inflammatory enzymes mean more plaque in vessels—and greater risk. The PLAC test could increase our ability to spot and treat potential heart attacks early in the process.[59]

Fish oil, flax, and other foods high in omega-3 have been recommended by the AHA and other groups for their anti-inflammatory properties, but newer research raises questions about the role of omega-3 in reducing risk of CHD and other cardiovascular problems.[60] In spite of conflicting reports, major professional organizations continue to recommend dietary omega-3 supplementation for risk reduction.[61] More research is necessary to determine the actual role that inflammation plays in increased risk of CVD or if there is something unique about inflammation that omega-3 may work to counter.[62]

**Homocysteine** In the last decade, an increasing amount of attention has been given to the role of homocysteine—an amino acid normally present in the blood—in increased risk for CVD. When present at high levels, homocysteine may be related to higher risk of coronary heart disease, stroke, and peripheral artery disease. Although more research is needed, scientists hypothesize that homocysteine works like C-reactive proteins—inflaming the inner lining of the arterial walls, promoting fat deposits on the damaged walls, and encouraging blood clot development.[63] When early studies indicated that folic acid and other B vitamins may help break down homocysteine in the body, food manufacturers responded by adding folic acids to a number of foods and touting the CVD benefits. With conflicting research, the jury is still out on the role of folic acid in CVD risk reduction. In fact, professional groups such as the American Heart Association do not currently recommend taking folic acid supplements to lower homocysteine levels and prevent CVD.[64] For now, a healthy diet is the best preventive action.

> **C-reactive protein (CRP)** A protein whose blood levels rise in response to inflammation.
>
> **homocysteine** An amino acid normally present in the blood that, when found at high levels, may be related to higher risk of cardiovascular disease.
>
> **electrocardiogram (ECG)** A record of the electrical activity of the heart; may be measured during a stress test.

## LO 5 | DIAGNOSING AND TREATING CARDIOVASCULAR DISEASE

Examine current strategies for diagnosis and treatment of cardiovascular disease.

Today, CVD patients have many diagnostic, treatment, prevention, and rehabilitation options that were not available a generation ago. Medications can strengthen heartbeat, control arrhythmias, remove fluids, reduce blood pressure, improve heart function, and reduce pain. Among the most common groups of drugs are *statins*, chemicals used to lower blood cholesterol levels; *ACE inhibitors*, which cause the muscles surrounding blood vessels to contract, thereby lowering blood pressure; and *beta-blockers*, which reduce blood pressure by blocking the effects of the hormone epinephrine. New treatment procedures and techniques are saving countless lives. Even long-standing methods of cardiopulmonary resuscitation (CPR) have been changed to focus primarily on chest compressions rather than mouth-to-mouth breathing. The thinking behind this is that people will be more likely to do CPR if the risk for exchange of body fluids is reduced—and any effort to save a person in trouble is better than inaction.

## Techniques for Diagnosing Cardiovascular Disease

Several techniques are used to diagnose CVD, including electrocardiogram, angiography, and positron emission tomography scans. An **electrocardiogram (ECG)** is a record of the electrical activity of the heart. Patients may undergo a *stress test*—standard exercise on a stationary bike or treadmill with an electrocardiogram and no injections—or a *nuclear stress test,* which involves injecting a radioactive dye and taking images of the heart to reveal problems with blood flow. In **angiography** (often referred to as *cardiac catheterization*), a needle-thin tube called a *catheter* is threaded through heart arteries, a dye is injected, and an X-ray image is taken to discover which areas are blocked. *Positron emission tomography (PET)* produces three-dimensional images of the heart as blood flows through it. Other tests include the following:

- **Magnetic resonance imaging (MRI).** This test uses powerful magnets to look inside the body. Computer-generated pictures can help physicians identify damage from a heart attack and evaluate disease of larger blood vessels such as the aorta.
- **Ultrafast computed tomography (CT).** This is an especially fast form of X-ray imaging of the heart designed to evaluate bypass grafts, diagnose ventricular function, and measure calcium deposits.
- **Cardiac calcium score.** This test measures the amount of calcium-containing plaque in the coronary arteries, a marker for overall atherosclerotic buildup. The greater amount of calcium, the higher your calcium score and the greater   your risk of heart attack. Concerns have been raised over higher than average exposure to radiation from these tests.

**angiography** A technique for examining blockages in heart arteries.

**coronary bypass surgery** A surgical technique whereby a blood vessel taken from another part of the body is implanted to bypass a clogged coronary artery.

**angioplasty** A technique in which a catheter with a balloon at the tip is inserted into a clogged artery; the balloon is inflated to flatten fatty deposits against artery walls and a stent is typically inserted to keep the artery open.

**thrombolysis** Injection of an agent to dissolve clots and restore some blood flow, thereby reducing the amount of tissue that dies from ischemia.

**5-year survival rates** The percentage of people in a study or treatment group who are alive 5 years after they were diagnosed with or treated for cancer.

**remission** A temporary or permanent period when cancer is responding to treatment and under control. This often leads to the disappearance of the signs and symptoms of cancer.

## Bypass Surgery, Angioplasty, and Stents

**Coronary bypass surgery** has helped many patients who suffered coronary blockages or heart attacks. In a coronary artery bypass graft (CABG), referred to as a "cabbage," a blood vessel is taken from another site in the patient's body (usually the saphenous vein in the leg or the internal thoracic artery in the chest) and implanted to bypass blocked coronary arteries and transport blood to heart tissue.

Another procedure, **angioplasty** (sometimes called *balloon angioplasty*), carries fewer risks. As in angiography, a thin catheter is threaded through blocked heart arteries. The catheter has a balloon at the tip, which is inflated to flatten fatty deposits against the artery walls, allowing blood to flow more freely. A stent (a mesh-like stainless steel tube) may be inserted to prop open the artery. Although highly effective, stents can lead to inflammation and tissue growth in the area that can actually lead to more blockage and problems. In about 30 percent of patients, the treated arteries become clogged again within 6 months. Newer stents are usually medicated to reduce this risk. Nonetheless, some surgeons argue that given this high rate of recurrence, bypass may be a more effective treatment. Newer forms of laser angioplasty and *atherectomy,* a procedure that removes plaque, are being done in several clinics.

## Aspirin and Other Drug Therapies

Although aspirin has been touted for its blood-thinning qualities and possibly reducing risks for future heart attacks among those who already have had MI events, the benefits of an aspirin regimen for otherwise healthy adults remains in question. New research and government recommendations seems to indicate that once daily, low-dose aspirin for otherwise healthy adults may not reduce CVD risk and, in fact, may do more harm than good. The FDA indicates it may be helpful to those who have had a heart attack or stroke in preventing a recurrence; however, it shouldn't be taken forever.[65] Furthermore, once a patient has taken aspirin regularly for possible protection against CHD, stopping this regimen may, in fact, increase his or her risk.[66]

If a victim reaches an emergency room and is diagnosed fast enough, a form of clot-busting therapy called **thrombolysis** can be performed. Thrombolysis involves injecting an agent such as *tissue plasminogen activator* (*tPA*) to dissolve the clot and restore some blood flow to the heart (or brain), thereby reducing the amount of tissue that dies from ischemia.[67] These drugs must be administered within 1 to 3 hours after a cardiovascular event.

## LO 6 | CANCER: AN EPIDEMIOLOGICAL OVERVIEW

Describe the impact of cancer on people in the United States and compare it to other major health problems in terms of morbidity/mortality, costs, and overall effectiveness of prevention and control.

After heart disease, cancer is the greatest killer in the United States.[68] Although there were over 589,000 deaths in 2015, the **5-year survival rates** (the relative rates for survival in persons living 5 years after diagnosis) are up dramatically from the virtual death sentences of many cancers in the early 1900s. Of course, there are often differences in stage of diagnosis, age of survivor, and other factors that may increase or decrease chances of survival. Today, of the approximately 1.7 million people diagnosed each year, nearly 68 percent will still be alive 5 years from now—an increase of nearly 20 percent since the 1970s—and survival rates for people diagnosed with many cancers in early stages approach 90 to 95 percent.[69] Some cancers will enter **remission**, which means the cancer is responding to treatment and under control. Others will be considered "cured," meaning that the people have no subsequent cancer in their bodies and can expect to live long and productive lives. Lifestyle, follow-up by health care providers, preventive treatments, environmental conditions, immune system functioning, and several other factors can influence the course of any cancer.

**Lifetime risk** of cancer refers to the probability that a person will develop or die from cancer. Although treatments and survival statistics have improved, nearly 1 in every 2 men and nearly 1 in 3 women will develop cancer in America.[70] In the following sections, we provide an overview of factors that increase risk of cancer and discuss ways to reduce them.

## LO 7 | WHAT IS CANCER?

Describe cancer, how it develops, and key risks for cancers overall.

**Cancer** is the general term for a large group of diseases characterized by the uncontrolled growth and spread of abnormal cells. If these cells aren't stopped, they can impair vital functions of the body and lead to death. When something interrupts normal cell function, uncontrolled growth and abnormal cellular development result in a **neoplasm,** a new growth of tissue serving no physiological function. This neoplasmic mass often forms a clumping of cells known as a **tumor.**

Not all tumors are **malignant** (cancerous); in fact, most are **benign** (noncancerous). Benign tumors are generally harmless unless they grow to obstruct or crowd out normal tissues. A benign tumor of the brain, for instance, is life threatening when it grows enough to restrict blood flow and cause a stroke. The only way to determine whether a tumor is malignant is through **biopsy,** or microscopic examination of cell development.

Benign and malignant tumors differ in several key ways. Benign tumors generally consist of ordinary-looking cells enclosed in a fibrous shell or capsule that prevents their spreading to other body areas. Malignant tumors are usually not enclosed in a protective capsule and can therefore spread to other organs (**FIGURE 12.5**). This process, known as **metastasis,** makes some forms of cancer particularly aggressive. By the time they are diagnosed, malignant tumors have frequently metastasized throughout the body, making treatment extremely difficult. Unlike benign tumors, which merely expand to take over a given space, malignant cells invade surrounding tissue, emitting clawlike protrusions that disturb the RNA and DNA within

**lifetime risk** The probability that a person will develop or die from cancer.

**cancer** A large group of diseases characterized by the uncontrolled growth and spread of abnormal cells.

**neoplasm** A new growth of tissue that serves no physiological function and results from uncontrolled, abnormal cellular development.

**tumor** A neoplasmic mass that grows more rapidly than surrounding tissue.

**malignant** Very dangerous or harmful; refers to a cancerous tumor.

**benign** Harmless; refers to a noncancerous tumor.

**biopsy** Microscopic examination of tissue to determine whether a cancer is present.

**metastasis** Process by which cancer spreads from one area to different areas of the body.

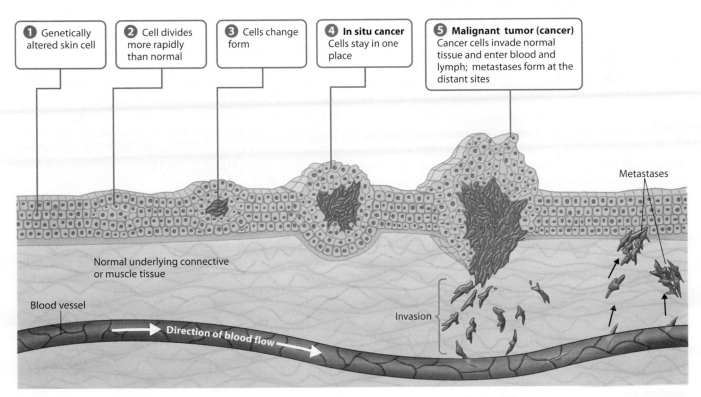

1 Genetically altered skin cell
2 Cell divides more rapidly than normal
3 Cells change form
4 **In situ cancer** Cells stay in one place
5 **Malignant tumor (cancer)** Cancer cells invade normal tissue and enter blood and lymph; metastases form at the distant sites

Metastases

Normal underlying connective or muscle tissue

Blood vessel

Direction of blood flow

Invasion

**FIGURE 12.5 Metastasis** A mutation to the genetic material of a skin cell triggers abnormal cell division and changes cell formation, resulting in a cancerous tumor. If the tumor remains localized, it is considered in situ cancer. If the tumor spreads, it is considered a malignant cancer.

VIDEO TUTOR
Metastasis

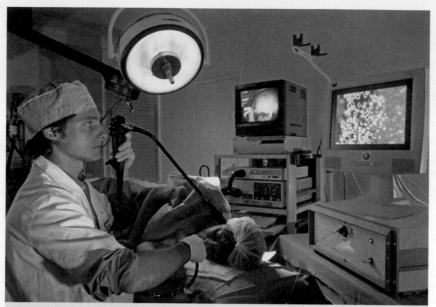

Physicians usually order biopsies of tumors, in which sample cells are taken from the tumor and studied under a microscope to determine whether they are cancerous. Newer techniques, like the minimally invasive "optical biopsy" shown here, allow for the microscopic examination of tissue without doing a physical biopsy.

normal cells. Disrupting these substances, which control cellular metabolism and reproduction, produces **mutant cells** that differ in form, quality, and function from normal cells.

**Cancer staging** is a classification system that describes how much a cancer has spread at the time it is diagnosed; it helps doctors and patients decide on appropriate treatments and estimate a person's life expectancy. Cancers are often staged based on the *TNM system* (*T*, the extent of the primary tumor, type of cells, size, and reach; *N*, the extent of spread to regional lymph nodes; and *M*, metastasis, the number of tumors, and grade/abnormality of cells). The most commonly known staging system assigns the numbers zero to four (see **TABLE 12.3**). However, some cancers, such as

**mutant cells** Cells that differ in form, quality, or function from normal cells.

**cancer staging** A classification system that describes how far a person's disease has advanced.

**carcinogens** Cancer-causing agents.

## TABLE **12.3** | Cancer Stages

| Stage | Definition |
|---|---|
| 0 | Early cancer, when abnormal cells remain only in the place they originated. |
| I | Higher numbers indicate more extensive disease: |
| II | Larger tumor size and/or spread of the cancer |
| III | beyond the organ in which it first developed to nearby lymph nodes and/or organs adjacent to the location of the primary tumor. |
| IV | Cancer has spread to other organs. |

**Source:** National Cancer Institute, National Institutes of Health, "Fact Sheet, Cancer Staging, 2015," January 6, 2015, www.cancer.gov/cancertopics/diagnosis-staging/staging/staging-fact-sheet

bone cancers and lymphomas are staged based on grade. Typically, the lower the stage and grade, the better the prognosis.[71]

## LO 8 | WHAT CAUSES CANCER?

Explain the suspected causes of cancer, and describe your own risks, based on genetics and lifestyle.

Causes of cancer are generally divided into two categories of risk factors: *hereditary* and *acquired* (environmental). Where hereditary factors cannot be modified, we have control over some environmental and behavioral factors, such as tobacco use, nutrition, physical activity, obesity, inflammation, certain infectious agents, certain medical treatments, drug and alcohol consumption, excessive sun exposure, and exposures to **carcinogens** (cancer-causing agents) in food. Where we live, the water we drink, the air we breathe and exposures in the workplace are often part of broader life choices.

## Lifestyle Risks

Anyone can develop cancer; however, most cases affect adults beginning in middle age. In fact, 78 percent of cancers are diagnosed at age 55 and above.[72] In order to determine why some people get cancer and others do not, scientists examine specific risks. *Relative risk* is a measure of the strength of the relationship between risk factors and a particular cancer. Basically, relative risk compares your risk if you engage in certain known risk behaviors with that of someone who does not engage in such behaviors. For example, men and women who smoke have 25 times the risk of lung cancer of a nonsmoker—a relative risk of 25.[73]

Over the years, researchers have found that diet, a sedentary lifestyle (and resultant obesity), overconsumption of alcohol, tobacco use, stress, and other lifestyle factors play a role in the incidence of cancer. Keep in mind that a high relative risk does not guarantee cause and effect, but it does indicate the likelihood of a particular risk factors or combination of factors being related to a particular outcome.

**Tobacco Use** Of all the potential risk factors for cancer, smoking is among the greatest. In the United States, tobacco is responsible for nearly 1 in 5 deaths annually, accounting for at least 30 percent of all cancer deaths and 80 percent of all lung cancer deaths.[74]. Smoking is associated with increased risk of at least 15 different cancers, including those of the nasopharynx, nasal cavity, paranasal sinuses, lip, oral cavity, pharynx, larynx, lung, esophagus, pancreas, uterine cervix, kidney, bladder, and stomach, and acute myeloid leukemia.

# 1/3

OF THE **CANCER** CASES THAT OCCUR IN DEVELOPED COUNTRIES ARE RELATED TO OVERWEIGHT OR OBESITY, PHYSICAL INACTIVITY, AND/OR POOR NUTRITION.

Surprisingly, women who smoke today have a greater risk of dying from lung cancer than during past decades. Several factors contribute to this risk, including women smoking more cigarettes, smoked over more years (*pack years*). Evidence also suggests that newly designed ventilated filters and increased levels of some chemicals in cigarettes may be factors in this increased risk.[75]

## Poor Nutrition, Physical Inactivity, and Obesity

Mounting scientific evidence suggests that about one third of the cancer deaths that occur in the United States each year may be due to lifestyle factors such as overweight or obesity, physical inactivity, and poor nutrition.[76] Dietary choices—particularly high-calorie, high-fat, and high-animal-protein diets—and physical activity are the most important modifiable determinants of cancer risk (besides not smoking). Several studies indicate a relationship between a high body mass index (BMI) and death rates from cancers of the esophagus, colon, rectum, liver, stomach, kidney, pancreas, and others.[77]

Just how great is the risk for someone with a high BMI? Women who gain 55 pounds or more after age 18 have almost a 50 percent greater risk of breast cancer compared to those who maintain their weight.[78] The relative risk of colon cancer in men is 40 percent higher for obese men than it is for non-obese men. The relative risks of gallbladder and endometrial cancers are five times higher in obese individuals than in individuals of healthy weight.[79] Numerous other studies support the link between various forms of cancer and obesity.[80]

## Genetic and Physiological Risks

Although there is still much uncertainty, scientists believe that between 5 and 10 percent of all cancers are strongly hereditary; some people may be more predisposed to the malfunctioning of genes that ultimately cause cancer.[81] Suspected cancer-causing genes are called **oncogenes**. While these genes are typically dormant, certain conditions such as age, stress, and exposure to carcinogens, viruses, and radiation may activate them. Once activated, they cause cells to grow and reproduce uncontrollably. Scientists are uncertain whether only people who develop cancer have oncogenes or whether we all have genes that can become oncogenes under certain conditions.

Certain cancers, particularly those of the breast, stomach, colon, prostate, uterus, ovaries, and lungs, are among those most likely to run in families. For example, a woman runs a much higher risk of breast cancer and/or ovarian cancer if her mother or sisters (primary relatives) have had the disease or if she inherits the breast cancer susceptibility genes (*BRCA1* or *BRCA2*). Hodgkin's disease and certain leukemias show similar familial patterns. The complex interaction of hereditary predisposition, lifestyle, and environment on the development of cancer makes it a challenge to determine a single cause. Even among those predisposed to genetic mutations, avoiding risks may decrease chances of cancer development.

## Reproductive and Hormonal Factors

The effects of reproductive factors on breast and cervical cancers have been well documented. Increased numbers of fertile or menstrual cycle years (early menarche, late menopause), not having children or having them later in life, recent use of birth control pills or hormone replacement therapy, and opting not to breast-feed, all appear to increase risks of breast cancer.[82] While the above factors appear to play a significant role in increased risk for non-Hispanic white women, they do not appear to have as strong an influence on Hispanic women, who may have more protective reproductive patterns (an overall lower age at first birth and greater number of births). They also use less hormone replacement therapy and have a lower utilization rate for mammograms, making comparisons difficult.[83]

## Inflammation and Cancer Risks

In recent years, several researchers have theorized that chronic inflammation can lead to increased risks for cancer, particularly cancer of the colon and digestive system. Theories hold that inflammation can damage cellular DNA, cause cells to divide more rapidly, and lead to an immune system that is weakened by having to cope with chronic inflammatory bombardment; infectious viruses, bacteria and parasitic invaders, and exposure to environmental irritants may lead to the inflammation that serves to initiate and/or promote cancer development.[84]

Although promising, more research is necessary to determine the exact role and mechanism that inflammation plays in cancer initiation and development, whether inflammation is the culprit or if other factors converge to increase risk.

## Occupational and Environmental Risks

Overall, workplace hazards account for only a small percentage of all cancers. However, various substances are known to cause cancer when exposure levels are high or prolonged. One is asbestos, a fibrous material once widely used in the construction, insulation, and automobile industries. Nickel, chromate, and chemicals such as benzene, arsenic, and vinyl chloride have been shown definitively to be carcinogens for humans. People who routinely work with certain dyes and radioactive substances may also have increased risks for cancer. Working with coal tars, as in mining, or with inhalants, as in the auto-painting business, is hazardous. So is working with herbicides and pesticides, although evidence is inconclusive for low-dose exposures. Several federal and state

**oncogenes** Suspected cancer-causing genes.

agencies are responsible for monitoring such exposures and ensuring that businesses comply with standards designed to protect workers.

**Radiation** Ionizing radiation (IR)—radiation from X-rays, radon, cosmic rays, and ultraviolet radiation (primarily ultraviolet B, or UVB, radiation)—is the only form of radiation proven to cause human cancer. Evidence that high-dose IR causes cancer comes from studies of atomic bomb survivors, patients receiving radiotherapy, and certain occupational groups (e.g., uranium miners). Virtually any part of the body can be affected by IR, but bone marrow and the thyroid are particularly susceptible. Radon exposure in homes can increase lung cancer risk, especially in cigarette smokers. To reduce the risk of harmful effects, diagnostic medical and dental X-rays are set at the lowest dose levels possible.

Nonionizing radiation produced by radio waves, cell phones, microwaves, computer screens, televisions, electric blankets, and other products has been a topic of great concern in recent years, but research has not proven excess risk to date. A wide range of studies has been conducted, and there is limited evidence (as compared to no evidence) that newer phones used for longer periods may increase cancer risks, particularly in children. Most of the key policymaking and health organizations have indicated that existing research does not support a cell phone–cancer link. Stay tuned; more studies are under way.[85] (See Chapter 15 for more on the potential environmental and health hazards of radiation.)

## Chemicals in Foods

Much of the concern about chemicals in foods centers on the possible harm caused by pesticide and herbicide residues. Although some of these chemicals cause cancer at high doses in experimental animals, the very low concentrations found in some foods are well within established government safety levels. Continued research regarding pesticide and herbicide use is essential, and scientists and consumer groups stress the importance of a balance between chemical use and the production of high-quality food products. Prevention efforts should focus on policies to protect consumers, develop low-chemical pesticides and herbicides, and reduce environmental pollution.

## Infectious Diseases and Cancer

Between 15 and 20 percent of cancers globally are believed to be caused by infectious viruses, bacteria, and parasites, particularly in the developing world.[86] Viruses are believed to inject their genes into host cells and cause them to grow uncontrollably. *Helicobacter pylori* (*H. pylori*) bacteria has long been associated with increased risk of stomach cancer.[87] Other pathogens can lead to inflammation that may prime cells for cancer development or overcome the immune system, leaving cells vulnerable to cancer growth.[88] (See **Focus On: Reducing Risks and Coping with Chronic Diseases and Conditions** for more on the role of infections in specific chronic diseases.)

### Hepatitis B, Hepatitis C, and Liver Cancer
Viruses such as hepatitis B (HBV) and C (HCV) are believed to stimulate the growth of cancer cells in the liver because they are chronic diseases that inflame liver tissue—potentially priming the liver for cancer or making it more hospitable for cancer development. Global increases in hepatitis B and C rates and concurrent rises in liver cancer rates seem to provide evidence of such an association.

### Human Papillomavirus and Cervical Cancer
Nearly 100 percent of women with cervical cancer have evidence of human papillomavirus (HPV) infection—a virus believed to be a major cause of cervical cancer. Fortunately, only a small percentage of HPV cases progress to cervical cancer.[89] Today, a vaccine is available to help protect young women from becoming infected with HPV and developing cervical cancer. (For more on the HPV vaccine, see the discussion in Chapter 13.)

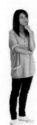

WHICH **PATH** WOULD YOU TAKE **?**

Scan the QR code to see how different health choices YOU make today can affect your risk for developing cardiovascular disease and cancer.

## LO 9 | TYPES OF CANCERS

Describe symptoms, populations at risk, and key methods of prevention for the most common types of cancer.

Cancers are grouped into four broad categories based on the type of tissue from which each arise.

- **Carcinomas.** Epithelial tissues (tissues covering body surfaces and lining most body cavities) are the most common sites for cancers called *carcinomas*. These cancers affect the outer layer of the skin and mouth as well as the mucous membranes. They metastasize through the circulatory or lymphatic system initially and form solid tumors.
- **Sarcomas.** Sarcomas occur in the mesodermal, or middle, layers of tissue—for example, in bones, muscles, and general connective tissue. They metastasize primarily via the blood in the early stages of disease. These cancers are less common but generally more virulent than carcinomas. They also form solid tumors.
- **Lymphomas.** Lymphomas develop in the lymphatic system—the infection-fighting regions of the body—and metastasize through the lymphatic system. Hodgkin's disease is an example. Lymphomas also form solid tumors.
- **Leukemias.** Cancer of the blood-forming parts of the body, particularly the bone marrow and spleen, is called leukemia. A nonsolid tumor, leukemia is characterized by an abnormal increase in the number of white blood cells.

| Estimated New Cases of Cancer* | | Estimated Deaths from Cancer* | |
| --- | --- | --- | --- |
| **Female** | **Male** | **Female** | **Male** |
| **Breast**<br>231,840 (29%) | **Prostate**<br>220,800 (26%) | **Lung & bronchus**<br>71,660 (26%) | **Lung & bronchus**<br>86,380 (28%) |
| **Lung & bronchus**<br>105,590 (13%) | **Lung & bronchus**<br>115,610 (14%) | **Breast**<br>40,290 (15%) | **Prostate**<br>27,540 (9%) |
| **Colon & rectum**<br>47,200 (6%) | **Colon & rectum**<br>45,890 (5%) | **Colon & rectum**<br>23,600 (9%) | **Colon & rectum**<br>26,100 (8%) |
| **Uterine corpus**<br>54,870 (8%) | **Urinary bladder**<br>56,3920 (6%) | **Pancreas**<br>19,850 (7%) | **Pancreas**<br>20,710 (7%) |
| **Thyroid**<br>47,230 (6%) | **Melanoma of the skin**<br>42,670 (5%) | **Ovary**<br>14,180 (5%) | **Liver & intrahepatic bile duct**<br>17,030 (5%) |
| **Non-Hodgkin lymphoma**<br>32,000 (4%) | **Kidney & renal pelvis**<br>38,270 (5%) | **Leukemia**<br>10,240 (4%) | **Leukemia**<br>14,210 (5%) |
| **Melanoma of the skin**<br>31,200 (4%) | **Non-Hodgkin lymphoma**<br>39,850 (5%) | **Uterine corpus**<br>10,170 (4%) | **Esophagus**<br>12,600 (4%) |
| **Kidney & renal pelvis**<br>23,290 (3%) | **Oral cavity & pharynx**<br>32,670 (4%) | **Non-Hodgkin lymphoma**<br>490 (1%) | **Urinary bladder**<br>11,510 (4%) |
| **Pancreas**<br>24,120 (3%) | **Leukemia**<br>30,900 (4%) | **Liver & intrahepatic bile duct**<br>7,520 (3%) | **Non-Hodgkin lymphoma**<br>11,480 (4%) |
| **Leukemia**<br>23,370 (3%) | **Pancreas**<br>24,840 (3%) | **Brain & other nervous system**<br>6,380 (2%) | **Kidney & renal pelvis**<br>9,070 (3%) |
| **All Sites**<br>810,170 (100%) | **All Sites**<br>848,200 (100%) | **All Sites**<br>277,280 (100%) | **All Sites**<br>312,150 (100%) |

*Excludes basal and squamous cell skin cancers and in situ carcinoma except urinary bladder. Percentages may not total 100% due to rounding.

**FIGURE 12.6** Leading Sites of New Cancer Cases and Deaths, 2015 Estimates

**Source:** Data from American Cancer Society, *Cancer Facts & Figures 2015* (Atlanta, GA: American Cancer Society, Inc.), table on page 9.

**FIGURE 12.6** shows the most common sites of cancer and the estimated number of new cases and deaths from each type in 2015. A comprehensive discussion of the many different forms of cancer is beyond the scope of this book, but we will discuss the most common types in the next sections.

## Lung Cancer

Lung cancer is the leading cause of cancer deaths for both men and women in the United States. Even as rates have decreased in recent decades, it still killed an estimated 221,200 Americans in 2015.[90] Since 1987, more women have died each year from lung cancer than from breast cancer, which over the previous 40 years had been the leading cause of cancer deaths in women. Although past reductions in smoking rates bode well for cancer and CVD statistics, there is growing concern about the number of youth, particularly young women and persons of low income and low educational level, who continue to pick up the habit. There is also concern about the increase in lung cancers among those who have never smoked—representing as many as 15 percent of all lung cancers. This type of lung cancer is believed to be related to exposure to secondhand smoke, radon gas, asbestos, wood-burning stoves, and aerosolized oils caused by cooking with oil and deep fat frying.[91]

### Detection, Symptoms, and Treatment

Symptoms of lung cancer include a persistent cough, blood-streaked sputum, chest pain, and recurrent attacks of pneumonia or bronchitis. Treatment depends on the type and stage of the cancer. Surgery, radiation therapy, and chemotherapy are all options. If the cancer is localized, surgery is usually the treatment of choice. If it has spread, surgery is combined with radiation and chemotherapy. Despite advances in medical technology, survival rates 1 year after diagnosis are only 44 percent overall. The 5-year survival rate for all stages combined is only 17 percent.[92] Newer tests, such as low-dose CT scans, molecular markers in sputum, and improved biopsy techniques, have helped improve diagnosis, but we still have a long way to go.

**Risk Factors and Prevention** Smokers, especially those who have smoked for more than 20 years, and people who have been exposed to secondhand smoke and industrial substances such as arsenic and asbestos or to radiation, are at the highest risk for lung cancer. Quitting smoking does reduce the risk,[93] but exposure to both secondhand cigarette smoke and radon gas is also believed to play an important role in lung cancer development.[94]

## Breast Cancer

Women have about a 1 in 8 chance of developing breast cancer in their lifetime. For women from birth to age 39, the chance is about a 1 in 202, with significantly higher rates after menopause.[95] In 2015, approximately 232,000 women and 2,400 men in the United States were diagnosed with invasive breast cancer for the first time. In addition, 60,000 new cases of in situ breast cancer, a more localized cancer, were diagnosed.

About 41,000 (and 440 men) died, making breast cancer the second leading cause of cancer death for women.[96] The good news is that death rates have dropped nearly 35 percent from peak rates in the 1990s. Earlier diagnosis and improved treatment are key factors in this decline.[97]

## Detection, Symptoms, and Treatment
The earliest signs of breast cancer are usually observable on mammograms, often before lumps can be felt. However, mammograms are not fool-proof and accuracy for younger women with dense breasts is lower.[98] Although mammograms detect between 80 and 90 percent of breast cancers in women without symptoms, a newer form of MRI appears to be more accurate, particularly in women with genetic risks for tumors.[99] In addition, MRIs may pick up an early form of *atypical hyperplasia* (also referred to as breast cancer *atypia*), in which precancerous cells are growing abnormally but would not show up in routine testing.

For decades monthly breast self-exams were also recommended for cancer screening. However, recent studies indicate that breast self-exams may lead to unnecessary worry, unnecessary tests, and increased health care costs. As a result, several groups downgraded the recommendation about breast self-exams from "do them and do them regularly" to "learn how to do them, and if you desire, do them to know your body and be able to recognize changes." **FIGURE 12.7** describes how to do a breast self-exam.

Once breast cancer has grown enough that it can be felt by palpating the area, many women will recognize the threat and seek medical care. Symptoms may include persistent breast changes, such as a lump in the breast or surrounding lymph nodes, thickening, dimpling, skin irritation, distortion, retraction or scaliness of the nipple, nipple discharge, or tenderness.

Treatments range from a lumpectomy to radical mastectomy to various combinations of radiation or chemotherapy. Among nonsurgical options, promising results have been noted among women using *selective estrogen-receptor modulators (SERMs)* such as tamoxifen and raloxifene, particularly women whose cancers appear to grow in response to estrogen. These drugs, as well as new *aromatase inhibitors,* work by blocking estrogen. The 5-year survival rate for people with localized breast cancer is 98 percent today; for higher stage cancer, the 5-year survival rate drops dramatically.[100]

## Risk Factors and Prevention
The incidence of breast cancer increases with age. Risk factors well supported by research include family history of breast cancer, menstrual periods that started early and ended late in life, weight gain after the age of 18, obesity after menopause, recent use of oral contraceptives or postmenopausal hormone therapy, never having children or having a first child after age 30, consuming two or more alcoholic drinks per day, and physical inactivity. Women with dense breasts, high bone mineral density, and exposure to high-dose radiation are also at increased risk.[101] Women who possess *BRCA1* and *BRCA2* gene mutations have a 60 to 80 percent risk of developing breast cancer by age 70, whereas women without the mutations have a 7 percent risk. Because these genes are rare, routine screening for them is not recommended unless there is a strong family history of breast cancer.[102]

International differences in breast cancer incidence correlate with variations in diet, especially fat intake, although a causal role for these dietary factors has not been firmly

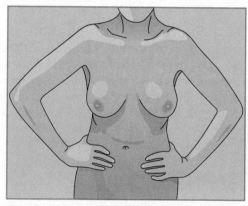

❶ Face a mirror and check for changes in symmetry.

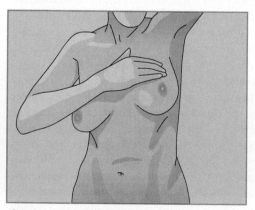

❷ Either standing or lying down, use the pads of the three middle fingers to check for lumps. Follow an up and down pattern on the breast to ensure all tissue gets inspected.

**FIGURE 12.7** Breast Self-Exam

**Source:** Adapted from Breast Self-Exam Illustration Series, National Cancer Institute Visuals Online Collection, U.S. National Institutes of Health, 1984.

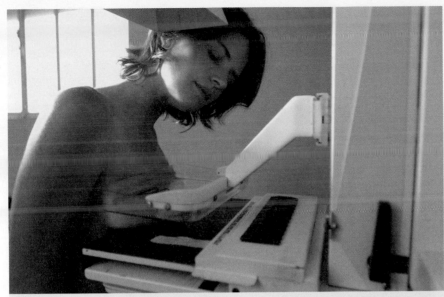
Early detection using the latest equipment with the lowest radiation exposure greatly increases a woman's chance of surviving breast cancer.

established. Sudden weight gain has also been implicated. Research also shows that regular exercise can reduce risk,[103] as may increasing dietary fiber intake.[104]

## Colon and Rectal Cancers

Colorectal cancers (cancers of the colon and rectum) continue to be the third most common cancer in both men and women, with just over 93,000 cases of colon and nearly 40,000 cases of rectal cancer diagnosed in the United States in 2013 and 49,700 deaths. Most cases occur in persons age 50 and over; however, new cases can occur at any age.[105] Younger men and women have approximately a 1 in 300 risk of developing colon and rectal cancer from birth to age 49. At age 50, risk for men is about 1 in 148 and 1 in 193 for women, increasing to about 1 in 26 by age 70.[106]

### Detection, Symptoms, and Treatment

Because colorectal cancer tends to spread slowly, the prognosis is quite good if it is caught in the early stages. While later stages may have symptoms such as stool changes, bleeding, cramping or pain in the lower abdomen, and unusual fatigue, colorectal cancers usually have no early symptoms. Regular screenings, such as colonoscopy or barium enemas, are recommended for those at high risk. Late in 2014, the FDA approved the first at home, noninvasive colon cancer test that detects blood and DNA mutations that indicate pre-cancer or cancer with over 90 percent accuracy; it may significantly increase early diagnosis and improve outcomes.[107] Treatment often consists of radiation or surgery. Chemotherapy, although not used extensively in the past, is increasingly used.

### Risk Factors and Prevention

Anyone can get colorectal cancer, but people over age 50, who are obese, smoke, who have a family history of colon and rectal cancer,

a personal or family history of polyps (benign growths) in the colon or rectum, or who have type 2 diabetes or inflammatory bowel problems such as colitis are at increased risk. Protective factors, such as increased physical activity, aspirin use, hormone replacement therapy, and removal of polyps appear to decrease risk of colon cancer. However, other factors, such as use of nonsteroidal anti-inflammatory drugs (NSAIDS), diet, vitamins, and calcium have shown conflicting results in studies.[108]

## Skin Cancer

Skin cancer is the most common form of cancer in the United States; however, since it is not reported, exact numbers are difficult to assess for the two most common, most curable forms of skin cancer—basal cell and squamous cell carcinoma—although estimates of 3.5 million cases are common.[109] **Malignant melanoma** affects nearly 74,000 Americans each year and kills over 10,000 per year, compared to 3,400 deaths for other forms of skin cancer.[110]

### Detection, Symptoms, and Treatment

Many people do not know what to look for when examining themselves for skin cancer. Fortunately, potentially cancerous growths are often visible as abnormalities on the skin. Basal and squamous cell carcinomas can be a recurrent annoyance, showing up most commonly on the face, ears, neck, arms, hands, and legs as warty bumps, colored spots, or scaly patches. Bleeding, itchiness, pain, or oozing are other symptoms that warrant attention.[111] Surgery may be necessary to remove them, but they are seldom life threatening.

> **malignant melanoma** A virulent cancer of the melanocytes (pigment-producing cells) of the skin.

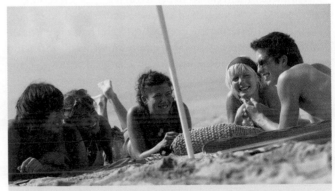
There is no such thing as a "safe" tan, because a tan is visible evidence of UV-induced skin damage. According to the American Cancer Society, tanned skin provides only about the equivalent of sun protection factor (SPF) 4 sunscreen—much too weak to be considered protective.

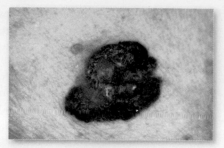

(a) Malignant melanoma

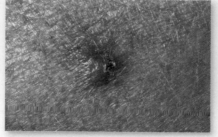

(b) Basal cell carcinoma

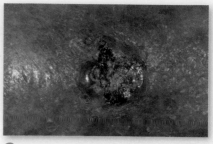

(c) Squamous cell carcinoma

**FIGURE 12.8 Types of Skin Cancers** Preventing skin cancer includes keeping a careful watch for any new pigmented growths and for changes to any moles. The ABCD warning signs of melanoma **(a)** include *asymmetrical* shapes, irregular *borders*, *color* variation, and an increase in *diameter*. Basal cell carcinoma **(b)** and squamous cell carcinoma **(c)** should be brought to your physician's attention, but are not as deadly as melanoma.

Melanoma, in contrast, is an invasive killer that may appear as a skin lesion that changes size, shape, or color and that spreads throughout organs of the body. While melanoma is less common than basal and squamous cell carcinomas, it is responsible for the majority of skin cancer deaths. Women are more likely to develop melanoma before age 50. After age 65, men have twice the risk of women.[112] Recreational sun exposure and occupational exposure are key risks. This is one of the few cancers that develops frequently in younger people, however, education and improved sunscreens appear to be factors in declining rates.[113] **FIGURE 12.8** shows melanoma compared to basal cell and squamous cell carcinomas. A simple *ABCD* rule outlines the warning signs of melanoma:

- **Asymmetry.** One half of the mole or lesion does not match the other half.
- **Border irregularity.** The edges are uneven, notched, or scalloped.
- **Color.** Pigmentation is not uniform. Melanomas may vary in color from tan to deeper brown, reddish black, black, or deep bluish black.
- **Diameter.** The diameter is greater than 6 millimeters (about the size of a pea).

Treatment of skin cancer depends on its seriousness. Surgery is performed in 90 percent of all cases. Radiation therapy, *electrodesiccation* (tissue destruction by heat), and *cryosurgery* (tissue destruction by freezing) are also common forms of treatment. For melanoma, treatment may involve surgical removal of the regional lymph nodes, radiation, or chemotherapy.

### Risk Factors and Prevention

Anyone overexposed to ultraviolet radiation without adequate protection is at risk for skin cancer. The risk is greatest for people who fit the following categories:

- Have fair skin; blonde, red, or light brown hair; blue, green, or gray eyes
- Always burn before tanning or burn easily and peel readily
- Don't tan easily but spend lots of time outdoors
- Use no or low sun protection factor (SPF) sunscreens or old, expired suntan lotions

- Have previously been treated for skin cancer or have a family history of skin cancer
- Have experienced severe sunburns during childhood

Preventing skin cancer is a matter of limiting exposure to harmful UV rays found in sunlight. What happens when you expose yourself to sunlight? Biologically, the skin responds to photodamage by increasing its thickness and the number of pigment cells (melanocytes), which produce the "tan" look. The skin's cells that ward off infection are also prone to photodamage, lowering the normal immune protection of our skin and priming it for cancer. Photodamage also causes wrinkling by impairing the elastic substances (collagens) that keep skin soft and pliable. Stay safe in the sun by limiting sun exposure when its rays are strongest, between 10:00 AM and 4:00 PM, and by applying an SPF 15 or higher sunscreen before going outside.

Despite the risk of skin cancer, many Americans are still "working on a tan," and many tanning salon patrons incorrectly believe that tanning booths are safer than sitting in the sun. The truth is that there is no such thing as a safe tan from *any* source! Every time you tan, you are exposing your skin to harmful UV light rays. All tanning lamps emit UVA rays, and most emit UVB rays as well; both types can cause long-term skin damage and contribute to cancer. Even worse, some salons do not calibrate the UV output of their tanning bulbs properly, which can cause more or less exposure than you paid for.

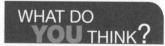

**WHAT DO YOU THINK?**

How do we determine whether a behavior or substance is a risk factor for a disease? Should programs be enacted to reduce the risk or stop the behavior?

- Do you think that there should be legislation banning tanning booths in all 50 states? Why or why not? Would you favor such a bill if it banned tanning for minors only?

## Prostate Cancer

Cancer of the prostate is the most frequently diagnosed cancer in American males today, excluding skin cancer, and is the second leading cause of cancer deaths in men after lung cancer. In 2015, about 221,000 new cases of prostate cancer were diagnosed in the United States, causing 27,500 deaths.[114] Fortunately, most cases of prostate cancer are diagnosed in earlier stages, resulting in survival rates of nearly 99 percent.[115]

**Detection, Symptoms, and Treatment** The prostate is a muscular, walnut-sized gland that surrounds part of a man's urethra, the tube that transports urine and sperm out of the body. As part of the male reproductive system, its primary function is to produce seminal fluid. Symptoms of prostate cancer include weak or interrupted urine flow; difficulty starting or stopping urination; feeling the urge to urinate frequently; pain upon urination; blood in the urine; or pain in the low back, pelvis, or thighs. Many men have no symptoms in the early stages.

Men over the age of 40 should have an annual digital rectal prostate examination. Another screening method for prostate cancer is the **prostate-specific antigen (PSA)** test, which is a blood test that screens for an indicator of prostate cancer. However, in 2011, a governmental panel called the United States Preventive Services Task Force made the recommendation that healthy men no longer receive the PSA test; overall, it does not save lives and may lead to painful, unnecessary cancer treatments. If you have a family history or other symptoms, consult with your physician.

**Risk Factors and Prevention** Chances of developing prostate cancer increase dramatically with age. More than 60 percent of prostate cancers are diagnosed in men over the age of 65, and 97 percent occur in men 50 or older.[116] The disease is discovered because it has progressed to the point of displaying symptoms, or more likely, men are seeing a doctor for other problems and get a screening test or PSA test.

Race is also a risk factor in prostate cancer. The highest prostate cancer incidence rates in the world are found in African American men and Jamaican men of African descent. They are also more likely to be diagnosed at more advanced stages than other racial groups.[117]

Having a father or brother with prostate cancer more than doubles a man's risk of getting prostate cancer. Risk is higher for men with an affected brother than it is for those with an affected father.[118]

Eating more fruits and vegetables, particularly those containing lycopene, a pigment found in tomatoes and other red fruits, may lower the risk of prostate cancer. The best advice is to follow the national dietary recommendations and maintain a healthy weight.

## Ovarian Cancer

Ovarian cancer is the fifth leading cause of cancer deaths for women, with about 21,300 diagnoses in 2015 and just over 14,000 deaths.[119] Ovarian cancer causes more deaths than any other cancer of the reproductive system because women tend not to discover it until the cancer is at an advanced stage, when 5-year survival is only 27 percent. Younger women (under the age of 65) are much more likely to survive 5 years compared to those 65 or older. For all stages, the 5-year survival is 45 percent.[120]

Ovarian cancer symptoms are often not obvious, and it is common for women to have no early symptoms at all. A woman may complain of feeling bloated, having pain in the pelvic area, feeling full quickly, or feeling the need to urinate more frequently. Some may experience persistent digestive disturbances, while other symptoms include fatigue, pain during intercourse, unexplained weight loss, unexplained changes in bowel or bladder habits, and incontinence.

Primary relatives (mother, daughter, sister) of a woman who has had ovarian cancer are at increased risk, as are those with a family or personal history of breast or colon cancer. Women who have never been pregnant are more likely to develop ovarian cancer than those who have had a child, and the use of fertility drugs may also increase a woman's risk.

General prevention strategies such as focusing on a healthy diet, exercise, sleep, stress management, and weight control are good ideas to lower your risk for any of the diseases discussed in this chapter. Getting annual pelvic examinations is important, and women over the age of 40 should have a cancer-related checkup every year.

> **prostate-specific antigen (PSA)** An antigen found in prostate cancer patients.
>
> **Pap test** A procedure in which cells taken from the cervical region are examined for abnormal activity.

## Cervical and Endometrial (Uterine) Cancer

Most uterine cancers develop in the body of the uterus, usually in the *endometrium* (lining). The rest develop in the cervix, located at the base of the uterus. In 2015, an estimated 12,900 new cases of cervical cancer and 54,870 cases of endometrial cancer were diagnosed in the United States, with nearly 10,200 deaths.[121] Increased estrogen levels as a result of menopausal estrogen therapy, being overweight/obese, and never having children may dramatically increase risk for endometrial cancer. In addition, risks are increased by treatment with tamoxifen for breast cancer, metabolic syndrome, late menopause, a history of polyps in the uterus or ovaries, a history of other cancers, and race (white women are at higher risk). Pregnancy, use of oral contraceptives or intrauterine devices, and physical activity are associated with reduced risk.

The overall incidence of cervical cancer has been declining steadily over the past decade, whereas the incidence of endometrial cancer has been increasing by nearly 2 percent per year.[122] The decline in cervical cancer may be due to more regular screenings of younger women using the **Pap test**, a procedure in which cells taken from the cervical region are examined for abnormal cellular activity.

**magnetic resonance imaging (MRI)** A device that uses magnetic fields, radio waves, and computers to generate an image of internal tissues of the body for diagnostic purposes without the use of radiation.

Although very effective for detecting early-stage cervical cancer, Pap tests are less effective for detecting cancers of the uterine lining. Early warning signs of uterine cancer include bleeding outside the normal menstrual period or after menopause or persistent unusual vaginal discharge. As of 2015, it is recommended women get a Pap test every 2 years beginning at age 21. Between ages 30 and 65, women should have an HPV and Pap test every 5 years and a Pap test alone every 3 years. Those with parents and/or siblings with breast cancer should talk with their doctor about having tests more frequently.

The primary cause of cervical cancer is infection with certain types of the human papillomavirus (HPV). Having sex at a young age and having multiple partners and unprotected sex can increase risks dramatically. Progression to cancer appears to be related to a weakened immune system, multiple births, cigarette smoking, and using oral contraceptives. Today, both young men and women have the option of getting vaccinated with either *Gardasil* or *Cervarix,* designed to protect against the two types of HPV that cause over 70 percent of cervical cancers. (See **Focus On: Reducing Risks and Coping with Chronic Diseases and Conditions** for more on these vaccines). Other sexually transmitted infections such as herpes may also increase risks.[123]

## Testicular Cancer

Testicular cancer is one of the most common types of solid tumors found in young adult men, affecting nearly 8,450 young men in 2015.[124] The average age at diagnosis is 33; however, teens and middle-aged men are often affected.[125] Still, with a 96 percent 5-year survival rate, it is one of the most curable forms of cancer. Although the cause of testicular cancer is unknown, several risk factors have been identified. Men with undescended testicles appear to be at greatest risk; HIV and a family history of testicular cancer are also possible risks.[126]

In general, testicular tumors first appear as an enlargement of one or both of the testis, a lump or thickening in testicular tissue. Some men report a heavy feeling, dull ache, or pain that extends to the lower abdomen or groin area. Testicular self-exams have long been recommended as a means of detecting testicular cancer (**FIGURE 12.9**). However, recent studies discovered that findings from monthly self-exams result in testing for noncancerous conditions and thus are not cost-effective. For this reason, the U.S. Preventive Services Task Force stopped recommending self-exams. Regardless, most cases of testicular cancer are discovered through self-exam; there is currently no other screening test for the disease.

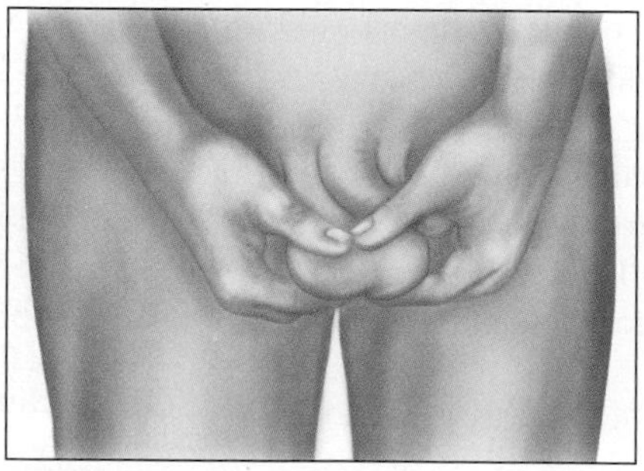

**FIGURE 12.9** Testicular Self-Exam

**Source:** From Michael Johnson, *Human Biology: Concepts and Current Issues*, 3rd ed. Copyright © 2006. Reprinted with permission of Pearson Education, Inc.

The testicular self-exam is best done after a hot shower, which relaxes the scrotum. Standing in front of a mirror, hold the testicle with one hand while gently rolling its surface between the thumb and fingers of your other hand. Feel underneath the scrotum for the tubes of the epididymis and blood vessels that sit close to the body. Repeat with the other testicle. Look for any lump, thickening, or pea-like nodules, paying attention to any areas that may be painful over the entire surface of the scrotum. When done, wash your hands with soap and water. Consult a doctor if you note anything that is unusual.

## Pancreatic Cancer: Deadly and on the Rise

Pancreatic cancer is one of the deadliest forms of cancer, with only 28 percent of patients surviving 1 year after diagnosis, and only 5 to 7 percent surviving 5 years.[127] Although most cases occur after age 50, there are increasing numbers of cases at earlier ages. Overall, rates are higher in men than women, in African Americans, and in populations with lower socioeconomic status and education levels.

Tobacco use appears to be a key risk factor, as is obesity, consumption of high levels of red meat, and high-fat diet. Family history, possible genetic links, and a history of chronic inflammation of the pancreas over the years (*pancreatitis*), seem to increase risk. Also, there appears to be a greater risk among diabetics and those who have had infections with hepatitis B and C and the *Helicobacter* bacteria. Because pancreatic cancer has few early symptoms, there is no reliable test to detect it in its early stages. Often, by the time it is diagnosed via CT or MRI examinations, it is too advanced to treat effectively.

## LO 10 | FACING CANCER

**Discuss cancer diagnosis and treatment, including radiotherapy and chemotherapy, and describe more recent developments in detection and treatment.**

The earlier cancer is diagnosed, the better the prospect for survival. Make a realistic assessment of your own risk factors; avoid behaviors that put you at risk; and increase healthy behaviors, such as improving your diet and exercise levels, reducing stress, and getting regular checkups. Even if you have significant risks, there are factors you can control. Do you have a family history of cancer? If so, what types? Make sure you know which symptoms to watch for, avoid known carcinogens—such as tobacco—and other environmental hazards, and follow the recommendations for self-exams and medical checkups outlined in **TABLE 12.4** on the next page.

The use of several high-tech imaging systems to detect cancer has become standard. **Magnetic resonance imaging (MRI)** uses a huge electromagnet to

## TABLE 12.4 | Screening Guidelines for the Early Detection of Cancer in Average-Risk Asymptomatic People

| Cancer Site | Screening Procedure | Age and Frequency of Test |
|---|---|---|
| Breast | Mammograms | The National Cancer Institute recommends that women in their forties and older have mammograms every 1 to 2 years. Women who are at higher-than-average risk of breast cancer should talk with their health care provider about whether to have mammograms before age 40 and how often to have them. |
| Cervix | Pap test (Pap smear) | Women should begin having Pap tests 3 years after they begin having sexual intercourse or when they reach age 21 (whichever comes first). Most women should have a Pap test at least once every 3 years. |
| Colon and rectum | *Fecal occult blood test:* Sometimes cancer or polyps bleed. This test can detect tiny amounts of blood in the stool. <br><br>*Sigmoidoscopy:* Checks the rectum and lower part of the colon for polyps. <br><br>*Colonoscopy:* Checks the rectum and entire colon for polyps and cancer. | People aged 50 and older should be screened. People who have a higher-than-average risk of cancer of the colon or rectum should talk with their doctor about whether to have screening tests before age 50 and how often to have them <br><br>Note: Although not part of recommendations, a new "at-home" blood/cancer DNA test is now FDA approved. |
| Prostate | Prostate-specific antigen (PSA) test | Some groups encourage yearly screening for men over age 50, and some advise men who are at a higher risk for prostate cancer to begin screening at age 40 or 45. Others caution against routine screening and encourage checking with your doctor. Currently, Medicare provides coverage for an annual PSA test for all men age 50 and older. |

**Sources:** National Cancer Institute, National Institutes of Health, "What You Need to Know About Cancer Screening," 2014, www.cancer.gov; National Cancer Institute, Fact Sheet, Prostate-Specific Antigen (PSA) Test, 2014, www.cancer.gov

detect hidden tumors by mapping the vibrations of the various atoms in the body on a computer screen. Another key weapon is the **computed tomography scan (CT scan)**, which uses X-rays to examine parts of the body. In both of these painless, noninvasive procedures, cross-sectioned pictures can reveal a tumor's shape and location more accurately than can conventional X-ray images. Exciting new tests are being explored for widespread use. These offer the promise of much earlier diagnosis and improved treatment for early cancer recurrence. New 3D mammogram machines offer significant improvements in imaging and breast cancer detection, but deliver nearly double the radiation risk of conventional mammograms.

## Cancer Treatments

Cancer treatments vary according to the type of cancer and the stage in which it is detected. Surgery, in which the tumor and surrounding tissue are removed, is one common treatment. New **stereotactic radiosurgery**, also known as **gamma knife surgery**, uses a targeted dose of gamma radiation to zap tumors with pinpoint accuracy without blood loss or need for a scalpel. **Radiotherapy** (the use of radiation) or **chemotherapy** (the use of drugs) to kill cancerous cells are also used. When cancer has spread throughout the body, chemotherapy is necessary.

Whether used alone or in combination, virtually all cancer treatments have side effects, including nausea, nutritional deficiencies, hair loss, and general fatigue. The more aggressive the cancer, the more likely there will be side effects from powerful drugs and invasive procedures. In the process of killing malignant cells, some healthy cells are also destroyed, and long-term damage to the cardiovascular system, kidneys, liver, and other body systems can be significant.

New ways of killing tumors and new chemotherapeutic drug cocktails are being developed regularly. Promising areas of research include *immunotherapy,* which enhances the body's own disease-fighting mechanisms, *cancer-fighting vaccines* to combat abnormal cells, *gene therapy* to increase the patient's immune response, and treatment with various substances that block cancer-causing events along the cancer pathway. Another promising avenue of potential treatment is *stem cell research,* although controversy around the use of stem cells continues to slow research. Because our knowledge of cancer treatment is constantly evolving, those who have been diagnosed with cancer and their loved ones should do their best to access information on the best cancer options for specific types of cancer, new treatments being developed, and whether or not they are eligible for new clinical trials and experimental treatments that might be available for particularly aggressive cancers.

**computed tomography scan (CT scan)** A scan by a machine that uses radiation to view internal organs not normally visible on X-ray images.

**stereotactic radiosurgery** A type of radiation therapy that can be used to zap tumors. Also known as *gamma knife surgery.*

**radiotherapy** Use of radiation to kill cancerous cells.

**chemotherapy** Use of drugs to kill cancerous cells.

# CVD and Cancer: What's Your Personal Risk?

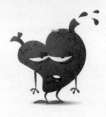

## 1 Evaluating Your CVD Risk

Complete each of the following questions and total your points in each section.

### A: Your Family Risk for CVD

| | Yes (1 point) | No (0 point) | Don't Know |
|---|---|---|---|
| 1. Do any of your primary relatives (parents, grandparents, siblings) have a history of heart disease or stroke? | ○ | ○ | ○ |
| 2. Do any of your primary relatives have diabetes? | ○ | ○ | ○ |
| 3. Do any of your primary relatives have high blood pressure? | ○ | ○ | ○ |
| 4. Do any of your primary relatives have a history of high cholesterol? | ○ | ○ | ○ |
| 5. Would you say that your family consumed a high-fat diet (lots of red meat, whole dairy, butter/margarine) during your time spent at home? | ○ | ○ | ○ |

Total points: _____

### B: Your Lifestyle Risk for CVD

| | Yes | No | Don't Know |
|---|---|---|---|
| 1. Is your total cholesterol level higher than it should be? | ○ | ○ | ○ |
| 2. Do you have high blood pressure? | ○ | ○ | ○ |
| 3. Have you been diagnosed as prediabetic or diabetic? | ○ | ○ | ○ |
| 4. Would you describe your life as being highly stressful? | ○ | ○ | ○ |
| 5. Do you smoke? | ○ | ○ | ○ |

Total points: _____

### C: Your Additional Risks for CVD

1. How would you best describe your current weight?
   a. Lower than what it should be for my height and weight (0 points)
   b. About what it should be for my height and weight (0 points)
   c. Higher than it should be for my height and weight (1 point)

2. How would you describe the level of exercise that you get each day?
   a. Less than what I should be exercising each day (1 point)
   b. About what I should be exercising each day (0 points)
   c. More than what I should be exercising each day (0 points)

3. How would you describe your dietary behaviors?
   a. Eating only the recommended number of calories each day (0 points)
   b. Eating less than the recommended number of calories each day (0 points)
   c. Eating more than the recommended number of calories each day (1 point)

4. Which of the following best describes your typical dietary behavior?
   a. I eat from the major food groups, especially trying to get the recommended fruits and vegetables. (0 points)
   b. I eat too much red meat and consume too much saturated and *trans* fats from meat, dairy products, and processed foods each day. (1 point)
   c. Whenever possible, I try to substitute olive oil or canola oil for other forms of dietary fat. (0 points)

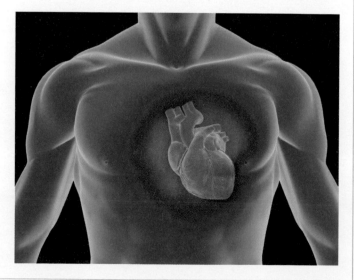

5. Which of the following (if any) describes you?

   a. I watch my sodium intake and try to reduce stress in my life. (0 points)

   b. I have a history of chlamydia infection. (1 point)

   c. I try to eat 5 to 10 mg of soluble fiber each day and try to substitute a non-animal source of protein (beans, nuts, soy) in my diet at least once each week. (0 points)

   Total points: _____

## Scoring Part 1

If you scored between 1 and 5 in any section, consider your risk. The higher the number, the greater your risk will be. If you answered Don't Know for any question, talk to your parents or other family members as soon as possible to find out if you have any unknown risks.

# 2 Evaluating Your Cancer Risk

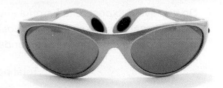

Read each question and circle the number corresponding to each with Yes or No. Individual scores for specific questions should not be interpreted as a precise measure of relative risk, but the totals in each section give a general indication of risk.

## A: Cancers in General

| | | Yes | No |
|---|---|---|---|
| 1. | Do you smoke cigarettes on most days of the week? | 2 | 1 |
| 2. | Do you consume a diet that is rich in fruits and vegetables? | 1 | 2 |
| 3. | Are you obese, or do you lead a primarily sedentary lifestyle? | 2 | 1 |
| 4. | Do you live in an area with high air pollution levels or work in a job where you are exposed to several chemicals on a regular basis? | 2 | 1 |
| 5. | Are you careful about the amount of animal fat in your diet, substituting olive oil or canola oil for animal fat whenever possible? | 1 | 2 |
| 6. | Do you limit your overall consumption of alcohol? | 1 | 2 |
| 7. | Do you eat foods rich in lycopenes (such as tomatoes) and antioxidants? | 1 | 2 |
| 8. | Are you "body aware" and alert for changes in your body? | 1 | 2 |
| 9. | Do you have a family history of ulcers or of colorectal, stomach, or other digestive system cancers? | 2 | 1 |
| 10. | Do you avoid unnecessary exposure to radiation and microwave emissions? | 1 | 2 |

Total points: _____

## B: Skin Cancer

| | | Yes | No |
|---|---|---|---|
| 1. | Do you spend a lot of time outdoors, either at work or at play? | 2 | 1 |
| 2. | Do you use sunscreens with an SPF rating of 15 or more when you are in the sun? | 1 | 2 |
| 3. | Do you use tanning beds or sun booths regularly to maintain a tan? | 2 | 1 |
| 4. | Do you examine your skin once a month, checking any moles or other irregularities, particularly in hard-to-see areas such as your back, genitals, neck, and under your hair? | 1 | 2 |
| 5. | Do you purchase and wear sunglasses that adequately filter out harmful sun rays? | 1 | 2 |

Total points: _____

## C: Breast Cancer

| | | Yes | No |
|---|---|---|---|
| 1. | Do you check your breasts at least monthly using breast self-exam procedures? | 1 | 2 |
| 2. | Do you look at your breasts in the mirror regularly, checking for any irregular indentations/lumps, discharge from the nipples, or other noticeable changes? | 1 | 2 |
| 3. | Has your mother, sister, or daughter been diagnosed with breast cancer? | 2 | 1 |
| 4. | Have you ever been pregnant? | 1 | 2 |
| 5. | Have you had a history of lumps or cysts in your breasts or underarm? | 2 | 1 |

Total points: _____

## D: Cancers of the Reproductive System

# Men

|   |   | Yes | No |
|---|---|---|---|
| 1. | Do you examine your penis regularly for unusual bumps or growths? | 1 | 2 |
| 2. | Do you perform regular testicular self-examinations? | 1 | 2 |
| 3. | Do you have a family history of prostate or testicular cancer? | 2 | 1 |
| 4. | Do you practice safe sex and wear condoms during every sexual encounter? | 1 | 2 |
| 5. | Do you avoid exposure to harmful environmental hazards such as mercury, coal tars, benzene, chromate, and vinyl chloride? | 1 | 2 |

Total points: _____

# Women

|   |   | Yes | No |
|---|---|---|---|
| 1. | Do you have regularly scheduled Pap tests? | 1 | 2 |
| 2. | Have you been infected with HPV, Epstein-Barr virus, or other viruses believed to increase cancer risk? | 2 | 1 |
| 3. | Has your mother, sister, or daughter been diagnosed with breast, cervical, endometrial, or ovarian cancer (particularly at a young age)? | 2 | 1 |
| 4. | Do you practice safer sex and use condoms with every sexual encounter? | 1 | 2 |
| 5. | Are you obese, taking estrogen, or consuming a diet that is very high in saturated fats? | 2 | 1 |

Total points: _____

### Scoring Part 2

Look carefully at each question for which you received a 2. Are there any areas in which you received mostly 2s? Did you receive total points of 11 or higher in A? Did you receive total points of 6 or higher in B through D? If so, you have at least one identifiable risk. The higher the score, the more risks you may have.

## YOUR PLAN FOR CHANGE

**ASSESS YOURSELF** activities evaluated your risk of heart disease and cancer. Based on your results, you may need to take steps to reduce your risk for these diseases and improve your future health.

### TODAY, YOU CAN:

☐ Get up and move! Take a walk in the evening, use the stairs, or ride your bike to class. Think of ways to incorporate more physical activity into your daily routine.

☐ Improve your dietary habits by reading labels and choosing low-sodium foods, low-fat foods, and nutrient-dense fruits and vegetables. Replace meat and processed foods with a serving of fresh fruit or soy-based protein and green leafy vegetables several times per week. Eat more monounsaturated fat and foods with lower cholesterol counts. Watch your total calorie consumption.

☐ Assess your personal risks for specific cancers, looking at lifestyle as well as your genetic risks. For which cancers might you be most at risk?

### WITHIN THE NEXT TWO WEEKS, YOU CAN:

☐ Buy a bottle of broad-spectrum sunscreen (with SPF 15 or higher). Apply it liberally as part of your daily routine. (Be sure to check the expiration date, particularly on sale items!) Also, stay in the shade when the sun is strongest, from 10 AM to 4 PM.

☐ Find out your family health history. Talk to your parents, grandparents, or an aunt or uncle to find out if family members have developed cancer or CVD. Ask if they know their latest cholesterol LDL/HDL levels. Do you have a family history of diabetes?

☐ Begin a regular exercise program. Set small goals and try to meet them. (See Chapter 9 for ideas.)

☐ Practice a new stress management technique. (See Chapter 3 for ideas for managing stress.)

☐ Make sure you get at least 8 hours of sleep per night.

### BY THE END OF THE SEMESTER, YOU CAN:

☐ Get a full lipid panel for yourself and have your blood pressure checked. Once you know your levels, you'll have a better sense of what risk factors to address. If your levels are high, talk to your doctor about how to reduce them.

☐ Stop smoking, avoid secondhand smoke, and limit your alcohol intake.

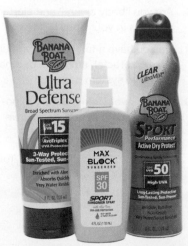

## CHAPTER REVIEW

To hear an MP3 Tutor Session, scan here or visit the Study Area in **MasteringHealth**.

### LO 1 | Cardiovascular Disease in the United States

- Cardiovascular disease is the leading cause of death in the United States, and it puts a huge economic burden on our society. African Americans have the highest rates of CVD deaths out of any other group in the United States. CVD is also a leading cause of death globally and is an increasing threat in the developing world.

### LO 2 | Understanding the Cardiovascular System

- The cardiovascular system consists of the heart and circulatory system and is a carefully regulated, integrated network of vessels that supplies the body with the nutrients and oxygen necessary to perform daily functions.

### LO 3 | Key Cardiovascular Diseases

- Cardiovascular diseases include atherosclerosis, coronary artery disease, peripheral artery disease, coronary heart disease, stroke, hypertension, angina pectoris, arrhythmias, congestive heart failure, and congenital and rheumatic heart disease.

### LO 4 | Reducing Your Risks

- *Cardiometabolic risks* refer to combined factors that increase a person's chances of CVD and diabetes. A person who possesses three or more cardiometabolic risk factors may have metabolic syndrome. Metabolic syndrome is increasing at all levels—among young and old, rich and poor, and in all ethnicities.
- Many risk factors for cardiovascular disease can be modified, such as cigarette smoking, high blood cholesterol and triglyceride levels, hypertension, lack of exercise, poor diet, obesity, diabetes, and emotional stress. Some risk factors, such as age, gender, and heredity, cannot be modified. The more risks you have: the greater your chances of developing CVD.

### LO 5 | Diagnosing and Treating Cardiovascular Disease

- Coronary bypass surgery is an established treatment for heart blockage; increasing numbers of angioplasty procedures and stents are being used with great success. Increasing numbers of pharmacological interventions such as statins are being used to reduce risk and prevent problems. Drug therapies can be used to prevent and treat CVD.

To hear an MP3 Tutor Session, scan here or visit the Study Area in **MasteringHealth**.

### LO 6 | Cancer: An Epidemiological Overview

- Cancer is the second most common cause of death in the United States. The current 5-year survival rates for cancer have greatly increased from those of previous generations.

### LO 7 | What Is Cancer?

- Cancer is a group of diseases characterized by uncontrolled growth and spread of abnormal cells. These cells may create tumors. Benign (noncancerous) tumors grow in size but do not spread; malignant (cancerous) tumors spread to other parts of the body.

### LO 8 | What Causes Cancer?

- Lifestyle factors for cancer include smoking and obesity as well as poor diet, lack of exercise, and other factors. Biological factors include inherited genes, age, and gender. Potential environmental carcinogens include asbestos, radiation, preservatives, and pesticides. Infectious agents may increase your risks for cancer; those that appear most likely to cause cancer are chronic hepatitis B and C, human papillomavirus, and genital herpes.

### LO 9 | Types of Cancers

- Each type of cancer poses different risks, depending on several factors. Common cancers include that of the lung, breast, colon and rectum, skin, prostate, testis, ovary, and uterus; leukemia; and lymphomas. Each has different strategies for prevention.

### LO 10 | Facing Cancer

- The most common treatments for cancer are surgery, chemotherapy, and radiation; newer therapies, including biologicals, smart drugs, and immunotherapy show promising results and should always be considered.
- Early diagnosis improves survival rate. Self-exams for breast, testicular, and skin cancer aid early diagnosis.

## POP QUIZ

Visit **MasteringHealth** to personalize your study plan with Chapter Review Quizzes and Dynamic Study Modules.

### LO 1 | Cardiovascular Disease in the United States

1. Which of the following is true about CVD?
   a. It's only a problem in developed nations.
   b. It claims the lives of more men than women every year.
   c. Risk factors are only an issue starting at age 50.
   d. It's the leading cause of death in America.

### LO 2 | Understanding the Cardiovascular System

2. Which type of blood vessels carry oxygenated blood away from the heart?
   a. Ventricles
   b. Arteries
   c. Pulmonary arteries
   d. Venules

## LO 3 | Key Cardiovascular Diseases

3. A stroke results
   a. when a heart stops beating.
   b. when cardiopulmonary resuscitation has failed to revive the stopped heart.
   c. when blood flow in the brain has been compromised, either due to blockage or hemorrhage.
   d. when blood pressure rises above 120/80 mm Hg.

## LO 4 | Reducing Your Risks

4. The "bad" type of cholesterol found in the bloodstream is known as
   a. high-density lipoprotein (HDL).
   b. low-density lipoprotein (LDL).
   c. total cholesterol.
   d. triglyceride.

## LO 5 | Diagnosing and Treating Cardiovascular Disease

5. The surgery in which a blood vessel is taken from another site in the patient's body and implanted to bypass the blocked artery and transport blood to the heart is called
   a. atherosclerosis surgery.
   b. thrombolysis.
   c. coronary bypass surgery.
   d. angioplasty.

## LO 6 | Cancer: An Epidemiological Overview

6. Overall, which cancer has the worst 5-year survival rate today?
   a. Prostate
   b. Pancreas
   c. Melanoma
   d. Breast

## LO 7 | What Is Cancer?

7. When cancer cells have *metastasized*,
   a. it has grown into a malignant tumor.
   b. it has spread to other parts of the body.

   c. the cancer is retreating and cancer cells are dying off.
   d. the tumor is localized and considered in situ.

## LO 8 | What Causes Cancer?

8. One of the biggest factors in increased risk for cancer is
   a. increasing age.
   b. not having children.
   c. being of long-lived parents.
   d. increased consumption of fruits and vegetables.

## LO 9 | Types of Cancers

9. The cancer that causes the most deaths for men and women in the United States is
   a. colorectal cancer.
   b. pancreatic cancer.
   c. lung cancer.
   d. stomach cancer.

## LO 10 | Facing Cancer

10. Which of the following treatment methods uses drugs to kill cancerous cells?
    a. Radiotherapy
    b. Chemotherapy
    c. Stem cell therapy
    d. Stereotactic radiosurgery

*Answers to the Pop Quiz can be found on page A-1. If you answered a question incorrectly, review the section identified by the learning outcome. For even more study tools, visit MasteringHealth.*

# THINK ABOUT IT!

## LO 1 | Cardiovascular Disease in the United States

1. Why do you think hypertension rates are rising among today's college students?

## LO 2 | Understanding the Cardiovascular System

2. What can your resting heart rate tell you about your overall health? What are some reasons a person's

resting heart rate might be higher or lower than the median?

## LO 3 | Key Cardiovascular Diseases

3. List the different types of CVD. Compare and contrast their symptoms, risk factors, prevention, and treatment.

## LO 4 | Reducing Your Risks

4. Discuss the role that exercise, stress management, dietary changes, medical checkups, sodium reduction, and other factors can play in reducing risk for CVD. What role might infectious diseases play in CVD risk?

## LO 5 | Diagnosing and Treating Cardiovascular Disease

5. Describe some of the diagnostic, preventive, and treatment alternatives for CVD. If you had a heart attack today, which treatment would you prefer? Explain why.

## LO 6 | Cancer: An Epidemiological Overview

6. What are some of the factors that account for the great increase in 5-year survival rates for people with cancer in recent years?

## LO 7 | What Is Cancer?

7. What is cancer? How does it spread? What is the difference between a benign tumor and a malignant tumor?

## LO 8 | What Causes Cancer?

8. List the likely causes of cancer. Which of these causes would be a risk for you, in particular? What can you do to reduce these risks? What risk factors do you share with family members? Friends?

## LO 9 | Types of Cancers

9. What are the differences between carcinomas, sarcomas, lymphomas, and leukemia? Which is the most common? Least common? Why is it important that you know the stage of your cancer?

## LO 10 | Facing Cancer

10. Why are breast and testicular self-exams especially important for college students? What factors keep you from doing your own self-exams? What could you do to make sure you do regular self-exams?

## ACCESS YOUR HEALTH ON THE INTERNET

The following websites explore further topics and issues related to CVD and cancer. For links to the websites below, visit **MasteringHealth**.

*American Heart Association*. This is the home page of the leading private organization dedicated to heart health. This site provides information, statistics, and resources regarding cardiovascular care, including an opportunity to test your risk for CVD. **www.heart.org**

*National Heart, Lung, and Blood Institute*. This valuable resource provides information on all aspects of cardiovascular health and wellness. **www.nhlbi.nih.gov**

*Global Cardiovascular Infobase*. This site contains epidemiological data and statistics for cardiovascular diseases for countries throughout the world, with a focus on developing nations. **www.cvdinfobase.ca**

*American Cancer Society*. This private organization is dedicated to cancer prevention. Here you'll find information, statistics, and resources regarding cancer. **www.cancer.org**

*National Cancer Institute*. On this site you will find valuable information on cancer facts, results of research, new and ongoing clinical trials, and the Physician Data Query (PDQ), a comprehensive database of cancer treatment information. **www.cancer.gov**

*Oncolink*. Sponsored by the University of Pennsylvania Cancer Center, this site educates cancer patients and their families by offering information on support services, cancer causes, screening, prevention, and common questions. **www.oncolink.com**

*Susan G. Komen for the Cure*. Up-to-date information about breast cancer, issues in treatment, and support groups are presented here, as well as a wealth of videos and information. This site is especially useful for diagnosed patients looking for additional support and advice. **www.komen.org**

*National Coalition for Cancer Survivorship*. Cancer survivors share their experiences advocating for themselves during and after cancer treatment. **www.canceradvocacy.org**

# Minimizing Your Risk for Diabetes

Your genetics play a key role in risk for diabetes, along with learned dietary patterns from parents and your own health behaviors.

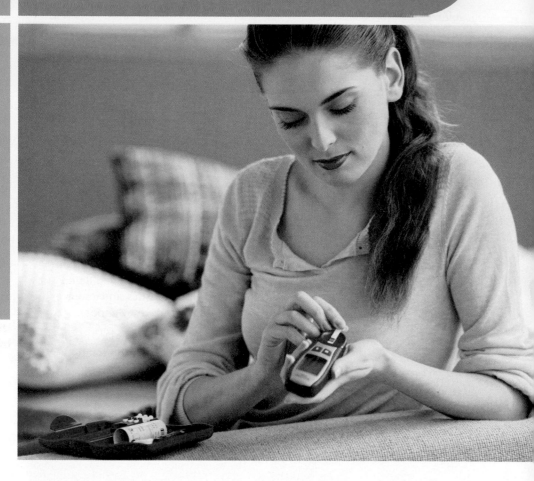

## LEARNING OUTCOMES

1 Differentiate among types of diabetes and identify common risk factors.
2 Describe the symptoms of, complications associated with, and main tests for diabetes.
3 Explain how diabetes can be prevented and treated.

**N**ora is overweight. She used to figure it was no big deal; but last week her mom called to tell Nora that she'd just been diagnosed with type 2 diabetes. Her voice sounded shaky as she reminded Nora about her own mother's death from kidney failure—a complication of diabetes—at age 52. Later, Nora searched online for information about her risk for diabetes. Her Hispanic ethnicity, family history, high stress level and lack of sleep, excessive weight, and sedentary lifestyle made her a prime candidate.

Nora made an appointment for a diabetes screening. She was instructed to fast the night before. At her visit, the nurse practitioner took a blood sample. A few days later, she called to tell Nora that her blood glucose was elevated, and although she wasn't diabetic yet, she needed to make changes to her diet and lifestyle to reduce her risk for developing type 2 diabetes, like her mom.

Over the past two decades, diabetes rates in the United States have increased dramatically[1] (see **FIGURE 1**). The Centers for Disease Control and Prevention (CDC) estimates that nearly 30 million people—almost 10 percent of the U.S. population—have diabetes, and another 86 million have *prediabetes*.[2] Experts predict that at current rates, more than 1 in 3 Americans will have diabetes by 2050. Diabetes kills more Americans each year than breast cancer and AIDS combined, and millions suffer the physical, emotional, and economic burdens of dealing with this difficult disease.[3]

Diabetes rates increase as age and weight increase. Among persons aged 20–44 years, approximately 4.1 percent have diabetes, compared to roughly 16.2 percent of those aged 45–64 and over 25.9 percent of those aged 65–74.[4] The economic burden of diagnosed diabetes, gestational diabetes, undiagnosed diabetes, and prediabetes was over $322 billion in 2012.[5] Costs for diagnosed diabetics averages nearly $11,000 per person per year, while undiagnosed diabetes averages just over $4,000.[6] For an explanation of the personal financial toll that comes with diabetes, read the **Money & Health** box on page 388.

## LO 1 | WHAT IS DIABETES?

**Differentiate among types of diabetes and identify common risk factors.**

**Diabetes mellitus** is a group of diseases, each with its own mechanism, all characterized by a persistently high level of glucose, a type of sugar, in the blood. One sign of diabetes is the production of an abnormal level of glucose in the urine, a fact reflected in its name: *Diabetes* derives from a Greek word meaning "to flow through," and *mellitus* is the Latin word for "sweet." The high blood glucose levels—or **hyperglycemia**—seen in diabetes can lead to serious health problems and premature death.

In a healthy person, the digestive system breaks down the carbohydrates we eat into glucose—one of our main energy sources—which it releases into the bloodstream for use by body cells. Our red blood cells can only use glucose to fuel functioning, and brain and other nerve cells prefer glucose over other fuels. When glucose levels drop below normal, you may feel unable to concentrate, and certain mental functions may be impaired. When more glucose is available than required to meet immediate needs, the excess is stored as glycogen in the liver and muscles for later use.

Glucose can't simply cross cell membranes on its own. Instead, cells have structures that transport glucose across in response to a signal generated by the **pancreas,** an organ located just beneath

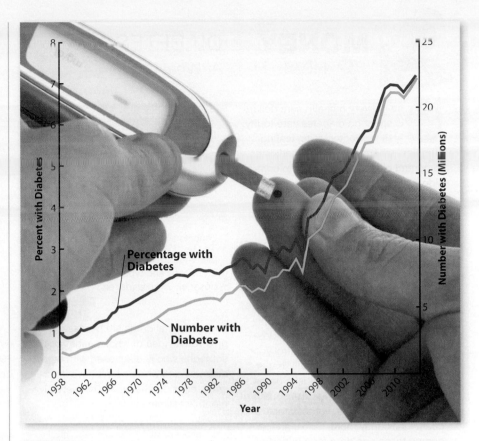

**FIGURE 1** Percentage and Number of U.S. Population with Diagnosed Diabetes, 1958–2013 Notice that these data are for diagnosed cases. Estimates of actual prevalence are higher.

**Source:** CDC, "Long-Term Trends in Diabetes," October 2014, www.cdc.gov/diabetes/statistics/slides/long_term_trends.pdf

the stomach. Whenever a surge of glucose enters the bloodstream, the pancreas secretes a hormone called **insulin.** Insulin stimulates cells to take up glucose from the bloodstream and carry it into the cell, where it's used for immediate energy. Conversion of glucose to glycogen for storage in the liver and muscles is also assisted by insulin. When levels of glucose fall, the pancreas stops secreting insulin—until the next influx of glucose arrives.

## Type 1 Diabetes

The more serious and less prevalent form of diabetes, called **type 1 diabetes** (or insulin-dependent diabetes), is an autoimmune disease in which the individual's immune system attacks and destroys the insulin-making cells in the pancreas. Destruction of those cells causes a dramatic reduction, or total cessation, of insulin production. Without insulin, cells cannot take up glucose, leaving blood glucose levels

permanently elevated. Only about 5 percent of diabetic cases are type 1.[7] European ancestry, a genetic predisposition, and certain viral infections all increase the risk.[8]

People with type 1 diabetes require daily insulin injections or infusions and must carefully monitor their diet and exercise levels. Often they face unique challenges as the "lesser known" diabetic type, with fewer funds available for research and fewer options for treatment.

**diabetes mellitus** A group of diseases characterized by elevated blood glucose levels.

**hyperglycemia** Elevated blood glucose level.

**pancreas** Organ that secretes digestive enzymes into the small intestine and hormones, including insulin, into the bloodstream.

**insulin** Hormone secreted by the pancreas and required by body cells for the uptake and storage of glucose.

**type 1 diabetes** Form of diabetes mellitus in which the pancreas is not able to make insulin, and therefore blood glucose cannot enter the cells to be used for energy.

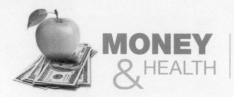

# MONEY & HEALTH

## DIABETES
### *At What Cost?*

One in every 5 health care dollars is spent on diabetes care today: fees for doctor visits, testing supplies, laboratory results, medicines to control glucose and others to control side effects, as well as the costs for other necessities often only partially covered, even for those with insurance. If you are underinsured or uninsured, the *diabetes drain* on your bank account could be major.

Costs of treatment varies tremendously; whether you have insurance, the nature of your deductibles and co-pays, proximity to pharmacies with a supply of generics, and the number and dosage of drugs necessary to control your blood glucose are all factors. What is known is that costs for diabetic drugs are on a rapid rise. Newer drugs may not be more effective, yet they may cost significantly more. Often, after a person takes one drug for a period of time, the drug becomes less effective

| Diabetic Health Care Need | Estimated Monthly Cost |
|---|---|
| Doctor visit for monitoring and testing | $200 |
| Lab tests: Fasting glucose blood test, glucose tolerance, A1C tests | $35–$200 |
| Home glucose meter, test strips | Meter= $35–$50<br>Test strips = roughly $1 each.<br>Average = $100/month |
| Lancets and lancing devices, alcohol wipes | $5–$10/month |
| Oral medications like *metformin* (depends on dosage and type); *Actos* (depends on dosage); *Januvia* (depends on dosage) | *Metformin:* $13–$15 at low end per month. Less at big box stores, more for different dosage; *Actos:* $220–$370/month; *Januvia:* $265/month |

and additional drugs are necessary. To give you an idea of what it might cost someone who is diagnosed with type 2 diabetes and who doesn't have insurance, consider these very conservative monthly estimates.

The American Diabetes Association estimates costs of between $350 and $900 per month for the typical type 2 diabetic. However, insulin-dependent diabetics may have costs that are two to three times higher.

**Sources:** American Diabetes Association, "Fast Facts: Data and Statistics about Diabetes," 2014, http://professional.diabetes.org/ResourcesForProfessionals.aspx?cid=91777; American Diabetes Association, "What Are My Options," March 2015, www.diabetes.org/living-with-diabetes/treatment-and-care/medication/oral-medications/what-are-my-options.html

# Type 2 Diabetes

**Type 2 diabetes** (non–insulin-dependent diabetes) accounts for 90–95 percent of all cases.[9] In type 2, either the pancreas does not make sufficient insulin, or body cells are resistant to its effects—a condition called **insulin resistance**—and don't use it efficiently (**FIGURE 2**).

## Development of Type 2 Diabetes

Type 2 diabetes usually develops slowly. In early stages, cells throughout the body begin to resist the effects of insulin; Over time, the body may not produce enough insulin. An overabundance of free fatty acids concentrated in a person's fat cells (as may be the case in an obese individual) inhibit glucose uptake by body cells and suppress the liver's sensitivity to insulin. As a result, the liver's ability to self-regulate its conversion of glucose into glycogen begins to fail, and blood levels of glucose gradually rise.

The pancreas attempts to compensate by producing more insulin, but it cannot maintain hyperproduction indefinitely. More and more pancreatic insulin-producing cells become nonfunctional, insulin output declines, and blood glucose levels rise high enough to warrant a diagnosis of type 2 diabetes.

## Nonmodifiable Risk Factors

Type 2 diabetes is associated with a cluster of nonmodifiable risk factors including age, ethnicity, and genetic and biological factors.

One in four adults over age 65 has type 2 diabetes. Although it used to be referred to as *adult-onset diabetes*, today it is increasingly diagnosed among children and teens.[10] Currently, diabetes is one of the leading chronic diseases in youth, affecting over 208,000 people under the age of 20, or 1 in every 400 youth.[11]

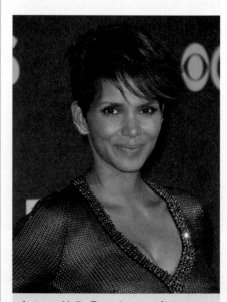

Actress Halle Berry is one of many Americans diagnosed with type 2 diabetes.

**type 2 diabetes** Form of diabetes mellitus in which the pancreas does not make enough insulin or the body is unable to use insulin correctly.

**insulin resistance** State in which body cells fail to respond to the effects of insulin; obesity increases the risk that cells will become insulin resistant.

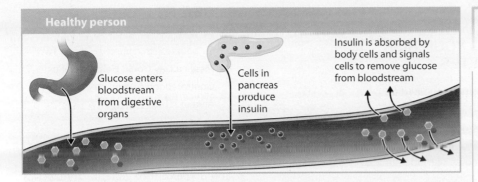

Healthy person

Glucose enters bloodstream from digestive organs

Cells in pancreas produce insulin

Insulin is absorbed by body cells and signals cells to remove glucose from bloodstream

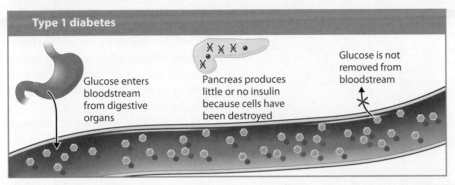

Type 1 diabetes

Glucose enters bloodstream from digestive organs

Pancreas produces little or no insulin because cells have been destroyed

Glucose is not removed from bloodstream

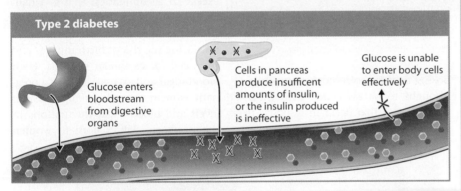

Type 2 diabetes

Glucose enters bloodstream from digestive organs

Cells in pancreas produce insufficent amounts of insulin, or the insulin produced is ineffective

Glucose is unable to enter body cells effectively

**FIGURE 2** Diabetes: What It Is and How It Develops

In a healthy person, a sufficient amount of insulin is produced and released by the pancreas and used efficiently by the cells. In type 1 diabetes, the pancreas makes little or no insulin. In type 2 diabetes, either the pancreas does not make sufficient insulin, or cells are resistant to insulin and are not able to use it efficiently.

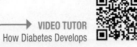

→ VIDEO TUTOR
How Diabetes Develops

Non-Hispanic whites, Native Americans, and non-Hispanic black youth have the highest rates, while Asian/Pacific Islanders have the lowest.[12] Having a close relative with type 2 diabetes is a significant risk factor. Most experts believe that type 2 diabetes is caused by a complex interaction between environmental factors, lifestyle, and genetic susceptibility. Although numerous genes have been identified as likely culprits in increased risk, the mechanisms by which inherited diabetes develops remains poorly understood.[13]

## Modifiable Risk Factors

Body weight, dietary choices, level of physical activity, sleep patterns, and stress level are all diabetes-related factors people have some control over. Type 2 diabetes is linked to overweight and obesity. In adults, a body mass index (BMI) of 25 or greater increases risks, with significantly higher risks for each 5 $kg/m^2$ increase.[14] In particular, excess weight carried around the waistline—a condition called *central adiposity*—and measured by waist circumference is a significant risk factor

**prediabetes** Condition in which blood glucose levels are higher than normal, but not high enough to be classified as diabetes.

for older women.[15] People with type 2 diabetes who lose weight and increase their physical activity can significantly improve their blood glucose levels.

Inadequate sleep may contribute to the development of both obesity and type 2 diabetes, possibly due to the fact that sleep-deprived people tend to engage in less physical activity.[16] People routinely sleep-deprived are also at higher risk for *metabolic syndrome* (discussed shortly), a cluster of risk factors that include poor glucose metabolism.[17] Recent data provides evidence of a link between diabetes and psychological or physical stress; however, a recent analysis of studies focused on the role of work-related stress on type 2 diabetes development showed mixed results.[18]

## Prediabetes

An estimated 86 million Americans age 20 or older—37 percent of the population over 20—and 51 percent of those over 65 —have **prediabetes**, a condition involving higher than normal blood glucose levels, but not high enough to be classified as diabetes. Nine out of ten people with prediabetes do not know they have it.[19] Current rates of prediabetes in college students are unknown; however, results from small studies as well as known increases in the rates of obesity, sedentary lifestyle, and metabolic risks point to a likely rise of rates on campus.[20]

Often, prediabetes is one of the risk factors linked to overweight and obesity that together constitute *metabolic syndrome*. Of the six conditions, prediabetes and central adiposity appear to be most dominant.[21] A person who has metabolic syndrome is five times more likely

**WHAT DO YOU THINK?**

**Why do you think type 2 diabetes is increasing in the United States?**

- Why is it increasing among young people?
- Do you think young people are generally aware of what diabetes is and their own susceptibility for it?

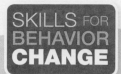
to develop type 2 diabetes than is a person without it.[22] Overall, Mexican Americans have the highest rates of metabolic syndrome, with white Americans and African Americans not far behind.[23] Women with uterine fibroids or ovarian cysts also are at increased risk.[24]

Without weight loss and increases in moderate physical activity, 15–30 percent of those with prediabetes will develop type 2 diabetes within 5 years.[25] Lack of knowledge—9 out of 10 people with prediabetes don't know they have it—poses a major challenge to slowing increasing diabetes rates.[26] A prediabetes diagnosis represents an opportunity to adjust your lifestyle. Increasing physical activity, improving diet, and losing weight can all prevent or delay a diabetes diagnosis.[27] See tips for halting or slowing the progression of diabetes in the **Skills for Behavior Change** box.

## Gestational Diabetes

**Gestational diabetes** is a state of high blood glucose levels during pregnancy, posing risks for both mother and child. Thought to be associated with metabolic stresses that occur in response to changing hormonal levels, as many as 18 percent of pregnancies are affected by gestational diabetes.[28] Between 40 and 50 percent of gestational diabetics may develop type 2 diabetes within a decade of initial diagnosis if they don't lose weight, improve diet, and exercise. If excess weight is never lost, higher "normal" weight increases risk of progression to type 2 diabetes with subsequent births.[29]

Women with gestational diabetes also have increased risk of high blood pressure, high blood acidity, increased infections, and death.[30] A result of the excess fat accumulation that is a hallmark sign of gestational diabetes, women can give birth to large babies—increasing the risk of birth injuries and the need for caesarean sections. High blood sugar and excess weight in a pregnant woman can trigger high insulin levels and blood sugar fluctuations in the newborn. Babies born to women

**gestational diabetes** Form of diabetes mellitus in which women who have never had diabetes have high blood sugar (glucose) levels during pregnancy.

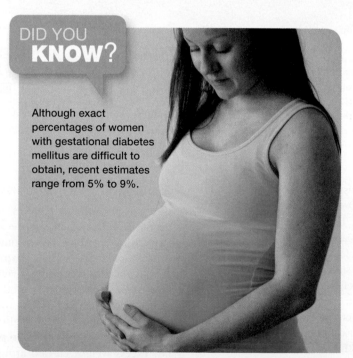

### DID YOU KNOW?

Although exact percentages of women with gestational diabetes mellitus are difficult to obtain, recent estimates range from 5% to 9%.

**Source:** C. Desisto et al., "Prevalence Estimates of Gestational Diabetes in the United States. Pregnancy Risk Assessment Monitoring System (PRAMS) 2007–2010," *Preventing Chronic Disease* 11 (2014): 130415, doi: http:11dx .doi.org/10.5888/pcd 11.130415

with gestational diabetes are also at risk for malformations of the heart, nervous system, and bones; respiratory distress; and fetal death.[31]

## LO 2 | WHAT ARE THE SYMPTOMS OF DIABETES?

Describe the symptoms of, complications associated with, and main tests for diabetes.

The symptoms of diabetes are similar for both type 1 and type 2, including:

- **Thirst.** Kidneys filter excessive glucose by diluting it with water. This can pull too much water from the body and result in dehydration.
- **Excessive urination.** For the same reason, increased need to urinate occurs.
- **Weight loss.** Because so many calories are lost in the glucose that passes into urine, a person with diabetes often feels hungry. Despite eating more, he or she typically loses weight.
- **Fatigue.** When glucose cannot enter cells, fatigue and weakness occur.
- **Nerve damage.** A high glucose concentration damages the smallest blood vessels of the body, including those supplying nerves in the hands and feet. This can cause numbness and tingling.
- **Blurred vision.** Too much glucose causes body tissues to dry out—particularly damaging to the eyes.
- **Poor wound healing and increased infections.** High levels of glucose can affect the body's ability to ward off infections and may affect overall immune system functioning.

## Complications of Diabetes

The main complications of poorly controlled diabetes include.[1]

- **Diabetic coma.** A coma from high blood acidity known as *diabetic ketoacidosis*

can occur when, in the absence of glucose, body cells break down stored fat for energy. The process produces acidic molecules called *ketones*. Too many ketones can raise blood acid level dangerously high. The diabetic person slips into a coma and, without medical intervention, will die.

- **Cardiovascular disease.** Because many diabetics are also overweight or obese, hypertension is often present. Blood vessels become damaged as glucose-laden blood flows sluggishly and essential nutrients and other substances are not transported as effectively.
- **Kidney disease.** Diabetes is the leading cause of kidney failure. The kidneys become scarred by overwork and the high blood pressure in their vessels. More than 240,000 Americans are currently living with kidney failure caused by diabetes.[33] In fact, 35 percent of those 20 years or older with diabetes have kidney failure.[34] Many of these people are on dialysis or waiting for a kidney transplant that may never come.
- **Amputations.** An impaired immune response combined with damaged blood vessels and neuropathy in hands and feet makes it easier for people with diabetes to not notice injury until damage is extensive. Lack of circulation to the area increases risk of infection and difficulty of treatment, leading to tissue death and amputation. More than 60 percent of nontraumatic amputations of legs, feet, and toes are due to diabetes[35] (see **FIGURE 3a**). In fact, each year nearly 73,000 nontraumatic lower-limb amputations are performed on people with diabetes (180 per day).[36]
- **Eye disease and blindness.** High blood glucose levels damage microvessels in the eye, leading to vision loss. Nearly 7.7 million people over the age of 40 have early-stage retinopathy, swelling of capillaries in the eye, which could lead to blindness without treatment (**FIGURE 3b**).[37]
- **Infectious diseases.** Persons with diabetes have increased risk of poor

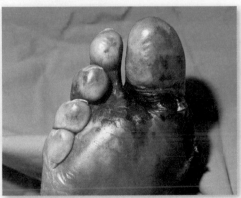

**a** Infections in the feet and legs are common in people with diabetes, and healing is impaired; thus, amputations are often necessary.

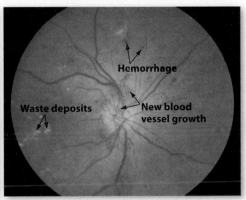

**b** Uncontrolled diabetes can damage the eye, causing swelling, leaking, and rupture of blood vessels; growth of new blood vessels; deposits of wastes; and scarring. All of these can progress to blindness.

Hemorrhage

Waste deposits

New blood vessel growth

**FIGURE 3** Complications of Uncontrolled Diabetes: Amputation and Eye Disease

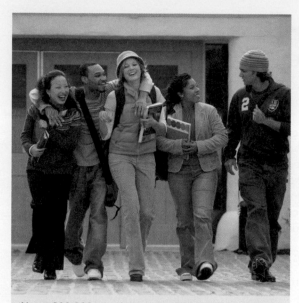

About 208,000 people younger than age 20 have type 1 or type 2 diabetes, with thousands more estimated to have prediabetes.

**Source:** American Diabetes Association, "Fast Facts: Data and Statistics about Diabetes," 2014, http://professional.diabetes.org

wound healing and greater susceptibility to infectious diseases, particularly influenza and pneumonia. Once infection occurs, it may be more difficult to treat.

■ **Tooth and gum diseases.** Research indicates that persons with diabetes are more susceptible to bacterial infections of the mouth that can lead to *gingivitis* (an early stage of gum disease) and *periodontitis*—a more serious inflammation of the gums that can lead to decay, tooth loss, and a variety of other health risks.[38] Emerging research suggests that the relationship between diabetes and gum disease may be a two way street, with those who have gum disease being more susceptible to problems with blood glucose control, increasing the risk of progression to diabetes.[39]

■ **Other complications.** Diabetics may have foot neuropathy and chronic pain that makes walking,

driving, and simple tasks more difficult. Persons with diabetes are more likely to suffer from depression, making intervention and treatment more difficult. Depressed individuals are 60 percent more likely to develop type 2 diabetes.

## Diagnosing Diabetes

Diabetes and prediabetes are diagnosed when a blood test reveals elevated blood glucose levels. Generally, a physician orders one of the following blood tests:

■ The *fasting plasma glucose (FPG) test* requires a patient to fast for 8 to 10 hours. Then, a small sample of blood is tested for glucose concentration. An FPG level greater than or equal to 100 mg/dL indicates prediabetes, and a level greater than or equal to 126 mg/dL indicates diabetes (**FIGURE 4**).

■ The *oral glucose tolerance test (OGTT)* requires the patient to drink

concentrated glucose. A sample of blood is drawn for testing 2 hours after drinking. A reading greater than or equal to 140 mg/dL indicates prediabetes; a reading greater than or equal to 200 mg/dL indicates diabetes.

■ A third test, *A1C* or *glycosylated hemoglobin test (HbA1C)*, doesn't require fasting and gives the average value of a patient's blood glucose over the past 2 to 3 months, instead of at one moment in time. In general, an A1C of 5.7 to 6.4 means high risk for diabetes or being prediabetic. If A1C is 6.5 or higher, then diabetes may be diagnosed.[40] **Estimated average glucose (eAG)** shows how A1C numbers correspond to blood glucose numbers. For example, someone with an A1C value of 6.1 would be able to look at a chart and see that his or her average blood glucose was around 128—a high level that should encourage healthy lifestyle modifications.

People with diabetes need to check blood glucose levels several times each day to ensure they stay within their target range. To check blood glucose, diabetics must prick their finger to obtain a drop of blood. A handheld glucose meter can then evaluate the blood sample.

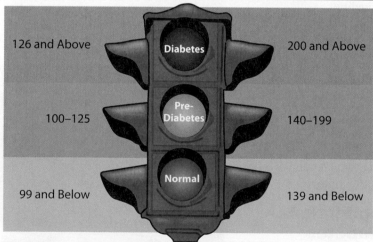

| FPG Levels | Diagnosis | OGTT Levels |
|---|---|---|
| 126 and Above | Diabetes | 200 and Above |
| 100–125 | Pre-Diabetes | 140–199 |
| 99 and Below | Normal | 139 and Below |

**FIGURE 4** Blood Glucose Levels in Prediabetes and Untreated Diabetes The fasting plasma glucose (FPG) test measures levels of blood glucose after a person fasts overnight. The oral glucose tolerance test (OGTT) measures levels of blood glucose after a person consumes a concentrated amount of glucose.

**Source:** American Diabetes Association, "Diagnosing Diabetes and Learning about Prediabetes," March 2014, www.diabetes.org/diabetes-basics/diagnosis

**estimated average glucose (eAG)** A method for reporting A1C test results that gives the average blood glucose levels for the testing period using the same units (milligrams per deciliter [mg/dL]) that patients are used to seeing in self-administered glucose tests.

## LO 3 | TREATING DIABETES

Explain how diabetes can be prevented and treated.

Treatment options for people with pre-diabetes and diabetes vary according to type and progression of the disease.

## Lifestyle Changes

Studies have shown that lifestyle changes can prevent or delay the development of type 2 diabetes by up to 58 percent.[41] Even for people with type 2 diabetes, lifestyle changes can sometimes prevent or delay the need for medication or insulin injections.

### Losing Weight

A landmark clinical trial, the *Diabetes Prevention Program (DPP)* study, showed that a loss of as little as 5 to 7 percent of current body weight and regular physical activity significantly lowered the risk of progressing to diabetes.[42] If you have diabetes, weight loss and exercise can improve your blood glucose and other health indicators.[43]

### Adopting a Healthy Diet

To prevent surges in blood sugar, people with diabetes must pay attention to the glycemic index and glycemic load of the foods they eat. Glycemic index compares the potential of foods containing the same amount of carbohydrate to raise blood glucose. The concept of glycemic load was developed by scientists to simultaneously describe the quality (glycemic index) and quantity of carbohydrate in a meal.[44] By learning to combine high—and low—glycemic index foods to avoid surges in blood glucose, diabetics can help control average blood glucose levels throughout the day.

## 35%
OF THOSE 20 YEARS OLD OR OLDER WITH DIABETES HAVE **KIDNEY FAILURE**.

Researchers have studied a variety of specific foods for their effect on blood glucose levels. Here is a brief summary of their findings:

- **Whole grains.** A diet high in whole grains may reduce a person's risk of developing type 2 diabetes.[45]
- **High-fiber foods.** Recent research indicates that eating high fiber foods may reduce diabetes risk.[46]
- **Fatty fish.** An impressive body of evidence has linked the consumption of fish high in omega-3 fatty acids with decreased progression of insulin resistance.[47] However, newer research has called omega-3's beneficial effects into question. More research is necessary to determine the role fatty acids play in diabetes risk reduction.[48]

## Increasing Physical Fitness

The DPP and other organizations recommend at least 30 minutes of physical activity 5 days a week to reduce your risk of type 2 diabetes.[49] Exercise increases sensitivity to insulin. The more muscle mass you have and the more you use your muscles, the more efficiently cells use glucose for fuel, meaning there will be less glucose circulating in the bloodstream. For most people, activity of moderate intensity can help keep blood glucose levels under control.

## Medical Interventions

Lifestyle changes are not always sufficient to control diabetes. Sometimes medication is necessary. In cases where medications are less effective, bariatric surgery may be an option for slowing or halting the progression of prediabetes and type 2 diabetes.

### Oral Medications

When lifestyle changes fail to control type 2 diabetes, oral medications may be prescribed. Some medications reduce glucose production by the liver, whereas others slow the absorption of carbohydrates from the small intestine. Other medications increase insulin production by the pancreas, whereas still others work to increase the insulin sensitivity of cells. The newest class of diabetes drugs is known as SGLT2

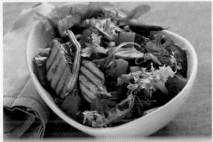

People with diabetes can occasionally indulge in sweets in moderation, particularly if they balance carbohydrates with protein. However, meals low in saturated and *trans* fats and high in fiber, like this salad of salmon and fresh vegetables, are recommended for helping to control blood glucose and body weight.

inhibitors. These drugs cause the kidneys to excrete more glucose, lowering levels of glucose circulating in the body.

Some people use diabetes medications without altering lifestyle, thinking the drugs are taking care of the problem. With time, medications become less effective and treatment options increasingly scarce. It is best to follow American Diabetes Association recommendations on diet, exercise, and lifestyle, in general.

### Weight Loss Surgery

People who undergo gastric/bariatric surgery for weight loss have shown remarkable reductions in blood glucose and diabetes symptoms for 2 to 3 years after surgery.[50] Those who combined gastric bypass or sleeve gastrectomy with intensive medical therapy had similar outcomes.[51] In many cases, former diabetics can stop taking medications for some of their cardiovascular risks, and stop diabetes symptoms altogether. Many professional groups are pushing for wider use of these more drastic weight loss methods.[52] Gastric bypass surgeries are not without risks, however, and can include death and serious complications. (See Chapter 10 for more on gastric bypass surgeries.)

### Insulin Injections

For people with type 1 diabetes, insulin injections or infusions are absolutely essential for daily functioning, because

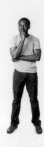

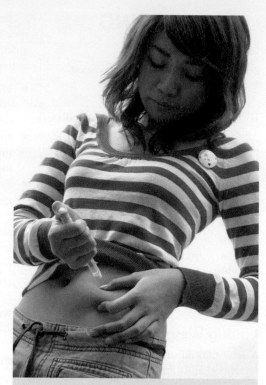

Some type 2 diabetics can control their condition with changes in diet and lifestyle habits or with oral medications. However, some type 2 diabetics and all type 1 diabetics require insulin injections or infusions.

their pancreases can no longer produce adequate amounts of insulin. In addition, people with type 2 diabetes whose blood glucose levels cannot be adequately controlled with other treatment options require insulin injections. Because insulin is a protein and would be digested in the gastrointestinal tract, it cannot be taken orally, and must be injected into the fat layer under the skin; from there, it is absorbed into the bloodstream.

People with diabetes used to need two or more daily insulin injections. Now, many use an *insulin infusion pump* to deliver minute amounts of insulin throughout the day. The external portion is only about the size of an MP3 player and can easily be hidden by clothes, while a thin tube and catheter is inserted under the patient's skin. Infusion over time is less painful and more effective than a few larger doses of insulin.

To overcome current insulin therapy limitations, researchers are working to link glucose monitoring and insulin delivery by developing an artificial pancreas. An artificial pancreas would mimic, as closely as possible, the way a healthy pancreas detects changes in blood glucose levels, responding automatically to secrete appropriate amounts of insulin. Although the first prototype devices received FDA approval, they cannot yet do the job of a fully functional pancreas.[53]

## Are You at Risk for Diabetes?

Certain characteristics place people at greater risk for diabetes. Nevertheless, many people remain unaware of the symptoms of diabetes until after the disease has begun to progress. Take the following quiz to help determine your risk for diabetes. If you answer yes to three or more of these questions, consider seeking medical advice.

|  | | Yes | No |
|---|---|---|---|
| 1. | Do any of your primary relatives (parents, siblings, grandparents) have diabetes? | ○ | ○ |
| 2. | Are you overweight or obese? | ○ | ○ |
| 3. | Do you smoke? | ○ | ○ |
| 4. | Have you been diagnosed with high blood pressure? | ○ | ○ |
| 5. | Are you typically sedentary (seldom, if ever, engage in vigorous aerobic exercise)? | ○ | ○ |
| 6. | Have you noticed an increase in your craving for water or other beverages? | ○ | ○ |
| 7. | Have you noticed that you have to urinate more frequently than you used to during a typical day? | ○ | ○ |
| 8. | Have you noticed any tingling or numbness in your hands and feet, which might indicate circulatory problems? | ○ | ○ |
| 9. | Do you often feel a gnawing hunger during the day, even though you usually eat regular meals? | ○ | ○ |
| 10. | Are you often so tired that you find it difficult to stay awake? | ○ | ○ |
| 11. | Have you noticed that you are losing weight but don't seem to be doing anything in particular to make this happen? | ○ | ○ |
| 12. | Have you noticed that you have skin irritations more frequently and that minor infections don't heal as quickly as they used to? | ○ | ○ |
| 13. | Have you noticed any unusual changes in your vision (blurring, difficulty in focusing, etc.)? | ○ | ○ |
| 14. | Have you noticed unusual pain or swelling in your joints? | ○ | ○ |
| 15. | Do you often feel weak or nauseated when you wake in the morning or if you wait too long to eat a meal? | ○ | ○ |
| 16. | If you are a woman, have you had several vaginal yeast infections during the past year? | ○ | ○ |

## YOUR PLAN FOR **CHANGE**

If the results of the **ASSESS YOURSELF** activity "Are You at Risk for Diabetes?" indicate you need to take further steps to decrease your risks, then follow this plan.

**TODAY,** YOU CAN:

☐ Talk to your parents and find out if there is a history of prediabetes or diabetes mellitus in your family.

☐ Take stock of other risk factors you may have for diabetes—do you exercise regularly and watch your weight? Do you eat healthfully? Have you ever had your blood glucose measured?

**WITHIN THE NEXT TWO WEEKS,** YOU CAN:

☐ Make an appointment with your health care provider to have your blood glucose levels tested.

☐ If you smoke, begin devising a plan to quit. (Chapter 8 can give you some ideas.)

**BY THE END OF THE SEMESTER,** YOU CAN:

☐ Pay attention to what you eat; increase your intake of whole grains, fruits, and vegetables; and decrease your consumption of saturated fats, *trans* fats, and sugar.

☐ Make physical activity and exercise part of your daily routine, aiming for at least 30 minutes 5 days a week.

## CHAPTER REVIEW

 To head an MP3 Tutor Session, scan here or visit the Study Area in **MasteringHealth**.

### LO 1 | What Is Diabetes?

- *Diabetes mellitus* is a group of diseases, each with its own mechanics. All are characterized by a persistently high level of glucose, a type of sugar, in the blood.
- Complications can range from cardiovascular disease to visual and gum problems, neuropathy, poor wound healing, and a host of other health problems.

### LO 2 | What Are the Symptoms of Diabetes?

- Symptoms of diabetes vary, but may include *polydypsia* (increased thirst), *polyphagia* (increased hunger), *polyuria* (increased urination), fatigue, blurred vision, nausea and lightheadedness, slow wound healing, numbness or tingling in hands and feet, frequent infections of the skin, tendency to bruise easily, among others.
- Key tests for diabetes include a fasting plasma glucose test taken after an 8- to 10-hour fast, an oral glucose tolerance test, taken 2 hours after consuming a concentrated glucose drink, and an estimated average glucose test.

### LO 3 | Preventing and Treating Diabetes

- Prevention of diabetes include lifestyle changes such as a healthy/balanced diet, healthy weight, regular exercise, sufficient sleep, and stress reduction.
- Treatment of diabetes may include oral or injectable medications such as insulin, use of infusion pumps and other technologies, appropriate visits to the doctor, monitoring of glucose levels, and possible weight loss surgery.

## POP QUIZ

Visit **MasteringHealth** to personalize your study plan with Chapter Review Quizzes and Dynamic Study Modules.

### LO 1 | What Is Diabetes?

1. Which of the following is *not* correct?
   a. Type 1 diabetes is an autoimmune disease in which the body does not produce insulin.
   b. Type 2 diabetes is a disease in which the body may not produce sufficient amounts of insulin, or it may not be utilized properly.
   c. Gestational diabetes is only a problem for the mother while she is pregnant.
   d. Increased weight gain, high stress, lack of sleep, and sedentary lifestyle are key contributors to risks for type 2 diabetes.

### LO 2 | What Are the Symptoms of Diabetes?

2. Which of the following is *not* an accurate match between blood glucose level and diabetes-related problems in adults?
   a. A fasting blood glucose of 100–126 mg/dL indicates prediabetes.
   b. A fasting blood glucose of 50–70 mg/dL is an ideal blood glucose level.
   c. A fasting blood glucose of less than 90–99 mgdL is normal.
   d. An A1C test of 5.7 is normal.

### LO 3 | Treating Diabetes

3. Which of the following statements is *correct*?
   a. People with type 2 diabetes must eliminate sweets or high sugar foods from their diets.
   b. Skipping meals and eating two high-protein meals/no-carbohydrate meals per day is the best way to control blood sugar.
   c. Regular exercise, weight control, a balanced diet, adequate sleep, and stress management are key factors in blood glucose prevention and control.
   d. Most people with prediabetes know they have it.

*Answers to the Pop Quiz questions can be found on page A-1. If you answered a question incorrectly, review the section identified by the Learning Outcome. For even more study tools, visit MasteringHealth.*

# 13

# Protecting against Infectious Diseases and Sexually Transmitted Infections

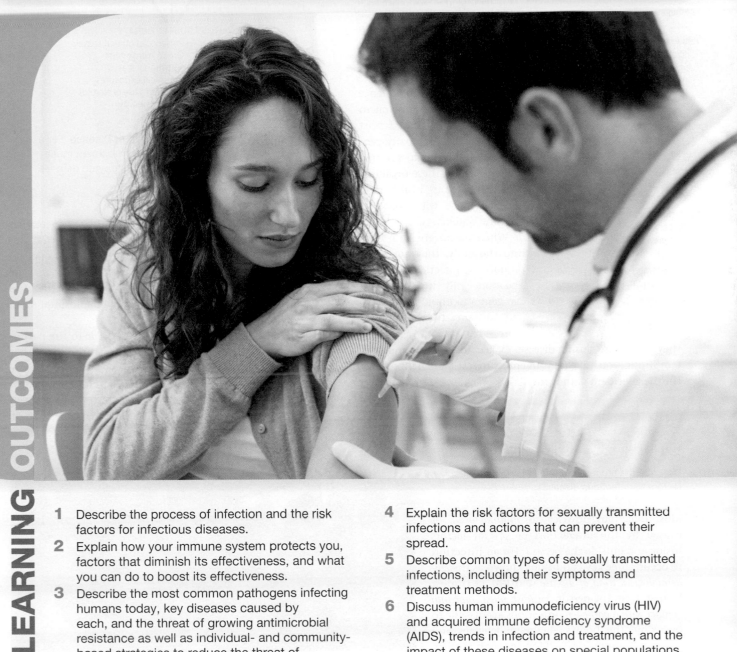

**P**athogens—disease-causing agents—are everywhere. We inhale them, swallow them, rub them in our eyes, and are constantly in a hidden, high-stakes battle with them. Although many pathogens have existed as long as there has been life on the planet, new varieties seem to emerge daily. Historically, infectious diseases have wiped out whole groups of people through **epidemics** such as the *Black Death*, or *bubonic plague*, which killed up to one third of the population of Europe in the 1300s. **Pandemics,** or global epidemics, continue to cause premature death throughout the world.

**pathogen** A disease-causing agent.

**epidemic** Disease outbreak that affects many people in a community or region at the same time.

**pandemic** Global epidemic of a disease.

**virulent** Strong enough to overcome host resistance and cause disease.

**infection** The state of pathogens being established in or on a host and causing disease.

**opportunistic infections** Infections that occur more often and with greater severity in people with compromised immune systems.

**immunocompromised** Having an immune system that is impaired.

**autoinoculate** Transmit a pathogen from one part of your body to another part.

Despite constant bombardment by pathogens, our immune systems are usually adept at protecting us. Millions of microorganisms live in and on our bodies all the time, usually in a symbiotic, peaceful coexistence, and exposure to invading microorganisms helps us build resistance to various pathogens. Generally harmless to someone in good health, these organisms can cause serious health problems in those with weakened immune systems.

When pathogens gain entry into the body, they are apt to produce an infection or illness. The more easily these pathogens can gain a foothold in the body and sustain themselves, the more **virulent**, or aggressive, they may be in causing disease. By keeping your immune system strong, you increase your ability to resist and fight off even the most virulent pathogen.

**HOSPITABLE ENVIRONMENT**
• Temperature
• Moisture/humidity
• Light
• Infection control protocols
• Ventilation/materials
• Building design

**AGENT INFECTIVITY**
• Virulence
• Ability to breech body defenses
• Unique pathogen characteristics

**DISEASE**

**HOST SUSCEPTIBILITY**
• Genetics
• Smoking
• Age
• Diabetes
• Stress
• Lack of sleep
• HIV or AIDS

• Presence of other diseases
• Organ transplants
• Nutritional status
• Chemical exposures
• Long-term use of steroids
• Chemotherapy

**FIGURE 13.1** Epidemiological Triad of Disease For a disease to occur, the agent, host, and environment must be conducive to overcoming the body's elaborate defense systems.

in an **opportunistic infection,** a normal pathogen overcomes an **immunocompromised** immune system—one that has been weakened or is nonfunctional. As an example, a person on antirejection drugs due to an organ transplant may be severely immunocompromised and would be vulnerable to any number of pathogens, be they lurking in a hospital room or carried in on well-wishing visitors.

Finally, the *environment* must be *hospitable* to the pathogen in terms of temperature, light, moisture, and other requirements. Although pathogens pose a threat if they

## LO 1 | THE **PROCESS** OF INFECTION

Describe the process of infection and the risk factors for infectious diseases.

-------------------------------------------------

Most infectious diseases are *multifactorial,* or caused by the interaction of several factors inside and outside the person. For an **infection** to occur, three key conditions known as the *epidemiological triad of disease* (**FIGURE 13.1**) must be met. First, the person, or *host, must come into contact with a pathogen* (infectious agent) able to overcome the body's elaborate defenses and capable of sustaining itself long enough to cause an infection.

Second, the *host must be susceptible,* or in some way vulnerable to infection. In other words, the pathogen must be so virulent that it overcomes a typical healthy immune system, or,

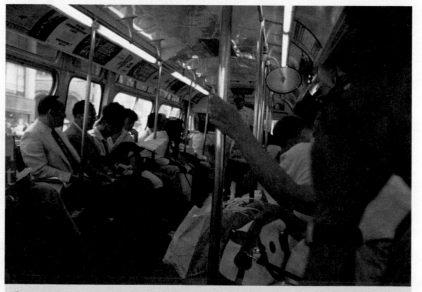

Crowded public transportation, trains, and airplanes are key areas where infectious diseases can be transmitted. Washing your hands and keeping hands from your face will help reduce risks.

## TABLE 13.1 | Routes of Disease Transmission

| Transmission Mode | Description |
|---|---|
| Contact | Either *direct* (e.g., skin or sexual contact) or *indirect* (e.g., infected blood or body fluid) |
| Food-borne or waterborne | Eating, drinking, washing, and unsanitary food preparation |
| Airborne | Infection spreads by inhaling droplets from an infected person's sneezes or coughs |
| Vector-borne | Blood-sucking insects such as mosquitoes, fleas, flies, or ticks pass along pathogens when they bite human victims. |
| Perinatal | Similar to contact infection; happens in the uterus, as the baby passes through the birth canal, or through breast-feeding |

gain entry and begin to grow in your body, the chances that they will do serious, long-term harm are actually quite small.

## Routes of Transmission

Pathogens may enter the body by *direct contact* between infected persons, or by *indirect contact,* like touching an object an infected person has touched. **TABLE 13.1** lists common routes of transmission. You may also **autoinoculate** yourself, or transmit a pathogen from one part of your body to another—for example, by touching a herpes sore on your lip and then touching your eye.

Your best friend may be the source of *animal-borne (zoonotic) infections.* Although rare in occurrence, dogs, cats, livestock, and wild animals can directly or indirectly spread viruses, bacteria, parasites, and fungi to each other and to humans. Companion animals like cats and dogs can carry fleas and ticks into homes; when these insects bite humans, disease such as *Lyme disease* can occur. Untreated puppies and dogs can be infested with worms that can be transmitted to humans via saliva, or through fecal residue on bedding, household carpets, or furniture. In 2015, when a form of influenza struck many dogs in the United States, people worried that they might get the flu from their dogs or transmit flu to their dogs. While some forms of influenza may be transmitted between humans and animals, this strain of influenza was not. Although *interspecies transmission*—transmission between humans and animals—can occur, with rabies being one of the most well-known zoonotic diseases in the United States, vaccination of pets, basic hygiene around pets, and care in contact with animal fluids is an important part of prevention.[1]

SKILLS FOR BEHAVIOR CHANGE

## REDUCE YOUR RISK OF INFECTIOUS DISEASE

▶ **Limit exposure to pathogens.** Don't drag yourself to classes or work and infect others when you are seriously ill. Also, don't share utensils or drinking glasses, and keep your toothbrush away from those of others. Keep hands away from your mouth, nose, and eyes. Use disposable tissues rather than reusable handkerchiefs.

▶ **Exercise regularly.** Regular exercise raises core body temperature and kills pathogens, and sweat and oil make the skin a hostile environment for many bacteria.

▶ **Get enough sleep.** Sleep allows the body time to refresh itself, produce necessary cells, and reduce inflammation. Even a single night without sleep can increase inflammatory processes and delay wound healing.

▶ **Stress less.** Rest and relaxation, stress management practices, laughter, and calming music have all been shown to promote healthy cellular activity and bolster immune functioning.

▶ **Optimize eating.** Enjoy a healthy diet, including adequate amounts of water, fruits and vegetables, protein, and complex carbohydrates. Eat more omega-3 fatty acids to reduce inflammation, and restrict saturated fats.

## Risk Factors You Can Control

Surrounded by pathogens, how can you be sure you don't get sick? Too much stress, poor diet, a low fitness level, lack of sleep, misuse or abuse of drugs, poor personal hygiene, and high-risk behavior significantly increase the risk for many diseases. In addition, college students are at higher risk because of their close living conditions; all these factors create higher risk for exposure to pathogens. The **Skills for Behavior Change** box lists some actions you can take to minimize risk of infection.

## Hard to Control Risk Factors

Unfortunately, some risk factors for certain diseases are hard or impossible to control. The following are the most common:

■ **Heredity.** Perhaps the single greatest factor influencing disease risk is genetics. It is often unclear whether

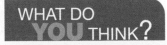

**WHAT DO YOU THINK?**

Do you have any risks for infectious disease that you were probably born with? Do you have any that are the result of your lifestyle?

■ What actions can you take to reduce your risks?

■ What behaviors do you or your friends engage in that might make you more susceptible to various infections?

■ Are your risks greater today than before you entered college? Why or why not?

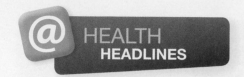
# ANTIBIOTIC RESISTANCE
*Bugs Versus Drugs*

Bacteria evolve and develop ways to survive drugs that previously killed them. Some microorganisms that were easily dealt with a few decades ago are becoming "superbugs" that cannot be stopped with existing medications.

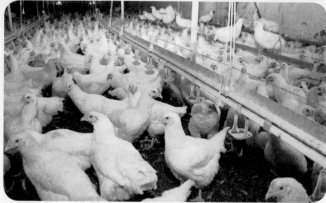

**Widespread use of antibiotics in industrial food production has been a key factor in antibiotic resistance.**

## Why Is Antibiotic Resistance on the Rise?

- **Overuse of antibiotics in food production.** About 70 percent of antibiotic production today is ingested by animals or fish living in crowded feedlots or fish farms to encourage their growth and fight off disease. Water runoff and sewage from feedlots can contaminate the water in rivers and streams with antibiotics. Antibiotic-resistant bacteria may also spread beyond farms via dried particles of animal manure that disperse in the wind.

- **Improper use of antibiotics by people** In the past, doctors were more inclined to give a patient antibiotics for ear infections, colds, and other ailments without verifying that bacteria was the true cause of the complaint and therefore a useful treatment. The Centers for Disease Control and Prevention (CDC) estimates that one third of the 150 million antibiotic prescriptions written each year are unnecessary, resulting in bacterial strains that are tougher than the drugs used to fight them. As resistance has become more widespread, many more doctors are asking patients to hold off on

antibiotics to see if the problem will clear up without antibiotics.

- **Misuse and overuse of antibacterial soaps and other cleaning products.** Preying on the public's fear of germs and disease, the cleaning industry adds antibacterial ingredients to many soaps and household products. Just how much these products contribute to overall resistance is difficult to assess; as with antibiotics, the germs these products do not kill may become stronger than before.

## What Can You Do?

- **Be responsible with medications.** Use antimicrobial drugs only for bacterial, not viral, infections. If you receive antibiotics, finish the entire prescription. If you stop taking the drug before finishing the prescription, the hardiest bacteria are the survivors, leading to drug-resistant microbes in the future.

Don't dump unused drugs down the toilet or sink. If you don't know where to take them, talk to your local pharmacist or waste disposal company

- **Use regular soap when washing your hands.** Research suggests that antibacterial agents contained in soaps actually may kill normal bacteria found on the skin that does not cause disease, thus creating an environment for resistant, mutated bacteria that are impervious to antibacterial cleaners and antibiotics to colonize the skin.

- **Avoid food treated with antibiotics.** Know where your food comes from. Buy organic meat and poultry, particularly those products that say that they have not been fed antibiotics or hormones. Look for farmed fish grown in U.S. coastal waters, where there is less likelihood of questionable fish-feeding practice and less chance of contaminated water and antibiotics or growth hormones.

**Sources:** CDC, "Fast Facts: Get Smart about Antibiotics," April 17, 2015, www.cdc.gov/getsmart/ community/about/index.html; Association for Professionals in Infection Control and Epidemiology, "Responsible Use of Antibiotics," 2013, www .apic.org; Association for Professionals in Infection Control and Epidemiology, "Antibiotics, Preserving Them for the Future," 2012, www.apic.org; Centers for Disease Control and Prevention, National Center for Emerging and Zoonotic Infectious Diseases, Division of Healthcare Quality Promotion, "Diseases/Pathogens Associated with Antimicrobial Resistance," Updated January 2013, www .cdc.gov

---

hereditary diseases are due to inherited genetic traits or to inherited insufficiencies in the immune system. Some believe that we may inherit the quality of our immune system, thus some people are naturally more resistant to disease and infection.

- Age. Thinning of the skin, reduced sweating, and other physical changes can make people more susceptible to disease as they age. The very young also tend to be particularly vulnerable to infectious diseases.

- Environmental conditions. A growing body of research points to climate change as a major contributor to infectious diseases. As temperatures rise, insect populations may rise, potentially increasing cases of malaria, which kills an estimated 584,000 people annually, and Dengue fever, which infects over 400 million people in the world each year.[2] Dwindling water supplies where there is little water turnover or flow contribute to more concentrated pathogen growth. When animals move to new environments in search of water and congregate near water sources, they are exposed to new species of animals with a new set of pathogens. In these environments, disease spreads quickly, as animals may have no acquired resistance to these particular pathogens. Scientists argue that changing environmental conditions, such as drought, flooding, fires, and other events may increase the rate of disease spread and may hasten interspecies transmission potential for humans.[3] In addition, natural disasters such as earthquakes, as well as long-term exposure to toxic chemicals, can significantly contribute to increasing numbers of infectious diseases.[4]

■ **Organism virulence and resistance.** Even tiny amounts of a particularly virulent organism may make the hardiest of us ill. Other organisms have mutated and become resistant to the body's defenses and to medical treatments. **Drug resistance** occurs when pathogens grow and proliferate in the presence of chemicals that would normally slow growth or kill them. See the **Health Headlines** box for more on drug resistance and superbugs.

## LO 2 | YOUR BODY'S DEFENSES AGAINST INFECTION

Explain how your immune system protects you, factors that diminish its effectiveness, and what you can do to boost its effectiveness.

- - - - - - - - - - - - - - - - - - - - - - - - - - - - - - - - - - - - - -

To gain entry into your body, pathogens must overcome barriers that prevent them from entering, mechanisms that weaken organisms, and substances that counteract the threat that these organisms pose. **FIGURE 13.2** summarizes some of the body's defenses against invasion and disease.

> **drug resistance** Occurs when microbes, such as bacteria, viruses, or other pathogens grow and proliferate in the presence of chemicals that would normally kill them or slow their growth.

## Physical and Chemical Defenses

Our most critical early defense system is the skin. Layered to provide an intricate web of barriers, the skin allows few pathogens to

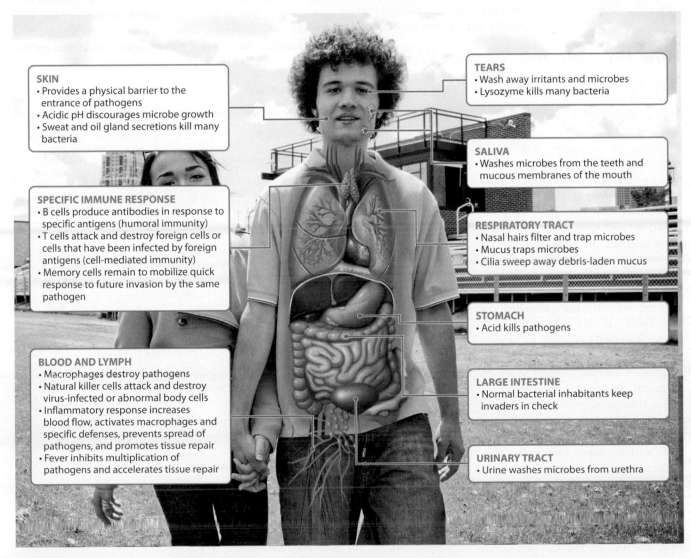

**SKIN**
- Provides a physical barrier to the entrance of pathogens
- Acidic pH discourages microbe growth
- Sweat and oil gland secretions kill many bacteria

**SPECIFIC IMMUNE RESPONSE**
- B cells produce antibodies in response to specific antigens (humoral immunity)
- T cells attack and destroy foreign cells or cells that have been infected by foreign antigens (cell-mediated immunity)
- Memory cells remain to mobilize quick response to future invasion by the same pathogen

**BLOOD AND LYMPH**
- Macrophages destroy pathogens
- Natural killer cells attack and destroy virus-infected or abnormal body cells
- Inflammatory response increases blood flow, activates macrophages and specific defenses, prevents spread of pathogens, and promotes tissue repair
- Fever inhibits multiplication of pathogens and accelerates tissue repair

**TEARS**
- Wash away irritants and microbes
- Lysozyme kills many bacteria

**SALIVA**
- Washes microbes from the teeth and mucous membranes of the mouth

**RESPIRATORY TRACT**
- Nasal hairs filter and trap microbes
- Mucus traps microbes
- Cilia sweep away debris-laden mucus

**STOMACH**
- Acid kills pathogens

**LARGE INTESTINE**
- Normal bacterial inhabitants keep invaders in check

**URINARY TRACT**
- Urine washes microbes from urethra

**FIGURE 13.2** The Body's Defenses against Disease-Causing Pathogens To protect against a steady onslaught by pathogens, the body has developed an elaborate defense system to keep invaders out!

**antigen** Substance capable of triggering an immune response.

**antibodies** Substances produced by the body that are individually matched to specific antigens.

**humoral immunity** Aspect of immunity that is mediated by antibodies secreted by white blood cells.

**toxins** Poisonous substances produced by certain microorganisms that cause various diseases.

**cell-mediated immunity** Aspect of immunity that is mediated by specialized white blood cells that attack pathogens and antigens directly.

**lymphocyte** A type of white blood cell involved in the immune response.

**macrophage** A type of white blood cell that ingests foreign material.

**autoimmune disease** Disease caused by an overactive immune response against the body's own cells.

enter. Enzymes in body secretions such as sweat provide additional protection, destroying microorganisms on skin surfaces by producing inhospitable pH levels. Only through cracks or breaks in the skin can pathogens gain easy access to the body.

The internal linings, structures, and secretions of the body provide another layer of protection. Mucous membranes in the respiratory tract, for example, trap and engulf invading organisms. Cilia, hairlike projections in the lungs and respiratory tract, sweep invaders toward body openings, where they are expelled. Nose hairs trap airborne invaders with a sticky film. Tears, earwax, and other secretions contain enzymes that destroy or neutralize pathogens.

immune response are **macrophages** (a type of phagocytic, or cell-eating, white blood cell).

Two forms of lymphocytes in particular, the *B lymphocytes* (B cells) and *T lymphocytes* (T cells), are involved in the immune response. *Helper T cells* are essential for activating B cells to produce antibodies. They also activate other T cells and macrophages. *Killer T cells* directly attack infected or malignant cells. *Suppressor T cells* turn off or suppress the activity of B cells, killer T cells, and macrophages. After a successful attack on a pathogen, some attacker T and B cells are preserved as *memory T and B cells,* enabling the body to recognize and respond quickly to subsequent attacks by the same kind of organism. Once people have survived certain infectious diseases, they will likely not develop them again. **FIGURE 13.3** provides a summary of the cell-mediated immune response.

## When the Immune System Misfires: Autoimmune Diseases

Sometimes the process for recognizing (and ignoring) the body's own cells goes awry, and the immune system targets its own tissues. This is known as **autoimmune disease** (*auto* means "self"). Common autoimmune disorders include *rheumatoid arthritis, lupus, type 1 diabetes, celiac disease,* and *multiple sclerosis.*

## How the Immune System Works

*Immunity* is a condition of being able to resist a particular disease by counteracting the substance that produces the disease. Any substance capable of triggering an immune response—a virus, a bacterium, a fungus, a parasite, a toxin, or a tissue or cell from another organism, or even chemicals from the environment—is called an **antigen**. When a pathogen breaches initial, outer defenses, the body first analyzes the antigen, verifying that it isn't part of the body itself. It then responds by forming **antibodies** specific to that antigen, much as a key is matched to a lock. Specific to each antigen, antibodies are designed to destroy or weaken the antigen. This process is part of a system called *humoral immune responses.* **Humoral immunity** is the body's major defense against many bacteria and the poisonous substances—**toxins**—they produce.

In **cell-mediated immunity**, specialized white blood cells called **lymphocytes** attack and destroy the foreign invader. Lymphocytes constitute the body's main defense against viruses, fungi, parasites, and some bacteria, and they are found in the blood, lymph nodes, bone marrow, and certain glands. Another key player in this

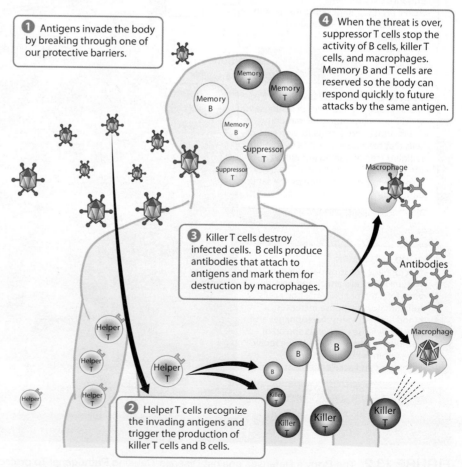

❶ Antigens invade the body by breaking through one of our protective barriers.

❷ Helper T cells recognize the invading antigens and trigger the production of killer T cells and B cells.

❸ Killer T cells destroy infected cells. B cells produce antibodies that attach to antigens and mark them for destruction by macrophages.

❹ When the threat is over, suppressor T cells stop the activity of B cells, killer T cells, and macrophages. Memory B and T cells are reserved so the body can respond quickly to future attacks by the same antigen.

**FIGURE 13.3** The Cell-Mediated Immune Response

# Inflammatory Response, Pain, and Fever

If an infection is localized, pus formation, redness, swelling, and irritation often occur. These symptoms are components of the body's inflammatory response and indicate the invading organisms are being fought. The four cardinal signs of inflammation are *redness, swelling, pain, and heat.*

*Pain* is often one of the earliest signs that an injury or infection has occurred. Pathogens kill or injure tissue at the site of infection, causing swelling that puts pressure on nerve endings in the area, resulting in pain. Although pain is unpleasant, it plays a valuable role in the body's response to injury or invasion by causing a person to avoid activity that may aggravate the injury and cause additional damage.

In addition to *inflammation,* another frequent indicator of infection is *fever,* or a body temperature above the average norm of 98.6°F. Caused by toxins secreted by pathogens that interfere with the control of body temperature, a fever also stimulates the body to produce more white blood cells. A mild fever is protective; raising body temperature by one or two degrees provides an environment that destroys some disease-causing organisms. As fever increases, more pathogens are destroyed. However, for babies and small children, when a fever goes higher than 101°F, medical attention should be sought. When fevers rise above 103°F for adults, medical attention is warranted.

# Vaccines Bolster Immunity

**Vaccination** is based on the principle that once people have been exposed to a specific pathogen and had a successful immune response, subsequent attacks will activate their "immune memory" and allow them to fight the pathogen off in the future.

A vaccine consists of killed or weakened versions of a disease-causing microorganism or an antigen that is similar to but less dangerous than the disease antigen. The dose given produces antibodies against future attacks—without actually causing the disease (or by causing a very minor case of it). Vaccines typically are given orally or by injection, and this form of immunity is termed *artificially acquired active immunity.* Concern about the safety of vaccines among certain Americans has led to a drop in vaccination rates and subsequent outbreaks of serious diseases such as the measles and pertussis—diseases that have rarely been seen in the United States since vaccines first became available beginning in the 1950s and 1960s (see the **Health Headlines** box on page 406).

**WHY SHOULD I CARE?**

An increasing number of chronic diseases are being linked to the inflammation that occurs when certain pathogens invade. Avoiding infections and their inflammatory side effects now has the added benefit that it may help you avoid certain chronic diseases later.

## TABLE 13.2 | Recommended Vaccinations for Teens and College Students

- Tetanus, diphtheria, pertussis vaccine (Td/Tdap)
- Meningococcal vaccine (booster at age 16)
- HPV vaccine series
- Hepatitis B vaccine series
- Polio vaccine series
- Measles-mumps-rubella (MMR) vaccine series
- Varicella (chickenpox) vaccine series
- Influenza vaccine
- Pneumococcal polysaccharide (PPV) vaccine
- Hepatitis A vaccine series (for high-risk groups)

**Source:** CDC, "Preteen and Teen Vaccines," July 2014, www.cdc.gov/vaccines/who/teens/vaccines/index.html; CDC, "Vaccine Information for Adults," September 2014, www.cdc.gov/vaccines/adults/rec-vac/index.html

Specific vaccination schedules have been established for various population groups. See **TABLE 13.2** for recommended vaccines for teens and college students ages 19 to 26. **FIGURE 13.4** shows the recommended vaccination schedule for the general adult population. Childhood vaccine schedules are available at the Centers for Disease Control and Prevention (CDC) website, as are requirements that vary by state.

**vaccination** Inoculation with killed or weakened pathogens or similar, less dangerous antigens, in order to prevent or lessen the effects of some disease.

Because of their close living quarters, high stress levels, and poor sleep habits, college students face a higher-than-average risk of infection from largely preventable diseases. Vaccines that should be a high priority among 20-somethings include *tetanus-diphtheria-pertussis vaccine (Tdap), meningococcal conjugate vaccine (MCV4), human papillomavirus (HPV),* and the yearly *influenza vaccine.*[5]

# LO 3 | TYPES OF PATHOGENS AND THE DISEASES THEY CAUSE

Describe the most common pathogens infecting humans today, key diseases caused by each, and the threat of growing antimicrobial resistance as well as individual- and community-based strategies to reduce the threat of infectious diseases.

Pathogens fall into six categories: bacteria, viruses, fungi, protozoans, parasitic worms, and prions. **FIGURE 13.5** shows several examples. Each has a particular route of transmission and characteristic elements that make it unique. In the following pages, we discuss each of these categories and give an overview of some diseases they cause that have a significant impact on public health.

| Vaccine | 19–21 years | 22–26 years | 27–49 years | 50–59 years | 60–64 years | 65+ years |
|---|---|---|---|---|---|---|
| Influenza (Flu)[1] | Get a flu vaccine every year | | | | | |
| Tetanus, diphtheria, pertussis (Td/Tdap)[2] | Get a Tdap vaccine once, then a Td booster vaccine every 10 years | | | | | |
| Varicella (Chickenpox)[3] | 2 doses | | | | | |
| HPV Vaccine for Women[3,4] | 3 doses | | | | | |
| HPV Vaccine for Men[3,4] | 3 doses | 3 doses | | | | |
| Zoster (Shingles)[5] | | | | | 1 dose | |
| Measles, mumps, rubella (MMR)[3] | 1 or 2 doses | | | | | |
| Pneumococcal (PCV13)[7] | 1-time dose | | | | | 1-time dose |
| Pneumococcal (PPSV23)[7] | 1 or 2 doses | | | | | 1 dose |
| Meningococcal | 1 or more doses | | | | | |
| Hepatitis A[3] | 2 doses | | | | | |
| Hepatitis B[3] | 3 doses | | | | | |
| *Haemophilus influenzae* type b (Hib) | 1 or 3 doses | | | | | |

1. Influenza vaccine: There are several flu vaccines available—talk to your health care professional about which flu vaccine is right for you.

2. Td/Tdap vaccine: Pregnant women are recommended to get tdap vaccine with each pregnancy in the third trimester to increase protection for infants who are too young for vaccination, but at highest risk for severe illness and death from pertussis (whooping cough). People who have not had Tdap vaccine since age 11 should get a dose of Tdap followed by TD booster doses every 10 years.

3. Varicella, HPV, MMR, hepatitis A, hepatitis B vaccine: These vaccines are needed for adults who didn't get these vaccines when they were children.

4. HPV vaccine: There are two HPV vaccines, but only one, HPV (Gardasilr), should be given to men. Gay men or men who have sex with men who are 22 through 26 years old should get HPV vaccine if they haven't already started or completed the series.

5. Zoster vaccine: You should get the zoster vaccine even if you've had shingles.

6. MMR vaccine: If you were born in 1957 or after, and don't have a record of being vaccinated or having had these infections, talk to your health care professional about how many doses you may need.

7. Pneumococcal vaccine: There are two different types of pneumococcal vaccines: PCV13 and PPSV23. Talk with your health care professional to find out if one or both pneumococcal vaccines are recommneded for you.

**If you travel outside of the United States, you may need additional vaccines. Ask your health care professional which vaccines you may need.**
**For more information, call toll free 1-800-CDC-INFO (1-800-232-4636) or visit http://www.cdc.gov/vaccines**

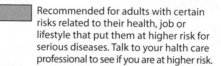

Recommended for all adults who have not been vaccinated, unless your health care professional tells you that you cannot safely receive the vaccine or that you do not need it.

Recommended for adults with certain risks related to their health, job or lifestyle that put them at higher risk for serious diseases. Talk to your halth care professional to see if you are at higher risk.

No recommendation

**FIGURE 13.4** Recommended Adult Immunization Schedule, by Vaccine and Age Group, 2015

**Source:** Centers for Disease Control and Prevention, "Recommended Adult Immunization Schedule—United States, 2015," Updated February 1, 2015, www.cdc.gov/vaccines/schedules/downloads/adult/adult-schedule.pdf
**Note:** Important explanations and additions to these recommendations should be checked by consulting the latest schedule at www.cdc.gov

# Bacteria

**Bacteria** (singular: *bacterium*) are simple, single-celled organisms. There are three major types of bacteria, classified by shape: *cocci, bacilli,* and *spirilla.* Although there are several thousand known species of bacteria (and many more unknown), only just over 100 are known to cause disease in humans. Often it is not the bacteria themselves that cause disease symptoms, but rather the toxins they produce.

Since the development of penicillin in 1928 by Alexander Fleming, bacteria were in a losing battle with their enemy: **antibiotics**. With each decade thereafter, newer, more potent and more specialized antibiotics decimated generation after generation of bacterial diseases. However, over half of antibiotics prescribed today are inappropriate, often given for viruses instead of bacteria. Patient misuse and improper prescription practices have contributed to a generation of "superbugs" as weaker bacteria have been killed and successive generations of bacteria mutate to become resistant. These resistant strains survive, mutate, and grow stronger. Today antibiotic resistance is one of the world's most pressing problems.[6] It is estimated that 4 out of 5 Americans receives at least one course of antibiotics a year, to a tune of nearly 260 million prescriptions.[7] Our current arsenal of antibiotics is becoming less effective and our supply of weapons declines each year. Refer back to the **Health Headlines** box on page 400 for more about superbugs and antibiotic resistance.

## Staphylococcal Infections

Staphylococci are present on the skin or in the nostrils of 20 to 30 percent of us at any given time and usually cause no problems for

**bacteria (singular: bacterium)**
Simple, single-celled microscopic organisms; about 100 known species of bacteria cause disease in humans.

**antibiotics** Medicines used to kill microorganisms, such as bacteria.

**staphylococci** A group of round bacteria, usually found in clusters, that cause a variety of diseases in humans and other animals.

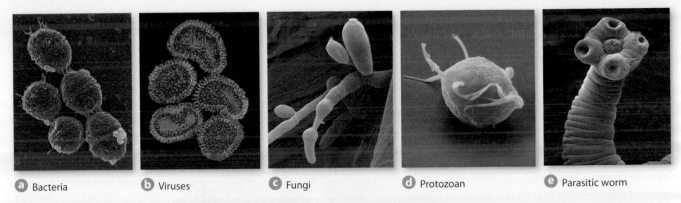

@ Bacteria     ⓑ Viruses     ⓒ Fungi     ⓓ Protozoan     ⓔ Parasitic worm

**FIGURE 13.5 Examples of Five Major Types of Pathogens (a)** Color-enhanced scanning electron micrograph (SEM) of *Streptococcus* bacteria, magnified 40,000×. **(b)** Colored transmission electron micrograph (TEM) of influenza (flu) viruses, magnified 32,000×. **(c)** Color SEM of *Candida albicans*, a yeast fungus, magnified 50,000×. **(d)** Color TEM of *Trichomonas vaginalis*, a protozoan, magnified 9,000×. **(e)** Color-enhanced SEM of a tapeworm, magnified 50×.

otherwise healthy persons. The presence of bacteria on or in a person without infection is called **colonization**. A colonized person may spread the bacteria to others, some of whom may develop infections, yet never develop the disease. For example, colonized persons can inadvertently touch their noses and spread those bacteria on a door handle, causing others who touch it to get sick. Likewise, when the pathogen is present on the skin surface, a cut or break in the skin can allow it to gain entry to the body, where **infection** develops. If you have ever suffered from acne, boils, styes (infections of the eyelids), or infected wounds, you have probably had a "staph" infection. If you pick at pimples and don't wash your hands, you can transmit those same bacteria to your eyes, or to other people. If you floss your teeth and don't wash your hands afterwards, your hands may be teeming with bacteria and other organisms that could infect others. Simple changes in your personal hygiene can make a huge difference in reducing risk.

One form of staph, **methicillin-resistant *Staphylococcus aureus* (MRSA)**, has come under intense international scrutiny as numerous cases have arisen around the world, especially in the United States. As the name implies, this bacteria has grown resistant to the class of drugs normally used to treat staph infections. Symptoms of MRSA infection often start with a rash or pimple-like skin irritation. Within hours, early symptoms may progress to redness, inflammation, pain, and deeper wounds. If untreated, MRSA may invade the blood, bones, joints, surgical wounds, heart valves, and lungs, and it can be fatal.

In the last decade, *health care–associated* or *health care–acquired MRSA* has been one of the leading **health care–associated infections (HAIs)** in the United States, being found in significant numbers in hospitals, nursing homes, and clinics where invasive treatments, infectious pathogens, and weakened immune systems converge. Today, 1 in 25 patients in a hospital has at least one HAI, with over 75,000 HAI patient deaths in 2013.[8] Many of these deaths were among patients with HA-MRSA, even though rates are on the decline due to intensive infection control methods.[9] While HA-MRSA is on the decline, *community-acquired MRSA (CA-MRSA)* is on the rise in the home, workplace, and other communities. Although the exact number of persons with CA-MRSA is not known, studies show that about 1 in 3 people carry staph in their nose, usually without any illness. Two in 100 people carry MRSA.[10]

Often, CA-MRSA appears as a skin infection that becomes red, inflamed, and painful and may be filled with pus or fluids. The initial irritated spot is often mistaken for a spider bite or boil, or an infection due to some type of injury, such as a cut or infected hair follicle. Although it can occur anywhere, irritation often appears in the groin area, beard, buttocks, underarm areas, or on the scalp. Because the initial site of infection may look like other things, many delay treatment until later in the infection process and unknowingly infect others.

Prevention of CA-MRSA involves keeping the hands away from the nose (since the nose often harbors the staph organism). Hand washing, good personal hygiene, not sharing razors, hankies, towels, pillows, or other personal products in the home, and careful attention to unusual sores on the body are all part of risk reduction.

Another type of MRSA appears to be spread among people who work closely with livestock in many regions of the world and is known as *livestock-associated MRSA*, or LA-MRSA.

### Clostridium difficile

Another bacterial disease that leads to major inflammation of the colon, complete with watery diarrhea, fever, pain, bloating and nausea, is *C. difficele or C. diff*. Ironically, the antibiotics used to treat bacterial infection are the major cause of *C. diff* development; when long-term antibiotic use occurs, some of the good bacteria that help keep

**SEE IT!** VIDEOS

This brief history of measles presents facinating facts from 1657 to the present day. Watch **A Brief History: Measles in America** in the Study Area of MasteringHealth™

**colonization** The process of bacteria or some other infectious organisms establishing themselves in a host without causing infection.

**methicillin-resistant *Staphylococcus aureus* (MRSA)** Highly resistant form of staph infection that is growing in international prevalence.

**health care–associated infections (HAIs)** Infections that patients acquire in a health care setting while receiving treatment for a different condition.

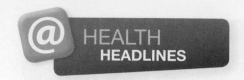
# VACCINE CONTROVERSY
*Should Parents Be Allowed to Opt Out?*

In 2000, the United States claimed victory over the measles, indicating that measles was no longer of concern on U.S. soil. In California last year, nearly 4 percent of children were allowed to skip measles vaccines. However, when a particularly nasty bout of measles was contracted in Disneyland, 169 people from over 20 states became ill. Most of those who got sick were unvaccinated. A 2014 outbreak of measles in Ohio among unvaccinated Amish children and the Disneyland outbreak has raised major concerns in many states.

In response, California recently passed one of the strictest laws in the country, mandating vaccinations of all school-age children. Several other states are examining their own policies about exemptions as rates of unvaccinated children in Washington, Oregon, Colorado, Wisconsin, and others grow yearly, with corresponding increases in vaccine-preventable diseases. Washington State passed a law requiring a doctor's signature to opt out of vaccinations. As rates of measles, pertussis, and other vaccine-preventable diseases skyrocket and large numbers of unvaccinated individuals travel to the United States putting people at all ages and stages of life at risk, more states are considering the rights of parents versus rights of the population as a whole.

Immunizations against widespread infectious diseases are one of the greatest public health success stories of all time—so successful, in fact, that most people have never seen or heard of anyone having diseases such as smallpox that once wiped out entire populations. Today, fear of the old "killer" diseases has waned and been replaced with distrust of the vaccines themselves, leading to a growing trend for parents to opt out of vaccinations for their children, even though failure to vaccinate puts children and communities at risk.

So why do people opt out? Typical reasons for vaccine exemptions include religious beliefs, personal beliefs, and

**Some parents have concerns over vaccination safety, but research shows that vaccines are safe and effective for most individuals, as well as crucial for maintaining good community health.**

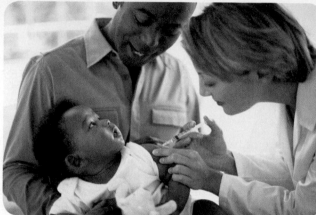

medical reasons, while others consider vaccinations to be a government intrusion into their individual rights. In some states, exemptions have been as easy to get as checking a box on a form. With the proliferation of misleading information about supposed dangers of vaccination, many mistakenly believe that they are doing the right thing by avoiding some or all vaccines.

Under-vaccination rates are particularly high in non-Hispanic, college-educated white families, with incomes above $75,000 a year and with health insurance. Although all 50 states require vaccinations, 48 states have religious or medical exemptions and several have personal belief options.

Much initial anxiety was fueled by an article in the medical journal *Lancet* in 1998, linking the MMR vaccine to increased risk of autism and bowel disease. The article prompted many to refuse the vaccine in the United States and elsewhere, and the resulting drop-off in immunizations led to increased cases of measles in many parts of the world. Over 10 years later, after a thorough investigation of ethical and factual issues with the research, *Lancet* retracted the article as being false. The lead author of the paper was later fired from his research position and had his license to practice revoked.

While research is ongoing, the Centers for Disease Control and Prevention (CDC)

has found *no* evidence to substantiate claims that vaccines lead to conditions like autism, multiple sclerosis, or sudden infant death syndrome.

Virtually all medical and public health organizations support vaccinations, pointing to stringent safety controls in the manufacturing and testing of vaccines, as well as ongoing safety monitoring and the long history of vaccines in wiping out killer diseases across the globe. If large numbers of people were to avoid vaccinations, old killers would be likely to reemerge, and those people who were already sick or weak from other conditions would be extremely vulnerable.

Today, the CDC's Immunization Safety Office monitors complaints and investigates potential problems with vaccines as they occur. Still, the danger of major complications from getting vaccinations is extremely low and generally pales in comparison to the effects of contracting the diseases that the vaccinations protect against.

**Sources:** R Seither et al., "Vaccination Coverage among Children in Kindergarten—United States, 2013–14 School Year," *MMWR* 63, no. 41 (2014): 913–920; CDC, "National Health Interview Survey," June 11, 2015, www.cdc.gov/nchs/nhis.htm; S. Omer et al., "Legislative Challenges to School Immunization Mandates, 2009–2012," *JAMA* 3111, no. 6 (2014): 620–21; Centers for Disease Control and Prevention, "Vaccine Safety: Concerns about Autism," modified March 2012, www.cdc.gov/vaccinesafety/Concerns/Autism/Index.html; The Editors of the *Lancet*, "Retraction—Ileal-lymphoid-nodular Hyperplasia, Non-specific Colitis, and Pervasive Development Disorder in Children," *Lancet* 375, no. 9713 (2010): 445; Centers for Disease Control and Prevention, National Immunization Survey, 2010–2011, accessed May 2014, www.cdc.gov/nchs/nis.htm; S. Robinson, H. Groom, and C. Young, "Frequency of Alternative Immunization Schedule Use in a Metropolitan Area," *Pediatrics* 130, no. 1 (2012): 32–38; S. Bean, *Vaccine Beliefs of Complementary and Alternative Medical (CAM) Providers in Oregon*, doctoral dissertation, Oregon State University, May 2014; V. Martinez-Sernandez and A. Figueiras, "Central Nervous System Demyelinating Disease and Recombinant Hepatitis B. Vaccinations: A Critical Systematic Review of Scientific Production," *Journal of Neurology* 260 (2013): 1951–1959.

the system running smoothly are often killed. The elderly, particularly those suffering from chronic conditions or living in nursing home or long-term care facilities, are at particular risk, with over 500,000 new cases annually, making *C. diff* the most common cause of health care–associated infections in the United States. Unnecessary antibiotic use and poor infection control are key culprits in *C. diff* spread.[11] Discontinuing antibiotic treatment and working to bolster the immune system are a key part of treatment.

## Streptococcal Infections

At least five types of the *Streptococcus* microorganism are known to cause bacterial infections. Group A streptococci (GAS) cause the most common diseases, such as streptococcal pharyngitis ("strep throat") and scarlet fever. One particularly virulent group of GAS can lead to a rare but serious disease called *necrotizing fasciitis* ("flesh-eating strep"). Group B streptococci can cause illness in newborn babies, pregnant women, older adults, and adults with illnesses such as diabetes or liver disease. Since about 1 in 4 pregnant women have group B strep in their rectum or vagina, the CDC recommends testing for it in the last weeks of pregnancy.[12] Expectant mothers who are group B positive can be treated with antibiotics to prevent problems in their newborn.

The species *Streptococcus pneumoniae* is responsible for thousands of cases of bacterial meningitis and pneumonia each year and is the primary culprit in most ear infections. While antibiotic treatments are still effective, an increasing number of cases are becoming resistant.

## Meningitis

Meningitis is an inflammation of the *meninges,* the membranes that surround the brain and spinal cord. There are a variety of causes, including bacterial, viral, parasitic, and fungal infections, as well as noninfectious causes such as trauma to the brain, cancer, lupus, drugs, or brain surgery.

One virulent form of bacterial meningitis prevalent on college campuses, *meningococcal meningitis* is the most serious

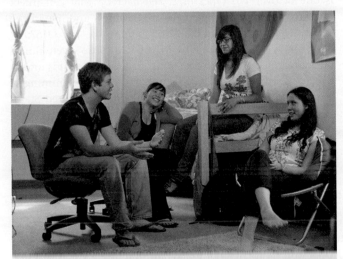

Close quarters, such as college dorms, are prime breeding grounds for some contagious diseases such as meningococcal meningitis.

infectious form. Spread through contact with saliva, nasal discharge, feces, or respiratory and throat secretions, it is highly contagious. Globally, it results in deaths for between 5 and 10 percent of those infected—despite treatment, within 24–48 hours.[13] In 2014, there were between 800 and 1,500 cases of meningococcal disease in the United States.[14] Adolescents and young adults are among those likely to contract the disease and have serious complications.[15]

A suspected student death from bacterial meningitis at San Diego State University and over 31 cases of viral meningitis at the University of Maryland in 2014 caused significant concern on college campuses throughout the country. *Bacterial meningitis* progresses rapidly, is life threatening, and needs immediate medical attention. *Viral meningitis* is much less dangerous and symptoms usually diminish in 3 to 5 days in otherwise healthy people. There is no vaccine or treatment for this form.

> ***Streptococcus*** A round bacterium, usually found in chain formation.
>
> **meningitis** An infection of the meninges, the membranes that surround the brain and spinal cord.
>
> **pneumonia** Inflammatory disease of the lungs characterized by chronic cough, chest pain, chills, high fever, and fluid accumulation; may be caused by bacteria, viruses, fungi, chemicals, or other substances.

Fortunately, vaccines exist for *pneumococcal meningitis,* the most common form of bacterial meningitis, and *meningococcal meningitis.* The other vaccine-preventable form of bacterial meningitis is *Haemophilus influenzae* type b (Hib). Check your immunization table for information regarding vaccination.

Typical signs of many forms of meningitis are sudden fever, severe headache, and a stiff neck, particularly stiffness that causes difficulty touching your chin to your chest. Persons who are suspected of having meningitis should receive immediate, aggressive medical treatment. Talk to the medical or health education staff at your local student health center to see if they have the vaccine most likely to protect you in your area.

Prevention of meningitis involves common sense infection control procedures such as frequent hand washing, using recommended cough/sneeze protocols such as sneezing into your arm and using disposable tissues rather than reusable hankies; keeping your hands away from your nose; and keeping "high touch" surfaces, such as phones, doorknobs, and remote controls clean.

## Pneumonia

Pneumonia is a general term for a wide range of conditions that result in inflammation of the lungs and difficulty breathing. It is characterized by chronic cough, chest pain, chills, high fever, fluid accumulation, and eventual respiratory failure. Although bacterial and viral pathogens are the most common culprits, pneumonia can also be caused by fungi, occupational exposure to chemicals, or trauma.

Bacterial pneumonia responds readily to antibiotic treatment in early stages, but can be deadly in more advanced stages. Forms of pneumonia caused by other organisms are more difficult to treat. Although medical advances have reduced the overall incidence of pneumonia, it continues to be a major threat in the United States and throughout the world.

## Tuberculosis (TB)

Only HIV/AIDS is a greater infectious agent killer than **tuberculosis** in the global population.[16] With about 9 million new cases and 1.5 million deaths in 2011, an astounding one third of the world's population is infected with TB.[17] Although infection rates decreased dramatically in the United States since the 1950s, there were still nearly 9,600 cases in 2013.[18] Tuberculosis is the number one infectious killer of women of reproductive age worldwide, as well as the leading cause of death among HIV-positive patients. Poverty and lack of access to treatment are also key risk factors.

Historically, people used the term *consumption* to refer to a bacterial respiratory disease with symptoms that include wasting/weight loss, fever, chronic cough and blood streaked sputum, fluid- and blood-filled lungs, and eventual spread throughout the body. The term is still used in some parts of the world today; however, TB is now widely recognized for these same symptoms. Airborne transmission via the respiratory tract is the primary mode of infection. Infected people can be contagious without showing symptoms and can transmit the disease while talking, coughing, sneezing, or singing.

The current recommended treatment for TB involves taking four drugs for 6 to 9 months; however, a new 12-dose regimen is available for high-risk populations.[19] Medications may cause side effects, ranging from minor stomach irritation to liver failure.[20] The side effects, lengthy treatment, and barriers to obtaining drugs and care in many developing areas leads to missed doses and treatments that end before the cure. This, in turn, breeds drug-resistant tuberculosis. **Multidrug-resistant TB (MDR-TB)** is currently resistant to at least two of the best anti-TB drugs in use today, and **extensively drug-resistant TB (XDR-TB)** is resistant to nearly all current TB drugs. These newer strains of tuberculosis are reaching epidemic proportions in over 58 countries.[21]

## Tick-borne Bacterial Diseases

In the past few decades, certain tick-borne diseases have become major health threats in the United States. The most noteworthy include two bacterially caused diseases. *Lyme disease* is present in many regions of the United States, particularly the upper Midwest. Symptoms of Lyme disease may range from none, to a rash or bull's-eye lesion and flu-like symptoms, to chronic arthritis, blindness, and long-term disability.

*Babesiosis* is a tick-borne disease garnering increased attention in the upper Midwest and Northeastern United States. When symptoms occur, they often mimic flu-like aches, headache, fatigue, and nausea.

**tuberculosis (TB)** A disease caused by bacterial infiltration of the respiratory system.

**multidrug-resistant TB (MDR-TB)** Form of TB that is resistant to at least two of the best antibiotics available.

**extensively drug-resistant TB (XDR-TB)** Form of TB that is resistant to nearly all existing antibiotics.

**rickettsia** A small form of bacteria that live inside other living cells.

Because the babesiosis parasite attacks and destroys red blood cells, anemia may result. The elderly and those whose immune systems are weakened are at greatest risk of complications.

Another tick-borne disease, *ehrlichiosis,* also has flu-like symptoms that may progress quickly to respiratory difficulties, and even death. Fortunately, antibiotics given early in the disease course are effective in preventing any serious threats from these diseases. The bottom line is, if you have flu-like symptoms in the typical non-flu months of the year, particularly if you have been in areas where ticks live, get yourself checked out.

**Rickettsia** are a small form of bacteria that produce toxins and multiply within small blood vessels, causing vascular blockage and tissue death. Rickettsia require an insect vector (carrier) for transmission to humans. Two common forms of human rickettsial disease are *Rocky Mountain spotted fever*, carried by a tick, and *typhus,* carried by a louse, flea, or tick. These diseases produce similar symptoms, including high fever, weakness, rash, and coma, and both can be life threatening.

The best protection against insect-borne diseases is to stay indoors at dusk and early morning to avoid hours of high insect activity. To prevent tick-borne diseases, remember to stay out of grass and woods during the times ticks are most active, from late spring to fall. Use insect repellents that contain 20 to 30 percent DEET, natural oils, or pyrethrins that you put on your clothing. Wear long sleeves and pants and tuck pants into socks. Do tick checks by examining genitals, buttocks, hair, and other body parts where ticks like to hide. Bathe or shower as soon as possible after coming indoors (within 2 hours) to wash off ticks. Also, do pet checks to make sure ticks don't crawl off your pets and onto you!

If you are traveling in areas of the world where insect-borne diseases such as malaria are prevalent, then bed nets, routine "tick checks," and other protective measures may be necessary. Consult a travel doctor; they may prescribe you with preventive medications.

## *Escherichia coli* O157:H7

*Escherichia coli* O157:H7 is one of over 170 types of *E. coli* bacteria that can infect humans. Most *E. coli* organisms are harmless and live in the intestines of healthy animals and humans. *E. coli* O157:H7, however, produces a lethal toxin and can cause severe illness or death. You can get it from eating ground beef that is undercooked, drinking unpasteurized milk or juice, or swimming in sewage-contaminated water. Outbreaks in the United States have been caused by foods like frozen pizza and quesadillas, organic spinach and spring mix lettuce, raw clover sprouts, romaine lettuce, bologna, cheese, and poultry.

A symptom of infection is non-bloody diarrhea, usually 2 to 8 days after exposure; however, asymptomatic cases have been noted. Children, older adults, and people with weakened immune systems are particularly vulnerable to serious side effects such as kidney failure, intestinal damage, or death.

Tick-borne diseases such as Lyme disease, Rocky Mountain spotted fever, and babesiosis are on the rise in many parts of the United States. Protect yourself with bug sprays and protective clothing.

Strengthened regulations on chlorine levels in pools and the cooking of meat have helped reduce *E. coli* infections. Difficulties in isolating the source of infections have prompted a close examination of labeling and distribution of food products. The U.S. Department of Agriculture (USDA) as well as the Environmental Protection Agency (EPA), Food and Drug Administration, and others are all involved in developing food and transportation policies designed to keep the food supply safe.

# Viruses

**Viruses** are the smallest known pathogens, approximately 1/500th the size of bacteria, and hundreds of viruses are known to cause diseases in humans. Essentially, a virus consists of a protein structure that contains either *ribonucleic acid* (*RNA*) or *deoxyribonucleic acid* (*DNA*). Viruses are incapable of carrying out any life processes on their own. To reproduce, they must invade and inject their own DNA or RNA into a host cell and force it to make copies of themselves. The new viruses then erupt out of the host cell and seek other cells to invade.

Viral diseases can be difficult to treat because many viruses can withstand heat, formaldehyde, and large doses of radiation with little effect on their structure. Some viruses have **incubation periods** (the length of time required to develop fully and cause symptoms in their hosts) that last for years, which delays diagnosis. Drug treatment for viral infections is also limited. Drugs powerful enough to kill viruses generally kill the host cells, too, although some medications block stages in viral reproduction without damaging the host cells.

**The Common Cold** Some experts claim there may be over 200 different viruses responsible for the common cold. Colds are the main reason for missed work and missed school in the United States, with millions of cases each year.[22] Although most colds occur in the winter and spring, you can actually get a cold any time. Adults have an average of two to three colds per year, and children have even more.[23] If you get a cold, the most likely cause is the rhinovirus, which causes 10 to 40 percent of all colds, followed by the coronavirus, responsible for 20 percent of all colds.[24] Colds are **endemic** (always present to some degree) throughout the world, with increasing prevalence in colder weather as people spend more time indoors. Otherwise healthy people carry cold viruses in their noses and throats most of the time, held in check until immune defenses are weakened. It is possible to "catch" a cold—through airborne transmission, touching skin-to-skin, or mucous membrane contact—and the hands are the greatest avenue for transmitting colds and other viruses. Obviously, then, covering your nose and mouth with a tissue, handkerchief, or even the crook of your elbow when sneezing is better than using your bare hand. Contrary to popular belief, you cannot catch a cold from getting a chill or being in the cold, but the chill may lower your immune system's resistance to a virus if one is present.

**Influenza** Influenza, or flu, is a contagious respiratory illness that includes fever and chills along with other cold symptoms. While death rates from the flu are only estimates since influenza is not a reportable disease, common estimates range from 3,000 per year to 49,000.[25] Although a rapid diagnosis flu test is available, doctors typically diagnose influenza based on symptoms.

Although many people don't realize it, there are actually many different types of influenza, including the most common *seasonal variety* and some other less common types. Fortunately most types of flu in the world are not readily transmitted to humans.

For seasonal flu, although symptoms are always more serious than a cold, most adolescents and adults recover after a week or two. However, seasonal flu can be deadly to the very young, people over age 65, and those who have weakened immune systems. Occasionally, a particularly deadly strain of influenza evolves and spreads rapidly, killing many.

Five to 20 percent of Americans get the flu each year, and of these, 200,000 will need hospitalization.[26] Once a person gets the flu, treatment is *palliative*—focused on relief of symptoms, rather than cure.

The best way to avoid the flu is to get an annual vaccination against it. Since there are numerous and constantly mutating flu strains, vaccines are formulated for the few strains most likely to be prevalent in an upcoming season. If researchers correctly predict strains, vaccines are thought to be 70 to 90 percent effective in healthy adults for about a year; if the prediction is off, a shot is less beneficial.[27]

In spite of minor risks, the CDC now recommends everyone over the age of 6 months get seasonal flu vaccine annually. Unfortunately, only about 68 percent of high-risk persons over the age of 65 and 47 percent of those between 6 months to 17 years are vaccinated each year.[28] Nearly 46.5 percent of those age 50-64 and only 29.6 percent of those 18 to 49 are vaccinated.[29] Flu shots take 2 to 3 weeks to become effective, so it's best to get shots in the fall, before the flu season begins. Today, you can choose to get a standard shot, a high-dose shot if you are over 65 or at risk, a nasal spray if you are between ages 2 and 49, a Flublok shot if you are allergic to the eggs used to produce vaccines, and several other options.

**Hepatitis** One of the most highly publicized viral diseases is **hepatitis**, a virally caused inflammation of the liver. Symptoms include fever, headache, nausea, loss of appetite, skin rashes, pain in the upper right abdomen, dark yellow (with brownish tinge) urine, and jaundice. Internationally, viral hepatitis is a major contributor to liver disease and accounts for high morbidity and mortality. Currently, there are several known forms (A, B, C, D, and E), with hepatitis A, B, and C having the highest rates of incidence.

**viruses** Minute microbes consisting of DNA or RNA that invade a host cell and use the cell's resources to reproduce themselves.

**incubation period** The time between exposure to a disease and the appearance of symptoms.

**endemic** Describing a disease that is always present to some degree.

**influenza** A common viral disease of the respiratory tract.

**hepatitis** A viral disease in which the liver becomes inflamed, producing symptoms such as fever, headache, and possibly jaundice.

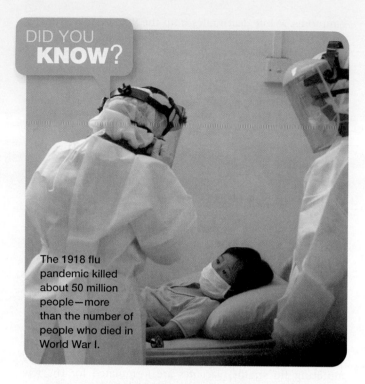

The 1918 flu pandemic killed about 50 million people—more than the number of people who died in World War I.

*Hepatitis A (HAV)* is contracted by eating food or drinking water contaminated with human feces. Since vaccinations became available, HAV rates had been steadily declining until 2013, when they again began to increase. In 2013, there were nearly 1,800 reported new cases of HAV.[30] Hepatitis A can also be spread through sexual contact with HAV-positive individuals or through the use of contaminated needles. Fortunately, individuals infected with HAV do not become chronic carriers, and vaccines for the disease are available. Many who contract HAV are asymptomatic (symptom-free).

*Hepatitis B (HBV)* is spread through body fluid exchange during unprotected sex, sharing needles when injecting drugs, through needlesticks on the job, or, in the case of a newborn baby, from an infected mother during birth. Hepatitis B can lead to chronic liver disease or liver cancer. Since vaccines became available in 1981, numbers of HBV cases have declined rapidly. Globally, HBV infections are on the decline, but over 240 million are chronically infected.[31] Needle exchange programs are believed to be an important part of risk reduction for HBV, HCV, and HIV infection in the last decade.[32]

Rates are also on the decline in the United States; however, an estimated 20,000 cases are reported each year, and nearly 1.4 million people are chronic carriers.[33] The highest rates of infection are among males ages 30 to 39, and black non-Hispanics; the lowest rates are among Asian Pacific Islanders and Hispanics.[34] Because the hepatitis B virus is considered 50 to 100 times more virulent than HIV, efforts to increase global vaccination rates have become a major priority.

**fungi** A group of multicellular and unicellular organisms that obtain their food by infiltrating the bodies of other organisms, both living and dead; several microscopic varieties are pathogenic.

**protozoans** Microscopic single-celled organisms that can be pathogenic.

**parasitic worms** The largest of the pathogens, most of which are more a nuisance than they are a threat.

*Hepatitis C (HCV)* infections are on an epidemic rise in many regions of the world as resistant forms emerge. Some cases can be traced to blood transfusions or organ transplants. An estimated 22,000 cases of HCV occurred in 2013, and the estimated number of chronic cases of HCV may be as high as 3.2 million.[35] Of those infected with the hepatitis C virus, 75 to 85 percent will develop chronic hepatitis C.[36] Of those who develop chronic liver disease, between 5 and 20 will develop cirrhosis of the liver.[37] One in 5 people will die from cirrhosis or liver cancer.[38] Although several vaccines are currently being tested and at least one is in early human trials, an actual vaccine is not yet available.

To prevent the spread of HBV and HCV use latex condoms correctly every time you have sex; don't share personal-care items that might have blood on them, such as razors or toothbrushes; get a blood test for HBV so you know your status; never share needles; and if you are having body art done, go only to reputable artists or piercers who follow established sterilization and infection-control protocols.

## Other Pathogens

While bacteria and viruses account for many common diseases, other organisms can also infect people. Among these are fungi, protozoans, parasitic worms, and prions.

**Fungi** Hundreds of species of **fungi** exist. While many of these multi- or unicellular organisms are beneficial—edible mushrooms, penicillin, and yeast used in bread—*candidiasis* (the cause of vaginal yeast infections, discussed later), athlete's foot, ringworm, jock itch, and toenail fungus are examples of common fungal diseases. With most fungal diseases, keeping the affected area clean and dry and treating it promptly with appropriate medications will generally bring relief. Fungal diseases typically transmit via physical contact, so avoid going barefoot in public showers, hotel rooms, and other areas where fungus may be present, and use care in choosing where you go for pedicures. Another key fungal disease that is increasing in the United States is *Valley Fever*—a potentially life-threatening respiratory disease common in the desert Southwest. Others may be spread to humans and pets via breathing in fungal spores.

**Protozoans** Protozoans are single-celled organisms that cause diseases such as malaria and African sleeping sickness and are largely controlled in the United States. A common waterborne protozoan disease in many regions of the country is *giardiasis*. Persons who drink contaminated water may be exposed to the *giardia* pathogen and will suffer intestinal pain and discomfort weeks after initial infection. Protection of water supplies is the key to prevention.

**Parasitic Worms** Parasitic worms are the largest pathogens. Ranging in size from small pinworms typically found in children to large tapeworms that can take up large portions of the human intestines, most are more nuisance than threat. Of special note are the worm infestations associated with eating raw fish (as in some forms of sushi). You can prevent worm infestations by cooking fish and other foods to temperatures sufficient to kill the worms and their eggs. Other preventive measures you can take include getting your pets checked, being careful while swimming in international areas known for these infections, and wearing shoes in parks or places where animal feces are present.

## Prions

A **prion** is a self-replicating, protein-based agent that can infect humans and other animals. One such prion is believed to be the underlying cause of spongiform diseases such as *bovine spongiform encephalopathy* (*BSE*, or "mad cow disease"). If humans eat contaminated meat from cattle with BSE, they may develop a mad cow–like disease known as *variant Creutzfeld-Jakob disease (vCJD)*. Symptoms of vCJD include loss of memory, tremors, and muscle spasms or "ticks." Over time, depression, difficulty walking, seizures, and severe dementia can ultimately lead to death in both cows and humans. An increasing number of infected cattle have been found in the United States and globally; however, to date, there have been no confirmed human infections from U.S. beef.

## Emerging and Resurgent Diseases

Although our immune systems are adept at responding to challenges, microbes and other pathogens constantly evolve and try to gain an edge. Within the past decade, rates for many infectious diseases have increased. This trend can be attributed to a combination of overpopulation, inadequate health care, increasing poverty, environmental changes, and drug resistance. At the same time, world travel and trade of goods has become increasingly fast and easy, giving many pathogens ample opportunity to hitch a ride to new locations.

In addition, significant increases in vaccine-preventable disease cases for pertussis, meningococcal meningitis, measles, chickenpox, hepatitis A, and other childhood diseases between 2013 and 2014 are causing concern throughout the country. Increased hospitalizations and deaths of children from vaccine-preventable diseases and more families using the "personal belief exemption" from vaccination prompted California to reinstate mandatory vaccinations of school-age children in May 2015.[39] Stay tuned as other states move to protect the population through similar vaccine mandates in schools.

### Measles and Mumps

The most well-known symptom of **mumps** is swelling of the salivary glands. In severe cases it can cause hearing loss or male sterility. **Measles**, known for its high fever and itchy red rash, is increasingly common—particularly on college campuses. Increased incidences of these and other vaccine-preventable diseases between 2013 and 2014 are reason for significant concern in many regions of the country. A growing number of children and young adults have not been vaccinated against measles or mumps because their parents believe the diseases are gone and the risk of a vaccine is greater than the risk of contracting the disease. See the **Health Headlines** box on page 406 for more on the growing vaccine controversy.

### West Nile Virus

Several thousand cases of West Nile virus occur in the United States each year. For most, symptoms are flu-like and can include a form of encephalitis (inflammation of the brain). With hundreds of individuals disabled and 45 deaths from the infection annually, the elderly and those with impaired immune systems bear the brunt of the disease burden.[40] Today, only Alaska and Hawaii remain free of the disease in the United States. Spread by infected mosquitoes, the best way to avoid infection is through mosquito eradication programs, wearing mosquito repellant, and avoiding mosquito-infested areas altogether, especially at peak mosquito feeding times. There is no vaccine or specific treatment.

> **prion** A recently identified self-replicating, protein-based pathogen.
>
> **mumps** A once common viral disease that is controllable by vaccination.
>
> **measles** A viral disease that produces symptoms such as an itchy rash and a high fever.

### Avian (Bird) Flu and Swine (Pig) Flu

*Avian influenza* is an infectious disease of birds. Birds infect other birds during migratory patterns, spreading the disease internationally as they fly among different locations. Strains capable of crossing the species barrier can cause severe illness in humans who come in contact with bird droppings or fluids. Bird flu appears to have originated in Asia and spread via migrating bird populations.[41] Although the virus has yet to mutate into a form highly infectious to humans, outbreaks in rural areas of the world (where people live in close proximity to poultry and other animals) have occurred. As of March 2013, the World Health Organization had recorded 468 cases of bird flu in humans, with 282 deaths.[42] Many health experts suggest that if the virus becomes easily transmissible between humans, it could become a major pandemic.[43]

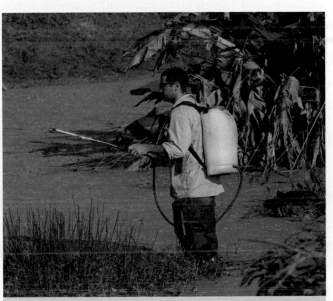

Careful monitoring and control of mosquito and other insect populations is important to combat emerging diseases such as West Nile virus.

*Swine flu*, also referred to as H1N1 or one of its variants, is a respiratory infection believed to initially be found primarily in pigs. In 2009, an outbreak of a virus that combined elements of a human flu virus and the pig virus occurred. Twelve cases were reported in the United States initially, primarily among people who had touched pigs or were in close proximity to them.[44] Today, H1N1 is one of the many possible viruses that humans can contract.

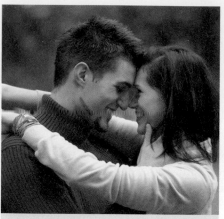

Decisions to be intimate should consider risks from highly infectious sexually transmitted diseases such as chlamydia and HPV, to name two.

## LO 4 | SEXUALLY TRANSMITTED INFECTIONS (STIS)

Explain the risk factors for sexually transmitted infections and actions that can prevent their spread.

Every year, there are at least 20 million new cases of **sexually transmitted infections (STIs)**, only some of which are curable.[45] While these numbers seem high, they are believed to capture only a fraction of the actual number of cases as many are not routinely reported.[46]

Sexually transmitted infections affect people of all backgrounds and socioeconomic levels, but they disproportionately affect women, minorities, and infants. Young people, aged 15 to 24 acquire half of all new STIs, making this age group the most at risk group for STIs overall.[47] Reasons for the higher rates of STIs in this population include a range of behavioral, biological, socioeconomic, and cultural reasons. Barriers to prevention and treatment, such as lack of access to affordable health care, confidentiality, and transportation, as well as peer norms and media influences, risk-taking behaviors, and social and cultural norms that promote and influence sexual interest and activity, are examples

**sexually transmitted infections (STIs)** Infections transmitted through some form of intimate, usually sexual, contact.

of some of the factors that put adolescents and young adults at risk.[48]

Early symptoms of an STI are often mild and unrecognizable: Without a thorough understanding of symptoms and risk, they may go untreated. Left untreated over time, some of these infections can have grave consequences, such as sterility, blindness, central nervous system destruction, disfigurement, and even death. Infants born to mothers carrying the organisms for these infections are at risk for a variety of health problems.

## What's Your Risk?

Generally, the more sexual partners a person has, the greater the risk for contracting an STI. Twenty-five percent of sexually active adolescent females are infected with an STI, such as chlamydia or human papillomavirus (HPV).[49] Shame and embarrassment often keep infected people from seeking treatment. Unfortunately, they usually continue to be sexually active, thereby infecting unsuspecting partners. People who are uncomfortable discussing sexual issues may also be less likely to use and ask their partners to use condoms to protect against STIs and pregnancy. Another reason proposed for the STI epidemic is our casual attitude about sex.

Ignorance—about the infections, their symptoms, and the fact that someone can be asymptomatic but still infected—is also a factor. A person who is infected but asymptomatic can unknowingly spread an STI to others who also ignore or misinterpret symptoms. By the time anyone seeks medical help, he or she may have infected several others. In addition, many people mistakenly believe that certain sexual practices—oral sex, for example—carry no risk for STIs. In fact, oral sex practices among young adults may be responsible for increases in herpes and other infections. **FIGURE 13.6** shows the continuum of disease risk for various sexual behaviors, and the **Skills for Behavior Change** box offers tips for ways to practice safer sex.

| High-risk behaviors | Moderate-risk behaviors | Low-risk behaviors | No-risk behaviors |
|---|---|---|---|
| Unprotected vaginal, anal, and oral sex—any activity that involves direct contact with bodily fluids, such as ejaculate, vaginal secretions, or blood—are high-risk behaviors. | Vaginal, anal, or oral sex with a latex or polyurethane condom and a water-based lubricant used properly and consistently can greatly reduce the risk of STI transmission.<br><br>Dental dams used during oral sex can also greatly reduce the risk of STI transmission. | Mutual masturbation, if there are no cuts on the hand, penis, or vagina, is very low risk.<br><br>Rubbing, kissing, and massaging carry low risk, but herpes can be spread by skin-to-skin contact from an infected partner. | Abstinence, phone sex, talking, and fantasy are all no-risk behaviors. |

**FIGURE 13.6 Continuum of Disease Risk for Various Sexual Behaviors** There are different levels of risk for various behaviors and various sexually transmitted infections (STIs); however, no matter what, any sexual activity involving direct contact with blood, semen, or vaginal secretions is high risk.

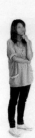

WHICH **PATH**
WOULD YOU TAKE **?**

Scan the QR code to see how different health choices YOU make today can affect your risk of contracting an infectious disease or sexually transmitted infection.

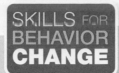

## Routes of Transmission

Sexually transmitted infections are generally spread through intimate sexual contact. Less likely modes of transmission include mouth-to-mouth contact or contact with fluids from body sores. Although each STI is a different infection caused by a different pathogen, all STI pathogens prefer dark, moist places, especially the mucous membranes lining reproductive organs. Most are susceptible to light, extreme temperature, and dryness, and many die quickly on exposure to air. Like other communicable infections, STIs have both pathogen-specific incubation periods and *periods of* communicability—times during which transmission is most likely.

## LO 5 | COMMON TYPES OF SEXUALLY TRANSMITTED INFECTIONS

Describe common types of sexually transmitted infections, including their symptoms and treatment methods.

There are more than 20 known types of STIs. Once referred to as *venereal diseases* and then *sexually transmitted diseases,* the current terminology is more reflective of the number and types of infections and of the fact that they are caused by pathogens. More virulent strains and antibiotic-resistant forms spell trouble in the days ahead. Here, we turn to some of the most common.

## Chlamydia

**Chlamydia,** an infection caused by the bacterium *Chlamydia trachomatis,* is the most commonly reported STI in the United States. In 2013, there were just over 1.4 million chlamydia infections reported in the United States, with nearly 950,000 of those cases occurring in the 15–24 age group.[50] The majority of these cases were among women.[51] Like other STIs, public health officials believe that actual figures could be higher because many cases go unreported.

**Signs and Symptoms** In men, early symptoms may include painful and difficult urination; frequent urination; and a watery, pus-like discharge from the penis. Symptoms in women may include a yellowish discharge, spotting between periods, and occasional spotting after intercourse. Women

are especially likely to be asymptomatic; many do not realize they have the disease, which can put them at risk for secondary damage.

**chlamydia** Bacterially caused STI of the urogenital tract.

# 110 MILLION

PEOPLE ARE LIVING WITH A **STI**
IN THE UNITED STATES.

**Complications** Men can suffer injury to the prostate gland, seminal vesicles, and bulbourethral glands, as well as arthritis-like symptoms and inflammatory damage to the blood vessels and heart. Men can also experience *epididymitis*—inflammation of the area near the testicles. In women, chlamydia-related inflammation can injure the cervix or fallopian tubes, causing sterility, and it can damage the inner pelvic structure, leading to **pelvic inflammatory disease (PID)**. If an infected woman becomes pregnant, she has a high risk for miscarriage and stillbirth. Women are at greater risks for urinary tract infections. Chlamydia may also be responsible for one type of *conjunctivitis,* an eye infection that affects not only adults but also infants, who can contract the disease from an infected mother during delivery. Untreated conjunctivitis can cause blindness.

> **pelvic inflammatory disease (PID)** Term used to describe various infections of the female reproductive tract.
>
> **gonorrhea** Second most common bacterial STI in the United States; if untreated, may cause sterility.

**Diagnosis and Treatment** A sample of urine or fluid from the vagina or penis is collected and tested to identify the presence of the bacteria. Unfortunately, chlamydia tests are not a routine part of many health clinics' testing procedures. If detected early, chlamydia is easily treatable with antibiotics such as tetracycline, doxycycline, or erythromycin.

## Gonorrhea

**Gonorrhea** is surpassed only by chlamydia in number of cases. The CDC estimates that there are over 333,000 cases per year, plus large numbers of cases that go unreported.[52] Although rates have declined in recent years, rates among men aged 20 to 24—the group with the highest rates overall—have increased.[53] Caused by the bacterial pathogen *Neisseria gonorrhoeae,* gonorrhea primarily infects the linings of the urethra, genital tract, pharynx, and rectum. It may spread to the eyes or other body regions by the hands or through body fluids, typically during vaginal, oral, or anal sex. It most frequently occurs in people in their early twenties.

**Signs and Symptoms** While some men are asymptomatic, a typical symptom is a white, milky discharge from the penis accompanied by painful, burning

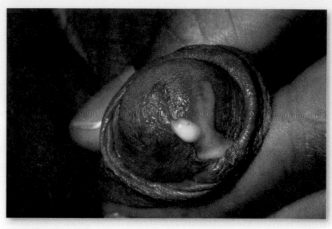

**FIGURE 13.7** Gonorrhea One common symptom of gonorrhea in men is a milky discharge from the penis, accompanied by burning sensations during urination. Whereas these symptoms will cause most men to seek diagnosis and treatment, women with gonorrhea are often asymptomatic, so they may not be aware they are infected.

urination 2 to 9 days after contact (**FIGURE 13.7**). Epididymitis can also occur as a symptom of infection.

Most women do not experience any symptoms, but others may have vaginal discharge or a burning sensation on urinating. The organism can remain in the woman's vagina, cervix, uterus, or fallopian tubes for long periods with no apparent symptoms other than an occasional slight fever. Thus a woman can be unaware that she has been infected and that she is infecting her sexual partners.

**Complications** Gonorrhea may spread to the prostate, testicles, urinary tract, kidneys, and bladder in men, and scar tissue may cause sterility. In some cases, the penis develops a painful curvature during erection. If the infection goes undetected in a woman, it can spread to the fallopian tubes and ovaries, causing sterility or severe inflammation and PID. The bacteria can also spread up the reproductive tract, through the blood, and infect the joints, heart valves, or brain. If an infected woman becomes pregnant, the infection can be transmitted to her baby during delivery, potentially causing blindness, joint infection, or a life-threatening blood infection.

**WHY SHOULD I CARE?**

Getting an STI can be painful, and you can infect your current partner with it. In the long term, it could affect the health of your children or your ability to have children.

**Diagnosis and Treatment** Diagnosis of gonorrhea requires a sample of either urine or fluid from the vagina or penis to detect the presence of the bacteria. In early stages gonorrhea is treatable with antibiotics, but it has begun to develop resistance. It is also important to recognize that chlamydia and gonorrhea often occur at the same time, but different antibiotics are needed to treat each infection separately.

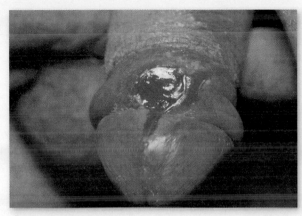

**a** Primary syphilis

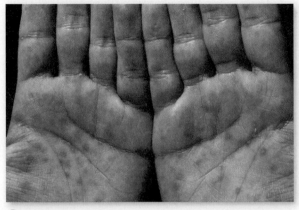

**b** Secondary syphilis

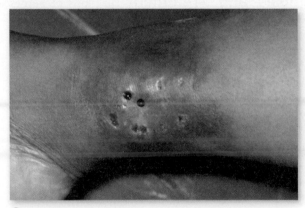

**c** Latent syphilis

**FIGURE 13.8 Syphilis** A chancre on the site of the initial infection is a symptom of primary syphilis **(a)**. A rash is characteristic of secondary syphilis **(b)**. Lesions called *gummas* are often present in latent syphilis **(c)**.

# Syphilis

**Syphilis** is caused by a bacterium called *Treponema pallidum*. The incidence of syphilis is highest in adults aged 20 to 29, and is particularly high among African Americans and men who have sex with men. There were 17,375 reported cases in 2013, a slight increase from 2012.[54] Because it is extremely delicate and dies readily on exposure to air, dryness, or cold, the organism is generally transferred only through direct sexual contact or from mother to fetus. The incidence of syphilis in newborns has continued to increase in the United States.[55]

**Signs and Symptoms** Syphilis is known as the "great imitator," because its symptoms resemble those of several other infections. It should be noted, however, that some people experience no symptoms at all. Syphilis can occur in four distinct stages:[56]

- **Primary syphilis.** The first stage of syphilis is often characterized by the development of a **chancre** (pronounced "shank-er"), a bacteria-oozing sore located at the infection site that usually appears about a month after initial infection (see **FIGURE 13.8**). In men, the site of the chancre tends to be the penis or scrotum; in women, the site of infection is often internal, on the vaginal wall or high on the cervix where the chancre is not readily apparent, making the likelihood of detection small. In both men and women, the chancre will disappear in 3 to 6 weeks.
- **Secondary syphilis.** If the infection is left untreated, a month to a year after the chancre disappears, secondary symptoms may appear, including a rash or white patches on the skin or on the mucous membranes of the mouth, throat, or genitals. Hair loss may occur, lymph nodes may enlarge, and the victim may develop a slight fever or headache. In rare cases, bacteria-containing sores develop around the mouth or genitals.
- **Latent syphilis.** After the secondary stage, if the infection is left untreated, the syphilis spirochetes begin to invade body organs, causing lesions called *gummas*. The infection now is rarely transmitted to others, except during pregnancy, when it can be passed to the fetus.
- **Tertiary/late syphilis.** Years after syphilis has entered the body, its effects become all too evident if still untreated. Late-stage syphilis indications include heart and central nervous system damage, blindness, deafness, paralysis, and dementia.

**Complications** Pregnant women with syphilis can experience premature births, miscarriages, stillbirths, or transmit the infection to her unborn child. An infected pregnant woman may transmit to her unborn child *congenital syphilis,* which can cause death; severe birth defects such as blindness, deafness, or disfigurement; developmental delays; seizures; and other health problems. Because in most cases the fetus does not become infected until after the first trimester, treatment of the mother during this time will usually prevent infection of the fetus.

**syphilis** One of the most widespread bacterial STIs; characterized by distinct phases and potentially serious results.

**chancre** Sore often found at the site of syphilis infection.

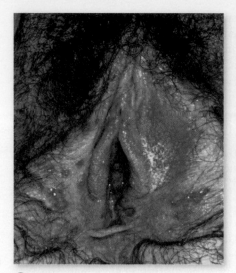

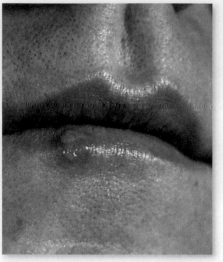

**ⓐ** Genital herpes is a highly contagious and incurable STI. It is characterized by recurring cycles of painful blisters on the genitalia.

**ⓑ** Oral herpes, caused by the same type of virus as genital herpes, is extremely contagious and can cause painful sores and blisters around the mouth.

**FIGURE 13.9** Herpes Both genital and oral herpes can be caused by either herpes simplex virus type 1 or 2.

**Diagnosis and Treatment** Syphilis can be diagnosed with a blood test or by collecting a sample from the chancre. It is easily treated with antibiotics, usually penicillin, for all stages except the late stage.

## Herpes

*Herpes* is a general term for a family of infections characterized by sores or eruptions on the skin caused by the *herpes simplex virus*. While herpes can be transmitted by sexual contact, kissing or sharing eating utensils can also transmit the infection. Herpes infections range from mildly uncomfortable to extremely serious. **Genital herpes** affects approximately 16 percent of the population aged 14 to 49 in the United States, with over 776,000 new cases overall each year in the United States.[57]

There are two types of herpes simplex virus. Only about 1 in 6 Americans currently has HSV-2; however, about half of adults have HSV-1, usually appearing as cold sores on their mouths and sometimes causing genital herpes infections.[58] Both types can infect any area of the body (**FIGURE 13.9**). Herpes simplex virus remains in certain nerve cells for life and can flare up when the body's ability to maintain itself is weakened.

**genital herpes** STI caused by the herpes simplex virus.

**human papillomavirus (HPV)** A group of viruses, many of which are transmitted sexually; some types of HPV can cause genital warts or cervical cancer.

**genital warts** Warts that appear in the genital area or the anus; caused by the human papillomavirus (HPV).

### Signs and Symptoms

The precursor phase of a herpes infection is characterized by a burning sensation and redness at the site of infection. By the second phase, a blister filled with a clear fluid containing the virus forms. If you pick at this blister or otherwise touch the site, you can autoinoculate other body parts. Particularly dangerous is the possibility of spreading the infection to your eyes, as blindness can occur.

Over a period of days, the unsightly blister will crust over, dry up, and disappear, and the virus will travel to the base of an affected nerve supplying the area and become dormant. Only when the victim becomes overly stressed, when diet and sleep are inadequate, when the immune system is overworked, or when excessive exposure to sunlight or other stressors occur will the virus become reactivated (at the same site every time) and begin the blistering cycle all over again. Each time a sore develops, it casts off (sheds) viruses that can be highly infectious, but a herpes site can shed the virus even when no overt sore is present.

**Complications** Many physicians recommend cesarean deliveries for infected pregnant women, as herpes can be passed to the baby during birth. Additionally, women with a history of genital herpes appear to have a greater risk of developing cervical cancer.

**Diagnosis and Treatment** Diagnosis of herpes can be determined by collecting a sample from the suspected sore or by performing a blood test. Although there is no cure for herpes at present, antiviral medications can prevent or shorten outbreaks. Certain prescription drugs like *acyclovir*, and over-the-counter medications like *Abreva* can be used to treat symptoms. The effectiveness of other treatments, such as L-lysine, is largely unsubstantiated. Other drugs, such as *famciclovir* (FAMVIR), may reduce viral shedding between outbreaks—potentially reducing risks to your sexual partners. Although vaccines are being tested, there is currently no commercially available vaccine that is protective against genital herpes.[59]

## Human Papillomavirus (HPV) and Genital Warts

**Human papillomavirus (HPV)** is one of a group of over 150 related viruses—each given a number indicating its type. HPV is the type that causes **genital warts** (also known as *venereal warts* or *condylomas*), and it is the most common sexually transmitted infection. Many are surprised to realize that HPV affects almost all sexually active men and women during their lives, even though many don't realize they are infected.[60] More than 40 types can actually infect the genital or anal areas of humans via skin-to-skin contact, making vaginal, anal, and oral sex all risky behaviors.[61] While genital warts are the most common result of the infection, HPV can also lead to cancer, particularly cervical cancer; however, cancer of the vulva, penis, anus, vagina, back of the throat, and tongue can occur. Because HPV is often asymptomatic in the early stages, the risk of infection is great, particularly among those who are immunocompromised, such as those with HIV or AIDS. Unfortunately, there is no diagnostic test to see if you have HPV, but a woman over the age of 30 can be screened for cervical cancer via a Pap test. Currently, about 79 million Americans are infected with HPV, and there are approximately 14 million new cases each year.[62]

## Signs and Symptoms

The typical incubation period is 6 to 8 weeks after contact. People infected with low-risk types of HPV may develop genital warts, a series of bumps or growths on the genitals, ranging in size from small pinheads to large cauliflower-like growths (**FIGURE 13.10**). Cancer may develop years after sexual contact and be symptomless for years.

## Complications

High-risk types of HPV (HPV-16 and -18) are responsible for an estimated 70 percent of cervical cancer cases.[63] In the United States, it is estimated that over 12,900 new cases and more than 4,100 deaths from cervical cancer will occur in 2015.[64] Exactly how high-risk HPV infection leads to cervical cancer is uncertain, though it may lead to *dysplasia*, or changes in cells that may lead to a precancerous condition. It is known that a Pap test done as routine screening for women aged 21 to 65 years old can help prevent cervical cancer.[65]

Of cases that become precancerous and are left untreated, the majority will eventually result in actual cancer. In addition, HPV may also pose a threat to a fetus that is exposed to the virus during birth. Cesarean deliveries may be considered in serious cases. Human papillomavirus can cause cancers—called "*oropharyngeal cancers*"—around the tonsils or the base of the tongue. Each year, approximately 8,400 Americans are diagnosed with HPV-caused cancers of the oropharynx, with over 80 percent of sexually active people aged 14 to 44 indicating they have had oral sex with a partner.[66] Men are about three times more likely to develop cancers of the oropharynx than are women.[67] See the **Student Health Today** box on page 418 for info on making oral sex safe.

New research has also implicated HPV as a possible risk factor for coronary artery disease, potentially causing an inflammatory response in the artery walls, leading to cholesterol and plaque buildup. (See Chapter 12 for more on the effects of inflammation and plaque buildup on arteries.)

## Diagnosis and Treatment

Diagnosis of genital warts from low-risk types of HPV is determined through a visual examination. High-risk types can be diagnosed in women through microscopic analysis of cells from a Pap smear or by collecting a sample from the cervix to test for HPV DNA. There is currently no HPV DNA test for men.

> **candidiasis** Yeast-like fungal infection often transmitted sexually; also called *moniliasis* or *yeast infection*.

Treatment is available only for the low-risk forms of HPV that cause genital warts. Most warts can be treated with topical medication or can be frozen with liquid nitrogen and then removed, but large warts may require surgical removal. There are currently two HPV vaccines that are licensed by the U.S. Food and Drug Administration (FDA) and recommended by the CDC. See the **Student Health Today** box on page 419 for more information about these vaccines.

## Candidiasis (Moniliasis)

Most STIs are caused by pathogens that come from outside the body; however, the yeast-like fungus *Candida albicans* is a normal inhabitant of the vaginal tract in most women. (See Figure 13.5c for a micrograph of this fungus.) Only when the normal chemical balance of the vagina is disturbed will these organisms multiply and cause the fungal disease **candidiasis,** also sometimes called *moniliasis* or a *yeast infection*.

## Signs and Symptoms

Symptoms of candidiasis include severe itching and burning of the vagina and vulva and a white, cheesy vaginal discharge. When this microbe infects the mouth, whitish patches form, and the condition is referred to as *thrush*. Thrush infection can also occur in men and is easily transmitted between sexual partners. Symptoms of candidiasis can be aggravated by contact with soaps, douches, perfumed toilet paper, chlorinated water, and spermicides.

## Diagnosis and Treatment

Diagnosis of candidiasis is usually made by collecting a vaginal sample and analyzing it to identify the pathogen. Antifungal drugs applied on the surface or by suppository usually cure candidiasis in just a few days.

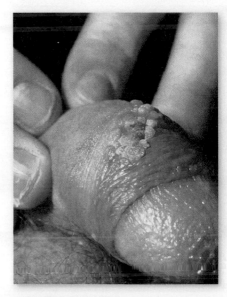
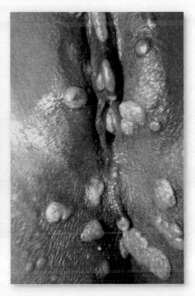

**FIGURE 13.10** **Genital Warts** Genital warts are caused by certain types of the human papillomavirus.

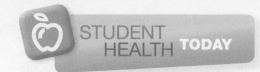

# MAKING ORAL SEX SAFE
## Condoms, Dental Dams, and Abstinence

Oral sex refers to orally stimulating the penis (fellatio), vagina and clitoris (cunnilingus), and/or anus (analingus). Many young people tend to believe that oral sex is safe, and while the risks of contracting an STI are lower with oral sex than with vaginal or anal intercourse, the risk is still not zero. It is entirely possible to contract HIV from oral sex, as well as herpes, gonorrhea, syphilis, genital warts, and other diseases. Beyond common STIs, it's also possible to spread or contract intestinal parasites, as well as hepatitis A and B. That being the case, here are a couple things you can do to minimize your risk:

- **Use a Condom Correctly.** Condom use during oral sex is especially important for HIV prevention. When performing or receiving fellatio, use a new latex condom each time. Check it for holes before using, and discard it after use. Never reuse a condom.
- **Use a Dental Dam.** A dental dam is essentially a small square of latex. While they were originally developed to be used during dental procedures, they are now commonly used as barriers when performing cunnilingus or analingus. Before using a dental dam, visually

check it for holes, and be sure to use a new one every time. Discard it after use, and never reuse a dental dam.

Lastly, keep in mind that condoms and dental dams provide less protection against STIs spread through contact with exposed sores, like HPV or herpes, than for other STIs. Abstinence is the only way to be 100 percent sure you don't transmit or contract an STI.

**Sources:** Centers for Disease Control and Prevention, "Oral Sex and HIV Risk," January 2014, www .cdc.gov/hiv/risk/behavior/oralsex .html; Centers for Disease Control and Prevention, "HIV Prevention," March 2014, www.cdc.gov/ hiv/basics/prevention.html; U.S. Department of Veterans Affairs, "Tips for Using Condoms and Dental Dams," www.hiv.va.gov/patient/ daily/sex/condom-tips.asp; Mayo Clinic, "Sexually Transmitted Diseases (STDs): Prevention," February 2013, www .mayoclinic.org/diseases-conditions /sexually-transmitted-diseases-stds/basics /prevention/con-20034128

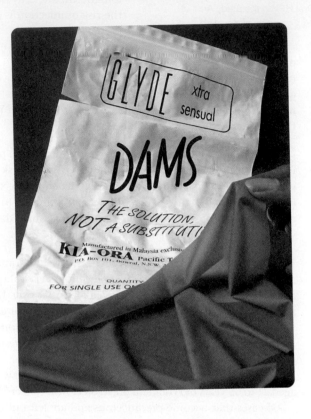

# Trichomoniasis

Unlike many STIs, **trichomoniasis** is caused by a protozoan, *Trichomonas vaginalis*. (See Figure 13.4d for a micrograph of this organism.) The "trich" organism can be spread by sexual contact and by contact with items that have discharged fluids on them. An estimated 3.4 million new cases occur in the United States each year, although only about one third of people who contract it experience symptoms.[68]

**trichomoniasis** Protozoan STI characterized by foamy, yellowish discharge and unpleasant odor.

**pubic lice** Parasitic insects that can inhabit various body areas, especially the genitals.

**Signs and Symptoms** Symptoms among women include a foamy, yellowish, unpleasant-smelling discharge accompanied by a burning sensation, itching, and painful urination. Most men with trichomoniasis do not have any symptoms, though some men experience irritation inside the penis, mild discharge, and a slight burning after urinating.[69]

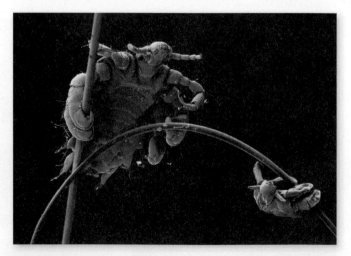

**FIGURE 13.11 Pubic Lice** Pubic lice, also known as "crabs," are small, parasitic insects that attach themselves to pubic hair; they may also move and end up infesting other body hair, even as far away as eyebrows or the hair on the head.

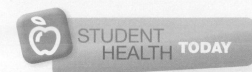
Most sexually active people will contract some form of human papillomavirus (HPV) at some time in their lives, though they may never even know it. There are about 40 types of sexually transmitted HPV, most of which cause no symptoms and go away on their own. Low-risk types can cause genital warts, but some high-risk types can cause cervical and other cancers. Every year in the United States, about 17,500 women and 9,300 men have one of several cancers caused by HPV, and 1 in 100 sexually active adults has genital warts.

- **Who should get the HPV vaccine?** There are two vaccines currently available—Cervarix and Gardasil. Human papillomavirus vaccines are recommended for 11- and 12-year-old girls, but can be given to girls as young as 9 years old. It is also recommended for girls and women ages 13 through 26 who have not yet been vaccinated or completed the vaccine series. Ideally, females should get a vaccine before they become sexually active. Females who are sexually active may get less benefit from it because they may have already contracted an HPV type targeted by the vaccines.

   One of the HPV vaccines, Gardasil, is also licensed, safe, and effective for males ages 9 through 26 years. The CDC recommends Gardasil for all boys 11 or 12 years old and for males ages

13 through 21 years who did not get any or all of the three recommended doses when they were younger. All men may receive the vaccine through the age of 26, but it is recommended that they should speak with their doctor to find out if getting vaccinated is right for them.

- **How are the two HPV vaccines, Cervarix and Gardasil, similar and different?** Both vaccines are very effective against high-risk HPV types 16 and 18, which cause 70 percent of cervical cancer cases. Both vaccines are given as shots and require three doses. But only Gardasil protects against low-risk HPV types 6 and 11. These HPV types cause 90 percent of cases of genital warts in females and males, so Gardasil is approved for use with males as well as females.

- **What do the two vaccines *not* protect against?** The vaccines do not protect against all types of HPV, so about 30 percent of cervical cancers will not be prevented by the vaccines. It will be important for women to continue getting screened for cervical cancer through regular Pap tests. Also, the vaccines do not prevent other sexually transmitted infections (STIs).

- **How safe are the HPV vaccines?** The vaccines are licensed by the FDA and approved by the CDC as safe and effective. They have been studied in thousands of females (ages 9 through 26) around the world, and their safety continues to be monitored by the CDC

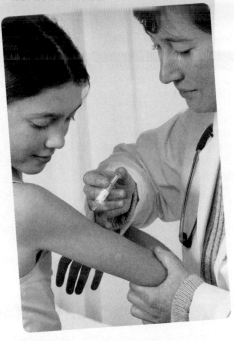

Ideally, females should get an HPV vaccine before they become sexually active. Males aged 9 through 26 can also be vaccinated.

and the FDA. Studies have found no serious side effects.

**Sources:** Centers for Disease Control and Prevention, "Vaccines and Preventable Diseases: HPV Vaccine—Questions & Answers," Reviewed July 2015, www.cdc.gov; American Cancer Society, "Human Papillomavirus (HPV), Cancer and HPV Vaccines—Frequently Asked Questions," 2015, www.cancer.org

**Diagnosis and Treatment** Diagnosis of trichomoniasis is determined by collecting fluid samples from the penis or vagina to test. Treatment includes oral metronidazole, usually given to both sexual partners to avoid the possible "ping-pong" effect of repeated cross-infection.

## Pubic Lice

**Pubic lice,** often called "crabs," are small parasitic insects that are usually transmitted during sexual contact (**FIGURE 13.11**). More annoying than dangerous, they have an affinity for pubic hair and attach themselves to the base of these hairs, where they deposit their eggs (nits). One to 2 weeks

later, these nits develop into adults that lay eggs and migrate to other body parts.

**Signs and Symptoms** Symptoms of pubic lice infestation include itchiness in the area covered by pubic hair, bluish-gray skin color in the pubic region, and sores in the genital area.

**Diagnosis and Treatment** Diagnosis of pubic lice involves an examination by a health care provider to identify the eggs in the genital area. Treatment includes washing clothing, furniture, and linens that may harbor the eggs, and usually takes 2 to 3 weeks to kill all larval forms.

## LO 6 | HIV/AIDS

Discuss human immunodeficiency virus (HIV) and acquired immune deficiency syndrome (AIDS), trends in infection and treatment, and the impact of these diseases on special populations.

Since **acquired immunodeficiency syndrome (AIDS)** was first recognized in the 1980s, approximately 78 million people worldwide have become infected with **human immunodeficiency virus (HIV)**, the virus that causes AIDS.[70] About 35.2 million people worldwide are living with HIV.[71] The vast majority of HIV-infected individuals (24.7 million) are in sub-Saharan Africa.[72] Globally, the numbers of people living with HIV have increased, even though the numbers of new infections have decreased in the last decade.[73] In the United States, there are over 1.2 million people infected with HIV and nearly 1 in 7 of these individuals aren't aware they are infected.[74] There are approximately 50,000 new HIV infections each year.[75] Since first discovered, over 650,000 people in the United States have died of AIDS, with about 13,000 deaths each year.[76]

**acquired immunodeficiency syndrome (AIDS)** A disease caused by a retrovirus, the human immunodeficiency virus (HIV), that attacks the immune system, reducing the number of helper T cells and leaving the victim vulnerable to infections, malignancies, and neurological disorders.

**human immunodeficiency virus (HIV)** The virus that causes AIDS by infecting helper T cells.

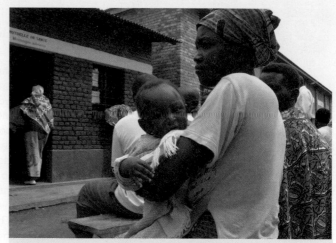

HIV/AIDS remains a devastating problem throughout the world. Over 23 million people live with HIV/AIDS in sub-Saharan Africa. The woman and child shown here await treatment outside a clinic in Rwanda.

**Source:** UNAIDS, "UNAIDS World AIDS Day Report 2012," 2012, Available at www.unaids.org

Men who have sex with men (MSM), particularly young black/African American MSM, are most seriously affected by HIV.[77] Overall, African Americans, Hispanic/Latinos, and white Americans bear the greatest burden of HIV infection in

## How HIV Is Transmitted

HIV typically enters the body when another person's infected body fluids (e.g., semen, vaginal secretions, blood) gain entry through a breach in body defenses. If there is a break in mucous membranes of the genitals or anus (as can occur during sexual intercourse, particularly anal intercourse), the virus enters and begins to multiply, invading the bloodstream and cerebrospinal fluid. It progressively destroys helper T cells, weakening the body's resistance to disease.

HIV/AIDS is not highly contagious. It cannot reproduce outside a living host, except in a laboratory, and does not survive well in open air. As a result, HIV cannot be transmitted through casual contact, including sharing food utensils, musical instruments, toilet seats, etc. Research also provides overwhelming evidence that insect bites do not transmit HIV.

### Engaging in High-Risk Behaviors
During the early days of the pandemic, it appeared that HIV infected only homosexuals, but it quickly became apparent that the disease was related to certain high-risk behaviors rather than groups of people. **FIGURE 13.12** shows the breakdown of sources of HIV infection among U.S. men and women.

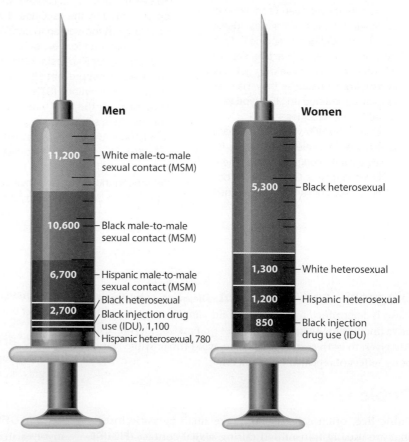

**Men**

11,200 — White male-to-male sexual contact (MSM)

10,600 — Black male-to-male sexual contact (MSM)

6,700 — Hispanic male-to-male sexual contact (MSM)

Black heterosexual

2,700 — Black injection drug use (IDU), 1,100

Hispanic heterosexual, 780

**Women**

5,300 — Black heterosexual

1,300 — White heterosexual

1,200 — Hispanic heterosexual

850 — Black injection drug use (IDU)

**FIGURE 13.12** Subpopulations of New HIV Infections in the United States by Sexual Orientation, Race, and Gender

**Source:** Data from Centers for Disease Control and Prevention, "Today's HIV/AIDS epidemic," March 2015, www.cdc.gov/nchhstp/newsroom/docs/hivfactsheets/todaysepidemic-508.pdf

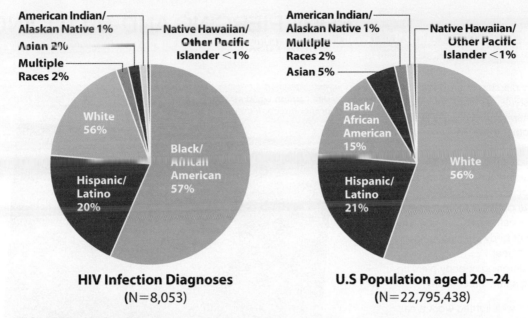

**American Indian/Alaskan Native 1%**

**Asian 2%**

**Multiple Races 2%**

**Native Hawaiian/Other Pacific Islander <1%**

White 56%

Black/African American 57%

Hispanic/Latino 20%

**HIV Infection Diagnoses**
**(N=8,053)**

**American Indian/Alaskan Native 1%**

**Multiple Races 2%**

**Asian 5%**

**Native Hawaiian/Other Pacific Islander <1%**

Black/African American 15%

White 56%

Hispanic/Latino 21%

**U.S Population aged 20–24**
**(N=22,795,438)**

**FIGURE 13.13** HIV Infections and Race in the United States Young Blacks and Hispanics (aged 20 to 24) have disproportionately higher rates of new HIV infections compared to their white peers.

**Source:** CDC, National Center for HIV/AIDS, Viral Hepatitis, STD & TB Prevention, "HIV Surveillance—Adolescents and Young Adults," www.cdc.gov/hiv/pdf/statistics_surveillance_Adolescents.pdf

the United States (see **FIGURE 13.13**). People of color have poorer HIV/AIDS outcomes than whites due to a number of social and economic barriers and challenges, such as lack of access to early diagnosis and treatment, discrimination, stigma, homophobia, and poverty.

The majority of HIV infections arise from the following:

- **Exchange of body fluids.** Substantial research indicates that blood, semen, and vaginal secretions are the major fluids of concern. Since the vaginal area is more susceptible to microtears, and because a woman is exposed to more semen than a man is to vaginal fluids, women are 4 to 10 times more likely than men to contract HIV through unprotected heterosexual intercourse. In fact, 80 percent of HIV in women is through heterosexual contact.[78] In rare instances, the virus has been found in saliva, but most health officials state that saliva is a less significant risk than other shared body fluids.

- **Contaminated needles.** Although users of illicit drugs are the most obvious members of this category, people with diabetes who inject insulin or athletes who inject steroids may also share needles. Sharing needles and engaging in high-risk sexual activities increases risks dramatically. Tattooing and body piercing can also be risky (see the **Student Health Today** box on page 422).

Prior to 1985, blood donations were not checked for HIV, and some people contracted the virus from transfusions. Because of massive screening efforts, the risk of receiving HIV-infected blood is now almost nonexistent in developed countries.

### Mother-to-Child (Perinatal) Transmission

Mother-to-child transmission of HIV can occur during pregnancy, during labor and delivery, or through breast-feeding.

Without antiretroviral treatment, approximately 15 to 45 percent of HIV-positive pregnant women will transmit the virus to their infant.[79]

## Signs and Symptoms of HIV/AIDS

A person may go for months or years after infection before any significant symptoms appear, and incubation time varies greatly from person to person. Without treatment, it takes an average of 8 to 10 years for the virus to cause the slow, degenerative changes in the immune system that are characteristic of AIDS. During this time, the person may experience *opportunistic infections* (infections that gain a foothold when the immune system is not functioning effectively). Colds, sore throats, fever, tiredness, nausea, night sweats, and other generally non–life-threatening conditions commonly appear and are described as pre-AIDS symptoms. Other symptoms of progressing HIV infection include wasting syndrome, swollen lymph nodes, and neurological problems. A diagnosis of AIDS, the final stage of HIV infection, is made when the infected person has either a dangerously low CD4 (helper T) cell count (below 200 cells per cubic milliliter of blood) or has contracted one or more opportunistic infections characteristic of the disease, such as Kaposi's sarcoma, tuberculosis, recurrent pneumonia, or invasive cervical cancer.

## Testing for HIV

Once antibodies have formed in reaction to HIV, a blood test known as the *ELISA*

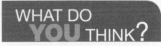

**WHAT DO YOU THINK?**

Do you think we have grown too apathetic about HIV/AIDS in the United States?

- Is HIV/AIDS prevention discussed on your campus?
- Are people as concerned with HIV as they are with other STIs?

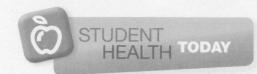
# BODY PIERCING AND TATTOOING
## *Potential Risks*

During body piercing or tattooing, the use of unsterile needles—which can transmit staph, HIV, hepatitis B and C, tetanus, and other diseases—poses a very real risk.

Laws and policies regulating body piercing and tattooing vary greatly by state. Because of the lack of universal regulatory standards and the potential for transmission of dangerous pathogens, anyone who receives a tattoo or body piercing cannot donate blood for 1 year.

If you opt for tattooing or body piercing, take the following safety precautions:

- Look for clean, well-lighted work areas, and inquire about sterilization procedures. Be wary of establishments that won't answer questions or show you their sterilization equipment.
- Packaged, sterilized needles should be used only once and then discarded. A piercing gun should not be used, because it cannot be sterilized properly. Watch that the artist uses new needles and tubes from a sterile package before your procedure begins. Ask to see the sterile confirmation logo on the bag itself.
- Immediately before piercing or tattooing, the body area should be carefully sterilized. The artist should wash his or her hands and put on new latex gloves for each procedure. Make sure the artist changes those gloves if he or she needs to touch anything else, such as the telephone, while working.
- Leftover tattoo ink should be discarded after each procedure. Do not

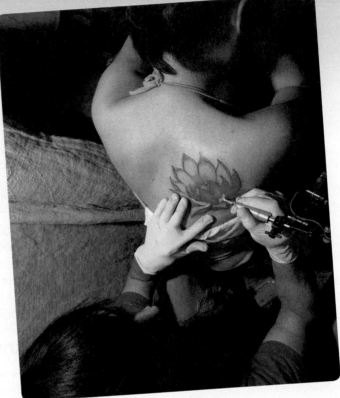

**Use caution when selecting a tattoo artist and facility to insure that proper infection control procedures are in place.**

allow the artist to reuse ink that has been used for other customers. Used needles should be disposed of in a "sharps" container, a plastic container with the biohazard symbol clearly marked on it.

Like any activity that involves bodily fluids, tattooing carries some risk of disease transmission.

**Source:** Mayo Clinic Staff, "Tattoos: Understand Risks and Precautions," March 2015, www.mayoclinic.com

---

(enzyme-linked immunosorbent assay) may detect their presence. It can take 3 to 6 months after initial infection for enough antibodies to show a positive test result, and individuals with negative test results should be retested within 6 months. When a person who previously tested *negative* (no HIV antibodies present) has a subsequent test that is *positive,* seroconversion is said to have occurred. In such a situation, the person would typically take another ELISA test, followed by a more precise test known as the *Western blot,* to confirm the presence of HIV antibodies.

A polymerase chain reaction (PCR) test detects the genetic material of HIV instead of the antibodies to the virus and can identify HIV within the first few weeks of infection. It is often performed on babies born to mothers who are HIV positive.

Rapid HIV tests using blood or oral fluids are also available and can produce results in 20 minutes. However, they require a confirmatory test with positive results, which may take up to several weeks. Home kits are also available, allowing a person to take a blood or saliva sample and anonymously send it to a laboratory. The person then calls a number to find out their results, with professional counselors available to provide support. Health officials distinguish between *reported* and *actual* cases of HIV infection because it is believed that many HIV-positive people avoid being tested for fear of knowing the truth, or recrimination from employers, insurance companies, and medical staff. However, early detection and reporting are important because immediate treatment in early stages is critical.

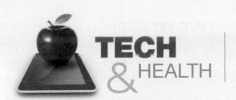

## SIMPLER TESTS CAN IMPROVE TREATMENT OUTCOMES FOR HIV AND TB PATIENTS

One of the side effects of AIDS antiviral therapy and tuberculosis treatment is liver failure due to the toxicity of the medication used to treat those diseases. In Africa that's been especially difficult to combat, as the tests routinely used to monitor liver function for signs of trouble require tubes of blood, laboratory facilities, time for processing results, as well as money for all of the above. In a place where poverty is widespread and patients are many, but skilled health care workers and equipment are scarce, liver function often goes unmonitored in those who are at greatest risk. It is estimated that in resource-poor countries, approximately 25 percent of HIV/AIDS patients lack access to diagnostic tools and die as a result of liver complications related to treatment. But a new cheap and simple test that determines liver function could change that.

The new test is a piece of specially treated paper the size of a stamp that costs around 10 cents. A small amount of blood or urine is applied, and then chemicals in the paper change color to show the result. As with diabetes or pregnancy home-testing kits, the test is designed to be simple enough so the person reading it doesn't need to be a trained medical professional to understand the results, and it doesn't need any external power or equipment. This test improves the odds for patients with tuberculosis or HIV/AIDS to able to withstand the side effects of their treatments successfully.

**Sources:** Diagnostics for All, "Liver Function Test," 2012, www.dfa.org/projects/liver-function. php; D. McNeil, "Far from Any Lab, Paper Bits Find Illness," September 27, 2011, *The New York Times*, www.nytimes.com/2011/09/27/health/27paper.html?_r=0; A. Maloney, "AlterNet's Top 20 Big Ideas that Don't Cost the Earth," January 7, 2011, *Thomson Reuters Foundation*, www.trust.org/alertnet/news/alertnets-top-20-big-ideas-that-dont-cost-the-earth

## New Hope and Treatments

New drugs have slowed the progression from HIV to AIDS and have prolonged life expectancies for most AIDS patients. In fact, since the 1990s, the U.S. death rate from AIDS is down nearly 83 percent.[80] The average cost for antiretroviral therapy (ART) is in excess of $23,000/year, with a lifetime estimated cost in excess of $380,000.[81]

Current treatments combine selected drugs, especially protease inhibitors and reverse transcriptase inhibitors. *Protease inhibitors* (e.g., amprenavir, ritonavir, and saquinavir) act to prevent the production of the virus in chronically infected cells that HIV has already invaded and seem to work best in combination with other therapies. Other drugs, such as AZT, ddI, ddC, d4T, and 3TC, inhibit the HIV enzyme *reverse transcriptase* before the virus has invaded the cell, thereby preventing the virus from infecting new cells. Combination treatments are still experimental, and no combination has proven effective for all people. Today, 44 new medicines, including antivirals, and vaccines are in testing.[82] See the **Tech & Health** box for more on potential benefits of simplified HIV testing.

# 36%

OF PEOPLE LIVING WITH HIV IN LOW- AND MIDDLE-INCOME COUNTRIES RECEIVE **TREATMENT**.

## Preventing HIV Infection

The only way to prevent HIV infection is through the choices you make in sexual behaviors and drug use and by taking responsibility for your own health and the health of your loved ones. You can't determine the presence of HIV by looking at a person; you can't tell by questioning the person, unless he or she has been tested recently and is giving an honest answer. So what should you do?

Of course, the simplest answer is abstinence. If you do decide to be intimate, the next best option is to use a condom.

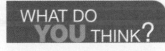

### WHAT DO YOU THINK?

**Why is HIV testing important?**

- Would you want any potential sexual partners to be tested for HIV or other STIs? How would you ask that person to get tested?
- How can you protect yourself from HIV?

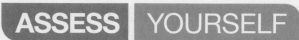

### STIs: Do You Really Know What You Think You Know?

The following quiz will help you evaluate whether your beliefs and attitudes about sexually transmitted infections (STIs) lead you to behaviors that increase your risk of infection. Indicate whether you believe the following items are true or false, then consult the answer key that follows.

| | | True | False |
|---|---|:---:|:---:|
| 1. | You can always tell when you've got an STI because the symptoms are so obvious. | ○ | ○ |
| 2. | Some STIs can be passed on by skin-to-skin contact in the genital area. | ○ | ○ |
| 3. | Herpes can be transmitted only when a person has visible sores on his or her genitals. | ○ | ○ |
| 4. | Oral sex is safe sex. | ○ | ○ |
| 5. | Condoms reduce your risk of both pregnancy and STIs. | ○ | ○ |
| 6. | As long as you don't have anal intercourse, you can't get HIV. | ○ | ○ |
| 7. | All sexually active females should have a regular Pap smear. | ○ | ○ |
| 8. | Once genital warts have been removed, there is no risk of passing on the virus. | ○ | ○ |
| 9. | You can get several STIs at one time. | ○ | ○ |
| 10. | If the signs of an STI go away, you are cured. | ○ | ○ |
| 11. | People who get an STI have a lot of sex partners. | ○ | ○ |
| 12. | All STIs can be cured. | ○ | ○ |
| 13. | You can get an STI more than once. | ○ | ○ |

## Answer Key

**1. False.** The unfortunate fact is that many STIs show no symptoms. This has serious implications: (a) you can be passing on the infection without knowing it, and (b) the pathogen may be damaging your reproductive organs without you knowing it.

**2. True.** Some viruses are present on the skin around the genital area. Herpes and genital warts are the main culprits.

**3. False.** Herpes is most easily passed on when the sores and blisters are present, because the fluid in the lesions carries the virus. But the virus is also found on the skin around the genital area. Most people contract herpes this way, unaware that the virus is present.

**4. False.** Oral sex is not safe sex. Herpes, genital warts, and chlamydia can all be passed on through oral sex. Condoms should be used on the penis. Dental dams should be placed over the female genitals during oral sex.

**5. True.** Condoms significantly reduce the risk of pregnancy when used correctly. They also reduce the risk of STIs. It is important to point out that abstinence is the only behavior that provides complete protection against pregnancy and STIs.

**6. False.** HIV is present in blood, semen, and vaginal fluid. Any activity that allows for the transfer of these fluids is risky. Anal intercourse is a high-risk activity, especially for the receptive (passive) partner, but other sexual activity is also a risk. When you don't know your partner's sexual history and you're not in a long-term monogamous relationship, condoms are a must.

**7. True.** A Pap smear is a simple procedure involving the scraping of a small amount of tissue from the surface of the cervix (at the upper end of the vagina). The sample is tested for abnormal cells that may indicate cancer. All sexually active women should have regular Pap smears.

**8. False.** Genital warts, which may be present on the penis, the anus, and inside and outside the vagina, can be removed. However, the virus that caused the warts will always be present in the body and can be passed on to a sexual partner.

**9. True.** It is possible to have many STIs at one time. In fact, having one STI may make it more likely that a person will acquire more STIs. For example, the open sore from herpes creates a place for HIV to be transmitted.

**10. False.** The symptoms may go away, but your body is still infected. For example, syphilis is characterized by various stages. In the first stage, a painless sore called a chancre appears for about a week and then goes away.

**11. False.** If you have sex once with an infected partner, you are at risk for an STI.

**12. False.** Some STIs are viruses and therefore cannot be cured. There is no cure at present for herpes, HIV/AIDS, or genital warts. These STIs are treatable (to lessen the pain and irritation of symptoms), but not curable.

**13. True.** Experiencing one infection with an STI does not mean that you can never be infected again. A person can be reinfected many times with the same STI. This is especially true if a person does not get treated for the STI and thus keeps reinfecting his or her partner with the same STI.

**Sources:** Adapted from Jefferson County Public Health, "STD Quiz," modified March 2009, www.co.jefferson.co.us/health/health_TTTT_R69.htm; Adapted from Family Planning Victoria, "Play Safe," updated July 2005, www.fpv.org.au/1_2_2.html.

# YOUR PLAN FOR **CHANGE**

After completing "STIs: Do Your Really Know What You Think You Know?," you can begin to change behaviors that may be putting you at risk for STIs and for infection in general.

### TODAY, YOU CAN:

☐ Put together an "emergency" supply of condoms. Outside of abstinence, condoms are your best protection against an STI. If you don't have a supply on hand, visit your local drugstore or health clinic. Remember that both men and women are responsible for preventing the transmission of STIs.

☐ To prevent infections in general, get in the habit of washing your hands regularly. After you cough, sneeze, blow your nose, use the bathroom, or prepare food, find a sink, wet your hands with warm water, and lather up with soap. Scrub your hands for about 20 seconds (count to 20 or recite the alphabet), rinse well, and dry your hands.

### WITHIN THE NEXT TWO WEEKS, YOU CAN:

☐ Talk with your significant other honestly about your sexual history. Make appointments to get tested if either of you think you may have been exposed to an STI.

☐ Adjust your sleep schedule so that you're getting an adequate amount of rest every night. Being well rested is one key aspect of maintaining a healthy immune system.

### BY THE END OF THE SEMESTER, YOU CAN:

☐ Check your immunization schedule and make sure you're current with all recommended vaccinations. Make an appointment with your health care provider if you need a booster or vaccine.

☐ If you are due for an annual pelvic exam, make an appointment. Ask your partner if he or she has had an annual exam and encourage him or her to make an appointment if not.

## CHAPTER REVIEW

To hear an MP3 Tutor Session, scan here or visit the Study Area in **MasteringHealth**.

### LO 1 | The Process of Infection

- For a person to become infected with a disease, he or she must come into contact with a pathogen, and the pathogen must get past the body's immune system defenses to establish infection.

### LO 2 | Your Body's Defenses against Infection

- The skin is the body's major barrier against infection, helped by enzymes and body secretions.
- If pathogens get inside the body, the immune system finds the foreign cells or particles and creates antibodies to destroy them. Inflammation and fever also play a role in defending the body against infections.
- Vaccines bolster the body's immune system against specific diseases.

### LO 3 | Types of Pathogens and the Diseases They Cause

- The major classes of pathogens are bacteria, viruses, fungi, protozoans, parasitic worms, and prions. Bacterial infections include staphylococcal infections, streptococcal infections, meningitis, pneumonia, tuberculosis, and tick-borne diseases. Major viral infections include the common cold, influenza, mononucleosis, and hepatitis.
- Emerging and resurgent diseases such as West Nile virus, and avian flu potentially pose significant threats for future generations. Many factors contribute to these risks.

### LO 4 | Sexually Transmitted Infections (STIs)

- Sexually transmitted infections (STIs) are spread through vaginal intercourse, oral-genital contact, anal intercourse, hand-genital contact, and sometimes through mouth-to-mouth contact.
- Every year, there are at least 20 million new cases of STIs in the United States. They affect people of all backgrounds and socioeconomic levels, but rates are disproportionately higher among young adults, women, minorities, and infants.
- Generally, the more sexual partners one has, the greater the risk of contracting an STI. Reduce risk of contraction by using condoms and dental dams and avoiding sexual activities that allow blood, semen, or other body fluid to enter breaks in the skin or breach mucous membranes.

### LO 5 | Common types of Sexually Transmitted Infections

- Major STIs include chlamydia, gonorrhea, syphilis, herpes, human papillomavirus (HPV) and genital warts, candidiasis, trichomoniasis, and pubic lice.

### LO 6 | HIV/AIDS

- Acquired immunodeficiency syndrome (AIDS) is caused by the human immunodeficiency virus (HIV). HIV/AIDS is a global pandemic.
- Anyone can get HIV by engaging in unprotected sexual activities or by injecting drugs (or by having sex with someone who does).

## POP QUIZ

Visit **MasteringHealth** to personalize your study plan with Chapter Review Quizzes and Dynamic Study Modules.

### LO 1 | The Process of Infection

1. Jennifer touched her viral herpes sore on her lip and then touched her eye. She ended up with the herpes virus in her eye as well. This is an example of
   a. acquired immunity.
   b. passive spread.
   c. autoinoculation.
   d. self vaccination.

2. One of the best ways to prevent contagious viruses from spreading is to
   a. wash your hands frequently.
   b. cover your mouth when sneezing, and dispose of your tissues.
   c. keep your hands away from your mouth and eyes.
   d. All of the above

### LO 2 | Your Body's Defenses against Infection

3. Which of the following do *not* assist the body in fighting disease?
   a. Antigens
   b. Antibodies
   c. Lymphocytes
   d. Macrophages

### LO 3 | Types of Pathogens and the Diseases They Cause

4. Which of the following is a *viral* disease?
   a. Hepatitis
   b. Pneumonia
   c. Malaria
   d. Streptococcal infection

5. Which of the following diseases is caused by a prion?
   a. Shingles
   b. Listeria
   c. Mad cow disease
   d. Trichomoniasis

### LO 4 | Sexually Transmitted Infections (STIs)

6. What type of environment do STI pathogens prefer?
   a. Any environment
   b. Dark, moist environments
   c. Light, dry places
   d. Cold, dry environments

### Common Types of Sexually Transmitted Infections

**LO 5**

7. Pelvic inflammatory disease (PID) is
   a. a sexually transmitted infection.
   b. a type of urinary tract infection.
   c. an infection of a woman's fallopian tubes or uterus.
   d. a disease that both men and women can get.

8. Which of the following STIs cannot be treated with antibiotics?
   a. Chlamydia
   b. Gonorrhea
   c. Syphilis
   d. Herpes

### HIV/AIDS

**LO 6**

9. Which of the following is *not* a true statement about HIV?
   a. You can tell if a potential sex partner has the virus by looking at him or her.
   b. The virus can be spread through semen or vaginal fluids.
   c. You cannot get HIV from a public restroom toilet seat.
   d. Unprotected anal sex increases risk of exposure to HIV.

10. After HIV/AIDS, which infectious disease kills more people than any other disease in the global population?
    a. Malaria
    b. Avian influenza
    c. Tuberculosis
    d. Hepatitis C

*Answers to the Pop Quiz can be found on page A-1. If you answered a question incorrectly, review the section identified by the Learning Outcome. For even more study tools, visit MasteringHealth.*

## THINK ABOUT IT!

### The Process of Infection

**LO 1**

1. What are three lifestyle changes you could make right now that would reduce your risk of developing an infectious disease? How can you help reduce antibiotic resistance in the world today?

### Your Body's Defenses against Infection

**LO 2**

2. What are pathogens, antigens, and antibodies? Discuss noncontrollable and controllable risk factors that can make you more or less susceptible to infectious pathogens in your immediate surroundings.

3. Explain why it is important to wash your hands often when you have a cold.

4. What is the difference between natural and acquired immunity? Discuss the importance of vaccinations in reducing societal risks for infectious diseases.

### Types of Pathogens and the Diseases They Cause

**LO 3**

5. What are some differences between bacteria and viruses?

### Sexually Transmitted Infections (STIs)

**LO 4**

6. What are the key risk factors for STI infections? What kind of behaviors should you avoid to cut down on the risk of contracting a sexually transmitted infection?

### Common Types of Sexually Transmitted Infections

**LO 5**

7. Identify five STIs and their symptoms. How are they transmitted? What are their potential long-term effects?

### HIV/AIDS

**LO 6**

8. Why are women more susceptible to HIV infection than men? What implication does this have for prevention, treatment, and research?

## ACCESS YOUR HEALTH ON THE INTERNET

Visit **MasteringHealth** for links to the websites and RSS feeds.

The following websites explore further topics and issues related to personal health. For links to the websites below, visit the Study Area in MasteringHealth.

*Centers for Disease Control and Prevention (CDC).* This government agency is dedicated to disease intervention and prevention. The site links to all the latest data and publications put out by the CDC. **www.cdc.gov**

*Association for Professionals in Infection Control and Epidemiology (APIC).* Excellent resource for health professionals and consumers covering a wide range of infectious disease issues in health care, workplaces, schools, and in personal environment. **www.apic.org**

*World Health Organization (WHO).* You'll gain access to the latest information on world health issues and direct access to publications and fact sheets at WHO's site. **www.who.int**

*American Sexual Health Association.* This site provides facts, support, and referrals about sexually transmitted infections and diseases. **www.ashastd.org**

*AVERT.* This is an international site with information on HIV/AIDS, global STI statistics, interactive quizzes, and graphics displaying current statistics for vulnerable populations. **www.avert.org**

# Reducing Risks for Chronic Diseases and Conditions

Behaviors you pursue now can put you at a greater risk for chronic diseases. Do you know if you're putting yourself at greater risk?

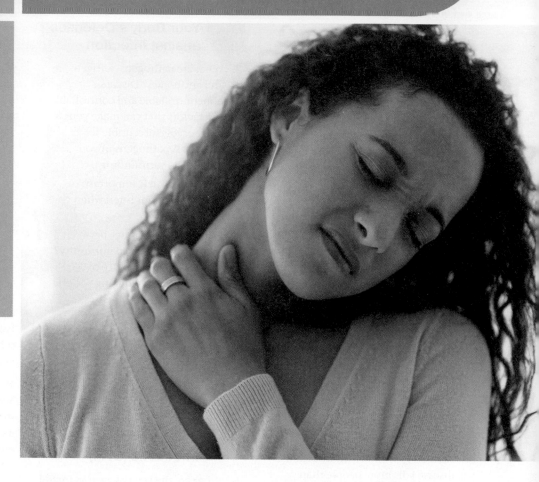

## LEARNING OUTCOMES

1 Describe the prevalence of, symptoms of, and risk factors for key respiratory diseases such as bronchitis, emphysema, and asthma.

2 Describe the allergic response and complications associated with allergies as well as who is susceptible to allergy development.

3 Explain common types of headaches, their risk factors, and possible causes.

4 Outline risk factors, symptoms, and strategies for preventing irritable bowel syndrome (IBS), Crohn's disease, and ulcerative colitis.

5 Explain the risk factors and symptoms of musculoskeletal problems and repetitive motion/stress disorders and suggest strategies for prevention.

**T**ypically, chronic diseases or conditions are those that take time to develop, cause progressive damage to the body, and are not easily cured. Most of the time, chronic diseases are not caused by pathogens or transmitted by any form of personal contact. Genetics, the environment, lifestyle, and personal health habits are often implicated as underlying causes; however, the causes of many chronic diseases and conditions remain a mystery. Healthy changes in lifestyle; public health efforts aimed at research, prevention, and control; and an ever-growing pharmaceutical arsenal can minimize the effects of these diseases. Policies that protect the environment and keep us safe from

chemicals can also make a difference. In this chapter we will highlight several chronic diseases, along with actions you can take to reduce your risks.

## LO **1** | CHRONIC LOWER RESPIRATORY (LUNG) DISEASES

Describe the prevalence of, symptoms of, and risk factors for key respiratory diseases such as bronchitis, emphysema, and asthma.

- - - - - - - - - - - - - - - - - - - - - - - - -

*Chronic lower respiratory diseases* (diseases of the lungs) are the third leading cause of death overall in the United

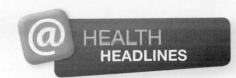
# BE ECO-CLEAN AND ALLERGEN FREE

Exposure to household chemicals, dust, and pet dander may exacerbate asthma, allergies, and other respiratory problems. You can reduce exposure to noxious household chemicals and create a clean, comfortable home by using cleaning supplies and household products that are less toxic to the home environment. Because some companies may want you to believe their product is greener than it actually is, read the labels carefully and look for independent certifications such as the Green Seal and the Environmental Protection Agency's (EPA's) Design for the Environment program.

- For a handy glass and surface cleaner, mix 1/2 cup of white vinegar or 2 tablespoons of lemon juice with 4 cups of water. Pour the solution into a spray bottle and keep the remainder for a quick and cheap refill.

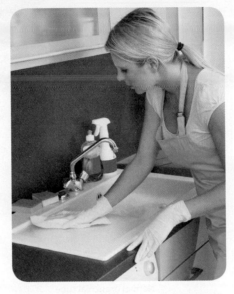

Using environmentally safe cleaning products and wearing gloves can reduce your risks from exposure to toxic chemicals in your home.

- Use baking soda to remove carpet odors and to scour sinks, toilets, and bathtubs.
- Instead of chlorine bleach, use 1/2 cup of hydrogen peroxide in your laundry or try oxygen-based bleaches.
- Make all-purpose cleaner with 1/2 cup of borax (found in the laundry aisle) and 1 gallon of hot water.
- For green air fresheners, use essential oils, such as lemon or lavender. Many store-bought air fresheners contain phthalates, often called "fragrance," that are related to respiratory problems and other noninfectious conditions. Place a few drops of essential oils on a piece of tissue paper, in a bowl of warm water, or in a store-bought diffuser.

---

States, killing nearly 150,000 people in 2015.[1] Today, more than 35 million Americans are living with chronic lung diseases such as asthma, emphysema, and bronchitis.[2]

A lung disease is any disease or disorder that impairs lung function. The lungs can be damaged by a single exposure to a toxic chemical or severe heat, or by years of inhaling the tar and chemicals in tobacco smoke. Occupational or home exposure to asbestos, silica dust, paint fumes and lacquers, pesticides,

## 35 MILLION

AMERICANS LIVE WITH **CHRONIC LUNG DISEASES** SUCH AS ASTHMA, EMPHYSEMA, AND BRONCHITIS.

and a host of other environmental substances can cause lung damage. When the lungs are impaired, a condition known as **dyspnea,** or breathlessness, can occur, even with mild exertion. As the lungs are oxygen deprived, the heart is forced to work harder and, over time, cardiovascular problems, suffocation, and death can occur.

## Chronic Obstructive Pulmonary Disease

Chronic obstructive pulmonary disease (COPD) is a general term that refers to lower respiratory diseases where some form of obstruction interferes with a person's ability to breathe. In the United States, the term COPD refers to two specific diseases, **chronic bronchitis** and **emphysema**, which often occur together and can lead to problems with inhalation and exhalation. Currently, nearly 15 million people aged 18 and over have impaired lung function caused by COPD; however, these numbers are believed to grossly underestimate the over 24 million people believed to have undiagnosed lung

impairment.[3] The majority of COPD sufferers either smoke or smoked in the past. Other risks include a history of *asthma*, occupational exposure to certain industrial fumes or gases, and exposure to dusts, extreme temperatures, and other lung irritants.[4]

There is no cure for COPD; however, there is much that can be done to prevent it. Quitting smoking, exercise, and avoiding obesity can all help your lungs function more effectively, as can avoiding secondhand smoke, toxic aerosols, radon, and other chemicals in the home. The **Health Headlines** box describes actions you can take to reduce risks from common exposures in your home.

---

**dyspnea** Shortness of breath, usually associated with disease of the heart or lungs.

**chronic obstructive pulmonary diseases (COPDs)** A collection of chronic lung diseases, including emphysema and chronic bronchitis, where some form of obstruction interferes with a person's ability to breathe.

**chronic bronchitis** An inflammation and eventual scarring of the lining of the bronchial tubes.

**emphysema** A respiratory disease in which the alveoli become distended or ruptured and are no longer functional.

At work, proper safety equipment and ventilation reduce risks. Policies that protect the environment (see Chapter 15) and restrict air pollution and other threats can have a major impact on risks for COPD. Even so, there is currently pressure to roll back many of the provisions of the Clean Air Act.

## Bronchitis

Bronchitis involves inflammation and eventual scarring of the lining of the bronchial tubes (*bronchi*) that connect the windpipe to the lungs. When the bronchi become inflamed or infected with bacteria, less air is able to flow from the lungs and heavy mucus begins to form. *Acute bronchitis* is the most common bronchial disease, and symptoms often improve in a week or two.

When the symptoms of bronchitis last for at least 3 months of the year for 2 consecutive years, the condition is considered *chronic bronchitis*. Over 10.1 million Americans, the majority of whom are women, suffer from chronic bronchitis; 33 percent are under age 45. In 2011, non-Hispanic black Americans experienced more chronic bronchitis than non-Hispanic white Americans for the first time. Highest rates of bronchitis and asthma occur in lowest income and education populations.[5]

## Emphysema

Emphysema involves the gradual, irreversible destruction of the alveoli (tiny air sacs through which gas exchange occurs) of the lungs. Over 4.7 million Americans suffer from emphysema. Over 90 percent of cases occur in people over the age of 45.[6] Today more women are diagnosed with emphysema than are men; in the last 5 years, emphysema rates have risen over 63 percent for women and declined 6 percent among men.[7] As the alveoli are destroyed, the affected person finds it more and more difficult to exhale, struggling to take in a fresh supply of air before the air held in the lungs has been expended. The

**asthma** a long-term, chronic inflammatory disorder characterized by attacks of wheezing, shortness of breath, and coughing spasms.

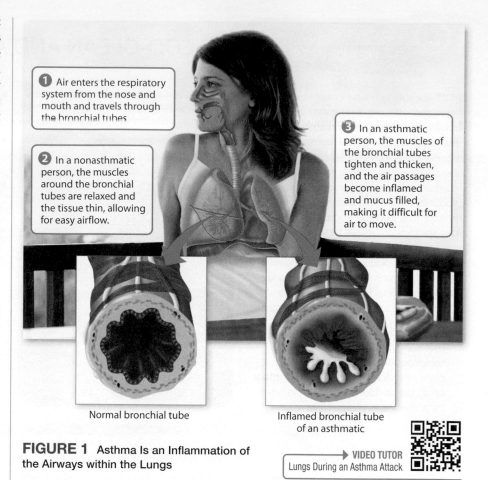

① Air enters the respiratory system from the nose and mouth and travels through the bronchial tubes

② In a nonasthmatic person, the muscles around the bronchial tubes are relaxed and the tissue thin, allowing for easy airflow.

③ In an asthmatic person, the muscles of the bronchial tubes tighten and thicken, and the air passages become inflamed and mucus filled, making it difficult for air to move.

Normal bronchial tube

Inflamed bronchial tube of an asthmatic

**FIGURE 1** Asthma Is an Inflammation of the Airways within the Lungs

→ **VIDEO TUTOR**
Lungs During an Asthma Attack

chest cavity gradually begins to expand, producing a barrel-shaped chest. (For more on emphysema and smoking, see Chapter 8.)

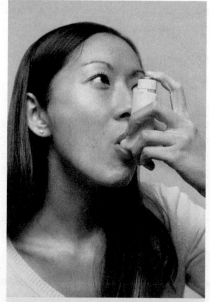

People with asthma can generally control their symptoms through the use of inhaled medications.

## Asthma

**Asthma** is a long-term, chronic disorder that inflames and narrows the airways of the lungs (see **FIGURE 1**). Tiny airways in the lungs overreact with spasms, resulting in wheezing, difficulty breathing, shortness of breath, and coughing spasms. Over 250 million people globally are living with asthma.[8] Although most asthma attacks are mild and non-life-threatening, nearly 10 percent of people with asthma have a severe, treatment-resistant form that can be life-threatening.[9]

Asthma falls into two distinctly different types. The more common form of asthma, known as *extrinsic or allergic asthma*, is typically associated with allergic triggers; it tends to run in families and develop in childhood. Often by adulthood, a person has few episodes or the disorder completely goes away. *Intrinsic or nonallergic asthma* may be triggered by anything except an allergy.

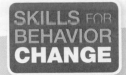

## SKILLS FOR BEHAVIOR CHANGE | PREVENTING ASTHMA ATTACKS

There is much that individuals and communities can do to reduce risk of asthma attacks:

▶ Purchase a good air filter for your home, and clean furnace filters regularly. Check wood-burning stoves regularly to make sure they're not spewing smoke and particulate matter.

▶ Wash pillows and sheets regularly. Use pillow protectors and mattress protectors. Don't purchase used mattresses, which may be teeming with mites.

▶ Try a nonshedding breed of dog or cat. Keep pets off your bed. Wash pets and their bedding weekly. Vacuum up shed hair regularly.

▶ Keep your home clean and pest free; cockroaches and other vermin have enzymes in their saliva or particles on their bodies that may trigger allergic reactions. Use a high-suction vacuum to reduce dust particles suspended in the air.

▶ Use antimold cleaners or run a dehumidifier to keep moisture levels down and reduce the growth of mold.

▶ Exercise regularly to keep your lungs functioning well.

▶ Avoid cigarette, cigar, and pipe smoke.

▶ Keep asthma medications handy. Let people close to you know that you are asthmatic, and educate them about what to do if you have an asthma attack.

Genetics may play a role in asthma development. If your mom or dad has asthma, or if family members have a history of allergies, asthma is more likely. Common asthma triggers vary from particular foods or medicines; to animal dander, common molds and fungi, and other allergens; to smoke and other pollutants; to anger, fear, and stress.[10] Certain fever reducers or anti-inflammatory drugs may also be triggers.[11]

Approximately 19 million adults and 8 million children in the United States have asthma.[12] The rate of asthma has increased over 30 percent in the last 20 years, with nearly 8 percent of the overall population in the United States affected.[13] Asthma is now the most common chronic illness in children—affecting 1 in 10—typically striking between infancy and age 5, with a spike in prevalence between ages 15 and 34, and tapering off after age 35.[14] In childhood, asthma strikes more boys than girls; in adulthood, it strikes more women than men. Poverty, low education, and risky home and work environments as well as limited access to health care lead to clear disparities in asthma treatment and control. Asthma cases are categorized by severity and assessed based on lung function. Even with advances in treatment, asthma deaths among young people have more than doubled, with over 3,600 deaths last year in the United States.[15] See the **Skills for Behavior Change** box for ways to avoid or reduce asthma attacks.

## LO 2 | ALLERGIES

Describe the allergic response and complications associated with allergies as well as who is susceptible to allergy development.

**Allergies** are characterized by an overreaction of the immune system to a foreign protein substance (**allergen** or *antigen*) that is swallowed, breathed into the lungs, injected, or touched.[16] When foreign pathogens such as bacteria or viruses enter the body, the body responds by producing *antibodies* to destroy these invaders. Normally, antibody production is a positive element in the body's defense system. However, for unknown reasons, sometimes the body develops an overly elaborate protective mechanism against relatively harmless substances. Most commonly, these *hypersensitivity*, or allergic, reactions occur as a response to environmental antigens such as molds, animal dander (hair and dead skin), pollen,

**allergy** Hypersensitive reaction to a specific antigen in which the body produces antibodies to a normally harmless substance in the environment.

**allergen** An antigen that induces a hypersensitive immune response.

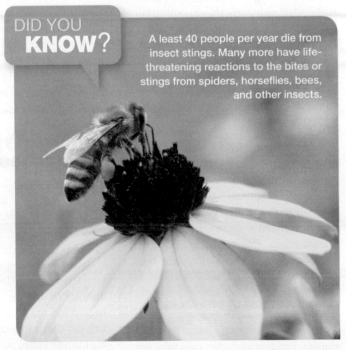

**DID YOU KNOW?**

A least 40 people per year die from insect stings. Many more have life-threatening reactions to the bites or stings from spiders, horseflies, bees, and other insects.

**Source:** Asthma and Allergy Foundation of America, "Allergy Facts and Figures," Accessed June 2015. http://www.aafa.org/display .cfm?id=9&sub=30#mort

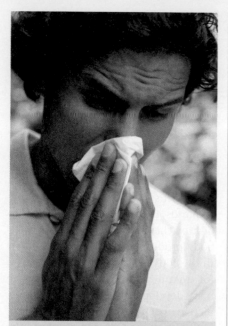

To minimize your exposure to hay fever, keep windows closed, stay indoors when pollen counts are highest (typically 10 A.M. to 4 P.M.), and change clothes after spending time outdoors.

ragweed, dust, and certain foods. Once excessive antibodies to allergens are produced, they trigger the release of **histamine,** a chemical that dilates blood vessels, increases mucus secretions, causes tissues to swell, and produces rashes, difficulty breathing, and sometimes *anaphylaxis*—a potentially life-threatening set of serious allergy symptoms. Many people have found that **immunotherapy** treatment, or "allergy shots," somewhat reduce the severity of their symptoms.

## Hay Fever

Hay fever, also known as *pollen allergy or allergic rhinitis,* is one of the most common chronic diseases in the United States, affecting nearly 18 million adults and 7 million children each year.[17] Usually considered a seasonal disease, it is

**histamine** Chemical substance that dilates blood vessels, increases mucous secretions, and produces other symptoms of allergies.

**immunotherapy** Treatment strategies based on the concept of regulating the immune system by administering antibodies or desensitizing shots of allergens.

**migraine** Throbbing headaches, often felt in one part of the head, with often debilitating symptoms such as nausia and light or sound sensitivity.

most prevalent when ragweed and flowers bloom. Hay fever attacks are characterized by sneezing and itchy, watery eyes and nose. As with other allergies, hay fever results from overzealous immune system reactions to certain substances. You are more likely to have hay fever if you have a family history of allergies or asthma, are male, or are exposed to allergens on a regular basis.

Typical over-the-counter treatment consists of antihistamines. These work well for mild cases, but may become less effective over time. Air-conditioning, whole house air filters, air purifiers, regular vacuuming, and wiping down surfaces with damp cloths can help relieve symptoms. To determine if you have pollen allergy, the best bet is to get tested by an *allergist*—a doctor specializing in allergies. Typical treatments include prescription medications and/or allergy shots. While allergy shots are one of the most effective ways of treatment, new tablets that dissolve under the tongue provide similar relief. See an allergist with questions about treatments best for you.[18]

## LO 3 | HEADACHES

Explain common types of headaches, their risk factors, and possible causes.

The fourth leading cause of emergency room visits, severe headaches or migraines affect over 14 percent of U.S adults 18 years or older.[19] Adults aged 18 to 44 are more likely to visit emergency rooms for headaches than other age group.[20] Major types of headaches include tension headaches, migraines, and cluster headaches.

## Tension-Type Headaches

Nearly 90 percent of women and 70 percent of men have *tension-type headaches* during their lives.[21] The most common type of headache, they are generally caused by muscle contractions or tension and pain in the neck or head, forehead, or temples; they can last for as little as 30 minutes or as long as a week.[22] Possible triggers include stress, depression and anxiety, jaw clenching, poor posture, or working in an awkward position. Red wine, lack of sleep, extreme fasting, hormonal changes, and certain food additives or

**SEE IT!** VIDEOS
Plagued by serious headaches? Watch **Migraine Breakthrough,** available on **MasteringHealth**™

preservatives have also been implicated.[23] Relaxation, hot water treatment, and massage are holistic treatments. Aspirin, ibuprofen, acetaminophen, and naproxen sodium can also help.

## Migraine Headaches

The prevalence of **migraines,** vascular headaches with often debilitating symptoms, is high, with 1 in 7 Americans affected annually.[24] Women are disproportionately affected, particularly during their reproductive years, leading to millions of visits to doctor's offices, outpatient clinics, and emergency rooms.[25] Migraine appears to run in families: If both your parents experience migraines, you have a 75 percent chance of experiencing them, too; if only one parent has them, you have a 50 percent chance.[26]

Symptoms vary greatly by individual, and attacks typically last anywhere from 4 to 72 hours, with distinct phases

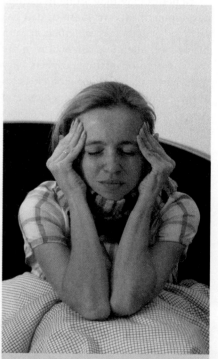

Patients report that migraines can be triggered by a litany of causes. What triggers a migraine in one person may relieve it in another.

of symptoms. Roughly, one third of people who get migraines can predict an attack based on a sensory warning sign called an *aura,* such as flashes of light, flickering vision, blind spots, tingling in arms or legs, or a sensation of odor or taste.[27] Sometimes nausea, vomiting, and extreme sensitivity to light and sound are present. Symptoms of migraine include excruciating pain behind or around one eye and usually occur on the same side of the head. Some people experience sinus pain, neck pain, or an aura without headache. Although vascular abnormalities in the brain have long been suspected as underlying causes, migraines may be triggered as a result of a complex biochemical and inflammatory process within the brain, possibly genetic.[28]

Treatment focuses on prevention of attacks and relief of symptoms. Drugs used for pain, epilepsy, depression, and high blood pressure may be used, along with stress management, trigger reduction, hormone therapies, and other medicines.

## Cluster Headaches

The pain of a cluster headache has been described as "killer" or "suicidal." Usually these headaches cause stabbing pain on one side of the head, behind the eye, or in one defined spot. Fortunately, cluster headaches are among the more rare forms of headache, affecting less than 1 percent of people, usually men. Adults in their twenties tend to be particularly susceptible.[29]

Cluster headaches can last for weeks and disappear quickly. More commonly, they last for 40 to 90 minutes in the middle of the night, usually during rapid eye movement (REM) sleep. Oxygen therapy, drugs, and even surgery have been used to treat severe cases.

## LO 4 | DIGESTION-RELATED DISORDERS

Outline risk factors, symptoms, and strategies for preventing irritable bowel syndrome (IBS), Crohn's disease, and ulcerative colitis.

Diseases of the gastrointestinal tract appear to be on the rise among adults young and old. We will focus on three of the more common "gut aches": *Irritable bowel syndrome (IBS) and the inflammatory bowel diseases (IBD) Crohn's disease and ulcerative colitis.*

## Irritable Bowel Syndrome (IBS)

**Irritable bowel syndrome (IBS)** includes a group of symptoms such as pain, bloating, discomfort in the abdomen, and fluctuations in bowel movements ranging from acute diarrhea to constipation. It is a form of *functional gastrointestinal (GI) disorder* where there is no apparent damage, but the GI tract, including muscular activities and food processing and elimination don't work normally.[30] An estimated 10 to 15 percent of U.S. adults suffer from IBS; often beginning in adolescence, IBS affects twice as many women as men, typically occurring in people under 45.[31] Because symptoms are so similar to many other gastrointestinal diseases, IBS is often diagnosed only after all others are ruled out.[32]

Although the cause is unknown, several factors, including problems with brain/gut signals, GI motility, pain sensitivity, infections, neurotransmitters and hormones, food sensitivity, anxiety, depression, stress, and genetic links are all being studied.[33] Treatment focuses on diet, medications to control symptoms, probiotics, and behavioral therapies including relaxation and stress management.[34]

## Crohn's Disease

**Crohn's disease** refers to a chronic inflammation of the small intestine and other areas of the GI tract, often referred to as an *inflammatory bowel disease (IBD).* Genes, environmental exposures, and an autoimmune reaction are among the most likely culprits.[35] Symptoms include diarrhea, abdominal pain and cramping, weight loss, fatigue, fever, and nausea/vomiting as well as skin problems, joint pain, and eye irritation. Irritation and inflammation can lead to perforations of the intestinal lining, leading to bleeding and life-threatening complications.[36] Like IBS, Crohn's disease tends to affect younger adults, although it can affect people of any ages, with increased risk among those who smoke and those with a family history of Crohn's.[37] Those diagnosed must carefully monitor diet to ensure adequate nutrition, be "tuned in" to their body and its changes, see their doctors if symptoms develop, and take medications to reduce inflammation and

# 10-15%

OF ADULTS IN THE UNITED STATES SUFFER FROM **IRRITABLE BOWEL SYNDROME**.

**irritable bowel syndrome** A functional bowel disorder caused by certain foods or stress that is characterized by nausea, pain, gas, or diarrhea.

**Crohn's disease** Type of inflammatory bowel disease (IBD) that can affect several parts of the GI tract as well has have significant affects on other body organs and systems.

prevent infection.[38] Surgery to remove damaged or obstructed portions of the bowel are sometimes necessary.

## Ulcerative Colitis

**Ulcerative colitis** is an IBD that affects the colon. It often first flares in the teens and can continue for life.[39] Symptoms may begin with loose stools and progress to pain, cramping, and bouts of bloody diarrhea. Nausea, vomiting, and fever may occur, and severe cases can affect the skin, joints, eyes, liver, and other organs. While the cause is unknown, ulcerative colitis appears to have a genetic component and is more common in males than females. Other risks appear to be exposure to a food-borne illness or allergy or infection in the GI tract.[40] Treatment focuses on relieving the symptoms by decreasing foods that are hard to digest; taking probiotics; and taking anti-inflammatory drugs, steroids, and other medications. Colon cancer risks are higher among those with ulcerative colitis, as is the risk of having to remove the colon if other treatment is ineffective.

## LO 5 | MUSCULOSK-ELETAL DISEASES

Explain the risk factors and symptoms of musculoskeletal problems and repetitive motion/stress disorders and suggest strategies for prevention.

- - - - - - - - - - - - - - - - - - - - - - - - - - -

**Musculoskeletal diseases** impact more than 1.7 billion people, making them the second largest cause of disability

**ulcerative colitis** An inflammatory bowel disease that affects the mucous membranes of the large intestine and can lead to ulcers, erosion of the outer lining of the colon, and serious bleeding.

**musculoskeletal diseases** Disorders affecting the musculoskeletal system, including muscles, tendons, nerves, and joints.

**arthritis** Painful inflammatory disease of the joints.

**osteoarthritis (OA)** Progressive deterioration of bones and joints that has been associated with the wear-and-tear theory of aging; also called *degenerative joint disease.*

**rheumatoid arthritis** Painful form of arthritis that occurs when the body's immune system attacks its own body cells.

**psoriatic arthritis** Form of inflammatory arthritis that causes acute pain and disability, often among those with a personal or family history of psoriasis.

globally.[41] In the United States, 1 in 2 (126.6 million) adults have musculoskeletal problems. Economic implications are staggering, with an estimated $874 billion (5.7% GDP) annual U.S. cost for treatment and lost wages.[42]

## Arthritis

Nearly 23 percent of Americans, or 53 million adults and 300,000 children, have one of the doctor-diagnosed forms of **arthritis**.[43] Arthritis consists of more than 100 conditions that wreak havoc on joints, bones, muscles, organs, cartilage, and connective tissues, leading to disability and pain. Arthritis affects people of all ages, sexes, and races. Two thirds of those with arthritis are under the age of 65.[44] Numbers of diagnosed cases are expected to exceed 67 million in the United States by 2030.[45]

Also called *degenerative joint disease,* **osteoarthritis (OA)** is the most common form of arthritis.[46] Before age 45, more men than women have osteoarthritis; after age 45, more women have it.[47] Although age, wear and tear, and injury are undoubtedly factors in osteoarthritis, heredity, abnormal joint use, diet and excess weight, abnormalities in joint structure, and impaired blood supply to the joint may also contribute. Weight loss; keeping active; strength, balance, and flexibility exercises; sleep; and healthy diet are important for arthritis management. For most people, anti-inflammatory drugs, over-the-counter and prescription pain relievers, and cortisone-related agents ease discomfort. In some sufferers, applications of heat and massage also relieve the pain. Surgical intervention can be necessary.

Other major forms include **rheumatoid arthritis**, in which a person's immune system attacks body tissues, including joints and other organs, causing inflammation, damage to affected areas, and pain/disability. **Psoriatic arthritis** is a disabling form of arthritis that can affect people with a family or personal history of *psoriasis*, a skin disease. Genetic and environmental factors may contribute to risk for both types.

## Low Back Pain

Approximately 85 percent of all Americans will experience low back pain (LBP)

at some point.[48] Not just for the elderly, a recent meta-analysis of LBP prevalence indicates between 3 and 35 percent of youth experience LBP each year.[49] A large survey of college students indicates low back pain to be the third most common problem treated on campus, after allergies and sinus infections.[50] Often, LBP is chronic and comes and goes with activities as varied as sneezing, bending over, and lifting heavy objects.[51] About 12 percent of those with LBP become permanently disabled.[52] Some episodes of low back pain result from muscular damage and are short lived and acute; others may involve dislocations, fractures, or problems with spinal vertebrae or discs, resulting in sciatica—intense pain and numbness in the leg or pain so severe that surgery is a last resort. Affecting over 632 million people and growing, LBP is the leading cause of disability.[53]

The vast majority of all back problems occur in the lumbar spine (lower back). You can avoid many problems by consciously maintaining good posture. Other things you can do to reduce risks of back pain are the following:

- Purchase a high-quality, supportive mattress, and avoid sleeping on your stomach.
- Avoid high-heeled shoes and wear shoes with good arch support.

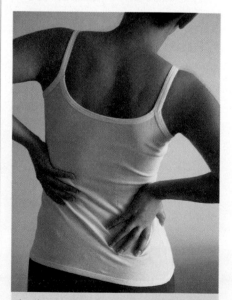

In the United States, low back pain is the major cause of disability for people of all ages.

- Avoid carrying heavy bags on one shoulder. Off-load some of the weight to your hips with a backpack.
- Control your weight.
- Warm-up and stretch before exercising or lifting heavy objects.
- When lifting something heavy, use your leg muscles and proper form. Do not bend from the waist or take the weight load on your back.
- Buy a chair with good lumbar support for desk work.
- Move your car seat forward so your knees are elevated slightly.
- Exercise regularly, particularly exercises that strengthen the core and abdominal muscles and stretch the back muscles.

# Repetitive Motion Disorders

*Repetitive motion disorders* (RMDs), also known as *"repetitive stress injuries (RSIs)"* include carpal tunnel syndrome, bursitis, tendonitis, ganglion cysts, and others.[54] Twisting of the arm or wrist, overexertion, and incorrect posture are usually contributors. Hands, wrists, elbows, and shoulders are most often affected, but the neck, back, hips, knees, feet, ankles, and legs can be affected, too. Over time, RMDs can cause permanent damage to nerves, soft tissue, and joints.

One of the most common RMDs is **carpal tunnel syndrome,** a product of spending hours typing at the computer,

**carpal tunnel syndrome** An occupational injury in which the median nerve in the wrist becomes irritated, causing numbness, tingling, and pain in the fingers and hands.

flipping groceries through computerized scanners, or other repeated hand and wrist movements. Such motions irritate the median nerve in the wrist, causing numbness, tingling, and pain in the fingers and hands. Better ergonomic workplace designs can eliminate many injuries of this nature. Physical and occupational therapy is an important part of treatment and eventual recovery.

Certain characteristics place people at greater risk for chronic illness. Examine areas below where you have checked *Yes*. If you have several risks for a given problem, think about how to reduce risks and talk with your doctor about possible concerns.

## 1 Chronic Lung Disease

|  | Yes | No |
|---|---|---|
| 1. As part of your daily routine, are you exposed to environmental toxins, such as tobacco smoke, air pollution, asbestos, or silica dust? | ◯ | ◯ |
| 2. Do you smoke? | ◯ | ◯ |
| 3. Does your family have a history of lung disease? | ◯ | ◯ |

## 2 Allergies

|  | Yes | No |
|---|---|---|
| 1. Were you exposed to cigarette smoke at home? | ◯ | ◯ |
| 2. Does your family have a history of allergies? | ◯ | ◯ |
| 3. Do you live in an area where pollen counts are high and/or air-quality levels are less than desirable? | ◯ | ◯ |

## 3 Headaches

|  | Yes | No |
|---|---|---|
| 1. Do you suffer from higher than normal levels of anxiety or stress? | ◯ | ◯ |
| 2. Is your desk or chair positioned such that you often have a stiff neck or unusual tension in your head/neck area? | ◯ | ◯ |
| 3. Does your family have a history of headaches? | ◯ | ◯ |

## 4 Digestion-Related Disorders

|  | Yes | No |
|---|---|---|
| 1. Do you suffer from bowel irregularity symptoms such as abdominal pain and/or bloating on a regular basis? | ◯ | ◯ |
| 2. Do you often experience heartburn, gas, or nausea? | ◯ | ◯ |
| 3. Does your family have a history of digestion-related disorders? | ◯ | ◯ |

## 5 Musculoskeletal Diseases

|  | Yes | No |
|---|---|---|
| 1. Are you overweight and/or not getting enough physical activity? | ◯ | ◯ |
| 2. Do you often carry a backpack or laptop thrown over one shoulder? | ◯ | ◯ |
| 3. Does your work require that you use one body part such as your wrist or elbow over and over again in the same motion? | ◯ | ◯ |
| 4. Do you have a family history of musculo-skeletal disease? | ◯ | ◯ |

## YOUR PLAN FOR CHANGE

Now that you have completed the **ASSESS YOURSELF** activity and considered your results, you may need to take further steps to understand and address your risks.

**TODAY, YOU CAN:**

☐ Make an appointment with your doctor to discuss symptoms or potential risk factors.

☐ Find out if your parents have had similar problems or know of anyone in your family who has.

**WITHIN THE NEXT TWO WEEKS, YOU CAN:**

☐ If you suffer from migraines, keep a diary of triggers. Create a routine that keeps you out of harm's way.

☐ If you suffer from irritable bowel syndrome, identify the foods or situations that bring it on.

**BY THE END OF THE SEMESTER, YOU CAN:**

☐ Adjust your routine to avoid environmental toxins. Avoid going to parties where people smoke, for example.

☐ Keep track of allergy-related symptoms to see if you can identify any likely triggers.

☐ Replace all cleaning products for your house, apartment, or dorm room with ones made from natural ingredients.

# STUDY PLAN

Customize your study plan—and master your health!—in the Study Area of MasteringHealth™

## CHAPTER REVIEW

To hear an MP3 Tutor Session, scan here or visit the Study Area in **MasteringHealth.**

### LO 1 | Chronic Lower Respiratory (Lung) Diseases

- Chronic lower respiratory disease (CLRD) (including bronchitis, emphysema, and asthma) is the third leading cause of death in the United States (right after heart disease and cancer).

### LO 2 | Allergies

- Allergies occur as the immune system responds to allergens. They can be triggered by pollens, foods, or other substances. Allergic rhinitis is more common among those with a family history of hay fever or other allergies.

### LO 3 | Headaches

- The most common types of headache are tension, migraine, and cluster. Prevention includes reducing triggers. Treatment includes medication, environmental changes, and behavioral strategies.

### LO 4 | Digestion-Related Disorders

- Irritable bowel syndrome (IBS) and other digestive problems affect increasing numbers of adults. Inflammatory bowel disease includes Crohn's disease and ulcerative colitis.

### LO 5 | Musculoskeletal Disorders

- Musculoskeletal problems such as arthritis, low back pain, and repetitive motion disorders cause significant pain and disability in millions of people. Many of these problems are preventable.

## POP QUIZ

Visit **MasteringHealth** to personalize your study plan with Chapter Review Quizzes and Dynamic Study Modules.

### LO 1 | Chronic Lower Respiratory (Lung) Diseases

1. Margaret experiences occasional wheezing, shortness of breath, and coughing spasms. What chronic respiratory disorder is she likely suffering from?
   a. Emphysema
   b. Bronchitis
   c. Asthma
   d. COPD

### LO 2 | Allergies

2. Julie has found that she cannot eat nuts without suffering from itching and nausea. What condition is she likely to be suffering from?
   a. Irritable bowel syndrome
   b. Ulcerative colitis
   c. Food allergy
   d. Diabetes mellitus

### LO 3 | Headaches

3. Which of the following is correct?
   a. Migraine incidence usually peaks in older adulthood (between ages 60 and 80).
   b. Women have more migraine headaches; men have more cluster headaches.
   c. Tension-type headaches are often preceded by an aura.
   d. If untreated, migraines can progress into epilepsy or another seizure-related disorder.

### LO 4 | Digestion-Related Disorders

4. Which of the following is correct?
   a. Inflammatory bowel syndrome often occurs before age 30, but can occur at any age.
   b. Crohn's disease and ulcerative colitis are examples of irritable bowel syndrome.
   c. Digestive diseases are on the decline in the United States due to improved dietary practices.
   d. Smokers have a lower risk of ulcerative colitis.

### LO 5 | Musculoskeletal Disorders

5. Which of the following conditions is currently the leading cause of disability throughout the world?
   a. Low back pain
   b. Upper respiratory infections
   c. Asthma
   d. On-the-job injuries

*Answers to the Pop Quiz can be found on page A-1. If you answered a question incorrectly, review the section identified by the Learning Outcome. For even more study tools, visit MasteringHealth.*

# 14 Preparing for Aging, Death, and Dying

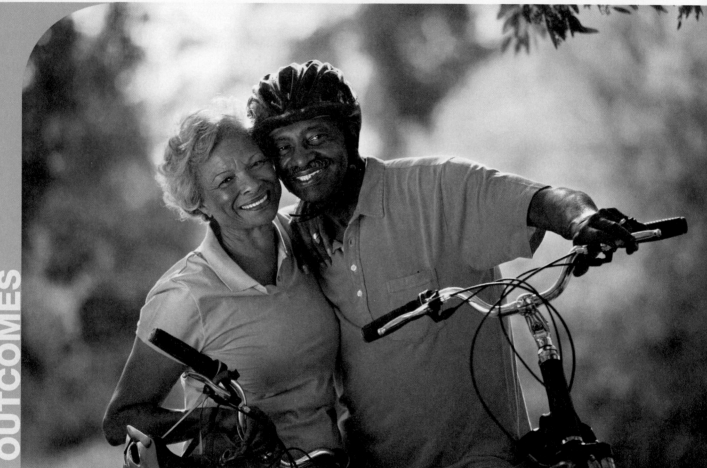

n a society that seems to worship youth, researchers have begun to offer good—even revolutionary—news about the aging process. Health promotion, disease prevention, and wellness-oriented activities can prolong vigor and productivity in older people, even among those who haven't always led model lifestyles or made healthful habits a priority. Numerous studies show that people who make even modest lifestyle changes can reap significant health benefits. In fact, getting older can mean getting better in many ways—particularly socially, psychologically, spiritually, and intellectually.

## LO 1 | AGING

Explain how the growing population of older adults will affect society, including considerations of economics, health care, living arrangements, and ethical and moral issues.

**Aging** has traditionally been described as the patterns of life changes that occur in members of all species as they grow older. Some believe that aging begins at the moment of conception. Others contend that it starts at birth. Still others believe that true aging does not begin until we reach our forties. The study of individual and collective aging processes, known as **gerontology**, explores the reasons for aging and the ways in which people cope with and adapt to this process. See the **Skills for Behavior Change** box for some characteristics shared among those who have aged well.

## Older Adults: A Growing Population

The United States and much of the developed world are on the brink of a *longevity revolution,* one that will affect society in

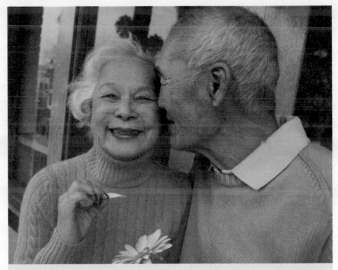

Grow old along with me!
The best is yet to be,
The last of life, for which the first was made . . .
—Robert Browning, *Rabbi Ben Ezra*

many ways. Medical care breakthroughs and improved understanding of fitness and nutrition have steadily increased life span. According to the latest statistics, life expectancy for a child born in 2014 is 79.5 years—more than 30 years longer than for a child born in 1900.[1] In 2013 there were 44.7 million people age 65 or older in the United States, making up over 14 percent of the total population.[2] In comparison, a mere 3 million people were age 65 and older in 1900 (see **FIGURE 14.1**).[3] Similar trends are true throughout the world, with the percentage of people over age 60 expected to double to 22 percent by 2050.[4]

Within the United States, the population of those over 65 will increase substantially over the next two decades due to the aging of the "baby boomer" generation, an especially large segment of the population who were born during the period of economic prosperity that began after World War II in the late 1940s and continued through the early 1960s. The oldest of the Baby Boomers are just beginning to retire, and their impact on the economy, housing market, health care system, and Social Security will be profound in coming decades.

**aging** The patterns of life changes that occur in members of all species as they grow older.

**gerontology** The study of individual and collective aging processes.

## Health Issues for an Aging Society

Meeting an older population's financial and medical needs, providing health care and adequate housing, and addressing end-of-life ethical considerations

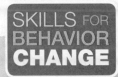
**HEAR IT!** PODCASTS

Want a study podcast for this chapter? Download **Life's Transitions: The Aging Process,** available on **MasteringHealth**™

are all of concern in an aging society. Many fear that the combination of fewer younger workers paying into the Social Security system and more older people drawing benefits for longer than ever before will result in tremendous government budget shortfalls and the potential bankruptcy of the system.

**Health Care Costs** Older Americans averaged $5,069 in out-of-pocket medical expenses in 2013, an increase of 35 percent since 2003.[5] About 66 percent of those costs, on average, went to pay for health insurance itself, whereas drugs or medical services not covered by insurance premiums accounted for roughly one third of the costs.[6] As people live longer, the chances of developing a costly chronic disease increase, and as technology improves, chronic illnesses that once were quickly fatal may now be treated successfully for years. Most older adults have at least one chronic condition: About 34 percent have hypertension, 49 percent have been diagnosed with arthritis, 31 percent have heart disease, 25 percent have cancer, and 21 percent have diabetes.[7]

**Housing and Living Arrangements** Most older adults never live in a nursing home. Many live with a spouse, partner, or alone; others live with family or friends or pay for home health services. An increasing number opt for assisted living in apartments, foster homes, or individual homes with supportive services like meals, help with housekeeping and medication, or other options that help seniors live independently (**FIGURE 14.2**). Other communities and facilities include 24/7 monitoring of unique needs, such as Alzheimer's cases or other disabilities. Newer, technologically advanced housing includes physiological monitoring that records heart rate and other life indicators to ensure prompt emergency services in case of problems. With increasing age comes an increased likelihood of some form of institutional setting, with just over 1 percent of those aged 65 to 74 years, 3 percent of

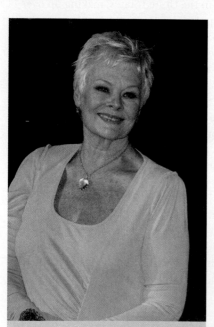

The people we often think of as aging gracefully—such as actress Dame Judi Dench—are those who continue to be active and productive; who are not frightened or ashamed of growing older; who adapt to the changing circumstances of their lives; and who strive to be healthy, vibrant, and alive at any age.

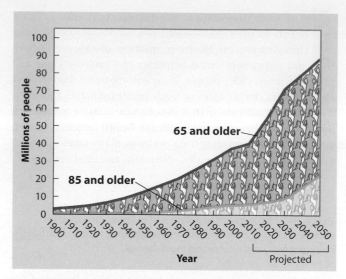

**FIGURE 14.1** Number of Americans 65 and Older (in millions), Years 1900–2008, and Projected 2010–2050

**Note:** Data for 2010–2050 are projections of the population.
**Source:** Data from U.S. Census Bureau, Decennial Census, Population Estimates and Projections, www.census.gov

those 75 to 85 years, and 10 percent of those over 85 years living in nursing homes.[8]

If you have the money, the sky's the limit in terms of care during your later years. Savings plans, long-term care insurance, supportive family members, and progressive communities provide many options for those who know how to maneuver in an increasingly complex, costly system. The average cost for institutional care varies tremendously by state and level of care, starting at more than $90,000 per year for a private room in a nursing home to $40,000 to $50,000 for an assisted living facility room.[9] Tremendous income-based disparities exist in caring for the elderly, and even with significant savings, many elderly budgets will be stretched to the limit. Many American seniors live on small fixed incomes, and in 2014 the *supplemental poverty measure* calculated by the government estimated that about 9.5 percent of seniors lived

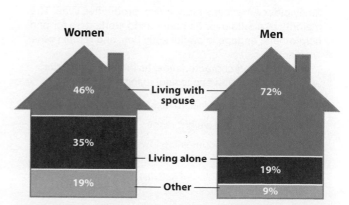

**FIGURE 14.2** Living Arrangements of Americans Age 65 and Older Percentages may not total 100% due to rounding.

**Source:** Administration on Aging, U.S. Dept. of Health and Human Services, "A Profile of Older Americans: Living Arrangements, 2014," 2015, www.aoa.acl.gov/Aging_Statistics/Profile/2014/docs/2014-Profile.pdf

# 3.4%

OF **SENIOR CITIZENS** LIVE IN SKILLED NURSING CARE FACILITIES.

in poverty in the United States.[10] Those without means are more likely to be shut out of all but the most meager care situations.

**Ethical and Moral Considerations** Difficult ethical questions arise when we consider the implications of an already overburdened health care system. The cost of care versus the quality and length of life it buys, particularly for terminally ill older people, is something each society must weigh. Is the prolonging of life at all costs a moral imperative, or will future generations devise a set of criteria for deciding who will be helped and who will not? Is one life worth more than another? If so, who should decide? Such debates leave much room for careful thought and discussion.

## LO 2 | PHYSICAL AND MENTAL CHANGES OF AGING

Describe the physical and mental changes associated with aging and the unique health challenges faced by older adults.

Although the physiological consequences of aging can differ in severity and timing, certain standard changes occur as a result of the aging process. Many of these changes are physical (see **FIGURE 14.3**), whereas others are mental or psychosocial.

### The Skin

As a normal part of aging, the skin becomes thinner and loses elasticity, particularly in the outer surfaces. Fat deposits, which add to the soft lines and shape of the skin, diminish. Starting at about age 30, lines develop on the forehead as a result of smiling, squinting, and other facial expressions. During the forties, these lines become more pronounced, with added "crow's feet" around the eyes. In a person's fifties and sixties, the skin begins to sag and lose color, which leads to pallor in the seventies. Body fat in underlying layers of skin continues to be redistributed away from the limbs and extremities into the body's trunk region. Age spots become

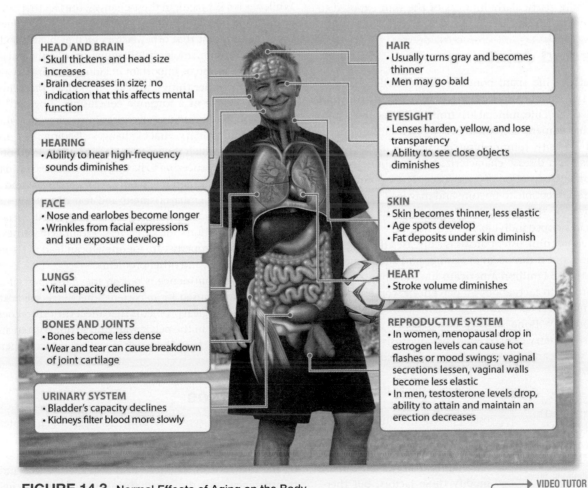

**HEAD AND BRAIN**
• Skull thickens and head size increases
• Brain decreases in size; no indication that this affects mental function

**HEARING**
• Ability to hear high-frequency sounds diminishes

**FACE**
• Nose and earlobes become longer
• Wrinkles from facial expressions and sun exposure develop

**LUNGS**
• Vital capacity declines

**BONES AND JOINTS**
• Bones become less dense
• Wear and tear can cause breakdown of joint cartilage

**URINARY SYSTEM**
• Bladder's capacity declines
• Kidneys filter blood more slowly

**HAIR**
• Usually turns gray and becomes thinner
• Men may go bald

**EYESIGHT**
• Lenses harden, yellow, and lose transparency
• Ability to see close objects diminishes

**SKIN**
• Skin becomes thinner, less elastic
• Age spots develop
• Fat deposits under skin diminish

**HEART**
• Stroke volume diminishes

**REPRODUCTIVE SYSTEM**
• In women, menopausal drop in estrogen levels can cause hot flashes or mood swings; vaginal secretions lessen, vaginal walls become less elastic
• In men, testosterone levels drop, ability to attain and maintain an erection decreases

**FIGURE 14.3** Normal Effects of Aging on the Body

➤ **VIDEO TUTOR**
Effects of Aging on Body

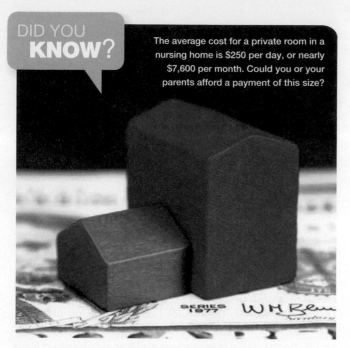
more numerous because of excessive pigment accumulation under the skin, particularly in areas of the skin exposed to heavy sun.

## Bones and Joints

Throughout the life span, bones are continually changing because of the accumulation and loss of minerals. By the third or fourth decade of life, mineral loss from bones becomes more prevalent than mineral accumulation, which results in a weakening and porosity (diminishing density) of bony tissue. **Osteoporosis** is a disease characterized by low bone density and structural deterioration of bone tissue. These porous, fragile bones are susceptible to fracture and may lead to crippling malformation of the spine characteristic of the dowager's hump seen in stooped individuals.

Many people think osteoporosis is a disease affecting only older women, but it can occur at any age and affects men, as well. More than 54 million Americans have low bone density or osteoporosis. In fact, about 50 percent of women and 25 percent of men over 50 years of age will break a bone because of osteoporosis.[11] Bone density scans using dual-energy X-ray absorptiometry can screen for osteoporosis. With early detection, steps can be taken to reverse bone loss and prevent fractures.

Some of the factors that predispose a person to developing osteoporosis are intrinsic and cannot be controlled, including gender, age, body size, ethnicity, and family history. You cannot modify these factors, but there *are* things you can do to prevent the disease. During your lifetime,

**osteoporosis** A degenerative bone disorder characterized by increasingly porous bones.

**urinary incontinence** Inability to control urination.

**cataracts** Clouding of the lens that interrupts the focusing of light on the retina, resulting in blurred vision or eventual blindness.

bone is constantly being added (formation) and being broken down and removed (reabsorption). At around age 30, a person reaches *peak bone mass*. After this point, a slow and steady decline occurs. Individuals who develop strong, dense, healthy bones through proper diet and exercise can minimize this decline and reduce their risk for osteoporosis.

Adequate calcium intake is important, as is vitamin D, which helps the body absorb and use calcium more efficiently. Bone is a living tissue that grows stronger with exercise and weight-bearing activity; therefore, bone loss can be slowed or prevented with regular weight-bearing exercise, such as walking, jogging, and dancing, as well as through strength training. Unhealthy behaviors that contribute to bone loss include smoking, excessive alcohol consumption, and anorexia nervosa.

Another bone condition that afflicts almost 27 million Americans is *osteoarthritis,* a progressive breakdown of joint cartilage that becomes more common with age and is a major cause of disability in the United States.[12]

## The Urinary Tract

For about two thirds of us, the thirties and forties bring a gradual decrease in the size and weight of the kidneys, effectively reducing blood filtering and other functions. In addition, shrinkage/thinning of the bladder and urinary tract affect urination.[13] While age is a key factor in these changes, the fact that one third of the aging population doesn't experience these declines supports the idea that that other factors such as high blood pressure, lead exposure, smoking, inflammation, obesity, and plaque formation may also be important in kidney and urinary risks. If so, like many other things, urinary and kidney problems may not be inevitable or a foregone conclusion of aging.[14] Some changes, such as hormonal decreases in women, may increase bladder and urinary tract changes leading to **urinary incontinence**, which ranges from passing a few drops of urine while laughing or sneezing to having no control over urination.

Incontinence can pose major social, physical, and emotional problems. Embarrassment and fear of wetting oneself may cause an older person to become isolated socially or increased frustrations for caregivers. Prolonged wetness and the inability to properly care for oneself can lead to tissue irritation, infections, and other problems.

However, incontinence is not an inevitable part of aging. Most cases are caused by persistent infections, medications, treatable neurological problems that affect the central nervous system, weakness in the pelvic wall, and so on. With treatment and exercises to strengthen pelvic wall, the incontinence is usually resolved.

## The Senses

With aging, the senses (vision, hearing, touch, taste, and smell) become less acute. By the time a person reaches age 30, the lens of the eye begins to harden, which can cause problems by the early forties. The lens also begins to yellow and lose transparency, and the pupil shrinks, allowing less light to penetrate. By age 60, depth perception declines, and farsightedness often develops. **Cataracts** (clouding of the lens) and

**glaucoma** (elevated pressure within the eyeball) become more likely. Eventually, a tendency toward color blindness may develop, especially for shades of blue and green. **Macular degeneration** is the breakdown of the light-sensitive area of the retina responsible for the sharp, direct vision needed to read or drive. Its effects can be devastating to independent older adults and causes are still being investigated.

*Presbycusis*, or age-related hearing loss, is one of the most common chronic conditions of the elderly—affecting an estimated 28 million Americans by 2030.[15] It appears that hearing loss may play a much greater role in maintaining health in the elderly than was thought. A new study has found that hearing loss and mental decline may be related—showing that older people with hearing deficits were more likely than those with normal hearing to develop problems with memory and thinking.[16]

With age, the ear structure also experiences changes and often deteriorates. The eardrum thickens and the inner ear bones are affected. The inner ear is the portion that controls balance (equilibrium). As a result, it often becomes difficult for a person to maintain balance. Studies have shown that exercises including resistance/strength training, yoga, and tai chi can improve balance in older adults.[17] The ability to hear high-frequency consonants (e.g., *s, t,* and *z*) also diminishes with age. Much of the actual hearing loss lies in the inability to distinguish extreme ranges of sound rather than in the inability to distinguish normal conversational tones.

## Sexual Function

As men age, they experience noticeable alterations in sexual function. Although the degree and rate of change vary greatly from man to man, several changes generally occur, including a slowed ability to obtain an erection, diminished ability to maintain an erection, and a decline in angle of the erection. Men may also experience a longer refractory period between orgasms and shortened duration of orgasm.

Women also experience several changes in sexual function as they age. Menopause usually occurs between the ages of 45 and 55. Women may experience hot flashes, mood swings, weight gain, development of facial hair, or other hormone-related symptoms. The walls of the vagina become less elastic, and the epithelium thins, possibly making intercourse painful. Vaginal secretions, particularly during sexual activity, diminish. The breasts become less firm, and loss of fat in various areas leads to fewer curves, with a decrease in the soft lines of body contours.

Although these physiological changes may sound discouraging, sex is still an essential component in the lives of those in their mid-fifties and older, and many people remain sexually active throughout their entire adult lives. According to a recent study, more than 80 percent of 50- to 90-year-olds are sexually active.[18] With the advent of drugs such as Viagra and medical interventions designed to treat sexual dysfunction, many older adults are able to be sexually active. However, older adults also report low percentages of condom use, signifying a need for education regarding the spread of STIs.

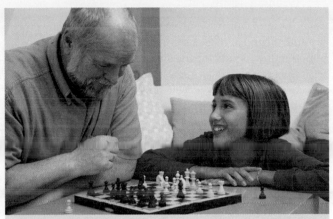

Certain physiological conditions or diseases may cause older people to experience memory loss, but in general the knowledge and memories gained through a lifetime remain intact.

## Mental Function and Memory

Given an appropriate length of time, older people learn and develop skills in a manner similar to that of younger people. Researchers have also determined that what many older adults lack in speed of learning they make up for in practical knowledge—that is, the "wisdom of age." Memory loss is not necessarily a normal part of aging; however, as a person ages, drug interactions, vascular deficiencies, hormonal or biochemical imbalances, and other physiological changes can make memory lapses occur more frequently. Although short-term memory may fluctuate on a daily basis, the ability to remember events from past decades seems to remain largely unchanged in the absence of disease.

### Dementias and Alzheimer's Disease

Memory failure, errors in judgment, disorientation, or erratic behavior can occur at any age and for various reasons, including nutrient deficiency (such as vitamin B deficiency), alcohol abuse, medication interactions, vascular problems, tumors, hormonal or metabolic imbalances, or any number of problems. Often, when the underlying issues are corrected, the memory loss and disorientation also improve. The terms *dementing diseases,* or **dementias,** are used to describe either reversible symptoms or progressive forms of brain malfunctioning.

Although there are many types of dementia, one of the most common forms is **Alzheimer's disease (AD).** Affecting an estimated 1 in 9 Americans over the age of 65 (5.3 million), this disease is one of the most painful and devastating conditions that families can endure.[19] Alzheimer's disease is a degenerative illness in which areas of the brain develop "tangles" that impair the way nerve cells communicate with one another, eventually

**glaucoma** Elevation of pressure within the eyeball, leading to hardening of the eyeball, impaired vision, and possible blindness.

**macular degeneration** Breakdown of the macula, the light-sensitive part of the retina responsible for sharp, direct vision.

**dementias** Progressive brain impairments that interfere with memory and normal intellectual functioning.

**Alzheimer's disease (AD)** A chronic condition involving changes in nerve fibers of the brain that results in mental deterioration.

causing them to die. This disease characteristically progresses in stages, each of which is marked by increasingly impaired memory and judgment. In later stages of the disease, these symptoms can be accompanied by agitation and restlessness (especially at night), loss of sensory perceptions, muscle twitching, and repetitive actions. Many patients become depressed, combative, and aggressive.

The final stage often includes complete disorientation, with patients becoming entirely dependent on the help of others to dress, eat, and perform other daily activities. Identity loss and speech problems are common. Eventually, control of bodily functions may be lost. Patients with AD live for an average of 4 to 6 years after diagnosis, although the disease can last for up to 20 years.[20]

The number of individuals with AD has significantly increased in the United States. Because of the growing number of people over age 65 in the United States, the annual number of new cases of Alzheimer's and other dementias is projected to almost triple by 2050.[21] An estimated 15 million family members and friends cared for a person with Alzheimer's disease or another dementia in 2010.[22] Caring for a person with AD can be a heavy financial burden; the average cost of full-time nursing care is about $80,000 each year.[23] Most people associate the disease with the aged, but AD has been diagnosed in people in their late forties.

Researchers are investigating several possible causes of the disease, including genetic predisposition, immune system malfunction, a slow-acting virus, chromosomal or genetic defects, chronic inflammation, uncontrolled hypertension, and neurotransmitter imbalance. There is no treatment that can stop the progression of AD, but there are medications that can prevent some symptoms from progressing for a short period of time or relieve symptoms such as sleeplessness, anxiety, and depression. Some researchers are looking at anti-inflammatory drugs, theorizing that AD may develop in response to an inflammatory ailment. Others are focusing on studying deposits of protein called plaques and their role in damaging and killing nerve cells.[24]

## WHY SHOULD I CARE?

Aging isn't a distant process somewhere in the future—it's something that is happening to every one of us every day of our lives. The way you live your life now has a direct impact on how you will live it in the future. Learning to cope with challenges and changes early in life develops attitudes and skills that contribute to a full and satisfying old age.

## LO 3 | STRATEGIES FOR HEALTHY AGING

List strategies for successful and healthy aging.

You can do many things to prolong and improve the quality of your life. To provide for healthy older years, make each of the following part of your younger years.

## Successful Aging

The key factors to living long and well include maintaining a healthy lifestyle. Maintaining a healthy lifestyle includes avoiding unhealthy habits such as smoking, excessive alcohol use, and obesity. Adherence to a healthy lifestyle can delay the onset of chronic illnesses.

## Improve Fitness

Just about any moderate-intensity exercise that gets your heart beating faster and increases strength and/or flexibility will maximize your physical health and functional years. One of the physical changes that the body undergoes is *sarcopenia,* age-associated loss of muscle mass. The less muscle you have, the less energy you will burn even while resting. The lower your metabolic rate, the more likely you will gain weight. With regular strength training, you can increase your muscle mass, boost your metabolism, strengthen your bones, prevent osteoporosis, and, in general, feel better and function more efficiently.

Both aerobic and muscle-strengthening activities are critical for healthy aging. TABLE 14.1 lists the basic recommendations for aerobic and strength-training exercises in older adults. In addition to these, the Centers for Disease Control and Prevention recommends that people who are at risk of falling perform regular balance exercises.[25] It is also recommended that older adults or adults with chronic conditions develop an activity plan with a health professional to manage risks and take therapeutic needs into account. This will maximize the benefits of physical activity and ensure your safety.

## TABLE 14.1 | Exercise Recommendations for Adults over Age 65

| Option 1 | Option 2 | Option 3 |
| --- | --- | --- |
| Moderate-intensity aerobic activity (e.g., brisk walking) at least 2 hours and 30 minutes every week | Vigorous-intensity aerobic activity (e.g., jogging or running) at least 1 hour and 15 minutes every week | An equal mix of moderate- and vigorous-intensity aerobic activity |
| *and* | *and* | *and* |
| muscle-strengthening activity, working all major muscle groups, 2 or more days a week | muscle-strengthening activity, working all major muscle groups, 2 or more days a week | muscle-strengthening activity 2 or more days a week |

**Source:** Centers for Disease Control, "How Much Physical Activity Do Older Adults Need?," 2014, www.cdc.gov

**SEE IT!** VIDEOS

What are the options to consider at the end of life? Watch **Opting Out of Old Age?** in the Study Area of MasteringHealth™

# 53,364

## Eat for Longevity

Although other chapters in this text provide detailed information about nutrition and weight control, certain nutrients are especially essential to healthy aging:

- **Calcium.** Bone loss tends to increase in women, particularly in the hip region, shortly before menopause. During perimenopause and menopause, this bone loss accelerates rapidly, with an average of about 3 percent skeletal mass lost per year over a 5-year period. The result is an increased risk for fracture and disability. Adequate consumption of calcium throughout one's life can help prevent bone loss.
- **Vitamin D.** Vitamin D is necessary for adequate calcium absorption, yet as people age, particularly in their fifties and sixties, they do not absorb vitamin D from foods as readily as they did in their younger years. If vitamin D is unavailable, calcium levels are also likely to be lower.
- **Protein.** As some older adults become concerned about cholesterol and fatty foods and others face a limited food budget, they often cut back on protein. Meat and seafood products cost more and have the "fat" stigma associated with animal products. Yet protein is necessary for muscle mass, and protein insufficiencies can spell trouble.

Other nutrients, including vitamin E, folic acid (folate), iron, potassium, and vitamin $B_{12}$ (cobalamin), are important to the aging process, and most of these are readily available in any diet that follows the U.S. Department of Agriculture's (USDA) MyPlate recommendations (www.choosemyplate.gov).

## Develop and Maintain Healthy Relationships

Social bonds lend vigor and energy to life. Be willing to give to others, and seek variety in your relationships rather than befriending only people who agree with you. By experiencing diverse people and points of view, we gain broader

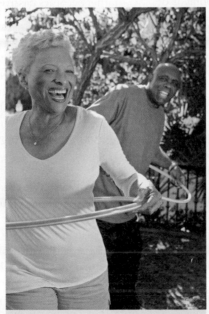

Many forms of activity can improve physical fitness.

perspective. Positive relationships are important for well-being at any age, but as people age, support systems decrease, making it particularly important to remain socially active.

## Enrich the Spiritual Side of Life

Although we often take the spiritual side of life for granted, cultivating a relationship with nature, the environment, a higher being, and yourself is a key factor in personal growth and development. Take time for thought and quiet contemplation, and enjoy the sunsets, sounds, and energy of life. Time set aside for yourself will leave you invigorated and refreshed—better able to cope with the ups and downs of life.

## LO 4 | UNDERSTANDING THE FINAL TRANSITIONS: DYING AND DEATH

Define death and discuss strategies for coping with death.

Throughout history, humans have attempted to determine the nature and meaning of death. Individuals' feelings about death vary widely, depending on many factors, including age, religious beliefs, family orientation, health, personal experience with death, and the circumstances of the death itself.

## Defining Death

According to the *Merriam Webster Dictionary,* **death** can be defined as the "a permanent cessation of all vital functions: the end of life."[26] This definition has become more significant as medical advances make it increasingly possible to postpone death. Legal and ethical issues led to the Uniform Determination of Death Act in 1981. This act, which several states have adopted, reads as follows: "An individual who has sustained either (1) irreversible cessation of circulatory and respiratory functions, or (2) irreversible cessation of all functions of the entire brain, including the brain stem, is dead. A determination of death must be made in accordance with accepted medical standards."[27]

> **death** The permanent ending of all vital functions.
>
> **brain death** The irreversible cessation of all functions of the entire brain stem.

The concept of **brain death,** defined as the irreversible cessation of all functions of the entire brain stem, has gained increasing credence. As defined by the Ad Hoc Committee of the Harvard Medical School, brain death occurs when the following criteria are met:[28]

- Unreceptivity and unresponsiveness—that is, no response even to painful stimuli
- No movement for a continuous hour after observation by a physician, and no breathing after 3 minutes off a respirator

- No reflexes, including brain stem reflexes; fixed and dilated pupils
- A "flat" electroencephalogram (EEG, which monitors electrical activity of the brain) for at least 10 minutes
- All of these tests repeated at least 24 hours later with no change
- Certainty that hypothermia (extreme loss of body heat) or depression of the central nervous system caused by use of drugs such as barbiturates are not responsible for these conditions

The Harvard report provides useful guidelines; however, the definition of death and all its ramifications continues to concern us.

## The Process of Dying

**Dying** is the process of decline in body functions that results in the death of an organism. It is a complex process that includes physical, intellectual, social, spiritual, and emotional dimensions. Now that we have examined the physical indicators of death, we must consider the emotional aspects of dying and "social death."

### Kübler-Ross and the Stages of Dying

Much of our knowledge about reactions to dying stems from the work of Elisabeth Kübler-Ross, a pioneer in **thanatology,** the study of death and dying. In 1969, Kübler-Ross published *On Death and Dying,* a sensitive analysis of the reactions of terminally ill patients. This pioneering work encouraged the development of death education as a discipline and prompted efforts to improve the care of dying patients. Kübler-Ross identified five psychological stages (**FIGURE 14.4**) that people coping with death often experience:[29]

**dying** Process of decline in body functions that results in the death of an organism.

**thanatology** The study of death and dying.

**social death** A seemingly irreversible situation in which a person is not treated like an active member of society.

1. **Denial.** ("Not me, there must be a mistake.") A person intellectually accepts the impending death but rejects it emotionally and feels a sense of shock and disbelief. The patient is too confused and stunned to comprehend "not being" and thus rejects the idea.
2. **Anger.** ("Why me?") The person becomes angry at having to face death when others, including loved ones, are healthy and not threatened. The dying person perceives the situation as unfair or senseless and may be hostile to friends, family, physicians, or the world in general.
3. **Bargaining.** ("If I'm allowed to live, I promise... .") The dying person may resolve to be a better person in return for an extension of life or may secretly pray for a short postponement of death in order to experience a special event, such as a family wedding or birth.

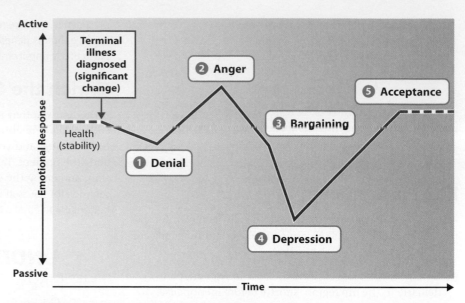

**FIGURE 14.4 Kübler-Ross's Stages of Dying** Kübler-Ross developed this model while working with terminally ill patients. She later expanded the model to apply to people experiencing grief or significant loss of any kind.

4. **Depression.** ("It's really going to happen to me, and I can't do anything about it.") Depression eventually sets in as vitality diminishes and the person begins to experience symptoms with increasing frequency. The person's deteriorating condition becomes impossible for him or her to deny. Common feelings experienced during this stage include doom, loss, worthlessness, and guilt over the emotional suffering of loved ones and arduous but seemingly futile efforts of caregivers.
5. **Acceptance.** ("I'm ready.") This is often the final stage. The patient stops battling with emotions and becomes tired and weak. With acceptance, the person does not "give up" and become sullen or resentfully resigned to death, but rather becomes passive.

Some of Kübler-Ross's contemporaries consider her stage theory too neat and orderly. Subsequent research has indicated that the experiences of dying people do not fit easily into specific stages, and patterns vary from person to person. While some people might remain emotionally calm, others may pass back and forth between the stages. Even if it is not accurate in all its particulars, however, Kübler-Ross's theory offers valuable insights for those seeking to understand or deal with the process of dying.

### Social Death

The need for recognition and appreciation within a social group is nearly universal. Loss of being valued or appreciated by others can lead to **social death**, a situation in which a person is not treated like an active member of society. Numerous studies indicate that people are treated differently when they are dying, leading them to feel

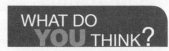

Why is there so much concern over the definition of *death*?

- How does modern technology complicate the understanding of when death occurs?

**SEE IT!** VIDEOS

Should families have group conversations about end-of-life decisions? Watch **The Conversation: A Family's Private Decision**, on **MasteringHealth**™

more isolated and unable to talk about their feelings: The dying person may be excluded from conversations or referred to as if he or she were already dead.[30] Dying patients are often moved to terminal wards and may be given minimal care; medical personnel may make degrading or impersonal comments about dying patients in their presence. In addition, inadequate pain control may contribute to patient suffering and anger or hostility, making caregiver assistance more difficult.

A decrease in meaningful social interaction often strips dying and bereaved people of their identity as valued members of society at a time when being able to talk, share, and make important decisions or say important things is critical.

## LO 5 | COPING WITH LOSS

Describe typical grief symptoms and the grieving process.

Coping with the loss of a loved one is extremely difficult. The dying person, as well as close family and friends, frequently suffers emotionally and physically from the loss of critical relationships and roles.

**Bereavement** is generally defined as the loss or deprivation that a survivor experiences when a loved one dies. In the lives of the bereaved or of close survivors, the loss of loved ones leaves "holes" and inevitable changes. Understanding normal reactions, time, patience, and support from loved ones can do much to help the bereaved heal and move on.

**Grief** occurs in reaction to significant loss, including one's own impending death, the death of a loved one, or a *quasi-death* experience (a significant loss such as the end of a relationship or job, which involves separation, rejection, or a change in personal identity). Grief may be experienced as a mental, physical, social, or emotional reaction, and often includes changes in patterns of eating, sleeping, working, and even thinking.

When a person experiences a loss that cannot be openly acknowledged, publicly mourned, or socially supported, coping may be much more difficult. This type of grief is referred to as *disenfranchised grief*. It may occur among people who experience a miscarriage, who are developmentally disabled, or who are close friends rather than blood relatives of the deceased. It may also include relationships that are not socially approved, such as extramarital affairs or homosexual relationships.

Symptoms of grief vary in severity and duration, depending on the situation and the individual. However, the bereaved person can benefit from emotional and social support from family, friends, clergy, employers, and traditional support organizations. The larger and stronger the support system, the easier readjustment is likely to be. See the **Skills for Behavior Change** box to learn about how you can best help a grieving friend.

The term *mourning* is often incorrectly equated with the term *grief*. As we have noted, *grief* refers to a wide variety of

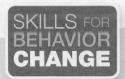

## SKILLS FOR BEHAVIOR CHANGE

### TALKING TO FRIENDS WHEN SOMEONE DIES

**DO ...**

▶ Let your genuine concern and caring show; say you are sorry about their loss and pain.

▶ Be available to listen, run errands, help with the children, or whatever else seems needed at the time.

▶ Allow them to express as much grief as they are feeling at the moment and are willing to share.

▶ Encourage them to be patient with themselves and not worry about things they should be doing.

▶ Allow them to talk about the person who has died as much and as often as they want to.

▶ Reassure them that they did everything they could, that the medical care given was the best, or whatever else you know to be true and positive about the care given.

**DON'T ...**

▶ Let your own sense of helplessness keep you from reaching out to those who are bereaved.

▶ Avoid them because you are uncomfortable.

▶ Say you know how they feel (unless you've suffered a similar loss, you probably don't).

▶ Say, "You ought to be feeling better by now" or anything else that implies judgment about their feelings or what they should be doing.

▶ Change the subject when they mention the person who has died.

feelings and actions that occur in response to bereavement. **Mourning**, in contrast, refers to culturally prescribed and accepted time periods and behavior patterns for the expression of grief. In Judaism, for example, *sitting shivah* is a designated mourning period of 7 days that involves prescribed rituals and prayers. Depending on a person's relationship with the deceased, various other rituals may continue for up to a year.

## What Is "Typical" Grief?

A bereaved person may suffer emotional pain and exhibit a variety of grief responses for many months after the death. Grief responses vary widely from person to person but frequently include periodic waves of prolonged physical distress, a feeling of tightness in the throat,

**bereavement** The loss or deprivation experienced by a survivor when a loved one dies.

**grief** An individual's reaction to significant loss, including one's own impending death, the death of a loved one, or a quasi-death experience; grief can involve mental, physical, social, or emotional responses.

**mourning** The culturally prescribed behavior patterns for the expression of grief.

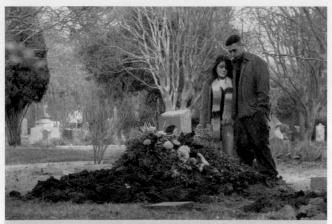

The most important thing you can do for a grieving friend is offer emotional support and a caring presence. Knowing what to say is less important than knowing how to listen.

choking and shortness of breath, a frequent need to sigh, feelings of emptiness and muscular weakness, or intense anxiety that is described as actually painful. Other common symptoms of grief include insomnia, memory lapses, loss of appetite, difficulty concentrating, a tendency to engage in repetitive or purposeless behavior, a feeling of being removed from reality, difficulty making decisions, lack of organization, excessive talking, social withdrawal or hostility, guilty feelings, and preoccupation with the image of the deceased. Susceptibility to disease increases with grief and may even be life threatening in severe and enduring cases.

**grief work** The process of accepting the reality of a person's death and coping with memories of the deceased.

**living will** A type of advance directive.

**advance directive** A document that stipulates an individual's wishes about medical care; used to make treatment decisions when and if the individual becomes physically unable to voice his or her preferences.

The rate of the healing process depends on the amount and quality of grief work that a person does. **Grief work** is the process of integrating the reality of the loss into everyday life and learning to feel better. Often, the bereaved person must deliberately and systematically work at reducing denial and coping with the pain that comes from remembering the deceased.

## Worden's Model of Grieving Tasks

William Worden, a researcher into the death process, developed an active grieving model that suggests four developmental tasks that a grieving person must complete in the grief work process:[31]

1. **Accept the reality of the loss.** This task requires acknowledging and realizing that the person is dead. Traditional rituals, such as the funeral, help many bereaved people move toward acceptance.
2. **Work through the pain of grief.** It is necessary to acknowledge and work through the pain associated with loss, or it will manifest itself through other symptoms or behaviors.

3. **Adjust to an environment in which the deceased is missing.** The bereaved may feel lonely and uncertain about a new identity without the person who has died. This loss confronts them with the challenge of adjusting their own sense of self.
4. **Emotionally relocate the deceased and move on with life.** Individuals never lose memories of a significant relationship. They may need help in letting go of the emotional energy that used to be invested in the person who has died, and they may need help in finding an appropriate place for the deceased in their emotional lives.

## LO 6 | LIFE-AND-DEATH DECISION MAKING

Explain the ethical concerns that arise from the concepts of the right to die and rational suicide.

When a loved one is dying, many complex and emotional—and often expensive—life-and-death decisions must be made during a highly distressing period in people's lives.

## The Right to Die

Few people would object to the right to a dignified death. Going beyond that concept, however, many people today believe that they should be allowed to die if their condition is terminal and their existence depends on mechanical life-support devices or artificial feeding or hydration systems. Artificial life-support techniques that may be legally refused by competent patients include electrical or mechanical heart resuscitation, mechanical respiration by machine, nasogastric tube feedings, int ravenous nutrition, gastrostomy (tube feeding directly into the stomach), and medications to treat life-threatening infections.

As long as a person is conscious and competent, he or she has the legal right to refuse treatment, even if this decision will hasten death. However, when a person is in a coma or otherwise incapable of speaking on his or her own behalf, medical personnel, family members, and administrative policy will dictate treatment. This issue has evolved into a battle involving personal freedom, legal rulings, health care administration policy, and physician responsibility. The **living will** and other **advance directives** were developed to assist in solving these conflicts.

Even young, apparently healthy people need a living will. Consider Terri Schiavo, who collapsed at age 26 from heart failure that led to irreversible brain damage. Schiavo, unable to survive without life support, never left any written guidelines about her wishes should she become incapacitated. After a 15-year legal battle between her parents, who wanted her to be kept alive, and her husband, who felt she should be allowed to die, the courts sided with her husband, and she was removed from life support.

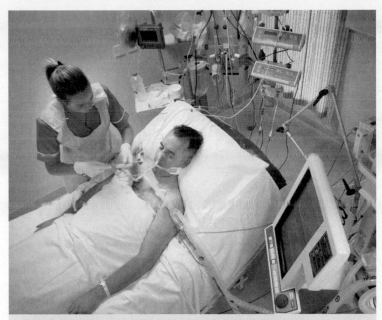

Today's sophisticated life-support technology can prolong a patient's life even in cases of terminal illness or mortal injury, yet not everyone would choose to have their life extended by such means. Living wills, advance directives, and health care proxies can protect your wishes and aid your loved ones should you become incapacitated.

# Rational Suicide and Euthanasia

It is estimated that thousands of terminally ill people every year decide to kill themselves rather than endure constant pain and slow decay. This alternative to the extended dying process is known as **rational suicide**. To these people, the prospect of an undignified death is unacceptable. This issue has been complicated by advances in death prevention techniques that allow terminally ill patients to exist in an irreversible disease state for extended periods of time.

Euthanasia is often referred to as "mercy killing." The term **active euthanasia** refers to ending the life of a person (or animal) who is suffering greatly and has no chance of recovery. This practice is currently illegal in the United States. **Passive euthanasia** refers to the intentional withholding of treatment that would prolong life. Deciding not to place a person with massive brain trauma on life support is an example of passive euthanasia. Advance directives, such as "do not resuscitate" orders, can provide legal justification for various forms of passive euthanasia.

According to public opinion polls, most Americans believe that suicide is morally wrong, but are divided on whether physician-assisted suicide is morally acceptable. See the **Points of View** box on the next page for a discussion of this topic.

**rational suicide** The decision to kill oneself rather than endure constant pain and slow decay.

**active euthanasia** "Mercy killing" in which a person or organization knowingly acts to end the life of a terminally ill person.

**passive euthanasia** The intentional withholding of treatment that would prolong life.

**hospice** A concept of end-of-life care designed to maximize quality of life and help dying people have peace, comfort, and dignity.

**palliative care** Any form of medical care focused on relieving the pain, symptoms, and stress of serious illness in order to improve the quality of life for patients and their families.

Many legal experts suggest that you take the following steps to ensure that your wishes are carried out:[32]

- **Be specific.** Complete an advance directive that permits you to make very specific choices about a variety of procedures, including cardiopulmonary resuscitation (CPR); being placed on a ventilator; being given food, water, or medication through tubes; being given pain medication; and organ donation.
- **Name a health care proxy.** You may want to also appoint a family member or friend to act as your agent, or *proxy*, by completing a form known as either a *durable power of attorney for health care* or a *health care proxy*. This allows the person you designate to make medical decisions for you in the event you are incapacitated.
- **Discuss your wishes.** Discuss your preferences in detail with your proxy and your doctor.
- **Deliver the directive.** Distribute several copies, not only to your doctor and your agent, but also to your lawyer and to immediate family members or a close friend. Make sure *someone* knows to bring a copy to the hospital in the event you are hospitalized.

One alternative to the traditional advance directive or living will is a document called "Five Wishes," which meets the legal requirements for advance directive statutes in most states. This document differs from most other living wills because it addresses personal, emotional, and spiritual needs, as well as medical needs.[33] It is available at low cost online at www.agingwithdignity.org.

## LO 7 | MAKING FINAL ARRANGEMENTS

Review the decisions that need to be made when someone is dying or has died, including hospice care, funeral arrangements, wills, and organ donation.

Caring for a dying person and his or her bereaved loved ones involves a wide variety of psychological, legal, social, spiritual, economic, and interpersonal issues.

## Hospice Care: Positive Alternatives

Since the mid-1970s, **hospice** programs in the United States have grown from a mere handful to more than 5,800 and are available in nearly every community.[34] These programs are a form of **palliative care** that focuses on

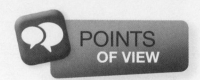
# Physician-Assisted Suicide
*Should It Be Legalized?*

*Physician-assisted suicide* (also known as *physician aid-in-dying*) refers to a practice in which the physician provides, after a terminally ill patient's request, a lethal dose of medication that the patient intends to use to end his or her own life. Currently, more than 30 states have statutes explicitly prohibiting assisted suicide. Only Oregon, Montana, New Mexico, Vermont, and Washington allow physician-assisted suicide under certain circumstances. The arguments for and against the legalization of physician-assisted suicide within individual states continue to be debated. Below are some of the major points from both sides of the issue.

## Arguments in Favor of Legalization of Physician-Assisted Suicide

- Decisions about time and circumstances regarding death are personal, and a competent person with a terminal illness should have the right to choose death.
- For some patients, treatment refusal does not lead to death quickly enough; therefore, their only option is to commit suicide.
- Many terminal conditions are accompanied by tremendous suffering and pain. Physician-assisted suicide is a compassionate response to unbearable suffering.
- Physician-assisted suicide already occurs, but behind closed doors and in secret. Legalization of physician-assisted suicide would promote open discussion of existing practices.
- Physician-assisted suicide is not a new phenomenon. It has been practiced in many societies throughout history and currently is legal in some European countries, such as Belgium and the Netherlands.

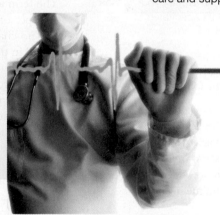

## Arguments against Legalization of Physician-Assisted Suicide

- It is unethical to take a human life, and historical, ethical traditions of medicine strongly oppose taking life. The Hippocratic Oath states that medical practitioners should not administer any deadly medicine or harm patients.
- Treatment refusal or withholding treatment equates to letting a patient die (passive) and is justifiable, whereas physician-assisted suicide equates to killing (active) and is not morally justifiable.
- Certain groups of terminally ill people, lacking access to care and support, may be pushed into assisted suicide.
- There may be uncertainty in the diagnosis and prognosis of the terminal illness. There may be errors in diagnosis and treatment of depression, or inadequate treatment of pain.

## WHERE DO YOU STAND?

- Do you think physician-assisted suicide should be legalized in your state?
- What criteria do you think should be used to monitor physician-assisted suicide if it were widely legalized?

- What are your feelings on physician-assisted suicide in general? Is it an appropriate option for patients diagnosed with devastating, terminal illnesses?

**Sources:** W. L. Carlson, T. D. Ong, "Suicide in Later Life: Failed Treatment or Rational Choice," *Clinics in Geriatric Medicine* 30, no. 3 (2014): 553–76; Oregon Department of Human Services, "FAQ's about the Death with Dignity Act," Updated May 2014, http://public.health.oregon.gov; International Task Force on Euthanasia and Assisted Suicide, "Assisted Suicide Laws," Updated February 2011, www.patientsrightscouncil.org

reducing pain and suffering while attending to the emotional and spiritual needs of dying individuals and their caregivers. Hospice may help survivors cope better with the death experience.

The primary goals of hospice programs are to relieve the dying person's pain; offer emotional support to the dying person and loved ones; and restore a sense of control to the dying person, family, and friends. Hospice programs also usually include the following characteristics:

- There is overall medical direction of the program, with all health care provided under the direction of a qualified physician. Emphasis is placed on symptom control, primarily the alleviation of pain.

- Services are provided by an interdisciplinary team.
- Coverage is provided 24 hours a day, 7 days a week, with emphasis on the availability of medical and nursing skills.
- Carefully selected and extensively trained volunteers who augment but do not replace staff service are an integral part of the health care team.
- Care of the family extends through the bereavement period.
- Patients are accepted on the basis of their health needs, not their ability to pay.

## Making Funeral Arrangements

Anthropological evidence indicates that all cultures throughout human history have developed some sort of funeral ritual. For this reason, social scientists agree that funerals assist survivors of the deceased in coping with their loss. In some faiths, the deceased may be displayed to formalize last respects and increase social support of the bereaved. This part of the funeral ritual is referred to as a *wake* or *viewing*. The funeral service may be held in a church, in a funeral chapel, or at the burial site. Some people choose to replace the funeral service with a simple memorial service held within a few days of the burial. Social interaction associated with funeral and memorial services is valuable in helping survivors cope with their losses.

In addition to details related to the type of funeral or memorial service and the method of burial or body disposition, loved ones must also consider the cost of funeral and memorial options. They usually have to contact friends and relatives, plan for the arrival of guests, choose markers, submit obituary information to newspapers, and deal with many other details. Even though funeral directors are available to facilitate decision making, the bereaved may experience undue stress, especially if the death is unexpected. People who make their own funeral arrangements ahead of time can save their loved ones the difficulty of having to make these decisions during a very stressful time.

## Wills

The issue of inheritance should be resolved before the person dies to reduce both conflict and needless expense. Unfortunately, many people are so intimidated by the thought of making a will that they never do so and die **intestate** (without a will). This is a mistake, especially because the procedure for establishing a legal will is relatively simple and inexpensive. If you don't make a will before you die, the courts (as directed by state laws) will make a will for you. Legal issues, rather than your wishes, will preside. Furthermore, settling an estate takes longer when a person dies without a will.

## Organ Donation

Organ donation takes healthy organs and tissues from one person for transplantation into another. Experts say that the organs from one donor can save or help as many as 50 people. You can donate internal organs (kidneys, heart, liver, pancreas, intestines, lungs); skin; bone and bone marrow; and corneas. Most organ and tissue donations occur after the donor has died, but some organs and tissues can be donated while the donor is alive.[35]

The number of patients waiting for organ donations greatly outnumbers available organs. Although some people are opposed to organ transplants and tissue donation, others experience personal fulfillment from knowing that their organs may extend and improve someone else's life after their own death. The most important step on the road to being an organ donor is to enroll in your state's donor registry. Go to www.organdonor.gov to sign up under your state. It is also a good idea to indicate your decision on your driver's license, tell your family and physician, and include the donation in your will and living will. Uniform donor cards are available through the U.S. Department of Health and Human Services and through many health care foundations and nonprofit organizations.

**intestate** Dying without a will.

How anxious or accepting are you about the prospect of your death? Indicate how well each statement describes your attitude.

Not True at All = ⓪    Mainly Not True = ❶    Not Sure = ❷
Somewhat True = ❸    Very True = ❹

1. I tend not to be very brave in times of crisis situations.  ⓪ ❶ ❷ ❸ ❹

2. I am something of a hypochondriac.  ⓪ ❶ ❷ ❸ ❹

3. I tend to be unusually frightened in airplanes at takeoff and landing.  ⓪ ❶ ❷ ❸ ❹

4. I would give a lot to be immortal in this body.  ⓪ ❶ ❷ ❸ ❹

5. I am superstitious that preparing for dying might hasten my death.  ⓪ ❶ ❷ ❸ ❹

6. My experience of friends and family dying has been wholly negative.  ⓪ ❶ ❷ ❸ ❹

7. I would feel easier being with a dying relative if he or she had not been told he or she was dying.  ⓪ ❶ ❷ ❸ ❹

8. I have fears of dying alone without friends around me.  ⓪ ❶ ❷ ❸ ❹

9. I have fears of dying slowly and suffering.  ⓪ ❶ ❷ ❸ ❹

10. I have fears of dying suddenly.  ⓪ ❶ ❷ ❸ ❹

11. I have fears of dying before my time or while my children are still young.  ⓪ ❶ ❷ ❸ ❹

12. I have fears of what could happen to my family after my death.  ⓪ ❶ ❷ ❸ ❹

13. I have fears of dying in a hospital or an institution.  ⓪ ❶ ❷ ❸ ❹

14. I have fears of not getting help with euthanasia.  ⓪ ❶ ❷ ❸ ❹

15. I have fears of dying without adequately having expressed my love to those I am close to.  ⓪ ❶ ❷ ❸ ❹

16. I have fears of being given unofficial and unwanted euthanasia.  ⓪ ❶ ❷ ❸ ❹

17. I have fears of getting insufficient pain control while dying.  ⓪ ❶ ❷ ❸ ❹

18. I have fears of being overmedicated and unconscious while dying.  ⓪ ❶ ❷ ❸ ❹

19. I have fears of being declared dead when not really dead or being buried alive.  ⓪ ❶ ❷ ❸ ❹

20. I have fears of what may happen to my body after death.  ⓪ ❶ ❷ ❸ ❹

Total points: _____

## Interpreting Your Score

If you are extremely anxious (scoring 38 or more), you might consider counseling or therapy; if you are unusually anxious (scoring between 24 and 37), you might want to find a method of meditation, philosophy, or spiritual practice to help experience, explore, and accept your feelings about death. Average anxiety is a score under 24.

# YOUR PLAN FOR CHANGE

The **ASSESS YOURSELF** activity encouraged you to explore your death-related anxiety. Now that you have considered your results, you may want to take steps to lessen your fears about death and dying.

### TODAY, YOU CAN:

☐ Learn about advance directives. Visit a low-cost legal clinic for information and a sample. You can also locate samples online, including the "Five Wishes" document, which is available at www.agingwithdignity.org.

☐ Fill out an organ donation card. Knowing that you may be able to prolong another person's life after your death can help you feel more at peace with your mortality.

### WITHIN THE NEXT TWO WEEKS, YOU CAN:

☐ Consider how you would like to be remembered. Are you living in a way that you want to be remembered? What actions can you take now to help ensure that your eulogy reflects your ideal life course?

☐ Talk to family members about their life goals. What have they achieved, and what do they wish they had done differently? What can you learn from their experiences?

### BY THE END OF THE SEMESTER, YOU CAN:

☐ Consider how you feel about various medical techniques that might be used in the event you become incapacitated. Do you feel comfortable being kept alive by a machine? Make your wishes on these matters known to family members and friends, and put them in writing.

☐ Talk to your parents or grandparents about the arrangements they prefer in the event of their death. Do they want a burial or cremation? A full funeral or a small service? Making these decisions now will save you and your loved ones stress later.

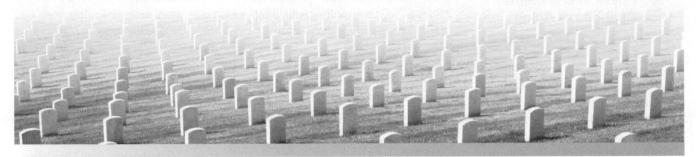

## CHAPTER REVIEW

To hear an MP3 Tutor Session, scan here or visit the Study Area in **MasteringHealth**.

### LO 1 | Aging

- Aging is the pattern of life changes that occur in members of all species as they grow older. The growing number of older adults (people aged 65 and older) has an increasing impact on society in terms of the economy, health care, housing, and ethical considerations.

### LO 2 | Physical and Mental Changes of Aging

- Aging changes the body and mind in many ways. Major physical concerns are osteoporosis, urinary incontinence, and changes in eyesight and hearing. Most older people maintain a high level of intelligence and memory. Potential mental problems include Alzheimer's disease.

### LO 3 | Strategies for Healthy Living

- Lifestyle choices we make today will affect health status later in life. Choosing to exercise, eat a healthy diet, foster lasting relationships, and enrich your spiritual side will contribute to healthy aging.

### LO 4 | Understanding the Final Transitions: Dying and Death

- *Death* can be defined biologically in terms of brain death or the cessation of vital functions. Dying is a multifaceted emotional process, and individuals may experience emotional stages of dying such as denial, anger, bargaining, depression, and acceptance. Social death results when a person is no longer treated as an active member of society.

### LO 5 | Coping with Loss

- Grief is the state of distress felt after loss. People differ in their responses to grief.

### LO 6 | Life-and-Death Decision Making

- Advanced directives assist people who believe they should allowed to die if their condition is terminal and their existence depends on mechanical life-support devices or artificial feeding or hydration systems.
- The right to die by rational suicide involves ethical, moral, and legal issues.
- Active euthanasia refers to ending the life of a person (or animal) who is suffering greatly and has no chance of recovery.

### LO 7 | Making Final Arrangements

- Hospice services are available to provide care for the terminally ill and their caregivers. After death, funeral arrangements must be made quickly and customs vary by family, region, religious affiliation, and cultural background. Decisions made in advance of illness and death, including wills and organ donation decisions, make the process easier for survivors.

## POP QUIZ

Visit **MasteringHealth** to personalize your study plan with Chapter Review Quizzes and Dynamic Study Modules.

### LO 1 | Aging

1. Which of the following is true?
   a. The majority of men aged 65 and older live with a spouse.
   b. The number of adults aged 65 and older is decreasing the United States.
   c. The majority of women aged 65 and older live alone.
   d. The majority of men and women aged 65 and older live in nursing homes.

### LO 2 | Physical and Mental Changes of Aging

2. The progressive breakdown of joint cartilage is known as
   a. osteoporosis.
   b. osteoarthritis.
   c. calcium loss.
   d. vitamin D deficiency.

3. Martha's ophthalmologist tells her that she has a condition that involves the breakdown of the light-sensitive area of the retina that is affecting her sharp, direct vision. What is this condition?
   a. Cataracts
   b. Glaucoma
   c. Macular degeneration
   d. Nearsightedness

4. What is the most common form of dementia in older adults?
   a. Alzheimer's disease
   b. Incontinence
   c. Depression
   d. Psychosis

### LO 3 | Strategies for Healthy Living

5. The keys to successful aging include
   a. Drinking red wine regularly
   b. Reducing protein intake
   c. Avoiding weight-bearing activities
   d. Eating sufficient calcium and vitamin D

### LO 4 | Understanding the Final Transitions: Dying and Death

6. The study of death and dying is called
   a. thanatology.
   b. gerontology.
   c. biology.
   d. a living will.

7. The Kübler-Ross stage of dying in which the individual rejects death emotionally and feels a sense of shock and disbelief is known as
   a. acceptance.
   b. bargaining.
   c. denial.
   d. anger.

## LO 5 | Coping with Loss

8. A culturally prescribed and accepted period of grief for someone who has died is known as
   a. bereavement.
   b. grief work.
   c. coping with loss.
   d. mourning.

## LO 6 | Life-and-Death Decision Making

9. Kerri's elderly grandmother is terminally ill and wants to die without medical intervention. Her family has agreed to withhold treatment that may prolong her life. This is called
   a. rational suicide.
   b. health care proxy.
   c. passive euthanasia.
   d. active euthanasia.

## LO 7 | Making Final Arrangements

10. Destiny's grandfather dies intestate. This means he
    a. had a health care proxy.
    b. did not have a will.
    c. received hospice care.
    d. did not have a trust.

*Answers to the Pop Quiz can be found on page A-1. If you answered a question incorrectly, review the section identified by the Learning Outcome. For even more study tools, visit MasteringHealth.*

# THINK ABOUT IT!

## LO 1 | Aging

1. As the older population grows, how will it affect your life? Would you be willing to pay higher taxes to support government social programs for older adults? Why or why not?

## LO 2 | Physical and Mental Changes of Aging

2. List the major physical and mental changes that occur with aging. Which of these, if any, can you change?

## LO 3 | Strategies for Healthy Living

3. How do the lifestyle choices we make now affect our health status later in life? What are some of the healthy choices and changes you could make today that will contribute to healthy aging later?

## LO 4 | Understanding the Final Transitions: Dying and Death

4. Discuss why so many of us deny death. How could death become a more acceptable topic to discuss?

## LO 5 | Coping with Loss

5. How do people differ in their responses to grief? What are some things you could do, and some things you shouldn't do, to support a friend or loved one who is grieving?

## LO 6 | Life-and-Death Decision Making

6. Discuss when you think people should start deciding whether to have an advance directive. What are some important considerations when preparing an advance directive?

## LO 7 | Making Final Arrangements

7. Are you an organ donor? What are some reasons why people decide to become organ donors? What might be some common hesitations?

# ACCESS YOUR HEALTH ON THE INTERNET

Visit **MasteringHealth** for links to the websites and RSS feeds.

The following websites explore further topics and issues related to personal health. For links to the websites below, visit the Study Area in MasteringHealth.

*Administration on Aging.* This U.S. Department of Health and Human Services link is dedicated to addressing the health needs of older adults. **www.aoa.gov**

*Alzheimer's Association.* This site includes media releases, position statements, fact sheets, and research on Alzheimer's disease. **www.alz.org**

*Grieving.com.* This forum site addresses all aspects of grief and loss, including terminal illness, non-death losses, and caregiving. **http://forums.grieving.com**

*National Hospice and Palliative Care Organization.* This site offers information on hospice care, including resources for finding a hospice, end-of-life issues, and advance directives. **www.nhpco.org**

*National Institute on Aging.* A site that provides information and research updates on aging related issues. **www.nia.nih.gov**

# 15 Promoting Environmental Health

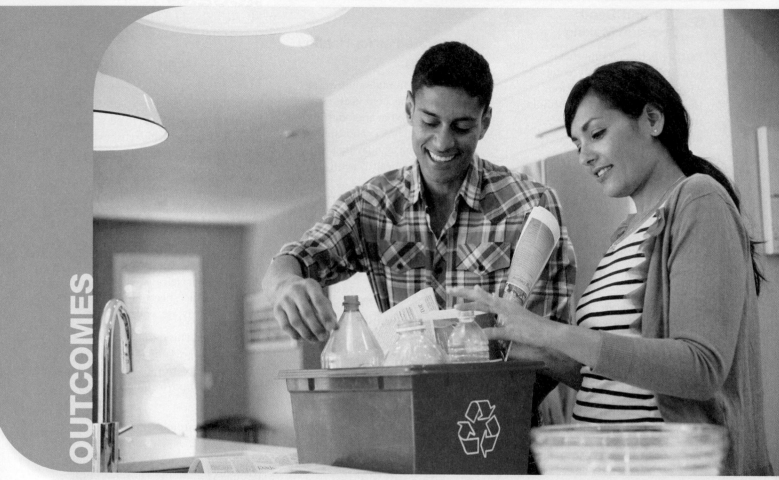

*"2014 was the planet's warmest year on record. Now, one year doesn't make a trend, but this does—14 of the 15 warmest years on record have all fallen in the first 15 years of this century."*

—Barack Obama, Excerpt from January 2015 State of the Union Address.

We live in an especially dangerous time. The global population has grown more in the past 50 years than at any other time in human history. More people pose a potentially devastating threat to the water we drink, the air we breathe, the food we eat, our natural resources, and the survival of all living things. Temperatures are rising, polar ice caps and glaciers are melting at rates that surpass even the most dire predictions of a decade ago, and threats of rising sea levels loom large. According to one report, we have lost half of the wild animals of the world in the last 40 years.[1] Drought, fires, floods and a host of other natural calamities are daily news. Clean water is becoming scarce, fossil fuels are being depleted, and the amount of solid and hazardous waste is growing. In short, our collective disregard for the planet's life-sustaining resources may ultimately put all living things in peril unless we take action now.

This chapter provides an overview of the factors contributing to the global environmental crisis. It also provides a blueprint for action—by individuals, communities, policymakers, and governments. Staying informed and becoming an advocate for a healthy environment are key things you can do to help.

## LO 1 | THE **THREAT** OF OVERPOPULATION

Explain the environmental impact associated with global population growth and our global ecological footprint.

**HEAR IT!** PODCASTS

Want a study podcast for this chapter? Download the podcast **Environmental Health,** available on MasteringHealth™

The United Nations projects that the world population will grow from its current level of 7 billion to 9.3 billion by 2050 and exceed all previous projections, swelling to between 11 and 12.3 billion by 2100 (**FIGURE 15.1**).[2] Tomorrow's population will be more industrialized, consume more resources, and produce even more waste than did previous generations unless actions are taken to control population growth.[3]

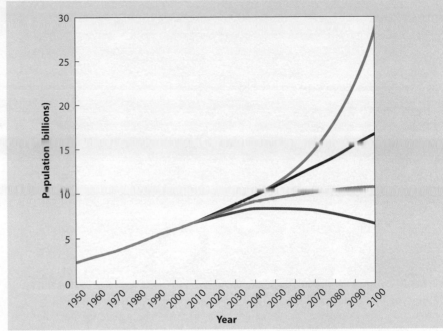

**Key:**
— Medium
— High
— Low
— Constant-fertility

**FIGURE 15.1** Estimated and Projected World Population Growth, 1950–2100

**Source:** United Nations, Department of Economic and Social Affairs, Population Division, "World Population Prospects: The 2010 Revision," http://esa.un.org, © 2011. Reprinted by permission.

## Bursting with People: Measuring the Impact

Currently our **ecological footprint**—a measure of the biologically productive land and water area an individual, a population or activity occupies and utilizes—is increasing at an unprecedented rate.[4] Realizing the growth in demand for finite resources, experts are analyzing the **carrying capacity of the earth**—the largest population that can be supported indefinitely, given the resources available in the environment.

Having doubled since 1961, our ecological footprint already exceeds Earth's capacity to support us; in fact, it would take 1.5 Earths to produce the resources necessary to support our current ecological footprint.[5] By 2030, it is estimated that it will take the resources of two planets to meet our growing demands.[6] Over half of our ecological footprint is from carbon dioxide emissions (carbon footprint). Whether we will be able to slow our rate of population growth

**ecological footprint** a measure of the biologically productive land and water area an individual, a population, or activity occupies and utilizes.

**carrying capacity of the earth** The largest population that can be supported indefinitely given the resources available in the environment.

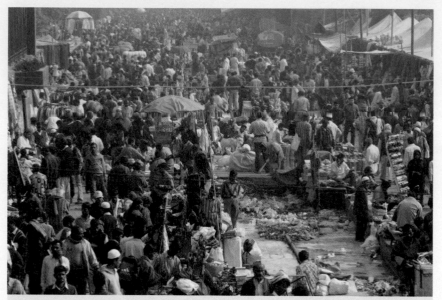

Every year the global population grows by 90 million, but Earth's resources are not expanding. Population increases are believed to be responsible for most of the current environmental stress.

and/or decrease our ecological footprint and restore the balance between humans and nature remains in question, even as we face an ever-increasing threat.

**ecosystem** Collection of physical (nonliving) and biological (living) components of an environment and the relationships between them.

**fossil fuel** Carbon-based material used for energy; includes oil, coal, and natural gas.

Per capita, countries with the largest ecological footprint include Qatar, Kuwait, United Arab Emirates, Singapore, Belgium, Denmark, the United States, Bahrain, and Sweden.[7] Evidence of the effects of unchecked population growth is everywhere:

- **Impact on other species.** Changes in the **ecosystem** are resulting in the mass destruction of many species and their habitats.[8] Over 477 vertebrae species have gone extinct since 1900—declining at rates that are over 100 times faster than normal rates of extinction would occur, prompting some scientists to predict the *sixth mass extinction of living creatures,* similar to the fifth extinction that occurred with the demise of the dinosaurs.[9] According to a recent report by the International Union for the Conservation of Nature (IUCN), nearly 25 percent of all mammals on Earth are threatened with extinction.[10] African elephants, black rhinos, and walruses are among those being ruthlessly killed for high-priced horns and tusks.[11] In spite of major efforts to stop poaching of elephants for ivory, nearly 35,000 African elephants are slaughtered each year—a rate that is outpacing the numbers

of births, ensuring extinction in the wild unless drastic measures are taken to prevent it.[12]

- **Impact on the food supply.** Recent research indicates that fish populations have declined by two thirds over the last century, with most of the decline occurring in the last 40 years; other research has reported that we are currently fishing the oceans at rates that are 250 percent more than they can regenerate, and scientists project a global collapse of all fish species by 2050.[13]

Today, our global quest for enough food means that increasing amounts of the earth's surface is used for agriculture. Because agriculture accounts for over 90 percent of our global water footprint, groundwater withdrawals have tripled in the last 50 years, which puts increased pressure on dwindling water reserves.[14]

- **Land degradation and contamination of drinking water.** The per capita availability of fresh water is declining rapidly, and contaminated water remains the greatest single environmental cause of human illness. Unsustainable land use is increasing land degradation, including erosion, toxic chemical infiltration, nutrient depletion, deforestation, and other problems that will inevitably affect human life.

- **Energy consumption.** "Use it *and* lose it" is an apt saying for our greedy use of nonrenewable **fossil fuels** (oil, coal, natural gas). The United States is the largest consumer of liquid fossil fuels and natural gas, and among the top four consumers of nuclear power, coal, and hydroelectric power.[15] In many developing regions of the world, movement toward greater industrialization and citizen affluence has also resulted in skyrocketing demand for limited fossil fuels.

## WHY SHOULD I CARE?

Imagine waking up in the morning to find you have no water for a shower, the electricity stops working throughout the day, gas stations have no fuel for sale, and basic necessities are either unavailable or unaffordable. Such scenarios are not science fiction. Major difficulties loom unless we take action to change our current rate of consumption of natural resources and unless the global community acts to enforce policies to check rampant population growth.

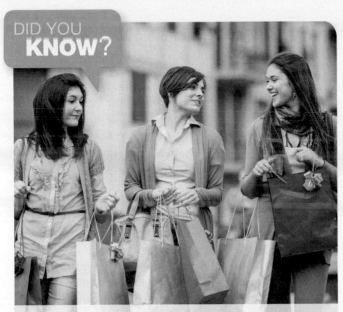

If everyone on Earth lived like the average American, it would take 3.9 Earths to meet our resource needs.

**DID YOU KNOW?**

is either not available or frowned upon, pregnancy rates continue to rise. However, as women become more educated, obtain higher socioeconomic status, and have more control over reproduction—as birth control becomes more accessible—fertility rates decline. Recognizing that population control will be essential in the decades ahead, many countries have enacted strict population control measures or have encouraged their citizens to limit the size of their families.

Mortality rates from chronic and infectious diseases have declined as a result of improved public health infrastructure, increased availability of drugs and vaccines, better disaster preparedness, and other factors. As people live longer, they add more years of resource consumption and add to the overall human footprint on the environment.

> **fertility rate** Average number of births a female in a certain population has during her reproductive years.

**SEE IT! VIDEOS**

What are the environmental and human costs of fashion and what's one solution? Watch **Actress Rosario Dawson's Mission for Sustainable Fashion** in the Study Area of **MasteringHealth™**

## Factors That Affect Population Growth

A number of factors have led to the world population's increase. Key indicators of growth patterns are fertility and mortality rates.

**Fertility rate** refers to how many births a woman has by the end of her reproductive life. Overall global fertility has declined to an average of 2.5 births per woman in 2013, even though rates remain much higher in certain regions.[16] While Europe, the United States, Mexico, China, and others have shown consistent declines in fertility rates in the last few decades, other countries, such as Niger (6.9 births per woman) and Somalia (6.1 births per woman) continue to have high fertility rates.[17] In 2014, the U.S. fertility rate was 2.1 births per woman—down significantly from 3.7 births per woman in the 1950s.[18] While some argue that lower fertility rates means slowing population growth, sheer population size can cause major increases, even if fertility rates remain constant or decline (**FIGURE 15.2**).

Historically, in countries where women have little education and little control over reproductive choices, and where birth control

### WHAT DO YOU THINK?

Should individuals get tax breaks for having fewer children?

- How would such policies compare to our current policies?
- Can you think of other policies that might be effective in encouraging population control and resource conservation in the United States?

## LO 2 | AIR POLLUTION

Discuss major causes of air pollution and the consequences of ozone depletion.

The term *air pollution* refers to the presence of substances (suspended particles, gases, and vapors) not found in perfectly clean air. From the beginning of time, natural events, living

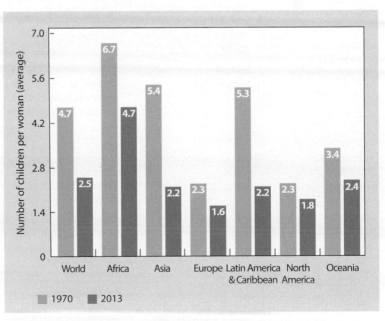

**FIGURE 15.2 Global Fertility Rates, by Region** Average fertility rates (births per woman) have declined in all regions since 1970.

pollutant Substance that contaminates some aspect of the environment and causes potential harm to living organisms.

smog Brownish haze that is a form of pollution produced by the photochemical reaction of sunlight with hydrocarbons, nitrogen compounds, and other gases in vehicle exhaust.

hydrocarbons Chemical compounds containing carbon and hydrogen.

temperature inversion Weather condition that occurs when a layer of cool air is trapped under a layer of warmer air.

creatures, and toxic by-products have polluted the environment. Air pollution is not new, but the vast array of **pollutants** that now exist and their potential interactive effects are.

Air pollutants are either *naturally occurring* or *anthropogenic* (caused by humans). Naturally occurring air pollutants include *particulate matter*, such as ash from volcanic eruptions, soil, and dust. Anthropogenic sources include those caused by *stationary sources* (e.g., power plants, factories, and refineries) and *mobile sources* such as vehicles.[19] According to U.S. Environmental Protection Agency estimates, mobile sources are major contributors of air pollutants like carbon monoxide (CO), sulfur oxides ($SO_x$), and nitrogen oxides ($NO_x$). Motor vehicles alone contribute nearly 30 percent of all $CO_2$ emissions in the United States.[20]

# Components of Air Pollution

Concern about air quality prompted Congress to pass the Clean Air Act in 1970 and to amend it several times since then. The act established standards for six of the most widespread air pollutants that seriously affect health: sulfur dioxide, particulates, carbon monoxide, nitrogen dioxide, ground level ozone, and lead. See **TABLE 15.1** for an overview of the sources and effects of these pollutants.

## Photochemical Smog
**Smog** is a brownish haze produced by the photochemical reaction of sunlight with **hydrocarbons**, nitrogen compounds, and other gases in vehicle exhaust. It is sometimes called *ozone pollution* because ground-level ozone is a main component of smog. Smog tends to form in areas that experience a **temperature inversion**, in which a cool layer of air is trapped under a layer of warmer air, preventing the air from circulating. Smog is more likely to occur in valley areas surrounded by hills or mountains, as in Los Angeles or Phoenix. The most noticeable adverse health effects of smog are difficulty breathing, burning eyes, headaches, and nausea. Long-term exposure

## TABLE 15.1 | Sources, Health Effects, and Environmental Impacts of Six Major Air Pollutants

| Pollutant | Description | Sources | Health Effects | Welfare Effects |
|---|---|---|---|---|
| Carbon monoxide (CO) | Colorless, odorless gas | Motor vehicle exhaust; indoor sources include kerosene and wood-burning stoves | Headaches, reduced mental alertness, heart attack, cardiovascular diseases, impaired fetal development, death | Contributes to the formation of smog |
| Sulfur dioxide ($SO_2$) | Colorless gas that dissolves in water vapor to form acid and interacts with other gases and particles in the air | Coal-fired power plants, petroleum refineries, manufacture of sulfuric acid, and smelting of ores containing sulfur | Eye irritation, wheezing, chest tightness, shortness of breath, lung damage | Contributes to the formation of acid rain, visibility impairment, plant and water damage, aesthetic damage |
| Nitrogen dioxide ($NO_2$) | Reddish brown, highly reactive gas | Motor vehicles, electric utilities, and other industrial, commercial, and residential sources that burn fuels | Susceptibility to respiratory infections, irritation of the lungs and respiratory symptoms (e.g., cough, chest pain, difficulty breathing) | Contributes to the formation of smog, acid rain, water quality deterioration, global warming, and visibility impairment |
| Ground-level ozone ($O_3$) | Component of smog | Vehicle exhaust and certain other fumes; formed from other air pollutants in the presence of sunlight | Eye and throat irritation, coughing, respiratory tract problems, asthma, lung damage | Plant and ecosystem damage, global warming |
| Lead (Pb) | Metallic element | Metal refineries, lead smelters, battery manufacturers, iron and steel producers | Anemia, high blood pressure, brain and kidney damage, neurological disorders, cancer, lowered IQ | Affects animals, plants, and the aquatic ecosystem |
| Particulate matter (PM) | Very small particles of soot, dust, or other matter, including tiny droplets of liquids | Diesel engines, power plants, industries, windblown dust, wood stoves | Eye irritation, asthma, bronchitis, lung damage, cancer, heavy metal poisoning, cardiovascular effects | Visibility impairment, atmospheric deposition, aesthetic damage |

**Source:** U.S. Environmental Protection Agency, "Air and Radiation: Air Pollutants," April. 2015, www.epa.gov

| When the AQI is in this range: | ... air quality conditions are | ... as symbolized by this color: |
| --- | --- | --- |
| 0 to 50 | Good | Green |
| 51 to 100 | Moderate | Yellow |
| 101 to 150 | Unhealthy for sensitive groups | Orange |
| 151 to 200 | Unhealthy | Red |
| 201 to 300 | Very unhealthy | Purple |
| 301 to 500 | Hazardous | Maroon |

**FIGURE 15.3** Air Quality Index (AQI) The EPA provides individual AQIs for ground-level ozone, particle pollution, carbon monoxide, sulfur dioxide, and nitrogen dioxide. All of the AQIs are presented using the general values, categories, and colors of this figure.

**Source:** U.S. Environmental Protection Agency, "Air Quality Index: A Guide to Air Quality and Your Health," Updated May 2014, www.airnow.gov/index.cfm?action=aqibasics.aqi

poses serious health risks, particularly for children, older adults, pregnant women, and people with chronic respiratory disorders.

**Air Quality Index** The Air Quality Index (AQI) is a measure of how clean or polluted the air is on a given day. The AQI focuses on health effects that can happen within a few hours or days after breathing polluted air.

The AQI runs from 0 to 500: The higher the AQI value, the greater the level of air pollution and associated health risks. An AQI value of 100 generally corresponds to the national air quality standard for the pollutant, which is the level the Environmental Protection Agency (EPA) has set to protect public health. When AQI values rise above 100, air quality is considered unhealthy—at certain levels for specific groups of people and at higher levels, for everyone.

As shown in **FIGURE 15.3**, the EPA has divided the AQI scale into six categories with corresponding color codes. National and local weather reports generally include information on the day's AQI.

## Acid Deposition

**Acid deposition** refers to the deposition of *wet* (rain, snow, sleet, fog, cloud water, and dew) and *dry* (acidifying particles and gases) acidic components that fall to the earth in dust or smoke.[21] When coal-powered plants, oil refineries, and other facilities burn these fuels, sulfur and nitrogen in the emissions combine with oxygen and sunlight to become sulfur dioxide and nitrogen oxide. Small acid particles are carried by the wind and combine with moisture to produce acidic rain or snow.[22]

**SEE IT!** VIDEOS

How far does China's extreme smog extend from its capital Beijing? Watch China Smog Creates What Some Call a Kind of Respiratory Nuclear Winter on MasteringHealth™

Acid deposition gradually acidifies ponds, lakes, and other bodies of water. Once the acid content of the water reaches a certain level, plant and animal life cannot survive.[23] Every year, acid deposition destroys millions of trees in Europe and North America. Scientists have concluded that much of the world's forestlands are now experiencing damaging levels of acid deposition.[24]

Acid deposition aggravates and may even cause bronchitis, asthma, and other respiratory problems, and people with emphysema or heart disease may suffer from exposure.[25] It may also be hazardous to fetuses. Acid deposition can cause metals such as aluminum, cadmium, lead, and mercury to **leach** out of the soil. If these metals make their way into water or food supplies, they can cause cancer in humans.

## Indoor Air Pollution

Mounting evidence indicates that air pollution levels within homes and other buildings, where we spend 90 percent of our time, may be two to five times higher than outdoor pollution levels.[26] Potentially dangerous chemical compounds can increase risks of cancer, contribute to respiratory problems, reduce the immune system's ability to fight disease, and increase problems with allergies and allergic reactions.

**acid deposition** Acidification process that occurs when pollutants are deposited by precipitation, clouds, or directly on the land.

**leach** To dissolve and filter through soil.

Indoor air pollution comes primarily from cooking stoves and furnaces, woodstoves and space heaters, household cleaners and solvents, mold, pesticides, asbestos, formaldehyde, radon, and lead. Today, more and more manufacturers are offering green building products and furnishings, such as natural fiber fabrics, untreated wood for furniture and floors, *low-VOC (volatile organic compound)* paints, and many other products in an attempt to reduce potential pollutants.

Multiple factors, including age, individual sensitivity, preexisting medical conditions, liver function, and the condition of the immune and respiratory systems contribute to a person's

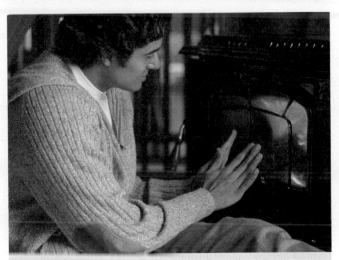

Inside air can be 10 to 40 times more hazardous than outside air. Indoor air pollution comes from woodstoves, furnaces, cigarette smoke, asbestos, formaldehyde, radon, lead, mold, and household chemicals.

## TABLE 15.2 | Indoor Air Pollutants, Their Sources, and Health Effects

| Pollutant | Sources | Health Effects |
|---|---|---|
| Asbestos | Deteriorating or damaged insulation; fireproofing, acoustical materials, and floor tiles | Long-term risk of chest and abdominal cancers and lung diseases. Smokers are at higher risk of developing asbestos-induced lung cancer. |
| Lead | Lead-based paint, contaminated soil, dust, and drinking water | At or above 80 μg/dL of blood (high levels) it can cause convulsions, coma, and death. Lower levels can cause central nervous system, kidney, and blood disorders. Blood lead levels as low as 10 μg/dL can impair mental and physical development. |
| Radon | Uranium in the soil or rock on which homes are built can lead to air exposure inside. Well water also can be a source. | A major nontobacco cause of lung cancer from air and drinking water exposure; it also has a synergistic effect with smoking exposure. |
| Environmental tobacco smoke | Smoke from the burning end of cigarettes, pipes, or cigars or smoke exhaled by a smoker; consists of a complex mixture of 4,000+ compounds | Over 40 compounds linked to increased risk of lung cancer; asthma, lower respiratory infections; sudden infant death syndrome (SIDS), and heart disease |
| Biological contaminants (molds, mildew, viruses, animal dander, cat saliva, dust mites, cockroaches, and pollen) | Improper ventilation and moisture buildup, lack of cleanliness/sanitation, contaminated heating systems, faulty construction, household pets, rodents, insects, damp carpets | Allergic reactions, including hypersensitivity, rhinitis, asthma, infectious illnesses, sneezing, watering eyes, coughing, shortness of breath, dizziness, lethargy, fever, digestive problems |
| Combustion products | Unvented kerosene heaters, woodstoves, fireplaces, gas stoves | Carbon monoxide causes headaches, dizziness, weakness, nausea, confusion and disorientation, chest pain, death. Nitrogen dioxide causes irritation of nose and eyes, respiratory distress. Particles cause lung damage and irritation. |
| Benzene | Paint, new carpet, new drapes, upholstery, fast-drying glues, caulks | Headaches, eye/skin irritation, fatigue, cancer |
| Formaldehyde | Tobacco smoke, plywood, cabinets, furniture, particleboard, new carpet and drapes, wallpaper, ceiling tile, paneling | Headaches, eye/skin irritation, drowsiness, fatigue, respiratory problems, memory loss, depression, gynecological problems, cancer |
| Chloroform | Paint, new drapes, new carpet, upholstery | Headaches, asthma attacks, dizziness, eye/skin irritations |
| Toluene | All paper products, most finished wood products | Headaches, eye/skin irritation, sinus problems, dizziness, cancer |
| Hydrocarbons | Tobacco smoke, gas burners and furnaces | Headaches, fatigue, nausea, dizziness, breathing difficulty |
| Ammonia | Tobacco smoke, cleaning supplies, animal urine | Eye/skin irritation, headaches, nosebleeds, sinus problems |
| Trichloroethylene | Paints, glues, caulking, vinyl coatings, wallpaper | Headaches, eye/skin irritation, upper respiratory irritation |

**Source:** U.S. Environmental Protection Agency, "The Inside Story: A Guide to Indoor Air Quality," Updated November 18, 2013, www.epa.gov/iaq/pubs/insidest.html

risk for being affected by indoor air pollution.[27] Those with allergies may be particularly vulnerable. Health effects may develop over years of exposure or may occur in response to toxic levels of pollutants, particularly in homes where air doesn't circulate freely as in some air-tight, draft free homes. Room temperature and humidity also play a role. **TABLE 15.2** lists major sources of indoor air pollution and possible health effects.

Preventing indoor air pollution should focus on three main areas: *source control* (eliminating or reducing contaminants), *ventilation improvements* (increasing the amount of outdoor air coming indoors), and *air cleaners* (removing particulates from the air).[28]

For ways to reduce your exposure to biological contaminants like mold, in particular, see the **Skills for Behavior Change** box.

## Ozone Layer Depletion

The ozone layer is a stratum in the stratosphere—the highest level of Earth's atmosphere, located 12 to 30 miles above the surface—that protects our planet and its inhabitants from ultraviolet B (UVB) radiation, a primary cause of skin cancer. Such radiation damages DNA and weakens human and animal immune systems. In the 1970s, scientists began to warn of a

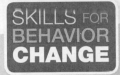
breakdown in the ozone layer. Certain chemicals, especially refrigerants, solvents, and aerosols called **chlorofluorocarbons (CFCs)**, were contributing to the ozone layer's rapid depletion.

The U.S. government banned the use of CFCs, and the discovery of an ozone "hole" over Antarctica led to treaties whereby the United States and other nations agreed to further reduce the use of CFCs and other ozone-depleting chemicals. Today, more than 197 United Nations countries have agreed to basic protocols designed to preserve and protect the ozone layer.[29] Although the ban on CFCs is believed to be responsible for slowing the depletion of the ozone layer, some CFC replacements may also cause damage by contributing to the enhanced greenhouse effect.

## LO 3 | CLIMATE CHANGE

Explain climate change and global warming, the underlying causes of each, impacts on health, and key actions for reducing risks.

**Climate change** refers to a shift in typical weather patterns across the world. These changes can include fluctuations in seasonal temperatures, rain or snowfall amounts, and the occurrence of catastrophic storms. **Global warming** is a type of climate change in which average temperatures increase. Over 97 percent of scientists now agree the planet is warming, and over the last 50 years, this warming has been driven largely by the burning of fossil fuels.[30] Over the last 100 years, the average temperature of the earth has increased by 1.5°F, with projections of another 2° to 11.5°F rise in the next 100 years.[31]

The *greenhouse effect* is a natural phenomenon in which greenhouse gases such as carbon dioxide ($CO_2$) form a layer in the atmosphere, allowing solar heat to pass through and trapping some of the heat close to the surface, where it warms the planet. The natural greenhouse effect is important for keeping the planet warm enough for life, but human activities have increased greenhouse gases in the atmosphere, resulting in the **enhanced greenhouse effect**, raising the planet's temperature higher than normal by trapping excess heat (see **FIGURE 15.4**).

According to data from U.S. and international sources, climate responds to changes in naturally occurring greenhouse gases as well as solar output and the earth's orbit; however, recent evidence points to unusual changes in climate that go beyond predictable natural causes. Consider the following:[32]

■ Global sea levels rose 6.7 inches in the last 100 years, mostly in the last decade.

■ Since 1981, 20 of the warmest years ever have occurred, and all of the 10 warmest years have been during the last 12 years.

■ Greenland is losing 36 to 60 cubic miles of ice per year; Antarctica is losing 36 cubic miles of ice per year.

■ Glaciers are receding at unprecedented and rapid rates.

Multiple reconstructions of the earth's climate history show that the amounts of greenhouse gases in the atmosphere went up dramatically around the time of the industrial revolution—when humans began burning fossil fuels on a large scale—and correlates very closely with temperature increases.[33] Studies also indicate that large changes in climate can occur in decades rather than centuries or thousands of years.[34]

## Reducing the Threat of Global Warming

Climate change problems are largely rooted in our energy, transportation, and industrial practices.[35] However, the problem isn't just one of increased $CO_2$ production. Rapid deforestation contributes to the rise in greenhouse gases. Trees take in carbon dioxide, transform it, store the carbon for food, and release oxygen into the air. As we lose forests at the rate of hundreds of acres per hour, we lose the capacity to store and dissipate carbon dioxide.[36] Population increases and human destruction of natural resources pose additional threats.

To slow climate change, most experts agree that reducing

**chlorofluorocarbons (CFCs)** Chemicals that contribute to the depletion of the atmospheric ozone layer.

**climate change** A shift in typical weather patterns that includes fluctuations in seasonal temperatures, rain or snowfall amounts, and the occurrence of catastrophic storms.

**global warming** A type of climate change in which average temperatures increase.

**greenhouse gases** Gases that accumulate in the atmosphere where they contribute to global warming by trapping heat near the Earth's surface.

**carbon dioxide ($CO_2$)** Gas created by the combustion of fossil fuels, exhaled by humans and animals, and used by plants for photosynthesis; the primary greenhouse gas in the atmosphere.

**enhanced greenhouse effect** Warming of Earth's surface as a direct result of human activities that release greenhouse gases into the atmosphere, trapping more of the sun's radiation than is normal.

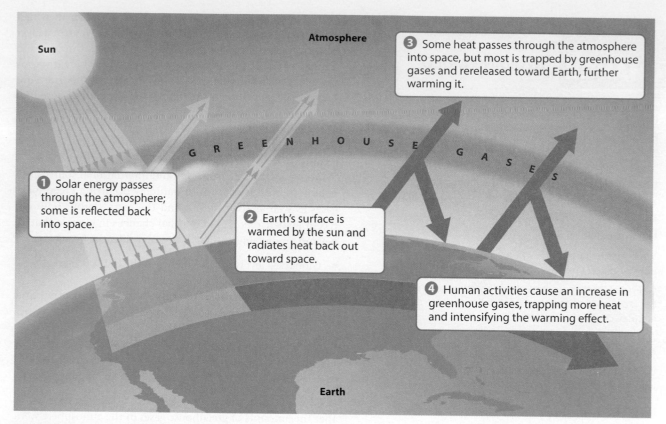

**1** Solar energy passes through the atmosphere; some is reflected back into space.

**2** Earth's surface is warmed by the sun and radiates heat back out toward space.

**3** Some heat passes through the atmosphere into space, but most is trapped by greenhouse gases and rereleased toward Earth, further warming it.

**4** Human activities cause an increase in greenhouse gases, trapping more heat and intensifying the warming effect.

Sun

Atmosphere

GREENHOUSE GASES

Earth

**FIGURE 15.4** The Enhanced Greenhouse Effect

The natural greenhouse effect is responsible for making Earth habitable; it keeps the planet 33°C (60°F) warmer than it would be otherwise. An increase in greenhouse gases resulting from human activities is creating the enhanced greenhouse effect, trapping more heat and causing dangerous global climate change.

**Source:** OzCoasts (Geoscience Australia), "The Enhanced Greenhouse Effect (Global Warming)," 2013, www.ozcoasts.gov.au/indicators/greenhouse_effect.jsp.

→ VIDEO TUTOR
Enhanced Greenhouse Effect

consumption of fossil fuels, shifting to alternative energy sources, and using mass transportation are all crucial; however, clean energy, green factories, improved energy efficiency, and governmental regulation are also key. The United Nations Conference on Sustainable Development (known as RIO+20) took place in 2012 in Rio de Janeiro and outlined a plan for protecting the environment (called "The World We Want") through **sustainable development**—development that meets the needs of the present without compromising the needs of future generations.[37] However, leaders of many nations, including the United States, France, Germany, and the United Kingdom opted not to attend, and the resulting plan includes a list of general goals to work toward, but without the "teeth" necessary to motivate nations to comply with sustainable development needs.

Although getting the nations of the world to come up with a plan that all can work toward may seem a bit like "herding cats," some glimmers of progress by individual nations may be occurring. Currently, the top three $CO_2$-emitting countries (China, 29%; United States, 15%; and the European Union, 11%) contribute 55 percent of all emissions.[38] While China increased its emissions by 4.2 percent and the United States increased emissions by 2.5 percent, the European Union actually decreased emissions by 1.4 percent in 2013.[39] The good news is that the rate of emission increases has begun to slow, with overall global emissions increasing by only 2 percent in 2014 compared to years of double-digit increases.[40]

Many U.S. cities and states have begun to consider a **carbon tax** similar to those in Ireland, Sweden, Australia, Great Britain, Quebec, and British Columbia. A carbon tax is the price a government charges for the carbon content in fuels. Diesel, gas, natural gas, jet fuel, and coal-fired electricity all emit percentages of carbon per unit of fuel. If you use more, you will pay more carbon tax. If your power is fueled by solar, wind, or hydro power, there is no $CO_2$ emission and no tax, incentivizing individuals to invest in noncarbon power generation—as well as drive less, turn down the heat, fly less, and reduce carbon footprints.

**sustainable development** Development that meets the needs of the present without compromising the ability of future generations to meet their own needs.

**carbon tax** A carbon tax is the price a government charges for the carbon content in fuels used by an individual, industry, or organization.

**SEE IT!** VIDEOS

How is climate change affecting the weather during winter? Watch **Snowstorms in the Forecast,** available on MasteringHealth™

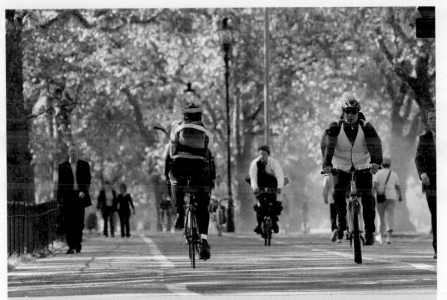

Making small changes such as driving less, riding your bike more, taking public transportation or carpooling, turning off lights, and recycling and composting can all help to reduce your carbon footprint.

Identify sources of pollution and chemical contaminants often found in water.

Seventy-five percent of Earth is covered with water, but less than 1 percent is freshwater easily accessible for human consumption in either surface water (lakes, rivers, swamps, etc.) or groundwater from underwater wells and aquifers.[43] The rest of our freshwater (approximately 1.5%) is locked in dwindling glaciers and ice caps.[44]

Although we have seen improvements in *gallons per capita per day (GPCD)* water usage from agriculture, thermoelectric power, municipal, and industrial sources in the United States—declining from 1,900 GPCD in 1900 to 1,100 GPCD in 2010—we continue to exceed most nations of the world in water consumption.[45] Residential use has also declined from nearly 120 GPCD in the 1980s to 88 GPCD in 2010.[46] Water-saving toilets, faucets, showerheads, washers, and dishwashers and drip irrigation options are responsible for much of this decline.[47] While these changes are laudable, it is important to note that the GPCD residential consumption in parts of Africa is closer to 5 gallons![48] At a time when over 1 billion of the earth's population has no access to clean water and where more than 4,500 children die every day from illnesses caused by lack of safe water, dwindling supplies of fresh water and devastating effects of climate change do not bode well for our water future.[49] Water issues will only get worse as demand for fresh water is projected to exceed current supply by over 40 percent by 2030.[50] The **Skills for Behavior Change** box on page 467 presents simple conservation measures you can adopt to save water where you live.

The city of Boulder, Colorado, was the first to implement a carbon tax, and others are considering doing so.

**Cap and trade** policies are designed to set limits, or caps, on how much carbon large industrial polluters can emit. Large emitters would be issued permits for allowable levels of pollutants and then taxed on overages, unless they were able to acquire/trade/pay for more allowances from companies that produced lower carbon emissions. Although controversial among those who are antitax and antigovernment, carbon taxes and cap and trade policies are mechanisms for incentivizing green behaviors and motivating those with large carbon footprints to reduce emissions.[41]

More wind, solar, and bioenergy use, reductions in natural gas prices due to production increases and weather, improved EPA ratings on vehicles, and more alternative energy sources may improve carbon emissions. Still, major fuel-hungry industry development in poorer regions of the world may offset some of the potential decreases in future years.[42]

Many communities and campuses have established plans to reduce their carbon footprint. Creating user-friendly bicycle lanes; more energy-efficient buses, trains, and commuter systems; incentives for buying hybrid or electric cars, bike-sharing programs, monitored bike garages to prevent theft/vandalism, and holding "bike to work" days, all motivate students to leave cars at home. Campus recycling programs at the end of the school year encourage reuse and recycling rather than having students dump their belongings to avoid paying shipping costs to send them home. Some campuses have raised fees for parking permits in the hopes of discouraging students from bringing cars to campus. You can participate in this effort by finding ways to reduce your own **carbon footprint**, or the amount of $CO_2$ emissions you contribute to the atmosphere in your daily life.

**cap and trade** Policies designed to set limits (caps) on how much carbon large industrial polluters can emit. Large emitters would be issued permits for allowable levels of pollutants and then taxed on overages unless they were able to acquire 'allowances' from other emitters.

**carbon footprint** Amount of greenhouse gases produced, usually expressed in equivalent tons of carbon dioxide emissions.

## Water Contamination

Fortunately, tap water in the United States is among the safest in the world. Under the Safe Drinking Water Act, the EPA sets standards for drinking water quality and oversees the states, localities, and water suppliers who implement those standards. Cities and municipalities have policies and procedures governing water treatment, filtration, and disinfection to screen out pathogens and microorganisms. However, their ability to filter out increasing amounts of chemical by-products and other substances is in question. According to a recent study of over 50 large wastewater sites in the United States, over half of the samples tested positive for at least 25 of the 56 prescription and over-the-counter drugs monitored![51] In another study, U.S. Geological Survey researchers discovered the presence of low levels of many chemical compounds in streams and watersheds throughout the United States.[52] Steroids, pharmaceuticals and personal care products, hormones, codeine, blood pressure and heart medications, insect repellent, and wastewater compounds were all detected.

Congress has coined two terms, *point source* and *nonpoint source,* to describe general sources of water pollution. **Point source pollutants** enter a waterway at a specific location such as a pipe, ditch, culvert, or other conduit. The two major sources of point source pollution are sewage treatment plants and industrial facilities. **Nonpoint source pollutants**—commonly known as *runoff* and *sedimentation*—drain or seep into waterways from broad areas of land. Nonpoint source pollution results from a variety of land use practices and includes soil erosion and sedimentation, construction and engineering project waste, pesticide and fertilizer runoff, urban street runoff, acid mine drainage, septic tank leakage, and sewage sludge. **TABLE 15.3** presents some of the pollutants causing the greatest potential harm.

## TABLE **15.3** | Water Pollutants, Health, and Ecosystem Effects

| Pollutant | Description | Health Effects |
|---|---|---|
| Gasoline and petroleum products | Leaks from underground storage tanks at filling stations; occupational exposures in processing plants and filling stations. Fumes can spark fires and cause respiratory issues. | Can affect nervous system, leading to headaches, dizziness, nausea; skin irritations and damage to kidneys and blood; benzene in gas linked to several cancers. Benzene can contaminate surface and groundwater sources leading to toxic results for humans, animals, birds, and aquatic life. |
| Organic solvents | Chemicals designed to dissolve grease and oil; dry-cleaning fluids, paints, antifreeze, etc. Consumers dump leftovers into the toilet or street drains; industries bury leftovers in barrels, which can corrode and leak. | Difficult to clean up; can cause cancer, damage to immune, nervous, and reproductive systems Harmful to aquatic life and animals that come in contact or ingest |
| Fracking by-products | Chemicals used in hydraulic fracking, a method of extracting natural gas from the ground by forcing pressurized liquids into underground rock | Linked to groundwater and surface water contamination; difficult to remediate; potentially harmful to animals, birds, humans; leads to air quality issues and difficulties with disposal; potential earthquake risk unclear |
| Polychlorinated biphenyls (PCBs) | Insulating materials in high-voltage electrical equipment such as transformers and fluorescent lights; no longer manufactured in the United States | Stored in the liver; associated with birth defects, cancer, and skin problems |
| Dioxins | Used as herbicides, produced during certain industrial processes | Accumulate in the body; long-term effects include possible immune system damage and increased risk of infections and cancer. Exposure to high concentrations for a short period of time can cause nausea, vomiting, diarrhea, painful rashes and sores, and chloracne. |
| Pesticides | Chemicals designed to prevent, mitigate, or kill any pest, including insects (insecticides) rodents, weeds (herbicides), and microorganisms (algaecides, fungicides, or bactericides) evaporate readily and can be dispersed by winds, water runoff, and food contamination. | Can accumulate in the body. Potential hazards include birth defects, cancer, liver and kidney damage, reproductive problems, nervous system and diseases in aquatic, animal, and bird populations; contamination of groundwater and food. |

**Sources:** Environmental Protection Agency. "Drinking Water Contaminants," 2014, http://water.epa.gov/drink/contaminants/; United States Geological Survey. "Contaminants Found in Ground Water," 2014, http://water.usgs.gov/edu/groundwater-contaminants.html; U.S. EPA, "Assessment of the Potential Impacts of Hydraulic Fracturing for Oil and Gas on Drinking Water Resources," (External Review Draft), (Washington, DC, 2015), EPA/600/R-15/047.

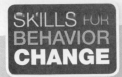

## WASTE LESS WATER!

### In the Kitchen

▶ Turn off the tap while washing dishes. Shut water off after a quick rinse.

▶ Repair leaky pipes and faucets. More than 3,000 gallons of water each year are lost to leaks.

▶ Equip faucets with aerators to reduce water use by 4 percent.

▶ Run dishwashers only when they are full, and use the energy-saving mode.

### In the Laundry Room

▶ Wash only full loads or use a washing machine that adjusts to allow a reduced water level for smaller loads.

▶ Upgrade to a high-efficiency washer to use 30 percent less water per load.

### In the Bathroom

▶ Detect and fix leaks. A leaky toilet can waste about 200 gallons of water per day.

▶ Replace old toilets with a high-efficiency models that use 60 to 80 percent less water per flush.

▶ Take showers instead of baths, and limit showers to the time it takes to lather up and rinse off. Ideally, get wet, shut off water, lather up, and turn on water to rinse.

▶ Replace old showerheads with efficient models that use 60 percent less water per minute.

▶ Turn off the tap while brushing your teeth to save up to 8 gallons of water per day.

# 31%

OF **PLASTIC BOTTLES** ARE RECOVERED/ RECYCLED EACH YEAR.

## LO 5 | **LAND** POLLUTION

Distinguish between municipal solid waste and hazardous waste and list strategies for reducing land pollution.

Much of the waste that ends up polluting water starts out polluting the land. Growing population creates more pressure on the land to accommodate increasing amounts of refuse, much of which is nonbiodegradable and some of which is directly harmful to living organisms.

### Solid Waste

Each day, every person in the United States generates nearly 4.4 pounds of **municipal solid waste (MSW)**, more commonly known as trash or garbage, totaling about 254 million tons of trash each year, with organic materials making up the largest share.[53] Of that 4.4 pounds per person per day, each person recycled and composted about 1.5 pounds of his or her waste.[54] Although experts believe that up to 90 percent of our trash is recyclable, we still fall far short of this goal (**FIGURE 15.5**). Currently, 34.3 percent of all MSW in the United States is recycled or composted, 12.9 percent is burned at combustion facilities, and the remaining 52.8 percent is disposed of in landfills.[55]

> **municipal solid waste (MSW)**
> Solid waste such as durable and nondurable goods; containers and packaging; food waste; yard waste; and miscellaneous waste from residential, commercial, institutional, and industrial sources.

The number of U.S. landfills has actually decreased in the past decade, but their sheer mass has increased. As communities run out of landfill space, it is becoming common to haul garbage to other states or to dump it illegally in woods, waterways, or oceans, where it contaminates ecosystems, or to ship it to landfills in developing countries, where it becomes someone else's problem. Communities, businesses, and individuals can adopt strategies to reduce solid waste:

■ *Source reduction (waste prevention)* involves altering the design, manufacture, or use of products and materials to reduce the amount and toxicity of waste.

■ *Recycling* involves sorting, collecting, and processing materials for reuse in new products and diverts items such

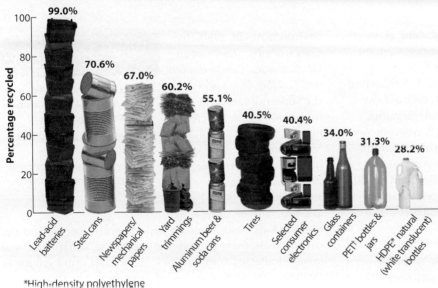

*High-density polyethylene
†Polyethylene terephthalate

**FIGURE 15.5** How Much Do We Recycle?

**Source:** EPA, "Advancing Sustainable Materials Management: 2013 Fact Sheet," June 2015, www.epa.gov/epawaste/nonhaz/municipal/pubs/2013_advncng_smm_fs.pdf

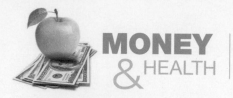
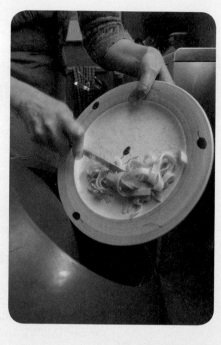

At a time when starvation, hunger, and food insecurity plague people throughout the world, a new study by Britain's Institute of Mechanical Engineers indicates that *up to half of the food produced worldwide never makes it into consumer's mouths.*

Global consumer behaviors in more affluent nations are responsible for much of the waste. Big box stores that promote "bigger size is cheaper" entice people to buy more than they can eat before it spoils. Freezers in homes encourage waste as food dries up before it is eaten while other food sits on shelves until past the expiration date.

It isn't just our behaviors in the home that contribute to the waste, however. When fresh produce is in surplus and demand is low, crops languish in fields. If weather or insects cause produce to be blemished, we reject it in stores and it is tossed in the trash. Americans are among the worst of the food wasters, wasting over 40 percent of all edible food. The average person in the United States dumps about 20 pounds of food each month, equivalent to between $28 and $43 per month. If we cut our food waste by just 15 percent, some estimate 26 million food-insecure people in the United States could be fed.

From an environmental perspective, when we waste food, we waste all of the time, effort, and resources that went into production and put unnecessary stress on the environment. By wasting less, we put less pressure on our vulnerable habitat.

What can you do?

- Be a better food planner. Make a list when shopping and only buy what you will use.
- Buy locally.
- Don't be picky. Buy fruit and vegetables even if they don't have a perfect shape, and eat them before they rot.
- Eat leftovers. Make a rule that you can't buy fast food or eat out when there is good food in your fridge.
- Eat lower on the food chain. By eating more vegetables and nuts, legumes, and other food crops and reducing consumption of meat, dairy and other animals, you have a smaller footprint stomping on the planet.

**Sources:** Institute of Mechanical Engineers, "Global Food: Waste Not, Want Not," 2013, www.imeche.org; J. Bloom, *American Wasteland* (Cambridge: DeCapo Press, 2010); National Resource Defense Council, "Food Facts: Your Scraps Add Up," March 2013, www.nrdc.org

---

**hazardous waste** Toxic waste that poses a hazard to humans or to the environment.

**Superfund** Fund established under the Comprehensive Environmental Response Compensation and Liability Act to be used for cleaning up toxic waste dumps.

as paper, cardboard, glass, plastic, and metals from the waste stream.

- *Composting* involves collecting organic waste, such as food scraps and yard trimmings, and allowing it to decompose with the help of microorganisms (mainly bacteria and fungi). This process produces a nutrient-rich substance used to fertilize gardens and for soil enhancement. Not all organic waste is composted. See the **Money & Health** box for more on the cost and prevalence of food waste.
- *Combustion with energy recovery* typically involves the use of boilers and industrial furnaces to incinerate waste and use the burning process to generate energy.

## Hazardous Waste

**Hazardous waste** is defined as waste with properties that make it capable of harming human health or the environment. In 1980, the *Comprehensive Environmental Response, Compensation and Liability Act*, known as the **Superfund**, was enacted to provide funds for cleaning up what are typically "abandoned" hazardous waste dump sites. Over the past three decades, the Superfund has located and assessed tens of thousands of hazardous waste sites, worked to protect people and the environment from contamination at the worst sites, and involved affected communities, states, and other groups in cleanup. The vast majority of sites have been cleared or "recovered."[56]

The large number of U.S. hazardous waste dump sites indicates the severity of our toxic chemical problem. American manufacturers and individuals generate around 40 million of tons of hazardous waste each year, including commercial

### WHAT DO YOU THINK?

Do you know anyone who throws recyclable items away rather than recycling them?

- What do you think motivates their behavior?
- What might encourage them to recycle more than they do now?

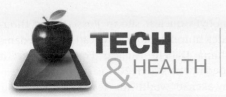
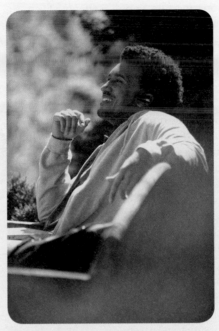

Given that cell phone use has skyrocketed and billions of people are hanging out with their phones 24/7, only the most apathetic wouldn't be concerned about *radio (RF) frequency.* But what is the real risk? In theory, RF energy has the potential to penetrate the skull, neck, and upper torso. For the very young, whose skulls have not yet sufficiently hardened, the risk might be even greater. However, after over a decade of research trying to prove a solid link to cell phone use and some type of disease, very little conclusive evidence exists. More research looking at superusers may provide the missing link. In the interim, it makes good sense to use caution. Go hands free. Check out the specific absorption rate (SAR) charts online or from your phone company before buying.

Cable or satellite TV box guzzling your electricity? While you are in class, out to dinner, or in bed sound asleep, your cable box is using more electricity than almost any appliance in your house! Surprised by that? A recent report indicates that a set-top cable or satellite box can consume as much as 35 watts of power and cost about

$8.00 a month in certain regions of the country. It is estimated that the nearly quarter of a million boxes currently in U.S. homes use as much electricity

together as four nuclear power plants generate. Even when turned off, hard drives keep running, downloading, and updating. Unplugging can help, but depending on location, it can require a long reboot when you want to use the system. The answer might be to use fewer boxes in your home or do more streaming on lower-energy-use devices such as laptops.

The global burden of e-waste (trashed computers, televisions, and other electronic devices) has also skyrocketed in recent years. Although there are many avenues for disposing of items like cell phones, hang on to your TV, phone, or other device for as long as possible. "Use it and *don't* lose it," so to speak. When you are thinking about *e-recycling,* check out www.ecycling-central.com for a state-by-state listing of e-recyclers in your area.

**A hands-free device lets you keep your phone—and any radio-frequency energy it may emit—away from your head.**

**Sources:** National Cancer Institute, Factsheet, "Cell Phones and Cancer Risk," 2013, www .cancer.gov/cancertopics/factsheet/Risk/ cellphones; R. Vartabedian, "Cable TV Boxes Become 2nd Biggest Energy Users in Many Homes," *LA Times,* June 19, 2014, www.latimes .com/nation/la-na-power-hog-20140617-story .html#page=1

chemical refuse, solvents and oils, petroleum-refining by-products, and household wastes such as batteries, cleaning products, and paints.[57] Many wastes are now banned from land disposal sites or are being treated to reduce their toxicity before they become part of land disposal sites. The EPA has developed protective requirements for land disposal facilities, such as double liners, detection systems for substances that may leach into groundwater, and groundwater monitoring systems.

## LO 6 | RADIATION

**Discuss the health concerns associated with ionizing and nonionizing radiation.**

Radiation is energy that travels in waves or particles. There are many different types of radiation, ranging from radio waves to gamma rays, all making up the electromagnetic spectrum. Exposure to radiation is an inescapable part of life on this planet, and only some of it poses a threat to human health.

## Nonionizing Radiation

**Nonionizing radiation** is radiation at the lower end of the electromagnetic spectrum. This radiation moves in relatively long wavelengths and has enough energy to move atoms around or to cause them to vibrate, but not enough to alter molecular structure. Examples of nonionizing radiation are radio waves, TV signals, microwaves, infrared waves, and visible light. Concerns have been raised about the safety of radio-frequency waves generated by cell phones (discussed in the **Tech & Health** box).

## Ionizing Radiation

**Ionizing radiation** is caused by the release of particles and electromagnetic rays from atomic nuclei during the normal process of disintegration. This type of radiation has enough energy to remove electrons from the

**nonionizing radiation** Electromagnetic waves having relatively long wavelengths and enough energy to move atoms around or cause them to vibrate.

**ionizing radiation** Electromagnetic waves and particles having short wavelengths and energy high enough to ionize atoms.

atoms it passes through. Some naturally occurring elements, such as uranium, emit ionizing radiation. The sun is another source of ionizing radiation, in the form of high-frequency ultraviolet rays.

Radiation exposure is measured in **radiation absorbed doses,** or **rads** (also called *roentgens*). Radiation can cause damage at doses as low as 100 to 200 rads. At this level, signs of radiation sickness include nausea, diarrhea, fatigue, anemia, sore throat, and hair loss. At 350 to 500 rads, these symptoms become more severe, and death may result as production of the white blood cells we need to fight disease is hindered. Doses above 600 to 700 rads are fatal.

Recommended maximum "safe" exposure ranges from 0.5 to 5 rads per year.[58] Approximately 50 percent of the radiation to which we are exposed comes from natural and human-made sources. Natural sources include radon gas in the air and cosmic radiation. Human-made sources include, but are not limited to, manufactured building materials. Another 45 percent comes from medical and dental x-rays. The remaining 5 percent is nonionizing radiation and includes light, heat, radar, microwaves, and radio waves. Unlike ionizing radiation, which can disrupt molecular bonds and affect cells and health, nonionizing radiation doesn't have sufficient energy to break molecular bonds or cause significant damage to cells.[59] Most of us are exposed to far less radiation than the safe maximum dosage per year. The effects of long-term exposure to relatively low levels of radiation are unknown.

## Nuclear Power Plants

Proponents of nuclear energy believe that it is a safe and efficient way to generate electricity. Initial costs of building nuclear power plants are high, but actual power generation is relatively inexpensive compared to other forms. Nuclear power also causes reductions in fossil fuel use in heating; however, it doesn't reduce fossil fuels used in transportation—our major source of fossil fuel usage. Also, nuclear reactors discharge fewer carbon oxides into the air than do fossil fuel–powered generators.

Although there are advantages to nuclear power, there are also clear disadvantages. Disposal of nuclear waste poses significant risks to our environment. In addition, a reactor core meltdown could pose serious threats to all living things.

A **nuclear meltdown** occurs when the temperature in the core of a nuclear reactor increases enough to melt both the nuclear fuel and its containment vessel. Most modern facilities seal the reactors and containment vessels in concrete buildings with pools of cold water at the bottom. If a meltdown occurs, the building and the pool are supposed to prevent radiation from escaping; however, a catastrophic 1986 fire and

explosion at Chernobyl's nuclear site in Russia killed thousands and left the area uninhabitable for decades.[60] The damage to the Fukushima Daiichi Nuclear Power Station in northern Japan caused by the March 2011 earthquake and tsunami has newly awakened worldwide fears about nuclear energy. Even so, the use of nuclear power worldwide is expected to double in the next 35 years, particularly in China and other parts of Asia.[61]

**radiation absorbed dose (rad)** Unit of measure of radiation exposure.

**nuclear meltdown** Accident that results when the temperature in the core of a nuclear reactor increases enough to melt the nuclear fuel and breach the containment vessel.

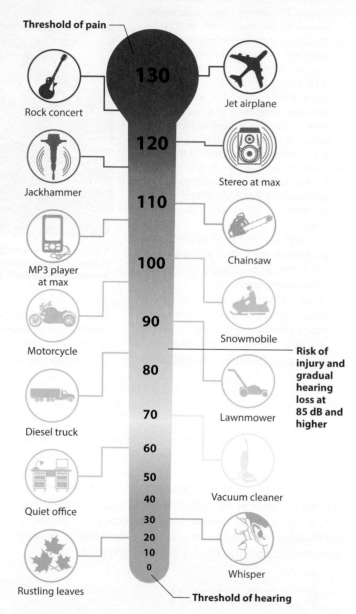

**Threshold of pain**

Rock concert — 130 — Jet airplane

120 — Stereo at max

Jackhammer — 110

MP3 player at max — 100 — Chainsaw

Motorcycle — 90 — Snowmobile

80 — **Risk of injury and gradual hearing loss at 85 dB and higher**

Diesel truck — 70 — Lawnmower

60

50

40 — Vacuum cleaner

Quiet office — 30

20

10

Rustling leaves — 0 — Whisper

**Threshold of hearing**

**FIGURE 15.6** Noise Levels of Various Sounds (in Decibels) Decibels increase logarithmically, thus each increase of 10 dB represents a tenfold increase in loudness.

**Source:** Adapted from National Institute on Deafness and Other Communication Disorders, "How Loud Is Too Loud? Bookmark," 2015, www.nidcd.nih.gov

## LO 7 | NOISE POLLUTION

Describe the physiological consequences of noise pollution and how to prevent or reduce its effects.

Our bodies have definite physiological responses to noise, and it can become a source of physical and mental distress. Sounds are measured in decibels. A sound with a decibel level of 110 is 10 times louder than one at 100 decibels (dB). A jet takeoff from 200 feet has a noise level of approximately 140 dB, whereas the human voice in normal conversation has a level of about 60 dB (**FIGURE 15.6**). Short-term exposure to loud noise reduces concentration and productivity and may affect mental and emotional health. Symptoms of noise-related distress include disturbed sleep patterns, headaches, and tension. Prolonged exposure to loud noise can lead to hearing loss, although risks depend on both the decibel level and the length of exposure.

Despite increasing awareness that noise pollution is more than just a nuisance, noise control programs have received low budgetary priority in the United States. According to the National Institute for Occupational Safety and Health, 30 million Americans are exposed to hazardous noise at work, and 10 million suffer from permanent hearing loss.[62] Here are some steps you can take to protect your hearing:

- Use headphones that go over, rather than inside, your ears, and don't crank up the volume on any sound system.
- Always use ear protection when using power equipment or firearms.
- Close windows to establish a barrier between yourself and outside noise.
- Wear earplugs when attending concerts, athletic events, races, and clubs, and avoid seats near speakers.

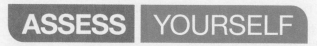
## Are You Doing All You Can to Protect the Environment?

Environmental problems often seem too big for the actions of one person to make a difference. Each day, however, there are things you can do. For each statement below, indicate how often you follow the described behavior.

| | | Always | Usually | Sometimes | Never |
|---|---|---|---|---|---|
| 1. | I walk or ride my bicycle rather than drive a car. | 1 | 2 | 3 | 4 |
| 2. | I carpool to school or work. | 1 | 2 | 3 | 4 |
| 3. | I read labels and buy products that have fewer chemicals in their ingredients whenever I buy food, personal care products, and household cleaners. | 1 | 2 | 3 | 4 |
| 4. | I use air conditioning only as needed on very hot days, and put on more clothes rather than crank up the furnace whenever possible. | 1 | 2 | 3 | 4 |
| 5. | I turn off the lights when a room is not being used. | 1 | 2 | 3 | 4 |
| 6. | I keep my cell phone and other electronics as long as they still work to reduce E-waste and conserve natural resources. | 1 | 2 | 3 | 4 |
| 7. | I have water-saving devices installed on my shower, toilet, and sinks. | 1 | 2 | 3 | 4 |
| 8. | I unplug my TV DVR/cable/satellite dish when gone for extended periods. | 1 | 2 | 3 | 4 |
| 9. | I use bath towels more than once before putting them in the wash. | 1 | 2 | 3 | 4 |
| 10. | I wear my clothes more than once between washings, when appropriate. | 1 | 2 | 3 | 4 |
| 11. | I limit my use of the clothes dryer and line dry my clothes as often as possible. | 1 | 2 | 3 | 4 |
| 12. | I purchase biodegradable soaps and detergents. | 1 | 2 | 3 | 4 |
| 13. | At home, I use dishes and utensils rather than Styrofoam or plastic. | 1 | 2 | 3 | 4 |
| 14. | When I buy prepackaged foods, I choose the ones with the least packaging. | 1 | 2 | 3 | 4 |
| 15. | I go paperless in my transactions whenever I can. | 1 | 2 | 3 | 4 |
| 16. | I use energy-efficient appliances. | 1 | 2 | 3 | 4 |
| 17. | I bring my own reusable bags to the grocery store. | 1 | 2 | 3 | 4 |
| 18. | I don't run water continuously when washing the dishes, shaving, or brushing my teeth. | 1 | 2 | 3 | 4 |
| 19. | I reuse the blank side of printed papers. | 1 | 2 | 3 | 4 |
| 20. | I try to reuse, recycle, donate, or sell household items when moving. | 1 | 2 | 3 | 4 |
| 21. | I bring my own beverage container and get refills instead of buying bottled water or coffee in paper cups. | 1 | 2 | 3 | 4 |
| 22. | I volunteer for cleanup days in my community. | 1 | 2 | 3 | 4 |
| 23. | I consider candidates' positions on environmental issues before casting my vote. | 1 | 2 | 3 | 4 |

## For Further Thought

Review your scores. Are your responses mostly 1s and 2s? If not, what actions can you take to become more environmentally responsible? Are there ways to help the environment on this list that you had not thought of? Are there behaviors not on the list that you are already doing?

# YOUR PLAN FOR CHANGE

The **ASSESS YOURSELF** activity gave you the chance to look at your behavior and consider ways to conserve energy, save water, reduce waste, and otherwise help protect the planet. Now that you have considered these results, you can take steps to become more environmentally responsible.

### TODAY, YOU CAN:

☐ Find out how much energy you are using. Visit http://footprint.wwf.org.uk/ to find out what your carbon footprint is and how your behaviors would affect the planet if others lived like you. Learn about things you can do to change your carbon footprint.

☐ Reduce paper waste in your mailbox. The Direct Marketing Association's Mail Preference Service site (www.dmachoice.org), 1-888-5-OPT-OUT, and www.catalogchoice.org are all free services that help cut down on unsolicited catalogs, credit card offers, and advertisements.

### WITHIN THE NEXT TWO WEEKS, YOU CAN:

☐ Look into joining a local environmental group, attending a campus environmental event, or taking an environmental science course.

☐ Take part in a local cleanup day or recycling drive to meet like-minded people while benefiting the planet.

### BY THE END OF THE SEMESTER, YOU CAN:

☐ Check if your campus dining hall composts or recycles. If it doesn't, ask the managers to start.

☐ Make a habit of recycling everything you can, from bottles to batteries.

☐ Let your legislators know how you feel about environmental issues and vote for candidates with pro-environment records.

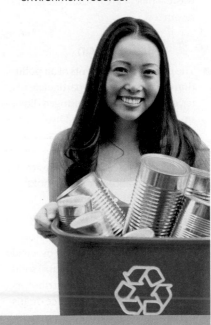

## CHAPTER REVIEW

 To hear an MP3 Tutor Session, scan here or visit the Study Area in **MasteringHealth.**

### LO 1 | The Threat of Overpopulation

- Population growth is the single largest factor affecting the environment. Demand for more food, water, and energy—as well as places to dispose of waste—places great strain on Earth's resources.

### LO 2 | Air Pollution

- The primary constituents of air pollution are sulfur dioxide, particulate matter, carbon monoxide, nitrogen dioxide, smog, carbon dioxide, and hydrocarbons. Indoor air pollution is caused primarily by tobacco smoke, woodstove smoke, furnace emissions, asbestos, formaldehyde, radon, lead, and mold.

### LO 3 | Climate Change

- Climate change is a major environmental threat and is caused by a wide range of factors. Air, water, and solid waste pollution are key contributors, as is our growing dependence on fossil fuels. Sustainable development should be an international goal.

### LO 4 | Water Pollution and Shortages

- Water pollution can be caused by either point sources (direct entry) or nonpoint sources (runoff or seepage). Major contributors to water pollution include petroleum products, organic solvents, polychlorinated biphenyl (PCBs), dioxins, pesticides, and lead.

### LO 5 | Land Pollution

- Municipal solid waste (MSW) includes household trash, plastics, glass, metals, and paper and other items. Many of these items can be recycled. Limited landfill space creates problems in dealing with growing volumes of MSW. Hazardous waste is toxic; improper disposal creates health hazards for people in surrounding communities.

### LO 6 | Radiation

- Nonionizing radiation comes from electromagnetic fields like those around power lines and is less disruptive to health. Ionizing radiation that results from x-rays and other sources can disrupt cellular activity and pose greater risks to health. The disposal and storage of radioactive waste from nuclear power plants pose potential public health problems.

### LO 7 | Noise Pollution

- Noise pollution can affect concentration and productivity and can also lead to hearing loss.

## POP QUIZ

Visit **MasteringHealth** to personalize your study plan with Chapter Review Quizzes and Dynamic Study Modules.

### LO 1 | The Threat of Overpopulation

1. The largest population that can be supported indefinitely given the resources available is known as the earth's
   a. maximum fertility rate.
   b. fertility capacity.
   c. maximum population growth.
   d. carrying capacity.

2. Human fertility rates go down when
   a. there is poverty and people can't afford to feed their families.
   b. governments subsidize families in the form of tax breaks.
   c. women have more education and power.
   d. environmental threats influence people to have fewer children.

### LO 2 | Air Pollution

3. The air pollutant that originates primarily from motor vehicle emissions is
   a. particulates.
   b. nitrogen dioxide.
   c. sulfur dioxide.
   d. carbon monoxide.

4. Which gas can potentially become cancer causing when it seeps into a home?
   a. Radon
   b. Carbon monoxide
   c. Hydrogen sulfide
   d. Ozone

5. The barrier that protects us from the sun's harmful ultraviolet rays is
   a. photochemical smog.
   b. the ozone layer.
   c. gray air smog.
   d. the greenhouse effect.

### LO 3 | Climate Change

6. When gases such as carbon dioxide, nitrous oxide, methane, CFCs, and hydrocarbons form a layer in the atmosphere, allowing solar heat to pass through and trapping some of the heat close to the surface to warm the planet, what is it called?
   a. Photochemical smog
   b. The ozone layer
   c. Gray air smog
   d. The enhanced greenhouse effect

### LO 4 | Water Pollution and Shortages

7. Some herbicides contain toxic substances called
   a. THMs.
   b. PCPs.
   c. dioxins.
   d. PCBs.

### LO 5 | Land Pollution

8. Looking for and buying products with little or no packaging is an

example of reducing municipal solid waste by

a. source reduction.
b. recycling.
c. cap and trade incentives.
d. incineration.

## LO 6 | Radiation

9. What is the recommended safe level of rads exposure per year?
   a. 0.5 to 5 rads
   b. 6 to 100 rads
   c. 101 to 200 rads
   d. 201 to 350 rads

## LO 7 | Noise Pollution

10. Intensity of (exposure to) sound is measured in
    a. foot candles.
    b. noise volume.
    c. hertz.
    d. decibels.

*Answers to the Pop Quiz can be found on page A-1. If you answered a question incorrectly, review the section identified by the Learning Outcome. For even more study tools, visit MasteringHealth.*

# THINK ABOUT IT!

## LO 1 | The Threat of Overpopulation

1. How are the rapid increases in global population and consumption of resources related? Is population control the best solution? Why or why not?

## LO 2 | Air Pollution

2. What are the primary sources of air pollution? What can be done to reduce air pollution?

## LO 3 | Climate Change

3. What are the causes and consequences of global warming? What can individuals and communities do to reduce the threat of global warming?

## LO 4 | Water Pollution and Shortages

4. What are point and nonpoint sources of water pollution? What can be done to reduce or prevent water pollution?

## LO 5 | Land Pollution

5. How do you think communities and governments could encourage recycling efforts?

## LO 6 | Radiation

6. What can be done, personally, to reduce your amount of radiation exposure? On the community level? On the national level?

## LO 7 | Noise Pollution

7. What are the physiological consequences of noise pollution? What are the greatest sources of noise pollution on campus? How can you lessen your exposure to it?

# ACCESS YOUR HEALTH ON THE INTERNET

Visit **MasteringHealth** for links to the websites and RSS feeds.

*Environmental Literacy Council.* This website is an excellent source of information about environmental issues in general. Topics range from how the ozone layer works to why the rain forests are important ecosystems. **www.enviroliteracy.org**

*Environmental Protection Agency (EPA).* The EPA is the U.S. government agency responsible for overseeing environmental regulation and protection issues. **www.epa.gov**

*National Center for Environmental Health (NCEH).* This site provides information on a wide variety of environmental health issues, including a series of helpful fact sheets. **www.cdc.gov/nceh**

*National Environmental Health Association (NEHA).* This organization provides educational resources and opportunities for environmental health professionals. **www.neha.org**

# 16 Making Smart Health Care Choices

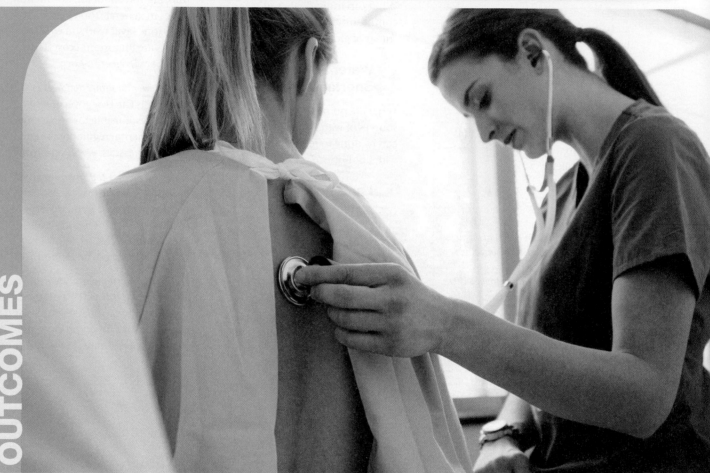

**LEARNING OUTCOMES**

1 Explain why it is important to be a responsible health care consumer, and identify several factors to consider when making health care decisions.

2 Describe and discuss conventional health care, including types of practitioners and the health care products and treatments available.

3 Describe the U.S. health care system in terms of types and availability of insurance and the changes related to health care reform.

4 Discuss issues facing our health care system today, including those related to cost, quality, and access to services.

Have you ever wondered whether you were sick enough to go to your campus health clinic? Have you left visits with your health care provider feeling that he or she didn't give a thorough exam or that you had more questions than you did when you arrived? Do you engage in risky behaviors, such as riding your bike without a helmet, and don't know where or how you would be treated if you were injured? Have you ever had to help a loved one make health care decisions? Are you one of the nearly 6 million young adults aged 19 to 34 in the United States without health insurance previously, who now have it –or- are you part of the nearly 18 percent of this age group who do not have health insurance?[1]

If the answer to any of these questions is yes, then you will find this chapter valuable for becoming a better health care consumer. Learning how to navigate the health care system is an important part of taking charge of your health.

## LO 1 | TAKING RESPONSIBILITY FOR YOUR HEALTH CARE

Explain why it is important to be a responsible health care consumer, and identify several factors to consider when making health care decisions.

Acting responsibly in times of illness can be difficult. If you are not feeling well, you must first decide whether you really need to seek medical advice. For ailments like colds or minor injuries, self-care may be the best course of action. In more serious cases, not seeking treatment, whether because of high costs or limited coverage, or trying to medicate yourself when a professional diagnosis and treatment are needed, is potentially dangerous. It's important to know the benefits and limits of self-care.

### Self-Care

Individuals can practice behaviors that promote health and reduce the risk of disease as well as treat minor afflictions without seeking professional help. Self-care consists of knowing your body, paying attention to its signals, and taking appropriate action to stop the progression of illness or injury. Common forms of self-care include the following:

- Diagnosing symptoms or conditions that occur frequently but may not require physician visits (e.g., the common cold, minor abrasions)
- Using over-the-counter remedies to treat mild, infrequent, and unambiguous pain and other symptoms
- Performing first aid for common, uncomplicated injuries and conditions
- Checking blood pressure, pulse, and temperature
- Performing monthly breast or testicular self-examinations
- Doing periodic checks for blood glucose, cholesterol, or other levels as prescribed by a physician
- Learning from reliable self-help books, websites, and videos
- Performing meditation and other relaxation techniques
- Maintaining a healthful diet, getting adequate rest, and exercising

In addition, a vast array of at-home diagnostic kits are now available to test for pregnancy, allergies, HIV, possible prediabetes and type 2 diabetes based on A1C levels, genetic disorders, and many other conditions. Caution is in order here: Diagnoses from these devices are not always accurate, or you may need professional interpretation to explain the ramifications of test results. Moreover, home health tests are not substitutes for regular, complete examinations by a trained practitioner.

Taking prescription drugs used for a previous illness to treat your current illness, using unproven self-treatment or using other people's medications are examples of inappropriate self-care. Using self-care methods appropriately takes effort, education, and the ability to make informed decisions based on scientific evidence.

## When to Seek Help

Effective self-care also means understanding when to seek medical attention rather than treating a condition yourself and knowing when and how to access the most cost effective and appropriate level of care. Generally, you should consult a physician if you experience *any* of the following:

- A serious accident or injury
- Sudden or severe chest pains, especially if they cause breathing difficulties

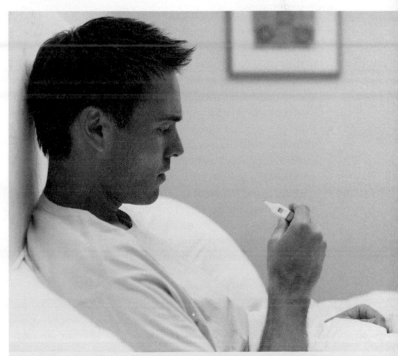

Deciding when to contact a physician can be difficult. Most people first try to diagnose and treat a minor condition themselves.

- Trauma to the head or spine accompanied by persistent headache, blurred vision, loss of consciousness, vomiting, convulsions, or paralysis
- Sudden high fever or recurring high temperature (over 102°F for children and 103°F for adults) and/or sweats
- Tingling sensation in the arm accompanied by slurred speech or impaired thought processes
- Adverse reactions to a drug or insect bite (shortness of breath, severe swelling, or dizziness)
- Unexplained sudden weight loss
- Persistent or recurrent diarrhea or vomiting
- Blue-tinted lips, eyelids, or nail beds
- Any lump, swelling, thickness, or sore that does not subside or that grows for over a month
- Any blood in the stool or urine, or significant pain, or marked, persistent change in bowel or bladder habits
- Yellowing of the skin or the whites of the eyes
- Sudden severe pain that has no apparent cause
- Any symptom that is unusual, persists, or recurs over time
- Pregnancy

See the **Skills for Behavior Change** box for pointers on taking an active role in your own health care.

## Assessing Health Professionals

Suppose you decide that you do need medical help. How should you go about assessing the qualifications of a health care provider? Numerous studies show that the most satisfied patients are those who feel their health care provider explains diagnosis and treatment options thoroughly and demonstrates competency as well as genuine concern.[2]

When evaluating health care providers, consider the following questions:

- Do they listen to you, respect you as an individual, and give you time to ask questions? Do you feel like they are in a rush to finish and move on to the next patient or are they "tuned in" to you? Do they return your calls, and are they available to answer questions between visits? How long would it take you to get in to see them if you really needed an appointment?
- What professional education and training have they had and what are their credentials? What license or board certification(s) do they hold? Note an important difference: *Board certified* indicates that the physician has passed the national board examination for his or her specialty (e.g., pediatrics) and has been certified as competent in that specialty. In contrast, *board eligible* merely means that the physician is eligible to take the exam, but not that he or she has passed it. Do they have a record of any malpractice claims?

# 35.1 MILLION

AMERICANS ARE ADMITTED TO THE HOSPITAL **EACH YEAR**.

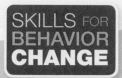

## SKILLS FOR BEHAVIOR CHANGE

### BE PROACTIVE IN YOUR HEALTH CARE

The following points help you communicate well with health care providers:

▶ Know your personal and family medical history.

▶ Research your condition—causes, physiological effects, possible treatments, and prognosis. Don't rely solely on the health care provider.

▶ Write out your questions in advance. Don't feel awkward asking them, and don't accept a defensive response. Asking questions is your right as a patient.

▶ Bring someone with you to appointments to listen, take notes, and ask for clarification if necessary. If you go alone, take notes.

▶ Ask the practitioner to explain the problem and possible tests, treatments, and medications. If you don't understand something, ask for clarification.

▶ If the health care provider prescribes any medications, ask whether you can take generic equivalents that cost less.

▶ Ask for a written summary of the results of your visit and any lab tests.

▶ Seek a second opinion about important tests or treatment recommendations.

▶ After your health care visit, you will likely receive an e-mail with a link to the provider's record of your visit. Read the record carefully, and contact the provider if you have any questions or concerns. Otherwise, store it with your other health care files. If your doctor doesn't provide this sort of service, write down an accurate account of what happened and what was said. Be sure to include the names of the provider and all other people involved in your care, the date, and the place.

▶ When filling prescriptions, read the pharmacist-provided drug information sheet that lists medical considerations and details about potential drug and food interactions.

- Are they affiliated with an accredited medical facility or institution? The Joint Commission is an independent nonprofit organization that evaluates and accredits more than 20,500 health care organizations and programs in the United States. Accreditation requires institutions to verify all education, licensing, and training claims of their affiliated practitioners.[3]
- Are they open to complementary or integrative strategies? Would they refer you for different treatment modalities if appropriate?
- Do they indicate possible treatment options clearly, the pros and cons of each, and the effectiveness of a given treatment in the short and long terms? What might be the side effects of a treatment and what possible symptoms might you expect?

- Who will be responsible for your care when your physician is on vacation or off call? Are they part of a practice group with colleagues who can help you when they are not available?
- Are there professional reviews and information on any lawsuits against them available online?

Being prepared for appointments and asking the right questions allow you to work in partnership with your health care provider. Many patients find that writing questions down before an appointment helps them get the answers they need. Don't accept a defensive or hostile response; if you are not satisfied with how a practitioner communicates, go elsewhere. It is also important that you provide honest answers to his or her questions about your symptoms, condition, lifestyle, and medical history.

Active participation in your treatment is the only sensible course in a health care environment that encourages *defensive medicine*, in which providers take certain actions primarily to avoid a **malpractice** claim. Only by taking an active and informed role in your own or loved ones health care and working with your providers can you help ensure the best health outcomes. Today, the third leading cause of death in America is preventable medical error: hospital errors, errors in diagnosis, injuries from medications, and other health care errors. In a complex, often over-taxed health care system, mistakes can happen. Being a savvy health care consumer is the best way to reduce your risks.[4]

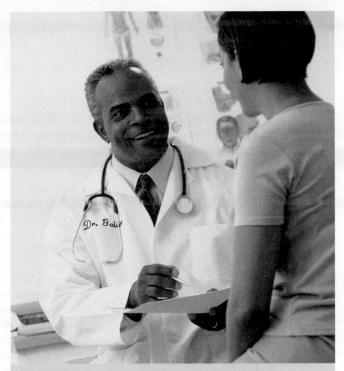

It's important to understand recommendations that your health care provider makes. Questions to ask include how often the practitioner has performed a procedure, the proportion of successful outcomes for the treatment or procedure, and why a test has been ordered.

### WHAT DO YOU THINK?

Do you believe that patients should have access to information about practitioners' and facilities' malpractice records?

- What about information on success and failure rates or outcomes of various procedures?

## Your Rights as a Patient

More than asking questions, being proactive in your health care also means being aware of your rights as a patient, as follows:[5]

1. The right of **informed consent** means that before receiving care, you should be fully informed of what is planned; risks and potential benefits; and possible alternative forms of treatment, including the option of no treatment. Your consent must be voluntary and without coercion. It is critical to read consent forms carefully and amend them as necessary before signing.
2. You are entitled to know whether the treatment you are receiving is standard or experimental. In experimental conditions, you have the legal and ethical right to know if any drug is being used as part of a research project for a purpose not approved by the Food and Drug

**SEE IT!** VIDEOS

Knowing your medical history can keep you informed of health risks. Watch **Your Medical History**, available on MasteringHealth™

Administration (FDA) and if the study is one in which some people receive treatment while others receive a **placebo**. (See the **Student Health Today** box on the next page for more on placebos and the placebo effect.)

3. You have the right to make decisions regarding the health care that is recommended by the physician.
4. You have the right to confidentiality, which includes the source of payment for treatment and care. It also means you have the right to make personal decisions concerning all reproductive matters.
5. You have the right to receive adequate health care, as well as to refuse treatment and to cease treatment at any time.
6. You are entitled to have access to all of your medical records and to have those records remain confidential.
7. You have the right to continuity of health care.
8. You have the right to seek the opinions of other health care professionals regarding your condition.
9. You have the right to courtesy, respect, dignity, responsiveness, and timely attention to health needs.

**malpractice** Improper or negligent treatment by a health practitioner that results in loss, injury, or harm to the patient.

**informed consent** Acknowledgment that you have been told of the potential risks and benefits of a recommended test or treatment, understand what you have been told, and agree to the care.

**placebo** Inactive substance used as a control in a clinical test to determine the effectiveness of a particular drug; the *placebo effect* occurs when patients given a placebo drug or treatment experience an improved state of health owing to the belief that they are receiving something that will be of benefit.

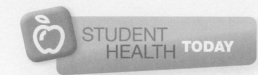
# THE PLACEBO EFFECT
## *Mind Over Matter?*

The *placebo effect* is an apparent cure or improved state of health brought about by a substance, product, or procedure that has no generally recognized therapeutic value. Patients often report improvements in a condition based on what they expect, desire, or were told would happen after receiving a treatment, even though the treatment was, for example, simple sugar pills instead of powerful drugs. Placebo-controlled studies are often used to determine the effectiveness of medications. Patients with a particular condition are given either the drug that is being tested or a placebo. If a significantly greater number of patients receiving the drug have a significantly better outcome than the patients receiving the placebo, the treatment can be considered effective. Most such studies are double-blind; that is, neither the patients nor the doctors involved are told until the study ends who had the real treatment.

There is also a *nocebo* effect, in which a practitioner's negative assessment of a patient's symptoms leads to a worsening of the condition, such as increased anxiety and pain. Similarly, a negative assessment of a treatment's potential efficacy induces a failure to respond to that treatment.

Researchers are investigating how and why expectation appears to change physiology. Evidence from pain studies suggests that use of a placebo for pain control causes the brain to release the same endogenous (natural) opioids it releases when the study participant uses a pain medication with an active ingredient. But pain is not the only factor to respond to expectation.

- A study of resting tremor (such as involuntary finger tapping) in patients with Parkinson's disease found that positive or negative expectations of a treatment's effectiveness reduced or increased patient tremor when they were given the same valid medication or the same placebo.
- A study of patients with clinical depression found no significant difference in effectiveness of a commonly prescribed antidepressant, an herbal remedy often used for depression, and a placebo after 26 weeks of therapy.
- Several studies have found a significant placebo effect in trials of medications to treat alcohol dependency; alcohol-dependent patients consume fewer alcoholic drinks and report less alcohol dependence and cravings, regardless of whether they are receiving the drug or a placebo.

If you're curious to learn more about the scientific evidence behind a drug prescribed for you, get online. A quick search using the exact name of the medication and the words "drug studies" should provide links to the information you're looking for.

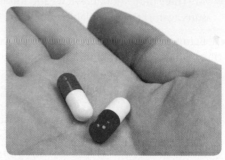

**Is it a real medicine or a placebo? In some cases, it may not make a difference.**

**Sources:** L. Colloca and C. Grillon, "Understanding Placebo and Nocebo Responses for Pain Management," *Current Pain and Headache Reports* 18, no. 6 (2014): 419, doi: 10.1007/s11916-014-0419-2; A. Keitel et al., "Expectation Modulates the Effect of Deep Brain Stimulation on Motor and Cognitive Function in Tremor-Dominant Parkinson's Disease," *PLoS One* 8, no. 12 (2013): e81878, doi: 10.1371/journal.pone.0081878; J. Sarris, M. Fava, I. Schweitzer, and D. Mischoulon, "St. John's Wort (*Hypericum perforatum*) versus Sertraline and Placebo in Major Depressive Disorder: Continuation Data from a 26-Week RCT," *Pharmacopsychiatry* 45, no. 7 (2012): 275–8, doi: 10.1055/s-0032-1306348; R. A. Litten et al., "The Placebo Effect in Clinical Trials for Alcohol Dependence: An Exploratory Analysis of 51 Naltrexone and Acamprosate Studies," *Alcoholism, Clinical and Experimental Research* 37, no. 12 (2013): 2128–37, doi: 10.1111/acer.12197; G. L. Petersen et al., "The Magnitude of Nocebo Effects in Pain: A Meta-Analysis," *Pain* (April 26, 2014), pii: S0304-3959(14)00195-X, doi: 10.1016/j.pain.2014.04.016

## LO 2 | CONVENTIONAL HEALTH CARE

Describe and discuss conventional health care, including types of practitioners and the health care products and treatments available.

Conventional health care, also called **allopathic medicine,** mainstream medicine, or traditional Western medical practice, is the dominant type of health care delivered in the United States, Canada, Europe, and much of the developed world. It is based on the premise that illness is a result of exposure to harmful environmental agents, or organic changes in the body. The prevention of disease and the restoration of health involve vaccines, drugs, surgery, and other treatments.

Be aware, however, that not all allopathic treatments have had the benefit of the extensive clinical trials and long-term studies of outcomes that would conclusively prove effectiveness in various populations. Even when studies appear to support the benefits of a particular treatment or product, other studies with equal or better scientific validity often refute earlier claims. Also, recommended treatments may change dramatically as new technologies and medical advances replace older practices. Like other professionals, medical doctors must keep up with new research and changing practices in their field(s) of specialty.

One of the ways health care providers ensure the quality of care they provide is by practicing **evidence-based medicine.** Decisions regarding patient care are based on clinical expertise, patient values, and current best scientific evidence.

**allopathic medicine** Conventional, Western medical practice; in theory, based on scientifically validated methods and procedures.

**evidence-based medicine** Decisions regarding patient care based on clinical expertise, patient values, and current best scientific evidence.

Clinical expertise refers to the clinician's cumulative experience, education, and clinical skills. The patient brings his or her own personal and unique concerns, expectations, and values. The best evidence is usually found in clinically relevant research conducted using sound methodology.

## Conventional Health Care Practitioners

Selecting a **primary care practitioner (PCP)**—a medical practitioner whom you can visit for routine ailments, preventive care, general medical advice, and appropriate referrals—is not an easy task. The PCP for most people is a family practitioner, an internist, or for women, an obstetrician-gynecologist (obgyn). Many people routinely see nurse practitioners or physician assistants who work for an individual doctor or a medical group, and others use nontraditional providers as their primary source of care. As a college student, you may opt to visit a PCP at your campus health center.

Doctors undergo rigorous training before they can begin practicing. After 4 years of undergraduate work, students typically spend 4 additional years studying for their doctor of medicine degree (MD). After this general training, some students choose a specialty, such as pediatrics, cardiology, oncology, radiology, or surgery, and spend another year in an internship and several years doing a residency. Some specialties also require a fellowship, so additional training after receiving a medical degree can take up to 8 years.

**Osteopaths** are general practitioners who receive training similar to that of a medical doctor but who place special emphasis on the skeletal and muscular systems. Their treatments may involve manipulation of the muscles and joints. Osteopaths receive the degree of doctor of osteopathy (DO) rather than an MD.

Eye care specialists can be either ophthalmologists or optometrists. An **ophthalmologist** holds a medical degree and can perform surgery and prescribe medications. An **optometrist** typically evaluates visual problems and fits glasses but is not a trained physician. If you have an eye condition requiring diagnosis and treatment, see an ophthalmologist.

**Dentists** diagnose and treat diseases of the teeth, gums, and oral cavity. They attend dental school for 4 years and receive the title of doctor of dental surgery (DDS) or doctor of medical dentistry (DMD). They must also pass both state and national board examinations before receiving their licenses to practice. The field of dentistry includes specialties; for example, *orthodontists* specialize in the alignment of teeth, *periodontists* treat diseases of the gums and other tissues surrounding the teeth, and *oral surgeons* perform surgical procedures to correct problems of the mouth, face, and jaw.

**Nurses** are trained health care professionals who provide a wide range of services for patients and their families, including patient education, counseling, providing community health and disease prevention information, and administration of medications. Registered nurses (RNs) in the United States complete either a 4-year program leading to a bachelor of science in nursing (BSN) degree or a 2-year associate degree program, and must also pass a national certification exam. Lower-level licensed practical or vocational nurses (LPN or LVN) complete a 1- to 2-year training program, which may be based in either a community college or hospital, and take a licensing exam.

**Nurse practitioners (NPs)** are nurses with advanced training obtained through either a master's degree program or a specialized nurse practitioner program. Nurse practitioners have the training and authority to conduct diagnostic tests and prescribe medications (in some states). They work in a variety of settings, including clinics and student health centers, and can specialize in areas such as pediatrics or acute care. Nurses and nurse practitioners may also earn the clinical doctor of nursing degree (ND), doctor of nursing science (DNS and DNSc degrees), or a research-based PhD in nursing.

**Physician assistants (PAs)** are licensed to examine and diagnose patients, offer treatment, and write prescriptions under a physician's supervision. An important difference between a PA and an NP is that the PA must practice under a physician's supervision. Like other health care providers, PAs are licensed by state boards of medicine.

**primary care practitioner (PCP)** Medical practitioner who provides preventive care and treats routine ailments, gives general medical advice, and makes appropriate referrals when necessary.

**osteopath** General practitioner who receives training similar to a medical doctor's but with an emphasis on the skeletal and muscular systems; may use spinal manipulation as part of treatment.

**ophthalmologist** Physician who specializes in the medical and surgical care of the eyes, including prescriptions for lenses.

**optometrist** Eye specialist whose practice is limited to prescribing and fitting lenses to correct vision problems.

**dentist** Physician who diagnoses and treats diseases of the teeth, gums, and oral cavity.

**nurse** Health professional who provides patient care in a variety of settings.

**nurse practitioner (NP)** Nurse with advanced training obtained through either a master's degree program or a specialized nurse practitioner program.

**physician assistant (PA)** Health care practitioner trained to handle most routine care under the supervision of a physician.

## Conventional Medication

Prescription drugs can be obtained only with a written prescription from a physician, while over-the-counter drugs can be purchased without a prescription (see Chapter 7). Making wise decisions about medication is an important aspect of responsible health care.

**Prescription Drugs** In about three fourths of doctor visits, the physician administers or prescribes at least one medication.[6] In fact, prescription drug use has increased steadily over the past decade, and over 68 percent of Americans now use one or more prescription drugs.[7] Even though these drugs are administered under medical supervision, the wise consumer still takes precautions. Adverse effects and complications arising from the use of prescription drugs are common, as is failure to respond to a medication.

Consumers have a variety of resources available to help them make educated decisions about whether to take a certain drug. One of the best resources is the U.S. FDA Center for Drug Evaluation and Research website (www.fda.gov/drugs), which provides current information for consumers on risks and

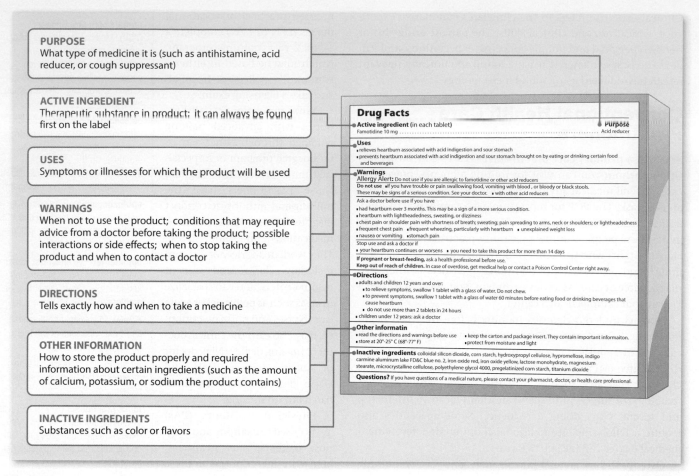

**PURPOSE**
What type of medicine it is (such as antihistamine, acid reducer, or cough suppressant)

**ACTIVE INGREDIENT**
Therapeutic substance in product; it can always be found first on the label

**USES**
Symptoms or illnesses for which the product will be used

**WARNINGS**
When not to use the product; conditions that may require advice from a doctor before taking the product; possible interactions or side effects; when to stop taking the product and when to contact a doctor

**DIRECTIONS**
Tells exactly how and when to take a medicine

**OTHER INFORMATION**
How to store the product properly and required information about certain ingredients (such as the amount of calcium, potassium, or sodium the product contains)

**INACTIVE INGREDIENTS**
Substances such as color or flavors

**Drug Facts**

**Active ingredient** (in each tablet) ... **Purpose**
Famotidine 10 mg .......................... Acid reducer

**Uses**
■ relieves heartburn associated with acid indigestion and sour stomach
■ prevents heartburn associated with acid indigestion and sour stomach brought on by eating or drinking certain food and beverages

**Warnings**
**Allergy Alert:** Do not use if you are allergic to famotidine or other acid reducers
**Do not use** ■ if you have trouble or pain swallowing food, vomiting with blood , or bloody or black stools. These may be signs of a serious condition. See your doctor. ■ with other acid reducers
**Ask a doctor before use if you have**
■ had heartburn over 3 months. This may be a sign of a more serious condition.
■ heartburn with lightheadedness, sweating, or dizziness
■ chest pain or shoulder pain with shortness of breath; sweating; pain spreading to arms, neck or shoulders; or lightheadedness
■ frequent chest pain ■ frequent wheezing, particularly with heartburn ■ unexplained weight loss
■ nausea or vomiting ■ stomach pain
Stop use and ask a doctor if
■ your heartburn continues or worsens ■ you need to take this product for more than 14 days
**If pregnant or breast-feeding,** ask a health professional before use.
**Keep out of reach of children.** In case of overdose, get medical help or contact a Poison Control Center right away.

**Directions**
■ adults and children 12 years and over:
■ to relieve symptoms, swallow 1 tablet with a glass of water. Do not chew.
■ to prevent symptoms, swallow 1 tablet with a glass of water 60 minutes before eating food or drinking beverages that cause heartburn
■ do not use more than 2 tablets in 24 hours
■ children under 12 years: ask a doctor

**Other informatin**
■ read the directions and warnings before use ■ keep the carton and package insert. They contain important informaiton.
■ store at 20°-25° C (68°-77° F) ■ protect from moisture and light

**Inactive ingredients** colloidal silicon dioxide, corn starch, hydroxypropyl cellulose, hypromellose, indigo carmine aluminum lake FD&C blue no. 2, iron oxide red, iron oxide yellow, lactose monohydrate, magnesium stearate, microcrystalline cellulose, polyethylene glycol 4000, pregelatinized corn starch, titanium dioxide

**Questions?** If you have questions of a medical nature, please contact your pharmacist, doctor, or health care professional.

**FIGURE 16.1** Over-the-Counter Medicine Label

**Source:** Consumer Healthcare Products Association, OTC Label. Courtesy of CHPA Educational Foundation, www.otcsafety.org

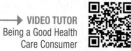

▶ VIDEO TUTOR
Being a Good Health Care Consumer

benefits of prescription drugs. Being knowledgeable can help ensure your safety.

**Generic drugs,** prescription medications sold under a chemical name rather than a brand name, contain the same active ingredients as brand-name drugs but are usually much less expensive. Not all drugs are available as generics. If your doctor prescribes medication, ask if a generic equivalent exists and if it would be safe and effective for you to try.

**generic drugs** Medications marketed by chemical names rather than brand names.

Although generic medications behave very similarly to brand-name versions and show a similar efficacy, there is some concern that substitutions made in minor ingredients might reduce a patient's response to the drug or cause side effects.[8] Always tell your doctor about any reactions you have to medications.

**Over-the-Counter Drugs** Medications available without a prescription are referred to as *over-the-counter (OTC)* drugs. American consumers spend billions of dollars yearly on OTC preparations for relief of everything from runny noses to ingrown toenails. Those most commonly used are pain relievers;

cold, cough, and allergy medications; stimulants; sleeping aids and relaxants; and dieting aids.

Despite a common belief that OTC products are safe and effective, indiscriminate use and abuse can occur with these drugs as with all others. For example, people who frequently use eye drops to "get the red out" or pop antacids after every meal are likely to become dependent. Many people also experience adverse side effects because they ignore warnings on drug interactions and other cautions printed on labels. The FDA has developed a standard label that appears on most OTC products (see **FIGURE 16.1**). It includes directions for use, active and inactive ingredients, warnings, and other useful information.

## LO 3 | **HEALTH** INSURANCE

Describe the U.S. health care system in terms of types and availability of insurance and the changes related to health care reform.

No matter how you're treated, chances are you'll use some form of health insurance to pay for your care. Insurance typically allows you, the consumer, to pay into a pool of funds and then bill the insurance carrier for covered charges you incur.

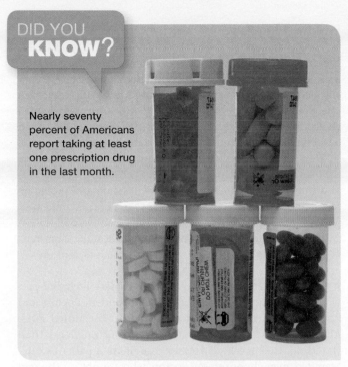
The fundamental principle of insurance underwriting is that the cost of health care can be predicted for large populations. This is how health care **premiums** are determined. Policyholders pay premiums into a pool from which insurance companies pay claims. When you are sick or injured, the insurance company pays your care provider out of the pool regardless of your total contribution. If you require a great deal of medical care, you may never pay anything close to the actual cost of that care. Or, if you are basically healthy, you may pay more in insurance premiums than the total cost of your medical bills. Health insurance is based on the idea that policyholders pay affordable premiums so they never have to face catastrophic bills. In profit-oriented systems, insurers prefer to have healthy people in their plans who pour money into risk pools without taking money out.

## Private Health Insurance

Originally, health insurance consisted solely of coverage for hospital costs (it was called *major medical*), but was gradually extended to cover routine physicians' treatment and other services, such as dental, vision care, and pharmaceuticals. These payment mechanisms laid the groundwork for today's steadily rising health care costs as hospitals were reimbursed for the costs of providing care plus an amount for profit. This system provided no incentive to contain costs, limit the number of procedures, or curtail capital investment in redundant equipment and facilities. Physicians were reimbursed on a fee-for-service (indemnity) basis determined by "usual, customary, and reasonable" fees. This system encouraged physicians to charge high fees, raise them often, and perform as many procedures as possible. Until the mid- to late-twentieth century, most insurance did not cover routine or preventive services, and consumers generally waited until illness developed to see a doctor instead of seeking preventive care. Consumers were also free to choose any provider or service they wished, including even inappropriate—and often expensive—levels of care.

To limit potential losses, private insurance companies began increasingly employing several mechanisms: cost sharing (in the form of deductibles, co-payments, and coinsurance), waiting periods, exclusions, "preexisting condition" clauses, and upper limits on payments:

- *Deductibles* are payments (which can range from about $500 to $5,000 annually) you make for health care before insurance coverage kicks in to pay for eligible services.
- *Co-payments* are set amounts that you pay per service or product received, regardless of the total cost (e.g., $20 per doctor visit or per prescription filled).
- *Coinsurance* is the percentage of costs that you must pay based on the terms of the policy (e.g., 20% of the total bill).
- Some group plans specify a *waiting period* that cannot exceed 90 days before they will provide coverage. Waiting periods do not apply to plans purchased by individuals.
- All insurers set some limits on the types of *covered services* (e.g., most exclude cosmetic surgery, private rooms, and experimental procedures).
- *Preexisting condition clauses* once limited the insurance company's liability for medical conditions that a consumer had before obtaining coverage. Under the 2010 Patient Protection and Affordable Care Act (ACA), no one can be discriminated against due to a preexisting condition.
- Some plans imposed an *annual upper limit* or *lifetime limit,* after which coverage would end. The ACA makes this practice illegal.

## Managed Care

Managed care describes a health care delivery system consisting of the following:

- A network of physicians, hospitals, and other providers and facilities linked contractually to deliver comprehensive health benefits within a predetermined budget and sharing economic risk for any budget deficit or surplus

**premium** Payment made to an insurance carrier, usually in monthly installments, that covers the cost of an insurance policy.

**managed care** Type of health insurance plan based on coordination of care and cost-reduction strategies; emphasizes health education and preventive care.

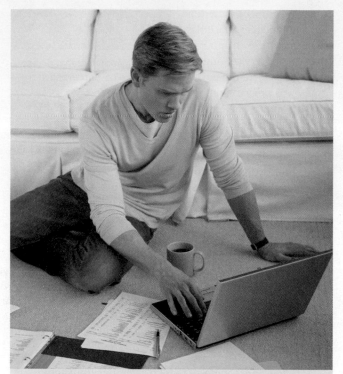

Choosing a health insurance plan can be confusing. Some things to think about include how comprehensive your coverage needs to be, how much you are willing to spend on premiums and co-payments, and whether the services of the plan meet your needs.

- A budget based on an estimate of the annual cost of delivering health care for a given population
- An established set of administrative rules regarding how services are to be obtained from participating health care providers under the terms of the health plan

Types of managed care plans include *health maintenance organizations* (HMOs), *preferred provider organizations* (PPOs), and *point of service* (POS). More than 73 million Americans are enrolled in HMOs, the most common type.[9]

Many managed care plans pay their contracted health care providers through **capitation**, a fixed monthly amount paid for each enrolled patient regardless of services provided. Some plans pay health care providers a salary, and some are still fee-for-service plans. Doctors participating in managed care networks are motivated (and sometimes incentivized) to keep their patient pool healthy and avoid preventable catastrophic ailments. Prevention and early intervention are often capstone components of such plans.

Managed care plans have grown steadily over the past several decades, and there has been a proportionate decline of enrollment in traditional indemnity plans. Indemnity insurance, which has no built-in incentives to control costs, has become unaffordable or unavailable for most Americans.

**capitation** Prepayment of a fixed monthly amount for each patient without regard to the type or number of services provided.

**Medicare** A federal health insurance program that covers people over the age of 65, permanently disabled people, and people with end-stage kidney failure.

## Health Maintenance Organizations

Health maintenance organizations provide a wide range of covered health benefits (e.g., physician visits, lab tests, surgery) for a fixed amount prepaid by the patient, the employer, Medicaid, or Medicare. Usually, HMO premiums are the least expensive form of managed care, but they are also the most restrictive (offering more limited choices of staff and health care facilities). There are low or no deductibles or coinsurance payments, and co-payments are small.

The downside of HMOs is that patients are required to use the plan's doctors and hospitals. Within an HMO, the PCP serves as a *gatekeeper*, coordinating the patient's care and providing referrals to specialists and other services. As more and more people enroll in HMOs, concerns have arisen about care allocation and access to services, profit-motivated medical decision making, and the degree of focus on prevention and intervention.

## Preferred Provider Organization

Preferred provider organizations are networks of independent doctors and hospitals that contract to provide care at discounted rates. Although they often offer more choices of providers than HMOs do, they are less likely to coordinate a patient's care. Members may choose to see doctors who are not on the preferred list at a higher percentage of out-of-pocket costs.

## Point of Service

Point of service (POS)—a hybrid of HMO and PPO plans—provides a more familiar form of managed care for people used to traditional indemnity insurance where services are directly reimbursed, which may explain why it is among the fastest growing of managed care plans. Under POS plans, members select an in-network PCP, but they can go to nonnetwork providers for care without a referral and must pay the extra cost.

## Independent Practice Association

*Independent practice associations* (IPAs) comprise independent physicians who maintain their own offices, but who also agree to enroll members of an organization for a negotiated fee for each assigned patient, or a negotiated fee-for-service basis. IPAs can help eliminate isolation, risks, and expenses associated with independent private practice.

## Exclusive Provider Organization

Exclusive provider organizations (EPOs) are a type of managed health care organization in which no coverage is typically provided for services received outside the EPO. Treatment or care received outside of the approved network must be paid by the patient.

No matter what type of plan you have, a special savings account for health-related expenses could save you money. See the **Money & Health** box to find out how they work and if they're right for you.

## Government-Funded Programs

The federal government, through programs such as Medicare and Medicaid, currently funds about 45 percent of the total U.S. health care spending.[10]

**Medicare** Medicare is a federal insurance program that employees and employers pay into over the course of a

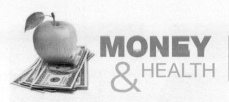

# MONEY & HEALTH | HEALTH CARE SPENDING ACCOUNTS

A Flexible Spending Account (FSA) for health care and a Health Savings Account (HSA) are savings plans that give you the opportunity to save money tax free to be used toward qualified health care expenses. As long as you're not claimed as a dependent on someone else's tax return, you can open either an FSA through your employer or an HSA through your bank.

If you're an employee, upon enrollment you identify the amount you want diverted from your paycheck into your FSA before taxes are withheld. The maximum you can contribute varies with different employers and health plans. One drawback to the FSA is that any funds still in the account at the end of the plan year are forfeited. This is known as the "use it or lose it" rule. Therefore, you need to estimate carefully what your out-of-pocket health expenses will be during the plan year.

With an HSA, there is no time limit on when the funds have to be used. Contributions to the account can be made from your paycheck by your employer as pre-tax deductions, or you can make them yourself, in which case you can claim them as an "above-the-line" deduction (a deduction from your gross income) when you file your tax return.

What expenses can you pay for with the money in your account? Deductibles, co-payments, eyeglasses, contact lenses, and prescription drugs are all allowed. Visits to approved health care providers, including dentists and optometrists, are also payable from your account if you have no health insurance coverage for them. You can even use the funds to pay for OTC drugs such as pain relievers or allergy medications as long as you have a written statement from your care provider.

If you currently pay out of pocket for more than one or two health care visits a year, for a few prescriptions, contact lenses, etc., and the money you use for these expenses comes from taxable income, then a health care savings plan might be worth a closer look. Contact your employee benefits specialist, your tax preparer, or a customer service provider at your bank.

---

person's working life, a form of long-term savings plan for health insurance and care, rather than the "entitlement" program. The funds are used to cover a broad range of services, except long-term care. Medicare covers citizens or permanent residents of the United States who are over the age of 65 and those 62 and older with a history of disability, amyotrophic lateral sclerosis (ALS), or permanent end-stage kidney damage. Currently, 52.3 million people receive Medicare. (43.5 million aged, and 8.8 million disabled persons.)[11] As the costs of medical care have continued to increase, Medicare has placed limits on the amount of reimbursement to providers. As a result, some providers no longer accept Medicare patients or those new to their practice.

Currently Medicare is divided into two major parts. Part A is the hospital insurance portion and helps pay for care while in hospitals, skilled nursing facilities, hospice care, and some home health care. Eligibility for Medicare begins at age 65, on the basis of having paid Medicare taxes while working. Typically, Medicare requires an annual deductible and may not pay all of a person's health care expenses depending on the state you live in and the type of Medicare plan you select (that is, *Original or an Advantage* plan).

Part B covers the services and supplies needed to diagnose and treat you and the preventive exams and services recommended based on your age and symptoms. Part B requires monthly payments by you, and these rates may vary, with higher income individuals paying more than lower income individuals. Typically, Part B covers most of your care as long as your provider or facility "*accepts assignment*"—meaning that they agree to only charge what Medicare says they should charge and will pay for.

To control hospital costs, the federal government set up a prospective payment system based on *diagnosis-related groups (DRGs)* for Medicare as well as other insurance plans. Nearly 500 groupings establish how much a hospital would be reimbursed for caring for a patient diagnosed with particular conditions. DRGs are based on the assumption that patients with similar health status and conditions require a similar amount of hospital resources. If the costs of treating a patient are less than the predetermined amount, the hospital can keep the difference. However, if a patient's care costs more than the set amount, the hospital must absorb the difference (with a few exceptions, this must be reviewed by a panel). This system motivates hospitals to discharge patients quickly, to provide more ambulatory care, and to admit patients classified into the most favorable (profitable) DRGs. Many private health insurance companies have also adopted reimbursement rates based on DRGs.

## WHY SHOULD I CARE?

The ultimate choice about health care remains with you. In order to make sound decisions about what is best for your health, you need to understand as much as you can about your options.

## Supplement or Medigap Plans

If providers charge more that Medicare allows, either you or a *supplement/Medigap* plan must make up the difference for these *Excess Medicare Part B* charges and other expenses such as deductibles and coinsurance by purchasing a group of supplemental insurance plans that cover charges that Medicare won't—things like additional international travel or additional stays in hospital.

**Advantage Plans** Medicare Advantage plans may replace original Medicare Part A and B—forming a sort of hybrid Medicare plan. Run by private companies, Advantage plans must provide the same benefit coverage as Medicare A and B. They vary beyond the minimum set of benefits and are often cheaper than Medigap. Some plans offer dental, vision, or prescription coverage. It is important to note that states differ in types of Advantage plans and coverage and that some health care organizations do not accept Medicare Advantage plans.

**Part D Medicare** In an era of rapidly increasing drug costs, prescription drug coverage is an essential part of any Medicare plan. Original Medicare (Part A and B) typically cover only minimal drugs, making the purchase of an additional drug plan (Part D) necessary. People who opt for Advantage plans must check to make sure their drugs are covered.

**Medicaid** In contrast to Medicare, **Medicaid**, covering approximately 72.2 million people, is a federal-state matching funds program that provides health insurance for people defined as low income, including many who are pregnant, blind, disabled, elderly, or eligible for Temporary Assistance for Needy Families (TANF). Because each state determines income eligibility, covered services, and payments to providers, there are vast differences in the way Medicaid operates from state to state. The ACA provides generous federal subsidies to states that expand Medicaid coverage to all Americans living below 133 percent of the federal poverty level (in 2015, the poverty level was $24,250 for a four person household).[12] Although states are responsible for only a small percentage of the funding to expand Medicaid, some have refused; however, those states complying with Medicaid expansion are expected to have increased enrollment by over 8.5 million Americans by 2016.[13]

**Medicaid** A federal-state matching funds program that provides health insurance to low-income people.

The Children's Health Insurance Program (CHIP) provides health insurance coverage to more than 8 million uninsured children whose family income is too high to qualify for Medicaid.[14] Like Medicaid, it is jointly funded by federal and state funds and is administered by state governments.

## Insurance Coverage by the Numbers

In 2015, the average family's annual health insurance premium was more than $16,000.[15] For workers employed in organizations that offer health care insurance, most of this cost is hidden: The worker pays 15 percent to 25 percent of the

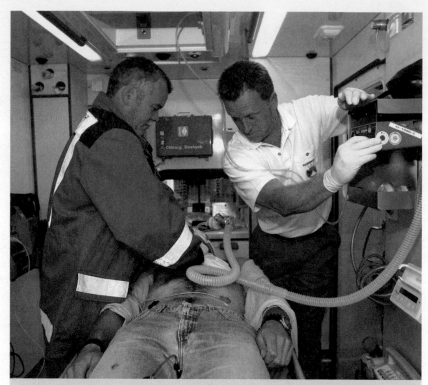

People without insurance can't gain access to preventive care, so they seek care only in an emergency or crisis. Because emergency care is extraordinarily expensive, they often are unable to pay, and the cost is absorbed by those who can pay—the insured or taxpayers.

full premium, usually as a deduction from his or her paycheck, and earns lower wages in return for the remaining cost of the coverage. However, people who are self-employed or work in companies that do not provide group health insurance must pay their premiums independently, often at extremely high rates. Millions of employed but uninsured Americans do not find them affordable. In total, about 25.8 million Americans are uninsured.[16] The vast majority of the uninsured work or are dependents of employed people.

Lack of health insurance has been associated with delayed health care and increased mortality. *Underinsurance* (i.e., the inability to pay out-of-pocket expenses despite having insurance) also may result in adverse health consequences. Among young adults ages 19 to 34, 18 percent do not have health insurance coverage.[17] College students as a group fare better than non-college adults when it comes to insurance. In a 2014 national survey of college students, 5 percent of respondents said they did not have health insurance.[18] People without adequate health care coverage are less likely than other Americans to have their children immunized, seek early prenatal care, obtain annual blood pressure checks and other screenings, and seek attention for symptoms of health problems. Forgoing preventative care because of cost, they tend to rely on emergency care at later stages of illness. Because emergency care is far more expensive than other types of care, uninsured and underinsured patients are often unable to pay, and the cost is absorbed by "the system" in the form of higher hospital costs, insurance premiums, and taxes for all.

# LO 4 | ISSUES FACING TODAY'S HEALTH CARE SYSTEM

Discuss issues facing our health care system today, including those related to cost, quality, and access to services.

In 2010, Congress passed the Patient Protection and Affordable Care Act (ACA) to provide a means for all Americans to obtain affordable health care. In addition to increasing access to care, the ACA is addressing the high cost of care and improving the overall quality of care.

## Access

The most significant factors in determining access to health care are the supply and proximity of providers and facilities and availability of insurance coverage.

### Access to Providers, Facilities, and Treatments

In 2014, there were almost 692,000 physicians in the United States.[19] However, there is an oversupply of higher-paid specialists and a shortage of lower-paid primary care physicians (family practitioners, internists, pediatricians, etc.). The majority of nongovernment hospitals in the United States are also located in urban areas, leaving many rural communities with a lack of facilities.[20]

Managed care health plans determine access on the basis of participating providers, health plan benefits, and administrative rules, which means that consumers have little say in who treats them or what facility they can use.

The ACA and other government investments have helped in the training many new health care providers, as well as encouraged primary care providers to set up their practices in high-need areas. Some of these efforts have included:

- Investing in new primary care training programs like the National Health Service Corps and the Graduate Medical Education program.
- Training new primary care providers through increased funding of medical training programs.
- Supporting mental and behavioral health training to boost numbers of those practicing in mental and behavioral health.

**Access to Quality Health Insurance** Not everyone has the same insurance (or any at all), and unfortunately that means not everyone gets the same level of care.[21] Key provisions in the ACA aim to increase access to quality health insurance among Americans. These include the following:

- Insurers are now required to cover several preventive services, such as health screenings for cancer, diabetes, and cardiovascular disease for patients at increased risk and counseling on topics such as losing weight, quitting smoking, treating depression, and reducing alcohol use.
- Insurers are required to cover young adults on a parent's plan through age 26.
- Coverage is in place for prescription medications, including psychotropic medications.
- Americans with preexisting conditions cannot be denied coverage.
- No annual and lifetime limits on benefits are allowed.
- Affordable Insurance Exchanges (AIEs) will facilitate consumer shopping and enrollment in plans with the same kinds of choices that members of Congress have.
- Small businesses, which typically paid as much as 18 percent more than large businesses, now qualify for special tax credits to help fund insurance plans.

Even before passage of the ACA, Congress provided assistance with insurance coverage for employees who change jobs. Under the Consolidated Omnibus Budget Reconciliation Act (COBRA), former employees, retirees, spouses, and dependents have the option to continue their insurance for up to 18 months at group rates. People who enroll in COBRA do pay a higher amount than they did when they were employed because they are covering both the personal premium and the amount previously covered by the employer.

## Cost

Both per capita and as a percentage of gross domestic product (GDP), the United States spends more on health care than any other nation (**FIGURE 16.2**). In 2014, our national health expenditures were projected to reach $2.9 trillion, nearly $9,150 for every man, woman, and child.[22] Health care expenditures are projected to grow by 5.7 percent each year, reaching over $5 trillion annually by 2023—nearly 20 percent of our projected GDP.[23]

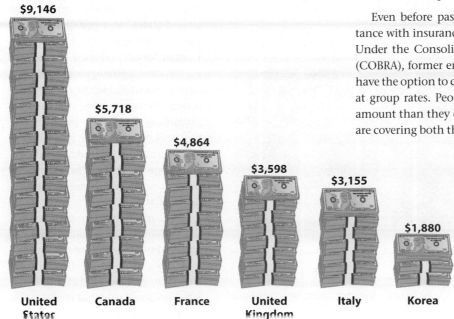

**$9,146** United States

**$5,718** Canada

**$4,864** France

**$3,598** United Kingdom

**$3,155** Italy

**$1,880** Korea

**FIGURE 16.2** Health Care Spending per Person, 2013

**Source:** The World Bank, "Health Care Expenditure Per Capita," 2015, http://data.worldbank.org/indicator/SH.XPD.PCAP

Why are U.S. health care costs so high? Many factors are involved: duplication of services; an aging population; growing rates of obesity, inactivity, and related health problems; demand for new diagnostic and treatment technologies; an emphasis on crisis-oriented care instead of prevention; physician overtreatment; and inappropriate use of services.

Our insurance system is also to blame. Currently, more than 2,000 companies provide health insurance in the United States, each with different coverage structures and administrative requirements. This lack of uniformity prevents our system from achieving the *economies of scale* (bulk purchasing at a reduced cost) and administrative efficiency realized in countries with a single-payer delivery system. According to the trade association for America's Health Insurance Plans (AHIP), commercial insurance companies commonly experience administrative costs greater than 12 percent of the total health care insurance premium.[24] These administrative expenses contribute to the high cost of health care and force companies to require their employees to share more of the costs, cut back on benefits, and drop some benefits altogether. See **FIGURE 16.3** for a breakdown of how health care dollars are spent.

The ACA's provision for Affordable Insurance Exchanges would increase bulk purchasing and reduce administrative costs, thus achieving some savings. Moreover, the ACA mandates that insurance companies that spend less than 80 percent of premium dollars on medical care in a given year now must send enrollees a rebate. All insurance companies now have to publicly justify their actions if they plan to raise rates by 10 percent or more, and tougher screening procedures and penalties are helping to reduce health care fraud, which should also cut down on ballooning costs.

AN ESTIMATED

# 440,000

PEOPLE **DIE** EACH YEAR FROM PREVENTABLE MEDICAL ERRORS IN HOSPITALS.

## Quality

The United States has several mechanisms for ensuring quality services: Providers are assessed according to education, licensure, certification/registration, accreditation, peer review, and the legal system of malpractice litigation. Over-the-counter and prescription medications, as well as medical devices, must be approved by the FDA. Insurance companies and government payers may also require a higher level of quality by linking payment to whether a practitioner is board certified, a facility is accredited, or a treatment is an approved therapy. In addition, most insurance plans now require prior authorization and/or second opinions, not only to reduce costs, but also to improve quality of care.

Although our health care spending far exceeds that of any other nation, we rank far below many other nations in key indicators of quality. For example, in 2015, the Central Intelligence Agency ranked the United States 42nd in life expectancy.[25] At a projected 79.5 years, U.S. life expectancy was a full decade below that of the top-ranked country, Monaco.[26] And our infant mortality rate, at 6.2 deaths per every 1,000 live births, is higher than that of 55 other nations.[27] The ACA is intended to improve the quality of health care in the United States. As a first step, in 2011 the Department of Health and Human Services released to Congress a National Strategy for Quality Improvement in Health Care. Its priorities include a new emphasis on promoting the safest, most preventive, and most effective care; increasing communication and coordination among providers; and ensuring that patients and families are engaged as partners in their care.[28]

Still, many health experts feel our system has failed and should be replaced (see the **Points of View** box for a discussion). As consumers, the best strategy is to read the accumulated evidence on what is and is not working in the health care system and base your decisions on a rational unbiased approach as we work to improve health care delivery in the United States.

**2013 total expenditures = $2.5 trillion**

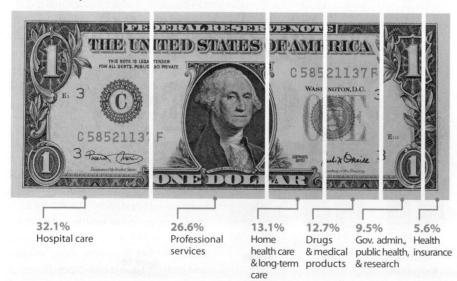

| 32.1% | 26.6% | 13.1% | 12.7% | 9.5% | 5.6% |
|---|---|---|---|---|---|
| Hospital care | Professional services | Home health care & long-term care | Drugs & medical products | Gov. admin., public health, & research | Health insurance |

**FIGURE 16.3** Where Do We Spend Our Health Care Dollars?

**Source:** U.S. Department of Health and Human Services, "Health, United States, 2014," National Center for Health Statistics, May 2015, www.cdc.gov/nchs/data/hus/hus14.pdf

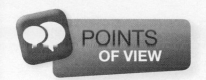

# POINTS OF VIEW

## National Health Care
*Is It a Government Responsibility?*

Whether universal health care coverage will—or should—be achieved in the United States and through what mechanism remain hotly debated topics. Proponents of reform argue that health care is a basic human right and should be available and affordable for everyone. They point to countries such as Canada, the United Kingdom, France, Israel, Taiwan, and Japan that currently provide health care to all citizens through a national service funded primarily through taxes. Opponents of health care reform feel that health care is not a right, but a commodity. They contend that the high cost of changing the system is more than the United States can afford and that the government should not interfere in what has been largely a free-market industry. In addition, lobbying efforts by the insurance industry, pharmaceutical manufacturers, the medical community, and special interest groups have all played a role in thwarting comprehensive reform.

In 2010, Congress passed the Patient Protection and Affordable Care Act (ACA)—a set of initial steps toward increasing the number of insured Americans. Still, it has been subjected to intense and often rancorous debate. The reforms mandated by the ACA are currently being implemented, and their actual effects are uncertain.

### Arguments for National Health Insurance

- Health care is a human right. Article 25 of the United Nations Universal Declaration of Human Rights states that "everyone has the right to a standard of living adequate for the health and well-being of oneself and one's family, including . . . medical care."
- Americans would be more likely to engage in health-promoting behaviors. People who are underinsured and uninsured forego preventive care checkups, wait to be seen about troubling symptoms, and fail to take prescribed medications because of cost concerns.
- Medical professionals could concentrate on the care of patients rather than on insurance procedures, malpractice liability, and other administrative distractions.
- Providing all citizens the right to health care is good for economic productivity because it allows them to live longer and healthier lives, thus contributing to society for a longer time.

### Arguments against National Health Insurance

- Health care is not a right, because it is not in the Bill of Rights in the U.S. Constitution, which lists rights that the government cannot infringe upon, not services or goods that the government must ensure for the people. Amending the U.S. Constitution to acknowledge a right to health care would be bad for economic productivity.
- It is the individual's responsibility, not the government's, to ensure personal health. Diseases and health problems can often be prevented by individuals choosing to live healthier lifestyles.
- Expenses for health care would have to be paid for with higher taxes or spending cuts in other areas, such as defense and education.

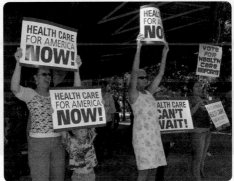

## WHERE DO YOU STAND?

- Do you think that the United States should move toward a system of national health care?
- Is health insurance a private or a public issue?

- Do you currently have health insurance? If you don't, what are the barriers that prevent you from having health insurance?
- If you do have health insurance, are you currently paying for it? If you are not paying for it, who is?

- Do you have a family member or close friend who lives in a country with a national health care system? If so, does this person support national health care or not, and why?

**Sources:** "The Universal Declaration of Human Rights" from The United Nations, 1948, www.un.org/en/ universaldeclaration-human-rights; P. Krugman, "The Medical Care," January 10, 2014, The New York Times; Right to Health Care ProCon.org, "Should All Americans Have the Right (Be Entitled) to Health Care?," Updated January 2014, http://healthcare.procon.org; The White House, "Health Care Reform: The Affordable Care Act," 2010, www.whitehouse.gov

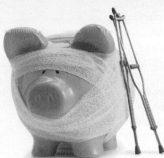

Answer the following questions to determine what you might do to become a better health care consumer.

|  |  | Yes | No | Not Applicable |
|---|---|:---:|:---:|:---:|
| 1. | Do you have health insurance? (If no, skip to 3) | ○ | ○ | ○ |
| 2. | Do you understand the coverage available to you? | ○ | ○ | ○ |
| 3. | Do you know which health care services are available for free or at a reduced cost at your student health center or local clinic? | ○ | ○ | ○ |
| 4. | In the last year have you received a prescription for medication? (If no, skip to 9) | ○ | ○ | ○ |
| 5. | When you received your prescription, did you ask the doctor or pharmacist if a generic brand could be substituted? | ○ | ○ | ○ |
| 6. | When you received your prescription, did you ask the doctor or pharmacist about potential side effects, including possible food and drug interactions? | ○ | ○ | ○ |
| 7. | If you experienced any unusual drug side effects, did you report them to your health care provider? | ○ | ○ | ○ |
| 8. | Did you take medication as directed? | ○ | ○ | ○ |
| 9. | When you receive a diagnosis, do you seek more information about the diagnosis and treatment? | ○ | ○ | ○ |
| 10. | If your health care provider recommends surgery or an invasive type of treatment, do you seek a second opinion? | ○ | ○ | ○ |
| 11. | Do you seek health information only from reliable and credible sources? | ○ | ○ | ○ |
| 12. | Do you read labels carefully before buying over-the-counter (OTC) medications? | ○ | ○ | ○ |
| 13. | Do you have a primary health care provider? | ○ | ○ | ○ |
| 14. | Do you think advertising plays a significant role in your decision to purchase health care products and services? | ○ | ○ | ○ |

# YOUR PLAN FOR **CHANGE**

Once you have considered your responses to the **ASSESS YOURSELF** questions, you may want to change or improve certain behaviors in order to get the best treatment from your health care provider and the health care system.

**TODAY,** YOU CAN:

☐ Research your insurance plan. Find out which health care providers and hospitals you can visit in your area, options for medical care outside your area, co-payment and premium costs, and plan drug coverage.

☐ Update your medicine cabinet. Dispose properly of any expired prescriptions or OTC medications. Keep on hand a supply of basic items, such as pain relievers, antiseptic cream, bandages, cough suppressants, and throat lozenges.

**WITHIN THE NEXT TWO WEEKS,** YOU CAN:

☐ Find a regular health care provider if you do not have one and make an appointment for a general checkup.

☐ Do some research on health conditions you have experienced or that run in your family. Write down any unanswered questions for discussion with your health care provider.

**BY THE END OF THE SEMESTER,** YOU CAN:

☐ Ask if a generic version is appropriate and available when filling your next prescription.

☐ Become informed about health care issues both in your state and the country. Write to your state and congressional legislators to express your opinions about needed reforms.

# STUDY PLAN

Customize your study plan—and master your health!—in the Study Area of MasteringHealth™

## CHAPTER **REVIEW**

 To hear an MP3 Tutor Session, scan here or visit the Study Area in **MasteringHealth**.

**LO 1 | Taking Responsibility for Your Health Care**

- Knowing when to take care of yourself and when to seek professional help will save you money and improve your health status. Advance planning can help you navigate health care treatment in unfamiliar situations or emergencies. Assess health professionals by considering their qualifications, their record of treating similar problems, and their ability to work with you.

**LO 2 | Conventional Health Care**

- In theory, conventional Western (allopathic) medicine is based on scientifically validated methods and procedures. Medical doctors, specialists of various kinds, nurses, physician assistants, and other health care professionals practice allopathic medicine.
- Prescription drugs are obtained through a written prescription from a physician, whereas over the-counter-drugs can be purchased without a prescription.

**LO 3 | Health Insurance**

- Health insurance is based on the concept of spreading risk. Insurance is provided by private insurance companies (which charge premiums) and the government Medicare and Medicaid programs (which are funded by taxes). Managed care (in the form of HMOs, PPOs, and POS plans) attempts to control costs by streamlining administrative procedures and promoting preventive care, among other initiatives.

**LO 4 | Issues Facing Today's Health Care System**

- Concerns about the U.S. health care system include access, cost, and quality. The Patient Protection and Affordable Care Act was passed by Congress in 2010 to address these issues. Many public health experts feel that it does not go far enough.

## POP **QUIZ**

Visit **MasteringHealth** to personalize your study plan with Chapter Review Quizzes and Dynamic Study Modules.

**LO 1 | Taking Responsibility for Your Health Care**

1. Of the following conditions, which would be appropriately managed by self-care?
   a. A persistent temperature of 104°F or higher
   b. Sudden weight loss of more than a few pounds without changes in diet or exercise patterns
   c. A sore throat, runny nose, and cough that persist for several days
   d. Yellowing of the skin or the whites of the eyes

2. A component of your rights as a patient includes *informed consent*. Informed consent means that before you receive any care you:
   a. should be fully informed of what is being planned.
   b. should know the risks and potential benefits.
   c. have the option to refuse treatment.
   d. all of the above.

**LO 2 | Conventional Health Care**

3. Which medical practice is based on treating the patient's symptoms using scientifically validated methods?
   a. Allopathic medicine
   b. Nonallopathic medicine
   c. Osteopathic medicine
   d. Chiropractic medicine

4. A specialist who diagnoses and treats diseases of the teeth, gums, and oral cavity is a(n)
   a. dentist.
   b. orthodontist.
   c. oral surgeon.
   d periodontist.

5. Which is a common type of over-the-counter drug?
   a. Antibiotics
   b. Hormonal contraceptives
   c. Antidepressants
   d. Antacids

**LO 3 | Health Insurance**

6. What is the term for an amount paid directly to a provider by a patient before his or her insurance carrier will begin paying for services?
   a. Coinsurance
   b. Cost sharing
   c. Co-payment
   d. Deductible

7. The most restrictive type of managed care is
   a. fee-for-service.
   b. health maintenance organizations.
   c. point of service.
   d. preferred provider organizations.

8. The federal health insurance program that covers 99 percent of adults over 65 years of age is
   a. Medicare.
   b. Medicaid.
   c. COBRA.
   d. HMO.

9. Deborah, 28, is a low-income single parent who receives Temporary Assistance for Needy Families (TANF). Her health insurance coverage is provided by a federal program known as
   a. CHIP.
   b. Social Security.
   c. Medicaid.
   d. Medicare.

**LO 4 | Issues Facing Today's Health Care System**

10. Which of the following is a key provision of the ACA?
    a. Insurers are required to cover only major medical emergencies.
    b. Lifetime limits on benefits are allowed if costs exceed a set amount.

c. Insurers are required to cover young adults on a parent's plan through age 21.
d. Americans with preexisting conditions can't be denied coverage.

*Answers to the Pop Quiz can be found on page A-1. If you answered a question incorrectly, review the section identifies by the Learning Outcome. For even more study tools, visit MasteringHealth.*

# THINK ABOUT IT!

## LO 1 | Taking Responsibility for Your Health Care

1. List several conditions for which you wouldn't need to seek medical help. When would you consider each condition to be bad enough to require medical attention? How would you decide where to go for treatment?

2. Describe your rights as a patient. Have you ever received treatment that violated these rights? If so, what action, if any, did you take?

## LO 2 | Conventional Health Care

3. What is the most common form of medicine practiced in Northern America? What is the scientific foundation for this form of medicine? What measures do practitioners take to help ensure quality of care?

## LO 3 | Health Insurance

4. What are the inherent benefits and risks of managed care health insurance plans?

5. Explain the differences between traditional indemnity insurance and managed health care. Should insurance companies dictate reimbursement rates for various medical tests and procedures in an attempt to keep prices down? Why or why not?

## LO 4 | Issues Facing Today's Health Care System

6. Discuss how the Affordable Care Act (ACA) has provided access to health care for Americans. What are the key provisions of the ACA?

# ACCESS YOUR HEALTH ON THE INTERNET

Visit **MasteringHealth** for links to the websites and RSS feeds.

The following websites explore further topics and issues related to personal health.

*Agency for Healthcare Research and Quality (AHRQ).* This provides links to sites that can address health care concerns and information on what questions to ask, what to look for, and what you should know when making critical decisions about personal care. **www.ahrq.gov**

*Food and Drug Administration (FDA).* This website provides news on the latest government-approved home health tests and other health-related products. **www.fda.gov**

*HealthGrades.* This company provides quality reports on physicians as well as hospitals, nursing homes, and other health care facilities. **www.healthgrades.com**

*National Committee for Quality Assurance (NCQA).* The NCQA assesses and reports on the quality of managed care plans, including HMOs. **www.ncqa.org**

*Healthcare.gov.* This website provides up-to-date information regarding health care reform in the United States. **www.healthcare.gov**

*Physician Compare.* The Affordable Care Act mandated this website be established to provide basic information on physicians for consumers to use to assist them in finding a doctor. **www.medicare.gov/find-a-doctor**

# Understanding Complementary and Integrative Health

Many American adults use some form of complementary therapy. What are the potential benefits and risks of these therapies?

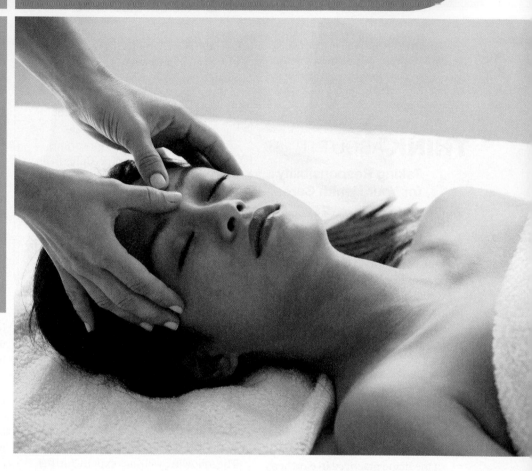

## LEARNING OUTCOMES

1 Distinguish between complementary health approaches, alternative health approaches, and integrative medicine.

2 Describe four complementary medical systems practiced in the United States.

3 Discuss several mind and body practices, including manipulative therapies and energy therapies.

4 Describe functional foods and dietary supplements and explain why caution is important when using these products.

Increasingly popular for both self-care and health promotion are a group of diverse medical systems, practices, and products developed outside of mainstream Western, or conventional, medicine.[1] Although these offer consumers a broader range of choices, and research suggests that some may be effective, the evidence of therapeutic benefits of others is not convincing, and a few have been associated with adverse effects.

**complementary health approaches** Practices and products that originated outside of but are used in conjunction with conventional medicine.

**alternative health approaches** Practices and products that originated outside of and are used in place of conventional medicine.

## LO 1 | WHAT IS COMPLEMENTARY AND INTEGRATIVE HEALTH?

Distinguish between complementary health approaches, alternative health approaches, and integrative medicine.

**Complementary health approaches** are practices and products commonly used together with conventional medicine.[2] A patient with chronic back pain, for example, may combine massage therapy with prescription medication. In contrast, **alternative health approaches** are used *in place of* conventional medicine, such as following a special diet or herbal remedy to treat cancer instead of

# 32%

OF 18- TO 44-YEAR-OLDS
REPORT HAVING USED
A **COMPLEMENTARY
HEALTH** APPROACH.

using surgery, radiation, or other conventional treatments. The National Center for Complementary and Integrative Health (NCCIH) reports that, in the United States, true alternative medicine is rare; most people who use nonmainstream approaches use them alongside conventional treatments.[3]

Doctors of medicine (MDs), doctors of osteopathy (DOs), nurses, and various allied health professionals practice conventional medicine. These practitioners may recommend massage therapy, specific vitamin or mineral supplements, or other complementary therapies for individual patients. However, some practitioners incorporate complementary therapies into their conventional health care in a coordinated, purposeful way. This approach is known as **integrative medicine**.[4]

A survey conducted by the NCCIH revealed that 33 percent of U.S. adults use one or more complementary therapies.[5] **FIGURE 1** identifies those most commonly used. Why do so many people

find complementary approaches appealing? Many people turn to these therapies to promote their general wellness or to relieve symptoms associated with a chronic disease or the side effects of conventional medicine.[6] They may also be seeking a **holistic** approach; that is, care that focuses on the mind and the whole body, rather than just an isolated symptom or body part. They may also desire a less invasive, more gentle approach to healing, one that allows them a measure of control over their treatment.

Although practitioners of most complementary health approaches spend many years in training, there is no national training or licensure standard, and states differ in their requirements and regulations. Each approach has a different set of training standards, guidelines for practice, and licensure procedures.

Before you consider using any complementary therapy, visit the website of the NCCIH, a division of the National Institutes of Health (NIH). Its mission is to study complementary health approaches using rigorous scientific methods, and build an evidence base regarding their safety and effectiveness. The organization serves as an information clearinghouse and conducts research, education, and outreach programs.

The NCCIH groups the complementary health approaches into three general categories of practice: natural products, mind and body practices, and other complementary health approaches—what we'll call complementary medical systems.

## LO 2 | COMPLE-MENTARY MEDICAL SYSTEMS

Describe four complementary medical systems practiced in the United States.

**Complementary medical systems** reflect specific theories of physiology, health, and disease that have developed outside the influence of conventional medicine. Many have been practiced throughout the world for centuries. For example, Native American, Aboriginal, African, Middle Eastern, South American, and Asian cultures have their own

**integrative medicine** Medical practice that brings conventional and complementary approaches together in a coordinated way.

**holistic** Relating to or concerned with the whole body and the interactions of systems, rather than treatment of individual parts.

**complementary medical systems** Approaches to health care that reflect specific theories of physiology, health, and disease that have developed outside the influence of conventional medicine.

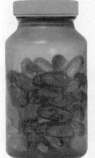

| 17.7% | 10.9% | 10.1% | 8.4% | 8.0% | 6.9% | 3.0% | 2.2% | 2.1% | 1.7% |
|---|---|---|---|---|---|---|---|---|---|
| Natural products | Deep breathing | Yoga, tai chi, or qi gong | Chiropractic & osteopathic | Meditation | Massage | Special diets | Homeopathic treatment | Progressive relaxation | Guided imagery |

**FIGURE 1** The Ten Most Common Complementary Therapies among U.S. Adults

**Source:** Data from T. C. Clarke, et al., "Trends in the Use of Complementary Health Approaches among Adults: United States, 2002–2012," *National Health Statistics Reports*, no. 79 (2015). February 2015. Available at www.cdc.gov/nchs/data/nhsr/nhsr079.pdf

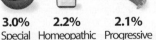

→ VIDEO TUTOR
CAM: Risks vs. Benefits

unique healing systems. Here, we discuss those most commonly available in the United States.

# Traditional Chinese Medicine

The concept of *qi* (pronounced "chee"), or vital energy, is foundational to **traditional Chinese medicine (TCM)**. When *qi* is in balance, the person is in a state of health; imbalance of *qi* results in disease. Diagnosis is based on personal history, observation of the body (especially the tongue), palpation, and pulse diagnosis, a detailed procedure requiring considerable skill. Techniques such as acupuncture, herbal medicine, massage, and *qigong* (a form of energy therapy) are among the TCM approaches to health and healing. TCM is complex, and research into its effectiveness is limited.[7]

Traditional Chinese medicine practitioners within the United States must have completed a graduate program in a college or university approved by the Accreditation Commission for Acupuncture and Oriental Medicine (ACAOM). Graduate programs usually involve an extensive 3- or 4-year clinical internship. In addition, the student must pass a certification and licensing examination by the National Commission for the Certification of Acupuncture and Oriental Medicine.

**traditional Chinese medicine (TCM)** Ancient comprehensive system of healing that uses herbs, acupuncture, massage, and qigong to bring vital energy, *qi*, into balance and to remove blockages of *qi* that lead to disease.

**Ayurveda (Ayurvedic medicine)** A comprehensive system of medicine, originating in ancient India, that places equal emphasis on the body, mind, and spirit and strives to restore the body's innate harmony through diet, exercise, meditation, herbs, massage, sun exposure, and controlled breathing.

**homeopathy (homeopathic medicine)** Unconventional Western system of medicine based on the principle that "like cures like" and the "law of minimum dose."

# Ayurveda

The "science of life," **Ayurveda (Ayurvedic medicine)** is one of the world's oldest medical systems, evolving over 3,000 years ago in India. Ayurveda seeks to integrate and balance the body, mind, and spirit to restore harmony in the individual.[8] Practitioners use techniques including questioning, observation, and pulse palpation to determine which of three vital energies, or *doshas,* is dominant in the patient. Treatment plans aim to bring the doshas into balance, thereby reducing symptoms. Dietary modification and herbal remedies drawn from the botanical wealth of the Indian subcontinent are common. Research into Ayurveda is limited, but studies have shown some of its herbal remedies to be effective for certain joint and digestive disorders.[9] However, some Ayurvedic remedies sold online have been found tainted with lead, mercury, or arsenic.[10] Treatments may also include certain yoga postures, meditation, massage, steam baths, changes in sleep patterns and sun exposure, and controlled breathing.

Training of Ayurvedic practitioners varies. There is no national standard for certification, although professional groups are working toward creating licensing guidelines.

# Homeopathy

**Homeopathy (homeopathic medicine)** is an unconventional Western system of medicine based on the principle that "like cures like." In other words, the same substance that in a large dose produces the symptoms of an illness—and may even be fatal—will in a small dose prompt the body's own defenses to cure the illness. Developed in the late 1700s by Samuel Hahnemann, a German physician, homeopathy follows the "law of minimum dose," which asserts that the lower the dose of a remedy, the greater its effectiveness. Thus, homeopathic remedies, which are derived from a wide range of natural, sometimes toxic, substances such as arsenic and belladonna, may be so diluted that no molecules of the original substance remain.[11] The NCCIH reports that little evidence supports homeopathy for treatment of any specific condition.[12]

Homeopathic training varies considerably, from diploma programs to correspondence courses. Only Arizona, Connecticut, and Nevada have homeopathic licensing boards. Requirements to practice vary from state to state.

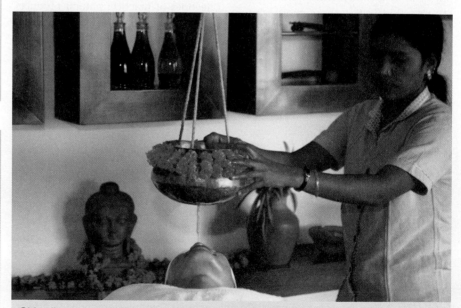

*Shirodhara*—a traditional Ayurvedic treatment in which warm herbalized oil is poured over the forehead in guided rhythmic patterns—is said to relieve stress and anxiety, treat insomnia and chronic headaches, and improve memory.

# Naturopathy

**Naturopathy (naturopathic medicine)** is a system of medicine that emphasizes the power of nature to restore health. Naturopathic physicians view their role as supporting the body's innate ability to maintain and restore health, typically by identifying and removing obstacles to these innate processes. They favor prevention and, when treatment is necessary, holistic, natural, and minimally invasive approaches.[13]

Specific approaches to care include diet; homeopathy; acupuncture; herbal medicine; spinal and soft-tissue manipulation; physical therapies involving electric currents, ultrasound, water, magnets, and color and light therapy; therapeutic counseling; and pharmacology. Only some of these therapies have been researched, and results have varied; moreover, the complexity of naturopathic care has made this system challenging to study. Limited research suggests that naturopathy may be more effective than conventional medicine for certain types of chronic pain. However, the efficacy and safety of some practices may not be supported by scientific evidence.[14]

Several major naturopathic schools in the United States and Canada provide training, conferring the *naturopathic doctor (ND)* degree on students who have completed a 4-year graduate program.

## LO 3 | MIND AND BODY PRACTICES

Discuss several mind and body practices, including manipulative therapies and energy therapies.

**Mind and body practices** are a large and diverse group of complementary health approaches that a trained practitioner or teacher often teaches or administers.[15] They include movement re-education therapies, as well as modalities in which the practitioner directly manipulates body tissues, attempts to shift the flow of body energy, or teaches the client techniques to promote relaxation or manage stress. Several relaxation techniques for stress management—including yoga, deep breathing, meditation, and progressive relaxation—are among the ten most commonly used complementary therapies in the United States (see Chapter 3).

# Manipulative Therapies

**Manipulative therapies** are approaches based on manipulation or movement of body tissues and structures.

## Chiropractic Medicine

**Chiropractic medicine** has been practiced for more than 100 years and focuses on disorders of the muscular and skeletal system and the use of various modalities to reduce health effects from these disorders.[16] Over the decades, allopathic medicine and chiropractic medicine have been in direct competition. Today, many health care providers work closely with chiropractors, and many insurance companies pay for chiropractic treatment, particularly if it is recommended by a medical doctor.

Chiropractic medicine is based on the principle that energy flows through the nervous system, including the spinal cord. If the spine is partly misaligned or dislocated, that force is disrupted. Chiropractors use a variety of techniques to manipulate the spine into proper alignment so energy can flow unimpeded. Typically chiropractors treat low-back pain; neck pain; pain in the arms, legs, and feet, as well as headaches. Chiropractic medicine appears to be beneficial in relieving low-back pain and may be helpful for neck pain, headaches, and some joint conditions.[17]

The average chiropractic training program includes intensive courses in biochemistry, anatomy, physiology, diagnostics, pathology, nutrition, and related topics, combined with hands-on clinical training. Increasing numbers of states require a 4-year undergraduate degree prior to entrance into a 4-year chiropractic program. Applicants must also pass an extensive licensing examination given by the National Board of Chiropractic Examiners. The practice of chiropractic is licensed and regulated in all 50 states.[18]

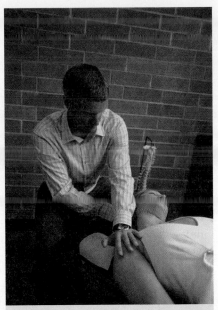

Chiropractic medicine is often used to treat pain. Chiropractors manipulate the alignment of the spine, allowing energy to flow freely throughout the body.

## Massage Therapy

References to massage exist in numerous ancient texts, including those of Greece, Rome, Japan, China, Egypt, and India.[19] **Massage therapy** is soft tissue manipulation by trained therapists for relaxation and healing. Therapists manipulate the patient's muscles and connective tissues to loosen the fibers and break up adhesions, improve the body's circulation, and remove waste products. The NCCIH reports that research evidence supports the effectiveness of massage

---

**naturopathy (naturopathic medicine)** System of medicine in which practitioners work to support the body's innate healing mechanisms and use treatment approaches such as diet, exercise, and massage that are minimally invasive.

**mind and body practices** A large and diverse group of complementary health approaches administered or taught by a trained practitioner or teacher.

**manipulative therapies** Treatments involving manipulation or movement of one or more body structures or the whole body.

**chiropractic medicine** System of treatment that involves manipulation of the spine and neuromuscular structures to promote proper energy flow.

**massage therapy** Soft-tissue manipulation by trained therapists for relaxation and healing.

therapy to temporarily relieve musculo-skeletal pain such as low-back and neck pain, and it may help to promote relaxation and relieve depression.[20]

The course of study in massage schools typically covers sciences such as anatomy and physiology as well as massage techniques, and business, ethical, and legal considerations.[21] For licensing, many states require a minimum of 500 hours of training and a passing grade on a national certification exam. Massage therapists work in private studios and health spas and in medical and chiropractic offices, hospitals, nursing homes, and fitness centers.[22]

## Movement Therapies

A broad range of Eastern and Western complementary health approaches use movement, including postural realignment, to increase physical, mental, and emotional well-being and reduce limitations in body functioning. Two commonly available approaches include:

- The *Alexander technique*, a movement education method designed to release harmful tension in the body to improve ease of movement, balance, and coordination.
- The *Feldenkrais method*, a system of gentle movements and exercises designed to improve movement, flexibility, coordination, and overall functioning through techniques that enhance the client's awareness and retrain the nervous system.

# Energy Therapies

**Energy therapies** focus either on energy fields thought to originate within the body (biofields) or from other sources (electromagnetic fields). The existence of these fields has not been experimentally proven. Popular

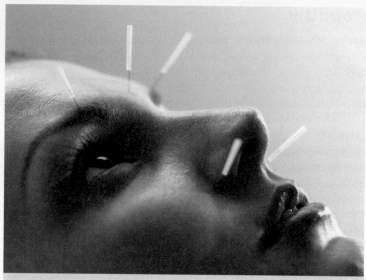

In acupuncture, long, thin needles are inserted into specific points along the body. This is thought to increase the flow of life-force energy, providing many physical and mental benefits.

examples of energy therapy include acupuncture, acupressure, qigong, Reiki, and therapeutic touch.

## Acupuncture and Acupressure

**Acupuncture**, one of the oldest and most popular TCM therapies, is used to relieve a wide variety of health conditions, from musculoskeletal dysfunction to depression. The therapist stimulates various points on the body with a series of precisely placed and extremely fine needles. The stimulation of these acupuncture points is thought to increase the flow of *qi* through the *meridians,* or energy pathways, in the body.

Following acupuncture, most participants in clinical studies report satisfaction with the treatment and improvement in their condition; however, extensive research has been inconclusive, and there is significant controversy over whether or not such results are simply a placebo response.[23] A 2014 study, for example, found acupuncture more effective than no treatment at all for relieving knee pain, but no better than a simulated (fake) acupuncture treatment used as a control.[24] In contrast, a 2014 meta-analysis did find a statistically significant increased response rate for acupuncture over a simulated treatment for back pain, neck pain, and chronic headaches.[25]

Most U.S. acupuncturists are state licensed; however, the licensing requirements vary by state. Most states require a diploma from the National Certification Commission for Acupuncture and Oriental Medicine for licensing. In addition, many conventional physicians and dentists practice acupuncture.[26]

**Acupressure** is based on the same principles of energy flow as acupuncture. Instead of inserting needles, however, the therapist applies pressure. The goal of the therapy is for *qi* to be evenly distributed and flow freely throughout the body. Practitioners typically have the same basic training and understanding of meridians and acupuncture points as do acupuncturists.

## Other Forms of Energy Therapy

*Qigong*, a technique of TCM, brings together movement, meditation, and regulation of breathing to increase the flow of *qi*, enhance blood circulation, and improve immune function. A 2015

**energy therapies** Therapies using energy fields, such as electromagnetic fields or biofields.

**acupuncture** Technique of traditional Chinese medicine that involves the placement of long, thin needles to affect flow of energy (*qi*) along energy pathways (meridians) within the body.

**acupressure** Technique of traditional Chinese medicine that uses application of pressure to selected points along meridians to balance energy.

systematic review of meta-analyses found that the practice of qigong and other meditative movement therapies was associated with statistically significant improvements in pain management and other aspects of health-related quality of life for people recovering from breast cancer, as well as people with low-back pain, heart failure, and other conditions.[27]

*Reiki* is a non-touch form of energy therapy that originated in Japan. The name is derived from the Japanese words representing "universal" and "vital energy," or *ki*. Reiki is based on the belief that by channeling *ki* to the patient, the practitioner facilitates healing. In two related non-touch energy therapies, *therapeutic touch* and *healing touch,* the therapist attempts to perceive, through his or her hands held just above the patient's body, imbalances in the patient's energy. The therapist promotes healing by increasing the flow of the body's energies and bringing them into balance. Although a 2014 systematic review found at least a partial therapeutic response from non-touch energy therapies, the variety of experimental designs and small size of the studies prevented the researchers from drawing conclusions about their effectiveness.[28]

## LO 4 | NATURAL PRODUCTS

Describe functional foods and dietary supplements and explain why caution is important when using these products.

Natural products, including functional foods and dietary supplements, are perhaps the most controversial category of complementary health approaches because of the sheer number of options available and the many claims that are made about their effects. Many of these claims have not been thoroughly investigated, and many of the products are not currently regulated.

## Functional Foods

Dietary changes are often part of complementary health approaches and

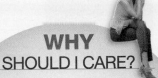

commonly involve consumption of certain *functional foods*—foods said to improve some aspect of physical or mental functioning beyond their specific nutrients. Both whole foods, such as broccoli and nuts, and modified foods, such as an energy shake said to enhance memory, are classified as functional foods.[29] Food producers sometimes refer to their functional foods as **nutraceuticals** to emphasize combined nutritional and pharmaceutical benefits.

Foods containing antioxidant phytochemicals are often marketed with claims about their health benefits. For example, the label on a package of cocoa may state that the product provides antioxidants that could help to reduce the risk of heart disease. The claim is backed up by research: Cocoa contains antioxidant phytochemicals called flavonoids, which have been shown to modestly reduce blood pressure and the formation of blood clots.[30] Many fruits, vegetables, soy products, red wine, and coffee and tea also contain flavonoids.

Fermented dairy foods such as yogurt and kefir that are rich in probiotics (beneficial bacteria) are another popular group of functional foods. They are commonly prescribed to improve gastrointestinal health, and the NCCIH reports strong evidence of their beneficial effect in reducing the duration and severity of diarrhea.[31] However, research into other health claims for probiotic foods is limited.[32]

Although the FDA does not have a specific definition of functional foods, they are regulated under the umbrella of conventional foods. The FDA regulates nutrient and health claims made on all food labels, but does not have the capacity to analyze the makeup of all food products.[33] Thus, their regulatory efforts focus on removing from the market products that have been found to be unsafe.

## Herbal Remedies and Other Dietary Supplements

The FDA defines a *dietary supplement* as a "product taken by mouth that contains a dietary ingredient intended to supplement the diet"; these dietary ingredients include vitamins, minerals, herbs, amino acids, enzymes, and other substances.[34] Dietary supplements can take the form of tablets, capsules, liquids, powders, or energy bars. No matter what form they take, they must be clearly labeled as a dietary supplement, not a conventional food, on the front panel.[35]

Herbal remedies, often referred to as *botanicals*, are derived from plant parts such as leaves, flowers, or seeds. People have been using herbal remedies for thousands of years, and they are key therapies within TCM, Ayurveda, and other traditional medical systems. Herbs were the original sources for compounds found in approximately 25 percent of the pharmaceutical drugs we use today, including aspirin (white willow bark), the heart medication digitalis (foxglove), and the cancer treatment Taxol (Pacific yew tree). In addition, scientists continue to make pharmacological advances by studying the herbal remedies used in cultures throughout the world.

It's tempting to assume herbal remedies are safe because they are natural, but the FDA has not developed a definition for the term *natural* and cautions consumers to avoid assuming that any

**nutraceuticals** Foods or food-based supplements that have combined nutritional and pharmaceutical benefits; used interchangeably with the term *functional foods*.

dietary supplement claiming to be "natural" is safe.[36] For example, in recent years, the NCCIH has warned that certain herbal products can cause a variety of health problems, such as liver damage, an abnormal increase in heart rate, miscarriage, and others. Some have been found to be contaminated with bacteria, and others with toxic metals or with grass, gluten, or other potential allergens. In 2015, the attorney general for the state of New York demanded that four retailers stopped selling numerous supplements after they were found to contain contaminants—and the majority of the products tested did not contain any of the herbs identified on their labels. Moreover, the NCCIH "Alerts and Advisories" web page continually releases notifications of herbs and other supplements containing hidden drug ingredients, including some that could promote a heart attack or stroke.[37] Finally, the NCCIH has reported that some herbal products can be dangerous when combined with prescription or over-the-counter drugs, can disrupt the normal action of the drugs, or can cause unusual side effects.[38]

Not all the supplements on the market today are directly derived from plant sources. In recent years, there have been increasing media claims about the health benefits of various hormones, enzymes, and other biological and synthetic compounds. Although a few products, such as melatonin (a hormone) or zinc lozenges (a mineral), have been widely studied, there is little quality research to support the claims of many others. TABLE 1 gives an overview of some of the most common dietary supplements on the market.

## Consumer Protection

The burgeoning popularity of functional foods and dietary supplements concerns many scientists and consumers. As noted previously, dietary supplements can be sold without FDA approval. This raises

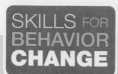

issues of consumer safety. Even when products are dispensed by licensed health care practitioners, the situation can be risky. Some herbalists and other practitioners who mix their own tonics may not use standardized measures and may not fully understand the potential interactions of their preparations. Products sold in "health food" stores and over the Internet may have varying levels of the active ingredient or may contain additives to which the consumer may have an adverse reaction.

As a result of such concerns, pressure has mounted to establish an approval process for dietary supplements similar to the process the FDA uses for drugs. In the meantime, if you're considering purchasing a dietary supplement, look for the United States Pharmacopeia (USP) Verified Mark on the label. The

USP does not regulate or determine the safety of medications, foods, or dietary supplements, but it does offer verification services to manufacturers of dietary supplement products. Dietary supplements bearing the USP Verified Mark on the label have met stringent standards for accurate labeling of ingredients in the identified amount and potency; purity and quality of ingredients, including absence of harmful levels of specified contaminants; and manufacture according to the FDA's Good Manufacturing Processes.[39]

Individuals must take an active role in their health care, which means staying educated. See the **Skills for Behavior Change** box for tips on how to make smart decisions about integrating complementary therapies into your health care.

TABLE 1 | Common Dietary Supplements: Benefits, Research, and Risks

| Herb | | Claims of Benefits | Research Findings | Potential Risks |
|---|---|---|---|---|
| | Echinacea (purple coneflower, *Echinacea purpurea, E. angustifolia, E. pallida*) | Stimulates the immune system and helps fight infection. Used to both prevent and treat colds and flu. | Some studies have provided preliminary evidence of its effectiveness in treating respiratory infections, but two recent studies found no benefit either for prevention or treatment. | Allergic reactions, including rashes, increased asthma, gastrointestinal problems, and anaphylaxis (a life-threatening allergic reaction). |
| | Flaxseed (*Linum usitatissimum*) and flaxseed oil | Used as a laxative and for hot flashes and breast pain, as well as to reduce cholesterol levels and risk of heart disease and cancer. | Flaxseed contains soluble fiber and may have a laxative effect. Study results are mixed on whether flaxseed decreases hot flashes. Insufficient data are available on the effect of flaxseed on cholesterol levels, heart disease, or cancer risks. | Delays absorption of medicines, but otherwise has few side effects. Oil taken in excess could cause diarrhea. Should be taken with plenty of water. |
| | Ginkgo (*Ginkgo biloba*) | Popularly used to prevent cognitive decline, dementia, and Alzheimer's disease, and general vascular disease. | Although some small studies have had promising results, the large Ginkgo Evaluation of Memory study found ginkgo did not reduce Alzheimer's disease or dementia, slow cognitive decline, or reduce blood pressure. | Gastric irritation, headache, nausea, dizziness, difficulty thinking, memory loss, and allergic reactions. Ginkgo seeds are highly toxic; only products made from leaf extracts should be used. |
| | Ginseng (*Panax ginseng*) | Claimed to increase resistance to stress, boost the immune system, lower blood glucose and blood pressure, and improve stamina and sex drive. | Some studies suggest that ginseng may improve immune function and lower blood glucose; however, research overall is inconclusive. | Headaches, insomnia, and gastrointestinal problems are the most commonly reported adverse effects. |
| | Green tea (*Camellia sinensis*) | Useful for lowering cholesterol and risk of some cancers, protecting the skin from sun damage, bolstering mental alertness, and boosting heart health. | Although some studies have shown promising links between green and white tea consumption and cancer prevention, recent research questions the ability of tea to significantly reduce the risk of breast, lung, or prostate cancer. | Insomnia, liver problems, anxiety, irritability, upset stomach, nausea, diarrhea, or frequent urination. |
| | Zinc (mineral) | Supports immune system; lozenges used to lessen duration and severity of cold symptoms. | Some research suggests that zinc lozenges can reduce the severity and duration of a cold if taken within 24 hours of onset of symptoms. | Use of zinc lozenges can cause nausea. Excessive use can reduce immune function. |

**Sources:** National Center for Complementary and Alternative Medicine, "Herbs at a Glance," January 2014, http://nccih.nih.gov/health/herbsataglance.htm; American Cancer Society, "Green Tea," May 2012, www.cancer.org; Office of Dietary Supplements, National Institutes of Health, "Dietary Supplement Fact Sheets," April 2014, http://ods.od.nih.gov/Health_Information/Information_About_Individual_Dietary_Supplements.aspx

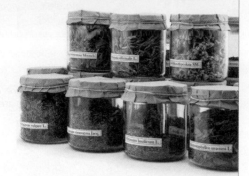

If you are like millions of Americans, you've already tried one or more complementary therapies (including supplements) or may be considering one. If so, assess yourself: For each item, indicate whether you do or do not practice the recommended safety strategy.

1. When considering a complementary therapy, do you research the scientific findings on safety and effectiveness of the specific therapy?　　Yes　　No

2. Before purchasing a dietary supplement, do you check the NCCIH Alerts and Advisories website?　　Yes　　No

3. If you buy dietary supplements, do you choose those with the USP Verified Mark on their label?　　Yes　　No

4. Do you tell all your health care providers about all of the complementary health approaches, including dietary supplements, you use, as well as all over-the-counter and prescription drugs?　　Yes　　No

5. Do you follow your practitioner's instructions and the instructions on the label of dietary supplements carefully?　　Yes　　No

6. Would you be able to articulate to a friend why a service or product labeled "natural" is not necessarily safe?　　Yes　　No

## Interpreting Your Score

If you are using, or considering using, any type of complementary health approach, you should be able to answer "Yes" to each question with confidence. "No" responses indicate actions that you can begin to take in order to use complementary approaches with greater safety. Ultimately, these six strategies can help you take responsibility for your health.

# YOUR PLAN FOR CHANGE

The **ASSESS YOURSELF** activity gave you the chance to evaluate your responsible use of complementary health approaches. Depending on the results of the assessment, and your own interest, you may consider investigating certain therapies further.

**TODAY,** YOU CAN:

☐ Close your eyes and think of a calm place or activity you enjoy for a few minutes. Perhaps you are lying on a beach or are curled up in front of a fireplace. Clear your mind of everything else and use relaxation to improve your health.

☐ Go to a credible website and look up information on a therapy you might be using or considering. What are the scientific findings? What are the benefits?

**WITHIN THE NEXT TWO WEEKS,** YOU CAN:

☐ Review your insurance documents or check with your carrier to see what complementary therapies are covered. Ask which expenses you'll be responsible for, and if you are limited to a certain network of practitioners.

☐ Check with your college's health clinic and find out what types of complementary therapies it offers.

**BY THE END OF THE SEMESTER,** YOU CAN:

☐ Schedule an appointment with your health care provider to discuss any complementary therapies you are considering.

☐ Make relaxation and stress-management techniques a part of your everyday life. This can mean practicing meditation, deep breathing, or even taking long walks in nature.

# STUDY PLAN

## CHAPTER REVIEW

### LO 1 | What Is Complementary and Integrative Health?

■ Both complementary and alternative health approaches originated outside of mainstream Western, or conventional, medicine. Complementary approaches are used together with conventional medicine, whereas alternative approaches are used in place of conventional medicine. Integrative medicine is a practice that incorporates complementary therapies into conventional care in a coordinated, purposeful way.

### LO 2 | Complementary Medical Systems

■ Complementary medical systems are comprehensive approaches to health care that reflect specific theories of physiology, health, and disease that have developed outside the influence of conventional medicine. They include traditional Chinese medicine, Ayurveda, and other culturally based systems, as well as homeopathy and naturopathy.

### LO 3 | Mind and Body Practices

■ As opposed to medical systems or natural products, mind and body practices are a large and diverse group of complementary health approaches administered or taught by a trainer, practitioner, or teacher. They include manipulative therapies such as chiropractic medicine, movement therapies such as the Alexander technique, energy therapies such as acupuncture, and relaxation and stress-management modalities such as yoga and meditation.

### LO 4 | Natural Products

■ Natural products include functional foods such as those containing anti-oxidant phytochemicals or probiotics, as well as dietary supplements, products containing vitamins, minerals, herbs, or other ingredients and taken by mouth. Consumers need to understand that the FDA does not study and approve dietary supplements before they are brought to market. Thus, there is no guarantee of their safety or effectiveness; moreover, a label claim that a product is "natural" does not mean that the product is safe to use. However, the USP Verified Mark on the label does indicate that a supplement has met certain criteria for ingredient accuracy, product purity, and manufacturing standards.

## POP QUIZ

### LO 1 | What Is Complementary and Integrative Health?

1. Complementary health approaches typically focus on treating the mind and the whole body, which makes them part of a
   a. natural approach.
   b. psychological approach.
   c. holistic approach.
   d. gentle approach.

### LO 2 | Complementary Medical Systems

2. What type of medicine addresses imbalances of *qi*?
   a. Chiropractic medicine
   b. Ayurvedic medicine
   c. Traditional Chinese medicine
   d. Homeopathic medicine

### LO 3 | Mind and Body Practices

3. Which of the following is a non-touch energy therapy?
   a. Acupressure
   b. Alexander technique
   c. Massage therapy
   d. Reiki

### LO 4 | Natural Products

4. Which of the following could be marketed as a functional food?
   a. Yogurt
   b. Green tea extract
   c. Multivitamins
   d. An iron tablet

*Answers to the Pop Quiz can be found on page A-1. If you answered a question incorrectly, review the section identified by the Learning Outcome. For even more study tools, visit MasteringHealth.*

## Chapter 1

1. b; 2. b; 3. d; 4. b; 5. a; 6. d; 7. a; 8. a; 9. a; 10. c

## Focus On: Improving Your Financial Health

1. c; 2. a; 3. b

## Chapter 2

1. b; 2. a; 3. b; 4. a; 5. c; 6. b; 7. b; 8. b; 9. b; 10. b

## Focus On: Cultivating Your Spiritual Health

1. c; 2. b; 3. b

## Chapter 3

1. c; 2. b; 3. c; 4. a; 5. d; 6. c; 7. d; 8. c; 9. b; 10. d

## Focus On: Improving Your Sleep

1. a; 2. c; 3. a; 4. d; 5. d

## Chapter 4

1. b; 2. a; 3. b; 4. d; 5. d; 6. c; 7. a; 8. b; 9. d; 10. c

## Chapter 5

1. b; 2. c; 3. c; 4. d; 5. b; 6. a; 7. a; 8. d; 9. b; 10. d

## Focus On: Understanding Your Sexuality

1. c; 2. b; 3. d; 4. c

## Chapter 6

1. c; 2. b; 3. d; 4. c; 5. a; 6. b; 7. d; 8. b; 9. a; 10. c; 11. a; 12. a

## Chapter 7

1. b; 2. b; 3. c; 4. c; 5. d; 6. a; 7. a; 8. b; 9. d; 10. a

## Chapter 8

1. c; 2. c; 3. b; 4. d; 5. b; 6. d; 7. c; 8. c; 9. b; 10. a

## Chapter 9

1. a; 2. b; 3. b; 4. a; 5. c; 6. b; 7. a; 8. d; 9. b; 10. d

## Chapter 10

1. b; 2. a; 3. c; 4. c; 5. b; 6. c; 7. b; 8. a; 9. d; 10. a

## Focus On: Enhancing Your Body Image

1. a; 2. b; 3. d

## Chapter 11

1. d; 2. c; 3. c; 4. b; 5. b; 6. b; 7. a; 8. c; 9. b; 10. a

## Chapter 12

1. d; 2. b; 3. c; 4. b; 5. c; 6. b; 7. b; 8. a; 9. c; 10. b

## Focus On: Minimizing Your Risk for Diabetes

1. c; 2. b; 3. c

## Chapter 13

1. c; 2. d; 3. a; 4. a; 5. c; 6. b; 7. c; 8. d; 9. a; 10. c

## Focus On: Reducing Risks for Chronic Diseases and Conditions

1. c; 2. c; 3. b; 4. a; 5. a

## Chapter 14

1. a; 2. b; 3. c; 4. a; 5. d; 6. a; 7. c; 8. d; 9. c; 10. b

## Chapter 15

1. d; 2. c; 3. d; 4. a; 5. b; 6. d; 7. c; 8. a; 9. a; 10. d

## Chapter 16

1. c; 2. d; 3. a; 4. a; 5. d; 6. d; 7. b; 8. a; 9. c; 10. d

## Focus On: Understanding Complementary and Integrative Health

1. c; 2. c; 3. d; 4. a

## Chapter 1: Accessing Your Health

1. K.D. Kochanek et al., "Mortality in the United States, 2013," *NCHS Data Brief*, No. 178 (2014), Available at www.cdc.gov/nchs/data/databriefs/db178.pdf

2. Centers for Disease Control and Prevention, "Achievements in Public Health, 1900–1999: Control of Infectious Diseases," *Morbidity and Mortality Weekly Report* 48, no. 29 (1999): 621–29, www.cdc.gov/mmwr/preview/mmwrhtml/mm4829a1.htm

3. Organization for Economic Cooperation and Development, *Health at a Glance 2013: OECD Indicators* (2013), doi:10.1787/health_glance-2013-en, Available at www.oecd.org/els/health-systems/Health-at-a-Glance-2013.pdf; S. H. Woolf and Laudan Aron, eds., *US Health in International Perspective: Shorter Lives, Poorer Health*, (Washington, DC: National Academies Press, 2013), Available at www.iom.edu/~/media/Files/Report%20Files/2013/US-Health-International-Perspective/USHealth_Intl_PerspectiveRB.pdf

4. U.S. Department of Health and Human Services (DHHS), *Healthy People 2020*, (Washington, DC: U.S. Government Printing Office, January 8, 2015), Available at www.healthypeople.gov/2020/topics-objectives/topic/health-related-quality-of-life-well-being

5. Centers for Disease Control and Prevention, "Adult Obesity Facts," September 2014, www.cdc.gov/obesity/data/adult.html.

6. World Health Organization (WHO), "Constitution of the World Health Organization," *Chronicles of the World Health Organization* (Geneva: WHO, 1947), www.who.int/governance/eb/constitution/en/index.html

7. R. Dubos, *So Human an Animal: How We Are Shaped by Surroundings and Events* (New York: Scribner, 1968), 15.

8. DHHS, *Healthy People 2020*, 2015.

9. Ibid.

10. Centers for Disease Control and Prevention, "Chronic Disease Prevention and Health Promotion," May 2014, www.cdc.gov/chronicdisease/overview/index.htm#2

11. U.S. Burden of Disease Collaborators, "The State of US Health, 1990–2010: Burden of Diseases, Injuries, and Risk Factors," *Journal of the American Medical Association* 310, no. 6 (2013): 591–606, doi:10.1001/jama.2013.13805; Centers for Disease Control and Prevention, "Alcohol Use and Health Fact Sheets," November 2014, www.cdc.gov/alcohol/fact-sheets/alcohol-use.htm; Centers for Disease Control and Prevention, "Smoking and Tobacco Use Fast Facts," February 2014, www.cdc.gov/tobacco/data_statistics/fact_sheets/fast_facts/

12. U.S. Burden of Disease Collaborators, "The State of US Health, " 2013.

13. Ibid.

14. CDC, "Alcohol Use and Health Fact Sheets," 2014.

15. CDC, "Smoking and Tobacco Use Fast Facts," 2014.

16. N.K. Mehta, J.S. House, and M.R. Elliott, "Dynamics of Health Behaviours and Socioeconomic Differences in Mortality in the USA," *Journal of Epidemiology and Community Health* (2015), doi: 10.1136/jech-2014-204248

17. U.S. DHHS, *Healthy People* 2020, 2015.

18. Agency for Healthcare Research and Quality, "2013 National Healthcare Disparities Report," *AHRQ Publication No. 14-0006* (2014), Available at www.ahrq.gov/research/findings/nhqrdr/nhdr13/2013nhdr.pdf

19. M.P. Doescher et al, "The Built Environment and Utilitarian Walking in Small U.S. Towns," *Preventive Medicine* 69 (2014): 80–86, doi: 10.1016/j.ypmed.2014.08.027; J. Sallis et al., "Role of Built Environments in Physical Activity, Obesity, and Cardiovascular Disease," *Circulation* 125 (2012): 729–37, Available at https://circ.ahajournals.org/content/125/5/729.full

20. J. A. Wasserman et al., "A Multi-Level Analysis Showing Associations between School Neighborhood and Child Body Mass Index," *International Journal of Obesity* 38, no. 7 (2014): 912–18, doi: 10.1038/ijo.2014.64; M. J. Trowbridge and T. L. Schmid, "Built Environment and Physical Activity Promotion: Place-Based Obesity Prevention Strategies," *Journal of Law, Medicine & Ethics*, Weight of the Nation Supplement, (Winter, 2013): 46–51, Available at www.aslme.org/media/downloadable/files/links/j/l/jlme-41-4-supp_trowbridge.pdf

21. S. Lindsay et al., "Monetary Matched Incentives to Encourage the Purchase of Fresh Fruits and Vegetables at Farmers Markets in Underserved Communities," *Preventing Chronic Disease* 10 (2013), doi: 10.5888/pcd10.130124; E. Weinstein et al., "Impact of a Focused Nutrition Educational Intervention Coupled with Improved Access to Fresh Produce on Purchasing Behavior and Consumption of Fruits and Vegetables in Overweight Patients with Diabetes Mellitus," *Diabetes Education* 40, no. 1 (2014): 100–106, doi: 10.1177/0145721713508823

22. The Commonwealth Fund, "Gaining Ground: Americans' Health Insurance Coverage and Access to Care After the Affordable Care Act's First Open Enrollment Period," July 10, 2014, www.commonwealthfund.org/publications/issue-briefs/2014/jul/health-coverage-access-aca

23. The Commonwealth Fund, "Are Americans Finding Affordable Coverage in the Health Insurance Marketplaces?" September 18, 2014, www.commonwealthfund.org/publications/issue-briefs/2014/sep/affordable-coverage-marketplace

24. The Commonwealth Fund, "Too High a Price: Out-of-Pocket Health Care Costs in the United States. Findings from the Commonwealth Fund Health Care Affordability Tracking Survey. September-October 2014," November 13, 2014, www.commonwealthfund.org/publications/issue-briefs/2014/nov/out-of-pocket-health-care-costs

25. I. Rosenstock, "Historical Origins of the Health Belief Model," *Health Education Monographs* 2, no. 4 (1974): 328–35.

26. A. Bandura, "Human Agency in Social Cognitive Theory," *American Psychologist* 44, no. 9 (1989): 1175–84.

27. P.J. Morgan, et al. "Associations between Program Outcomes and Adherence to Social Cognitive Theory Tasks: Process Evaluation of the SHED-IT Community Weight Loss Trial for Men," *International Journal of Behavioral Nutrition and Physical Activity* 11, no. 1 (2014): 89, doi: 10.1186/s12966-014-0089-9

28. M. C. Snead, et al., "Relationship between Social Cognitive Theory Constructs and Self-Reported Condom Use: Assessment of Behaviour in a Subgroup of the Safe in the City Trial," *BMJ Open* 4, no. 12 (2014): e006093, doi: 10.1136/bmjopen-2014-006093

29. J. O. Prochaska and C. C. DiClemente, "Stages and Processes of Self-Change of Smoking: Toward an Integrative Model of Change," *Journal of Consulting and Clinical Psychology* 51 (1983): 390–95.

30. J. Huang, F. J. Chaloupka, and G. T. Fong, "Cigarette Graphic Warning Labels and Smoking Prevalence in Canada: A Critical Examination and Reformulation of the FDA Regulatory Impact Analysis," *Tobacco Control* 23, Supplement 1 (2014): i7–i12, doi: 10.1136/tobaccocontrol-2013-051170

31. K. Simmen-Janevska, V. Brandstatter, and A. Maercker. "The Overlooked Relationship between Motivational Abilities and Posttraumatic Stress: A Review," *European Journal of Psychotraumatology* 10, no. 3 (2012), doi:10.3402/ejpt.v3i0.18560

32. A. Ellis and M. Benard, *Clinical Application of Rational Emotive Therapy* (New York: Plenum, 1985).

33. National Institute on Drug Abuse, "Drugs, Brains, and Behavior: The Science of Addiction: Treatment and Recovery," July 2014, www.drugabuse.gov/publications/drugs-brains-behavior-science-addiction/treatment-recovery

34. American Cancer Society, "Staying Smoke-Free," February 6, 2014, www.cancer.org/healthy/stayawayfromtobacco/guidetoquittingsmoking/guide-to-quitting-smoking-staying-smoke-free

### Why Should I Care?

page 3, S.B. Almadani et al., "Effects of Inflammatory Bowel Disease on Students' Adjustment to College," *Clinical Gastroenterology Hepatology* 12, no. 12 (2014), doi: 10.1016/j.cgh.2014.03.032; C.J. Bryan et al., "Depression, Posttraumatic Stress Disorder, and Grade Point Average among Student Service Members and Veterans," *Journal of Rehabilitation Research and Development* 51, no. 7 (2014), doi: 10.1682/JRRD.2014.01.0012.

### Pulled Statistics:

page 3, World Health Organization, "Life Expectancy Data by Country," Global Health Observatory Data Repository, 2014, http://apps.who.int/gho/data/node.main.688.

page 10, The Commonwealth Fund, "Gaining Ground: Americans' Health Insurance Coverage and Access to Care After the Affordable Care Act's First Open Enrollment Period," July 10, 2014, www.commonwealthfund.org/publications/issue-briefs/2014/jul/health-coverage-access-aca.

## Focus On: Improving Your Financial Health

1. W. Evans, B. Wolfe, and N. Adler, "The Income-Health Gradient," *Institute for Research on Poverty: Focus* 30, no. 1 (2013), Available at www.irp.wisc.edu/publications/focus/pdfs/foc301b.pdf; Institute for Health Metrics and Evaluation, "U.S County Profiles," Accessed February 3, 2015, www.healthdata.org/us-county-profiles

2. World Health Organization, "Social Determinants of Health: Key Concepts," *Commission on Social Determinants of Health, 2005–2008*, Accessed April 2014, www.who.int/social_determinants/thecommission/finalreport/key_concepts/en

3. OECD, *How's Life? 2013: Measuring Well-being* (Paris: OECD Publishing, 2013). doi: http://dx.doi.org/10.1787/9789264201392-en

4. R. Hiscock et al., "Socioeconomic Status and Smoking: A Review," *Annals of the New York Academy of Sciences* 1248, no. 1 (2012): 107–23, doi:10.1111/j.1749-6632.2011.06202.x

5. Ibid.

6. A. Carlsson et al., "Financial Stress in Late Adulthood and Diverse Risks of Incident Cardiovascular Disease and All-Cause Mortality in Women and Men," *BMC Public Health* 14, no. 1 (2014): 17, doi:10.1186/1471-2458-14-17

7. Pruchno et al., "Neighborhood Food Environment and Obesity in Community-Dwelling Older Adults: Individual and Neighborhood Effects," *Journal of Public Health* 104, no. 5 (2014); D. Viola et al., "Overweight and Obesity: Can We Reconcile Evidence about Supermarkets and Fast Food Retailers for Public Health Policy?," *Journal of Public Health Policy* 34, no. 3 (2013): 424–38, doi: 10.1057/jphp.2013.19

8. Centers for Disease Control and Prevention, "Food Deserts," Updated June 2013, www.cdc.gov/healthcommunication/toolstemplates/entertainmented/tips/fooddesert.html

9. E. R. Cheng and D. A. Kindig, "Disparities in Premature Mortality Between High- and Low-Income US Counties," *Preventing Chronic Disease* 9 (2012): 110120, doi: http://dx.doi.org/10.5888/pcd9.110120

10. N. Spencer, T. M. Thanh, and S. Louise, "Low Income/Socio-Economic Status in Early Childhood and Physical Health in Later Childhood/Adolescence: A Systematic Review," *Maternal Child Health Journal* 17, no. 3 (2013): 424–31, doi: 10.1007/s10995-012-1010-2

11. College Board, Trends in Higher Education, "Tuition and Fee and Room and Board Charges over Time," Accessed January 2015, http://trends.collegeboard.org/college-pricing/figures-tables/tuition-fees-room-board-time

12. National Survey of Student Engagement, *NSSE Annual Results 2012: Promoting Student Learning and Institutional Improvement: Lessons from NSSE at 13* (Bloomington, IN: Indiana University Center for Postsecondary Research, 2012).

13. American College Health Association, *American College Health Association-National College Health Assessment II (ACHA-NACHA II): Undergraduate Students, Reference Group Data Report, Spring 2014* (Hanover, MD: American College Health Association, 2014).

14. K. Eagan et al., *The American Freshman: National Norms for Fall 2013* (Los Angeles: Higher Education Research Institute, UCLA, 2014).

15. Sallie Mae and Ipsos, *How America Pays for College 2014: A National Study*, Accessed January 2015, http://news.salliemae.com/research-tools/america-pays-2014

16. The White House, Office of the Press Secretary, "FACT SHEET on the President's Plan to Make College More Affordable: A Better Bargain for the Middle Class," August 22, 2013, www.whitehouse.gov/the-press-office/2013/08/22/fact-sheet-president-s-plan-make-college-more-affordable-better-bargain

17. Sallie Mae and Ipsos, *How America Pays for College 2014*, 2015.

18. American Council on Education, "National Study of Non-First-Time Students Shows Disturbing Completion Rates," Accessed February 3, 2015, www.insidetrack.com/2014/10/27/national-study-non-first-time-students-shows-disturbing-completion-rates/

19. National Center for Education Statistics, "Annual Earnings of Young Adults," *The Condition of Education 2014* (NCES 2014-083), May, 2014, http://nces.ed.gov/programs/coe/indicator_cba.asp

20. M. Heron, "Deaths: Leading Causes for 2012, Table 9," *National Vital Statistics Reports* 63, no. 9 (2014), www.cdc.gov/nchs/data/nvsr/nvsr63/nvsr63_09.pdf

21. Healthcare.gov, "Why Should I Have Health Coverage?," Accessed April 2014, www.healthcare.gov/why-should-i-have-health-coverage

22. Bankruptcy Abuse Prevention and Consumer Protection Act of 2005, Pub.L. 109–8, 109th Cong. (2005). Full text available at www.govtrack.us.

23. Federal Reserve Bank of New York, Research and Statistics Group, Microeconomic Studies, "Quarterly Report on Household Debt and Credit," November 2014, www.newyorkfed.org

24. Ibid.

25. Credit Card Accountability Responsibility and Disclosure Act, The CARD Act of 2009, Pub.L. 111–24, 111th Cong. (2009). Full text available at www.gpo.gov.

26. Javelin Strategy & Research, "The 2014 Identity Fraud Report: Card Data Breaches and Inadequate Consumer Password Habits Fuel Disturbing Fraud Trends," February 2014, www.javelinstrategy.com/brochure/314

27. Ibid.

28. Federal Trade Commission, Consumer Information, "Lost or Stolen Credit, ATM, and Debit Cards," August 2012, www.consumer.ftc.gov/articles/0213-lost-or-stolen-credit-atm-and-debit-cards

**Pulled Statistics:**

page 31, Nerd Wallet, "American Household Credit Card Debt Statistics: 2014," December 2014, www.nerdwallet.com/blog/credit-card-data/average-credit-card-debthousehold

page 33, Javelin Strategy & Research, "The 2014 Identity Fraud Report: Card Data Breaches and Inadequate Consumer Password Habits Fuel Disturbing Fraud Trends," February 2014, www.javelinstrategy.com

## Chapter 2: Promoting and Preserving Your Psychological Health

1. K. Neff, *Self Compassion: The Proven Power of Being Kind to Yourself* (New York: Harper Collins, 2011).

2. A. H. Maslow, *Motivation and Personality*, 2nd ed. (New York: Harper and Row, 1970).

3. D. J. Anspaugh and G. Ezell, *Teaching Today's Health*, 10th ed. (Boston: Pearson, 2013).

4. X. Wang et al., "Social Support Moderates Stress Effect on Depression," *International Journal of Mental Health Systems* 8, no. 1 (2014): 1–5; J. Holt-Lunstad, T. B. Smith, and J. B. Layton, "Social Relationships and Mortality Risk: A Meta-Analytic Review," *PLoS Medicine* 7, no. 7 (2010): e1000316, doi: 10.1371/journal.pmed.1000316; N. I. Eisenberger and S. W. Cole, "Social Neuroscience and Health: Neurophysiological Mechanisms Linking Social Ties with Physical Health," *Nature Neuroscience* 15 (2012): 669–74, doi:10.1038/nn.3086; Y. Luo et al., "Loneliness, Health, and Mortality in Old Age: A National Longitudinal Study," *Social Science & Medicine* 74, no. 6 (2012): 907–14.

5. C. Carter, *Raising Happiness: 10 Simple Steps for More Joyful Kids and Happier Parents* (New York: Ballantine Publishing, 2010).

6. X. Wang et al., "Social Support Moderates Stress Effect," 2014; W. Cheng, W. Ickes, and L. Verhofstadt, "How is Family Support Related to Students' GPA Scores? A Longitudinal Study," *Higher Education* 64, no. 3 (2012): 399–420; L. Rice et al., "The Role of Social Support in Students' Perceived Abilities and Attitudes toward Math and Science," *Journal of Youth and Adolescence* 42, no. 7 (2013): 1028–40; J. Cullum et al., "Ignoring Norms with a Little Help from my Friends: Social Support Reduces Normative Influence on Drinking Behavior," *Journal of Social & Clinical Psychology* 32, no. 1 (2013): 17–33; J. Hirsch and A. Barton, "Positive Social Support, Negative Social Exchanges, and Suicidal Behavior in College Students," *Journal of American College Health* 59, no. 5 (2011): 393–98; I. Yalcin, "Social Support and Optimism as Predictors of Life Satisfaction of College Students," *International Journal for the Advancement of Counseling* 33, no. 2 (2011): 79–87.

7. National Cancer Institute, "Spirituality in Cancer Care," Revised 2012, www.cancer.gov/cancertopics/pdq/supportivecare/spirituality/patient

8. M. Seligman, *Helplessness: On Depression, Development, and Death* (New York: W. H. Freeman, 1975).

9. P. Salovey and J. Mayer, "Emotional Intelligence," *Imagination, Cognition, and Personality* 9, no. 3 (1989): 185–211.

10. A. Martins, N. Ramalho, and E. Morin, "A Comprehensive Meta Analysis of the Relationship between Emotional Intelligence and Health," *Personality and Individual Differences* 49, no. 6 (2010): 554–64.

11. D. Goleman, R. Boyatzis, and A. McKee, *Primal Leadership: Unleashing the Power of Emotional Intelligence* (Boston: Harvard Business Review Press, 2013); M. A. Brackett, S. E. Rivers, and P. Salovey, "Emotional Intelligence: Implications for Personal, Social, Academic, and Workplace Success," *Social and Personality Psychology Compass* 5, no. 1 (2011): 88–103.

12. K. Huffman and C. A. Sanderson, *Real World Psychology* (Hoboken, NJ: Wiley, 2014).

13. Ibid.

14. S. Rimer, Harvard School of Public Health, "The Biology of Emotion—And What It May Teach Us about Helping People to Live Longer," 2012, www.hsph.harvard.edu/news/hphr/chronic-disease-prevention/happiness-stress-heart-disease/

15. Ibid; Steptoe, C. de Oliveira, P. Demakakos, and P. Zaninotto, "Enjoyment of Life and Declining Physical Function at Older Ages: A Longitudinal Cohort Study," *Canadian Medical Association Journal* 186, no. 4 (2014): e150–56.

16. Ibid; E. A. Wheeler, "Amusing Ourselves to Health: A Selected Review of Lab Findings," in *Positive Psychology: Advances in Understanding Adult Motivation*, ed. J. D. Sinnott (New York: Springer, 2013).

17. B. Fredrickson, et al., "A Functional Genomic Perspective on Human Well-Being," *Proceedings of the National Academy of Sciences* 110, no. 33 (2013): 13684–89.

18. E. Diener, "Subjective Well-Being: A Primer for Reporters and Newcomers," Accessed February 2015, http://internal.psychology.illinois.edu/~ediener/faq.html; L. Tay, M. Herian, and E. Diener, "The Metrics of Societal Happiness," *Social Indicators Research* 117, no. 2 (2014): 577–600.

19. E. Roysamb et al., "Well-Being: Heritable and Changeable," *Stability of Happiness Theories and Evidence on Whether Happiness Can Change* (San Diego: Academic Press, 2014): 9–35.

20. M. Seligman, *Flourish: A Visionary New Understanding of Happiness and Well-Being* (New York: Free Press, 2011).

21. Medline Plus, "Mental Disorders," February 12, 2015, www.nlm.nih.gov/medlineplus/mentaldisorders.html.

22. Ibid.

23. R. Karg, et al. "Past Year Mental Health Disorders among Adults in the U.S.: Results from the

2008–2012 Mental Health Surveillance Study," *Center for Behavioral Health Statistics and* Quality (2014), Available at www.samhsa.gov/data/sites/default/files/NSDUH-DR-N2MentalDis-2014-1/Web/NSDUH-DR-N2MentalDis-2014.htm

24. National Alliance on Mental Illness, "Mental Illness Factors and Numbers," March 2013, Available at www2.nami.org/factsheet/mentalillness_factsheet.pdf; Substance Abuse and Mental Health Services Administration, "Results from the 2012 National Survey on Drug Use and Health: Mental Health Findings," NSDUH Series H-47, HHS Publication no. (SMA) 13-4805 (Rockville, MD: Substance Abuse and Mental Health Services Administration, 2013).

25. L. Szabo, "Cost of Not Caring: Nowhere to Go," *USA Today*, May 5, 2014, www.usatoday.com/story/news/nation/2014/05/12/mental-health-system-crisis/7746535/; H. A. Whiteford et al., "Global Burden of Disease Attributable to Mental and Substance Use Disorders: Findings from the Global Burden of Disease Study 2010," *The Lancet* 382, no. 9904 (2013): 1575–86.

26. L. Szabo, "Cost of Not Caring," 2014.

27. American Psychological Association, "College Students' Mental Health is a Growing Concern, Survey Finds," June 2013, www.apa.org/monitor/2013/06/college-students.aspx; D. Gruttadaro and D. Crudo, *College Students Speak: A Survey Report on Mental Health* (Arlington, VA: National Alliance on Mental Health, 2012), Available at www.nami.org/Content/NavigationMenu/Find_Support/NAMI_on_Campus1/NAMI_Survey_on_College_Students/collegereport.pdf

28. American College Health Association, *American College Health Association–National College Health Assessment II (ACHA–NCHA II): Reference Group Data Report Spring 2014* (Hanover, MD: American College Health Association, 2014), Available at www.acha-ncha.org/reports_ACHA-NCHAII.html

29. Ibid.

30. National Alliance on Mental Illness, "Mental Illness Factors and Numbers," 2013.

31. R. Karg, et al. "Past Year Mental Health Disorders among Adults in the U.S.," 2014.

32. Ibid.

33. National Institute of Mental Health, "Depression," Accessed February 2014, www.nimh.nih.gov/health/topics/depression/index.shtml

34. Ibid.

35. American College Health Association, *American College Health Association II): Reference Group Data Report Spring 2014,* 2014.

36. HelpGuide.org, "Depression in Men," 2014, www.helpguide.org/mental/depression_men_male.htm

37. A. Shah et al., "Sex and Age Differences in the Association of Depression with Obstructive Coronary Artery Disease and Adverse Cardiovascular Events," Journal of the American Heart Association 3, no. 3 (2014): e000741.

38. R. Karg, et al. "Past Year Mental Health Disorders among Adults," 2014; Mayo Clinic, "Depression in Women: Understanding the Gender Gap," January 19, 2013, www.mayoclinic.org/diseases-conditions/depression/in-depth/depression/art-20047725

39. A. Gurian, "Depression in Adolescence: Does Gender Matter?," *NYU Child Study Center*, Accessed February 23, 2015, www.aboutourkids.org/articles/depression_in_adolescence_does_gender_matter#

40. D. Johnson and M. Whisman, "Gender Differences in Rumination: A Meta-Analysis," *Personality and Individual Differences* 55, no. 4 (2013.): 367–74.

41. R. Uher, "Persistent Depressive Disorder, Dysthymia, and Chronic Depression: Update on Diagnosis, Treatment," *Psychiatric Times*, July 2014, www.psychiatrictimes.com/special-reports/persistent-depressive-disorder-dysthymia-and-chronic-depression/page/0/3

42. WebMD, "Seasonal Depression (Seasonal Affective Disorder)," Accessed February 23, 2015, www.webmd.com/depression/guide/seasonal-affective-disorder

43. American Psychiatric Association, "Seasonal Affective Disorder," Accessed February 23, 2015, www.psychiatry.org/seasonal-affective-disorder; Cleveland Clinic, "Seasonal Depression," Accessed February 2015, http://my.clevelandclinic.org/services/neurological_institute/center-for-behavioral-health/disease-conditions/hic-seasonal-depression

44. SAMHSA, "Mental Disorders: Bipolar and Related Disorders," October 10, 2014, www.samhsa.gov/disorders/mental; R. C. Kessler et al., "Twelve-Month and Lifetime Prevalence and Lifetime Morbid Risk of Anxiety and Mood Disorders in the United States," *International Journal of Methods in Psychiatric Research* 21, no. 3 (2012): 169–84.

45. SAMHSA, "Treatments for Mental Disorders," October 9, 2014, www.samhsa.gov/treatment/mental-disorders

46. Mayo Clinic Staff, MayoClinic.com, "Depression: Causes," 2013, www.mayoclinic.org/diseases-conditions/depression/basics/causes/con-20032977

47. PsychGuides.com, "Mood Disorder Symptoms, Causes and Effects," Accessed 2015, www.psychguides.com/guides/mood-disorder-symptoms-causes-and-effect/

48. SAMSHA, "Mental Disorders: Anxiety Disorders," October 10, 2014, www.samhsa.gov/disorders/mental; R. Karg, et al., "Past Year Mental Health Disorders among Adults in the U.S.," 2014; K. R. Merikangas et al., "Lifetime Prevalence of Mental Disorders in U.S. Adolescents: Results from the National Comorbidity Survey Replication—Adolescent Supplement (NCS-A)," *Journal of the American Academy of Child and Adolescent Psychiatry* 49, no. 10 (2010): 980–89, doi: 10.1016/j.jaac.2010.05.017

49. American College Health Association, *National College Health Assessment III: Reference Group Data Report Spring 2014,* 2014.

50. National Institute of Mental Health, "Anxiety Disorders," Accessed February 2015, www.nimh.nih.gov/health/publications/anxiety-disorders/index.shtml#pub7

51. American College Health Association, *National College Health Assessment II: Reference Group Data Report Spring 2014,* 2014.

52. Mayo Clinic Staff, MayoClinic.com, "Panic Attacks and Panic Disorder: Symptoms," May 31, 2012, www.mayoclinic.org/diseases-conditions/panic-attacks/basics/symptoms/con-20020825

53. Web MD, "Anxiety and Panic Disorders Health Center: Specific Phobias," Accessed February 23, 2015, www.webmd.com/anxiety-panic/specific-phobias

54. Ibid.

55. Mayo Clinic, "Generalized Anxiety Disorder: Causes," Accessed February 2014, www.mayoclinic.org/diseases-conditions/generalized-anxiety-disorder/basics/causes/con-20024562

56. National Institute of Mental Health, "Obsessive Compulsive Disorder: Prevalence," Accessed February 23, 2015, www.nimh.nih.gov/health/statistics/prevalence/obsessive-compulsive-disorder-among-adults.shtml

57. National Institute of Mental Health, "Obsessive Compulsive Disorder," Accessed February 23, 2015, www.nimh.nih.gov/health/topics/obsessive-compulsive-disorder-ocd/index.shtml

58. Anxiety and Depression Association of America, "Facts and Statistics," Accessed February 23, 2015, www.adaa.org/about-adaa/press-room/facts-statistics

59. U.S. Dept. of Veterans Affairs, "PTSD: National Center for PTSD," November 10, 2014, www.ptsd.va.gov/public/PTSD-overview/basics/how-common-is-ptsd.asp; R. H. Pietrzak et al., "Prevalence and Axis I Comorbidity of Full and Partial PTSD in the U.S.: Results from Wave 2 of the National Epidemiologic Survey on Alcohol and Related Conditions," *Journal of Anxiety Disorders* 25, no. 3 (2011): 456–65.

60. U.S. Department of Veterans Affairs, "PTSD: National Center for PTSD," November 10, 2014, www.ptsd.va.gov/public/PTSD-overview/basics/how-common-is-ptsd.asp

61. National Institute of Mental Health, "Post-Traumatic Stress Disorder," Accessed February 23, 2015, www.nimh.nih.gov/health/topics/post-traumatic-stress-disorder-ptsd/index.shtml#part4

62. R. H. Pietrzak et al., "Prevalence and Axis I Comorbidity of Full and Partial PTSD in the U.S.," 2011; J. Gradus, U.S. Department of Veterans Affairs, National Center for PTSD, "Epidemiology of PTSD," January 2014, www.ptsd.va.gov/professional/PTSD-overview/epidemiological-facts-ptsd.asp; S. Staggs, PsychCentral, "Myths and Facts about PTSD," February 2014, http://psychcentral.com/lib/myths-and-facts-about-ptsd

63. American Psychiatric Association, *Diagnostic and Statistical Manual of Mental Disorders (DSM-5)*, 5th ed. (Washington, DC: American Psychiatric Association, 2013).

64. R. A. Sansone and L. A. Sansone, "Personality Disorders: A Nation-Based Perspective on Prevalence," *Innovations in Clinical Neuroscience* 8, no. 4 (2011): 13–18.

65. J. Twenge, *The Narcissism Epidemic: Living in the Age of Entitlement* (San Jose, CA: Atria Books, 2010).

66. American Psychiatric Association, *DSM-5*, 2013.

67. Mayo Clinic Staff, MayoClinic.com, "Borderline Personality Disorder," Accessed February 23, 2015, www.mayoclinic.org/diseases-conditions/borderline-personality-disorder/basics/definition/con-20023204

68. SAMHSA, "Report to Congress on Borderline Personality Disorder," HHS Pub. No. SMA-11-4644, 2011, Available at http://store.samhsa.gov/shin/content//SMA11-4644/SMA11-4644.pdf

69. Ibid.

70. National Institute of Mental Health, "Schizophrenia," Accessed February 23, 2015, www.nimh.nih.gov/health/topics/schizophrenia/index.shtml

71. Ibid.

72. Ibid.

73. World Health Organization, "Preventing Suicide: A Global Imperative," 2014, Available at www.who.int/mental_health/suicide-prevention/world_report_2014/en/)

74. Ibid.

75. Ibid.

76. M. Heron, "Deaths: Leading Causes for 2010," *National Vital Statistics Reports* 62, no. 6 (2013), Available at www.cdc.gov/nchs/data/nvsr/nvsr62/nvsr62_06.pdf

77. Centers for Disease Control and Prevention, "National Suicide Statistics at a Glance," January 2014, www.cdc.gov/violenceprevention/suicide/statistics/index.html

78. A. P. Haas et al., "Suicide and Suicide Risk in Lesbian, Gay, Bisexual, and Transgender Populations: Review and Recommendations," *Journal of Homosexuality* 58, no. 1 (2011): 10–51.

79. D. Reynolds and P. Schneider, "An Overview of Suicide Risks among Lesbian, Gay, Bisexual, Transgender and Questioning (LGBTQ) Youth," Social Workers Help Starts Here, blog, December 9, 2009, www.helpstartshere.org/mind-spirit/suicide-prevention/an-overview-of-suicide-risks-among-lesbian-gay-bisexual-transgender-and-questioning-lgbtq-youth.html

80. Ibid; E. Mereish, C. O'Clerigh, and J. Bradford, "Interrelationships between LGBT-Based Victimization, Suicide, and Substance Use Problems in a Diverse Sample of Sexual and Gender Minority Men and Women," *Psychology, Health & Medicine* 19, no. 1 (2014): 1–13

81. Centers for Disease Control and Prevention, "Suicide Facts at a Glance," 2012, Available at www.cdc.gov/violenceprevention/pdf/Suicide-DataSheet-a.pdf

82. Centers for Disease Control and Prevention, "National Suicide Statistics at a Glance," January 2015, www.cdc.gov/violenceprevention/suicide/statistics/mechanism02.html

83. American Foundation for Suicide Prevention, "Suicide Warning Signs," Accessed February 23, 2015, www.afsp.org/preventing-suicide/suicide-warning-signs

84. Ibid.

85. American Foundation for Suicide Prevention, "Frequently Asked Questions," Accessed February 23, 2015, www.afsp.org/preventing-suicide/frequently-asked-questions

86. Substance Abuse and Mental Health Services Administration, *Results from the 2012 National Survey on Drug Use and Health: Mental Health Findings*, NSDUH Series H-47, HHS Publication No. (SMA) 13-4805, (Rockville, MD: Substance Abuse and Mental Health Services Administration, 2013), Available at www.samhsa.gov/data/sites/default/files/2k12MH_Findings/2k12MH_Findings/NSDUHmhfr2012.pdf

87. Ibid.

88. MentalHealth.gov, "Mental Health Myths and Facts," Accessed February 23, 2015, www.mentalhealth.gov/basics/myths-facts/

89. A. Lasalvia et al., "Global Pattern of Experienced and Anticipated Discrimination Reported by People with Major Depressive Disorder: A Cross-Sectional Survey," *The Lancet* 381, no. 9860 (2013): 55–62, doi: 10.1016/S0140-6736(12)61379-8

90. K. Huffman and C. A. Sanderson, *Real World Psychology* (Hoboken, NJ: Wiley, 2014).

91. Ibid.

92. Mayo Clinic, Cognitive Behavioral Therapy, February 2013, www.mayoclinic.com/health/cognitive-behavioral-therapy/MY00194

93. National Institute of Mental Health, "Antidepressant Medications for Children and Adolescents: Information for Parents and Caregivers," Accessed February 23, 2015, www.nimh.nih.gov/health/topics/child-and-adolescent-mental-health/antidepressant-medications-for-children-and-adolescents-information-for-parents-and-caregivers.shtml

94. B. K. Hölzel et al., "Mindfulness Practice Leads to Increases in Regional Brain Gray Matter Density," *Psychiatry Research: Neuroimaging* 191, no. 1 (2011): 36–43; Mayo Clinic, "St. John's Wort (*Hypericum perforatum*)," November 2013, www.mayoclinic.org/drugs-supplements/st-johns-wort/background/HRB-20060053

**Pulled Statistics:**

Page 45, Substance Abuse and Mental Health Services Administration, *Results from the 2012 National Survey on Drug Use and Health: Mental Health Findings*, NSDUH Series H-47, HHS Publication no. (SMA) 13-4805 (Rockville, MD: Substance Abuse and Mental Health Services Administration, 2013).

Page 53, National Alliance on Mental Illness, "College Students Speak: A Survey Report on Mental Health," 2012, Available at: www.nami.org/Content/NavigationMenu/Find_Support/NAMI_on_Campus1/collegereport.pdf

## Focus On: Cultivating Your Spiritual Health

1. K. Eagan et al., *The American Freshman: National Norms Fall 2014* (Los Angeles: Higher Education Research Institute, UCLA, 2014), Available at http://heri.ucla.edu/monographs/TheAmerican-Freshman2014-Expanded.pdf

2. Ibid.

3. H. G. Koenig, "Religion, Spirituality and Health: The Research and Clinical Implications," *ISRN Psychiatry* (2012), doi: 10.5402/2012/27830

4. K. Eagan et al., *The American Freshman,* 2014.

5. Ibid.

6. B. L. Seaward, *Managing Stress: Principles and Strategies for Health and Well Being*, 7th ed. (Sudbury, MA: Jones and Bartlett, 2012).

7. DanahZohar.com, "Learn the Qs," Accessed January 2014, http://dzohar.com/?page_id=622

8. C. Wigglesworth, "Spiritual Intelligence and Why It Matters," Deep Change, 2011, www.deepchange.com/SpiritualIntelligenceEmotionalIntelligence2011.pdf

9. NIH, NCCIH, Research Results, accessed March 2015, https://nccih.nih.gov/research/results

10. B. C. Bock et al., "Yoga as a Complementary Treatment for Smoking Cessation in Women," *Journal of Women's Health* 21, no. 2 (2012): 240–48; L. Carim-Todd, S. H. Mitchell, and B. S. Oken, "Mind-Body Practices: An Alternative, Drug-Free Treatment for Smoking Cessation? A Systematic Review of the Literature," *Drug and Alcohol Dependence* 132, no. 3 (2013): 399–410; V. Conn, "The Power of Being Present: The Value of Mindfulness Interventions in Improving Health and Well-Being," *Western Journal of Nursing Research* 33 (2011): 993–95; Y. Matchim, J. Armer, and B. Stewart, "Effects of Mindfulness-Based Stress Reduction on Health among Breast Cancer Survivors," *Western Journal of Nursing Research* 33, no. 8 (2011): 996–1016.

11. National Cancer Institute (NCI), "Spirituality in Cancer Care," July 3, 2014, www.cancer.gov/cancertopics/pdq/supportivecare/spirituality/HealthProfessional/page1

12. C. Lysne and A. Wachholtz, "Pain, Spirituality and Meaning Making: What Can We Learn from the Literature?," *Religions*, no. 2 (2011): 1–16, doi:10.3390/rel2010001; H. Koenig and A. Bussing, "Spiritual Needs of Patients with Chronic Diseases." *Religions* 1, no. 1 (2010): 18–27.

13. R. E. Wells et al., "Complementary and Alternative Medicine Use among U. S. Adults with Common Neurological Conditions," *Journal of Neurology* 257, no. 11 (2010): 1822–11, Available at www.ncbi.nlm.nih.gov

14. ClinicalTrials.gov, "Mind–Body Interventions in Cardiac Patients," January 2011, http://clinicaltrials.gov/ct2/show/NCT01270568

15. P. Rajguru et al. "Use of Mindfulness Meditation in the Management of Chronic Pain: A Systematic Review of Randomized Controlled Trials," *American Journal of Lifestyle Medicine* (2014), doi: 10.1177/1559827614522580

16. G. Lucchetti, A. Lucchetti, and H. Koenig, "Impact of Spirituality/Religiosity on Mortality: Comparison with Other Health Interventions," *The Journal of Science and Healing* 7, no. 4 (2011): 234–38.

17. C. Aldwin et al., "Differing Pathways between Religiousness, Spirituality, and Health: A Self-Regulation Perspective," *Psychology of Religion and Spirituality* 6, no. 1 (2014): 9–21.

18. NCI, "Spirituality in Cancer Care," 2014.

19. A. Wachholtz and M. Rogoff, "The Relationship between Spirituality and Burnout among Medical Students," *Journal of Contemporary Medical Education* 1, no. 2 (2013): 83–91, doi: 10.5455/jcme.20130104060612

20. National Center for PTSD, "Spirituality and Trauma: Professionals Working Together," January 3, 2014, www.ptsd.va.gov/professional/provider-type/community/fs-spirituality.asp

21. Ibid.; NCCAM, "Prayer and Spirituality in Health: Ancient Practices, Modern Science," *CAM at the NIH: Focus on Complementary and Alternative Medicine* 12, no. 1 (2005), www.jpsych.com/pdfs/NCCAM%20-%20Prayer%20and%20Spirituality%20in%20Health.pdf; NCI, "Spirituality in Cancer Care," 2014.

22. D. R. Vago and D. A. Silbersweig, "Self-Awareness, Self-Regulation, and Self-Transcendence (S-ART): A Framework for Understanding the Neurobiological Mechanisms of Mindfulness," *Human Neuroscience* 6, no. 269 (2012), Available at www.ncbi.nlm.nih.gov/pmc/articles/PMC3480633/

23. G. Desbordes et al., "Effects of Mindful-Attention and Compassion Meditation Training on Amygdala Response to Emotional Stimuli in an Ordinary, Non-meditative State," *Frontiers in Human Neuroscience* 6, no. 292 (2012), doi: 10.3389/fnhum.2012.00292

24. National Center for Complementary and Integrative Health (NCCIH), "Research Spotlight: Meditation May Increase Empathy," Modified January 2012, https://nccih.nih.gov/research/results/spotlight/060608.htm

25. G. Desbordes et al., "Effects of Mindful-Attention and Compassion Meditation," 2012.

26. F. Zeidan et al., "Neural Correlates of Mindfulness Meditation-Related Anxiety Relief," *Social Cognitive and Affective Neuroscience* 9, no. 6 (2014): 751–59, doi: 10.1093/scan/nst041; G. Desbordes et al., "Effects of Mindful-Attention," 2012; J.C. Ong et al., "A Randomized Controlled Trial of Mindfulness Meditation for Chronic Insomnia," *Sleep* 37, no. 9 (2013): 1553–63; NCCIH, "Research Spotlight," 2014; A. Chiesa and A. Serretti, "Mindfulness-Based Stress Reduction for Stress Management in Healthy People," *Journal of Alternative and Complementary Medicine* 15, no. 5 (2009): 593–600.

27. S. Keng et al. "Effects of Mindfulness on Psychological Health: A Review of Empirical Studies," *Clinical Psychology Review* 31, no. 6 (2011); 1041–1056; E. Hoge et al., "Randomized Controlled Trial of Mindfulness Meditation for Generalized Anxiety Disorder: Effects on Anxiety and Stress Reactivity," *The Journal of Clinical Psychiatry* 74, no. 8 (2013): 786–92; S. Jedel et al., "A Randomized Controlled Trial of Mindfulness-Based Stress Reduction to Prevent Flare-Up in Patients with Inactive Ulcerative Colitis," *Digestion* 89, no. 2 (2014): 142–55.

28. W. Marchand, "Neural Mechanisms of Mindfulness and Meditation: Evidence From Neuroimging Studies," *World Journal of Radiology* 6, no. 7 (2014): 471–70, doi: 10.4329/wjr.v6.i7.471

29. S. Keng et al. "Effects of Mindfulness on Psychological Health," *Clinical Psychology Review* 31, no. 6 (2011); 1041–56.

30. W. Marchand, "Neural Mechanisms of Mindfulness and Meditation," 2014; B. Holzel et al., "Neural Mechanisms of Symptom Improvements in Generalized Anxiety Disorder Following Mindfulness Training," *Neuroimage: Clinical* 2 (2013): 448–58; B. Holzel et al., "Mindfulness Practice Leads to Increases in Regional Brain Gray Matter Density," *Psychiatry Research: Neuroimaging* 191, no. 1 (2011): 36–43; B. Holzel et al., "Stress Reduction Correlates with Structural Changes in the Amygdala," *Social Cognitive and Affective Neuroscience* 5 (2009): 11–17.

31. American Cancer Society, "Spirituality and Prayer," December 2012, www.cancer.org/treatment/treatmentsandsideeffects/complementaryandalternativemedicine/mindbodyandspirit/spirituality-and-prayer; University of Minnesota Center for Spirituality and Healing, "What Is Prayer?," August 2013, www.takingcharge.csh.umn.edu/explore-healing-practices/prayer

32. R. Jahnke et al., "A Comprehensive Review of Health Benefits of Qigong and Tai Chi," *American Journal of Health Promotion* 24, no. 6 (2010): e1–e25, www.ncbi.nlm.nih.gov/pubmed/20594090; American Tai Chi Association, "Psychiatric Expert: Tai Chi and Qigong Can Improve Mood in Older Adults, September 6, 2013, www.americantaichi.net/TaiChiQigongForHealthArticle.asp?cID=2&sID=10&article=chi_201309_1&subject=MentalHealth

33. M. Rudd and J. Aakers, "How to Be Happy by Giving to Others," *Scientific American*, July 8, 2014, www.scientificamerican.com/article/how-to-be-happy-by-giving-to-others/

34. F. Warneken and M. Tomasello, "The Roots of Human Altruism," *British Journal of Psychology* 100, no. 3 (2009): 455–71; C. Carter, *Raising Happiness: 10 Simple Steps for More Joyful Kids and Happier Parents* (New York: Ballantine Publishing, 2010); R. I. Dunbar et al., "Social Laughter Is Correlated with an Elevated Pain Threshold," *Proceedings of the Royal Society*, September 14, 2011, doi: 10.1098/rspb.2011.1373.39%

**Pulled Statistics:**

Page 61, K. Eagan et al., *The American Freshman: National Norms Fall 2014* (Los Angeles: Higher Education Research Institute, UCLA, 2014), Available at http://heri.ucla.edu/monographs/TheAmericanFreshman2014-Expanded.pdf

Page 63, Higher Education Research Institute, "Attending to Student's Inner Lives," April 2011, Available at http://spirituality.ucla.edu/docs/white%20paper/white%20paper%20final.pdf

Page 67, *Yoga Journal*, "New Study Finds More Than 20 Million Yogis in U.S.," December 5, 2012, http://blogs.yogajournal.com/yogabuzz/2012/12/new-study-find-more-than-20-million-yogis-in-u-s.html

## Chapter 3: Managing Stress and Coping with Life's Challenges

1. American Psychological Association, "Stress in America Annual Survey: Are Teens Adopting Adults' Stress Habits?" February 11, 2014, Available at www.apa.org/news/press/releases/stress/2013/stress-report.pdf; American Psychological Association (APA), "Stress in America: Missing the Health Care Connection," February 2013, www.apa.org/news/press/releases/stress/2012/full-report.pdf; S. Bethune, "Health-care Falls Short on Stress Management," *Monitor on Psychology* 44, no. 4 (2013): 22.

2. American Psychological Association, "A Stress Snapshot: Women Continue to Face an Uphill Battle with Stress," Accessed January 30, 2015, http://apa.org/news/press/releases/stress/2013/snapshot.aspx

3. American Psychological Association, "Stress: The Different Kinds of Stress," Accessed February 2014, www.apa.org

4. B. L. Seaward, *Managing Stress: Principles and Strategies for Health and Well-Being*, 8th ed. (Sudbury, MA: Jones and Bartlett, 2013), 8; National Institute of Mental Health (NIMH), "Stress Fact Sheet," Accessed January 2014, www.nimh.nih.gov

5. H. Selye, *Stress without Distress* (New York: Lippincott Williams & Wilkins, 1974), 28–29.

6. W. B. Cannon, *The Wisdom of the Body* (New York: Norton, 1932).

7. M. P. Picard and D. M. Turnbull, "Linking the Metabolic State and Mitochondrial DNA in Chronic Disease, Health and Aging," *Diabetes* 62, no. 3 (2013), Available at http://diabetes.diabetesjournals.org/content/62/3/672.full; S. Cohen et al., "Chronic Stress, Glucocorticoid Receptor Resistance, Inflammation and Disease Risk," *Proceedings of the National Academy of Sciences of the United States of America* 109, no. 16 (2012): 5995–99, doi: 10.1073/pnas.1118355109

8. S. Taylor, *The Tending Instinct: Women, Men and the Biology of Our Relationships* (New York: Time Books, Henry Holt and Company, 2002).

9. C. Cardodosa et al., "Stress-Induced Negative Mood Moderates the Relation between Oxytocin Administration and Trust: Evidence for the Tend-and-Befriend Response to Stress?" *Pschoneuroendocrinology* 38, no. 11 (2013): 2800–804.

10. J. Lee and V. R. Harley, "The Male Fight-Flight Response: A Result of SRY Regulation of Catecholamines?," *BioEssays* 34, no. 6 (2012): 454–57, doi: 10.1002/bies.201100159

11. A. Crum, P. Salovey, and S. Achor, "Rethinking Stress: The Role of Mindsets in Determining the Stress Response," *Journal of Personality and Social Psychology* 104, no. 4 (2013): 716–33.

12. P. Thoits, "Stress and Health: Major Findings and Policy Implications," *Journal of Health and Social Behavior* 51, no. 1, supplement (2010): S54–55, doi: 10.1177/0022146510383499; K. M. Scott et al., "Associations between Lifetime Traumatic Events and Subsequent Chronic Physical Conditions: A Cross-National, Cross-Sectional Study," *PLoS One* 8, no. 11 (2013), doi: 10.1371/journal.pone.0080573

13. K. M. Scott et al., "Associations between Lifetime Traumatic Events and Subsequent Chronic Physical Conditions: A Cross-National, Cross-Sectional Study," *PLoS One* 8, no. 11 (2013), doi: 10.1371/journal.pone.0080573

14. Robert Scaer, *The Body Bears the Burden: Trauma, Dissociation, and Disease*, 3rd ed. (New York: Routledge Press, 2014).

15. A. Steptoe and M. Kivimaki, "Stress and Cardiovascular Disease: An Update on Current Knowledge," *Annual Review of Public Health* 34 (2013): 337–54.

16. N. Aggarwal et al., "Perceived Stress Is Associated with Subclinical Cerebrovacular Disease in Older Adults," *The American Journal of Geriatric Psychiatry* 22, no. 1 (2014): 53–62; A. Steptoe and M. Kivimaki, "Stress and Cardiovascular Disease: An Update on Current Knowledge," *Annual Review of Public Health* 34 (2013): 337–54; S. Richardson et al., "Meta-Analysis of Perceived Stress and Its Association with Incident Coronary Heart Disease," *American Journal of Cardiology* 110, no. 12 (2012): 1711–17; A. Steptoe and M. Kivimaki, "Stress and Cardiovascular Disease," *Nature Reviews Cardiology* 9, no. 6 (2012): 360–70.

17. M. Kivimaki et al., "Job Strain as a Risk Factor for Coronary Heart Disease: A Collaborative Meta-Analysis of Individual Participants," *The Lancet* 380, no. 9852 (2012): 1491–97; E. Mostofsky et al., "Risk of Acute Myocardial Infarction After the Death of a Significant Person on One's Life. The Determinants of Myocardial Infarction Onset Study," *Circulation* 125,no. 3 (2012): 491–96, doi: 10.1161/CIRCULATIONAHA.111.061770

18. K. Scott, S. Melhorn, and R. Sakai. "Effects of Chronic Social Stress on Obesity," *Current Obesity Reports Online First* 1, no. 1 (2012): 16–25, doi: 10.1007/s13679-011-0006-3; F. Ippoliti, N. Canitano, and R. Businare, "Stress and Obesity as Risk Factors in Cardiovascular Diseases: A Neuroimmune Perspective," *Journal of Neuroimmune Pharmacology* 8, no. 1 (2013): 212–26; S. Pagota et al., "Association of Post-Traumatic Stress Disorder and Obesity in a Nationally Representative Sample," *Obesity* 20, no. 1 (2012): 200–205.

19. Mayo Clinic, "Stress and Hair Loss: Are They Related?," January 2014, www.mayoclinic.com/health/stress-and-hair-loss/AN01442

20. American Diabetes Association, "How Stress Affects Diabetes," 2013, www.diabetes.org/living-with-diabetes/complications/mental-health/stress.html; A. Pandy et al., "Alternative Therapies Useful in the Management of Diabetes: A Systematic Review," *Journal of Bioallied Science* 3, no. 4 (2011): 504–12.

21. C. Lee et al., "Increases in Blood Glucose in Older Adults: The Effects of Spousal Health," *Journal of Aging and Health* 26 (2014): 932–68.

22. M. Virtanen et al., "Psychological Distress and Incidence of Type 2 Diabetes in High Risk and Low Risk Populations: The Whitehall II Cohort Study," *Diabetes Care* 37, no. 8 (2014): 2091–97.

23. National Digestive Diseases Information Clearinghouse (NDDIC), "Irritable Bowel Syndrome: How Does Stress Affect IBS?," October 2013, http://digestive.niddk.nih.gov/ddiseases/pubs/ibs/#stress

24. H. F. Herlong, "Digestive Disorders White Paper–2013," *Johns Hopkins Health Alerts*, 2013, www.johnshopkinshealthalerts.com

25. E. Carlsson et al., "Psychological Stress in Children May Alter the Immune Response," *Journal of Immunology* 192, no. 5 (2014): 2071–81; G. Marshall, ed., "Stress and Immune-Based Diseases," *Immunology and Allergy Clinics of North America* 31, no. 1 (2011): 1–148; L. Christian, "Psychoneuroimmunology in Pregnancy: Immune Pathways Linking Stress with Maternal Health, Adverse Birth Outcomes and Fetal Development," *Neuroscience and Biobehavioral Reviews* 36, no. 1 (2012): 350–61, doi: 10.1016/j.neubiorev.2011.07.005; A. Pedersen et al., "Influence of Psychological Stress on Upper Respiratory Infection: A Meta-Analysis of Prospective Studies," *Psychosomatic Medicine* 72, no. 8 (2010): 823–32.

26. M. Kondo, "Socioeconomic Disparities and Health: Impacts and Pathways," *Journal of Epidemiology* 22, no. 1 (2012): 2–6; T. Theorell, "Evaluating Life Events and Chronic Stressors in Relation to Health: Stressors and Health in Clinical Work," *Advances in Psychosomatic Medicine* 32 (2012): 58–71; J. Gouln and J. Kiecolt-Glaser, "The Impact of Psychological Stress on Wound Healing: Methods and Mechanisms," *Immunology and Allergy Clinics of North America* 31, no. 1 (2011): 81–93.

27. American College Health Association (ACHA), *American College Health Association–National College Health Assessment II (ACHA-NCHA II): Reference Group Data Report Spring, 2014* (Hanover, MD: American College Health Association, 2014).

28. Ibid.

29. M. Marin et al., "Chronic Stress, Cognitive Functioning and Mental Health," *Neurobiology of Learning and Memory* 96, no. 4 (2011): 583–95; R. M. Shansky and J. Lipps, "Stress-Induced Cognitive Dysfunction: Hormone-Neurotransmitter Interactions in the Prefrontal Cortex," *Neuroscience and Biobehavioral Reviews* 7 (2013): 123, Available at www.ncbi.nlm.nih.gov/pmc/articles/PMC3617365

30. E. Dias-Ferreira et al., "Chronic Stress Causes Frontostriatal Reorganization and Affects Decision-Making," *Science* 325, no. 5940 (2009): 621–25; D. de Quervan et al., "Glucocorticoids and the Regulation of Memory in Health and Disease," *Frontiers in Neuroendocrinology* 30, no. 3 (2009): 358–70.

31. L. Johansson, "Can Stress Increase Alzheimer's Disease Risk in Women?," *Expert Review of Neurotherapeutics* 14, no. 2 (2014): 123–25, doi: 10.1586/14737175.2014.878651; P. J. Lucassen et al., "Neuropathology of Stress," *Acta Neuropathologica* 127, no. 1 (2014): 109–35.

32. T. Frodi and V. O'Keane, "How Does the Brain Deal with Cumulative Stress? A Review with Focus on Developmental Stress, HPA Axis Function and Hippocampal Structure in Humans," *Neurobiology of Disease* 52 (2013): 24–37; P. S. Nurius, E. Uehara, and D. F. Zatzick, "Intersection of Stress, Social Disadvantage, and Life Course Processes: Reframing Trauma and Mental Health," *American Journal of Psychiatric Rehabilitation* 16 (2013): 91–114; K. Scott et al., "Association of Childhood Adversities and Early-Onset Mental Disorders with Adult-Onset Chronic Physical Conditions," *Archives of General Psychiatry* 68, no. 8 (2011): 833–44.

33. American Psychological Association, "Stress in America: Paying with Our Health," 2015, Accessed April 2015, http://www.apa.org/news/press/releases/stress/2014/stress-report.pdf

34. S. Charles et al., "The Wear and Tear of Daily Stressors on Mental Health," *Psychological Science* 24, no. 5 (2013): 733–41; J. R. Piazza et al., "Affective Reactivity to Daily Stressors and Long-Term Risk of Reporting a Chronic Physical Health Condition," *Annals of Behavioral Medicine* 45, no. 1 (2013): 110–20, doi: 10.1007/s12160-012-9423-0; C. Aldwin et al., "Do Hassles Mediate between Life Events and Mortality in Older Men?: Longitudinal Findings from the VA Normative Aging Study," *Experimental Gerontology* 59 (2014): 74–80.

35. C. Aldwin et al., "Do Hassles Mediate between Life Events and Mortality?," 2014; S. O'Neill et al., "Affective Reactivity to Daily Interpersonal Stressors as a Prospective Predictor of Depressive Symptoms," *Journal of Social and Clinical Psychology* 23, no. 2 (2004): 172–94, doi 10.1521/jscp.23.2.172.31015.

36. K. M. Krajnak, "Potential Contribution of Work-Related Psychosocial Stress to the Development of Cardiovascular Disease and Type II Diabetes: A Brief Review," *Environmental Health Insights* 8, Supplement 1 (2014): 41–45, doi: 10.4137/EHI.S15263.e; N. Vurtanen, S. T. Nyberg, and G. D. Batty, "Perceived Job Insecurity as a Risk Factor for Incident Coronary Heart Disease: Systematic Review and Meta-Analysis," *BMJ* 347 (2013): f4746. doi:10.116/bmj.f4746; K. Toren et al., "A Longitudinal General Population-Based Study of Job Strain and Risk for Coronary Heart Disease and Stroke in Swedish Men," *BMJ Open* 4, no. 3 (2014): e004355, doi: 10:1136/bmjopen-2013-004355

37. American College Health Association, *National College Health Assessment II: Reference Group Data Report Spring, 2014*, 2014.

38. S. Schwartz et al., "Acculturation and Well-Being among College Students from Immigrant Families," *Journal of Clinical Psychology* (2012): 1–21, doi: 10.1002/jclp21847; A. Pieterse et al., "An Exploratory Examination of the Associations among Racial and Ethnic Discrimination, Racial Climate, and Trauma-Related Symptoms in a College Student Population," *Journal of Counseling Psychology* 57, no. 3 (2010): 255–63; A. McAleavey, L. Castonguay, and B. Locke, "Sexual Orientation Minorities in College Counseling: Prevalence, Distress, and Symptom Profiles," *Journal of College Counseling* 14, no. 2 (2011): 127–42.

39. K. Brown, *Predictors of Suicide Ideation and the Moderating Effects of Suicide Attitudes*, Master's thesis, University of Ohio, 2011, http://etd.ohiolink.edu; J. Gomez, R. Miranda, and L Polanco, "Acculturative Stress, Perceived Discrimination and Vulnerability to Suicide Attempts among Emerging Adults," *Journal of Youth and Adolescence* 40, no. 11 (2011): 1465–76.

40. B. L. Seaward, *Managing Stress: Principles and Strategies for Health and Well-Being*, 7th ed. (New York: Barnes and Noble, 2012).

41. J. Twenge, *Generation Me–Revised and Updated: Why Today's Young Americans Are More Confident, Assertive, Entitled and More Miserable Than Ever* (New York, Simon and Schuster, 2014).

42. A. Peng, J. Schaubroeck, and J. Xie, "When Confidence Comes and Goes: How Variation in Self-Efficacy Moderates Stressor–Strain Relationships," *Journal of Occupational Health Psychology*, Jan. 19, 2015: No Pagination Specified, http://dx.doi.org/10.1037/a0038588; R. Fida, et al. "'Yes I can'": The Protective Role of Personal Self Efficacy in Hindering Counterproductive Work Activity Under Stressful Conditions," *Anxiety, Stress and Coping*, 2014: 1–21, doi: 10.1080/10615806.2014.969718

43. A. Peng, J. Schaubroeck, and J. Xie, "When Confidence Comes and Goes," 2015.

44. I. Bragard et al., "Efficacy of a Communication and Stress Management Training on Medical Resident's Self Efficacy, Stressful Communication and Burnout," *Journal of Health Psychology* 15, no. 7 (2010): 1075–84; M. Komarraju and D. Nadler, "Self Efficacy and Academic Achievement: Who Do Implicit Beliefs, Goals and Effort Regulation Matter?," *Learning and Individual Differences* 25 (2013): 67–72.

45. P. N. von der Embse and S. Witmer, "High-Stakes Accountability: Student Anxiety and Large-Scale Testing," *Journal of Applied School Psychology* 30, no. 2 (2014): 132–56, doi: 10.1080/15377903.2014.888529

46. A. Zuffiano et al., "Academic Achievement: The Unique Contribution of Self Efficacy Beliefs in Self-Regulated Learning beyond Intelligence, Personality Traits and Self-esteem," *Learning and Individual Differences* 23 (2013): 158–62.

47. M. Friedman and R. H. Rosenman, *Type A Behavior and Your Heart* (New York: Knopf, 1974).

48. M. Whooley and J. Wong, "Hostility and Cardiovascular Disease," *Journal of the American College of Cardiology* 58, no. 12 (2011): 1228–30; J. Newman et al., "Observed Hostility and the Risk of Incident Ischemic Heart Disease: A Perspective Population Study from the 1995 Canadian Nova Scotia Health Survey," *Journal of the American College of Cardiology* 58, no. 12 (2011): 1222–28; T. Smith et al., "Marital Discord and Coronary Artery Disease: A Comparison of Behaviorally Defined Discrete Groups," *Journal of Consulting and Clinical Psychology* 80, no. 1 (2012): 87–92.

49. G. Mate, *When the Body Says No: Understanding the Stress-Disease Connection* (Hoboken, NJ: John Wiley and Sons, 2011).

50. H. Versteeg, V. Spek, and S. Pedersen, "Type D Personality and Health Status in Cardiovascular Disease Populations: A Meta-Analysis of Prospective Studies," *European Journal of Cardiovascular Prevention and Rehabilitation* 19, no. 6 (2011): 1373–380, doi: 10.1177/1741826711425338; F. Mols and F. J. Denollet, "Type D Personality in the General Population: A Systematic Review of Health Status, Mechanisms of Disease and Work-Related Problems," *Health and Quality of Life Outcomes* 8, no. 9 (2010): 1–10, Available from www.hqlo.com

51. S. Kobasa, "Stressful Life Events, Personality, and Health: An Inquiry into Hardiness," *Journal of Personality and Social Psychology* 37, no. 1 (1979): 1–11.

52. C. D. Schetter and C. Dolbier, "Resilience in the Context of Chronic Stress and Health in Adults," *Social and Personality Psychology Compass* 5, no. 9 (2011): 634–52, doi: 10.1111/j.1751-9004.2011.00379.x

53. C. Ryff et al., "Psychological Resilience in Adulthood and Later Life: Implications for Health," *Annual Review of Gerontology and Geriatrics* 32, no. 1 (2012): 73–92.

54. The American Psychological Association, "The Road to Resilience: What Is Resilience?," Accessed February 2014, www.apa.org/helpcenter/road-resilience.aspx

55. E. Chen et al., "Protective Factors for Adults from Low-Childhood Socioeconomic Circumstances: The Benefits of Shift-and-Persist for Allostatic Load," *Psychosomatic Medicine* 74, no. 2 (2012): 178–86, doi: 10.1097/PSY.0B013e31824206fd

56. Higher Education Research Institute, "A Year of Change: First Year," Accessed January 30, 2015, www.heri.ucla.edu/infographics/YFCY-2014-Infographic.pdf; J. K. Eagen, et al., *The American Freshman: National Norms Fall 2014–Expanded Edition* (Los Angeles: Higher Education Research Institute, 2015),www.heri.ucla.edu/monographs/TheAmericanFreshman2014-Expanded.pdf

57. Ibid.; K. Eagen, *The American Freshman*, 2015.

58. B. L. Seaward, *Managing Stress*, 2012.

59. J. Moskowitz et al., "A Positive Affect Intervention for People Experiencing Health-related Stress: Development and Non-randomized Pilot Test," *Journal of Health Psychology* 17, no. 5 (2012): 676–92, doi: 10.1177/1359105311425275; P. Thoits, "Mechanisms Linking Social Ties and Support to Physical and Mental Health," *Journal of Health and Social Behavior* 52, no. 2 (2011): 145–61; B. Lake and E. Oreheck, "Relational Regulation Theory: A New Approach to Explain the Link between Perceived Social Support and Mental Health," *Psychological Review* 118, no. 3 (2011): 482–95.

60. B. L. Seaward, *Managing Stress*, 2012.

61. M. A. Stults-Kolehmainen and R. Sinha, "The Effect of Stress on Physical Activity and Exercise," *Sports Medicine* 44, no. 1 (2014): 81–121; G. Colom, C. Alcover, C. Sanchez-Curto, and J. Zarate-Osuna, "Study of the Effect of Positive Humour as a Variable That Reduces Stress. Relationship of Humour with Personality and Performance Variables," *Psychology in Spain* 15, no. 1 (2011): 9–21.

62. L. Poole et al., "Associations of Objectively Measured Physical Activity with Daily Mood Ratings and Psychophysiological Stress Responses in Women," *Psychophysiology* 48 (2011): 1165–72, doi: 10.1111/j.1469-8986.2011.01184.x; D. A. Girdano, D. E. Dusek, and G. S. Everly, *Controlling Stress and Tension*, 9th ed. (San Francisco: Benjamin Cummings, 2012), 375.

63. M. A. Stults-Kolehmainen and R. Sinha, "The Effect of Stress on Physical Activity and Exercise," 2014; E. M. Jackson, "Stress Relief: The Role of Exercise in Stress Management," *ACSM Health and Fitness Journal* 17, no. 3 (2013), doi, 10.1249/FIT.0b013e31828cb1c9

64. P. M. Gollwitzer and G. Oettingen, "Implementation Intentions.," in *Encyclopedia of Behavioral Medicine* (Part 9), eds. M. Gellman and J. R. Turner (New York: Springer-Verlag, 2013), 1043–48; C. Stern et al. "Effects of Implementation Intention on Anxiety, Perceived Proximity and Motor Performance," *Personality and Social Psychology Bulletin* 39, no. 5 (2013): 623–35; A. Dalton and S. Spiller, "Too Much of a Good Thing: The Benefits of Implementation Intentions Depend on the Number of Specific Goals," *Journal of Consumer Research* 39, no. 3 (2012): 600–14.

65. National Center for Complementary and Integrative Health."Nationwide Survey reveals widespread use of mind and body practices." February 2015. http://www.nih.gov/news/health/feb2015/nccih-10a.htm

66. NIH Medline Plus, "What Yoga Can and Can't Do for You," December 2013, www.nlm.nih.gov/medlineplus/news/fullstory_143813.html; J. Kiecolt-Glaser et al., "Stress, Inflammation, and Yoga Practice," *Psychosomatic Medicine* 72, no. 2 (2010): 113–21.

67. R. D. Brook et al., "Beyond Medications and Diet: Alternative Approaches to Lowering Blood Pressure: A Scientific Statement from the American Heart Association," *Hypertension* 61, no. 6 (2013): 1360–83.

68. National Center for Complementary and Integrative Health, "Massage Therapy for Health Purposes: What You Need to Know," February 2014, http://nccam.nih.gov/health/massage/massageintroduction.htm

**Pulled Statistics:**

Page 72, American Psychological Association, "Stress in America: Missing the Health Care Connection," 2013, Accessed January 2015, https://www.apa.org/news/press/releases/stress/2012/full-report.pdf

Page 80, American College Health Association, *American College Health Association-National College*

*Health Assessment II: Reference Group Executive Summary Spring, 2014* (Hanover, MD: American College Health Association, 2014), www.acha.org

Page 84, American Psychological Association. "Stress in America—Are Teens Adopting Adults' Stress Habits?," 2013, Accessed on January 29, 2015, www.apa.org/news/press/releases/stress/2013/teen-stress.aspx

## Focus On: Improving Your Sleep

1. National Heart, Lung, and Blood Institute, "Sleep Disorders & Insufficient Sleep: Improving Health through Research," Accessed January 2015, www.nhlbi.nih.gov/news/spotlight/fact-sheet/sleep-disorders-insufficient-sleep-improving-health-through-research.html

2. The Philips Center for Health and Well-Being, "Philips Index for Health and Well-Being: A Global Perspective Report 2010," October 2011, www.newscenter.philips.com/pwc_nc/main/standard/resources/corporate/press/2010/Global%20Index%20Results/20101111%20Global%20Index%20Report.pdf

3. American College Health Association, *American College Health Association–National College Health Assessment II (ACHA–NCHA II): Reference Group Data Report Spring 2014* (Hanover, MD: American College Health Association, 2014), Available at www.achancha.org/reports_ACHA-NCHAII.html

4. S. Hershner and R. Chevin. "Causes and Consequences of Sleepiness Among College Students," *Nature and Science of Sleep* 6 (2014): 73-84, doi: 10.2147/NSS.S62907; A. Wald et al., "Associations between Healthy Lifestyle Behaviors and Academic Performance in U.S. Undergraduates: A Secondary Analysis of the American College Health Association's National College Health Assessment II, " *American Journal of Health Promotion* 28, no. 5 (2014): 298-305, doi: http://dx.doi.org/10.4278/ajhp.120518-QUAN-265; K. Ahrberg et al., "Interaction between Sleep Quality and Academic Performance," *Journal of Psychiatric Research* 46, no. 12 (2012): 1618-22.

5. S. Hershner and R. Chevin. "Causes and Consequences of Sleepiness among College Students," *Nature and Science of Sleep* 6 (2014): 73-84, doi: 10.2147/NSS.S62907; A. Wald et al., "Associations between Healthy Lifestyle Behaviors, " 2014.

6. National Sleep Foundation, "2011 Sleep in America Poll: Communications Technology and Sleep," March 2011, www.sleepfoundation.org/article/sleep-america-polls/2011-communications-technology-use-and-sleep

7. National Sleep Foundation, "Excessive Sleepiness," Accessed February 5, 2015, http://sleepfoundation.org/sleep-disorders-problems/excessive-sleepiness

8. Harvard University Radcliff Institute for Advanced Study, "Drowsy Driving," Accessed February 5, 2015, www.radcliffe.harvard.edu/news/radcliffe-magazine/drowsy-driving

9. C-SPAN, "Awake, Alert, Alive: Overcoming the Dangers of Drowsy Driving–NTSB Conference Opening Panel," October 21, 2014, www.c-span.org/video/?322228-1/discussion-combating-drowsy-driving

10. National Sleep Foundation, "Who's at Risk?, " Accessed February 5, 2015, http://drowsydriving.org/about/whos-at-risk/

11. L. Culpepper, "The Social and Economic Burden of Shift-Work Disorder," *The Journal of Family Practice* 59, no. 1, Supplement (2010): S3-S11; S. Rajaratname et al., "Sleep Loss and Circadian Disruption in Shift Work: Health Burden and Management, " *The Medical Journal of Australia* 199, no. 8 (2013): 11-15; F. P. Cappuccio et al., "Sleep Duration and All-Cause Mortality: A Systematic

Review and Meta-Analysis of Prospective Studies," *Sleep* 33, no. 5 (2010): 585-92.

12. National Sleep Foundation, "Who's at Risk?," 2015.

13. G. Hertz et al., "Sleep Dysfunction in Women," *Medscape* (2014), http://emedicine.medscape.com/article/1189087-overview

14. S. Tregear et al., "Obstructive Sleep Apnea and Risk of Motor Vehicle Crash: Systematic Review and Meta-Analysis," *Journal of Clinical Sleep Medicine* 5, no. 6 (2009): 573-81; K. Ward, et al. "Excessive Daytime Sleepiness Increases the Risk of Motor Vehicle Crash in Obstructive Sleep Apnea," *Journal of Clinical Sleep Medicine* 9, no. 10 (2013):1013-21

15. M. Meeker and L. Wu, "How Much Time Do We Really Spend on Our Smartphones Every Day?," *Business Insider,* June 6, 2013, www.businessinsider.com.au/how-much-time-do-we-spend-on-smartphones-2013-6; Marketing Charts, "College Students Own an Average of 7 Tech Devices," June 2013, www.marketingcharts.com/wp/topics/demographics/college-students-own-an-average-of-7-tech-devices-30430

16. Anne-Marie Chang et al., "Evening Use of Light-Emitting eReaders Negatively Affects Sleep, Circadian Time, and Next Morning Alertness," *Proceedings of the National Academy of Sciences* (2014), doi: 10.1073/pnas.1418490112]

17. N. Rod et al., "The Joint Effect of Sleep Duration and Disturbed Sleep on Cause-Specific Mortality: Results from the Whitehall II Cohort Study," *PLoS ONE* 9, no. 4 (2014): e91965, doi:10.1371/journal.pone.0091965; National Heart Lung and Blood Institute, "Why Is Sleep Important?," February 2012, www.nhlbi.nih.gov/health/health-topics/topics/sdd/why.html; F. P. Cappuccio et al., "Sleep Duration and All-Cause Mortality," 2010.

18. K. M. Orzech et al., "Sleep Patterns Are Associated with Common Illness in Adolescents," *Journal of Sleep Research* (2013), doi: 10.1111/jsr.12096; J. M. Krueger and J. A. Majde, "Sleep and Host Defense," in *Principles and Practice of Sleep Medicine,* eds. M. H. Kryger, T. Roth, and W. C. Dement (St. Louis, MO: Saunders 2011), 261-90; M. Manzer and M. Hussein, "Sleep-Immune System Interaction: Advantages and Challenges of Human Sleep Loss Model," *Frontiers of Neurology* 3, no. 2 (2012), doi: 10.3389/fneur.2012.00002

19. X. Yu et al., "TH17 Cell Differentiation Is Regulated by Circadian Clock," *Science* 342, no. 6159 (2013): 727-30; A. Bollinger, A. Bollinger, H. Oster, and W. Scolbach, "Sleep, Immunity and Circadian Clocks: A Mechanistic Model," *Gerontology* 56, no. 6 (2010): 574-80, doi: 10.1159/000281827

20. F. Heredia et al., "Self-Reported Sleep Duration, White Blood Cell Counts and Cytokine Profiles in European Adolescents: The Helena Study, " *Sleep Medicine* 15, no. 10 (2014). 1251-58.

21. F. Sofi et al., "Insomnia and Risk of Cardiovascular Disease: A Meta-Analysis," *European Journal of Preventive Cardiology* 21, no. 1 (2014): 57-64; R. Lanfranchi, F. Prince, D. Filipini, and J. Carrier, "Sleep Deprivation Increases Blood Pressure in Healthy Normotensive Elderly and Attenuates the Blood Pressure Response to Orthostatic Challenges," *Sleep* 34, no. 3 (2010): 335-39; F. Cappucio, D. Cooper, and D. Lanfranco, "Sleep Duration Predicts Cardiovascular Outcomes: A Systematic Review and Meta-Analysis of Prospective Studies," *European Heart Journal,* first published online February 7, 2011, doi: 10.1093/eurheart

22. M. A. Miller and F. P. Cappuccio, "Biomarkers of Cardiovascular Risk in Sleep Deprived People," *Journal of Human Hypertension* 27, no. 10 (2013): 583-88; S. Agarwal, N. Bajaj, and

C. Bae, "Association between Sleep Duration and Cardiovascular Disease: Results from the National Health and Nutrition Examination Survey (NHANES 2005-2008)," *Journal of the American College of Cardiology* 59, no. 13, Supplement 1 (2012): e1514; F. Sofi et al., "Insomnia and Risk of Cardiovascular Disease: A Meta-Analysis," *European Journal of Preventive Cardiology* 21, no. 1 (2014): 51-67.

23. M. A. Miller et al., "Sustained Short Sleep and Risk of Obesity. Evidence in Children and Adults," in *Handbook of Obesity,* 3rd ed., vol. 1, eds. G. A. Bray and C. Bouchard (Boca Raton, FL: CRC Press, Taylor & Francis Group, 2014), 397-41; Q. Xiao et al., "A Large Prospective Investigation of Sleep Duration, Weight Change and Obesity in the NIH-AARP Diet and Health Study," *American Journal of Epidemiology* 178, no. 11 (2013): 1600-10.

24. M. A. Miller et al., "Sustained Short Sleep and Risk of Obesity," 2014; Q. Xiao et al., "A Large Prospective Investigation of Sleep Duration," 2013; L. Nielson, T. Danielson, and A. Serensen, "Short Sleep Duration as a Possible Cause of Obesity: Critical Analysis of the Epidemiological Evidence," *Obesity Reviews* 12, no. 2 (2011): 78-92; National Sleep Foundation, "Obesity and Sleep," Accessed January 2014, www.sleepfoundation.org/article/sleep-topics/obesity-and-sleep

25. C. L. Jackson et al., "Association between Sleep Duration and Diabetes in Black and White Adults," *Diabetes Care* 36, no. 11 (2013): 3557-65; E. G. Holliday et al., "Short Sleep Duration Is Associated with Risk of Future Diabetes but Not Cardiovascular Disease: A Prospective Study and Meta-Analysis," *PLoS ONE* 8, no. 11 (2013): e82305, doi: 10.1371/journal.pone.0082305; American Diabetes Association, "Too Little Sleep Linked to Higher A1C," January 2014, www.diabetesforecast.org/2014/Jan/too-little-sleep-linked-to.html

26. National Institutes of Health (NIH), "Teacher's Guide–Information about Sleep," Accessed January 2015, http://science.education.nih.gov/supplements/nih3/sleep/guide/info-sleep.htm

27. National Institutes of Health, "Information about Sleep," Accessed January 2015, http://science.education.nih.gov/supplements/nih3/sleep/guide/info-sleep.htm; C. Peri and M. Smith, "What Lack of Sleep Does to Your Mind," WebMD, January 2013, www.webmd.com/sleep-disorders/excessive-sleepiness-10/emotions-cognitive

28. A. Chatburn, et al. "Complex Associative Memory Processing and Sleep: A Systematic Review and Meta-Analysis of Behavioural Evidence and Underlying EEG Mechanisms." *Neuroscience and Biobehavioral Reviews* 47 (2014): 645-55; E. Fortier-Brochu, S. Beauliew-Bonneau, H. Ivers, and C. Morin, "Insomnia and Daytime Cognitive Performance: A Meta-Analysis," *Sleep Medicine Reviews* 16, no. 1 (2011), doi: 10-1016/j.smrv.2011.03.008; W. Klemm, "How Sleep Helps Memory," *Psychology Today,* March 11, 2011, www.psychologytoday.com/blog/memory-medic/201103/how-sleep-helps-memory; M. A. Miller et al., "Chapter: Sleep and Cognition," in *Sleep Disorders* (2014), in press.

29. A. Gomes, J. Tavares, and M. Azevedo, "Sleep and Academic Performance in Undergraduates: A Multi-Measure, Multi-Predictor Approach," *Chronobiology* 28, no. 9 (2011): 786-801, doi:10.3109/07420528.2011.606518; Yu-Chih Chiang, "The Effects of Sleep on Performance of Undergraduate Students Working in the Hospitality Industry as Compared to Those Who Are Not Working in the Industry," 2013, http://lib.dr.iastate.edu/cgi/viewcontent.cgi?article=4067&context=etd

30. Z. Terpening et al., "The Contributors of Nocturnal Sleep to the Consolidation of Motor Skill Learning in Healthy Aging and Parkinson's Disease," *Journal of Sleep Research* 22, no. 4 (2013): 398–405; L. Genzel et al., "Complex Motor Sequence Skills Profit from Sleep," *Neuropsychobiology* 66, no. 4 (2012): 237–43, doi: 10.1159/000341878

31. Centers for Disease Control and Prevention, "Drowsy Driving: Asleep at the Wheel," 2014, Accessed February 2015, http://www.cdc.gov/Features/dsDrowsyDriving/

32. National Sleep Foundation, "Young People More Likely to Drive Drowsy," November 2012, www.sleepfoundation.org/alert/young-people-more-likely-drive-drowsy.

33. Centers for Disease Control and Prevention, "Insufficient Sleep is a Public Health Epidemic," January 13, 2014, www.cdc.gov/features/dssleep/; National Highway Traffic Safety Administration, "Drowsy Driving and Automobile Crashes," February 2014, www.nhtsa.gov/people/injury/drowsy_driving1/Drowsy.html#NCSDR/NHTSA

34. Ibid.; Centers for Disease Control and Prevention, "Drowsy Driving—19 States and the District of Columba. 2009–2010," *Morbidity and Mortality Weekly Report* 61, no. 51 (2013): 1033–37, Available at www.cdc.gov/mmwr/preview/mmwrhtml/mm6151a1.htm

35. H. Oster, "Does Late Sleep Promote Depression?" *Expert Reviews of Endocrinology and Metabolism* 7, no. 1 (2012): 27–29, www.expert-reviews.com/doi/abs/10.1586/eem.11.80;C. Baglioni et al., "Insomnia as a Predictor of Depression: A Meta-Analytic Evaluation of Longitudinal Epidemiological Studies," *Journal of Affective Disorders* 135, no. 1 (2011): 10–19.

36. National Institute of General Medical Sciences, "Circadian Rhythms Fact Sheet," Accessed February 5, 2015, www.nigms.nih.gov/Education/Pages/Factsheet_CircadianRhythms.aspx.

37. E. Carlson et al., "Tick Tock: New Clues About Biological Clocks and Health," *Inside Life Science,* November 1, 2012, http://publications.nigms.nih.gov/insidelifescience/biological-clocks.html; M. Vitaterna, J. Takahashi, and F. Turek, "Overview of Circadian Rhythms," National Institute on Alcohol Abuse and Alcoholism, 2014, http://pubs.niaaa.nih.gov/publications/arh25-2/85-93.htm

38. NIH, "Teacher's Guide–Information about Sleep," Accessed February 2014, http://science.education.nih.gov/supplements/nih3/sleep/guide/info-sleep.htm

39. B. Rasch and J. Born, "About Sleep's Role in Memory," *Physiological Reviews* 93, no. 2 (2013): 681–766.

40. Centers for Disease Control and Prevention, "Insufficient Sleep is a Public Health Epidemic," January 13, 2014, www.cdc.gov/features/dssleep/; F. Cappuccio et al. "Sleep Duration and All-Cause Mortality: Systematic Review," *Sleep* 33, no. 5 (2010): 585–92.

41. NIH, "Teacher's Guide–Information About Sleep," 2014.

42. E. Mezick et al., "Sleep Duration and Cardiovascular Responses to Stress in Undergraduate Men." *Psychophysiology* 51, no. 1 ( 2014): 88–96.

43. E. Carlson et al., "Tick Tock," 2012; CDC, "Insufficient Sleep Is a Public Health Epidemic," 2014, www.cdc.gov/features/dssleep/

44. N. Rod, M Kumari, and T. Lange et al. "The Joint Effect of Sleep Duration and Disturbed Sleep on Cause-Specific Mortality: Results from the Whitehall II Cohort Study," *PLoS ONE* 9, no. 4 (2014): e91965, doi:10.1371/journal.pone.0091965; Q. Xiao et al., "A Large Prospective Investigation of Sleep Duration, Weight Change, and Obesity in the NIH-AARP Diet and Health Study Cohort," *American Journal of Epidemiology* 178, no. 11 (2013): 1600–10; C .L. Jackson et al., "Association Between Sleep Duration and Diabetes in Black and White Adults," *Diabetes Care* 36, no. 11 (2013): 3557–65; F. Cappuccio et al., "Sleep Duration Predicts Cardiovascular Outcomes: A Systematic Review and Meta-Analysis of Prospective Studies," *European Heart Journal* 32, no. 12 (2011): 1484–92.

45. National Sleep Foundation, "Napping," Accessed February 5, 2015, http://sleepfoundation.org/sleep-topics/napping; National Sleep Foundation, "Drowsy Driving—Is There a Perfect Time to Take a Nap?," Accessed January 15, 2015; B. Faraut et al., "Benefits of Napping and an Extended Duration of Recovery Sleep on Alertness and Immune Cells After Acute Sleep Restriction," *Brain, Behavior and Immunity* 25, no. 1 (2011): 18–24, doi: 10.1016/j.bbi.2010.08.001

46. Vanderbilt University Medical Center Reporter, "Take a Walk in the Sun to Ease Time Change Woes, Sleep Expert Says, " October 30, 2014, http://news.vanderbilt.edu/2014/10/take-a-walk-in-the-sun-to-ease-time-change-woes-says-vanderbilt-sleep-expert/

47. National Sleep Foundation, "Exercise and Sleep," Accessed February 5, 2015, www.sleepfoundation.org/article/sleep-america-polls/2013/exercise-and-sleep

48. National Sleep Foundation, "What You Breathe While You Sleep Can Affect How You Feel the Next Day," Accessed February 5, 2015, http://sleepfoundation.org/bedroom/smell.php

49. E. Carlson et al., "Tick Tock," 2012.

50. American College Health Association, *National College Health Assessment II: Reference Group Data Report Spring 2014*, 2014.

51. National Sleep Foundation, "Caffeine and Sleep," Accessed February 2014, www.sleepfoundation.org; American College Health Association, *National College Health Assessment II: Reference Group Data Report Spring 2014,* 2014.

52. National Sleep Foundation, Insomnia, Accessed February 5, 2015, http://sleepfoundation.org/sleep-disorders-problems/insomnia

53. Ibid.

54. Ibid.

55. Ibid.

56. American College Health Association, *National College Health Assessment II: Reference Group Data Report Spring 2014*, 2014.

57. Society of Behavioral Medicine, "Adult Insomnia," Accessed February 5, 2014, http://www.behavioralsleep.org/adultinsomnia.aspx

58. Y. Chong, C. D. Fryar, and Q. Gu, "Prescription Sleep Aid Use among Adults: United States, 2005–2010," *NCHS Data Brief,* no. 127 (2013), Available at www.cdc.gov/nchs/data/databriefs/db127.htm

59. National Sleep Foundation, "Sleep Apnea," Accessed January 2015, www.sleepfoundation.org/article/sleep-related-problems/obstructive-sleep-apnea-and-sleep.

60. Sleep Disorders Guide, "Sleep Apnea Statistics," Accessed January 2015, www.sleepdisordersguide.com/sleepapnea/sleep-apnea-statistics.html

61. National Sleep Foundation, "Sleep Apnea," 2015.

62. Ibid.

63. Ibid.

64. National Institute of Neurological Disorders and Stroke, "Restless Legs Syndrome Fact Sheet," updated July 25, 2014, www.ninds.nih.gov/disorders/restless_legs/detail_restless_legs.htm

65. Ibid.

66. National Institute of Neurological Disorders and Stroke, "Narcolepsy Fact Sheet," updated January 5, 2015, www.ninds.nih.gov/disorders/narcolepsy/detail_narcolepsy.htm

67. National Sleep Foundation, "Narcolepsy and Sleep," 2014, www.sleepfoundation.org/article/sleep-related-problems/narcolepsy-and-sleep

**Pulled Statistics:**

Page 100, American College Health Association, American College Health Association— National College Health Assessment II: Reference Group Executive Summary, Spring 2014 (Hanover, MD: American College Health Association, 2014).

Page 102, American College Health Association, American College Health Association— National College Health Assessment II: Reference Group Executive Summary, Spring 2014 (Hanover, MD: American College Health Association, 2014).

## Chapter 4: Preventing Violence and Injury

1. Voltaire, "Semiramis," V.1, trans. by J. K. Hoyt, in *The Cyclopaedia of Practical Quotations*, 1896. New York: Funk & Wagnalls Company.

2. World Health Organization (WHO), *Global Status Report on Violence Prevention* (Geneva: World Health Organization, 2014), Available at www.undp.org/content/dam/undp/library/corporate/Reports/UNDP-GVA-violence-2014.pdf

3. Centers for Disease Control and Prevention, "Deaths, Percent of Total Deaths, and Death Rates for the 15 Leading Causes of Death: United States and Each State, 1999–2013," December 31, 2014, Available at www.cdc.gov/nchs/data/dvs/LCWK1_2013.pdf

4. WHO, *Global Status Report on Violence Prevention* 2014.

5. Ibid.

6. Ibid.

7. U.S. Department of Justice, Federal Bureau of Investigation, *Crime in the United States, Preliminary Semiannual Uniform Crime Report for January–June 2013*, May 2014, www.fbi.gov/about-us/cjis/ucr/crime-in-the-u.s/2013/preliminary-semiannual-uniform-crime-report-january-june-2013; J. Rudolph, "Violent Crime up in the U.S. for the First Time in Nearly 2 Decades, Despite FBI Claims," *Huffington Post,* October 17, 2012, www.huffingtonpost.com/2012/10/17/violent-crime-bureau-justice-statistics_n_1974123.html

8. C. Barnett-Ryan, L. Langton, M. Planty, "The Nation's Two Crime Measures," September 18, 2014, *Bureau of Justice Statistics,* www.bjs.gov/index.cfm?ty=pbdetail&iid=5112; Bureau of Justice Statistics, "Reporting Crimes to Police," February 11, 2015, www.bjs.gov/index.cfm?ty=tp&tid=96

9. J. Langton and J. Truman. "Criminal Victimization, 2013 (Revised)," *Bureau of Justice Statistics*, September 18, 2014, www.bjs.gov/index.cfm?ty=tp&tid=96

10. U.S. Department of Justice. Bureau of Justice Statistics. "Criminal Victimization, 2013." 2014. http://www.bjs.gov/content/pub/pdf/cv13.pdf

11. Ibid.

12. American College Health Association, *American College Health Association—National College Health Assessment II: Reference Group Data Report, Spring 2014* (Hanover, MD: American College Health Association, 2014), Available at www.acha-ncha.org/reports_ACHA-NCHAII.html

13. Ibid.

14. Ibid.

15. National Criminal Justice Reference Service, "Section 6: Statistical Overviews," *NCVRW Resource Guide*, 2014, http://ovc.ncjrs.gov/ncvrw2014/pdf/StatisticalOverviews.pdf.

16. Center for Public Integrity, "Sexual Assault on Campus: A Frustrating Search for Justice," Updated February 2013, www.publicintegrity.org/accountability/education/sexual-assault-campus

17. World Health Organization Violence Prevention Alliance, "The Ecological Framework," 2015, www.who.int/violenceprevention/approach/ecology/en/index.html; World Health Organization, Global Status Report on Violence Prevention, (Geneva: World Health Organization, 2014), Available at www.undp.org/content/dam/undp/library/corporate/Reports/UNDP-GVA-violence-2014.pdf; Centers for Disease Control and Prevention, National Center for Injury Prevention and Control, "Understanding School Violence: Fact Sheet—2015," 2015, www.cdc.gov/violenceprevention/pdf/school_violence_factsheet-a.pdf

18. Substance Abuse and Mental Health Services Administration, "The NSDUH Report: Violent Behaviors and Family Income among Adolescents," August 19, 2010, Newsletter, www.oas.samhsa.gov

19. Centers for Disease Control and Prevention, "Intimate Partner Violence: Risk and Protective Factors," February 11, 2015, www.cdc.gov/violenceprevention/intimatepartnerviolence/riskprotectivefactors.html; D. M. Capaldi et al., "A Systematic Review of Risk Factors for Intimate Partner Violence," *Partner Abuse* 2, no. 2 (2012): 231–80, Available at www.ncbi.nlm.nih.gov

20. World Health Organization Violence Prevention Alliance, "The Ecological Framework," 2015, www.who.int/violenceprevention/approach/ecology/en/index.html; J. H. Derzon, "The Correspondence of Family Features with Problem, Aggressive, Criminal and Violent Behaviors: A Meta-Analysis," *Journal of Experimental Criminology* 6, no. 3 (2010): 263–92, doi: 10.1007/s11292-010-9098-0; L. Kiss et al., "Gender-Based Violence and Socioeconomic Inequalities: Does Living in More Deprived Neighborhoods Increase Women's Risk of Intimate Partner Violence?," *Social Science and Medicine* 74, no. 8 (2012): 1172–79; H. Beydoun et al., "Intimate Partner Violence against Adult Women and Its Association with Major Depressive Disorder, Depressive Symptoms and Postpartum Depression: A Systematic Review and Meta-Analysis," *Social Science & Medicine* 75, no. 6 (2012): 959–75, doi: 10.1016/j.socscimed.2012.04.025

21. M. L. Hunt, A. W. Hughey, and M. G. Burke, "Stress and Violence in the Workplace and on Campus: A Growing Problem for Business, Industry and Academia," *Industry and Higher Education* 26, no. 1 (2012): 43–51; K. Devries et al., "Intimate Partner Violence and Incident Depressive Symptoms and Suicide Attempts: A Systematic Review of Longitudinal Studies," *PLoS Medicine* 10, no. 5 (2013): e1001439.

22. T. Frisell et al., "Violent Crime Runs in Families: A Total Population Study of 12.5 Million Individuals," *Psychological Medicine* 41, no. 1 (2010): 97–105, doi:10.1017S0023329170000462; T. Dishion, "A Developmental Model of Aggression and Violence: Microsocial and Macrosocial Dynamic within an Ecological Framework," in *Handbook of Developmental Psychpathology* (New York: Springer, 2014), 449–66; M. Lee et al., "Exposure to Family Violence and Attachment Styles as Predictors of Dating Violence Perpetuation among Men and Women: A Mediation Model," , *Journal of Interpersonal Violence* 29, no. 1 (2014): 120–43. doi: 10.1177/0886260513504644

23. K. Makin-Byrd and K. L. Bierman, "Individual and Family Predictors of the Perpetration of Dating Violence and Victimization in Late Adolescence," *Journal of Youth Adolescence* 42, no. 4 (2013): 536–50, doi: 10.1007/s10964-012-9810-7; J. H. Derzon, "The Correspondence of Family Features," 2010; C. Cook et al., "Predictors of Bullying and Victimization in Childhood and Adolescence: A Meta-Analytic Investigation," *School Psychology Quarterly* 25, no. 2 (2010): 65–83.

24. R. Puff and J. Segher, *The Everything Guide to Anger Management: Proven Techniques to Understand and Control Anger* (Avon, MA: Adams Media, Inc. A Division of F. and W. Media, 2014).

25. C. J. Ferguson, "Genetic Contributions to Antisocial Personality and Behavior: A Meta-Analytic Review from an Evolutionary Perspective," *The Journal of Social Psychology* 150, no. 2 (2010): 160–80; D. Boisvert and J. Vaske, "Genetic Theories of Criminal Behavior," *The Encyclopedia of Criminology and Criminal Justice* (Boston, MA: Wiley-Blackwell, 2014), 1–6.

26. R. Kendra, K. Bell, and J. Guimond, "The Impact of Child Abuse History, PTSD and Anger Arousal on Dating Violence Perpetrators among College Women," *Journal of Family Violence* 27, no. 3 (2012): 165–75; C. Sousa et al., "Longitudinal Study on the Effects of Child Abuse and Children's Exposure to Domestic Violence, Parent-Child Attachments and Antisocial Behavior in Adolescence," *Journal of Interpersonal Violence* 26, no. 1 (2011): 111–36.

27. W. Gunter and B. Newby, "From Bullied to Deviant: The Victim-Offender-Overlap among Bullying Victims," *Youth Violence and Juvenile Justice* (2014), doi: 10.1177/1541204014521250, (Epub ahead of print.); M. M. Ttofi, D. P. Farrington, and F. Lösel, "School Bullying as a Predictor of Violence Later in Life: A Systematic Review and Meta-Analysis of Prospective Longitudinal Studies," *Aggression and Violent Behavior* 17, no. 5 (2012): 405–18.

28. K. M. Devries et al., "Intimate Partner Violence Victimization and Alcohol Consumption in Women: A Systematic Review and Meta-Analysis," *Addiction* 109 (2014): 379–91, doi: 10.1111/add.12393; A. Abbey, "Alcohol's Role in Sexual Violence Perpetration: Theoretical Explanations, Existing Evidence and Future Directions," *Drugs and Alcohol Review* 30, no. 5 (2012): 481–85; J. M. Boden, D. M. Fergusen, and L. J. Horwood, "Alcohol Misuse and Violent Behavior: Findings from a 30-Year Longitudinal Study," *Drugs and Alcohol Dependence* 122, (2012): 135–41; United Nations Office on Drugs and Crime, "World Drug Report," 2013, www.unodc.org/unodc/secured/wdr/wdr2013/World_Drug_Report_2013.pdf; A. Sanderlund et al. "The Association between Sports Participation, Alcohol Use and Aggression and Violence: A Systematic Review," *Journal of Science and Medicine in Sport* 17, no. 1 (2014): 2–7.

29. P. H. Smith et al., "Intimate Partner Violence and Specific Substance Use Disorders. Findings from the National Epidemiologic Survey on Alcohol and Related Conditions," *Psychology of Addictive Behaviors* 26, no. 2 (2012): 236–45; J. Kuhns et al., "The Prevalence of Alcohol-Involved Homicide Offending: A Meta-Analytic Review," *Homicide Studies* 18, no. 3 (2014): 251–270, doi:10.1177/1088767913493629

30. A. Abbey, "Alcohol's Role in Sexual Violence Perpetration," 2011.

31. Ibid; S. Gervais, et al., "Understanding the Link between Men's Alcohol Use and Sexual Violence Perpetration: The Mediating Role of Sexual Objectification," *Psychology of Violence* 4, no. 2 (2014): 150–69.

32. C. Love et al., "Understanding the Connection between Suicide and Substance Abuse: What the Research Tells Us," SAMHSA Webinar Series, September 11, 2014, http://captus.samhsa.gov/sites/default/files/capt_resource/webcast_suicide_and_substance_abuse_part_1_sept_11_2014_final.pdf; Mary McMurran, ed., *Alcohol-Related Violence Prevention and Treatment* (West Sussex, UK: John Wiley and Sons, 2013); K. Graham et al., "Alcohol-Related Negative Consequences among Drinkers around the World," *Addiction* 106, no. 8 (2011): 1391–1405.

33. American Psychological Association, "Violence in the Media—Psychologists Study TV and Video Game Violence for Potential Harmful Effects," November 2013, www.apa.org/research/action/protect.aspx; V. Pozios et al., "Does Media Violence Lead to the Real Thing?," *New York Times*, August 23, 2013, www.nytimes.com/2013/08/25/opinion/sunday/does-media-violence-lead-to-the-realthing.html; T. Greitemer, "Video Games Do Affect Social Outcomes: A Meta-Analytical Review of the Effects of Violent and Prosocial Video Game Play," *Personality and Social Psychology Bulletin* 40, no. 5 (2014): 578–89

34. W. Gunter and K. Daley, "Causal or Spurious? Using Propensity Score Matching to Detangle the Relationship between Violent Video Games and Violent Behavior," *Computers in Human Behavior* 4, no. 28 (2012): 1348–55.

35. T. Greitemeyer and D. Mugge, "Video Games Do Affect Social Outcomes: A Meta-Analytic Review of the Effects of Violent and Prosocial Video Game Play," *Personality and Social Psychology Bulletin* 40, no. 5 (2014): 578–89; C. J. Ferguson et al, "Not Worth the Fuss After All? Cross-Sectional and Prospective Data on Violent Video Game Influences on Aggression, Visuospatial Cognition and Mathematics Ability in a Sample of Youth," *Journal of Youth and Adolescence* 42, no. 1 (2013): 109–22; J. Perlus et al. "Trends in Bullying, Physical Fighting, and Weapon Carrying among 6th-through 10th-Grade Students from 1998 to 2010: Findings from a National Study," *American Journal of Public Health* 104, no. 6 (2014): 110–6.

36. M. Elson and C. Ferguson, "Twenty-Five Years of Research on Violence in Digital games and Aggression: Empirical Evidence, Perspectives, and a Debate Gone Astray," *European Psychologist* 19, no. 1 (2014): 33–46.

37. C. J. Ferguson et al, "Not Worth the Fuss After All?," 2013.

38. R. A. Ramos et al., "Comfortably Numb or Just Yet Another Movie? Media Violence Exposure Does NOT Reduce Viewer Empathy for Victims of Real Violence among Primarily Hispanic Viewers," *Psychology of Popular Media Culture* 2, no. 1 (2013): 2–10.

39. World Health Organization, "Definitions and Typology of Violence," 2015, www.who.int/violenceprevention/approach/definition/en/

40. Centers for Disease Control and Prevention, "Youth Violence: Definitions," December 2013, www.cdc.gov/violenceprevention/youthviolence/definitions.html; L. L. Dahlberg and E. G. Krug, "Violence: A Global Public Health Problem," in *World Report on Violence and Health* (Geneva: World Health Organization, 2002), 1–21.

41. World Health Organization, "Definitions and Typology of Violence," 2015.

42. Centers for Disease Control and Prevention, "Health, United States, 2013," May 2014, www.cdc.gov/nchs/data/hus/hus13.pdf

43. Centers for Disease Control and Prevention, "Deaths: Preliminary Data for 2013," *National Vital Statistics Reports* 61, no. 6 (2012), Available at www.cdc.gov/nchs/data/nvsr/nvsr61/nvsr61_06.pdf; Centers for Disease Control and Prevention, "Faststats: Assault or Homicide," December 2013, www.cdc.gov/nchs/fastats/homicide.htm

44. U. S. Department of Justice, Federal Bureau of Investigation, "Expanded Homicide Data Table 10," *Crime in the United States 2013,* Available at www.fbi.gov/about-us/cjis/ucr/crime-in-the-u.s/2013/crime-in-the-u.s.-2013/offenses-known-to-law-enforcement/expanded-homicide/expanded_homicide_data_table_10_murder_circumstances_by_relationship_2013.xls

45. A. Cooper and E. Smith, "Homicide in the U.S. Known to Law Enforcement, 2011," *Bureau of Justice Statistics,* December 30, 2013, Available at www.bjs.gov/index.cfm?ty=pbdetail&iid=4863

46. Ibid.

47. Ibid.

48. Ibid.

49. Federal Bureau of Investigation, "Hate Crime Statistics, 2013," February 2015, Available at www.fbi.gov/about-us/cjis/ucr/hate-crime/2013

50. Bureau of Justice Statistics, "Hate Crime Victimization-2004-2012-Statistical Tables," February 2014, www.bjs.gov/index.cfm?ty=pbdetail&iid=4883

51. Ibid.

52. U.S. Department of Justice, "Juvenile Justice Fact Sheet—Highlights of the 2012 National Youth Gang Survey," December 2014, www.ojjdp.gov/pubs/248025.pdf; Federal Bureau of Investigation, "2013 National Gang Threat Assessment-Emerging Trends," February 2015, www.fbi.gov/stats-services/publications/national-gang-report-2013

53. National Gang Center, "National Youth Survey Analysis," February 2015, www.nationalgangcenter.gov/Survey-Analysis

54. FB I, "2013 National Gang Threat Assessment," 2015.

55. D. McDaniel, "Risk and Protective Factors Associated with Gang Affiliation among High-Risk Youth: A Public Health Approach," *Injury Prevention,* January 11, 2012, Available at http://injuryprevention.bmj.com/content/early/2012/01/04/injuryprev-2011-040083.full.pdf+html

56. U.S. Code of Federal Regulations, Title 28CFR0.85.

57. U.S. Department of Homeland Security, "The Internet as a Terrorist Tool for Recruitment and Radicalizaton of Youth-White Paper," April 24, 2009, Available at www.homelandsecurity.org/docs/reports/Internet_Radicalization.pdf

58. P. Lin and J. Gill, "Homicides of Pregnant Women," *Journal of Forensic Medicine and Pathology* (2010), doi: 10-1097/PAF.obo13e3181d3dc3b. (Epub ahead of print.)

59. Violence Policy Center, *American Roulette: Murder-Suicide in the United States,* 4th ed. (Washington, DC: Violence Policy Center, 2012), Available at www.vpc.org

60. S. Catalano, "Intimate Partner Violence: Attributes of Victimization, 1993-2011" *Bureau of Justice Statistics,* November 13, 2013, Available at www.bjs.gov/index.cfm?ty=pbdetail&iid=4801

61. M. C. Black et al., *The National Intimate Partner and Sexual Violence Survey (NISVS): 2010 Summary Report* (Atlanta, GA: National Center for Injury Prevention and Control, Centers for Disease Control and Prevention, 2011), Available at www.cdc.gov

62. L. Walker, *The Battered Woman* (New York: Harper and Row, 1979).

63. L. Walker, *The Battered Woman Syndrome,* 3rd ed. (New York: Springer, 2009).

64. Psychiatric Times, "Battered Woman Syndrome," July 2009, www.psychiatrictimes.com/trauma-and-violence/battered-woman-syndrome

65. Child Welfare Information Gateway, *Definitions of Child Abuse and Neglect* (Washington, DC: U.S. Department of Health and Human Services, Children's Bureau, 2014), Available at www.childwelfare.gov/topics/systemwide/laws-policies/statutes/define/; U. S. Department of Health and Human Services Administration for Children and Families, "Definitions of Child Abuse and Neglect," February 2011, www.childwelfare.gov/systemwide/laws_policies/statutes/define.cfm

66. R. Gilbert and C. Spatz Widom et al. "Burden of Child Maltreatment in 'High Income' Countries," *Lancet* 373, no. 9657 (2009): 68–81; GAO, *Child Maltreatment: Strengthening National Data on Child Fatalities Could Aid in Prevention* (Washington, D.C.: U.S. Government Printing Office, 2011), Available at www.gao.gov/assets/330/320774; Childhelp, National Child Abuse Statistics, "Child Abuse in America–2013," 2013, www.childhelp.org/pages/statistics; National Children's Alliance, "National Statistics on Child Abuse," 2015, www.childhelp.org/child-abuse-statistics

67. Childhelp, "Child Abuse Statistics and Facts," 2015.

68. M. Lachs and J. Berman, " Under the Radar: New York State Elder Abuse Prevalence Study," New York City Department for Aging, May 2011, Available at www.ocfs.state.ny.us/main/reports/Under%20the%20Radar%2005%2012%2011%20final%20report.pdf; Centers for Disease Control and Prevention, "Elder Abuse Prevention," June 2014, www.cdc.gov/Features/ElderAbuse/; National Institute on Aging, "Elder Abuse," February 2015. www.nia.nih.gov/health/publication/elder-abuse

69. J. Grohol, "DSM-5 Changes: PTSD, Trauma and Stress-Related Disorders," *Psych Central-Professional,* May 28, 2013, http://pro.psychcentral.com/dsm-5-changes-ptsd-trauma-stress-related-disorders/004406.html

70. M. Breiding et al., "Prevalence and Characteristics of Sexual Violence, Stalking, and Intimate Partner Violence Victimization—National Intimate Partner and Sexual Violence Survey, United States, 2011," *Morbidity and Mortality Weekly Report* 63, no. SS08 (September 5, 2014), 1–18, Available at www.cdc.gov/mmwr/preview/mmwrhtml/ss6308a1.htm?s_cid=ss6308a1_e

71. Ibid.

72. Ibid.

73. Ibid; C. MaCaskill, "Sexual Violence on Campus: How Too Many Institutions of Higher Education Are Failing to Protect Students," July 9, 2014, www.mccaskill.senate.gov/SurveyReportwithAppendix.pdf; White House Task Force to Protect Students from Sexual Assault, *Not Alone: First Report of White House Task Force to Protect Students from Sexual Assault,* April 2014, www.whitehouse.gov/sites/default/files/docs/report_0.pdf

74. J. Carr, *American College Health Association Campus Violence White Paper* (Baltimore: American College Health Association, 2005), Available at www.acha.org

75. National Criminal Justice Reference Service, "School and Campus Crime," *Resource Guide,* 2013, http://ovc.ncjrs.gov

76. Centers for Disease Control and Prevention, National Center for Injury Prevention and Control, "Understanding Sexual Violence Fact Sheet," 2014, www.cdc.gov

77. Jeanne Clery Act Information, "The Campus Sexual Violence Elimination Act," 2014, www.cleryact.info/campus-save-act.html

78. White House Task Force to Protect Students from Sexual Assault, *Not Alone: First Report of White House Task Force to Protect Students from Sexual Assault,* April 2014, www.whitehouse.gov/sites/default/files/docs/report_0.pdf

79. SB-967, "Student Safety: Sexual Assault," 2013–2014, https://leginfo.legislature.ca.gov/faces/billNavClient.xhtml?bill_id=201320140SB967

80. B. Chappell, "California Enacts 'Yes means Yes' Law, Defining Sexual Consent,"September 29, 2014, www.npr.org/blogs/thetwo-way/2014/09/29/352482932/california-enacts-yes-means-yes-law-defining-sexual-consent

81. R. Bergen and E. Barnhill, National Online Resource Center on Violence Against Women, "Marital Rape: New Research and Directions," National Resource Center on Domestic Violence, 2011.

82. D. Finkelhor and K. Yllö, *License to Rape: Sexual Abuse of Wives* (New York: The Free Press, 1985).

83. Ibid.

84. National Online Resource Center, Violence Against Women, "Marital Rape: New Research and Directions," 2011, www.vawnet.org/applied-research-papers/print-document.php?doc_id=248

85. Association of Title IX Administrators, "The Challenge of Title IX Responses to Campus Relationship and Intimate Partner Violence: The 2015 White Paper, 2015," 2015, Available at www.atixa.org/wordpress/wp-content/uploads/2012/01/Challenge-of-TIX-with-Author-Photos.pdf

86. U.S. Equal Employment Opportunity Commission, "Sexual Harassment," February 2015, www.eeoc.gov/laws/types/sexual_harassment.cfm

87. U.S. Department of Education, "U.S. Department of Education Releases List of Higher Education Institutions with Open Title IX Sexual Violence Investigations," May 1, 2014, www.ed.gov/news/press-releases/us-department-education-releases-list-higher-education-institutions-open-title-ix-sexual-violence-investigations

88. Centers for Disease Control, "Sexual Violence, Stalking, and Intimate Partner Violence Widespread in the US," NISVS 2010 Summary Report, Press Release, December 2011.

89. Centers for Disease Control and Prevention, "Sexual Violence, Stalking, and Intimate Partner Violence Widespread in the US," 2011; National Criminal Justice Reference Service (NCVRW), "Crime Victimization in the United States: Statistical Overviews," in *NCVRW Resource Guide-2012,* June 2014, www.ncjrs.gov/ovc_archives/ncvrw/2012/pdf/StatisticalOverviews.pdf

90. M. Breiding et al., "Prevalence and Characteristics of Sexual Violence, Stalking, and Intimate Partner Violence Victimization," 2014.

91. Centers for Disease Control and Prevention, "Sexual Violence, Stalking, and Intimate Partner Violence Widespread in the US," 2011; NCVRW, "Crime Victimization in the United States," 2014.

92. M. Stoltenborgh et al., "The Current Prevalence of Child Sexual Abuse Worldwide: A Systematic Review and Meta-Analysis," *International Journal of Public Health* 58, no. 3 (2013): 469–83; L. P. Chen et al., "Sexual Abuse and Lifetime Diagnosis of Psychiatric Disorders: Systematic Review and Meta-Analysis," *Mayo Clinic Proceedings* 85, no. 7 (2010): 618–29; Childhelp, "Child Abuse Statistics and Facts," 2015; U.S. Department of Health and Human Services, Children's Bureau, "Child Maltreatment," 2013, www.acf.hhs.gov/sites/default/files/cb/cm2012.pdf

93. U.S. Department of Justice, "Sexual Assault of Young Children as Reported to Law Enforcement: Victim, Incident, and Offender Characteristics," *Bureau of Justice Statics,* March 2015, www.bjs.gov/content/pub/pdf/saycrle.pdf

94. Childhelp, "Child Abuse Statistics and Facts," 2015, www.childhelp.org/pages/statistics; L. P. Chen et al., "Sexual Abuse and Lifetime Diagnosis of Psychiatric Disorders," 2010; M. Stoltenborgh et al., "The Current Prevalence of Child Sexual Abuse Worldwide, 2013; T. Hilberg, C. Hamilton-Giachrtsis, and L. Dixon, "Review of Meta-Analyses on the Association between Child Sexual Abuse and Adult Mental Health Difficulties: A Systematic Approach," *Trauma, Violence, Abuse* 12, no. 1 (2011): 38–49.

95. Childhelp, "Child Abuse in America–2012," 2014.

96. K. Kochanek et. al., "Mortality in the United States, 2013," *NCHS Data Brief* 178, December 2014, www.cdc.gov/nchs/data/databriefs/db178.htm#what

97. Centers for Disease Control and Prevention, "10 Leading Causes of Death by Age Group, United States–2012," November 2014, Available at www.cdc.gov/injury/wisqars/pdf/leading_causes_of_death_by_age_group_2012-a.pdf

98. Centers for Disease Control and Prevention, "Wide-Ranging Online Data for Epidemiologic Research (WONDER)," May 2013, http://wonder.cdc.gov/mortsql.html

99. NHTSA, "The Fatality Analysis Reporting System (FARS) and the National Automotove Sampling System (NASS) General Estimates System (GES)," *Data Webinar*, January 15, 2015 www.nrd.nhtsa.dot.gov/Pubs/13WPPP.pdf; National Highway Traffic Safety Administration, "Traffic Safety Facts: 2012 Data," 2014.

100. NHTSA, "The Fatality Analysis Reporting System (FARS) and the National Automotive Sampling System (NASS)," 2015.

101. Ibid.

102. Ibid.

103. National Highway Traffic Safety Administration, "Traffic Safety Facts, 2013 Data: Alcohol-Impaired Driving," December 2014, www-nrd.nhtsa.dot.gov/Pubs/812102.pdf

104. National Institute on Drug Abuse, "Drug Facts: Drugged Driving," Revised December 2014, www.drugabuse.gov/publications/drugfacts/drugged-driving

105. S. Salomonsen-Sautel et al., "Trends in Fatal Motor Vehicle Crashes Before and After Marijuana Commercialized in Colorado," *Drug and Alcohol Dependence* 140 (2014): 137–44

106. Centers for Disease Control and Prevention, "Drowsy Driving: Asleep at the Wheel," 2014, www.cdc.gov/features/dsDrowsyDriving/index.html

107. Centers for Disease Control and Prevention, "Distracted Driving," October, 2014, www.cdc.gov/motorvehiclesafety/distracted_driving/.

108. NHTSA, "The Fatality Analysis Reporting System (FARS) and the National Automotive Sampling System (NASS)," 2015.; National Highway Traffic Safety Administration, "What Is Distracted Driving? Key Facts and Statistics," February 2015, www.distraction.gov/get-the-facts/facts-and-statistics.html

109. Centers for Disease Control and Prevention, "Distracted Driving," 2014.

110. National Highway Traffic Safety Administration, "What Is Distracted Driving?," 2015.

111. Governors Highway Safety Association, "Distracted Driving Laws," March 2015, www.ghsa.org/html/stateinfo/laws/cellphone_laws.html

112. Centers for Disease Control and Prevention, "Policy Impact: Seat Belts," Updated January 2014, www.cdc.gov/Motorvehiclesafety/seatbeltbrief

113. National Highway Traffic Safety Administration, "Traffic Safety Facts: 2012 Data," March 2014, www-nrd.nhtsa.dot.gov/Pubs/811892.pdf

114. NHTSA, "The Fatality Analysis Reporting System (FARS) and the National Automotove Sampling System (NASS)," 2015.

115. National Highway Traffic Safety Administration, "Traffic Safety Facts: 2012 Data / Bicyclists and Other Cyclists," April 2014, www-nrd.nhtsa.dot.gov/Pubs/812018.pdf

116. Ibid.

117. Ibid.

118. Centers for Disease Control and Prevention, "Unintentional Drowning: Get the Facts," October 24, 2014, www.cdc.gov/HomeandRecreationalSafety/Water-Safety/waterinjuries-factsheet.html

119. Ibid.

120. Ibid.

121. Ibid.

122. U. S. Coast Guard, "Coast Guard News: U.S. Coast Guard Releases 2013 Recreational Boating Statistics Report," May 2014, http://coastguardnews.com/u-s-coast-guard-releases-2013-recreational-boating-statistics-report/2014/05/14/?utm_source=feedburner&utm_medium=feed&utm_campaign=Feed%3A+CoastGuardNews+(Coast+Guard+News)

123. Ibid.

124. Ibid.

125. U. S. Coast Guard, "Boating Safety Resource Center: BUI Initiatives," April 2014, www.uscgboating.org/recreational-boaters/boating-under-the-influence.php

126. American Boating Association, "Boating Safety—It Could Mean Your Life," 2013, www.americanboating.org/safety.asp

127. Centers for Disease Control and Prevention, "National Vital Statistics System Mortality Data," March 4, 2015, www.cdc.gov/nchs/deaths.htm

128. Centers for Disease Control and Prevention, "Prescription Drug Overdose," October 2014, www.cdc.gov/homeandrecreationalsafety/overdose/index.html

129. J. B. Mowry et al., "2012 Annual Report of the American Association of Poison Control Centers' National Poison Data System (NPDS): 30th Annual Report," *Clinical Toxicology* 51, no. 10 (2013): 949–1229, doi: 10.3109/15563650.2013.863906

130. American Association of Poison Control Centers, "Prevention," February 2015, www.aapcc.org/prevention

131. Centers for Disease Control and Prevention, "Falls among Older Adults: An Overview," December 2014, www.cdc.gov/homeandrecreationalsafety/falls/adultfalls.html

132. U.S. Fire Administration, "U.S. Fire Deaths, Fire Death Rates, and Risks of Dying in a Fire," November 4, 2014, www.usfa.fema.gov/data/statistics/fire_death_rates.html

133. U.S. Fire Administration, "Campus Fire Safety: Safety Tips for Students and Parents," March 2014, www.usfa.fema.gov/citizens/college

134. Ibid.

135. Ibid.

**Pulled Statistics:**

Page 118, CDC, "The National Intimate Partner and Sexual Violence Survey (NISVS): 2010 Summary Report," February 26, 2014, www.cdc.gov/

Page 120, White House Task Force to Protect Students from Sexual Assault, "Not Alone: First Report of White House Task Force to Protect Students from Sexual Assault," April 2014, www.whitehouse.gov/sites/default/files/docs/report_0

Page 127, American College Health Association, American College Health Association—National College Health Assessment II: Reference Group Executive Summary Spring 2014 (Hanover, MD: American College Health Association, 2014).

## Chapter 5: Connecting and Communicating in the Modern World

1. J. T. Cacioppo, *Rewarding Social Connections Promote Successful Aging*, American Association for the Advancement of Science Annual Meeting, Chicago, Illinois, 2014.

2. Y. Luo et al., "Loneliness, Health, and Mortality in Old Age: A National Longitudinal Study," *Social Science and Medicine* 71, no. 6 (2012): 907–14.

3. J. T. Cacioppo and B. Patrick, *Loneliness: Human Nature and the Need for Social Connection*. (New York: W. W. Norton, 2008).

4. Ibid.

5. M. T. Frías, A. Brassard, and P. R. Shaver,"Childhood Sexual Abuse and Attachment Insecurities as Predictors of Women's Own and Perceived-Partner Extradyadic Involvement," *Child Abuse and Neglect* (2014), http://dx.doi.org.proxy.lib.uni.edu/10.1016/j.chiabu.2014.02.009; A. Lowell, K. Renk, and A. H. Adgate, "The Role of Attachment in the Relationship between Child Maltreatment and Later Emotional and Behavioral Functioning," *Child Abuse and Neglect* (2014), http://dx.doi.org.proxy.lib.uni.edu/10.1016/j.chiabu.2014.02.006

6. R. Sternberg, "A Triangular Theory of Love," *Psychological Review* 93 (1986): 119–35.

7. R. Sternberg, *Cupid's Arrow: The Course of Love through Time* (Boston: Cambridge University Press, 1998).

8. H. Fisher, *Why We Love* (New York: Henry Holt, 2004); H. Fisher et al., "Defining the Brain System of Lust, Romantic Attraction, and Attachment," *Archives of Sexual Behavior* 31, no. 5 (2002): 413–19.

9. Ibid.

10. L. Festinger, S. Schachter, and K. Back, *Social Pressures in Informal Groups: A Study of Human Factors in Housing* (Stanford, CA: Stanford University Press, 1950); E. J. Finkel and R. F. Baumeister, "Attraction and Rejection," in *Advanced Social Psychology: The State of the Science,* eds. R. F. Baumeister and E. J. Finkel (New York: Oxford University Press, 2010), 419–59.

11. S. Levay and J. Baldwin, *Human Sexuality*, 4th ed. (Sunderland, MA: Sinauer Associates, 2012).

12. L. Lee et al., "If I'm Not Hot, Are You Hot or Not? Physical-Attractiveness Evaluations and Dating Preferences as a Function of One's Own Attractiveness," *Psychological Science* 19, no. 7 (2008): 669–77.

13. J. Holt-Lunstad, T. Smith, and J. Layton, "Social Relationships and Mortality Risk: A Meta-Analytic Review," *PLoS Medicine* 7, no. 7 (2010); J. L. Kohn and S. L. Averett, "The Effect of Relationship Status on Health with Dynamic Health and Persistent Relationships," *Journal of Health Economics* 36 (2014): 69–83.

14. J. Holt-Lunstad, T. Smith, and J. Layton, "Social Relationships and Mortality Risk: A Meta-Analytic Review," *PLoS Medicine* 7, no. 7 (2010): e1000316; M. Ferris, "Social Connectedness and Health," (St. Paul, MN: Wilder Foundation, 2012).

15. J. Holt-Lunstad, T. Smith, and J. Layton, "Social Relationships and Mortality Risk: A Meta-Analytic Review," *PLoS Medicine* 7, no. 7 (2010): e1000316.

16. E. Robinson, J. Thomas, P. Aveyard, and S. Higgs, "What Everyone Else is Eating: A Systematic Review and Meta-Analysis of the Effect of Informational Eating Norms on Eating Behavior," *Journal of the Academy of Nutrition and Dietetics* 114, no. 3 (2014) 414–29; N. A. Christakis and J. H. Fowler, "Social Contagion Theory: Examining Dynamic Social Networks and Human Behavior," *Statistics in Medicine* 32, no. 4 (2013): 556–77.

17. S. Cohen and T. A. Wills, "Stress, Social Support, and the Buffering Hypothesis," *Psychological Bulletin* 98 (1985): 310–57.

18. S. Schnall, K. D. Harber, J. K. Stefanucci, and D. R. Proffitt, "Social Support and the Perception of Geographical Slant," *Journal of Experimental Social Psychology*, 44, no. 5 (2008): 1246–255.

19. K. Hampton, L. S. Goulet, L. Rainie, and K. Purcell, "Social Networking Sites and Our Lives," *Pew Internet and American Life Project,* June 16, 2011, Available at www.pewinternet.org/files/old-media//Files/Reports/2011/PIP%20-%20Social%20networking%20sites%20and%20our%20lives.pdf

20. L. F. Berkman, I. Kawachi, and M. Glymour, eds. *Social Epidemiology* (Oxford University Press, 2014).

21. J. T. Cacioppo and B. Patrick, *Loneliness: Human Nature and the Need for Social Connection.* (New York: W. W. Norton, 2008).

22. K. Hampton, L. S. Goulet, L. Rainie, et al., "Social Networking Sites and Our Lives," *Pew Internet and American Life Project,* 2011.

23. C. R. Rogers, "Interpersonal Relationship: The Core of Guidance," in *Person to Person: The Problem of Being Human,* eds. C. R. Rogers and B. Stevens (Lafayette, CA: Real People Press, 1967).

24. B. Hurn and B. Tomalin, *Cross-Cultural Communication: Theory and Practice* (London: Pagrave-Macmillan, 2013).

25. Ibid.

26. Ibid.

27. J. Wood, *Interpersonal Communication: Everyday Encounters,* 7th ed. (Belmont, CA: Cengage, 2012).

28. Ibid.

29. R. E. Jack et al., "Facial Expressions of Emotion are not Culturally Universal," *Proceedings of the National Academy of Sciences* 109, no. 19 (2012): 7241–244.

30. K. Hampton, L. S. Goulet, L. Rainie, and K. Purcell, "Social Networking Sites and our Lives," Pew Internet and American Life Project.

31. Ibid.

32. Ibid.

33. Ibid.

34. Ibid.

35. Ibid.

36. Ibid.

37. Ibid.

38. E. C. Tandoc, P. Ferrucci, and M. Duffy, "Facebook Use, Envy, and Depression among College Students: Is Facebooking Depressing?," *Computers in Human Behavior* 43, (2015): 139–46.

39. M. Meeker and L. Wu, "2013 Internet Trends," *KPCB,* May 19, 2013, Available at www.kpcb.com/blog/2013-internet-trends

40. J. A. Roberts, L. Yaya, and C. Manolis, "The Invisible Addiction: Cell-phone Activities and Addiction among Male and Female College Students," *Journal of Behavioral Addiction* 3, no. 4 (2014): 254–65.

41. Ibid.

42. K. M. Hertlein and K. Ancheta, "Advantages and Disadvantages of Technology in Relationships: Findings from an Open-Ended Survey," *The Qualitative Report* 19, no. 22 (2014): 1–11.

43. Y. T. Uhls et al., "Five Days at Outdoor Education Camp without Screens Improves Preteen Skills with Nonverbal Emotion Cues," *Computers in Human Behavior* 39, (2014): 387–92.

44. N. Carr, *The Shallows: What the Internet Is Doing to Our Brains* (New York: W. W. Norton, 2011).

45. T. Worley, "Exploring the Association between Relational Uncertainty, Jealousy about Partner's Friendships, and Jealousy Expression in Dating Relationships," *Communication Studies* 65, no. 4 (2014): 370–88; B. Sagarin et al., "Sex Differences in Jealousy: A Meta-Analytic Examination," *Evolution and Human Behavior* 33, no. 6 (2012): 595–614.

46. United States Department of Labor, Bureau of Labor Statistics, "American Time Use Survey Summary–2013 Results," June 2014, www.bls.gov/news.release/atus.t01.htm

47. The Gottman Institute, "Research FAQs," www.gottman.com/research/research-faqs

48. G. F. Kelly, *Sexuality Today,* 11th ed. (New York, NY: McGraw-Hill, 2014).

49. F. Newport and J. Wilke, "Most in U.S. Want Marriage, but Its Importance Has Dropped," *Gallup,* August 2, 2013, www.gallup.com/poll/163802/marriage-importance-dropped.aspx

50. D. B. Elliot, K. Krivickas, and M. W. Brault, "Historical Marriage Trends from 1890–2010: A Focus on Race Differences," Annual Meeting of the Population Association of America, 2012, www.census.gov/hhes/socdemo/marriage/data/acs/ElliottetalPAA2012paper.pdf

51. G. Livingston, "Four-in-Ten Couples are Saying 'I Do' Again," *Pew Research Center,* November 14, 2014, www.pewsocialtrends.org/2014/11/14/four-in-ten-couples-are-saying-i-do-again/

52. U.S. Census Bureau, "Families and Living Arrangements: 2014, Table MS-2 Estimated Median Age at First Marriage, by Sex: 1890 to the Present," www.census.gov/hhes/families/data/marital.html

53. M. Banschick, "The High Failure Rate of Second and Third Marriages," *Psychology Today,* February 6, 2012, www.psychologytoday.com/blog/the-intelligent-divorce/201202/the-high-failure-rate-second-and-third-marriages

54. K. Heller, "The Myth of the High Rate of Divorce," *Psych Central,* April 2, 2014, http://psychcentral.com/lib/2012/the-myth-of-the-high-rate-of-divorce

55. R. M. Kreider and R. Ellis, "Number, Timing, and Duration of Marriages and Divorces: 2009," *Current Population Reports,* P70-125 (Washington, DC: U.S. Census Bureau, 2011), Available at www.census.gov/prod/2011pubs/p70–125.pdf

56. Ibid.

57. A. J. Cherlin, "Americans Prefer Serial Monogamy to Open Relationships," *New York Times* Blog, May 21, 2013, http://www.nytimes.com/roomfordebate/2012/01/20/the-gingrich-question-cheating-vs-open-marriage/americans-prefer-serial-monogamy-to-open-relationships

58. I. Siegler et al., "Consistency and Timing of Marital Transitions and Survival During Midlife: The Role of Personality and Health Risk Behaviors," *Annals of Behavioral Medicine* 45, no. 3 (2013): 338–47, doi: 10.1007/s12160-012-9457-3; A. A. Aizer et al., "Marital Status and Survival in Patients with Cancer," *Journal of Clinical Oncology* 31, no. 31 (2013): 3869–3876, doi: 10.1200/JCO.2013.49.6489

59. C. C. Miller, "Study Finds More Reasons to Get and Stay Married," *New York Times,* January 8, 2015, www.nytimes.com/2015/01/08/upshot/study-finds-more-reasons-to-get-and-stay-married.html?rref=upshot&abt=0002&abg=0&_r=2

60. K. Williams, "Has the Future of Marriage Arrived? A Contemporary Examination of Gender, Marriage, and Psychological Well-Being." *Journal of Health and Social Behavior* 44.4 (2003): 470–87.

61. U.S. Department of Health and Human Services, Vital and Health Statistics, "Health Behaviors of Adults: United States, 2008–2010," DHHS Pub 10, No. 257 (2013): 7–78, Available at www.cdc.gov/nchs/data/series/sr_10/sr10_257.pdf

62. Ibid.

63. Ibid.

64. U.S. Department of Health and Human Services, Division of Vital Statistics, "First Premarital Cohabitation in the United States: 2006–2010 National Survey of Family Growth," *National Health Statistics Report* 64 (2013), Available at www.cdc.gov/nchs/data/nhsr/nhsr064.pdf

65. Ibid.

66. A. Kuperberg, "Age at Co-Residence, Premarital Cohabitation and Marriage Dissolution: 1985–2009," *Journal of Marriage and Family,* 76 no. 2 (2014): 352–69.

67. U.S. Department of Health and Human Services, "First Premarital Cohabitation in the United States," 2013.

68. U.S. Census Bureau, "Characteristics of Same-Sex Households: 2013," 2013, www.census.gov/hhes/samesex/

69. Obergefell v. Hodges, 576 U.S. (2015).

70. Ibid

71. Ibid.

72. A. Blinder and T. Lewin, "Clerk in Kentucky Chooses Jail Over Deal on Same-Sex Marriage," September 3, 2015, http://www.nytimes.com/2015/09/04/us/kim-davis-same-sex-marriage.html?_r=0; Krishnadev Calamur, "In Some States Defiance of Supreme Court's Same-Sex Ruling," June 29, 2015, http://www.npr.org/sections/thetwo-way/2015/06/29/418600672/in-some-states-defiance-over-supreme-courts-same-sex-marriage-ruling.

73. U.S. Census Bureau, "Marital Status: 2007–2011 American Community Survey, 5-Year Estimates, Table S1201," http://factfinder2.census

**Pulled Statistics:**

Page 147, A. Smith and M. Duggan, "Online Dating and Relationships," Pew Research (2013), www.pewinternet.org/2013/10/21/online-dating-relationships/

Page 150, K. Parker, W. Wang, and M. Rohol, "Record Share of Americans Have Never Married," Pew Research (2014), www.pewsocialtrends.org/files/2014/09/2014-09-24_Never-Married-Americans.pdf

## Focus On: Understanding Your Sexuality

1. I. A. Hughes et al., "Consensus Statement on Management of Intersex Disorders," *Journal of Pediatric Urology* 2, no. 3 (2006): 148–62; Intersex Society of North America, "How Common Is Intersex?," 2008, www.isna.org.

2. G. M. Herek and K. A. McLemore, "Sexual Prejudice," *Annual Review of Psychology* 64 (2013): 309–33.

3. Federal Bureau of Investigation, "Hate Crime Statistics, 2013," (Fall 2014), www.fbi.gov/about-us/cjis/ucr/hate-crime/2013/topic-pages/incidents-and-offenses/incidentsandoffenses_final.pdf

4. M. Rosario and E. Schrimshaw, "Theories and Etiologies of Sexual Orientation," *APA Handbook of Sexuality and Psychology* 1 (2014): 555–96.

5. S. M. Cabrera et al., "Age of Thelarche and Menarche in Contemporary U.S. Females: A Cross-Sectional Analysis," *Journal of Pediatric Endocrinology and Metabolism* 27, 1–2 (2014): 47–51.

6. S. Levay and J. Baldwin, *Human Sexuality,* 4th ed. (Sunderland, MA: Sinauer Associates, 2012).

7. Womenshealth.gov, "Premenstrual Symptoms Fact Sheet," December 23, 2014, http://womenshealth.gov/publications/our-publications/fact-sheet/premenstrual-syndrome.html#e

8. Ibid.

9. Ibid.

10. Mayo Clinic Staff, "Diseases and Conditions: Menstrual Cramps," May 8, 2014, www.mayoclinic.org/diseases-conditions/menstrual-cramps/basics/definition/con-20025447

11. National Institute on Aging, "Menopause", January 22, 2015, Available at www.nia.nih.gov/health/publication/menopause

12. National Institutes of Health, "WHI Follow-Up Study Confirms Risk of Long-Term Combination

Hormone Therapy Outweigh Benefits for Postmenopausal Women," News Release, March 4, 2008, www.public.nhlbi.nih.gov/newsroom/home/; National Heart, Lung, and Blood Institute (NHLBI), "WHI Study Data Confirm Short-Term Health Disease Risks of Combination Hormone Therapy for Postmenopausal Women," News Release, February 15, 2010, www.nih.gov/news/health/feb2010/nhlbi-15.htm

13. M. Beck, "Benefits of Hormone-Replacement Therapy Outweigh Risks, Reviews of Studies Show," Health blog, *The Wall Street Journal*,May 22, 2012, http://blogs.wsj.com/health/2012/05/22/benefits-of-hormone-replacement-therapy-out-weigh-risks-reviews-of-studies-show

14. M. Owings, S. Uddin, and S. Williams, "Trends in Circumcision for Male Newborns in U.S. Hospitals: 1979–2010," August 2013, www.cdc.gov/nchs/data/hestat/circumcision_2013.pdf

15. American Academy of Pediatrics, "2012 Technical Report, Male Circumcision," *Pediatrics* 130, no. 3 (2012): e756–e785, doi: 10.1542/peds.2012-1990

16. Ibid.

17. G. F. Kelly, *Sexuality Today*, 11th ed. (New York, NY: McGraw-Hill, 2014).

18. Ibid.

19. American College Health Association, *American College Health Association–National College Health Assessment II (ACHA-NCHA II) Reference Group Data Report, Spring 2014* (Hanover, MD: American College Health Association, 2014), Available at www.acha-ncha.org/docs/ACHA-NCHA-II_ReferenceGroup_DataReport_Spring2014.pdf

20. S. Caron, *The Sex Lives of College Students: Two Decades of Attitudes and Behaviors,* (Orono, ME: Maine College Press, 2014).

21. American College Health Association, *American College Health Association–National College Health Assessment II: Reference Group Data Report, Spring 2014,* 2014..

22. Ibid.

23. Ibid.

24. C. Harte and C. Meston. "Recreational Use of Erectile Dysfunction Medications and Its Adverse Effects on Erectile Function in Young, Healthy Men: The Mediating Role of Confidence in Erectile Ability." *Journal of Sexual Medicine.* 2012. 9(7):(1852–59)

25. G. Prestage et al., "Australian Gay and Bisexual Men's Use of Erectile Dysfunction Medications During Recent Sexual Encounters," *The Journal of Sexual Medicine* 11, no. 3, (2014): 809–19; D. J. Snipes and E. G. Benotsh, "High-Risk Cocktails and High-Risk Sex: Examining the Relation between Alcohol Mixed with Energy Drink Consumption, Sexual Behavior, and Drug Use in College Students," *Addictive Behaviors* 38, no. 1 (2013): 1418–23.

26. J. Bliss, "Police, Experts: Alcohol Most Common in Sexual Assaults," *USA Today*, October 28, 2013, www.usatoday.com/story/news/nation/2013/10/28/alcohol-most-common-drug-in-sexual-assaults/3285139

**Pulled Statistics:**

Page 164, Data from American College Health Association, American College Health Association—National College Health Assessment II (ACHA-NCHA II): Reference Group Data Report Spring 2014 (Hanover, MD: American College Health Association, 2014).

## Chapter 6: Considering Your Reproductive Choices

1. American College Health Association, *American College Health Association—National College Health Assessment III (ACHA-NCHA III): Reference Group Data Report, Spring 2014* (Hanover, MD: American College Health Association, 2014), Available at www.achancha.org/docs/ACHA-NCHA-II_ReferenceGroup_DataReport_ Spring2014.pdf

2. L. B. Finer and M. R. Zolna, "Shifts in Intended and Unintended Pregnancies in the United States, 2001–2008," *American Journal of Public Health* 104, no. S1 (2014): S44–S48.

3. J. Trussell, "Contraceptive Efficacy," in *Contraceptive Technology*, 20th rev. ed., eds. R. A. Hatcher et al. (New York: Ardent Media, 2011).

4. World Health Organization, "Nonoxynol-9 Ineffective in Preventing HIV Infection," Press Release, June 28, 2002, www.who.int/mediacentre/news/releases/who55/en/

5. J. Trussell, "Contraceptive Efficacy," 2011.

6. Ibid.

7. Ibid.

8. Mayo Clinic Staff, "Tests and Procedures: Spermicide," January 2013, www.mayoclinic.org/tests-procedures/spermicide/basics/risks/prc-20012597; World Health Organization, "Nonoxynol-9 Ineffective in Preventing HIV Infection," 2002.

9. World Health Organization, "Nonoxynol-9 Ineffective in Preventing HIV Infection," 2015, www.who.int/mediacentre/news/notes/release55/en

10. J. Trussell, "Contraceptive Efficacy," 2011.

11. Ibid.

12. Ibid.

13. American College Health Association, *National College Health Assessment III): Reference Group Data Report, Spring 2014*, 2014.

14. J. Trussell, "Contraceptive Efficacy," 2011.

15. Ibid.

16. O. Lidegaard et al., "Thrombotic Stroke and Myocardial Infarction with Hormonal Contraception," *New England Journal of Medicine* 366, no. 24 (2012): 2257–66, doi: 10.1056/NEJMoa1111840

17. J. Trussell, "Contraceptive Efficacy," 2011.

18. E. G. Raymond, "Progestin-Only Pills," in *Contraceptive Technology*, 20th rev. ed., eds. R. A. Hatcher et al. (New York: Ardent Media, 2011).

19. Janssen Pharmaceuticals, "OrthoEvra," October 2012, www.orthoevra.com; Drugs.com, "Xulane," April 2015, www.drugs.com/pro/xulane.html

20. J. Trussell, "Contraceptive Efficacy," 2011.

21. Janssen Pharmaceuticals, "Important Safety Update for U.S. Health Care Professionals ORTHO EVRA," March 2011, www.orthoevra.com/isi-hcp.html

22. J. Trussell, "Contraceptive Efficacy," 2011.

23. Ibid.

24. Pfizer, "Depo-subQ Provera," September 2013, www.depo-subqprovera104.com

25. J. Trussell, "Contraceptive Efficacy," 2011.

26. Merck & Co., Inc., "Nexplanon," Accessed April 2015, www.merck.com/product/usa/pi_circulars/n/nexplanon/nexplanon_pi .pdf

27. J. Jones, W. Mosher, and K. Daniels, "Current Contraceptive Use in the United States, 2006–2010, and Changes in Pattern of Use Since 1995," *National Health Statistics Reports* 60 (2012): 1–25.

28. The American Congress of Obstetricians and Gynecologists, "ACOG Committee Opinion-Adolescents and Long-Acting Reversible Contraception: Implants and Intrauterine Devices," Number 539, October 2012, www.acog.org/Resources_And_Publications/Committee_Opinions/Committee_on_Adolescent_Health_Care/Adolescents_and_Long-Acting_Reversible_Contraception

29. J. Trussell, "Contraceptive Efficacy," 2011.

30. American College Health Association,*National College Health Assessment III: Reference Group Data Report Spring, 2014*, 2014.

31. J. Trussell, "Contraceptive Efficacy," 2011.

32. American College Health Association, *National College Health Assessment III: Reference Group Data Report Spring, 2014*, 2014.

33. J. Trussell, "Contraceptive Efficacy," 2011.

34. Office of Population Research & Association of Reproductive Health Professionals, The Emergency Contraception Website, "Answers to Frequently Asked Questions about Effectiveness," Updated July 2014, http://ec.princeton.edu/questions/eceffect.html

35. American College Health Association, *National College Health Assessment II: Undergraduate Students Reference Group Data Fall 2014*, 2014.

36. K. Daniels, J. Daugherty, and J. Jones, "Current Contraceptive Status among Women Aged 15–44: United States 2011–2013," *National Health Statistics Data Brief*, no. 173 (Hyattsville, MD: National Center for Health Statistics, 2014).

37. J. Trussell, "Contraceptive Efficacy," 2011.

38. Guttmacher Institute, "Fact Sheet: Induced Abortion in the United States," July 2014, www.guttmacher.org/pubs/fb_induced_abortion.html

39. American Psychological Association (APA), Task Force on Mental Health and Abortion, *Report of the Task Force on Mental Health and Abortion* (Washington, DC: American Psychological Association, 2008), Available at www.apa.org/pi/wpo/mental-health-abortion-report.pdf

40. *Roe v. Wade*, 410 U.S. 113 (1973).

41. L. Saad, "Abortion," *Gallup Politics*, Blog, January 22, 2013, www.gallup.com/poll/160058/majority-americans-support-roe-wade-decision.aspx

42. Guttmacher Institute, "In Just the Last Four Years, States Have Enacted 231 Abortion Restrictions," January 2015, https://guttmacher.org/media/inthenews/2015/01/05/index.html

43. APA, *Report of the Task Force*, 2008; J. R. Steinberg, C. E. McCulloch, and N. E. Adler, "Abortion and Mental Health: Findings from the National Comorbidity Survey-Replication," *Obstetrics & Gynecology* 123, no. 2 (2014): 263–70.

44. Ibid.

45. Ibid.

46. Guttmacher Institute, "Fact Sheet: Induced Abortion in the United States," 2014.

47. Ibid.

48. Ibid.

49. Planned Parenthood, "The Abortion Pill (Medication Abortion)," www.plannedparenthood.org/health-topics/abortion/abortion-pill-medication-abortion-4354.asp

50. K. Cleland et al., "Significant Adverse Events and Outcomes After Medical Abortion," *Obstetrics and Gynecology* 121, no. 1 (2013): 166–171.

51. K. Cleland et al., "Significant Adverse Events and Outcomes After Medical Abortion," 2013.

52. M. Lino, *Expenditures on Children by Families, 2013* (Alexandria, VA: U.S. Department of Agriculture, Center for Nutrition Policy and Promotion, 2014), www.cnpp.usda.gov/ExpendituresonChildrenbyFamilies

53. Truven Health Analytics, "The Cost of Having a Baby in the United States," January 2013, http://transform.childbirthconnection.org/wp-content/uploads/2013/01/Cost-of-Having-a-Baby1.pdf

54. T. J. Mathews and B. E. Hamilton, "*First Births to Older Women Continue to Rise*," National Center for Health Statistics Data Brief, No. 152, May 2014, www.cdc.gov/nchs/data/databriefs/db152.pdf

55. J. A. Martin et al., U.S. Department of Health and Human Services, National Center for Health Statistics, "Births: Final Data for 2012," *National Vital Statistics Reports* 62, no. 9 (2013), Available at www.cdc.gov/nchs/data/nvsr/nvsr62/nvsr62_09 .pdf#table01

56. American Pregnancy Association, "Miscarriage," Updated June 2014, http://americanpregnancy.org/pregnancycomplications/miscarriage.html

57. Committee on Gynecologic Practice of American College of Obstetricians and Gynecologists; Practice Committee of American Society for Reproductive Medicine, "Age-Related Fertility Decline: A Committee Opinion," *Fertility and Sterility*, 90, Supplement 5 (2008): S154–55.

58. Centers for Disease Control and Prevention (CDC), "Preconception Care and Health Care: Women," January 2015, www.cdc.gov/preconception/women.html

59. bid.

60. S. M. Schrader and K. L. Marlow, "Assessing the Reproductive Health of Men with Occupational Exposures," *Asian Journal of Andrology* 16, no. 1 (2014): 23–30; CDC, "Preconception Health and Healthcare," September 2014, www.cdc.gov/preconception/careformen/exposures.html

61. B. M. D'Onofrio et al., "Paternal Age at Childbearing and Offspring Psychiatric and Academic Morbidity," *Journal of the American Medical Association Psychiatry*, 71 no. 4 (2014): 432–38; E. Calloway, "Fathers Bequeath More Mutations as They Age," *Nature*, 488 no. 7412 (2012): 439.

62. Planned Parenthood, "Pregnancy Tests," Accessed April 2015, www.plannedparenthood.org/health-topics/pregnancy/pregnancy-test-21227.asp

63. Committee on Obstetric Practice, "Committee Opinion no. 548, American Congress of Obstetricians and Gynecologists: Weight Gain During Pregnancy," *Obstetrics and Gynecology* 121, no. 1 (2013): 210–12, doi: 10.1097/01.AOG.0000425668.87506.4c

64. The American Congress of Obstetricians and Gynecologists, "Tobacco, Alcohol, Drugs, and Pregnancy," December 2013, www.acog.org/~/media/For%20Patients/faq170.pdf?dmc=1&ts=20140516T2242271513

65. National Center for Chronic Disease Prevention and Health Promotion, "Tobacco Use and Pregnancy," *Reproductive Health*, Updated August 2014, www.cdc.gov/Reproductivehealth/TobaccoUsePregnancy/index.htm; The American Congress of Obstetricians and Gynecologists, "Tobacco, Alcohol, Drugs, and Pregnancy," 2013.

66. CDC, "Facts about Cleft Lip and Cleft Palate," 2014, www.cdc.gov/ncbddd/birthdefects/cleftlip.html

67. B. E. Hamilton et al., "Births: Preliminary Data for 2013," 2014, www.cdc.gov/nchs/data/nvsr/nvsr63/nvsr63_02.pdf

68. J. Christensen, *CNN News*, "Why So Many C-Sections Have Medical Groups Concerned," May 8, 2014, www.cnn.com/2014/05/08/health/c-section-report

69. E. Puscheck, "Early Pregnancy Loss," *Medscape Reference: Drugs, Diseases & Procedures*, Updated October 2014, http://reference.medscape.com/article/266317-overview

70. V. P. Sepilian et al., "Ectopic Pregnancy," *Medscape Reference*, Updated September 2014, http://emedicine.medscape.com/article/2041923-overview

71. What to Expect, "Stillbirth," Accessed April 2015, www.whattoexpect.com/pregnancy/pregnancy-health/complications/stillbirth.aspx

72. K. L. Wisner et al., "Onset Timing, Thoughts of Self-harm, and Diagnoses in Postpartum Women with Screen-Positive Depression Findings," *JAMA Psychiatry* 70, no. 5 (2013): 1–9, doi:10.1001/jama-psychiatry.2013.87

73. American Academy of Pediatrics, "Benefits of Breastfeeding for Mom," Updated July 2014, www.healthychildren.org/English/ages-stages/baby/breastfeeding/pages/Benefits-of-Breastfeeding-for-Mom.aspx

74. CDC, "Sudden Unexpected Infant Death and Sudden Infant Death Syndrome," January 2015, www.cdc.gov/sids

75. Ibid.

76. Ibid.

77. CDC, "Infertility FAQs," Reproductive Health, updated June 2013, www.cdc.gov/reproductive-health/Infertility/

78. MayoClinic.com, "Infertility: Causes," July 2014, www.mayoclinic.com/health/infertility/DS00310/DSECTION=causes

79. U.S. Department of Health and Human Services, "Polycystic Ovary Syndrome (PCOS) Fact Sheet," December 2014, www.womenshealth.gov/publications/our-publications/fact-sheet/polycystic-ovary-syndrome.html

80. B. Kumbak, E. Oral, and O. Bukulmez, "Female Obesity and Assisted Reproductive Technologies," *Seminars in Reproductive Medicine* 30, no. 6 (2012): 507–16, doi: 10.1055/s-0032-1328879

81. CDC, "Pelvic Inflammatory Disease CDC Fact Sheet," Sexually Transmitted Diseases, Updated July 2014, www.cdc.gov/std/PID/STDFact-PID.htm

82. CDC, "Infertility: FAQs," June 2013, www.cdc.gov/reproductivehealth/Infertility/index.htm#4

83. Ibid.; S. Cabler, A. Agarwal, and S. S. du Plessis, "Obesity and Male Fertility," *Male Infertility* 33 (2012): 349–60.

84. CDC, "Infertility: FAQs," 2013.

85. Ibid.

86. WebMD Medical Reference, "Fertility Drugs," July 2012, www.webmd.com/infertility-and-reproduction/guide/fertility-drugs

87. American Society for Reproductive Medicine, "Fertility Drugs and the Risk for Multiple Births," Accessed March 2015, www.asrm.org/uploadedFiles/ASRM_Content/Resources/Patient_Resources/Fact_Sheets_and_Info_Booklets/fertilitydrugs_multiplebirths.pdf

88. WebMD, "Using a Surrogate Mother, What You Need to Know," September 2013, www.webmd.com/infertility-and-reproduction/guide/using-surrogate-mother.

89. R. M. Kreider and D. A. Loftquist, *Adopted Children and Stepchildren: 2010*, U.S. Census Bureau, April 2014, www.census.gov/content/dam/Census/library/publications/2014/demo/p20-572.pdf

90. Intercountry Adoption, U.S. Department of State, "FY 2013 Annual Report on Intercountry Adoption," Accessed March 2015, http://travel.state.gov/content/dam/aa/pdfs/fy2013_annual_report.pdf

91. Adoption.com, "Adoption Costs," Accessed March 2015, http://costs.adoption.com

**Pulled Statistics:**

Page 174, W. D. Mosher and J. Jones, "Use of Contraception in the United States: 1982–2008," *Vital and Health Statistics* 23, no. 29 (2010), www.cdc.gov/nchs/data/nhsr/nhsr062.pdf

Page 189, Gallup, "U.S. Still Split on Abortion: 47% Pro-Choice, 46% Pro-Life," 2014, www.gallup.com/poll/170249/split-abortion-pro-choice-pro-life.aspx

## Chapter 7: Recognizing and Avoiding Addiction and Drug Abuse

1. J. Grant et al., "Introduction to Behavioral Addictions," *American Journal of Behavioral Addictions* 36, no. 5 (2010): 233–41; National Institute on Drug Abuse, National Institutes of Health (NIH), U.S. Department of Health and Human Services, *Drugs, Brains, and Behavior: The Science of Addiction,* NIH Publication no. 07-5605 (Bethesda, MD: National Institute on Drug Abuse, Revised 2010), Available at www.drugabuse.gov

2. American Society of Addiction Medicine, "Definition of Addiction," April 2011, www.asam.org/for-the-public/definition-of-addiction

3. D. E. Smith, "Editor's Note: The Process Addictions and the New ASAM Definition of Addiction," *Journal of Psychoactive Drugs* 44, no. 1 (2012); National Institute on Drug Abuse, NIH, *Drugs, Brains, and Behavior*, 2010.

4. National Council on Problem Gambling, "Problem Gambling: Have the Conversation in March," February 19, 2015, www.ncpgambling.org/wp-content/uploads/2014/04/PGAM-Press-Release-General-FINAL.pdf

5. American Psychiatric Association, *Diagnostic and Statistical Manual of Mental Disorders,* 5th ed. (Arlington, VA: American Psychiatric Publishing, 2013), p. 585.

6. M. N. Potenza, "Neurobiolgoy of Gambling Behaviors," *Current Opinion in Neurobiology* 23, no.4 (2013): 660–67.

7. Ibid.

8. National Center for Responsible Gambling, "College Students: Facts and Stats," www.collegegambling.org/just-facts/gambling-college-campuses

9. Ibid.

10. H. Hatfield, "Shopping Spree or Addiction?," *WebMD*, 2014, www.webmd.com/mental-health/features/shopping-spree-addiction; M. Lejoyeux and A. Weinstein, "Compulsive Buying," *The American Journal of Drug and Alcohol Issues* 36, no.5 (2010): 248–53.

11. H. Hatfield, "Shopping Spree or Addiction?,"2014; M. Lejoyeux and A. Weinstein, "Compulsive Buying," 2010.

12. B. Cook and H. A. Hausenblas, "The Role of Exercise Dependence for the Relationship between Exercise Behavior and Eating Pathology: Mediator or Moderator?" *Journal of Health Psychology* 13, no. 4 (2008): 495–502.

13. K. Berczik et al., "Exercise Addiction: Symptoms, Diagnosis, Epidemiology and Etiology," *Substance Use and Misuse* 47 (2012): 403–17.

14. A. Alexander, "Internet Addiction Statistics 2012," April 24, 2012, http://ansonalex.com/infographics/internet-addiction-statistics-2012-infographic

15. J. Anthony et al., "Problematic Internet Use and Other Risky Behaviors in College Students: An Application of Problem-Behavior Theory," *American Psychological Association* 27 no. 1 (2012): 133–41.

16. American College Health Association, *American College Health Association—National College Health Assessment II: Reference Group Data Report Spring 2014* (Hanover, MD: American College Health Association, 2014).

17. Substance Abuse and Mental Health Services Administration, *Results from the 2013 National Survey on Drug Use and Health: Summary of National Findings*, NSDUH Series H-48, HHS Publication No. (SMA) 14-4863 (Rockville, MD: Substance Abuse and Mental Health Services Administration, 2014).

18. L. D. Johnston et al., *Monitoring the Future National Results on Drug Use: 2015 Overview, Key Findings on Adolescent Drug Use* (Ann Arbor: Institute for Social Research, The University of Michigan, 2015).

19. Ibid.

20. National Institute of Drug Abuse, "Drug Facts: Nationwide Trends," NIDA, January 2014, www.drugabuse.gov/publications/drugfacts/nationwide-trends

21. National Drug Intelligence Center, "National Drug Threat Assessment 2011," 2011, www.justice.gov

22. L. D. Johnston et al., *Monitoring the Future National Results on Drug Use,* 2015.

23. Erowid, The DXM Vault, 2011, www.erowid.org
24. Substance Abuse and Mental Health Services Administration, *Results from the 2013 National Survey*, 2014.
25. Ibid.
26. Ibid.
27. L. D. Johnston et al., *Monitoring the Future National Results on Drug Use*, 2013, http://www.monitoringthefuture.org/pubs/monographs/mtf-overview2013.pdf.
28. American College Health Association, *American College Health Association–National College Health Assessment*, 2014.
29. Ibid.
30. Ibid.
31. Ibid.
32. L. M. Garnier-Dykstra et al., "Nonmedical Use of Prescription Stimulants during College: Four-Year Trends in Exposure Opportunity, Use, Motives, and Sources," *Journal of American College Health* 60, no. 3 (2012): 226–34.
33. Substance Abuse and Mental Health Services Administration, *Results from the 2013 National Survey*, 2014.
34. Ibid
35. Ibid.
36. L. D. Johnston et al., *Monitoring the Future National Survey Results on Drug Use,* 2013.
37. A. Arria, et al., "Drug Use Patterns and Continuous Enrollment in College: Results from a Longitudinal Study," *Journal of Studies on Alcohol and Drugs* 74, (2013): 71–83.
38. A. Arria et al., "Drug Use Patterns in Young Adulthood and Post-College Employment," *Drug and Alcohol Dependence* 127, no. 1–3 (2013): 23–30.
39. Substance Abuse and Mental Health Services Administration, *Results from the 2013 National Survey*, 2014.
40. Addiction Center, "Drinking and Drug Abuse is Higher among Greeks," February 15, 2015, www.addictioncenter.com/college/drinking-drug-abuse-greek-life/
41. Ibid.
42. National Center on Addiction and Substance Abuse at Columbia University, "Wasting the Best and the Brightest: Substance Abuse at America's Colleges and Universities," May 28, 2007, , www.casacolumbia.org
43. Substance Abuse and Mental Health Services Administration, *Results from the 2013 National Survey*, 2014.
44. L. D. Johnston et al., *Monitoring the Future National Results on Drug Use,* 2014, http://www.monitoringthefuture.org/pubs/monographs/mtf-overview2014.pdf.
45. CPDD Community Website, "Methamphetamine Abuse and Parkinson's Disease," July 31, 2011, www.cpddblog.com
46. NIH, National Institute on Drug Abuse, "Meth amphetamine: What are the long term effects of Methamphetamine Abuse?" September 2013. www.drugabuse.gov/publications/research-reports/methamphetamine/what-are-long-term-effects-methamphetamine-abuse
47. N. Volkow, "Bath Salts: Emerging and Dangerous Products," *National Institute on Drug Abuse*, February 2011, www.drugabuse.gov/about-nida/directors-page/messages-director/2011/02/bath-salts-emerging-dangerous-products
48. S. Melton, "Bath Salts: An 'Ivory Wave' Epidemic?" *Medscape*, August 26, 2011, www.medscape.com/viewarticle/748311
49. Ibid.
50. D. C. Mitchell et al., "Beverage Caffeine Intakes in the U.S.," *Food and Chemical Toxicology*, 63 (2014): 136–42.

51. Ibid.
52. Ibid.
53. Harvard Health Letter, "What Is It about Coffee," January 2012, www.health.harvard.edu
54. National Institute on Drug Abuse, "DrugFacts: Khat," April 2013, www.drugabuse.gov/publications/drugfacts/khat
55. Ibid.
56. Ibid.
57. Substance Abuse and Mental Health Services Administration, *Results from the 2013 National Survey*, 2014.
58. Ibid.
59. National Institute on Drug Abuse, "Drug Facts: Marijuana," January 2014, www.drugabuse.gov/publications/drugfacts/marijuana
60. M. Asbridge et al., "Acute Cannabis Consumption and Motor Vehicle Collision Risk: Systematic Review of Observational Studies and Meta-analysis," *British Medical Journal* 344 (2012): 1–9, doi:10.1136/bmj.e536
61. National Institute on Drug Abuse, "Drug Facts: Marijuana," 2014.
62. Ibid.
63. S. Lev-Ran et al., "The Association between Cannabis Use and Depression: A Systematic Review and Meta-Analysis of Longitudinal Studies," *Psychological Medicine* 44 (2014), doi: 10.1017/S0033291713001438; L. R. Pacek et al., "The Bidirectional Relationships between Alcohol, Cannabis, Co-occurring Alcohol and Cannabis Use Disorders with Major Depressive Disorder: Results from a National Sample," *Journal of Affective Disorders* 148, no. 2 (2013):188–95, doi: 10.1016/j.jad.2012.11.059
64. L. R. Pacek et al., "The Bidirectional Relationships between Use Disorders with Major Depressive Disorder," 2013.
65. L. Degenhardt et al., "The Persistence of the Association between Adolescent Cannabis Use and Common Mental Disorders into Young Adulthood," *Addiction* 108, no. 1 (2013): 124–33.
66. J. Copeland, "Changes in Cannabis Use among Young People: Impact on Mental Health," *Current Opinion in Psychiatry* 26, no. 4 (2013): 325–29.
67. National Institute on Drug Abuse, Marijuana: Facts for Teens," October 2013, www.drugabuse.gov/publications/marijuana-facts-teens; Science Daily; "Marijuana Use Prior to Pregnancy Doubles Risk of Premature Birth," July 17, 2012, www.sciencedaily.com
68. National Institute on Drug Abuse (NIDA), "Drug Facts: Spice," December 2012, www.drugabuse.gov/publications/drugfacts/spice-synthetic-marijuana
69. Ibid.; L. D. Johnston et al., *Monitoring the Future National Survey Results on Drug Use, 1975–2012: Volume I, Secondary School Students,* 2013.
70. NIDA, "Spice," March 2015
71. Ibid.
72. Ibid.
73. National Institutes of Health, National Institute on Drug Abuse, "Drug Facts: Spice," 2012.
74. The Partnership at Drugfree.org, "GHB," www.drugfree.org/drug-guide/ghb
75. Substance Abuse and Mental Health Services Administration, "Results from the 2012 National Survey," 2013, http://archive.samhsa.gov/data/NSDUH/2012SummNatFindDetTables/Index.aspx.
76. National Institutes on Drug Abuse, "Heroin: What is the Scope of Heroin Use in the United States?" November, 2014, www.drugabuse.gov/publications/research-reports/heroin/scope-heroin-use-in-united-states
77. Ibid.
78. T. Cicero, "The Changing Face of Heroin Use in the United States: A Retrospective Analysis of the Past 50 Years," *JAMA* 71, no. 7 (2014): 821–26.

79. Substance Abuse and Mental Health Services Administration, "Results from the 2012 National Survey," 2013.
80. L. D. Johnston et al., *Monitoring the Future National Survey Results on Drug Use,* 2014.
81. National Institute on Drug Abuse, "NIDA InfoFacts: MDMA (Ecstasy)," September 2013, www.drugabuse.gov/infofacts/ecstasy.html
82. The Partnership at DrugFree.org, "Experts: People Who Think They Are Taking "Molly" Don't Know What They Are Getting," June 24, 2013, www.drugfree.org/join-together/drugs/experts-people-who-think-they-are-taking-molly-dont-know-what-theyre-getting
83. National Institute on Drug Abuse, "DrugFacts: Salvia," April 2013, www.drugabuse.gov/publications/drugfacts/salvia
84. Ibid.
85. Ibid.
86. Ibid.
87. The National Collegiate Athletic Association, "NCAA National Study of Substance Use Habits of College Student Athletes—Final Report 2014," August 2014, www.ncaa.org/sites/default/files/Substance%20Use%20Final%20Report_FINAL.pdf
88. H. G. Pope et al., "The Lifetime Prevalence of Anabolic-Androgenic Steroid Use and Dependence in Americans: Current Best Estimates," *American Journal on Addictions* (2013), doi: 10.1111/j.1521-0391.2013.12118.x
89. Ibid.
90. Substance Abuse and Mental Health Services Administration, "Results from the 2013 National Survey," 2014.
91. Office of National Drug Control Policy, "How Illicit Drug Use Affects Business and the Economy," *Executive Office of the President,* www.whitehouse.gov/ondcp/ondcp-fact-sheets/how-illicit-drug-use-affects-business-and-the-economy
92. Ibid.

**Pulled Statistics:**

Page 212, American College Health Association. *American College Health Association—National College Health Assessment II: Reference Group Executive Summary, Spring 2014* (Hanover, MD: American College Health Association, 2014).

Page 219, Substance Abuse and Mental Health Services Administration, Results from the 2013 National Survey on Drug Use and Health: Summary of National Findings , NSDUH Series H-48, HHS Publication No. (SMA) 14-4863 (Rockville, MD: Substance Abuse and Mental Health Services Administration, 2014).

# Chapter 8: Drinking Alcohol Responsibly and Ending Tobacco Use

1. M. Stahre et al., "Contribution of Excessive Alcohol Consumption to Death and Years of Potential Life Lost in the United States," *Prevention of Chronic Disease* 11 (2014): 130293, www.cdc.gov/pcd/issues/2014/13_0293.htm
2. U.S. Department of Health and Human Services, *The Health Consequences of Smoking—50 Years of Progress: A Report of the Surgeon General* (Atlanta, GA: U.S. Centers for Disease Control and Prevention, Office on Smoking and Health, 2014), Available at www.surgeongeneral.gov/library/reports/50-years-of-progress/exec-summary.pdf; Centers for Disease Control and Prevention, "Current Cigarette Smoking among Adults—United States 2005–2013," *Morbidity and Mortality Weekly* 63, no. 47 (2014):1108–1112.

3. T. Naimi et al., "Confounding and Studies of 'Moderate' Alcohol Consumption: The Case of Drinking Frequency and Implications for Low Risk Drinking Guidelines," *Addiction* 108, no. 9 (2013): 1534–543; J. Marrone et al., "Moderate Alcohol Intake Lowers Biochemical Markers of Bone Turnover in Postmenopausal Women," *Journal of the North American Menopause Society* 19, no. 9 (2012): 974–79; C. Stockley, "Is It Merely a Myth That Alcoholic Beverages Such as Red Wine Can Be Cardioprotective?," *Society of Chemical Industry* 92 (2012): 1815–821, doi: 10.1002/jsfa.5696; A. Klatsky, "Alcohol and Cardiovascular Health," *Physiology and Behavior* 100, no. 1 (2010): 76–81, doi: 10.1016/j.physbeh.2009

4. National Center for Health Statistics, "Summary Health Statistics for U.S. Adults: National Health Interview Survey, 2012," *Vital and Health Statistics* 10, no. 260 (2014): 34.

5. Ibid.

6. D. J. Rohsenow et al., "Hangover Sensitivity after Controlled Alcohol Administration as Predictor of Post-College Drinking," *Journal of Abnormal Psychology* 121, no. 1 (2012): 270–75, doi: 10.1037/a0024706

7. K. Jackson et al., "Role of Tobacco Smoking in Hangover Symptoms among University Students," *Journal of Studies on Alcohol and Drugs* 74 (2013): 41–9.

8. M. A. White et al., "Hospitalizations for Alcohol and Drug Overdoses in Young Adults Ages 18–24 in the United States, 1999–2008: Results from the Nationwide Inpatient Sample," *Journal of Studies on Alcohol and Drugs* 72, no. 5 (2011): 774–876.

9. National Institute on Alcohol Abuse and Alcoholism, "Drinking Can Put a Chill on Your Summer Fun," 2012, http://pubs.niaaa.nih.gov; Centers for Disease Control and Prevention, "Unintentional Drowning: Get the Facts," November 2012, www.cdc.gov

10. Centers for Disease Control and Prevention, "Injury Prevention and Control: Home and Recreational Safety: Fire Deaths and Injuries: Fact Sheet," October 2011, www.cdc.gov

11. U.S. Department of Health and Human Services (HHS) Office of the Surgeon General and National Action Alliance for Suicide Prevention, "2012 National Strategy for Suicide Prevention: Goals and Objectives for Action," September 2012, www.surgeongeneral.gov

12. Ibid.

13. American College Health Association, *American College Health Association—National College Health Assessment II: Reference Group Executive Summary Spring 2014* (Hanover, MD: American College Health Association, 2014), Available at www.acha-ncha.org/reports_ACHA-NCHAII.html

14. N. Barnett, et al., "Description and Predictors of Positive and Negative Alcohol-Related Consequences in the First Year of College," *Journal of Studies on Alcohol and Drugs* 75, no.1 (2014): 103–14; M. Bersamin et al., "Young Adults and Casual Sex: The Relevance of College Settings," *Journal of Sex Research* 49, no. 2–3 (2012): 274–81.

15. S. Lawyer et al., "Forcible, Drug-Facilitated, and Incapacitate Rape and Sexual Assault among Undergraduate Women," *Journal of American College Health* 58, no. 5 (2010): 453–60, doi: 10.1080/07448480903540515

16. C. Stappenbeck, "A Longitudinal Investigation of Heavy Drinking and Physical Dating Violence in Men and Women," *Addictive Behaviors* 35, no. 5 (2010): 479–85, doi: 10.1016/j.addbeh.2009.12.027

17. Centers for Disease Control and Prevention, "Ten Leading Causes of Death by Age Group," August 2013, www.cdc.gov/injury/wisqars/leading-causes.html

18. Centers for Disease Control and Prevention, "Vital Signs: Drinking and Driving, a Threat to Everyone—October 2011," October 2013, www.cdc.gov/vitalsigns/drinkinganddriving

19. Ibid.; National Highway Traffic Safety Administration, "Traffic Safety Facts: 2012 Data Alcohol-Impaired Driving," December 2013, www-nrd.nhtsa.dot.gov/Pubs/811870.pdf

20. American College Health Association, *National College Health Assessment II: Reference Group Data Report, Spring 2014,* 2014.

21. Insurance Institute for Highway Safety, "Alcohol-Impaired Driving—2013," www.iihs.org/iihs/topics/t/alcohol-impaired-driving/fatalityfacts/alcohol-impaired-driving/2013

22. Ibid.

23. Ibid.

24. M. Silveri, "Adolescent Brain Development and Underage Drinking in the United States: Identifying Risks of Alcohol Use in College Populations," *Harvard Review of Psychiatry* 20, no. 4 (2012): 189–200.

25. Ibid.

26. S. J. Nielsen et al., "Calories Consumed from Alcoholic Beverages by U.S. Adults, 2007–2010," *NCHS Data Brief,* no. 110 (2012), Available at www.cdc.gov

27. L. Arriola et al., "Alcohol Intake and the Risk of Coronary Heart Disease in Spanish EPIC Cohort Study," *Heart* 96, no. 10 (2010): 124–30; T. Wilson et al., "Should Moderate Alcohol Consumption Be Promoted?," in *Nutrition and Health: Nutrition Guide for Physicians* (New York: Humana Press, 2010): 107–14; The American Heart Association, "Alcohol and Cardiovascular Disease," 2011, www.heart.org

28. Ibid.

29. The American Heart Association, "Alcohol and Heart Health," 2015, www.heart.org

30. J. Abraham et al., "Alcohol Metabolism in Human Cells Causes DNA Damage and Activates the Fanconi Anemia—Breast Cancer Susceptibility (FA-BRCA) DNA Damage Response Network," *Alcoholism: Clinical & Experimental Research* 35, no.12 (2011), doi: 10.1111/j.1530-0277.2011.01563.x

31. W. Y. Chen et al., "Moderate Alcohol Consumption during Adult Life, Drinking Patterns, and Breast Cancer Risk," *Journal of the American Medical Association* 306, no. 17 (2011): 1884–890, doi:10.1001/jama.2011.1590

32. C. S. Berkey et al., "Prospective Study of Adolescent Alcohol Consumption and Risk of Benign Breast Disease in Young Women," *Pediatrics* 125, no. 5 (2010): e1081–87.

33. SAMHSA, "18 Percent of Pregnant Women Drink Alcohol During Early Pregnancy," *The NSDUH Report,* September 9, 2013, www.samhsa.gov/data/sites/default/files/spot123-pregnancy-alcohol-2013/spot123-pregnancy-alcohol-2013.pdf; Y. Liu et al., "Alcohol Intake between Menarche and First Pregnancy: Prospective Study of Breast Cancer Risk," *Journal of the National Cancer Institute* 105, no. 20 (2013): 1571–78.

34. Centers for Disease Control and Prevention, "Fetal Alcohol Spectrum Disorders (FASDs): Alcohol Use During Pregnancy," April 17, 2014, www.cdc.gov/ncbddd/fasd/alcohol-use.html

35. Centers for Disease Control and Prevention, "Fetal Alcohol Spectrum Disorders (FASDs:) Data and Statistics," Updated January 28, 2015, www.cdc.gov/ncbddd/fasd/data.html

36. Ibid.

37. Fetal Alcohol Spectrum Disorders (FASD) Center for Excellence, "What Is FASD?," March 2014, www.Fasdcenter.samhsa.gov

38. American College Health Association, *National College Health Assessment II: Reference Group Executive Summary Spring 2014,* 2014.

39. Substance Abuse and Mental Health Services Administration, "Results from the 2013 National Survey on Drug Use and Health: Summary of National Findings 2013," September 2014, www.samhsa.gov

40. U.S. Department of Health and Human Services, National Institute on Alcohol Abuse and Alcoholism, "Moderate and Binge Drinking," 2012, www.niaaa.nih.gov/alcohol-health/overview-alcohol-consumption/moderate-binge-drinking

41. A. White and R. Hingson, "The Burden of Alcohol Use: Excessive Alcohol Consumption and Related Consequences among College Students," *Alcohol Research: Current Reviews*, 35, no. 2 (2014), Available at http://pubs.niaaa.nih.gov/publications/arcr352/201-218.htm

42. C. Neighbors et al., "Event Specific Drinking among College Students," *Psychology of Addictive Behaviors* 25, no. 4 (2011): 702–707, doi: 10.1037/a0024051

43. M. A. Lewis et al., "Use of Protective Behavioral Strategies and Their Association to 21st Birthday Alcohol Consumption and Related Negative Consequences: A Between and Within Person Evaluation," *Psychology of Addictive Behaviors* 26, no. 2 (2012), 179–86, doi: 10.1037/a0023797

44. National Institute on Alcohol Abuse and Alcoholism, "Fall Semester: A Time for Parents to Revisit Discussions about College Drinking," June 2012, www.collegedrinkingprevention.gov

45. American College Health Association, *National College Health Assessment II: Reference Group Executive Summary Spring 2014,* 2014.

46. C. Foster et al., "National College Health Assessment Measuring Negative Consequences among College Students," *American Journal of Public Health Research* 2, no.1 (2014): 1–5

47. American College Health Association, *National College Health Assessment II: Reference Group Executive Summary Spring 2014,* 2014.

48. S. Onyper et al., "Class Start Times, Sleep and Academic Performance in College: A Path Analysis," *Chronobiology* 29, no. 3 (2012): 318–35; S. Kenney et al., "Global Sleep Quality as a Moderator of Alcohol Consumption and Consequences in College Students," *Addictive Behaviors* 37, no. 4 (2012): 507–12.

49. R. Hingson et al., "Magnitude of Alcohol-Related Mortality and Morbidity among U.S. College Students Ages 18–24," 2009.

50. Ibid.

51. J. W. LaBrie et al., "Are They All the Same? An Exploratory, Categorical Analysis of Drinking Game Types," *Addictive Behaviors* 38, no. 5 (2013): 2133–39; N. P. Barnett et al., "Predictors and Consequences of Pregaming Using Day and Week-Level Measures," *Psychology of Addictive Behaviors* 27, no. 4 (2013): 921.

52. B. Zamboanga et al., "Knowing Where They're Going: Destination-Specific Pregaming Behaviors in a Multiethnic Sample of College Students," *Journal of Clinical Psychology* 69, no. 4 (2013): 383–96.

53. N. P. Barnett et al., "Predictors and Consequences of Pregaming, ," 2013.

54. J. Alfonso et al., "Do Drinking Games Matter? An Examination by Game Type and Gender in a Mandated Student Sample," *The American Journal of Drug and Alcohol Abuse* 39, no. 5 (2013): 312–19; J. W. LaBrie et al., "Are They All the Same?," 2013.

55. N. P. Barnett et al., "Predictors; and Consequences of Pregaming," 2013.

56. R. Hingson et al., "Magnitude of Alcohol-Related Mortality and Morbidity among U.S. College Students Ages 18–24," 2009.

57. Ibid.

58. A. Barry et al. "Drunkorexia: Understanding the Co-occurrence of Alcohol Consumption and Eating/Exercise Weight Management Behaviors," *Journal of American College Health Association* 60, no. 3 (2012): 236–43, doi: 10.1080/07448481.2011.587487

59. M. Eisenberg and C. Fitz, "'Drunkorexia': Exploring the Who and Why of a Disturbing Trend in College Students' Eating and Drinking Behaviors," *American Journal of College Health* 62, no. 8 (2014):570–77.

60. Ibid.

61. Ibid.

62. Ibid.

63. G. DiFulvio et al., "Effectiveness of the Brief Alcohol and Screening Intervention for College Students (BASICS) Program for Mandated Students," *Journal of American College Health* 60, no. 4 (2012): 269–80.

64. Medline Plus, "Alcoholism and Alcohol Abuse," February 2014, www.nlm.nih.gov/medlineplus/ency/article/000944.htm

65. Center of Behavioral Health Statistics and Quality, "Nearly Half of College Student Treatment Admissions Were for Primary Alcohol Abuse," *Data Spotlight* (2012), www.samhsa .gov

66. K. Beck et al., "Social Contexts of Drinking and Subsequent Alcohol Use Disorder Among College Students," *American Journal of Alcohol Abuse* 39, no.1 (2012): 38–43.

67. A. Arria, "College Student Success: The Impact of Health Concerns and Substance Abuse," Lecture presented at NASPA Alcohol and Mental Health Conference (Fort Worth, TX: January 19, 2013).

68. M. Waldron et al., "Parental Separation and Early Substance Involvement: Results from Children of Alcoholic and Cannabis Twins,"*Drug and Alcohol Dependence* 134 (2014): 78–84.

69. A. Levin, "Determining Alcoholism Proves Complicated Endeavor," *Psychiatric News* 47, no. 24 (2012): 20, doi: 10.1176/appi .pn.2012.12b13

70. D. Stacey, "RASGRF2 Regulates Alcohol-Induced Reinforcement by Influencing Mesolimbic Dopamine Neuron Activity and Dopamine Release," *Proceedings of the National Academy of Sciences* 109, no. 51 (2012): 21128–33, doi: 10.1073/pnas.1211844110

71. J. Niels Rosenquist et al., "The Spread of Alcohol Consumption Behavior in a Large Social Network," *Annals of Internal Medicine* 152, no. 7 (2010): 426–33.

72. Centers for Disease Control and Prevention, Fact Sheet, "Excessive Alcohol Use and Risks to Women's Health," November 19, 2014, www.cdc.gov/alcohol/fact-sheets/womens-health.htm

73. Centers for Disease Control and Prevention, "The High Cost of Excessive Drinking to States," February 2015, www.cdc.gov/features/CostsOfDrinking

74. Ibid.

75. Underage Drinking Enforcement Training Center, Underage Drinking Costs, "Underage Drinking," September 2011, www.udetc.org/UnderageDrinkingCosts.as

76. Ibid.

77. Ibid.

78. Substance Abuse and Mental Health Services Administration, "The NSDUH Report—Alcohol Treatment: Need, Utilization, and Barriers," April 2009, www.samhsa.gov

79. A. Laudet et al., "Collegiate Recovery Community Programs: What Do We Know and What Do We Need to Know?," *Journal of Social Work Practice in the Addictions* 14 (2014): 84–100; A. Laudet, et al., "Characteristics of Students Participating in Collegiate Recovery Programs: A National Survey," *Journal of Substance Abuse Treatment* 51 (2014): 38–46.

80. J. Liang and R. Olsen, "Alcohol Use Disorders and Current Pharmacological Therapies: The Role of GABA Receptors," *Acta Pharmacologica Sinica* 35, no. 8 (2014): 981–93.

81. U.S. Department of Health and Human Services, *The Health Consequences of Smoking—50 Years of Progress*, 2014.

82. CDC, "Fast Facts: Tobacco," April 2015, www .cdc.gov/tobacco/data_statistics/fact_sheets/fast_facts/index.htm

83. Substance Abuse and Mental Health Services Administration, "Results from the 2012 National Survey on Drug Use and Health: Summary of National Findings," U.S. Department of Health and Human Services Series H-46, No. (SMA) 13-4795 (Rockville, MD: Substance Abuse and Mental Health Services Administration, 2013), Available at www.samhsa.gov/data/NSDUH/2012SummNatFindDetTables/National-alFindings/NSDUHresults2012.pdf

84. Centers for Disease Control and Prevention, "50th Anniversary of the First Surgeon General's Report on Smoking and Health," January 2014, www.cdc.gov/mmwr/preview/mmwr .html/mm6302a1.htm?s_cid=mm6302a1_w

85. Campaign for Tobacco-Free Kids, "Toll of Tobacco in the United States of America,"February 2014, www.tobaccofreekids.org/research/factsheets/pdf/0072.pdf?utm_source=factsheets_finder&utm_medium=link&utm_campaign=analytics

86. American Lung Association, "General Smoking Facts," June 2011, www.lung.org

87. Tobacco Free Providence, "Sweet Deceit Survey Results," January 2012, www .tobaccofreeprovidence.org

88. American Cancer Society, "Cancer Facts & Figures 2015," April 2015, www.cancer.org/acs/groups/content/@editorial/documents/document/acspc-044552.pdf

89. U.S. Department of Health and Human Services, *The Health Consequences of Smoking—50 Years of Progress*, 2014.

90. Campaign for Tobacco-Free Kids, "Toll of Tobacco in the United States of America," 2014.

91. Campaign for Tobacco-Free Kids, "State Cigarette Excise Tax Rates & Rankings," December 2013, www.tobaccofreekids.org/research/factsheets/pdf/0097.pdf

92. American College Health Association, *American College Health Association–National College Health Assessment II: Reference Group Data Report, Spring 2014*, 2014.

93. Ibid.

94. Substance Abuse and Mental Health Services Administration, "Results from the 2012 National Survey on Drug Use and Health: Summary of National Findings," 2013.

95. Y. Choi et al., "I Smoke but I Am Not a Smoker": Phantom Smokers and the Discrepancy between Self-identity and Behavior," *Journal of American College Health* 59, no. 2 (2011): 117–25.

96. E. Sutfin et al., "Tobacco Use by College Students: A Comparison of Daily and Nondaily Smokers," *American Journal of Health Behavior* 36, no. 2 (2012): 218–29, doi: 10.5993/AJHB.36.2.7

97. U.S. Department of Health and Human Services, *The Health Consequences of Smoking—50 Years of Progress*, 2014.

98. Tobacco-Free Kids, "1998 State Tobacco Settlement 15 Years Later, February 2014, www .tobaccofreekids.org/what_we_do/state_local/tobacco_settlement

99. 111th Congress of the United States of America, *Family Smoking Prevention and Tobacco Control Act of 2009*, HR 1256, www.govtrack.us

100. U.S. Department of Health and Human Services, *The Health Consequences of Smoking—50 Years of Progress*, 2014; U.S. Department of Health and Human Services, "How Tobacco Smoke Causes Disease: The Biology and Behavioral Basis for Smoking Attributable Disease: A Report of the Surgeon General," 2010, Available at www.ncbi.nlm.nih.gov

101. American Cancer Society, "Child and Teen Tobacco Use," March 6, 2015, www .cancer.org/acs/groups/cid/documents/webcontent/002963-pdf.pdf

102. National Institute on Drug Abuse Research Report Series, "Tobacco Addiction," *NIH Publication no. 12-4342*, 2012, Available at www .drugabuse.gov

103. American Cancer Society, "Who Smokes Cigars?" February 19, 2014, www.cancer .org/cancer/cancercauses/tobaccocancer/cigarsmoking/cigar-smoking-who-smokes-cigars

104. K. Sterling et al., "Factors Associated with Small Cigar Use Among College Students," *American Journal of Health Behavior* 37, no. 3 (2013): 325–33.

105. Centers for Disease Control and Prevention, "Smoking and Tobacco Use: Bidis and Kreteks," Updated July 2013, www.cdc.gov/tobacco/data_statistics/fact_sheets/tobacco_industry/bidis_kreteks

106. Centers for Disease Control and Prevention, "Smoking and Tobacco Use: Bidis and Kreteks," June 2011, www.cdc.gov

107. American Cancer Society, "Questions about Smoking, Tobacco, and Health: What about More Exotic Forms of Smoking Tobacco, Such as Clove Cigarettes, Bidis, and Hookahs?," January 2013, www.cancer.org

108. American Cancer Society, "Questions about Smoking, Tobacco, and Health: What about More Exotic Forms of Smoking Tobacco, Such as Clove Cigarettes, Bidis, and Hookahs?," February 2014, www.cancer.org/cancer/cancercauses/tobaccocancer/questionsaboutsmokingtobaccoandhealth/questions-about-smoking-tobacco-and-health-other-forms-of-smoking

109. Centers for Disease Control and Prevention, "Youth and Tobacco Use," February 2014, www .cdc.gov/tobacco/data_statistics/fact_sheets/youth_data/tobacco_use

110. Campaign for Tobacco Free Kids, "Toll of Tobacco in the United States of America," 2014.

111. National Cancer Institute, "Lung Cancer Prevention," February 2014, www.cancer .gov/cancertopics/pdq/prevention/lung/HealthProfessional/page2

112. American Cancer Society, "Cancer Facts & Figures 2015," www.cancer.org/acs/groups/

content/@editorial/documents/document/
acspc-044552.pdf

113. Ibid.

114. American Cancer Society, "What Are Oral Cavity and Oropharyngeal Cancers?," February 2014, www.cancer.org/cancer/oralcavityandoropharyngealcancer/detailedguide/oral-cavity-and-oropharyngeal-cancer-what-is-oral-cavity-cancer

115. American Cancer Society, "Cancer Facts & Figures 2015," 2015.

116. Ibid.

117. American Heart Association, *Heart Disease and Stroke Statistics—2015 Update* (Dallas, TX: American Heart Association, 2015), Available at http://circ.ahajournals.org/content/early/2014/12/18/CIR.0000000000000152.full.pdf

118. Ibid.

119. Ibid.

120. Ibid.

121. American Heart Association, "Stroke Risk Factors," October 2012, www.strokeassociation.org/STROKEORG/AboutStroke/UnderstandingRisk/Understanding-Risk_UCM_308539_SubHomePage.jsp; CDC, "Health Effects of Cigarette Smoking," February 2014, www.cdc.gov/tobacco/data_statistics/fact_sheets/health_effects/effects_cig_smoking

122. U.S. Department of Health and Human Services, *The Health Consequences of Smoking—50 Years of Progress: A Report of the Surgeon General*, 2014.

123. Johns Hopkins Health Alerts, "Emphysema: Symptoms and Remedies," March 2012, www.johnshopkinshealthalerts.com

124. C. B. Harte et al., "Association between Cigarette Smoking and Erectile Tumescence: The Mediating Role of Heart Rate Variability," *International Journal of Impotence Research* (2013): doi: 10.1038/ijir.2012.43

125. Centers for Disease Control and Prevention, "Tobacco Use and Pregnancy," Modified January 2014, www.cdc.gov/reproductivehealth/TobaccoUsePregnancy

126. Ibid.

127. Centers for Disease Control and Prevention, "Current Cigarette Smoking among Adults—United States 2005–2013," *Morbidity and Mortality Weekly* 63, no. 47 (2014): 1108–12; M. Thun et al., "50-Year Trends in Smoking-Related Mortality in the United States," *The New England Journal of Medicine* 368 (2013): 351–64, doi: 10.1056/NEJMsa1211127; American Cancer Society, "Women and Smoking: An Epidemic of Smoking-Related Cancer and Disease in Women," Revised February 2014, www.cancer.org/Cancer/CancerCauses/TobaccoCancer/WomenandSmoking/women-and-smoking-intro

128. American Academy of Periodontology, "Gum Disease Risk Factors, www.perio.org/consumer/risk-factors

129. I. Moreno-Gonzalez, et al., "Smoking Exacerbates Amyloid Pathology in a Mouse Model of Alzheimer's Disease," *Nature Communications* 4 (2013), www.nature.com/ncomms/journal/v4/n2/abs/ncomms2494.html; J. Cataldo et al., "Cigarette Smoking Is a Risk Factor of Alzheimer's Disease: An Analysis Controlling for Tobacco Industry Affiliation," *Journal of Alzheimer's Disease* 19, no. 2 (2010): 465–80, doi: 10.3233/JAD-2010-1240

130. Centers for Disease Control and Prevention, "Smoking and Tobacco Use Facts: Secondhand Smoke," April 2014, www.cdc.gov/tobacco/data_statistics/fact_sheets/secondhand_smoke/general_facts

131. Ibid

132. Ibid.

133. Ibid.

134. Ibid.

135. National Cancer Institute, "Secondhand Smoke and Cancer," January 2011, www.cancer.gov/cancertopics/factsheet/Tobacco/ETS

136. U.S. Department of Health and Human Services, *The Health Consequences of Involuntary Exposure to Tobacco Smoke*, November 2011; Centers for Disease Control and Prevention, "Smoking and Tobacco Use Fact Sheet," February 2014, www.cancer.org/docroot/ped/content/ped_10_2x_secondhand_smoke-clean_indoor_air.asp

137. Centers for Disease Control and Prevention, "Tobacco Use: Smoking Cessation," February 2014, www.cdc.gov/tobacco/data_statistics/fact_sheets/cessation/quitting/index.htm#quitting

138. American Lung Association, "Benefits of Quitting," March 2012, www.lungusa.org

139. N. Hopper, "What a Pack of Cigarettes Costs Now, State by State," *The Awl*, August 1, 2014, www.theawl.com/2014/08/how-much-a-pack-of-cigarettes-costs-state-by-state

140. American Cancer Society, "Guide to Quitting Smoking: A Word about Quitting Success Rates," February 2014, www.cancer.org/Healthy/StayAwayfromTobacco/GuidetoQuittingSmoking/guide-to-quitting-smoking-success-rates

141. Everyday Health, "A Guide to Using the Nicotine Patch," May 2011, www.everydayhealth.com

142. U.S. Food and Drug Administration, "Public Health Advisory: FDA Requires New Boxed Warnings for the Smoking Cessation Drugs Chantix and Zyban," July 2009, http://www.fda.go

**Pulled Statistics:**

Page 232, National Institute on Alcohol Abuse and Alcoholism, "Drinking Facts and Statistics," 2014, www.niaaa.nih.gov/alcohol-health/overview-alcohol-consumption/alcohol-facts-and-statistics.

Page 238, www.niaaa.nih.gov/alcohol-health/overview-alcohol-consumption/alcohol-facts-and-statistics

## Chapter 9: Nutrition: Eating for a Healthier You

1. L. L. Wilkinson et al., "Attachment Anxiety, Disinhibited Eating and Body Mass Index in Adulthood," *Appetite* 57, no. 2 (2011): 543.

2. U.S. Department of Agriculture, "Part D: Section 6: Sodium, Potassium, and Water," *Report of the Dietary Guidelines Advisory Committee on the Dietary Guidelines for Americans, 2010* (Washington, DC.: U.S. Department of Agriculture, Agricultural Research Service, 2010).

3. S. C. Killer, A. K. Blannin, and A. E. Jeukendrup, "No Evidence of Dehydration with Moderate Daily Coffee Intake: A Counterbalanced Cross-Over Study in a Free-Living Population," *PLoS ONE* 9, no. 1 (2014): e84154, doi:10.1371/journal.pone.0084154

4. American College of Sports Medicine (ACSM), "Selecting and Effectively Using Hydration for Fitness," 2011, www.acsm.org/docs/brochures/selecting-and-effectively-using-hydration-for-fitness.pdf

5. U.S. Department of Agriculture, *What We Eat in America*, NHANES 2009–2010, 2010

6. Food and Nutrition Board, Institute of Medicine, *Dietary Reference Intakes for Energy, Carbohydrate, Fiber, Fat, Fatty Acids, Cholesterol, Protein, and Amino Acids (Macronutrients)*, (Washington, DC: National Academies Press, 2005), Available at www.nap.edu/openbook.php?isbn=0309085373

7. S. M. Phillips and L. J. C. van Loon, "Dietary Protein for Athletes: From Requirements to Optimum Adaptation," *Journal of Sports Science* 29, no. S1 (2011): S29–S38.

8. Institute of Medicine of the National Academies, "Dietary, Functional, and Total Fiber," *Dietary Reference Intakes for Energy, Carbohydrate, Fiber, Fat, Fatty Acids, Cholesterol, Protein, and Amino Acids* (Washington, DC: The National Academies Press, 2005), 339–421, Available at www.nap.edu/openbook.php?isbn=0309085373

9. Ibid.

10. Ibid.

11. C. E. Ramsden et al., "Use of Dietary Linoleic Acid for Secondary Prevention of Coronary Heart Disease and Death: Evaluation of Recovered Data from the Sydney Diet Heart Study and Updated Meta-Analysis," *British Medical Journal* 346 (2013): e8707, doi: http://dx.doi.org/10.1136/bmj.e8707; L. Gillingham, S. Harris-Janz, and P. Jones, "Dietary Monounsaturated Fatty Acids Are Protective against Metabolic Syndrome and Cardiovascular Disease Risk Factors," *Lipids* 46, no. 3 (2011): 209–28, doi: 10.1007/s11745-010-3524-y

12. W. Willet, "Dietary Fats and Coronary Heart Disease," *Journal of Internal Medicine*, no. 1 (2012): 13–24; N. Bendson et al., "Consumption of Industrial and Ruminant Trans Fatty Acids and Risk of CHD: A Systemic Review and Meta-Analysis of Cohort Studies," *European Journal of Clinical Nutrition* 65 (2011): 773–83.

13. U.S. Food and Drug Administration, "FDA Targets Trans Fats in Processed Foods," FDA Consumer Updates, December 2013, www.fda.gov/ForConsumers/ConsumerUpdates/ucm372915.htm

14. Ibid.

15. H. J. Silver et al., "Consuming a Balanced High Fat Diet for 16 Weeks Improves Body Composition, Inflammation and Vascular Function Parameters in Obese Premenopausal Women," *Metabolism* (January 17, 2014), doi: 10.1016/j.metabol.2014.01.004; Z. Shadman, "Association of High Carbohydrate versus High Fat Diet with Glycated Hemoglobin in High Calorie Consuming Type 2 Diabetics," *Journal of Diabetes and Metabolic Disorders* 12, no. 1 (2013): 27.

16. Food and Nutrition Board, Institute of Medicine, *Dietary Reference Intakes for Energy, Carbohydrate, Fiber, Fat, Fatty Acids, Cholesterol, Protein, and Amino Acids (Macronutrients)* (Washington, DC: National Academies Press, 2005), Available at www.nap.edu/openbook.php?isbn=0309085373.

17. National Institutes of Health Office of Dietary Supplements, "Dietary Supplement Fact Sheet: Vitamin D," June 2011, http://ods.od.nih.gov/factsheets/VitaminD-HealthProfessional

18. Institute of Medicine Committee to Review Dietary Reference Intakes for Vitamin D and Calcium, *Dietary Reference Intakes for Calcium and Vitamin D*, eds. A. Ross, C. Taylor, A. Yaktine, H. Del Valle (Washington, DC: National Academies Press, 2011), Available at www.iom.edu/Reports/2010/Dietary-Reference-Intakes-for-Calcium-and-Vitamin-D.aspx

19. Ibid.

20. U.S. Department of Agriculture, *What We Eat in America*, 2010.

21. Ibid.; C. Ayala et al., "Application of Lower Sodium Intake Recommendations to Adults—United States, 1999–2006," *Morbidity and Mortality Weekly (MMWR)* 58, no. 11 (2009): 281–83.

22. American Heart Association, "Sodium (Salt)," February 2014, www.heart.org/HEARTORG/GettingHealthy/NutritionCenter/HealthyDietGoals/Sodium-Salt-or-Sodium-Chloride_UCM_303290_Article.jsp

23. R. L. Bailey et al., "Estimation of Total Usual Calcium and Vitamin D Intakes in the United States," *Journal of Nutrition* 140, no. 4 (2010): 817–22, doi: 10.3945/jn.109.118539

24. S. A. McNaughton et al., "An Energy-Dense, Nutrient-Poor Dietary Pattern Is Inversely Associated with Bone Health in Women," *Journal of Nutrition* 141, no. 8 (2011): 1516–23, doi: 10.3945/jn.111.138271

25. World Health Organization, "Micronutrient Deficiencies: Iron Deficiency Anemia," 2014, www.who.int/nutrition/topics/ida/en/index.html

26. U.S. Centers for Disease Control and Prevention (CDC), "Iron and Iron Deficiency," *Nutrition for Everyone*, February 23, 2011, www.cdc.gov/nutrition/everyone/basics/vitamins/iron.html

27. C. Geissler and M. Singh, "Iron, Meat, and Health," *Nutrients* 3, no. 3 (2011): 283–316, doi: 10.3390/nu3030283

28. Academy of Nutrition and Dietetics, "Position of the Academy of Nutrition and Dietetics: Functional Foods" *Journal of the Academy of Nutrition and Dietetics*, 113 (2013): 1096–1103.

29. Ibid.

30. Ibid.

31. M. E. Obrenovich, et al., "Antioxidants in Health, Disease, and Aging," *CNS & Neurological Disorders Drug Targets* 10, no. 2 (2011): 192–207; V. Ergin, R. E. Hariry, and C. Karasu, "Carbonyl Stress in Aging Process: Role of Vitamins and Phytochemicals as Redox Regulators," *Aging and Disease* 4, no. 5 (2013): 276–94, doi: 10.14336/AD.2013.0400276

32. E. A. Klein et al., "Vitamin E and the Risk of Prostate Cancer: The Selenium and Vitamin E Cancer Prevention Trial (SELECT)," *Journal of the American Medical Association* 306, no. 14 (2011): 1549–56, doi: 10.1001/jama.2011.1437

33. U.S. Department of Agriculture, Economic Research Service, "Loss-Adjusted Food Availability Documentation: Overview: Calories," November 2, 2012, www.ers.usda.gov

34. D. Grotto and E. Zied, "The Standard American Diet and Its Relationship to the Health Status of Americans," *Nutrition in Clinical Practice* 25, no. 6 (2010): 603–12, doi: 10.1177/0884533610386234

35. U.S. Department of Agriculture and U.S. Department of Health and Human Services, *Dietary Guidelines for Americans, 2010*, 7th ed. (Washington, DC: U.S. Government Printing Office, 2010), Available at www.cnpp.usda.gov/publications/dietaryguidelines/2010/policydoc/policydoc.pdf

36. Ibid.

37. Ibid.

38. U.S. Department of Agriculture, "Empty Calories: How Do I Count the Empty Calories I Eat?," June 4, 2011, www.choosemyplate.gov/foodgroups/emptycalories_count_table.html

39. U.S. Food and Drug Administration, "Nutrition Facts Label: Proposed Changes Aim to Better Inform Food Choices," February 2014, www.fda.gov/ForConsumers/ConsumerUpdates/ucm387114.htm

40. U.S. Food and Drug Administration, "Label Claims for Conventional Foods and Dietary Supplements," December 2013, www.fda.gov/Food/IngredientsPackagingLabeling/LabelingNutrition/ucm111447.htm

41. The Vegetarian Resource Group, "How Often Do Americans Eat Vegetarian Meals? And How Many Adults in the U.S. Are Vegan?" May 18, 2012, www.vrg.org/journal/vj2011issue4/vj2011issue-4poll.php

42. F. Newport, "In U.S. 5% Consider Themselves Vegetarians," *Gallup*, July 26, 2012, www.gallup.com/poll/156215/Consider-Themselves-Vegetarians.aspxw

43. Y. Yokoyama et al., "Vegetarian Diets and Blood Pressure: A Meta-Analysis," *Journal of the American Medical Association Internal Medicine*, February 2014, doi:10.1001/jamainternmed.2013.14547

44. C. G. Lee et al., "Vegetarianism as a Protective Factor for Colorectal Adenoma and Advanced Adenoma in Asians," *Digestive Diseases and Science* (2013), doi: 10.1007/s10620-013-2974-5

45. Office of Dietary Supplements, "Frequently Asked Questions," July 2013, http://ods.od.nih.gov/Health_Information/ODS_Frequently_Asked_Questions.aspx#; V. A. Moyer, "Vitamin, Mineral, and Multivitamin Supplements for the Primary Prevention of Cardiovascular Disease and Cancer: U.S. Preventive Services Task Force Recommendation Statement," *Annals of Internal Medicine* 160, no. 8 (2014): 558–64, doi:10.7326/M14-0198

46. R. Chowdhury et al., "Association between Fish Consumption, Long Chain Omega 3 Fatty Acids, and Risk of Cerebrovascular Disease: Systematic Review and Meta-Analysis," *British Medical Journal* 345 (2012): e6698, www.ncbi.nlm.nih.gov/pmc/articles/PMC3484317

47. Office of Dietary Supplements, "Vitamin A Fact Sheet for Consumers," June 2013, http://ods.od.nih.gov/factsheets/VitaminA-QuickFacts/; Office of Dietary Supplements, "Vitamin E Fact Sheet for Consumers," June 2013, http://ods.odnih.gov/factsheets/list-all/VitaminE-QuickFacts/; Office of Dietary Supplements, "Vitamin D Fact Sheet for Consumers," June 2013, http://ods.od.nih.gov/factsheets/VitaminD-QuickFacts

48. Academy of Nutrition and Dietetics, "It's About Eating Right: Dietary Supplements," January 2013, www.eatright.org/public/content.aspx?id=7918

49. U.S. Department of Health and Human Services, "Food Safety Modernization Act (FSMA)," November 2013, www.fda.gov/Food/GuidanceRegulation/FSMA/ucm304045.htm

50. The Organic Trade Association, "Eight in Ten U.S. Parents Report They Purchase Organic Products," April 2013, www.ota.com/news/press-releases/17124

51. USDA Economic Research Service, "Organic Market Overview," April 7, 2014, www.ers.usda.gov/topics/natural-resources-environment/organic-agriculture/organic-market-overview.aspx

52. K. Brandt et al., "Agroecosystem Management and Nutritional Quality of Plant Foods: The Case of Organic Fruits and Vegetables," *Critical Reviews in Plant Sciences* 30, no. 1–2 (2011): 177–97; C. Smith-Spangler et al., "Are Organic Foods Safer or Healthier Than Conventional Alternatives? A Systematic Review," *Annals of Internal Medicine* 157, no. 5 (2012): 348–66, doi:10.7326/0003-4819-157-5-201209040-00009

53. U.S. Environmental Protection Agency, "Pesticides and Foods: Health Problems Pesticides May Pose," May 2012, www.epa.gov/pesticides/food/risks.htm

54. U.S. Department of Agriculture, Pesticide Data Program: 21st Annual Summary, Calendar Year 2011, Agricultural Marketing Service, February 2013, www.ams.usda.gov/AMSv1.0/getfile?dDocName=stelprdc5102692

55. CDC, "Estimates of Food-Borne Illnesses in the United States," January 2014, www.cdc.gov/foodborneburden/index.html

56. CDC, "Trends in Foodborne Illness in the United States, 2012,"April 2013, www.cdc.gov/features/dsfoodnet2012

57. CDC, "Listeria (Listeriosis)," March 16, 2015, www.cdc.gov/listeria

58. Ibid.

59. Ibid.

60. Ibid.

61. R. Johnson, "The U.S. Trade Situation for Fruit and Vegetable Products," Congressional Research Service, January 2014, www.fas.org/sgp/crs/misc/RL34468.pdf

62. S. Clark et al., "Frequency of US Emergency Department Visits for Food-related Acute Allergic Reactions," *Journal of Allergy Clinical Immunology* 127, no. 3, (2011): 682–83, doi: 10.1016/j.jaci.2010.10.040

63. National Institute of Allergy and Infectious Diseases, "Food Allergy," August 2013, www.niaid.nih.gov/topics/foodallergy/Pages/default.aspx

64. R. S. Gupta et al., "The Prevalence, Severity, and Distribution of Childhood Food Allergy in the United States," *Journal of Pediatrics* 128, no. 1 (2011): e9–e17, doi: 10.1542/peds.2011-0204

65. National Institute of Allergy and Infectious Diseases, "Food Allergy," August 2013, www.niaid.nih.gov/topics/foodallergy/Pages/default.aspx

66. U.S. Food and Drug Administration, "Food Allergies: What You Need to Know," April 2013, www.fda.gov/food/resourcesforyou/consumers/ucm079311.htm

67. A. Rubio-Tapia et al., "The Prevalence of Celiac Disease in the United States," *American Journal of Gastroenterology* 107 (2012):1 538–44

68. Panel, NIAID-Sponsored Expert, "Guidelines for the Diagnosis and Management of Food Allergy in the United States: Report of the NIAID-sponsored Expert Panel," *Journal of Allergy and Clinical Immunology* 126, no. 6 (2010): S1–S58.

69. J. N. Keith et al., "The Prevalence of Self-Reported Lactose Intolerance and the Consumption of Dairy Foods among African American Adults Less than Expected," *Journal of the National Medical Association* 103 (2011): 36–45.

70. G. Pinholster, "AAAS Board of Directors: Legally Mandating GM Food Labels Could 'Mislead and Falsely Alarm Consumers,'" American Association for the Advancement of Science News, October 2012, www.aaas.org/news/aaas-board-directors-legally-mandating-gm-food-labels-could-mislead-and-falsely-alarm; World Health Organization, "20 Questions on Genetically Modified Foods," Accessed March 2014, www.who.int/foodsafety/publications/biotech/20questions/en

**Pulled Statistics:**

Page 276, C. Ogden, B. Kit, M. Carroll, S. Park, "Consumption of Sugar Drinks in the United States, 2005–2008," *NCHS Data Brief*, no. 71. (Hyattsville, MD: National Center for Health Statistics, 2011), www.cdc.gov/nchs/data/databriefs/db71.htm.

Page 281, K. Heidal, S. Colby, G. Mirabella, et al., "Cost and Calorie Analysis of Fast Food Consumption in College Students," *Food and Nutrition Sciences* 3, no. 7, (2012): 942–46, doi:10.4236/fns.2012.37124

# Chapter 10: Reaching and Maintaining a Healthy Weight

1. M. Ng et al., " Global, Regional, and National Prevalence of Overweight and Obesity in Children and Adults during 1980–2013: A Systematic Analysis for the Global Burden of Disease Study 2013," *Lancet* 384, no. 9945 (2014): 766–81; C. L. Ogden et al., "Prevalence of Childhood and Adult Obesity in the United States, 2011–2012," *Journal of the American Medical Association* 311, no. 8 (2014): 806–14, doi:10.1001/jama.2014.732; C. L. Ogden et al., "Prevalence of Obesity among Adults: United States, 2011-2012," *National Center for Health Statistics Data Brief* 131 (2013), www.cdc.gov/nchs/data/databriefs/db131.htm

2. Centers for Disease Control and Prevention (CDC), "Health, United States, 2013." Figure 10. Overweight and Obesity among Adults Aged 20 and Over by Sex, United States, 1988-1994, then, 2009-2012, May 2014, www.cdc.gov/nchs/data/hus/hus13.pdf

3. C. L. Ogden et al., "Prevalence of Obesity among Adults: United States, 2011–2012," *NCHS Data Brief* no 131 (Hyattsville, MD: National Center for Health Statistics, 2013).

4. D. Mozaffarian et al., "Heart Disease and Stroke Statistics—2015 Update: A Report From the American Heart Association," *Circulation* 131, no. 4 (2015): 434–41.

5. Ibid.

6. Ibid.

7. Ibid.

8. Ibid.

9. World Health Organization (WHO), "Obesity and Overweight Fact Sheet," January 2015, www.who.int/mediacentre/factsheets/fs311/en

10. Ibid.; International Obesity Taskforce, "Obesity–The Global Epidemic," 2014, www.iaso .org/iotf/obesity/obesitytheglobalepidemic; M. Ng et al., "Global, Regional, and National Prevalence of Overweight and Obesity in Children and Adults, 2014.

11. K. M. Flegal et al., "Association of All-Cause Mortality with Overweight and Obesity Using Standard Body Mass Index Categories: A Systematic Review and Meta-Analysis," *Journal of the American Medical Association* 309, no. 1 (2013): 71–82.

12. American Heart Association, "With a Very Heavy Heart: Obesity and Cardiovascular Disease," February 2014, www.heart.org/idc/groups/heart-public/@wcm/@adv/documents/downloadable/ucm_461353.pdf

13. American Diabetes Association, "Statistics about Diabetes and Pre-diabetes," February 19, 2015, www.diabetes.org/diabetes-basics/statistics

14. C. L. Himes and S. L. Reynolds. "Effect of Obesity on Falls, Injury, and Disability," *Journal of the American Geriatrics Society* 60, no. 1 (2012): 124–29; L. A. Schaap, A. Koster, and M. Visser, "Adiposity, Muscle Mass, and Muscle Strength in Relation to Functional Decline in Older Persons," *Epidemiologic Reviews* 35, no. 1 (2013): 1.

15. D. Spruijt-Metz, "Etiology, Treatment, and Prevention of Obesity in Childhood and Adolescence: A Decade in Review," *Journal of Research on Adolescence* 21 (2011): 129–52, doi: 10.1111/j.1532-7795.2010.00719.x; S. A. Affenito et al., "Behavioral Determinants of Obesity: Research Findings and Policy Implications," *Journal of Obesity* 2012 (2012), www.hindawi .com/journals/jobes/2012/150732

16. K. Silventoinen et al., "The Genetic and Environmental Influences on Childhood Obesity: A Systematic Review of Twin and Adoption Studies," *International Journal of Obesity* 34, no. 1 (2010): 29–40; D. Cummings and M. Schwartz, "Genetics and Pathophysiology of Human Obesity," *Annual Review of Medicine* 54 (2003): 453–71.

17. T. Tanaka, J. S. Ngwa, and F. J. van Rooij, "Genome-Wide Meta-Analysis of Observational Studies Shows Common Genetic Variants Associated with Macronutrient Intake," *American Journal of Clinical Nutrition* 97, no. 6 (2013): 1395–402; M. M. Hetherington and J. E. Cecil, "Gene-Environment Interactions in Obesity," *Forum Nutrition* 63 (2010): 195–203; M. Graff, J. S. Ngwa, and T. Workalemahu, "Genome-Wide Analysis of BMI in Adolescents and Young Adults Reveals Additional Insights into the Effects of the Genetic Loci over the Life Course," *Human Molecular Genetics* 22, no. 17 (2013): 3597–607.

18. D. Withers, et al., "A Link between FTO, Ghrelin and Impaired Brain Food-cue Responsivity," *The Journal of Clinical Investigation* 123, no. 8 (2013): 3339–351, doi: 10.1172/JC144403

19. M. Graff, J. S. Ngwa and T. Workalemahu, "Genome-Wide Analysis of BMI in Adolescents and Young Adults Reveals Additional Insights," 2013.

20. T. O. Kilpelainen et al., "Physical Activity Attenuates the Influence of *FTO* Variants on Obesity Risk: A Meta-Analysis of 218,166 Adults and 19,268 Children," *PLoS Medicine* 8, no.11 (2012): e1001116, doi:10.1371/journal.pmed.1001116; A. S. Richardson et al., "Moderate to Vigorous Physical Activity Interactions with Genetic Variants and Body Mass Index in a Large US Ethnically Diverse Cohort," *Pediatric Obesity* 9, no. 2 (2013): e35–46, doi: 10.1111/j.2047-6310.2013.00152

21. J. C. Wells, "The Evolution of Human Adiposity and Obesity: Where Did It All Go Wrong?," *Disease Models and Mechanisms* 5, no. 5 (2012): 595–607, doi:10.1242/dmm.009613; J. R. Speakman et al., " Evolutionary Perspectives on the Obesity Epidemic: Adaptive, Maladaptive, and Neutral Viewpoints," *Annual Review of Nutrition* 33 (2013): 289–317.

22. A. Tremblay et al., "Adaptive Thermogenesis Can Make a Difference in the Ability of Obese Individuals to Lose Body Weight," *International Journal of Obesity* 37 (2013): 759–64.

23. J. Buss et al., "Associations of Ghrelin with Eating Behaviors, Stress, Metabolic Factors, and Telomere Length among Overweight and Obese Women: Preliminary Evidence of Attenuated Ghrelin Effects in Obesity," *Appetite* 76, no. 1 (2014): 84–94; B. Biondi, "Thyroid and Obesity: An Intriguing Relationship," *Journal of Clinical Endocrinology and Metabolism* 95, no. 8 (2010): 3614–17; T. Reinehr, "Obesity and Thyroid Function," *Molecular and Cellular Endocrinology* 316, no. 2 (2010): 165–71.

24. D. E. Cummings et al., "Plasma Ghrelin Levels After Diet-Induced Weight Loss or Gastric Bypass Surgery," *New England Journal of Medicine* 346, no. 21 (2002): 1623–30.

25. M. Khatib et al., "Effect of Ghrelin on Regulation of Growth Hormone Release: A Review," *The Health Agenda* 2, no. 1 (2014), Available at www.healthagenda.net/wp-content/uploads/2013/11/Effect-of-ghrelin-on-regulation-of-growth-hormone-release-A-review.pdf; C. DeVriese et al., "Focus on the Short- and Long-Term Effects of Ghrelin on Energy Homeostasis," *Nutrition* 26, no. 6 (2010): 579–84; T. Castaneda et al., "Ghrelin in the Regulation of Body Weight and Metabolism," *Frontiers in Neuroendocrinology* 31, no. 1 (2010): 44–60.

26. P. Marzullo et al. "Investigations of Thyroid Hormones and Antibodies in Obesity: Leptin Levels Are Associated with Thyroid Autoimmunity Independent of Bioanthropometric, Hormonal and Weight-Related Determinants," *The Journal of Clinical Endocrinology and Metabolism* 95, no. 8 (2010): 3965–72; H. Feng et al., "Review: The Role of Leptin in Obesity and the Potential for Leptin Replacement Therapy," *Endocrine* 44 (2013): 33–39.

27. L. K. Mahan and S. Escott-Stump, *Krause's Food, Nutrition, and Diet Therapy,* 13th ed. (New York: W. B. Saunders, 2012).

28. USDA Economic Research Service, "Food Availability (per capita) Data System," March 2014, www.ers.usda.gov/data-products/food-availability

29. E. Ford and W. Dietz, "Trends in Energy Intake among Adults in the United States: Findings from NHANES," *American Journal of Clinical Nutrition,* April 2013, http://bit.ly/XUJ7Dq

30. Centers for Disease Control and Prevention, "Facts about Physical Activity," May 2014, http://www.cdc.gov/physicalactivity/data/facts.htm

31. M. Wang, L. Pbert, and S. Lemon, "Influence of Family, Friend and Co-worker Social Support and Social Undermining on Weight Gain Prevention among Adults," *Obesity* 22, no. 9 (2014): 1973–80; T. Lehey, J. LaRose, J. Fave, and R. Wing, "Social Influences Are Associated with BMI and Weight Loss Intentions in Young Adults," *Obesity* 19, no. 6 (2011): 1157–62.

32. C. Gillespie et al., "The Growing Concern of Poverty in the United States: An Exploration of Food Prices and Poverty on Obesity Rates for Low-Income Citizens," *Undergraduate Economic Review* 8, no. 1 (2012): 1–38.

33. J. F. Sallis et al., "Role of Built Environments in Physical Activity, Obesity and Cardiovascular Disease," *Circulation* 125, no. 5 (2012): 729–37; J. Kolodziejczyk et al., "Influence of Specific Individual and Environmental Variables on the Relationship between Body Mass Index and Health-related Quality of Life in Overweight and Obese Adolescents," *Quality of Life Research* 24, no. 1 (2015): 251–61.

34. CDC, "About BMI for Adults," February 2015, www.cdc.gov/healthyweight/assessing/bmi/adult_bmi/index.html

35. J. I. Mechanick et al., "Clinical Practice Guidelines for the Perioperative Nutritional, Metabolic and Nonsurgical Support of the Bariatric Surgery Patient—2013 Update," *Endocrine Practice* 19, no. 2 (2013): e1–36, www.aace.com/files/publish-ahead-of-print-final-version.pdf

36. C. L. Ogden, M. D. Carroll, B. K. Kit, K. M. Flegal, "Prevalence of childhood and adult obesity in the United States, 2011–2012," *JAMA,* 2014, 311(8):806–814

37. American Heart Association, "Body Composition Tests," April 2013, www.heart.org/HEARTORG/GettingHealthy/NutritionCenter/Body-Composition-Tests_UCM_305883_Article.jsp; S. J. Mooney, A. Baecker, and A. G. Rundel, "Comparison of Anthropometric and Body Composition Measures as Predictors of Components of the Metabolic Syndrome in the Clinical Setting," *Obesity Research and Clinical Practice* 7, no. 1 (2013): e55–e66.

38. C. L. Ogden et al., "Prevalence of Childhood and Adult Obesity in the United States," 2014; National Center for Health Statistics, "Health, United States, 2011: With Special Features on Socioeconomic Status and Health," Hyattsville, MD; U.S. Department of Health and Human Services, 2012, Available at www.cdc.gov/nchs/data/hus/hus11.pdf

39. R. Puhl, "Weight Stigmatization toward Youth: A Significant Problem in Need of Societal Solutions," *Childhood Obesity* 7, no. 5 (2011): 359–63; S. A. Mustillo, K. Budd, and K. Hendrix, "Obesity, Labeling, and Psychological Distress in Late-Childhood and Adolescent Black and White Girls: The Distal Effects of Stigma," *Social Psychology Quarterly* 76, no. 3 (2013): 268–89.

40. L. Goh et al., "Anthropometric Measurements of General and Central Obesity and the Prediction of Cardiovascular Disease Risk in Women: A Cross sectional Study," *BMJ Open* 4, (2014): e004138, doi:10.1136/bmjopen-2013-004138; M. Bombelli et al., "Impact of Body Mass Index and Waist Circumference on the Long Term Risk of Diabetes Mellitus, Hypertension and Cardiac Organ Damage," *Hypertension* 58, no. 6 (2011): 1029–35; S. Czernichow et al., "Body Mass Index, Waist Circumference and Waist-Hip Ratio: Which is the Better Discriminator of Cardiovascular Disease Mortality Risk? Evidence from an Individual-Participant Meta-Analysis of 82,864 Participants from Nine Cohort Studies," *Obesity Reviews* 12, no. 9 (2011): 1467–78.

41. National Heart, Lung, and Blood Institute, "Classification of Overweight and Obesity by BMI, Waist Circumference and Associated Disease Risks," 2012, www.nhlbi.nih.gov/health/public/heart/obesity/lose_wt/bmi_dis.htm

42. University of Maryland Medical Center, Rush University, "Waist to Hip Ratio Calculator," March 2014, www.healthcalculators.org/calculators/waist_hip.asp

43. P. Brambilla et al., "Waist Circumference-to-Height Ratio Predicts Adiposity Better than Body Mass Index in Children and Adolescents," *International Journal of Obesity* 37, no. 7 (2013): 943–46.

44. L. Gray, N. Cooper, A. Dunkley et al., "A Systematic Review and Mixed Treatment Comparison of Pharmacological Interventions for the Treatment of Obesity," *Obesity Reviews* 13, no. 6 (2012): 483–98.

45. ConsumerSearch, "Diet Pills: Reviews," 2012, www.consumersearch.com/diet-pills

46. U.S. Food and Drug Administration, "Fen-Phen Safety Update Information," December 2014, www.fda.gov

47. C. E. Weber et al., "Obesity and Trends in Malpractice Claims for Physicians and Surgeons," *Surgery* 154, no. 2 (2013): 299–304.

48. Mayo Clinic, "Gastric Bypass Surgery," April 7, 2014, www.mayoclinic.com/health/gastric-bypass/MY00825

49. John's Hopkins Health Library, "BPD/DS Weight-Loss Surgery," March 2014, www.hopkinsmedicine.org/healthlibrary/test_procedures/gastroenterology/bpdds_weight-loss surgery_135,64

50. F. Rubino et al., "Metabolic Surgery to Treat Type 2 Diabetes: Clinical Outcomes and Mechanisms of Action," *Annual Review of Medicine* 61 (2010): 393–411; S. Brethauer et al., "Can Diabetes Be Surgically Cured? Long-Term Metabolic Effects of Bariatric Surgery in Obese Patients with Type 2 Diabetes Mellitus," *Annals of Surgery* 258, no. 4 (2013): 628–37.

**Pulled Statistics:**

Page 298, C. D. Fryar and R. B. Ervin, "Caloric Intake from Fast Food among Adults: United States, 2007–2010," *NCHS Data Brief*, No. 114. (2013), www.cdc.gov

Page 308, Centers for Disease Control and Prevention, "Adult Obesity Facts: Obesity Affects Some Groups More than Others," September 2014, www.cdc.gov/obesity/data/adult.html

## Focus On: Enhancing Your Body Image

1. University of the West of England, "30% of Women Would Trade at Least One Year of Their Life to Achieve Their Ideal Body Weight and Shape," March 2011, http://info.uwe.ac.uk/news/UWENews/news.aspx?id=1949

2. M. Bucchianeri et al., "Body Dissatisfaction from Adolescence to Young Adulthood: Findings from a 10-year Longitudinal Study," *Body Image* 10, no. 1 (2013): 1–7.

3. University of Minnesota Health Talk, "Social Media May Inspire Unhealthy Body Image," May 2013, www.healthtalk.umn.edu/2013/05/15/thigh-gap-and-social-media

4. Ibid.

5. Centers for Disease Control and Prevention, "FASTSTATS: Obesity and Overweight," April 29, 2015, www.cdc.gov/nchs/fastats/obesity-overweight.htm

6. J. B. Webb et al., "Do You See What I See?: An Exploration of Inter-Ethnic Ideal Body Size Comparisons among College Women," *Body Image* 10, no. 3 (2013): 369–79.

7. V. Swami et al., "The Attractive Female Body Weight and Female Body Dissatisfaction in 26 Countries across 10 World Regions: Results of the International Body Project I," *Personality and Social Psychology Bulletin* 36, no. 3 (2010): 309–25.

8. Mayo Clinic Staff, "Body Dysmorphic Disorder," May 2013, www.mayoclinic.com/health/body-dysmorphic-disorder/DS00559

9. J. D. Feusner et al., "Abnormalities of Object Visual Processing in Body Dysmorphic Disorder," *Psychological Medicine* 41, no. 11 (2011): 2385–97, doi: 10.1017/S0033291711000572

10. Body Image Health, "The Model for Healthy Body Image and Weight," March 2014, http://bodyimagehealth.org/model-for-healthy-body-image

11. I. Ahmed et al., "Body Dysmorphic Disorder," *Medscape Reference*, January 2014, http://emedicine.medscape.com/article/291182-overview

12. Mayo Clinic Staff, "Body Dysmorphic Disorder," 2013; KidsHealth, "Body Dysmorphic Disorder," May 2013, http://kidshealth.org/parent/emotions/feelings/bdd.html

13. I. Ahmed et al., "Body Dysmorphic Disorder," 2014.

14. J. Reel, *Eating Disorders: An Encyclopedia of Causes, Treatment and Prevention*, (New York: Greenwood Publishing, 2013); A. Taheri et al., "The Relationship between Social Physique Anxiety and Anthropometric Characteristics of the Non-athletic Female Students," *Annals of Biological Research* 3, no. 6 (2012): 2727–29; A. Sicilia et al., "Exercise Motivation and Social Physique Anxiety in Adolescents," *Psychologica Belgica* 54, no. 1 (2014): 111–29, doi: http://dx.doi.org/10.5334/pb.ai

15. American Psychiatric Association, *Diagnostic and Statistical Manual of Mental Disorders*, 5th ed. (Washington, DC: American Psychiatric Association, 2013).

16. National Eating Disorders Association, "Get the Facts on Eating Disorders," May 2015, www.nationaleatingdisorders.org/get-facts-eating-disorders

17. D. A. Gagne et al., "Eating Disorder Symptoms and Weight and Shape Concerns in a Large Web-Based Convenience Sample of Women Ages 50 and Above: Results of the Gender and Body Image (GABI) Study," *International Journal of Eating Disorders* 45, no. 7 (2012): 832–44, doi: 10.1002/eat.22030

18. American College Health Association, *National College Health Assessment II: Undergraduates Reference Group Executive Summary Spring 2014* (Hanover, MD: American College Health Association, 2014), Available at www.acha-ncha.org/reports_ACHA-NCHAII.html

19. L. M. Gottschlich, "Female Athlete Triad," *Medscape Reference, Drugs, Diseases & Procedures*, January 25, 2012, http://emedicine.medscape.com/article/89260-overview#a0156

20. Alliance for Eating Disorder Awareness, "What Are Eating Disorders?," 2013, www.allianceforeatingdisorders.com/portal/what-are-eating-disorders#.Uycs4_Pn9IY

21. Ibid.

22. National Eating Disorders Association, "Anorexia Nervosa," April 2014, www.nationaleatingdisorders.org/anorexia-nervosa

23. S. A. Swanson et al., "Prevalence and Correlates of Eating Disorders in Adolescents: Results from the National Comorbidity Survey Replication Adolescent Supplement," *Archives of General Psychiatry* 68, no. 7 (2011): 714–23, doi: 10.1001/archgenpsychiatry.2011.22

24. P. Crocker et al., "Body-Related State Shame and Guilt in Women: Do Causal Attributions Mediate the Influence of Physical Self-concept and Shame and Guilt Proneness," *Body Image* 11, no. 1 (2013): 19–26; A. R. Smith, T. E. Joiner, and D. R. Dodd, "Examining Implicit Attitudes toward Emaciation and Thinness in Anorexia Nervosa," *International Journal of Eating Disorders* 47, no. 2 (2013): 138–47; R. N. Carey, N. Donaghue, and P. Broderick, "Concern among Australian Adolescent Girls: The Role of Body Comparisons with Models and Peers," *Body Image* 11, no. 1 (2014): 81–84.

25. A.D.A.M. Medical Encyclopedia, U.S. National Library of Medicine, "Anorexia Nervosa," February 13, 2012, www.ncbi.nlm.nih.gov; B. Suchan et al., "Reduced Connectivity between the Left Fusiform Body Area and the Extrastriate Body Area in Anorexia Nervosa Is Associated with Body Image Distortion," *Behavioural Brain Research* 241 (2013): 80–85, doi: 10.1016/j.bbr.2012.12.002; G. Frank et al., "Anorexia Nervosa and Obesity Are Associated with Opposite Brain Reward Response," *Neuropsychopharmacology* 37, no. 9 (2012): 2031–46, doi: 10.1038/npp.2012.51

26. R. Kessler et al., "The Prevalence and Correlates of Binge Eating Disorder in the World Health Organization World Mental Health Surveys," *Biological Psychiatry* 73, no. 9 (2013): 904–14, doi: 10.1016/j.biopsych.2012.11.020

27. National Institute of Mental Health, "Eating Disorders," January 2013, www.nimh.nih.gov/health/topics/eating-disorders/index.shtml

28. T. A. Oberndorfer et al., "Altered Insula Response to Sweet Taste Processing After Recovery from Anorexia and Bulimia Nervosa," *American Journal of Psychiatry* 170, no. 10 (2013): 1143–51.

29. Mayo Clinic, "Binge-Eating Disorder," April 2012, www.mayoclinic.com/health/binge-eating-disorder/DS00608

30. R. Kessler et al., "The Prevalence and Correlates of Binge Eating Disorder," 2013.

31. National Eating Disorder Association, "Other Specified Feeding or Eating Disorder," March 2014, www.nationaleatingdisorders.org/other-specified-feeding-or-eating-disorder

32. K. N. Franco, Cleveland Clinic Center for Continuing Education, "Eating Disorders," 2011, www.clevelandclinicmeded.com/medicalpubs/diseasemanagement/psychiatry-psychology/

eating-disorders; Mirasol Eating Disorder Recovery Centers, "Eating Disorder Statistics," March 2014, www.mirasol.net/eating-disorders/information/eating-disorder-statistics.php

33. M. Smith, L. Robinson, and J. Segal, "Helping Someone with an Eating Disorder," Helpguide.org, February 2014, www.helpguide.org/mental/eating_disorder_self_help.htm; C. Biggs, "On the Outside: Helping a Friend through an Eating Disorder," Act: Every Action Counts, February 28, 2013, http://act.mtv.com/posts/neda-week-helping-a-friend-through-an-eating-disorder

34. National Eating Disorder Association, "Find Help and Support," March 2014, www.nationaleating-disorders.org/find-help-support

35. H. Goodwin, E. Haycraft, and C. Meyer, "The Relationship between Compulsive Exercise and Emotion Regulation in Adolescents," British Journal of Health Psychology 17, no. 4 (2012): 699–710.

36. J. J. Waldron, "When Building Muscle Turns into Muscle Dysmorphia," Association for Sport Applied Psychology, March 2014, www.appliedsportpsych.org/resource-center/health-fitness-resources/when-building-muscle-turns-into-muscle-dysmorphia

37. M. Silverman, "What is Muscle Dysmorphia?" Massachusetts General Hospital, February 18, 2011, https://mghocd.org/what-is-muscle-dysmorphia; J. J. Waldron, "When Building Muscle Turns into Muscle Dysmorphia," 2014.

38. L. M. Gottschlich et al., "Female Athlete Triad," 2014.

**Pulled Statistics:**

Page 318, C. Ross, "Why Do Women Hate Their Bodies?" World of Psychology, Blog, Psych Central, June 2, 2012, http://psychcentral.com/blog/archives/2012/06/02/why-dowomen-hate-their-bodies

## Chapter 11: Improving Your Personal Fitness

1. Centers for Disease Control and Prevention (CDC), "Behavioral Risk Factor Surveillance System Prevalence and Trends Data," March 2014, http://apps.nccd.cdc.gov/BRFSS/display .asp?yr=2012&state=US&qkey=8041&grp=0&SUBMIT3=Go

2. Ibid.

3. Ibid.

4. C. E. Garber et al., "American College of Sports Medicine Position Stand: Quantity and Quality of Exercise for Developing and Maintaining Cardiorespiratory, Musculoskeletal and Neuromotor Fitness in Apparently Healthy Adults: Guidance for Prescribing Exercise," Medicine and Science in Sports and Exercise 33, no. 7 (2011): 1334–59, doi: 10.1249/MSS.0b013e318213fefb

5. American College Health Association, American College Health Association-National College Health Assessment II (ACHA-NCHA II): Reference Group Executive Summary, Spring 2014 (Hanover, MD: American College Health Association, 2014), Available at www.acha-ncha.org/docs/ACHA-NCHAII_ReferenceGroup_ExecutiveSummary_Spring2014.pdf

6. Lee et al., "Impact of Physical Inactivity on the World's Major Non-communicable Diseases," Lancet 380, no. 9838 (2012): 219–29.

7. S. Plowman and D. Smith, Exercise Physiology for Health, Fitness, and Performance, 3rd ed. (Philadelphia, PA: Lippincott Williams & Wilkins,2011).

8. 8S. Grover et al., "Estimating the Benefits of Patient and Physician Adherence to Cardiovascular Prevention Guidelines: The MyHealth-Checkup Survey," Canadian Journal of Cardiology 27, no. 2 (2011): 159–66, doi: 10.1016/j .cjca.2011.01.007

9. American Heart Association, "About Cholesterol," Updated July 31, 2014, www.heart.org

10. L. Montesi et al., "Physical Activity for the Prevention and Treatment of Metabolic Disorders," Internal and Emergency Medicine 8, no. 8 (2013): 655–66.

11. Ibid.

12. D. C. Lee et al., "Changes in Fitness and Fatness on the Development of Cardiovascular Disease Risk Factors Hypertension, Metabolic Syndrome, and Hypercholesterolemia," Journal of the American College of Cardiology 59, no. 7 (2012): 665–72, doi: 10.1016/j.jacc.2011.11.013

13. M. Uusitupa, J. Tuomilehto, and P. Puska, "Are We Really Active in the Prevention of Obesity and Type 2 Diabetes at the Community Level?," Nutrition and Metabolism in Cardiovascular Diseases 21, no. 5 (2011): 380–89, doi: 10.1016/j.numecd.2010.12.007

14. National Diabetes Information Clearinghouse, U.S. Department of Health and Human Services, Diabetes Prevention Program (DPP), (Bethesda, MD: National Diabetes Information Clearinghouse, 2008), NIH Publication no. 09–5099, Available at http://diabetes.niddk.nih.gov

15. J. Erdrich, X. Zhang, E. Giovannucci, and W. Willet, "Proportion of Colon Cancer Attributable to Lifestyle in a Cohort of US Women," Cancer, Causes & Control (2015), doi: 10.1007/s10552-015-0619-z (Epub ahead of print); M. Harvie, A. Howell, and D. Evans, "Can Diet and Lifestyle Prevent Breast Cancer: What is the Evidence?" ASCO Educational Book 35, (2015): e66–73, doi: 10.14694/EdBook_AM.2015.35.e66

16. World Cancer Research Fund/American Institute for Cancer Research, Policy and Action for Cancer Prevention. Food, Nutrition, and Physical Activity: A Global Perspective (Washington, DC: American Institute for Cancer Research, 2009), Available at www.dietandcancerreport.org

17. Ibid.; F. Canches-Gomas et al., "Physical Inactivity and Low Fitness Deserve More Attention to Alter Cancer Risk and Prognosis," Cancer Prevention Research 8 (2015): 105–110; D. Schmid and M. Leitzman, "Association between Physical Activity and Mortality among Breast Cancer and Colorectal Cancer Survivors: A Systematic Review and Meta-analysis," Annals of Oncology 25, no. 7 (2014):1293–1311, doi:10.1093/annonc/mdu012; D. Brenner et al., "Physical Activity After Breast Cancer: Effect on Survival and Patient-reported Outcomes," Current Breast Cancer Reports 6 (2014): 193–204.

18. C. Denlinger, et al. "Survivorship: Health Lifestyles," Journal of National Comprehensive Cancer Network 12, no. 9 (2014): 122–27; D. Brenner et al. "Physical Activity After Breast Cancer," 2014.

19. M. Nilsson et al., "Increased Physical Activity Is Associated with Enhanced Development of Peak Bone Mass in Men: A Five Year Longitudinal Study," Journal of Bone and Mineral Research 27, no. 5 (2012): 1206–14, doi: 10.1002/jbmr.1549; M. Callréus et al., "Self-Reported Recreational Exercise Combining Regularity and Impact Is Necessary to Maximize Bone Mineral Density in Young Adult Women: A Population-Based Study of 1,061 Women 25 Years of Age," Osteoporosis International 23, no. 10 (2012): 2517–26, doi: 10.1007/s00198-011-1886-5

20. R. Rizzoli, C. A. Abraham, and M. L. Brandi, "Nutrition and Bone Health: Turning Knowledge and Beliefs in Healthy Behavior," Current Medical Research & Opinion 30, no. 1 (2014): 131–41.

21. V. A. Catenacci et al., "Physical Activity Patterns Using Accelerometry in the National Weight Control Registry," Obesity 19, no. 6 (2011): 1163–70, doi: 10.1038/oby.2010.264

22. T. L. Gillum et al., "A Review of Sex Differences in Immune Function After Aerobic Exercise," Exercise Immunology Review 17 (2011): 104–20.

23. MedLine Plus, National Institutes of Health, "Exercise and Immunity," Updated May 13, 2012, www.nlm.nih.gov

24. N. P. Walsh et al., "Position Statement. Part Two: Maintaining Immune Health," Exercise and Immunology Review 17 (2011): 64–103.

25. M. W. Kakanis et al., "The Open Window of Susceptibility to Infection After Acute Exercise in Healthy Young Male Elite Athletes," Exercise Immunology Review 16 (2010): 119–37.

26. C. Huang et al., "Cardiovascular Reactivity, Stress, and Physical Activity," Frontiers in Physiology 4 (2013): 1–13, doi:10.3389/fphys.201300314

27. S. Covell et al. "Physical Activity Level and Future Risks of Mild Cognitive Impairment or Dementia: A Critically Appraised Topic," Neurologist 19, no. 3 (2015): 89–91; T. M. Burkhalter and C. H. Hillman, "A Narrative Review of Physical Activity, Nutrition, and Obesity to Cognitive and Scholastic Performance across the Human Lifespan," Advances in Nutrition: An International Review Journal 2, no. 2 (2011): 201S –206S; C. Hogan, "Exercise Holds Immediate Benefits for Affect and Cognition in Younger and Older Adults," Psychology of Aging 28, no. 2 (2013): 587–94.

28. M. Daly, D. McMinn, and J. Allan, "A Bidirectional Relationship between Physical Activity and Executive Function in Older Adults," Frontiers in Human Neuroscience 8 (2014): 1–9.

29. J. Hu et al., "Exercise Improves Cognitive Function in Aging Patients," International Journal of Clinical and Experimental Medicine 7, no. 10 (2014): 3144–49.

30. M. Beckett et al., "A Meta-analysis of Prospective Studies in the Role of Physical Activity and the Prevention of Alzheimer's Disease in Older Adults," BMC Geriatrics 15, no. 9 ( 2015), doi:10.10.1186/s12877-015-0007-2

31. J. Woodcock, O. Franco, N. Orsini, and I. Roberts, "Non-Vigorous Physical Activity and All-Cause Mortality: Systematic Review and Meta-Analysis of Cohort Studies," International Journal of Epidemiology 40, no. 1 (2011): 121–38.

32. J. Berry et al., "Lifetime Risks for Cardiovascular Disease Mortality by Cardiorespiratory Fitness Levels Measured at Ages 45, 55, and 65 Years in Men: The Cooper Center Longitudinal Study," Journal of the American College of Cardiology 57, no. 15 (2011): 1604–10, doi: 10.1016/j.jacc.2010.10.056

33. D. Dunlop et al., "Sedentary Time in US Older Adults Associated with Disability in Activities of Daily Living Independent of Physical Activity," Journal of Physical Activity and Health 12, no. 1(2015): 93–101.

34. American College of Sports Medicine, ACSM's Guidelines for Exercise Testing and Prescription, 9th ed. (Baltimore, MD: Lippincott Williams & Wilkins, 2014).

35. C. E. Garber et al., "American College of Sports Medicine Position Stand: Quantity and Quality of Exercise for Developing and Maintaining Cardiorespiratory, Musculoskeletal and Neuromotor Fitness in Apparently Healthy Adults: Guidance for Prescribing Exercise," Medicine and Science in Sports and Exercise 43, no. 7 (2011): 1334–59.

36. Ibid.

37. Ibid.

38. American College of Sports Medicine, *ACSM's Resource Manual for Guidelines for Exercise Testing and Prescription* (Philadelphia, PA: Lippincott Williams & Wilkins, 2014).

39. W. Micheo, L. Baerga, and G. Miranda, "Basic Principles Regarding Strength, Flexibility, Flexibility, and Stability Exercises," *Physical Medicine & Rehabilitation* 4, no. 11 (2012): 805–11, doi: 10.1016/j.pmrj.2012.09.583

40. Ibid.

41. M. Pahor et al., "Effect of Structured Physical Activity on Prevention of Major Mobility Disability in Older Adults: The LIFE Study Randomized Clinical Trial," *JAMA* 311, no. 23 (2014): 2387–96, doi:10.1001/jama.2014.5616

42. American College of Sports Medicine, *Guidelines for Exercise Testing and Prescription*, 2014.

43. Ibid.

44. D. G. Behm and A. Chaouachi, "A Review of the Acute Effects of Static and Dynamic Stretching on Performance," *European Journal of Applied Physiology* 111, no. 11 (2011): 2633–51, doi: 10.1007/s00421-011-1879-2

45. K. C. Huxel Bliven and B. E. Anderson, "Core Stability Training for Injury Prevention," *Sports Health: A Multidisciplinary Approach* 5, no.6 (2013): 514–22.

46. Ibid.

47. D. G. Behm and J. C. Colao Sanchez, "Instability Resistance Training Across the Exercise Continuum," *Sports Health: A Multidisciplinary Approach* 5, no. 6 (2013): 500–3.

48. Ibid.

49. M. N. Sawka et al., "American College of Sports Medicine Position Stand: Exercise and Fluid Replacement," *Medicine and Science in Sports and Exercise* 39, no. 2 (2007): 377–90.

50. Ibid.

51. K. Pritchett and R. Pritchett, "Chocolate Milk: Post-Exercise Recovery Beverage for Endurance Sports," *Medicine and Sports Science* 59 (2011): 127–34.

52. K. B. Fields et al., "Prevention of Running Injuries," *Current Sports Medicine Reports* 9, no. 3 (2010): 176–82, doi: 10.1249/JSR.0b013e3181de7ec5

53. American Academy of Ophthalmology, "Eye Health in Sports and Recreation," March 2014, www.aao.org/eyesmart/injuries/eyewear.cfm

54. Ibid.

55. Bicycle Helmet Safety Institute, "Helmet-Related Statistics from Many Sources," January 2014, www.helmets.org/stats.htm

56. American College Health Association, *National College Health Assessment II: Reference Group Data Report, Spring 2013*, 2013.

57. Bicycle Helmet Safety Institute, "Helmet-Related Statistics from Many Sources," 2014.

58. N. G. Nelson et al., "Exertional Heat-Related Injuries Treated in Emergency Departments in the U.S., 1997–2006," *American Journal of Preventive Medicine* 40, no. 1 (2011): 54–60, doi: 10.1016/j.amepre.2010.09.031

59. E. E. Turk, "Hypothermia," *Forensic Science Medical Pathology* 6, no. 2 (2010): 106–115, doi: 10.1007/s12024-010-9142-4

60. Ibid.

61. American Council on Exercise, "Exercising in the Cold," Fit Facts, Blog, 2010, www.acefitness.org

**Pulled Statistics:**

Page 330, Centers for Disease Control and Prevention–Division of Nutrition, Physical Activity and Obesity, "How Much Physical Activity Do Adults Need?" *Physical Activity for Everyone,* June 2015, www.cdc.gov/physicalactivity/basics/adults/index.htm

Page 334, Centers for Disease Control and Prevention (CDC), "Nutrition, Physical Activity and Obesity: Data, Trends, and Maps," June 30, 2015, www.cdc.gov/nccdphp/DNPAO/index.html

## Chapter 12: Reducing Your Risk of Cardiovascular Disease and Cancer

1. M. Naghavi et al., "Global, Regional, and National Age-Sex Specific All-Cause and Cause-Specific Mortality for 240 Causes of Death, 1990–2013: A Systematic Analysis for the Global Burden of Disease Study 2013," *The Lancet* 117, no. 171 (2015): 385

2. Ibid.

3. World Health Organization, "10 Facts on the State of Global Health," April 2015, www.who.int/features/factfiles/global_burden/facts/en/index3.html

4. American Cancer Society, *Cancer Facts and Figures 2015* (Atlanta, GA: American Cancer Society, 2015), Available at www.cancer.org/acs/groups/content/@editorial/documents/document/acspc-044552.pdf

5. Ibid.

6. Ibid.

7. D. Mozaffarian et al., "Heart Disease and Stroke Statistics, 2015 Update," *Circulation* 131 (2015): e29–2322.

8. Ibid.

9. Ibid.

10. Ibid.

11. Ibid.

12. Ibid.

13. Ibid.

14. American Heart Association, "Cardiovascular Health," April 2015, www.heart.org/idc/groups/heart-public/@wcm/@sop/@smd/documents/downloadable/ucm_462014.pdf; D. M. Lloyd-Jones et al., "Defining and Setting National Goals for Cardiovascular Health Promotion and Disease Reduction: The AHA's Strategic Impact Goal through 2020 and Beyond," *Circulation* 121 (2010): e14–e31.

15. American Heart Association, "Cardiovascular Health," 2015; D. Mozaffarian et al., "Heart Disease and Stroke Statistics," 2015.

16. D. Mozaffarian et al., "Heart Disease and Stroke Statistics," 2015.

17. H. Ning et al., "Status of Cardiovascular Health in US Children Up to 11 Years of Age. The National Health and Nutrition Examination Surveys 2003–2010." *Circulation: Cardiovascular Quality and Outcomes* 8, no. 2 (2015): 164–171, doi: 10.1161/CIRCOUTCOMES.114.001274); L. Hayman and S. Camhi. "Ideal Cardiovascular Health in Adolescence is Associated with Reduced Risks of Hypertension, Metabolic Syndrome and High Cholesterol," *Evidence Based Nursing* 16, no. 1 (2013): 24–5, doi:10.1136/eb-2012-100887

18. American Heart Association, "Why Blood Pressure Matters," August 2014, www.heart.org/HEARTORG/Conditions/HighBloodPressure/WhyBloodPressureMatters/Why-Blood-Pressure-Matters_UCM_002051_Article.jsp

19. D. Mozaffarian et al., "Heart Disease and Stroke Statistics," 2015.

20. Ibid.

21. Ibid.

22. Ibid.

23. L. Rutten-Jacobs et al., "Cardiovascular Disease Is the Main Cause of Long-Term Excess Mortality after Ischemic Stroke in Young Adults," *Hypertension* 65, no. 3 (2015): 670–75.

24. D. Mozaffarian et al., "Heart Disease and Stroke Statistics," 2015.

25. Centers for Disease Control and Prevention, "High Blood Pressure Facts," February 19, 2015, www.cdc.gov/bloodpressure/facts.htm

26. C. Rosendorf et al., "Treatment of Hypertension in Patients with Coronary Artery Disease: A Scientific Statement from the American Heart Association, American College of Cardiology, and American Society of Hypertension," *Journal of the American College of Cardiology* 65, no. 18, (2015): 1998–2038; P. James et al., "2014 Evidence-Based Guideline for the Management of High Blood Pressure in Adults: Report From the Panel Members Appointed to the Eighth Joint National Committee (JNC 8)," *Journal of American Medical Association,* 311, no. 5 (2014): 507–20, doi:10.1001/jama213.284427

27. D. Mozaffarian et al., "Heart Disease and Stroke Statistics," 2015; American Heart Association, About Peripheral Artery Disease, August 2014, www.heart.org/HEARTORG/Conditions/More/PeripheralArteryDisease/About-Peripheral-Artery-Disease-PAD_UCM_301301_Article.jsp

28. Ibid.

29. D. Mozaffarian et al., "Heart Disease and Stroke Statistics," 2015.

30. American Heart Association, "Angina in Women Can Be Different than Men," April 2015, www.heart.org/HEARTORG/Conditions/HeartAttack/WarningSignsofaHeartAttack/Angina-in-Women-Can-Be-Different-Than-Men_UCM_448902_Article.jsp

31. D. Mozaffarian et al., "Heart Disease and Stroke Statistics," 2015; American Heart Association, "Angina (Chest Pain)," April 2015, www.heart.org/HEARTORG/Conditions/HeartAttack/SymptomsDiagnosisofHeartAttack/Angina-Chest-Pain_UCM_450308_Article .jsp; American Heart Association, "Angina in Women," 2015.

32. D. Mozaffarian et al., "Heart Disease and Stroke Statistics," 2015.

33. Ibid.

34. B. M. Kissel et al., "Age at Stroke: Temporal Trends in Stroke Incidence in a Large, Biracial Population," *Neurology* 79 (2012): 1781–87.

35. Ibid.

36. American Stroke Association, "Stroke Treatments," May 2013, www.strokeassociation.org/STROKEORG/AboutStroke/Treatment/Stroke-Treatments_UCM_310892_Article.jsp

37. C. J. L. Murray et al., "The State of US Health, 1990–2010 Burden of Diseases, Injuries, and Risk Factors," *Journal of the American Medical Association* 310, no. 6 (2013): 591–608.

38. D. Mozaffarian et al., "Heart Disease and Stroke Statistics," 2015; A. Noortie, "Ischaemic Stroke in Young Adults: Risk Factors and Long-term Consequences," *Nature Reviews Neurology* 10, no. 6 (2014):315–25; S. Saydah, "Cardiometabolic Risk Factors among US Adolescents and Young Adults and Risk of Early Mortality," *Pediatrics* 131 (2013): e679–86.

39. L. Nelson et al., "Hypertension and Inflammation in Alzheimer's Disease: Close Partners in Disease Development and Progression!," *Journal of Alzheimer's Disease* 41, no. 2 (2014): 331–33; S. Sharp et al., "Hypertension Is a Potential Risk Factor for Vascular Dementia: Systematic Review," *International Journal of Geriatric Psychiatry* 26, no. 7, (2011): 661–69.

40. H. Beltrain-Sanchez et al., "Prevalence and Trends in Metabolic Syndrome in the Adult U.S. Population, 1999–2010," *Journal of the American*

*College of Cardiology* 62, no. 8, (2013): 607–703; D. Mozaffarian et al., "Heart Disease and Stroke Statistics," 2015.

41. D. Mozaffarian et al., "Heart Disease and Stroke Statistics," 2015; S. Grundy et al., "Definition of Metabolic Syndrome. Report of the National Heart, Lung, and Blood Institute/American Heart Association Conference on Scientific Issues Related to Definition," *Circulation* 109, no. 2, (2011): 433–38.

42. A. Noortie. "Ischaemic Stroke in Young Adults," 2014; S. Saydah, "Cardiometabolic Risk Factors among US Adolescents and Young Adults and Risk of Early Mortality," 2013.

43. D. Mozaffarian et al., "Heart Disease and Stroke Statistics," 2015.

44. Ibid.

45. National Cancer Institute, "Fact Sheet: Harms of Smoking and Benefits of Quitting," January 2011, www.cancer.gov

46. D. Keene et al., "Effect on Cardiovascular Risk of High Density Lipoprotein Targeted Drug Treatments Niacin, Fibrates, and CETP Inhibitors: Meta-analysis of Randomised Controlled Trials Including 117,411 Patients," *British Medical Journal* 349 (2014): g4379, doi: http://dx.doi.org/10.1136/bmj.g4379; G. Schwarts et al., "Effects of Dalcetrapib in Patients with a Recent Acute Coronary Syndrome," *New England Journal of Medicine* 367 (2012): 2089–99; C. Zheng and M. Aikawa, "High Density Lipoproteins: From Function to Therapy," *American College of Cardiology* 60, no. 23 (2012): 2380–83.

47. D. Mozaffarian et al., "Heart Disease and Stroke Statistics," 2015.

48. National Center For Health Statistics, "Health, United States, 2011: With Special Features on Socioeconomic Status and Health," 2012, www.cdc.gov

49. D. Mozaffarian et al., "Heart Disease and Stroke Statistics," 2015.

50. Ibid.; Y. Chida and A. Steptoe, "Greater Cardiovascular Responses to Laboratory Mental Stress Are Associated with Poor Subsequent Cardiovascular Risk Status: A Meta-Analysis of Prospective Evidence," *Hypertension* 55 (2010): 1026–32.

51. T. Kotchen, A. Cowley and E. Frohlich, "Salt in Health and Disease–A Delicate Balance," *New England Journal of Medicine* 368 (2013): 1229–37.

52. A. Steptoe and M. Kivimaki, "Stress and Cardiovascular Disease: An Update on Current Knowledge," *Annual Review of Public Health* 34 (2013): 337–54, doi: 10.1146/annurev-publhealth-031912-114452; C. Vlachopoulous, P. Xaplanteris, and C. Stefanadis, "Mental Stress, Arterial Stiffness, Central Pressures and Cardiovascular Risk," *Hypertension* 56, no. 3 (2010): e28–e30.

53. A. Steptoe and M. Kivimaki, "Stress and Cardiovascular Disease," 2013; R. C. Thurston, M. Rewak, and L.D. Kubzansky, "An Anxious Heart: Anxiety and the Onset of Cardiovascular Diseases," *Progress in Cardiovascular Diseases* 55, no. 6 (2013):524–37.

54. D. Mozaffarian et al., "Heart Disease and Stroke Statistics," 2015.

55. T Huang and F. Hu, "Gene-Environmental Interactions and Obesity: Recent Developments and Future Directions," *BMC Medical Genomics* 8, Supplement 1 (2015): S2; G. Thanassoulis et al., "A Genetic Risk Score Is Associated with Incident Cardiovascular Disease and Coronary Artery Calcium," *Circulation: Cardiovascular Genetics* 5, no. 1 (2012): 113–21; C. Chow et al., "Parental History

and Myocardial Infarction Risk across the World: The Interheart Study," *Journal of the American College of Cardiology* 57 (2011): 619–27.

56. D. Mozaffarian et al., "Heart Disease and Stroke Statistics," 2015.

57. Ibid.

58. The Emerging Risk Factors Collaboration, "C-Reactive Protein, Fibrinogen and CVD Prediction," *New England Journal of Medicine* 367 (2012). 1310–20.

59. "The PLAC Test: Predicting Heart Attack Risk in People with No Symptoms." *Scientific American-Health After 50*, 27, no. 2 (2015): 1–2.

60. R. Chowdhury et al., "Association of Dietary, Circulating, and Supplement Fatty Acids with Coronary Risk: A Systematic Review and Meta Analysis," *Annals of Internal Medicine* 160, no. 6 (2014): 398–406, doi:10.7326?M13-1788; The ORIGIN Trial Investigators, "n–3 Fatty Acids and Cardiovascular Outcomes in Patients with Dysglycemia," *New England Journal of Medicine* 367 (2012): 309–18, doi: 10.1056/NEJMoa1203859

61. American Heart Association, "Fish and Omega 3 Fatty Acids," May 14, 2014, www.heart.org/HEARTORG/General/Fish-and-Omega-3-Fatty-Acids_UCM_303248_Article.jsp

62. B. Keavney, "C-reactive Protein and the Risk for Cardiovascular Disease," British Medical Journal 342 (2011): d144; The Emerging Risk Factors Collaboration, "C-reactive Protein Concentration and Risk of Coronary Heart Disease, Stroke, and Mortality: An Individual Participant Meta-analysis," The Lancet 375, no. 9709 (2010): 132–140.

63. D. Wald, J. Morris, and N. Wald, "Reconciling the Evidence on Serum Homocysteine and Ischemic Heart Disease: A Meta-Analysis," *PLoS ONE* 6, no. 2: e16473; J. Abraham and L. Cho, "The Homocysteine Hypothesis: Still Relevant to the Prevention and Treatment of Cardiovascular Disease?," *Cleveland Clinic Journal of Medicine* 77, no. 12 (2010): 911–18.

64. American Heart Association, "Homocysteine, Folic Acid, and Cardiovascular Disease," March 18, 2014., www.heart.org

65. FDA, "Can an Aspirin a Day Help Prevent a Heart Attack?," May 5, 2014, www.fda.gov/ForConsumers/ConsumerUpdates/ucm390539.htm; Y. Ikeda et al., "Low-Dose Aspirin for Primary Prevention of Cardiovascular Events in Japanese Patients 60 Years or Older with Atherosclerotic Risk Factors: A Randomized Clinical Trial," *Journal of the American Medical Association* 312, no. 23 (2014): 2510–20; C. M. Rembold, "ACP Journal Club Review: Aspirin Does Not Reduce CHD or Cancer Mortality but Increases Bleeding," *Annals of Internal Medicine* 156, no. 12 (2012): JC6–3.

66. American Heart Association, "Prevention and Treatment of Heart Attack," August 2014, www.heart.org

67. D. Mozaffarian et al., "Heart Disease and Stroke Statistics," 2015.

68. American Cancer Society, *Cancer Facts and Figures*, 2015, www.cancer.org

69. American Cancer Society, "Cancer Treatment and Survivorship–Facts and Figures 2014–2015," 2014, www.cancer.org/acs/groups/content/@research/documents/document/acspc-042801.pdf

70. American Cancer Society, *Cancer Facts and Figures*, 2015.

71. National Cancer Institute, "Fact Sheet: Cancer Staging, 2015," January 6, 2015, www.cancer.gov/cancertopics/diagnosis-staging/staging/staging-fact-sheet

72. American Cancer Society, *Cancer Facts and Figures*, 2015.

73. Ibid.

74. American Cancer Society, *Cancer Facts and Figures*, 2015; Centers for Disease Control and Prevention, Smoking and Cancer, April 2015, www.cdc.gov/tobacco/data_statistics/sgr/50th-anniversary/pdfs/fs_smoking_cancer_508.pdf

75. M. Thun et al., "50 Year Trends in Smoking-Related Mortality in the U.S.," *New England Journal of Medicine* 368, (2013): 351–64.

76. American Cancer Society, *Cancer Facts and Figures*, 2015.

77. C. Eheman et al., "Annual Report to the Nation on the Status of Cancer, 1975–2008, Featuring Cancers Associated with Excess Weight and Lack of Sufficient Physical Activity," *Cancer* 118, no. 9 (2012): 2338–66, doi: 10.1002/cncr.27514/full; American Cancer Society, "Nutrition and Physical Activity Research Highlights," April 2015, www.cancer.org/research/acsresearchupdates/nutrition-and-physical-activity-research-highlights; W. Blot and R Tarone, "Doll and Peto's Quantitative Estimates of Cancer Risks: Holding Generally True for 35 Years," *Journal of the National Cancer Institute* 107, no. 4, (2015): djr044, http://jnci.oxfordjournals.org/content/107/4/djv044.full

78. H. R. Harris et al., "Body Fat Distribution and Risk of Premenopausal Breast Cancer in the Nurses' Health Study II," *Journal of the National Cancer Institute* 103, no. 3 (2011): 373–78.

79. R. Kaaks and T. Kuhn, "Epidemiology: Obesity and Cancer—The Evidence is Fattening Up," *Nature Reviews Endocrinology* 10 (2014): 644–45.

80. K. Bhaskaran et al., "Body-mass Index and Risk of 22 Specific Cancers: A Population-based Cohort Study of 5.24 million UK Adults," *The Lancet* 384 (2014): 755–65; C. Eheman et al., "Annual Report to the Nation on the Status of Cancer," 1975–2008, 2012.

81. American Cancer Society, "Family Cancer Syndromes," June 25, 2014, www.cancer.org/cancer/cancercauses/geneticsandcancer/heredity-and-cancer

82. American Cancer Society, "Breast Cancer Overview: What Causes Breast Cancer?," February 26, 2015, www.cancer.org/Cancer/BreastCancer/DetailedGuide/breast-cancer-what-causes

83. American Cancer Society, "Cancer Facts and Figures for Hispanic/Latinos," 2012–2014, April 2015, www.cancer.org/acs/groups/content/@epidemiologysurveilance/documents/document/acspc-034778.pdf; M. Banegas et al., "The Risk of Developing Invasive Breast Cancer in Hispanic Women," *Cancer* 119, no. 7 (2013): 1373–80.

84. O. Kiraly et al., "Inflammation-Induced Cell Proliferation Potentiates DNA Damage-Induced Mutations in Vivo," *PLoS Genetics* 11, no. 2 (2015): e1004901; S. Sebastian et al., "Colorectal Cancer in Inflammatory Bowel Disease: Results of the 3rd ECCO Pathogenesis Scientific Workshop (I)," *Journal of Crohn's and Colitis* 8, no. 1 (2014): 5–18.

85. National Cancer Institute, "Cell Phones and Cancer Risk," March 2013, www.cancer.gov; S. Joachim et al., "Cellular Telephone Use and Cancer Risk: Update of a Nationwide Danish Cohort," *Journal of the National Cancer Institute* 98, no. 23 (2006): 1707–13.

86. American Cancer Society, "Can Infections Cause Cancer?," September 24, 2014, www.cancer.org/cancer/cancercauses/othercarcinogens/infectiousagents/infectiousagentsandcancer/infectious-agents-and-cancer-intro; American Cancer Society, "Infectious Agents and Cancer," March 2013, www.cancer.org

87. American Cancer Society, "Can Infections Cause Cancer," 2014.

88. American Cancer Society, *Cancer Facts and Figures*, 2015.

89. National Cancer Institute, "Cervical Cancer," April 2015, www.cancer.gov

90. American Cancer Society, *Cancer Facts and Figures*, 2015.

91. American Cancer Society, "Lung Cancer Risks for Non-Smokers," October 31, 2014, www .cancer.org/cancer/news/why-lung-cancer-strikes-nonsmokers

92. American Cancer Society, *Cancer Facts and Figures*, 2015.

93. American Cancer Society, "When Smokers Quit, What Are the Benefits Over Time?," February 2014, www.cancer.org/healthy/stayawayfrom-tobacco/guidetoquittingsmoking/guide-to-quitting-smoking-benefits

94. American Cancer Society, *Cancer Facts and Figures*, 2015.

95. Ibid.

96. Ibid.

97. American Cancer Society, "Statistics Report: 1.5 million Cancer Deaths Avoided in 2 Decades," December 31, 2014, www.cancer.org/cancer/news/news/facts-figures-report-cancer-deaths-avoided-in-2-decades

98. American Cancer Society, *Cancer Facts and Figures*, 2015.

99. Ibid.

100. Ibid.

101. Ibid.

102. Susan G. Komen for the Cure, "Genetic Testing for BRCA1 and BRCA2 Gene," January 2015, ww5.komen.org/BreastCancer/GeneMutationsampGeneticTesting.html

103. I. Lahart et al., "Physical Activity, Risk of Death and Recurrence in Breast Cancer Survivors: A Systematic Review and Meta-analysis of Epidemiological Studies," *Acta Oncologica* 54, no. 5 (2015): 635–54, doi:10.3109/0284186X.2014.998275; Y. Wu et al., "Physical Activity and Risk of Breast Cancer: A Meta-analysis of Prospective Studies," *Breast Cancer Research and Treatment* 137, no. 3 (2013): 869–82; R. Patterson, L. Cadmus, and T. Emond, "Physical Activity, Diet, Adiposity and Female Breast Cancer Prognosis: A Review of Epidemiological Literature," *Maturitas* 66 (2010): 5–15.

104. Y. Wu et al., "Meta-Analysis of Studies on Breast Cancer Risk and Diet in Chinese Women," *International Journal of Clinical and Experimental Medicine* 8, no. 11 (2015): 73–85; D. Aune et al., "Dietary Fiber and Breast Cancer Risks: A Systematic Review and Meta Analysis of Prospective Studies," *Annals of Oncology* 23, no. 6. (2012): 1394–402, doi: 10.1093/annuls/mdr589

105. American Cancer Society, *Cancer Facts and Figures*, 2015.

106. Ibid.

107. FDA, "FDA Approves 1st Non-invasive DNA Screening for Colorectal Cancer," August 11, 2014, www.fda.gov/NewsEvents/Newsroom/PressAnnouncements/ucm409021.htm

108. Ibid.; National Cancer Institute, "Colorectal Cancer Prevention," 2015, www.cancer.gov/cancertopics/pdq/prevention/colorectal/Patient/page3#_139

109. American Cancer Society, *Cancer Facts and Figures*, 2015.

110. Ibid.

111. Ibid.

112. Ibid.

113. Ibid.

114. Ibid.

115. Ibid.

116. Ibid.

117. Ibid.

118. American Cancer Society, "Prostate Cancer," April, 2015, www.cancer.org

119. American Cancer Society, *Cancer Facts and Figures*, 2015.

120. Ibid.

121. Ibid.

122. Ibid.

123. Ibid.

124. Ibid.; American Cancer Society, "Testicular Cancer," 2015, www.cancer.org/acs/groups/cid/documents/webcontent/003142-pdf.pdf

125. National Cancer Institute, "Testicular Cancer," 2013, www.cancer.gov

126. American Cancer Society, "Testicular Cancer," 2015.

127. American Cancer Society, *Cancer Facts and Figures*, 2015.

**Pulled Statistics:**

Page 356, D. Mozaffarian et al., "Heart Disease and Stroke Statistics, 2015 Update," *Circulation* 131 (2015): e29–2322.

Page 359, D. Mozaffarian et al., "Heart Disease and Stroke Statistics, 2015 Update," *Circulation* 131 (2015): e29–2322.

Page 371, American Cancer Society, *Cancer Facts and Figures 2015* (Atlanta, GA: American Cancer Society, 2015), Available at www.cancer.org/acs/groups/content/@editorial/documents/document/acspc-044552.pdf

## Focus On: Minimizing Your Risk for Diabetes

1. E. Selvin et al., "Trends in Prevalence and Control of Diabetes in the United States, 1988–1994 and 1999–2010," *Annals of Internal Medicine* 160, no. 8 (2014): 517–25.

2. Centers for Disease Control and Prevention, "National Diabetes Statistics Report, 2014," May 2015, www.cdc.gov/diabetes/pubs/statsreport14/national-diabetes-report-web .pdf; American Diabetes Association, "Fast Facts," March 2015, http://professional.diabetes.org/admin/UserFiles/0%20-%20Sean/Documents/Fast_Facts_3-2015.pdf; Centers for Disease Control and Prevention, "Early Release of Selected Estimates Based on Data from the National Health Interview Survey–January to June, 2014," May 2015, www .cdc.gov/nchs/data/nhis/earlyrelease/earlyrelease201412.pdf

3. Centers for Disease Control and Prevention, "National Diabetes Statistics Report, 2014," May 2015.

4. Centers for Disease Control and Prevention, "Summary Health Statistics for U.S. Adults: National Health Interview Survey, 2012," *Vital and Health Statistics* 10, no. 260 (2014), available at www.cdc.gov/nchs/products/series/series10.htm

5. T. Dall et al., "The Economic Burden of Elevated Blood Glucose Levels in 2012: Diagnosed and Undiagnosed Diabetes, Gestational Diabetes Mellitus, and Prediabetes," *Diabetes Care* 37, no. 12, (2014): 3172–79.

6. Ibid.

7. American Diabetes Association, "Diabetes Basics: Type 1," May 2014, www.diabetes.org/diabetesbasics/type-1

8. Ibid.

9. Centers for Disease Control and Prevention, "National Diabetes Statistics Report, 2014," May 2015.

10. Ibid.

11. R. Hamman et al., "The SEARCH for Diabetes in Youth Study: Rationale, Findings, and Future Directions," *Diabetes Care* 37, no. 12 (2014): 3336–44, doi: 10.2337/dc14-0574

12. D. J. Pettitt et al., "Prevalence of Diabetes in U.S. Youth in 2009: The SEARCH for Diabetes in Youth Study," *Diabetes Care* 37, no. 2 (2014): 402–08.

13. R. Mihaescu et al., "Genetic Risk Profiling for Prediction of Type 2 Diabetes," *PLoS Currents* 3 (2011): doi: 10.1371/currents.RRN1208, www.ncbi.nlm.nih.gov/pmc/articles/PMC3024707; E. Nizami, R. Evangelia, and F. Kavvoura, "Genetic Risk Factors for Type 2 Diabetes: Insights from the Emerging Genomic Evidence," *Current Vascular Pharmacology* 10, no. 2 (2012): 147–55; K. Colclough et al., "Clinical Utility Gene Card: Maturity-Onset Diabetes of the Young," *European Journal of Human Genetics* (2014): doi: 10.1038/ejhg.2014.14

14. J. Logue et al., "Association between BMI Measured within a Year After Diagnosis of Type 2 Diabetes and Mortality," *Diabetes Care* 36, no. 4 (2013): 887–93; M. Ashwell, P. Gunn, and S. Gibson, "Waist-to-Height Ratio Is a Better Screening Tool than Waist Circumference and BMI for Adult Cardiometabolic Risk Factors: Systematic Review and Meta-Analysis," *Obesity Reviews* 13, no. 3 (2012): 275–86.

15. M. Schulze et al., "Body Adiposity Index, Body Fat Content and Incidence of Type 2 Diabetes," *Diabetologia* (2012), doi: 10.1007/s00125-012-2499-z

16. L. Bromley et al., "Sleep Restriction Decreases the Physical Activity of Adults at Risk for Type 2 Diabetes," *Sleep* 35, no. 7 (2012): 977–84, doi: 10.5665/sleep.1964

17. R. Hancox and C. Landlus, "Association between Sleep Duration and Haemoglobin A1C in Young Adults," *Journal of Epidemiology and Community Health* 66, no. 10 (2011): 957–61; H. C. Hung et al., "The Association between Self-Reported Sleep Quality and Metabolic Syndrome," *PLoS One* 8, no. 1 (2013): e54304, doi:10.1371/journal.pone.0054304; T. Ohkuma et al., "Impact of Sleep Duration on Obesity and the Glycemic Level in Patients with Type 2 Diabetes," *Diabetes Care* 36, no. 3 (2013): 611–17.

18. M. Cosgrove, L. Sargeant, R. Caleyachetty, and S. Griffin, "Work Related Stress and Type 2 Diabetes: A Systematic Review and Meta-Analysis," *Occupational Medicine* (2012), doi: 10.1093/occmed/kqs002; T. Monk and D. J. Buysse, "Exposure to Shiftwork as a Risk Factor for Diabetes," *Journal of Biological Rhythms* 28, no. 5 (2013): 356–59; M. Novak et al., "Perceived Stress and Incidence of Type 2 Diabetes: A 35 Year Follow up Study of Middle Aged Swedish Men," *Diabetic Medicine* 30, no. 1 (2013): e8-3-16.

19. Centers for Disease Control and Prevention (CDC), "National Diabetes Statistics Report, 2014"; CDC, "Prediabetes: Could It Be You?," 2014, www.cdc.gov/diabetes/pubs/statsreport14/prediabetes-infographic.pdf

20. N. Yahia et al., Assessment of College Students' Awareness and Knowledge about Conditions Relevant to Metabolic Syndrome," *Diabetology & Metabolic Syndrome* 6, no. 1 (2014): 111; J. M. Schilter and L. C. Dalleck, "Fitness and Fatness: Indicators of Metabolic Syndrome and Cardiovascular Disease Risk Factors in College Students?," *Journal of Exercise Physiology Online* 13, no. 4 (2010): 29–39.

21. American Heart Association, "Metabolic Syndrome," May 2014, www.heart.org/HEARTORG/Conditions/More/MetabolicSyndrome/Metabolic-Syndrome_UCM_002080_SubHomePage.jsp

22. National Heart Lung and Blood Institute, "What Is Metabolic Syndrome?," November 2011, www.nhlbi.nih.gov/health/dci/Diseases/ms/ms_whatis.html

23. National Heart, Lung, and Blood Institute, "Who Is at Risk for Metabolic Syndrome?," November 2011, www.nhlbi.nih.gov/health/health-topics/topics/ms/atrisk.html

24. Ibid.

25. CDC, "Prediabetes: Could It Be You?," 2014.

26. Centers for Disease Control and Prevention, "Diabetes in the United States – A Snapshot," June, 2014, http://www.cdc.gov/media/dpk/2014/images/diabetes-report/Infographic1-web.pdf

27. L. S. Geiss et al., "Diabetes Risk Reduction Behaviors among U.S. Adults with Prediabetes," *Journal of Preventive Medicine* 38, no. 4 (2010): 403–09; Centers for Disease Control, "National Diabetes Prevention Program: About the Program," October 2012, www.cdc.gov

28. American Diabetes Association, "What Is Gestational Diabetes?," June 2014, www.diabetes .org/diabetes-basics/gestational/what-is-gestational-diabetes.html

29. Ibid; C. Kim et al., "Gestational Diabetes and the Incidence of Type 2 Diabetes: A Systematic Review," *Diabetes Care* 25, no. 10 (2002): 1862–68; G. Chodick et al., "The Risk of Overt Diabetes Mellitus among Women with Gestational Diabetes: A Population-Based Study," *Diabetic Medicine* 27, no. 7 (2010): 779–85.

30. National Healthy Mothers, Healthy Babies Coalition, "The Lasting Impact of Gestational Diabetes on Mother and Children," May 2015, www .hmhb.org/virtual-library/interviews-with-experts/gestational-diabetes

31. P. M. Catalano et al., "The Hyperglycemia and Adverse Pregnancy Outcome Study: Associations of GDM and Obesity with Pregnancy Outcomes," *Diabetes Care* 35, no. 4 (2012): 780, doi: 10.2337/dc11-1790

32. Centers for Disease Control and Prevention, "National Diabetes Statistics Report, 2014," May 2015; American Diabetes Association, "Living with Diabetes: Complications," May 2014, www .diabetes.org/living-with-diabetes/complications/; K. Weinspach et al., "Level of Information about the Relationship between Diabetes Mellitus and Periodontitis—Results from a Nationwide Diabetes Information Program," *European Journal of Medical Research* 18, no. 1 (2013): 6, doi: 10.1186/2047-783X-18-6

33. National Kidney Foundation, "Fast Facts," February 2015, www.kidney.org/news/newsroom/factsheets/FastFacts.cfm

34. Ibid.

35. Centers for Disease Control and Prevention. "National Diabetes Statistics Report, 2014," May 2015.

36. Ibid.

37. Prevent Blindness America, "Diabetic Retinopathy Prevalence by Age," May 2014, www .visionproblemsus.org/diabetic-retinopathy/diabetic-retinopathy-by-age.html

38. American Diabetes Association, "Diabetes and Oral Health Problems," October 2014, www .diabetes.org/living-with-diabetes/treatment-and-care/oral-health-and-hygiene/diabetes-and-oral-health.html

39. Ibid.

40. K. Behan, "New ADA Guidelines for Diagnosis, Screening of Diabetes," *Advance Laboratory* 20, no. 1 (2011): 22, available at http://laboratory-manager.advanceweb.com

41. American Diabetes Association, "Diagnosing Diabetes and Learning about Prediabetes," March 2014, www.diabetes.org/diabetes-basics/diagnosis

42. Diabetes Prevention Program Research Group, "Reduction in the Incidence of Type 2 Diabetes with Lifestyle Intervention or Metformin," *New England Journal of Medicine* 345 (2002): 393–403.

43. American Diabetes Association, "Healthy Weight Loss," 2013, www.diabetes.org; W. Knowles et al., "10 Year Follow-Up of Diabetes Incidence and Weight Loss in the DPP Outcomes Study," *The Lancet* 374, no. 9702 (2009): 1677–86.

44. Linus Pauling Institute, "Glycemic Index and Glycemic Load," April 2014, http://lpi .oregonstate.edu/infocenter/foods/grains/gigl .html

45. S. Jonnalagadda et al., "Putting the Whole Grain Puzzle Together: Health Benefits Associated with Whole Grains—Summary of American Society for Nutrition 2010 Satellite Symposium," *Journal of Nutrition* 41, no. 5 (2011): 10115–25.

46. R. Post et al., "Dietary Fiber for the Treatment of Type 2 Diabetes Mellitus: A Meta Analysis," *Journal of the American Board of Family Medicine* 25, no. 1 (2012): 16–23; S. Bhupathiraju et al., "Glycemic Index, Glycemic Load and Risk of Type 2 Diabetes: Results from 3 Large US Cohorts and an Updated Meta-Analysis," *Circulation* 129, Supplement 1 (2014): AP140; A. Olubukola, P. English, and J. Pinkney, "Systematic Review and Meta-Analysis of Different Dietary Approaches to the Management of Type 2 Diabetes," *The American Journal of Clinical Nutrition* 97, no. 3 (2013): 505–16.

47. Wallin et al., "Fish Consumption, Dietary Long-Chain N-3 Fatty Acids, and the Risk of Type 2 Diabetes: Systematic Review and Meta Analysis of Prospective Studies," *Diabetes Care* 35, no. 4 (2012): 918–29; L. Djousse et al., "Dietary Omega-3 Fatty Acids and Fish Consumption and Risk of Type 2 Diabetes," *American Journal of Clinical Nutrition* 93, no. 1 (2011): 113–50.

48. Jeppesen, K. Schiller, and M. Schultze, "Omega-3 and Omega-6 Fatty Acids and Type 2 Diabetes," *Current Diabetes Reports* 13, no. 2 (2013): 279–88.

49. American Diabetes Association, "What We Recommend," December 2013, www.diabetes .org/food-and-fitness/fitness/types-of-activity/what-we-recommend.html; National Diabetes Information Clearing House, "Diabetes Prevention Program," September 2013, http://diabetes.niddk.nih.gov/dm/pubs/preventionprogram/index.aspx

50. S. R. Kashyap et al., "Metabolic Effects of Bariatric Surgery in Patients with Moderate Obesity and Type 2 Diabetes," *Diabetes Care* 36, no. 8 (2013): 2175–82.

51. P. R. Schauer et al., "Bariatric Surgery versus Intensive Medical Therapy for Diabetes–3 Year Outcomes," *New England Journal of Medicine* 370 (2014): 2002–13, doi: 10.1056/NEJMoa1401329

52. P. Poirier et al., on behalf of the American Heart Association Obesity Committee of the Council on Nutrition, Physical Activity, and Metabolism, "Bariatric Surgery and Cardiovascular Risk Factors: A Scientific Statement from the American Heart Association," *Circulation* 123, no. 15 (2011): 1683–701, doi: 10.1161/CIR.0b013e3182149099

53. Medtronic, "Medtronic Gains Approval of First Artificial Pancreas Device System with Threshold Suspend Automation," September 2013, http://newsroom.medtronic .com/phoenix.zhtml?c=251324&p=irol-newsArticle&id=1859361

**Pulled Statistics:**

Page 393, National Kidney Foundation, "Diabetes and Kidney Disease," Accessed May 2015, www.kidney .org/news/newsroom/factsheets/Diabetes-And-CKD

## Chapter 13: Protecting against Infectious Diseases and Sexually Transmitted Infections

1. M. Day et al., "Surveillance of Zoonotic Infectious Disease Transmitted by Small Companion Animals," *Emerging Infectious Diseases* (2012), wwwnc.cdc.gov/eid/article/18/12/12-0664_article

2. World Health Organization (WHO), "Factsheet on the World Malaria Report–2014," December 2014, www.who.int/malaria/media/world_malaria_report_2014/en/; Centers for Disease Control and Prevention, "Dengue," March 26, 2015, www.cdc.gov/Dengue/

3. E. Hoberg and D. Brooks, "Evolution in Action: Climate Change, Biodiversity Dynamics and Emerging Infectious Disease," *Philosophical Transactions of the Royal Society of London B: Biological Sciences* 370, no. 1665 (2015), doi: 10.1098/rstb.2013.0553; S. Altizer et al., "Climate Change and Infectious Diseases: From Evidence to a Predictive Framework," *Science* 341, no. 6145 (2013): 514–19; WHO, "Climate Change and Infectious Disease," May 2015, www.who.int/globalchange/publications/climatechangechap6.pdf; J. Remais et al., "Convergence of Non-communicable and Infectious Diseases in Low- and Middle-Income Countries," *International Journal of Epidemiology* 42, no. 1 (2013): 221–27, doi: 10.1093/ije/dys135; Environmental Protection Agency, "Climate Impacts on Human Health," April 2013, www. epa.gov/climatechange/effects/health.html

4. B. T. Kerridge et al., "Conflict and Diarrheal and Related Diseases: A Global Analysis," *Journal of Epidemiology and Global Health* 3, no. 4 (2013): 269–77; K. F. Cann et al., "Extreme Water-Related Weather Events and Waterborne Disease," *Epidemiology and Infection* 141, no. 4 (2013): 671–86.

5. Centers for Disease Control and Prevention (CDC), "Birth–18 years and 'Catch-Up' Immunization Schedules," May 26, 2015, www.cdc .gov/vaccines/schedules/hcp/child-adolescent .html

6. CDC, "Get Smart: Know When Antibiotics Work," April 17, 2015, www.cdc.gov/getsmart/community/about/index.html

7. L. Hicks et al., "U.S. Outpatient Antibiotic Prescribing, 2010," *New England Journal of Medicine* 368, no. 15 (2013): 1468–69.

8. CDC, "Health-Associated Infections," January 12, 2015, www.cdc.gov/HAI/surveillance/; S. Magill et al., "Multistate Point-Prevalence Survey of Health Care–Associated Infections," *New England Journal of Medicine* 370, no. 13 (2014):1198–208.

9. CDC, "Health-Associated Infections," 2015; S. Magill et al., "Multistate Point-Prevalence Survey," 2014.

10. CDC, "General Information about MRSA in the Community," September 2013, www.cdc.gov/mrsa/community/index.html

11. Centers for Disease Control and Prevention-Newsroom, "Nearly Half a Million Americans Suffered from *Clostridium difficile* Infections in a Single Year," February 2015, www.cdc.gov/media/releases/2015/p0225-clostridium-difficile.html

12. CDC, "Group B Streptococcus (Group B Strep) and Pregnancy," January 2011, www.cdc.gov/pregnancy/infections-groupb.html

13. CDC, "Chapter 8: Meningococcal Disease: Manual for the Surveillance of Vaccine Preventable Disease," April 1, 2014, Available at www.cdc.gov/vaccines/pubs/surv-manual/chpt08-mening.html

14. Ibid.

15. Ibid.

16. WHO, "Tuberculosis Fact Sheet," March 2015, www.who.int/mediacentre/factsheets/fs104/en/

17. CDC, "Tuberculosis (TB): Data and Statistics," April 2014, www.cdc.gov/tb/statistics/

18. Ibid.

19. CDC, "Tuberculosis," April 2015, www.cdc.gov/tb/

20. CDC, "Tuberculosis (TB): Treatment," August 2012, www.cdc.gov/tb/topic/treatment/default.htm

21. Ibid.

22. CDC, "Common Colds: Protect Yourself and Others," February 2015, www.cdc.gov/features/rhinoviruses/

23. Ibid.

24. Web MD, "Causes of the Common Cold," January 2015, www.webmd.com/cold-and-flu/cold-guide/common_cold_causes; CDC, "Common Colds: Protect Yourself and Others," February 2015.

25. M. G. Thompson et al., "Updated Estimates of Mortality Associated with Seasonal Influenza through the 200--2007 Influenza Season," *MMWR* 59, no. 33 (2010): 1057–62.

26. CDC, "Seasonal Influenza: Key Facts about Influenza (Flu) and Flu Vaccine," February 2013, www.cdc.gov

27. CDC, "Selecting the Viruses in the Seasonal Influenza (Flu) Vaccine," February 2014, www.cdc.gov/flu/about/season/vaccine-selection.htm

28. J. S. Schiller, B. W. Ward, G. Freeman, "Early Release of Selected Estimates Based on Data from the 2013 National Health Interview Survey," CDC, National Center for Health Statistics, June 2014, www.cdc.gov/nchs/nhis.htm

29. Ibid.

30. CDC, "Viral Hepatitis Surveillance, United States, Disease Burden from Viral Hepatitis A, B, and C in the United States–2013," April 2015, www.cdc.gov/hepatitis/Statistics/index.htm; CDC, "Reported Cases of Acute Hepatitis A, by State, United States, 2007–2011," August 2013, www.cdc.gov/hepatitis/Statistics/2011Surveillance/Table2.1.htm; World Health Organization, "Global Policy Report on Prevention and Control of Viral Hepatitis in WHO Member States," July 2013, http://www.who.int/hiv/pub/hepatitis/global_report/en/

31. CDC, "Viral Hepatitis Surveillance-United States-2013," 2015; CDC, "Reported Cases of Acute Hepatitis A, by State," 2013, www.cdc.gov/hepatitis/Statistics/2011Surveillance/Table2.1.htm; WHO, "Global Policy Report on Prevention and Control of Viral Hepatitis," 2013.

32. E. Aspinall et al., "Are Needle and Syringe Programmes Associated with a Reduction in HIV Transmission among People Who Inject Drugs: A Systematic Review and Meta-analysis," *International Journal of Epidemiology*, 43, no. 1 (2014): 235–48, doi: 10.1093/ije/dyt243 (Epub ahead of print December 12, 2013); A. Dutta et al., "Key Harm Reduction Interventions and Their Impact on Reduction of Risky Behavior and HIV Incidence among People Who Inject Drugs in Low-Income and Middle-Income Countries," *Current Opinion HIV AIDS* 7, no. 4 (2012): 362–8, doi: 10.1097/COH.0b013e328354a0b5

33. CDC, "Viral Hepatitis Surveillance, United States, Disease Burden from Viral Hepatitis A, B, and C in the United States-2013," April 2015, www.cdc.gov/hepatitis/Statistics/index.htm

34. CDC, "Viral Hepatitis Statistics and Surveillance–2011," August 2013, www.cdc.gov/hepatitis/Statistics/2011Surveillance/Commentary.htm#hepB

35. CDC, "Hepatitis C FAQs for the Public," April 2015, www.cdc.gov/hepatitis/C/cFAQ.htm#cFAQ21; CDC, "Viral Hepatitis Surveillance United States, Disease Burden from Viral Hepatitis A, B, and C," 2015.

36. CDC, "Hepatitis C FAQs," April 2015.

37. Ibid.

38. Ibid.

39. R. Seither et al., "Vaccination Coverage among Children in Kindergarten–United States 2013-2014 School Year," *MMWR* 63, no. 41 (2014): 913–20; California Department of Public Health, "Vaccine Preventable Disease Surveillance in California- Annual Report-2013," 2014, www.cdph.ca.gov/programs/immunize/Documents/VPD-DiseaseSummary2013.pdf

40. CDC, "West Nile Virus (WNV) Activity Reported to ArboNET, by State, United States, 2011," April 2012, www.cdc.gov

41. WHO, "Cumulative Number of Confirmed Human Cases of Avian Influenza A (H5N1) Reported to WHO," 2013, www.who.int

42. Ibid.

43. CDC, "Avian Influenza A (H7N9) Virus," April 2013, www.cdc.gov; CDC, "Highly Pathogenic Asian-Origin Avian Influenza A (H5N1) Virus," May 2015, www.cdc.gov/flu/avianflu/h5n1-virus.htm

44. CDC, "The 2009 H1N1 Pandemic," August 2010, www.cdc.gov/h1n1flu/cdcresponse.htm

45. CDC, "2013 Sexually Transmitted Disease Surveillance," March 2015, www.cdc.gov/std/stats13/; CDC, "Fact Sheet-Reported STDs in the United States," December 2014, www.cdc.gov/nchhstp/newsroom/docs/std-trends-508.pdf

46. CDC, "Fact Sheet–Reported STDs in the United States," December 2014, www.cdc.gov/nchhstp/newsroom/docs/std-trends-508.pdf

47. CDC, "STDs in Adolescents and Young Adults," December 2014, www.cdc.gov/std/stats13/adol.htm

48. Ibid.

49. Ibid.

50. CDC, "Chlamydia—CDC Fact Sheet, Detailed Version," December 2014, www.cdc.gov/std/chlamydia/STDFact-chlamydia-detailed.htm

51. Ibid.

52. CDC, "CDC Fact Sheet–Reported STDS in the United States–2013 National Data for Chlamydia, Gonorrhea, and Syphilis," December 2014, www.cdc.gov/nchhstp/newsroom/docs/std-trends-508.pdf

53. Ibid; CDC, "STDS in Adolescents and Young Adults," December 2014, www.cdc.gov/std/stats13/adol.htm

54. CDC, "CDC Fact Sheet–National Data for Chlamydia, Gonorrhea, and Syphilis," 2014.

55. Ibid.

56. Ibid.

57. CDC, "Genital Herpes–CDC Fact Sheet (Detailed)," December 2014, www.cdc.gov/std/herpes/stdfact-herpes-detailed.htm

58. Ibid; American Sexual Health Association, "Herpes: Fast Facts," May 2015, www.ashasexualhealth.org/stdsstis/herpes/fast-facts-and-faqs/

59. CDC, "Genital Herpes–CDC Fact Sheet," 2014.

60. CDC, "Genital HPV Infection–CDC Fact Sheet," February 2015, www.cdc.gov/std/HPV/STDFact-HPV.htm

61. CDC, "What is HPV?," January 22, 2015, www.cdc.gov/hpv/whatishpv.html

62. CDC, "Genital HPV Infection Fact Sheet," 2015; American Sexual Health Association, "HPV: Fast Facts," April 2014, www.ashasexualhealth.org/stdsstis/hpv/fast-facts/; CDC, "What is HPV?," 2015.

63. National Women's Law Center, "Pap Smears," 2010, http://hrc.nwlc.org; CDC, "Cervical Cancer," March 2013, www.cdc.gov

64. The Henry J. Kaiser Foundation, "The HPV Vaccine: Access and Use in the U.S.," February 26, 2015, http://kff.org/womens-health-policy/fact-sheet/the-hpv-vaccine-access-and-use-in/

65. CDC, "What is HPV?," 2015; CDC, "What Should I Know About Screening?," January 2015, www.cdc.gov/cancer/cervical/basic_info/screening.htm; CDC, "Cervical Cancer," May 2015, www.cdc.gov/cancer/cervical

66. CDC, "Human Papillomavirus (HPV) and Oropharyngeal Cancer–Fact Sheet," November 2013, www.cdc.gov/std/hpv/stdFact-HPVandoralcancer.htm

67. Ibid.

68. CDC, "Trichomoniasis: CDC Fact Sheet," April 2015, www.cdc.gov/std/trichomonas/stdfact-trichomoniasis.htm

69. Ibid.

70. UNAIDS, "Global HIV/AIDS Fact Sheet–2014," May 2015, www.unaids.org/sites/default/files/en/media/unaids/contentassets/documents/factsheet/2014/20140716_FactSheet_en.pdf

71. UNAIDS, "Global HIV/AIDS Fact Sheet–2014," May 2015; Joint United Nations Programme on HIV/AIDS (UNAIDS) and World Health Organization (WHO), *2013 UNAIDS Report on the Global AIDS Epidemic* (Geneva: UNAIDS, 2013), Available at www.unaids.org/en/resources/publications/2013/name,85053,en.asp

72. UNAIDS, "Global HIV/AIDS Fact Sheet–2014," May 2015.

73. CDC, "HIV in the United States: At a Glance," December 2013, www.cdc.gov/hiv/resources/factsheets/us.htm; Care.org, "HIV&AIDS: Facts," January 2014, www.care.org/work/health/hiv-aids/hiv-aids-facts; Joint UNAIDS and WHO, *2013 UNAIDS Report*, 2013, Available at www.unaids.org/en/resources/publications/2013/name,85053,en.asp

74. CDC, "HIV in the United States," 2015; CDC, "Today's HIV/AIDS Epidemic," March 2015, www.cdc.gov/nchhstp/newsroom/docs/hivfactsheets/todaysepidemic-508.pdf

75. CDC, "HIV in the United States," 2015; CDC, "Today's HIV/AIDS Epidemic," 2015.

76. Ibid.

77. CDC, "Today's HIV/AIDS Epidemic," 2015.

78. CDC, "HIV among Women," March 2015, www.cdc.gov/HIV/risk/gender/women/facts/index.html

79. WHO, "Mother to Child Transmission of HIV," April 2014, www.who.int/hiv/topics/mtct/en

80. Pharmaceutical Research and Manufacturers of America, "Medicine in Development: 2014 Report," May 2015, www.phrma.org/sites/default/files/pdf/2014-meds-in-dev-hiv-aids.pdf

81. Ibid.

82. Ibid.

**Pulled Statistics:**

Page 414, CDC, "Incidence, Prevalence, and Cost of Sexually Transmitted Infections in the United States," February 2013, www.cdc.gov/std/stats/sti-estimates-fact-sheet-feb-2013.pdf

Page 423, WHO, "HIV/AIDS," November 2014, www.who.int/mediacentre/factsheets/fs360/en/

## Focus On: Reducing Risks for Chronic Diseases and Conditions

1. American Lung Association, "Estimated Prevalence and Incidence of Lung Disease," May 2014, www.lung.org/finding-cures/our-research/trend-reports/estimated-prevalence.pdf; Centers for Disease Control and Prevention, "Leading Causes of Death," February 6, 2015, www.cdc.gov/nchs/fastats/leading-causes-of-death .htm
2. American Lung Association, "Chronic Obstructive Pulmonary Disease (COPD) Fact Sheet," May 2014, www.lung.org/lung-disease/copd/resources/facts-figures/COPD-Fact-Sheet.html
3. Ibid.
4. American Lung Association, "Chronic Obstructive Pulmonary Disease," 2014; Centers for Disease Control and Prevention, "Chronic Obstructive Pulmonary Disease Among Adults—United States, 2011," November 2012, www.cdc .gov
5. American Lung Association, "Chronic Obstructive Pulmonary Disease," 2014; American Lung Association, "Trends in COPD," 2013, www .lung.org/finding-cures/our-research/trend-reports/copd-trend-report.pdf
6. American Lung Association, "Trends in COPD," 2013.
7. Ibid.
8. National Institute of Allergy and Infectious Diseases, "Asthma-Common Fungus Promotes Airway Sensitivity in Asthma," April 10, 2015, www.niaid.nih.gov/topics/asthma/research/Pages/FungalAllergenFeature.aspx
9. Ibid.
10. American Lung Association, "Reduce Asthma Triggers," June 2015, www.lung.org/lung-disease/asthma/taking-control-of-asthma/reduce-asthma-triggers.html
11. American Lung Association, "Reduce Asthma Triggers," 2015; U. Gohil, A. Modan, and P. Gohil, "Aspirin-Induced Asthma–A Review," *Global Journal of Pharmacology* 4, no. 1 (2010): 19–30.
12. Centers for Disease Control and Prevention, "Most Recent Asthma Data," April 23, 2015, www.cdc.gov/asthma/most_recent_data.htm; Centers for Disease Control and Prevention, "Early Release of Selected Estimates Based on Data From the National Health Interview Survey, January–September 2014," March 2015, www .cdc.gov/nchs/data/nhis/earlyrelease/earlyrelease201503_15.pdf; Centers for Disease Control and Prevention, "Faststats: Asthma," May 14, 2015, www.cdc.gov/nchs/fastats/asthma.htm; American Lung Association, "Estimated Prevalence and Incidence of Lung Disease," May 2014, www.lung.org/finding-cures/our-research/trend-reports/estimated-prevalence.pdf
13. Centers for Disease Control and Prevention, "Early Release of Selected Estimates," 2015.
14. Ibid.; Centers for Disease Control and Prevention, "Faststats: Asthma," 2015.
15. Centers for Disease Control and Prevention, "Faststats: Asthma," 2015.
16. National Institute of Allergy and Infectious Diseases, "Allergic Diseases," May 2015, www .niaid.nih.gov/topics/allergicdiseases/Pages/default.aspx
17. Ibid.; Centers for Disease Control and Prevention, "Allergies and Hay Fever," February 2014, www.cdc.gov/nchs/fastats/allergies.htm
18. National Institute of Allergy and Infectious diseases, "Pollen Allergy," January 2012, www .niaid.nih.gov
19. R. Burch et al., "The Prevalence and Burden of Migraine and Severe Headache in the United States: Updated Statistics from Government Health Surveillance Studies," *Headache: The Journal of Head and Face Pain* 55, no. 1 (2015): 21–34, doi: 10.1111/head.12482
20. J. Lucado, K. Paez, and A. Elixhauser, "Headaches in U.S. Hospitals and Emergency Departments, 2008," *HCUP Statistical Brief*, no. 111 (2011), Available at www.hcup-us.ahrq.gov
21. National Headache Foundation, "Press Kits: Categories of Headache," June 2014, www .headaches.org/press/NHF_Press_Kits/Press_Kits_-_Categories_Of_Headache
22. WebMD, "Migraines and Headache Health Center: Tension Headaches," 2013, www .webmd.com
23. Mayo Clinic, "Tension Headache: Basics and Symptoms," July 2013, www.mayoclinic.org/diseases-conditions/tension-headache/basics/definition/con-20014295
24. R. Burch et al., "The Prevalence and Burden of Migraine and Severe Headache in the United States," 2015, doi: 10.1111/head.12482; National Institute of Neurological Disorders and Stroke, "NINDS Migraine Information Page," February 23, 2015, www.ninds.nih.gov/disorders/migraine/migraine.htm; National Headache Foundation, "Migraine," June 2015, www .headaches.org/education/Headache_Topic_Sheets/Migraine
25. R. Burch et al., "The Prevalence and Burden of Migraine and Severe Headache," 2015; National Institute of Neurological Disorders and Stroke, "NINDS Migraine Information Page," 2015.
26. National Headache Foundation, "Migraines," 2015.
27. National Institute of Neurological Disorders and Stroke, NINDS Migraine Information Page, 2015.
28. Ibid.
29. National Headache Foundation, "Cluster Headaches," 2013, www.headaches.org
30. National Institute of Diabetes and Digestive and Kidney Diseases. "Definition and Facts for Irritable Bowel Syndrome," June 2015, www .niddk.nih.gov/health-information/health-topics/digestive-diseases/irritable-bowel-syndrome/Pages/definition-facts.aspx
31. National Institute of Diabetes and Digestive and Kidney Diseases, "Irritable Bowel Syndrome," 2015; H. F. Herlong, *Digestive Disorders*. *The Johns Hopkins White Papers*. Baltimore, MD: Johns Hopkins Medicine, 2013.
32. National Institute of Diabetes and Digestive and Kidney Diseases, "Irritable Bowel Syndrome," 2015.
33. Ibid.
34. National Digestive Diseases Information Clearinghouse, "Irritable Bowel Syndrome," 2015; H. F. Herlong, *Digestive Disorders*, 2013.
35. National Institutes of Diabetes and Digestive and Kidney Diseases. "Crohn's Disease," September 2014, www.niddk.nih.gov/health-information/health-topics/digestive-diseases/crohns-disease
36. Centers for Disease Control and Prevention, "Inflammatory Bowel Disease," May 2014, www .cdc.gov/ibd
37. National Institutes of Diabetes and Digestive and Kidney Diseases, "Crohn's Disease," 2014.; National Digestive Diseases Information Clearinghouse, " Irritable Bowel Syndrom," 2015.
38. Centers for Disease Control and Prevention, "Inflammatory Bowel Disease (IBD)," 2014.
39. H. F. Herlong, *Digestive Disorders*, 2013.
40. Ibid.
41. "Global Burden of Diseases, Injuries and Risk Factors Study 2013," *The Lancet*, June 2015, www .thelancet.com/themed/global-burden-of-disease
42. Bone and Joint Initiative-USA, "The Burden of Musculoskeletal Diseases in the United States: Prevalence, Societal and Economic Cost," May 2015, www.boneandjointburden.org/facts-brief
43. Centers for Disease Control, "Data and Statistics, Arthritis," March 11, 2015, www.cdc.gov/arthritis/data_statistics
44. Centers for Disease Control, "Arthritis: National Statistics," February 23, 2015, www .cdc.gov/arthritis/data_statistics/national-statistics.html; Arthritis Foundation, "The Heavy Burden of Arthritis in the U.S.," March 2012, www.arthritis.org/files/images/AF_Connect/Departments/Public_Relations/Arthritis-Prevalence-Fact-Sheet--3-7-12.pdf
45. Centers for Disease Control, "National Arthritis Statistics: Future Burden of Arthritis," February 2015, www.cdc.gov/arthritis/data_statistics/national-statistics .html#FutureArthritisBurden
46. Arthritis Foundation, "Arthritis Facts," June 2015, www.arthritis.org/about-arthritis/understanding-arthritis/arthritis-statistics-facts.php; National Institute of Arthritis and Musculoskeletal and Skin Disease, "Handout on Health: Osteoarthritis," April 2015, www .niams.nih.gov/Health_Info/Osteoarthritis/default.asp
47. National Institute of Arthritis and Musculoskeletal and Skin Disease, "Handout on Health: Osteoarthritis," 2015.
48. Calvo-Munoz, "Prevalence of Low Back Pain in Children and Adolescents: A Meta-analysis," *BMC Pediatrics* 13, no 1 (2013): 14, doi:10.1186/2431-13-14
49. Ibid.
50. American College Health Association, *American College Health Association-National College Health Assessment II: Reference Group Executive Summary*, Spring, 2014 (Hanover, MD): American College Health Association.
51. F. Balague et al., "Non-Specific Low Back Pain," *The Lancet* 379, no. 9814 (2012): 482–91, doi: 10.1016/S0140-6736(11)60610-7; National Information Institute of Neurological Disorders and Stroke, "NINDS Back Pain Information Page," April 2014, www.ninds.nih.gov/disorders/back-pain/backpain.htm
52. F. Balague et al., "Non-Specific Low Back Pain," 2012; National Information Institute of Neurological Disorders and Stroke, "NINDS Back Pain Information Page," 2015; R. Shri et al., "Obesity as a Risk Factor for Sciatica: A Meta-analysis," *American Journal of Epidemiology* (2014): doi:10.1093/aje/Kwn007
53. National Institute of Neurological Disorders and Stroke, "Low Back Pain Fact Sheet," April 2015, http://www.ninds.nih.gov/disorders/backpain/detail_backpain.htm; M. Mehra et al., "The Burden of Chronic Low Back Pain with and without a Neuropathic Component: A Healthcare Resource Use and Cost Analysis," *Journal of Medical Economics* 15, no. 2 (2011): 245–52.
54. National Institute of Neurological Disorders, "NINDS Repetitive Motion Disorders Information Page," October 2011, www.ninds.nih.gov

**Pulled Statistics:**

Page 429, American Lung Association, "Chronic Obstructive Pulmonary Disease (COPD) Fact Sheet," March 2015. www.lung.org

Page 433, National Institute of Diabetes and Digestive and Kidney Diseases, "Definition and Facts for Irritable Bowel Syndrome," September 2014, www.niddk.nih.gov/health-information/health-topics/digestive-diseases/irritable-bowel-syndrome

## Chapter 14: Preparing for Aging, Death, and Dying

1. Central Intelligence Agency, *The World Factbook. Country Comparisons: Life Expectancy at Birth,* 2014, www.cia.gov/library/publications/the-world-factbook/rankorder/2102rank.html
2. Administration on Aging, U.S. Department of Health and Human Services, "A Profile of Older Americans: 2014," 2014, www.aoa.acl.gov/Aging_Statistics/Profile/2014/docs/2014-Profile.pdf
3. Federal Interagency Forum on Aging-Related Statistics, "Older Americans 2012: Key Indicators of Well-Being," June 2012, www.agingstats.gov
4. Central Intelligence Agency, *The World Factbook,* 2014.
5. Administration on Aging, "A Profile of Older American," 2014.
6. Ibid.
7. Ibid.
8. Ibid.
9. Genworth, "Compare Long-Term Care Costs Across the United States," February 2015, www.genworth.com/corporate/about-genworth/industry-expertise/cost-of-care.html
10. Administration on Aging, "A Profile of Older Americans," 2014.
11. National Osteoporosis Foundation, "Debunking the Myths," June 2015, http://nof.org/OPmyths
12. Centers for Disease Control and Prevention, "Arthritis-Related Statistics," March 2014, www.cdc.gov/arthritis/data_statistics/arthritis_related_stats.htm
13. J. Weinstein et al., "The Aging Kidney," *NIH-Advanced Chronic Kidney Disease* 17, no. 4 (2011): 302–307; Merck Manual Consumer Version, "Effects of Aging on Urinary Tract," June 2015, www.merckmanuals.com
14. Ibid.
15. National Institute on Deafness and Other Communication Disorders, "Age-Related Hearing Loss," November 2013, www.nidcd.nih.gov/health/hearing/Pages/Age-Related-Hearing-Loss.aspx; F. Lin et al., "Hearing Loss and Cognitive Decline in the Elderly," *Journal of American Medical Association-Internal Medicine* 173, no. 4 (2013): 293–99, doi: 10.1001/jamainternmed.2013.1868
16. J. Solheim et al., "Daily Life Consequences of Hearing Loss in the Elderly," *Disability Rehabilitation* 33, no. 23–24 (2011): 2179–85, doi: 10.3109/09638288.2011.563815; F. Lin et al., "Hearing Loss and Cognitive Decline," 2013.
17. T. E. Howe et al., "Exercise for Improving Balance in Older People," *Cochrane Database of Systematic Reviews* (2012), www.cochrane.org/CD004963/MUSKINJ_exercise-for-improving-balance-in-older-people
18. M. N. Lochlainne et al., "Sexual Activity and Aging," *Journal of American Medical Directors Association* 14, no. 8 (2013): 565–72; R. von Simson et al., "Sexual Health and the Older Adult," *Student BMJ* 20 (2012): e688, doi: 10.1136/sbmj.e688
19. Alzheimer's Association, "2015 Alzheimer's Disease Facts and Figures," 2015, www.alz.org
20. Ibid.
21. L. Hebert et al., "Alzheimer Disease in the United States (2010–2050) Estimated Using the 2010 Census," *Neurology* 80, no. 19 (2013), doi: 10.1212/WNL.0b013e31828726f5
22. Ibid.
23. Ibid.
24. Alzheimer's Association, "What Is Alzheimer's?" 2015, www.alz.org
25. Centers for Disease Control and Prevention, "Making Physical Activity a Part of an Older Adult's Life," November 2011, www.cdc.gov
26. By permission. From *Merriam-Webster's Collegiate® Dictionary,* 11th Edition © 2013 by Merriam-Webster, Inc., Available at www.Merriam-Webster.com
27. President's Commission on the Uniform Determination of Death, *Defining Death: Medical, Ethical and Legal Issues in the Determination of Death* (Washington, DC: U.S. Government Printing Office, 1981).
28. Ad Hoc Committee of the Harvard Medical School to Examine the Definition of Brain Death, "A Definition of Irreversible Coma," *Journal of the American Medical Association* 205 (1968): 377.
29. Elisabeth Kübler-Ross, *On Death and Dying* (New York: Scribner, 2014).
30. Victorian Government Health Information, "Death and Dying," July 2014, www.health.vic.gov
31. Behavioural Neuropathy Clinic, "Grief and the grieving process," 2015, www.adhd.com.au/grief.htm
32. American Bar Association Commission on Law and Aging, *Consumer's Tool Kit for Health Care Advance Planning,* 2d ed., 2012, www.americanbar.org/content/dam/aba/uncategorized/2011/2011_aging_bk_consumer_tool_kit_bk.authcheckdam.pdf
33. Aging with Dignity, "Five Wishes," 2013, www.agingwithdignity.org
34. National Hospice and Palliative Care Organization, "NHPCO Facts and Figures: Hospice Care in America, 2014 Edition," 2014, www.nhpco.org
35. U.S. Department of Health and Human Services, "The Need Is Real," June 2015, www.organdonor.gov/about/data.html

**Pulled Statistics:**

Page 441, Administration on Aging, U.S. Dept. of Health and Human Services, "A Profile of Older Americans: 2014," 2015, www.aoa.gov/Aging_Statistics/Profile/2014/docs/2014_Profile.pdf

Page 445, U.S. Census Bureau, "2010 Census Shows 65 and Older Population Growing Faster than Total U.S. Population," November 2011, www.census.gov

## Chapter 15: Promoting Environmental Health

1. World Wildlife Fund, "Living Planet Index," July 2015, wwf.panda.org/about_our_earth/all_publications/living_planet_report/living_planet_index2/
2. P. Gerland et al., "World Population Stabilization Unlikely This Century," *Science* 346, no. 6206 (2014): 231–37; Worldwatch Institute, "U.N. Raises 'Low' Population Projections for 2050," June 2014, www.worldwatch.org/node/6038
3. United Nations, "Global Environment Outlook: Environment for Development (GEO 5): Summary for Policy Makers," 2012, www.uncsd2012.org; United Nations, "UNEP Yearbook: Emerging Issues in our Global Environment, 2014," 2015, www.unep.org/yearbook/2014/
4. World Wildlife Fund, "Living Planet Index," 2015.
5. Ibid.
6. Ibid.
7. Ibid.
8. United Nations, "UNEP Yearbook, 2014," 2015.
9. G. Ceballos et al., "Accelerated Modern Human-induced Species Losses: Entering the Sixth Mass Extinction," *Science Advances* 1, no. 5 (2015): e1400253, doi: 10.1126/sciadv.1400253
10. The IUCN Red List of Threatened Species, "IUCN Red List Status: Mammals," June 2015, www.iucnredlist.org/initiatives/mammals/analysis/red-list-status
11. Ibid., J. Croxall et al., "Seabird Conservation Status, Threats and Priority Actions: A Global Assessment," *Bird Conservation International* 22 (2012): 1–34, doi: 10.1017/S0959270912000020
12. G. Whillemyer et al., "Illegal Killing for Ivory Drives Global Decline in African Elephants," *Proceedings of the National Academy of Sciences* 111, no. 36 (2014): 13117–121; W. Ripple, et al., "Collapse of the World's Largest Herbivores," *Science Advances* 1, no. 4 (2015): e1400103.
13. United Nations Environmental Program, "Towards a Green Economy: Pathways to Sustainable Development and Poverty Eradication," June 2015, www.unep.org/greeneconomy/greeneconomyreport/tabid/29846/default.aspx; V. Christenson et al., "A Century of Fish Biomass Decline in the Ocean," *Marine Ecology Program Series* 512 (2014): 155–166, doi: 10.3354/meps10946
14. United Nations, "UNEP Yearbook, 2014," 2015.
15. U.S. Energy Information Administration, "Independent Statistics and Analysis," 2013, www.eia.gov
16. Central Intelligence Agency, "The World Factbook, Country Comparison: Total Fertility Rate," June 2014, www.cia.gov/library/publications/the-world-factbook/rankorder/2127rank.html; C. Haub and T. Kaneda, "2014 World Population Data Sheet," Population Reference Bureau, World Population, 2014, www.prb.org/Publications/Datasheets/2014/2014-world-population-data-sheet/data-sheet.aspx
17. C. Haub and T. Kaneda, "2014 World Population Data Sheet," 2014.
18. Population Reference Bureau, "The Decline in U.S. Fertility," 2014, www.prb.org/Publications/Datasheets/2014/2014-world-population-data-sheet/us-fertility-decline-factsheet.aspx; Central Intelligence Agency, "The World Factbook: Country Comparison: Total Fertility Rate," 2014.
19. U.S. Environmental Protection Agency, "Air Enforcement," June 2014, www2.epa.gov/enforcement/air-enforcement
20. U.S. Environmental Protection Agency, "Overview of Greenhouse Gases: Emissions and Trends: Carbon Dioxide," April 2014, www.epa.gov/climatechange/ghgemissions/gases/co2.html
21. A. Soos, "Acid Rain Change," *Environmental News Network,* 2013, www.enn.com
22. U.S. Environmental Protection Agency, "Reducing Acid Rain," 2012, www.epa.gov
23. U.S. Environmental Protection Agency, "Acid Rain: Effects of Acid Rain—Surface Waters and Aquatic Animals," 2012, www.epa.gov
24. Ibid.; A. Soos, "Acid Rain Change," 2013.
25. U.S. Environmental Protection Agency, "Acid Rain: Effects of Acid Rain—Human Health," 2012, www.epa.gov
26. U.S. Environmental Protection Agency, "Questions About Your Community: Indoor Air," 2013, www.epa.gov/region1/communities/indoorair.html
27. U.S. Environmental Protection Agency, "An Introduction to Indoor Air Quality," Updated November 2014, www.epa.gov/iaq/ia-intro.html
28. Ibid.
29. U.S. Environmental Protection Agency, "Ozone Layer Depletion: Ozone Science: Brief Questions and Answers on Ozone Depletion," Updated February 2010, www.epa.gov; Environment, Health and Safety Online, "Ozone Depletion and UV Radiation," 2013, www.ehso.com; National Aeronautics and Space Administration, "Ozone Hole Watch," 2013, http://ozonewatch.gsfc.nasa.gov

30. White House, "Remarks by the President on Climate Change-Georgetown University," Press Release, June 2013, www.whitehouse.gov/the-press-office/2013/06/25/remarks-president-climate-change

31. U.S. Global Change Research Group, "Climate Change Impacts in the United States," May 2014, http://nca2014.globalchange.gov/downloads/report; NASA, "Global Climate Change. Evidence of Change: How Do We Know?," June 2014, http://climate.nasa.gov/evidence; U.S. Environmental Protection Agency, "Climate Change Facts: Answers to Common Questions," 2014; J. C. L. Olivier et al., "Trends in Global $CO_2$ Emissions–2013 Report," October 2013, www.pbl.nl/en/publications/trends-in-global-co2-emissions-2013-report

32. NASA, "Global Climate Change," 2014; Environmental Protection Agency, "Climate Change Facts: Answers to Common Questions," 2014; J. C. L Olivier et al., "Trends in Global $CO_2$ Emissions–2013 Report," 2013.

33. NASA, "Global Climate Change," 2014.

34. Ibid; J. C. L. Olivier et al., "Trends in Global $CO_2$ Emissions-2013 Report," 2013.

35. Ibid; U.S. Environmental Protection Agency, "National Greenhouse Gas Emissions Data," April 2014, www.epa.gov/climatechange/ghgemissions/usinventoryreport.html

36. Ibid.

37. World Commission on Environment and Development, *Our Common Future* (Oxford: Oxford University Press, 1987): 27.

38. J. C. L. Olivier et al., "Trends in Global $CO_2$ Emissions–2014 Report," 2014.

39. Ibid.

40. Ibid.

41. Environmental Defense Fund, "Cap and Trade—How Cap and Trade Works, 2015, www.edf.org/climate/how-cap-and-trade-works

42. Ibid.

43. The Water Information Program, "Water Facts," June 2015, www.waterinfo.org/resources/water-facts

44. Ibid.

45. Pacific Institute, "Water Use Trends in the United States," April 2015, http://pacinst.org/wp-content/uploads/sites/21/2015/04/Water-Use-Trends-Report.pdf

46. Ibid.

47. Ibid.

48. The Water Information Program, "Water Facts," June 2015, www.waterinfo.org/resources/water-facts

49. Department of National Intelligence, "Worldwide Threat Assessment of the Intelligence Community," January 9, 2014, www.dni.gov/files/documents/Intelligence%20Reports/2014%20WWTA%20%20SFR_SSCI_29_Jan.pdf; Department of National Intelligence, "Global Water Security," February 2012, www.dni.gov/files/documents/Special%20Report_ICA%20Global%20Water%20Security.pdf

50. World Economic Forum, "Global Agenda Council on Water Security 2012–2014," June 2015, www3.weforum.org/docs/GAC/2013/Connect/WEF_GAC_WaterSecurity_2012-2014_Connect.pdf; Water Information Program. "Water Facts," 2015.

51. M. Kostich, A. Batt, and J. Lazorcheck, "Concentrations of Prioritized Pharmaceuticals in Effluents from 50 Large Wastewater Treatment Plants in the U.S. and Implications for Risk Estimation," *Environmental Pollution* 184 (2014): 354–59.

52. U.S. Geological Survey, "National Water Quality Assessment Program" June 2015, http://water.usgs.gov/nawga/

53. U.S. Environmental Protection Agency, "Advancing Sustainable Materials Management 2013 Fact Sheet—Assessing Trends in Material Generation, Recycling and Disposal in the United States," June 2015, www.epa.gov/epawaste/nonhaz/municipal/pubs/2013_advncng_smm_fs.pdf

54. Ibid.

55. Ibid.

56. U.S. Environmental Protection Agency, "Superfund: Superfund National Accomplishments Summary, Fiscal Year 2013," June 2014, www.epa.gov/superfund/accomp/pdfs/FY_2013_SF_EOY_accomp_sum_FINAL.pdf

57. U.S. Environmental Protection Agency, "Hazardous Waste," June 2015, www.epa.gov/osw/basic-hazard.htm; U.S. Environmental Protection Agency, "Household Hazardous Waste," 2014, www.epa.gov/osw/conserve/materials/hhw.htm

58. U.S. Nuclear Regulatory Commission, "Radiation Basics," 2014, www.nrc.gov/about-nrc/radiation/health-effects/radiation-basics.html

59. Ibid.

60. Reuters, "Factbox: Key Facts on Chernobyl Nuclear Accident," March 2011, www.reuters.com

61. International Atomic Energy Agency, "IAEA Issues Projections for Nuclear Power from 2020–2050," May 12, 2015, www.iaea.org/newscenter/news/iaea-issues-projections-nuclear-power-2020-2050; U.S. Energy Information Administration, "Independent Statistics and Analysis," 2012, www.eia.gov

62. National Institute for Occupational Safety and Health, "Workplace Safety and Health Topics: Noise and Hearing Loss Prevention," 2011, www.cdc.gov

**Pulled Statistics:**

Page 458, Population Reference Bureau, "2014 World Population Data Sheet," 2014, www.prb.org/pdf14/2014-world-population-data-sheet_eng.pdf

Page 467, EPA, "Advancing Sustainable Materials Management: 2013 Fact Sheet," June 2015, www.epa.gov/epawaste/nonhaz/municipal/pubs/2013_advncng_smm_fs.pdf

# Chapter 16: Making Smart Health Care Choices

1. S. Collins, P. Rasmussen, and M. Doty, "Gaining Ground: Americans' Health Insurance Coverage and Access to Care After the Affordable Care Act's First Open Enrollment Period," July 2014, www.commonwealthfund.org/publications/issue-briefs/2014/jul/health-coverage-access-aca

2. M. A. Hillen et al., " How Can Communication by Oncologists Enhance Patients' Trust? An Experimental Study," *Annals of Oncology* 25, no. 4 (2014): 896–901.

3. The Joint Commission, "About The Joint Commission," 2015, www.jointcommission.org

4. J. James, "New Evidence-Based Estimates of Patient Harms Associated with Hospital Care," *Journal of Patient Safety* 9, no. 3 (2013): 122–28.

5. Consumer Health, "Patient Rights: Informed Consent," March 2013, www.emedicinehealth.com/patient_rights/article_em.htm#patient_rights

6. Centers for Disease Control and Prevention, "Therapeutic Drug Use," May 14, 2015, www.cdc.gov/nchs/fastats/drug-use-therapeutic.htm

7. W. Zhong et al., "Age and Sex Patterns of Drug Prescribing in a Defined American Population," *Mayo Clinic Proceedings* 88, no. 7 (2013): 697–707.

8. L. Gallelli et al., "Safety and Efficacy of Generic Drugs with Respect to Brand Formulation," *Journal of Pharmacology and Pharmacotherapeutics* 4, Supplement 1 (2013): S110–14.

9. Kaiser Family Foundation, "Total HMO Enrollment, July 2012," May 2014, http://kff.org/other/state-indicator/total-hmo-enrollment

10. Centers for Medicare and Medicaid Services, "National Health Expenditure Projections 2013–2023," 2013, www.cms.gov/Research-Statistics-Data-and-Systems/Statistics-Trends-and-Reports/NationalHealthExpendData/Downloads/Proj2013.pdf

11. National Committee to Preserve Social Security and Medicare, "Fast Facts About Medicare," February 2015, www.ncpssm.org/Medicare/MedicareFastFacts

12. U.S. Department of Health & Human Services, "2015 Poverty Guidelines," January 2015, http://aspe.hhs.gov/poverty/15poverty.cfm

13. Centers for Medicare and Medicaid Services, "National Health Expenditure Projections," 2013.

14. Centers for Medicare and Medicaid Services, "Children's Health Insurance Program," July 2015, www.medicaid.gov/chip/chip-program-information.html

15. National Conference of State Legislators, "Health Insurance: Premiums and Increases," June 2015, www.ncsl.org/issues-research/health/health-insurance-premiums.aspx

16. The Rand Corporation, "The Affordable Care Act in Depth," April 8, 2015, www.rand.org/health/key-topics/aca/in-depth.html

17. S. Collins, P. Rasmussen, and M. Doty, "Gaining Ground: Americans' Health Insurance Coverage," 2014.

18. American College Health Association, *American College Health Association–National College Health Assessment II: Reference Group Executive Summary. Spring 2014* (Hanover, MD: American College Health Association, 2014).

19. Bureau of Labor Statistics, U.S. Department of Labor, "Occupational Outlook Handbook: Physicians and Surgeons," January 2014, www.bls.gov/ooh/healthcare/physicians-and-surgeons.htm

20. American Hospital Association, "Fast Facts on U.S. Hospitals," January 2014, www.aha.org/research/rc/stat-studies/fast-facts.shtml

21. O. W. Brawley, *How We Do Harm: A Doctor Breaks Ranks about Being Sick in America* (New York: St. Martin's Press, 2011).

22. Centers for Medicare and Medicaid Services, "National Health Expenditure Projections 2013–2023," 2013.

23. Ibid.

24. America's Health Insurance Plans, "Fast Check: Administrative Costs," November 2012, www.ahip.org/ACA-Toolbox/Documents/Communications-Toolkit/Fact-Check-Administrative-Costs.aspx

25. Central Intelligence Agency, "Country Comparison: Life Expectancy at Birth. CIA World Factbook," June 2015, www.cia.gov/library/publications/the-world-factbook/rankorder/2102rank.html

26. Ibid.

27. Central Intelligence Agency, "Country Comparison: Infant Mortality Rate. CIA Factbook," June 2015, www.cia.gov/library/publications/the-world-factbook/rankorder/2091rank.html

28. Department of Health and Human Services, "Report to Congress: National Strategy for Quality Improvement in Health Care," 2011, www.ahrq.gov/workingforquality/nqs/nqs2011annlrpt.htm

**Pulled Statistics:**

Page 482, Centers for Disease Control and Prevention, "Hospital Utilization," 2015, www.cdc.gov

Page 492, J. John, "A New, Evidence-based Estimate of Patient Harms Associated with Hospital Care," Journal of Patient Safety 9, no. 3 (2013): 122–28

## Focus On: Understanding Complementary and Integrative Health

1. National Center for Complementary and Integrative Health, "Complementary, Alternative, or Integrative Health: What's in a Name?," March 2015, https://nccih.nih.gov/health/integrative-health#types
2. Ibid.
3. Ibid.
4. Ibid.
5. T. C. Clarke et al., "Trends in the Use of Complementary Health Approaches among Adults: United States, 2002–2012," National Health Statistics Reports, no. 79 (Hyattsville, MD: National Center for Health Statistics), February 2015. Available at www.cdc.gov/nchs/data/nhsr/nhsr079.pdf
6. Ibid.
7. National Center for Complementary and Integrative Health, "Traditional Chinese Medicine: An Introduction," October 2013, http://nccam.nih.gov/health/whatiscam/chinesemed.htm
8. National Center for Complementary and Integrative Health, "Ayurvedic Medicine: An Introduction," NCCIH Publication no. D287, January 2015, http://nccam.nih.gov/health/ayurveda/introduction.htm
9. Ibid.
10. Ibid.
11. National Center for Complementary and Integrative Health, "Homeopathy: An Introduction," NCCIH Publication no. D439, April 2015, http://nccih.nih.gov/health/homeopathy
12. Ibid.
13. National Center for Complementary and Integrative Health, "Naturopathy: An Introduction," NCCIH Publication no. D372, March 2012, https://nccih.nih.gov/health/naturopathy/naturopathyintro.htm
14. Ibid.
15. National Center for Complementary and Integrative Health, "Complementary, Alternative, or Integrative Health: What's in a Name?" 2015.
16. American Chiropractic Association, "About Chiropractic," Accessed June 2015, www.acatoday.org/level1_css.cfm?T1ID=42
17. NIH-National Center for Complementary and Integrative Health, "Spinal Manipulation," January 28, 2015, https://nccih.nih.gov/health/spinalmanipulation
18. Ibid.
19. National Center for Complementary and Integrative Health, "Massage Therapy for Health Purposes: What You Need to Know," NCCIH Publication no. D327, updated February 2014, http://nccih.nih.gov/health/massage/massageintroduction.htm
20. Ibid.
21. Ibid.
22. Bureau of Labor Statistics, U.S. Department of Labor, "Massage Therapists," Occupational Outlook Handbook, 2012–2013 Edition, January 2014, www.bls.gov/ooh/Healthcare/Massage-therapists.htm
23. National Center for Complementary and Integrative Health, "Acupuncture: What You Need to Know," NCCIH Publication no. D404, November 2014, http://nccih.nih.gov/health/acupuncture/introduction.htm
24. R. S. Hinman et al., "Acupuncture for Chronic Knee Pain. A Randomized Clinical Trial," Journal of the American Medical Association 312, no. 13 (2014): 1313–22.
25. A. J. Vickers and K. Linde, "Acupuncture for Chronic Pain," Journal of the American Medical Association 311, no. 9 (2014): 955–56.
26. National Center for Complementary and Integrative Health, "Acupuncture: What You Need to Know, 2014.
27. G. A. Kelley and K. S. Kelley, "Meditative Movement Therapies and Health-Related Quality-of-Life in Adults: A Systematic Review of Meta-Analyses," PLoS ONE 10, no.6 (2015): e0129181, doi: 10.1371/journal.pone.0129181
28. R. Hammerschlag, B. L. Marx, and M. Alckin, "Nontouch Biofield Therapy: A Systematic Review of Human Randomized Controlled Trials Reporting Use of Only Nonphysical Contact Treatment," Journal of Alternative and Complementary Medicine 20, no. 12 (2014): 881–92, doi: 10.1089/acm.2014.0017
29. Academy of Nutrition and Dietetics, "Position of the Academy of Nutrition and Dietetics: Functional Foods," Journal of the Academy of Nutrition and Dietetics 113, no. 8 (2013): 1096–1103.
30. A. Kerimi and G. Williamson, "The Cardiovascular Benefits of Dark Chocolate," Vascular Pharmacology 15 (2015), doi: 10.1016/j.vph.2015.05.011
31. National Center for Complementary and Integrative Health, "Oral Probiotics: An Introduction," NCCIH Publication no. D345, December 2012, https://nccih.nih.gov/health/probiotics/introduction.htm
32. Ibid.
33. U. S. Food and Drug Administration, "Questions and Answers on Dietary Supplements," April 2015, www.fda.gov/Food/DietarySupplements/QADietarySupplements/default.htm
34. Ibid.
35. Ibid.
36. Ibid.
37. National Center for Complementary and Integrative Health, "Alerts and Advisories," June 2015, https://nccih.nih.gov/news/alerts
38. National Center for Complementary and Integrative Health, "Using Dietary Supplements Wisely," NCCIH Publication no. D426, updated June 2014, https://nccih.nih.gov/health/supplements/wiseuse.htm
39. U. S. Pharmacopeial Convention, "Dietary Supplements," 2015, www.usp.org/usp-consumers/dietary-supplements-consumers

**Pulled Statistics:**

Page 495, T. C. Clarke et al., "Trends in the Use of Complementary Health Approaches among Adults: United States, 2002–2012," National Health Statistics Reports 79 (Hyattsville, MD: National Center for Health Statistics), February 2015. Available at www.cdc.gov/nchs/data/nhsr/nhsr079.pdf

# PHOTO CREDITS

Note: Page references followed by *f* indicate an illustrated figure; by *t* a table; and by *p* a photograph.